PROGRESS IN CLINICAL AND BIOLOGICAL RESEARCH

TUMOR CELL SURFACES AND MALIGNANCY

TUMOR CELL SURFACES AND MALIGNANCY

Proceedings of the ICN-UCLA Symposium
held at Keystone, Colorado
March 18—March 23, 1979

Editors

RICHARD O. HYNES
Massachusetts Institute of Technology
Cambridge, Massachusetts

C. FRED FOX
University of California
Los Angeles, California

Alan R. Liss, Inc. • New York

Library of Congress Cataloging in Publication Data

Main entry under title:

Tumor cell surfaces and malignancy.

    (Progress in clinical and biological research; v. 41)
    Includes index.
    1. Cancer — Congresses. 2. Cancer cells — Congresses.
3. Plasma membranes — Congresses. I. Hynes, Richard O.
II. Fox, C. Fred. III. ICN Pharmaceuticals, inc. IV. California.
University. University at Los Angeles. V. Series. [DNLM:
1. Cell membrane — Pathology — Congresses. 2. Cell
transformation, Neoplastic — Congresses WI PR668E v. 41 /
QZ202 T923 1979]   RC261.A1T85   616.99'4071
80-7798
ISBN 0-8451-0041-6

Pages 1–736 of this volume are reprinted from Journal of Supramolecular Structure, Volumes 11 and 12. The Journal is the only appropriate literature citation for these articles. The page numbers in the table of contents, author index, and subject index of this volume correspond to the page numbers at the foot of these pages.

The **table of contents** does not necessarily follow the actual pattern of the plenary sessions but, rather, reflects the thrust of the meeting as it evolved from the combination of plenary and poster sessions culminating in the final collection of invited and submitted papers. The actual order of the articles appearing in this volume does not follow the order in which the articles are cited in the table of contents. Many articles were submitted for consideration by Journal of Supramolecular Structure and are reprinted here. These articles are included in the text in the order in which they were accepted for publication and then published in the Journal, and they are followed by invited papers which were submitted solely for publication in the proceedings and did not receive editorial review.

Contents

xii   Contents

Preface

The meeting from which the papers in this book arise was held in Keystone, Colorado, in March 1979. The major focus of the meeting was the role of cell surfaces in the altered beahvior of malignant cells. The program was organized to bring together scientists working in a number of different areas related to this problem and to promote interactions among them. To provide context for considering possible roles of cell surface changes in malignancy, there were contributions addressed to defining the cell biological properties of transformed and malignant cells, to the question of growth control in normal cells, and to the products of the transforming genes of oncogenic viruses. Our challenge is to find out how the latter gene products bring about the phenotypic alterations characteristic of malginant cells and, in particular, the contribution of cell surface alterations to these phenotypic changes.

In recent years a lot of attention has been paid to the roles of cell surface proteins, in particular fibronectin in the behavior of cells, and the significant progress which has been made was reflected in the program. The study of hormone-receptor interactions is also adavancing rapidly, and their possible involvement in transformation was considered. Interactions between the surface membrane and the cytoskeleton inside the cell were another area of discussion.

While it is clear that new insights into a number of problems are available, we still do not undersantd the mechanisms by which changes at the level of the genome bring about surface changes and how these in turn cause phenotypic alterations. Nor do we fully understand how a hormone binding at the cell surface triggers events inside the cell. However, the meeting left the impression that several areas of research relevant to these problems are in a state of rapid advance, and that new avenues for productive investigation are being opened up and avidly exploited.

Our thanks are due to the Symposia staff at UCLA for their essential help in organizing the program. We are particularly grateful to the NIH for Contract No. 263-79C-0352, which was sponsored jointly by the National Cancer Institute, National Institute of Aging, National Institute of Allergy and Infectious Disease, and Fogarty International Center. In addition, we wish to thank ICN Pharmaceuticals for the ongoing support they have contributed to the ICN-UCLA Symposia series.

We hope that the meeting and this collection of papers will help to promote future research.

Richard O. Hynes
C. Fred Fox

Journal of Supramolecular Structure 10:25—31 (1979)
Tumor Cell Surfaces and Malignancy 1—7

Flow Cytometry Analysis of Early DNA Content Changes in Human and Monkey Cells Following Infection With Simian Virus 40

John M. Lehman, Iris B. Klein, and L. Scott Cram

Department of Pathology, University of Colorado School of Medicine, Denver, Colorado 80262 (J.M.L., I.B.K.), and Biophysics and Instrumentation Group, Los Alamos Scientific Laboratory, Los Alamos, New Mexico 87545 (L.S.C.)

Simian virus 40 (SV_{40}) is capable of inducing cellular DNA synthesis in permissive and nonpermissive cells. Utilizing flow cytometry, we analyzed the DNA content changes in two diploid human cell strains and two monkey cell lines. The osteogenesis imperfecta (OI) human skin fibroblasts were induced into DNA synthesis, and within one to two cell generations, a polyploid cell population was produced. With WI-38 phase II cells, a similar pattern of increased cycling of cells into DNA synthesis was observed; however, the majority ($\sim 60\%$) of the cells were blocked in the $G_2 + M$ phase of the cell cycle. At later time intervals, an increase in the G_1 population was demonstrated. The two monkey cell lines responded to SV_{40} virus with an accumulation of cells in the $G_2 + M$ phase of the cell cycle. Thus, two diploid human cell strains exhibited different cell cycle kinetics early after infection with SV_{40} virus. The one strain (WI-38) behaved similarly to the two monkey cell lines studied. The other strain (OI) responded similarly to nonpermissive (transforming) cells infected with SV_{40} virus.

Key words: simian virus 40, flow cytometry, DNA synthesis induction, transformation, human diploid cells

SV_{40} virus is capable of transforming numerous strains of diploid rodent and human cells. Previous studies with diploid mouse and Chinese hamster embryo cells demonstrated the production of a tetraploid-polyploid population within 24—48 h after infection that resulted from two or more consecutive S periods without a mitosis [1, 2]. Therefore, the early changes observed in cellular DNA synthesis regulation may be an important step in the mechanism of neoplastic transformation.

Human diploid fibroblasts infected with SV_{40} virus may replicate the virus, which

Received April 30, 1979; accepted May 17, 1979.

0091-7419/79/1101-0025$01.70 © 1979 Alan R. Liss, Inc.

leads to lysis, or some cells may be transformed. Changes in human cells were first detected 4–6 weeks after infection, which is prior to morphological transformation. These changes included an increase in the tetraploid population and an increase in chromosome breaks. There was no evidence of chromosome changes early on (1–2 days) [3, 4]; however, cellular DNA synthesis as measured by ^{3}H-thymidine incorporation was observed within the first week after infection [5]. Monkey cells permit the complete replication of SV_{40} virus and are induced into the S phase of the cell cycle [6, 7].

This paper reports the early DNA content distribution of monkey cells and human cells following infection with SV_{40} virus. These analyses were performed with flow cytometry which allowed a quantitation of DNA content per cell and was capable of measuring a large population of cells within the first few cell generations following infection.

MATERIALS AND METHODS

The strains of human cells used in this study were obtained from patients with osteogeneis imperfecta (OI) and from WI-38 at passage 20–30 in vitro. Three strains of OI cells at the 20–25th passage were used for these studies (C, H, J) and all strains responded similarly. The infection and DNA content studies were performed at two passages for each cell strain. The monkey cell lines (BSC-1 and CV-1) at passage 30–40 were obtained from American Type Tissue Culture Collection. All cells were maintained in minimal essential medium (Gibco) supplemented with 5% fetal calf serum (Microbiological Associates). Confluent cultures were subcultivated with 0.25% trypsin–0.1% versene in phosphate-buffered saline (minus Ca^{++} and Mg^{++}). The RH-911 strain of SV_{40} virus was used for infection and was grown in CV-1 cells [1]. Cells and virus pools were checked for the presence of mycoplasma [8]. Assays for the SV_{40}-specific intranuclear T antigen and viral antigen were performed as previously reported [1].

The cells were subcultured into T-75 Costar flasks, infected 24 h later, and harvested at the various time intervals for DNA content measurement. DNA content measurements were performed with the flow cytometry system developed at the Los Alamos Scientific Laboratory. The cells were harvested as previously described by Tobey et al [9] and stained with acriflavin-Feulgen or mithramycin [9, 10]. Stained cells were introduced into the laminar flow stream of the flow cytometer, where they crossed an argon-ion laser beam at the rate of 5×10^4 cells per minute. The fluorescent intensity of the acriflavin or mithramycin dye was measured for each cell with a photomultiplier tube and recorded in a multichannel pulse-height analyzer. Details of this instrumentation have been previously described [11].

RESULTS

The OI (C, J, H) and WI-38 cells were infected with a multiplicity of 200 plaque-forming units (PFU) per cell and the monkey cells were infected with a multiplicity of 10 PFU per cell. Within 48–72 h, 40–50% of the human cells (OI and WI-38) were expressing the SV_{40}-specific intranuclear T antigen and 10–20% of the cells were producing virion capsid antigen. At 24 h after infection 80–85% of the cells of both monkey cell lines were expressing T antigen and 20–30% were expressing V antigen. Within this time period, a large percentage of the OI cells and WI-38 cells were infected with

SV$_{40}$ virus, thus allowing an analysis of the changes in the cell cycle resulting from SV$_{40}$ infection.

Figure 1 shows the DNA content distribution of control and infected cells (OIC) at 48 and 96 hours after infection. A semilog plot was employed to emphasize the cells in the polyploid range. The G$_1$ (2C) peaks of both control and infected cultures were normalized and plotted in semilog to emphasize the cells in S, G$_2$ + M, and tetraploid G$_2$. It was evident at the earliest time point, 48 h, that there were more cells in the S phase (2C to 4C) of the cell cycle in the infected population. The G$_2$ + M population (4C) was also considerably greater in the infected population and there was a twofold to fourfold

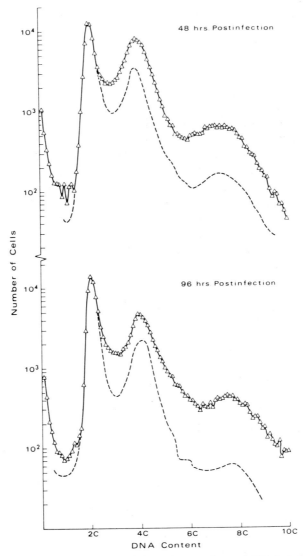

Fig. 1. DNA content distribution of control (- - -) and infected (△-△-△) OI-infected cells at 48 and 96 h after infection. The cells were dispersed, fixed, stained with mithramycin, and measured with the flow cytometer. The data are presented in semilog to emphasize the S and G$_2$ + M populations.

increase in the number of cells with DNA content between 4C and 8C. The tetraploid G_2 + M cells (8C) in the infected population were increased (threefold to fourfold) over the control (Table I). The other cell strains of OI (H and J) were analyzed for this DNA content shift and showed a similar pattern to the OIC. Thus, SV_{40} virus induced these human cells into DNA synthesis and increased the number of polyploid cells within 3–4 days following infection.

TABLE I. Percentage of OI Cells in Various Phases of the Cell Cycle Following Infection With Simian Virus 40

Cells	Hours after infection	Between 4C and 8C	8C
OI control	48	3.9	1.3
OI infected	48	8	3.1
OI control	72	2.2	0.68
OI infected	72	9.1	2.8
OI control	96	2.1	0.83
OI infected	96	8.7	3.7

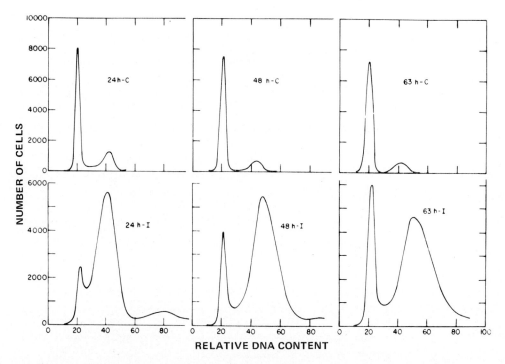

Fig. 2. DNA content distribution of control (upper) and infected (lower) WI-38 cells 24, 48, and 63 h after infection. The cells were dispersed, fixed, stained with mithramycin, and measured with the flow cytometer.

TABLE II. Percentage of WI-38 and BSC-1 Cells in Various Phases of the Cell Cycle Following Infection With Simian Virus 40

Cells	Hours after infection	G$_1$	S	G$_2$ + M
WI-38 control	24	66.7	10.0	23.3
WI-38 infected	24	14.1	3.7	82.2
WI-38 control	48	78.1	5.6	16.3
WI-38 infected	48	15.2	4.7	80.1
WI-38 control	63	82.4	2.7	14.9
WI-38 infected	63	21.8	5.3	72.9
BSC-1 control	48	64.9	9.8	25.4
BSC-1 infected	48	16.4	5.1	78.5

When the DNA content distributions of WI-38 control and infected cells were measured at 24, 48, and 63 h after infection, a pattern different from the OI cells was detected (Fig. 2). The mock-infected cells at all times had a normal DNA content distribution for G$_1$, S, and G$_2$ + M cells (Table II). The infected population at 24 h had a DNA content distribution markedly different from the control cells. There was a large increase in the number of cells in S and G$_2$ + M phases of the cell cycle (85%), and a decrease in the G$_1$ population (Fig. 2, Table II). At 48 and 63 h, there was an increase in the G$_1$ population; however, a considerable percentage of cells were in the G$_2$ + M phase. The WI-38 cells responded with a stimulation of DNA synthesis following SV$_{40}$ virus infection; however, the majority of the cells were apparently blocked in the G$_2$ + M phase. The G$_2$ + M peak at 48 and 63 h was shifted to the right when compared to the 24-hour time point (40 vs 50), indicating an increase in DNA content in the G$_2$ + M phase. When later times — 2 weeks and 4 weeks — were assayed for DNA content distribution, the infected cultures were similar to the controls.

To determine whether the WI-38 cells in the G$_2$ + M phase were blocked in mitosis, we assayed for the number and type of mitotic figures at 48 and 96 h after infection. Similar multiplicities of virus were used, and a comparable number of cells producing T and V antigen were observed as described above. At 48 h the control culture had 0.5% mitotic cells and the infected culture contained 1.1%. The control and infected cultures at 96 h had 0.05% and 1.3% mitotic figures, respectively. A higher mitotic index was observed in the infected cultures; however, all stages of the mitotic cycle were observed, which suggests that the mitotic cells were cycling and not blocked in a particular stage of mitosis. These results suggest that the cells are probably blocked in the G$_2$ phase of the cell cycle.

The two lines of monkey cells (CV-1 and BSC-1), which are permissive to SV$_{40}$ replication exhibited an increase in the G$_2$ + M peak (78.5% vs 25.4% for the control) (Fig. 3, Table II). At later time intervals (>72 h), the majority of cells were dead. Both CV-1 and BSC-1 cells responded similarly. Stimulation of DNA synthesis was determined by autoradiography following 6-h pulses of ^{3}H-thymidine. Both the CV-1 and the BSC-1 used in these studies exhibited a stimulation of DNA synthesis with approximately 20–50% more cells in DNA synthesis. Grain counts were compared to minimize the background of viral DNA synthesis.

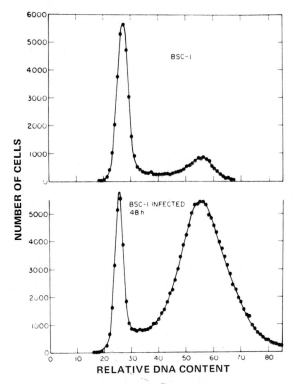

Fig. 3. DNA content distribution of control (upper) and infected (lower) BSC-1 cells at 48 h after infection.

DISCUSSION

Two strains of human diploid fibroblasts were induced into cellular DNA synthesis following infection with SV_{40} virus; however, these two human cell strains exhibited different DNA content distributions. The majority of the OI-infected cells were initially induced into DNA synthesis. A second round of DNA synthesis was induced in some cells, producing a tetraploid population similar to what has been observed with diploid Chinese hamster and mouse cells [1, 12, 13]. The WI-38 cells exhibited a DNA content distribution different from that observed for the three OI cell strains. There was a decrease in the G_1 population with a concomitant increase in the S and G_2 + M population. A portion of the G_2 + M cells were capable of mitosis, since at later time intervals an increase in the G_1 population was observed, suggesting that mitosis was possible in certain of the G_2 + M population. These different responses must be unique to the cell strains, since the same pool and multiplicity of virus were utilized. The monkey cells (CV-1 and BSC-1) exhibited an increase in the number of cells in the G_2 + M phase of the cell cycle similar to that of the WI-38 cells.

At present, there is no definitive explanation for this difference in distribution of cells about the cell cycle following SV_{40} infection. Both cell strains are fibroblastic but they are obtained from different sites. The WI-38 cells were cultured from the lung of a fetus [14] and the OI cell strains were initiated from skin biopsies of newborns. Whether age of the patient or site from which the cells were obtained is an important factor in the response of these cells to induction of DNA synthesis with SV$_{40}$ virus will be answered by an analysis of the responses of numerous strains of human cells to SV$_{40}$ infection. Another explanation may involve the replication of the viral DNA (whole virion) and subsequent block of cells in the G$_2$ phase. The monkey cells which are permissive to SV$_{40}$ replication accumulated cells in the G$_2$ phase; however, WI-38 cells assayed for virion antigen exhibited no increase above the OI cells. This can be explained if a significant amount of viral DNA was replicated without late protein synthesis. At present, this explanation cannot be validated unless the G$_2$ population was isolated and characterized for replicating viral DNA. The fact that these cells responded differently to virus-induced cellular DNA synthesis may be useful in defining steps in the neoplastic transformation of human cells with SV$_{40}$ virus [15].

ACKNOWLEDGMENTS

This study was supported in part by grants CA-16030, CA-13419, and CA-15823 from the National Cancer Institute, and by the US Energy Research and Development Administration.

REFERENCES

1. Lehman JM, Defendi V: J Virol 6:738, 1970.
2. Horan PK, Jett JH, Romaro A, Lehman JM: Int J Cancer 14:514, 1974.
3. Moorhead PS, Saksela E: Hereditas 52:271, 1965.
4. Girardi AJ, Weinstein D, Moorhead PS: Ann Med Exp Fenn 44:242, 1966.
5. Sauer G, Defendi V: Proc Natl Acad Sci USA 56:452, 1966.
6. Sweet BH, Hilleman MR: Proc Soc Exp Biol Med 105:420, 1960.
7. Ritzi E, Levine AJ: J Virol 5:686, 1970.
8. Hayflick L: Texas Rep Biol Med 23:285, 1965.
9. Tobey RA, Crissman HA, Kraemer PM: J Cell Biol 54:638, 1972.
10. Crissman HA, Tobey RA: Science 21:1297, 1974.
11. Holm DM, Cram LS: Exp Cell Res 80:105, 1973.
12. Lehman JM, Mauel J, Defendi V: Exp Cell Res 67:230, 1971.
13. Lehman JM: Int J Cancer 13:164, 1974.
14. Hayflick L: Exp Cell Res 37:614, 1965.
15. Aarsonson SA, Todaro GJ: Virology 36:254, 1968.

Journal of Supramolecular Structure 11:33—49 (1979)
Tumor Cell Surfaces and Malignancy 9—25

Nuclear Control of Tumorigenicity in Cells Reconstructed by PEG-Induced Fusion of Cell Fragments

Jerry W. Shay and Mike A. Clark

The University of Texas Health Science Center at Dallas, Department of Cell Biology, Dallas, Texas 75235

The techniques of somatic cell hybridization have provided a valuable means of studying mechanisms of regulation of mammalian cell differentiation and transformation. Most previous studies have indicated that fusions between tumorigenic and nontumorigenic cells result in hybrid cells that are usually tumorigenic. In recent years it has been demonstrated that the phenotypic expression of tumorigenicity is at least partially due to the extensive chromosome loss that occurs in most interspecific and some intraspecific hybrid cells. In the present study we have utilized enucleation techniques that permit cells to be divided into nuclear (karyoplast) and cytoplasmic (cytoplast) cell fragments. Even though these nuclear and cytoplasmic fragments are metabolically stable for short periods of time, in our hands they ultimately degenerate. Viable cells can be reconstructed by PEG-induced fusion of karyoplasts to cytoplasts. Since reconstructed cells apparently do not segregate chromosomes, they may provide a clearer understanding of the interactions between the nucleus and the cytoplasm in the control of the expression of tumorigenicity. We have reconstructed cells using karyoplasts from the tumorigenic Y-1 cell line and cytoplasts from a nontumorigenic cell line, A-MT-BU-A1. In addition we have reconstructed cells containing Y-1 cytoplasts and A-MT-BU-A1 karyoplasts. The reconstructed cells produced were assayed for tumorigenicity by their ability to grow in soft agar and in nude mice. The results of these experiments indicate that the reconstructed cells containing a tumorigenic nucleus and a nontumorigenic cytoplasm ultimately are tumorigenic and conversely the reconstructed cells containing a nontumorigenic nucleus and a tumorigenic cytoplasm are nontumorigenic. These experiments support the concept that with these cell lines the nucleus (karyoplast) is sufficient to control the phenotypic expression of tumorigenicity.

Key words: cell enucleation, cell reconstruction, nuclear control of tumorigenicity

Hybrid cells produced by fusing tumorigenic and nontumorigenic cells from different species in most instances are tumorigenic. The tumorigenic phenotypes expressed in such hybrids have been partially explained by the extensive chromosome losses that occur in

Abbreviations used: PEG — polyethylene glycol; HAT — hypoxanthine, aminopterin, thymidine; CAP — chloramphenicol; ACTH — adrenocoricotrophic hormone; BrdU or BUDR — bromodeoxyuridine.

Received March 18, 1979; accepted May 25, 1979.

interspecific and some intraspecific hybrid cells. There have been reports that such fusions cause suppression of the tumorigenic phenotype but in these cases chromosome loss was not extensive [1]. In intraspecific hybrids there is little chromosome segregation and when tumorigenic and nontumorigenic cells from the same species are produced, the non-tumorigenic phenotype is frequently but not always retained [1, 2]. These studies suggest that there is some factor present in nontumorigenic cells that is capable of suppressing the tumorigenicity of the other cells and when this factor is lost, as a result of chromosome loss or possibly some epigenetic factor, the tumorigenic phenotype is expressed. Thus, the conflicting results from different experiments may simply reflect the chromosomal instability of the hybrid cells. Interspecific whole-cell fusion studies are probably not ideal for investigating certain aspects of the etiology of the suppression or expression of the tumorigenic state.

In an attempt to overcome the difficulties with the interpretation of such experiments, we and others have been developing techniques for the enucleation of mammalian cells in culture, using the drug cytochalasin B in combination with mild centrifugation [3–5]. Such techniques permit the separation of cells into nuclear (karyoplast) and cytoplasmic (cytoplast) fragments [6], which are incapable of regenerating into whole cells under our conditions unless recombined by standard hybridization techniques. Such reconstructed cells are viable, capable of indefinite growth in cell culture [5, 7], and do not appear to segregate chromosomes. Analysis of reconstructed cells may provide a clearer understanding of the nuclear and cytoplasmic contributions to certain aspects of the expression or suppression of the tumorigenic state.

In the present study we report the reconstruction of a tumorigenic karyoplast with a nontumorigenic cytoplast. In addition, using the same cell lines we report a new technique for identifying reconstructed cells of a nontumorigenic karyoplast with a tumorigenic cytoplast. The results of these experiments indicate that with these cell lines the nucleus (karyoplast) is sufficient to control the phenotypic expression of tumorigenicity.

METHODS

Cell Lines

The tumorigenic Y-1 line was originally derived from a murine adrenal tumor [8]. The nontumorigenic A-MT-BU-A1 cell line (hereafter designated AMT) was originally derived from MT-29240 in Dr. Coon's laboratory and is a murine transplantable tumor that arose spontaneously in a female Balb/c mouse. The AMT cell line is contact-inhibited and is chloramphenicol- and BrdU-resistant, and although it contains intracisternal A virus particles, it is not tumorigenic as tested by lack of growth in soft agar and nude mice. (We thank Drs. Malech and Wivel for providing the AMT cell line). Both parental cell lines, hybrids, and reconstructed cells were found to be free from mycoplasma contamination by three different assays [9–11].

Enucleation

The Y-1 cells are flat and epitheloid, while the AMT are fibroblastoid. Both are strongly adherent to Falcon 3013 25-cm^2 tissue culture flasks (Falcon Plastics, Oxnard, California) and are therefore easily enucleated with a high efficiency by means of techniques previously described [12]. Briefly, almost confluent flasks of Y-1 and AMT cells are

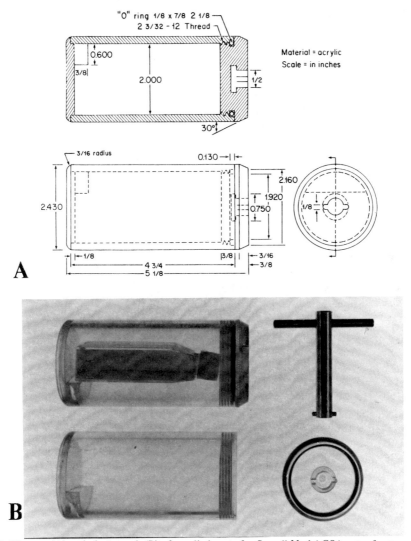

Fig. 1. Diagram (A) and photograph (B) of acrylic inserts for Sorvall Model GSA rotor for use with culture flask enucleation procedure.

completely filled with Dulbecco's modified Eagle's medium (DMEM) containing 10 μg/ml of cytochalasin B and centrifuged in a GSA rotor for 20–30 min at 20,000g at 37° in acrylic holders (Fig. 1a, b) using a Sorvall RC5 superspeed centrifuge. Equally successful enucleation is accomplished without the acrylic inserts by placing 150 ml of H_2O into the GSA rotor opening and placing the flasks directly into the rotor. Enucleation efficiencies of 95–99% or better are obtained with these cell lines without substantial cell detachment. A second centrifugation can be undertaken that results in even higher efficiencies of enucleation. The resulting procedure produces a population of Y-1 karyoplasts and cytoplasts and AMT karyoplasts and cytoplasts. Using the procedures described by Lucas and Kates [39], the amount of cytoplasm retained in the Y-1 and AMT karyoplasts ranges from 2% to 6%, as determined by the amount of ribosomal RNA.

Fusion

The karyoplasts and cytoplasts are mixed and fused using polyethylene glycol 400 MW as previously described for whole cells [13]. Essentially the mixture of karyoplasts and cytoplasts (2×10^6 cells) are centrifuged at 500g for 2 min in a 15-ml conical centrifuge tube. Most of the culture medium is removed without disturbing the pellet, 1 ml of a 50% PEG-400MW solution, which is liquid at room temperature, is carefully added to the pellet, and the cells are lightly mixed for 1 min at room temperature. The solution is then diluted with 10 ml of complete growth medium and immediately centrifuged at 500g for 2 min. The supernate is removed, 2 ml of complete growth medium is added, and centrifugation is repeated. The resulting fused cell fragments are then plated out in culture flasks at densitites of less than 2×10^4 cells per cm^2.

Selection of Hybrids and Reconstructed Cells

Three types of experiments were undertaken and are diagrammatically illustrated in Figures 2–4. The first experiment we undertook was to fuse whole Y-1 cells with whole AMT cells. As previously mentioned, the AMT cells have both nuclear (BrdU-resistant, HAT^S) and cytoplasmic (chloramphenicol-resistant, CAP^r) genetic markers. The Y-1 cells are HAT^r and CAP^S. As is illustrated in Figure 2, after fusion the heterokaryons, homokaryons, and unfused parentals are plated out in HAT medium containing 50 μg/ml of

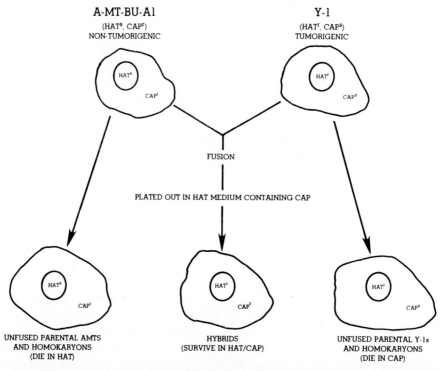

Fig. 2. Schematic representation of the experimental design to select whole-cell hybrids between the nontumorigenic AMT and tumorigenic Y-1 cells. The unfused parental cells and homokaryons die in HAT/CAP, whereas the heterokaryons survive.

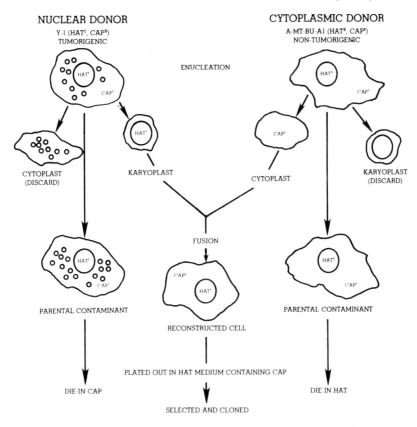

Fig. 3. Schematic representation of the experimental design to select reconstructed cells between karyoplasts derived from the tumorigenic Y-1s and cytoplasts derived from the nontumorigenic AMT cells. See Methods section for a more complete description of the selection procedures.

chloramphenicol. Under these selection conditions only the hybrid cells will survive in both HAT and CAP. The unfused AMT cells will die because of the HAT, while the unfused Y-1 cells will be killed by the CAP. Karyotyping after selection indicated the hybrid nature of the surviving clones.

The reconstruction experiment combining Y-1 karyoplasts to AMT cytoplasts used the selection procedure illustrated in Figure 3. The Y-1 cells were incubated prior to enucleation in the presence of latex spheres, as previously described [7, 41]. The Y-1 karyoplasts fused to AMT cytoplasts survive in HAT medium containing CAP, while the small percentage of whole Y-1 cells and AMT cells die in the presence of CAP and HAT, respectively. Immediately after fusion the single reconstructed cells were isolated on glass fragments and placed in multiwell chambers. Only the reconstructed cells not containing latex spheres were considered reconstructed, since both cytoplasmic hybrids (cybrids) and whole-cell fusions would contain latex spheres and would survive in HAT/ CAP. The clones not containing latex spheres that grew were then analyzed for chromosome constitution to separate whole-cell hybrids from reconstructed cells, and then only reconstructed cells were further analyzed for the tumorigenic properties.

The reconstruction experiments fusing the AMT karyoplasts to Y-1 cytoplasts are illustrated in Figure 4. Essentially BrdU-resistant AMT karyoplasts are fused to CAP^S

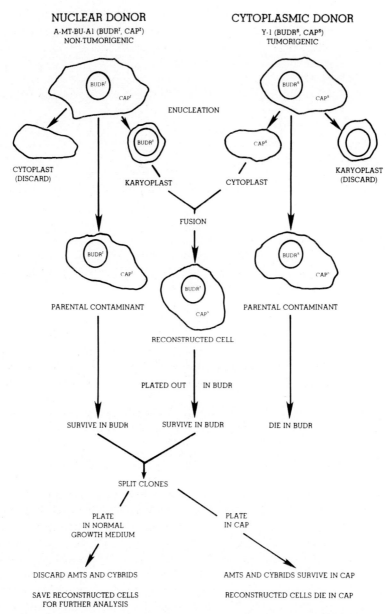

Fig. 4. Schematic representation of the experimental design to select reconstructed cells between karyoplasts derived from the nontumorigenic AMTs and cytoplasts derived from the tumorigenic Y-1 cells. See Methods section for a more complete description of the selection procedures.

Y-1 cytoplasts. The Y-1 cells that have not enucleated and whole-cell hybrids die in the presence of BrdU. The surviving BrdU-resistant reconstructed cells, AMT parentals, and cybrids (AMT whole cells × Y-1 cytoplasts) are then isolated and each growing clone is split; one half of each clone is placed in complete growth medium and the other half is placed in growth medium containing CAP. A clone that survives in medium containing CAP must have been derived from either a whole AMT cell or a cybrid. Clones that die in

CAP (but have survived the BrdU treatment) must be reconstructed cells. Thus the AMTs and cybrid clones are identified and eliminated from further study. The replicate CAP-sensitive clones, which have been maintained in normal growth medium, are then analyzed.

Electron Microscopy

The isolated hybrid and reconstructed cells were analyzed not only for their tumorigenic properties but also for their ultrastructural properties, by means of transmission electron microscopy. The AMT cells contain intracisternal A virus particles (IAP), which are excellent morphologic markers. These particles are not shed from the cells but are only transmitted vertically (that is, by mitosis) [14, 15]. The techniques for electron microscopy are standard procedures previously described [3, 16]. Thin sections were examined on a JEOL 100-B transmission electron microscope and the surface morphology of cells was observed in a JEOL U-3 scanning electron microscope.

Cell Cycle Analysis

Cell cycle analysis was done using the method described by Crissman and Tobey [17]. The cells were observed and analyzed with a Becton-Dickinson cell sorter (FACS III) using a laser wavelength of 488 nm.

In Vitro and In Vivo Tumor Assays

The parental cell lines and clones of hybrids and reconstructed cells were studied for their ability to grow in soft agar by the technique described by Miller et al [18]. This procedure consisted of first adding 10 ml of DMEM plus 10% fetal calf serum plus 3% agar into a 10-cm petri dish. After this solution had solidified another 10 ml of DMEM plus 10% fetal calf serum plus 1.5% agar and 1,000 cells were poured on top of the solidified mixture. These dishes were then incubated at $37°C$ in a humidified atmosphere containing 95% air and 5% CO_2 for two weeks. At the end of this time discrete clones of cells were readily identified and counted.

We also tested the ability of cells to grow and produce tumors in nude mice. The nude mice used in this experiment were obtained from Dr. John Porter (University of Texas Health Science Center at Dallas) and were 2–3 months old. Cells to be injected were trypsinized from the growth substrata, the trypsin was then neutralized with complete growth medium and the cells were diluted to a final concentration of 2×10^6 per ml. A total of six animals were used to test each cell line and reconstructed clone. Two animals were inoculated with 0.5×10^6, 1×10^6, or 2×10^6 cells. The cells were injected subcutaneously using a 21-gauge needle. When tumors reached approximately 1 cm (usually 3–4 weeks) the animals were sacrificed, and the tumor was excised and placed in cell culture. Once the resulting cultures were of sufficient size they were tested for their ability to respond to ACTH and to grow in HAT, BUDR, and CAP. In all instances the cells originating from the tumor were found to have the characteristics of the cells injected. If the animals failed to have a tumor in 8 weeks we considered the clone non-tumorigenic.

RESULTS

Experimental Design

The experimental designs for these studies are illustrated in Figures 2–4, as described in the Methods section. Essentially, hybrids were produced and selected be-

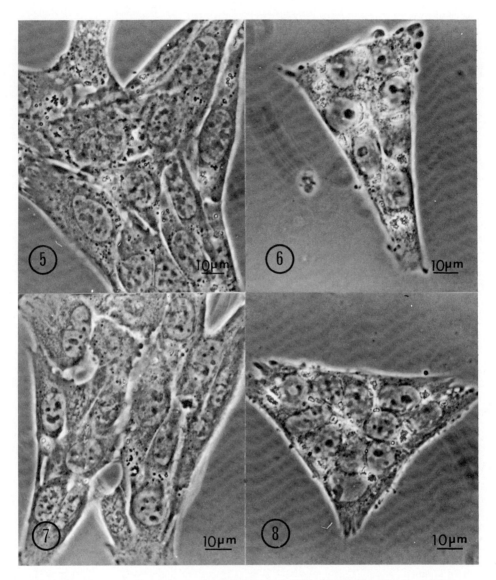

Figs. 5–8. Phase-contrast photomicrographs of the parental AMTs (Fig. 5), Y-1 (Fig. 6), and the reconstructed cells AMT(k) × Y-1(c) (Fig. 7) and Y-1(k) × AMT(c) (Fig. 8). Note that the overall morphology of the reconstructed cells resembles the morphology of the nuclear donor. ×700.

tween the nontumorigenic AMT and tumorigenic Y-1 cells (Fig. 2). The cell reconstruction experiments are illustrated in Figures 3 and 4. Reconstructed cells containing a tumorigenic nucleus and a nontumorigenic cytoplasm were produced and identified as illustrated in Figure 3. Reconstructed cells containing a nontumorigenic nucleus and a tumorigenic cytoplasm were produced and identified as illustrated in Figure 4. After selection the hybrids and reconstructed cells were further analyzed for morphology (light microscopy and transmission and scanning electron microscopy) and for in vitro and in vivo tumor production.

Morphology

Phase contrast. Figures 5 and 6 illustrate parental AMT (Fig. 5) and Y-1 (Fig. 6)

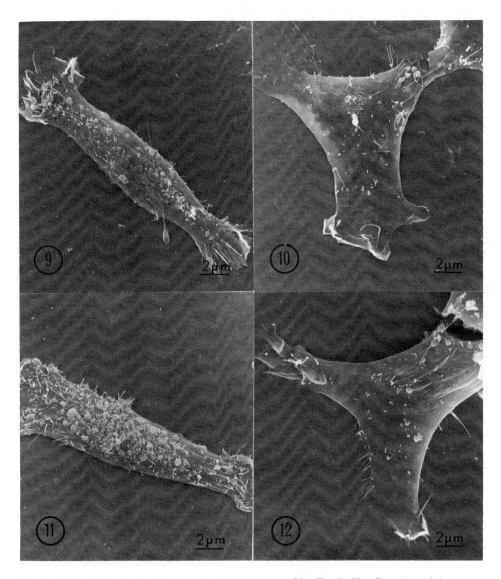

Figs. 9–12. Scanning electron micrographs of the parental AMT (Fig. 9), Y-1 (Fig. 10), and the reconstructed cells AMT(k) × Y-1(c) (Fig. 11) and Y-1(k) × AMT(c) (Fig. 12). As with the phase-contrast photomicrographs, the reconstructed cell surface topography resembles the morphology of the nuclear donor. ×1,600.

cells. The nontumorigenic AMT cells are fibroblastic in morphology and have a modal chromosome number of 65 (Fig. 5), while the tumorigenic Y-1 cells are epithelioid in morphology and have a modal chromosome number of 40 (Fig. 6). A minimum of 25 chromosome spreads were counted for each cell line. The AMT cells frequently contain numerous nucleoli, while the Y-1 cells usually contain a single prominent nucleolus. The reconstructed cells consisting of an AMT karyoplast and a Y-1 cytoplast, designated AMT(k) × Y-1(c), are depicted in Figure 7 and have a modal chromosome number of 65 while the reconstructed cells consisting of a Y-1 karyoplast and an AMT cytoplast, designated Y-1(k) × AMT(c), are depicted in Figure 8 and have a modal chromosome number of 40. As the photomicrographs in Figures 7 and 8 clearly illustrate, the overall morphology

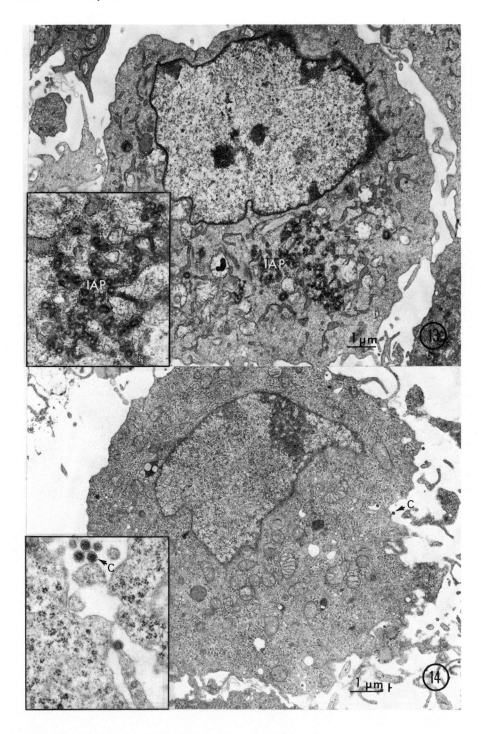

Figs. 13, 14. Transmission electron micrographs of AMT parentals (Fig. 13), containing intracisternal A particles (IAPs) (insert), and of Y-1 parentals (Fig. 14), containing C-type virus particles (insert). ×9,000.

of the selected reconstructed cells is essentially identical to that of the nuclear donor; the morphology of the AMT(k) $\times$ Y-1(c) reconstructed cells resembles the AMT parental morphology, while the morphology of the Y-1(k) $\times$ AMT(c) reconstructed cells resembles the Y-1 parental morphology.

Scanning electron microscopy. Figures 9–12 illustrate the surface topography and overall cell shape of the parental and reconstructed cells. AMT cells and reconstructed cells containing an AMT(k) $\times$ Y-1(c) are depicted in Figures 9 and 11. The fibroblastic shape of isolated cells is clearly different from the Y-1 cells. The surfaces of the fibroblastic cells contain considerably more blebs and microvilli than the epithelioid cells. Y-1 cells and reconstructed cells containing a Y-1(k) $\times$ AMT(c) are depicted in Figures 10 and 12. The epithelial shape of isolated cells is similar to those seen in clusters (Figs. 6, 8), and the surfaces of the cells contain a few blebs and microvilli. Figures 7, 8, 11, and 12 indicate that the shape and surface features of the reconstructed cells are essentially controlled by the nucleus. Even though enucleated cells (cytoplasts) can maintain the shape of the whole cell for short periods of time, it is clear that once rescued by another nucleus the cytoskeletal elements within the cytoplasm do not appear to maintain their independence but are directed by the host nucleus.

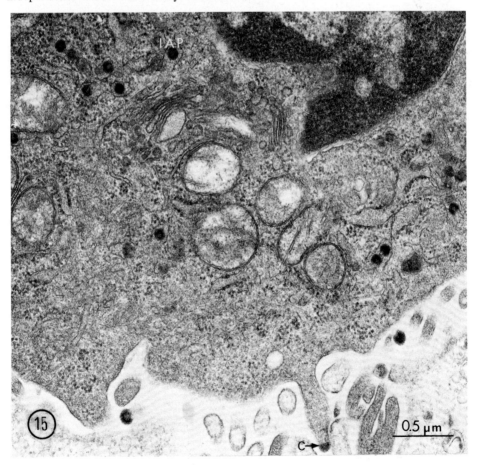

Fig. 15. Transmission electron micrograph of a hybrid cell produced by fusing AMTs to Y-1 cells. Note the presence of both intracisternal A and C-type virus particles. $\times$ 36,000.

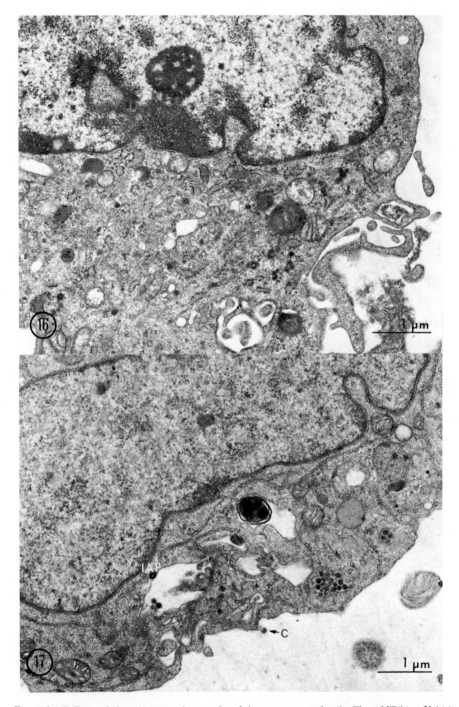

Figs. 16, 17. Transmission electron micrographs of the reconstructed cells. The AMT(k) × Y-1(c) reconstructed cells (Fig. 16) contain intracisternal A particles, but C-type particles have not been observed. The Y-1(k) × AMT(c) (Fig. 17) contain both types of particles. ×17,000.

Transmission electron microscopy. The most striking ultrastructural difference between the Y-1 parentals and the AMT parentals is shown in Figures 13 and 14. The Y-1 cells contain numerous C-type virus particles, which are shed from the cell surface (Fig. 14 and insert) and are both vertically and horizontally transmitted. The AMT cells, though originally derived from a murine mammary tumor, are nontumorigenic in vivo but contain numerous intracisternal A-type virus particles (Fig. 13). These A-type virus particles reside within the cisternae of the endoplasmic reticulum and are only vertically transmitted (ie, by mitosis), as shedding does not occur. As previously reported, cocultivation of AMT cytoplasts with other whole cells does not result in transfer of intracisternal A particles to the other cells. However, when whole-cell hybrids are produced by AMT and Y-1 cells, both types of particles are present (Fig. 15). The ultrastructure of the reconstructed cells are depicted in Figures 16 and 17. The AMT(k) × Y-1(c) reconstructed cells contain intracisternal A particles, but C-type particles in these cells have not been observed (Fig. 16). It is possible that the nuclei in these reconstructed cells cannot incorporate the C-type virus genome but definitive information on this is not yet available. The Y-1(k) × AMT(c) reconstructed cells contain both C-type and intracisternal A-type virus particles (Fig. 17). However, considerably fewer intracisternal A-type virus particles were observed in the reconstructed cells than in the parental AMTS.

In Vitro and In Vivo Tumor Assays

The parentals, hybrids, and reconstructed cells were studied for their ability to grow in soft agar. In six different experiments in which 1,000 Y-1 parentals or Y-1(k) × AMT(c) originating from a single pure clone were placed in soft agar, 22–26% of the cells would develop into viable colonies consisting of greater than 50 cells in 3 weeks. This is in contrast to the results obtained from the AMT parentals and AMT(k) × Y-1(c). When 1,000 of these cells were placed in soft agar, none of the cells developed into viable colonies consisting of greater than 50 cells in 2–3 weeks. In each instance the reconstructed cell behaved identically with the parental cell line from which the nucleus was derived.

The AMT × Y-1 whole-cell hybrid clones varied widely in their ability to grow in soft agar. Some of the hybrid clones behaved like the AMT cells in that they failed to grow in agar while some of the clones grew just as efficiently as, but none more efficiently than, Y-1 cells. In addition a few of the clones grew in soft agar with an intermediate efficiency.

When Y-1 cells or Y-1(k) × AMT(c) cells were injected into nude mice, each of the six mice injected developed large tumors in 4 weeks even at the lower inoculation. This is in direct contrast with the results obtained from the inoculation of AMT cells or AMT(k) × Y-1(c) cells. In these instances none of these mice produced tumors even when allowed to survive for 8 weeks. These data correlated very closely with the soft agar data.

Hybrid cells formed from the fusion of an AMT × Y-1 were also tested for their ability to produce tumors. For this experiment we chose three different clones. One clone had a plating efficiency in soft agar of 25%, another had a plating efficiency of less than 0.5%, and the third had a plating efficiency of 5% in soft agar. Approximately 2×10^6 cells taken from each clone were injected into nude mice. By 8 weeks only the mouse that was injected with cells taken from the clone that grew best in soft agar produced a tumor. The other two clones did not produce tumors by 8 weeks.

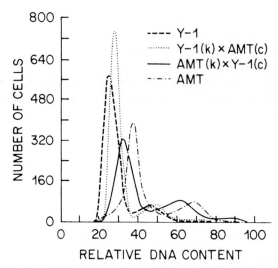

Fig. 18. Cell cycle analysis of the parental and reconstructed cells by means of a fluorescence-activated cell sorter. As to the percentage of cells in various stages of the cell cycle, the reconstructed cells lie between the parental cells, but overall the reconstructed cells have a cell-cycle profile closer to that of the nuclear donor.

Cell-Cycle Analysis

The results obtained from the cell sorter showing the distribution of DNA content of the reconstructed and parental cells illustrated are in Figure 18. The larger peaks represent the various cell lines in the G_1 phase of the cell cycle (prior to DNA replication), while the smaller peaks represent cells in the G_2 or M phase of the cell cycle. The cells in S phase (during DNA replication) lie between the two peaks. The parental Y-1 and AMT cells differ dramatically in the percentage of cells in various stages of the cell cycle, while the reconstructed cells lie between the parentals. Even though the reconstructed cells behave somewhat differently from the parentals, they do have a cell-cycle profile closer to that of the nuclear donor. The approximate percentage of the parental and reconstructed cells in various stages of the cell cycle is as follows: Y-1 [G_1 = 84%, S = 7%, G_2 + M = 9%]; Y-1(k) $\times$ AMT(c) [G_1 = 81%, S = 6%, G_2 + M = 13%], AMT(k) $\times$ Y-1(c) [G_1 = 65%, S = 12%, G_2 + M = 23%]; AMT [G_1 = 69%, S = 11%, G_2 + M = 20%].

DISCUSSION

Several approaches to elucidating the genetic basis of tumorigenesis are available but the most popular has been the production of somatic cell hybrids between tumorigenic and nontumorigenic cells. More recently the use of cytoplasmic hybrids (cybrids) has also been available for studying certain aspects of tumorigenesis. Both of these methods have provided useful information concerning the control mechanisms in the expression or suppression of tumorigenesis but few widely supported generalizations have been derived from such studies. Technical developments for producing reconstructed cells (eg, nuclear transplantation) have also been progressing in recent years and this report illustrates the utility of using such reconstructed cells for analyzing nuclear and cytoplasmic control mechanisms in the expression or suppression of the tumorigenic state. The following discussion will review some of the results of fusion experiments involving whole cells and cytoplasmic hybrids, which will illustrate that, even though these approaches result in the acquisition of useful information, elucidation of the mechanisms involved in tumorigenesis have not been unequivocally resolved with these techniques.

There have been numerous reports on the fusion and characterization of hybrid cells produced between tumorigenic and nontumorigenic cells [1, 2, 19–34] and this discussion is not meant to be exhaustive but only to highlight some of the main points. The most important variable in fusing whole cells in attempting to study the underlying genetic basis of tumorigenesis has been the selection of appropriate cell types. Essentially two types of experiments have been utilized. The first involves interspecific hybrids that rapidly segregate chromosomes, and the results of these experiments have not elucidated any generalized mechanisms. Most but not all interspecific hybrids produced by fusing a tumorigenic with a nontumorigenic cell result in expression of the tumorigenic phenotype. These experiments cannot clearly differentiate between instability of the chromosome constitution in such hybrids and specific genetic or epigenetic factors that may be involved in the control of tumorigenesis events. The second type of whole-cell hybrid experiment involves intraspecific crosses, which segregate fewer chromosomes and have provided interesting insights into certain aspects of the expression of the tumorigenic state. Even though there are exceptions to the following statement it does appear to have substantial support from a variety of laboratories. Essentially in intraspecific crosses between tumorigenic and nontumorigenic cells there is an initial suppression of the tumorigenic state provided by some factor in the nontumorigenic cells. This suppression is then removed when a certain chromosome or possibly some epigenetic factor is lost. This was illustrated in a recent report by Sager and Kovac [2], who produced intraspecific hybrids both of which had a stable diploid chromosome constitution, and their results indicated an initial suppression of the tumorigenic state followed by a reexpression of the tumorigenic state along with chromosomal instability. These studies with whole-cell hybrids are consistent with the ones we report in this communication in that intraspecific hybrids are capable of expressing both the tumorigenic and nontumorigenic phenotype. This type of experiment does not, however, allow one to distinguish between genetic and epigenetic factors that may be of fundamental importance. Since hybrids containing almost complete sets of chromosomes from the parental cells can either suppress or express the tumorigenic phenotype, experiments have recently been reported in which cytoplasmic hybrids have been used to try to determine if epigenetic factors may be involved in either the suppression or expression of the tumorigenic state [15, 35, 36].

In brief, the results of such experiments are as follows: Using diploid intraspecific cells, Howell and Sager [35] showed that fusing a nontumorigenic cell with a tumorigenic cytoplasm did not result in expression of the tumorigenic phenotype. They did interpret some of their results to indicate that when a tumorigenic cell was fused with a nontumorigenic cytoplasm, a partial suppression occurred in some of the cybrid clones, indicating that the cytoplasm may be capable of transmitting some suppression factor. Ziegler [36], on the other hand, reported that the cell cytoplasm did not have any effect on the supression or expression of the tumorigenic state in cybrids, which would indicate that independent cytoplasmic control does not play a major role in tumorigenesis. However, Ziegler did report that the cytoplasm could affect the saturation density of cybrids, which is consistent with the observations we previously reported [15]. In those experiments, we fused tumorigenic murine SV-403T3 cells to nontumorigenic murine A-MT-BU-A1 cytoplasms and the resulting cybrids grew to higher saturation densities than the parental SV403T3 cells, and were capable of making tumors in nude mice at lower inoculation densities than the SV-403T3 cells. As with the whole-cell hybrids, broad generalizations concerning the control of the tumorigenic state with cytoplasmic hybrids have not appeared. Again the choice of cells lines and selection procedures for studying these phenomena appear to be of major importance.

In this report we have illustrated the techniques for producing reconstructed cells between tumorigenic and nontumorigenic parental components and have analyzed these reconstructed cells for their ability to grow in soft agar and in nude mice. As far as we were able to determine, this is the first report of the use of reconstructed cells to analyze factors that may be important in controlling the expression or suppression of the tumorigenic phenotype, even though several reports and procedures are available for producing such reconstructed cells [7, 37, 38, 40, 41]. The results of these initial experiments are consistent with the idea that the nucleus (karyoplast) is sufficient to control the expression or suppression of the tumorigenic state.

ACKNOWLEDGMENTS

This study was supported in part by US Public Health Service funds (HL20643, HL00422) and a grant from the Muscular Dystrophy Association.

The excellent photographic assistance of Ms Mary Tobleman is gratefully acknowledged. We also wish to thank Mr. Mike Glover for his help in the design and construction of the acrylic inserts used for the enucleation experiments and Dr. Woodridge E. Wright for valuable discussions.

REFERENCES

1. Stanbridge EJ: Nature 260:17, 1976.
2. Sager R, Kovac PE: Somat Cell Genet 4:375, 1978.
3. Shay JW, Porter KR, Prescott DM: Proc Natl Acad Sci USA 71:3059, 1974.
4. Wright WE, Hayflick L: Exp Cell Res 74:187, 1972.
5. Prescott DM, Myerson D, Wallace J: Exp Cell Res 71:480, 1972.
6. Shay JW, Porter KR, Prescott DM: J Cell Biol 59(2):311a, 1973.
7. Veomett G, Prescott DM, Shay J, Porter KR: Proc Natl Acad Sci USA 71:1999, 1974.
8. Buonassisi V, Sato G, Cohen AI: Proc Natl Acad Sci USA 48:1184, 1962.
9. Schneider EL, Stanbridge EJ, Epstein CJ: Exp Cell Res 84:311, 1976.
10. Brown S, Teplitz M, Revel JP: Proc Natl Acad Sci USA 71:464, 1974.
11. Chanock RM, Hayflick L, Barile MF: Proc Natl Acad Sci USA 48:41, 1962.
12. Veomett G, Shay J, Hough PVC, Prescott DM: In Prescott DM (ed): "Methods in Cell Biology." New York: Academic, 1976, pp 1–6.
13. Clark MA, Crenshaw AH, Shay JW: Tissue Culture Assoc Man 4:801, 1978.
14. Malech HL, Wivel NA: Cell 9:383, 1976.
15. Shay JW, Peters TT, Fuseler JW: Cell 14:835, 1978.
16. Shay JW, Gershenbaum MR, Porter KR: Exp Cell Res 94:47, 1975.
17. Crissman HA, Tobey RA: Science 184:1297, 1974.
18. Miller CL, Fuseler JW, Brinkley BR: Cell 12:319, 1977.
19. Lyons LB, Thompson EB: J Cell Physiol 90:179, 1976.
20. Foa C, Simonetti J, Berebbi M, Fischer P, Vetterlein M: Oncology 35:58, 1978.
21. Jha KK, Cacciapuoti J, Ozer HL: J Cell Physiol 97:147, 1978.
22. Marshall CJ, Dave H: J Cell Sci 33:171, 1978.
23. Stanbridge EJ, Wilkinson J: Proc Natl Acad Sci USA 75:1466, 1978.
24. Bregula U, Klein G, Harris H: J Cell Sci 8:673, 1971.
25. Harris H, Miller OJ, Klein G, Worst P, Tachibana T: Nature 223:363, 1969.
26. Jonasson J, Povey S, Harris H: J Cell Sci 24:217, 1977.
27. Jonasson J, Harris H: J Cell Sci 24:255, 1977.

28. Klein G, Bregula U, Wiener F, Harris H: J Cell Sci 8:659, 1971.
29. Miller CL, Fuseler JW, Brinkley BR: Cell 12:319, 1977.
30. Straus DS, Jonasson J, Harris H: J Cell Sci 25:73, 1977.
31. Wiener F, Klein G, Harris H: J Cell Sci 8:681, 1971.
32. Wiener F, Klein G, Harris H: J Cell Sci 12:253, 1973.
33. Wiener F, Klein G, Harris H: J Cell Sci 15:177, 1974.
34. Wiener F, Klein G, Harris H: J Cell Sci 16:189, 1974.
35. Howell AN, Sager R: Proc Natl Acad Sci USA 75:2358, 1978.
36. Ziegler ML: Somat Cell Genet 4:477, 1978.
37. Ege T, Krondahl U, Ringertz NR: Exp Cell Res 88:428, 1974.
38. Ege T, Ringertz NR: Exp Cell Res 94:469, 1975.
39. Lucas JJ, Kates JR: Cell 7:397, 1976.
40. Krondahl U, Bols N, Ege T, Linder S, Ringertz NR: Proc Natl Acad Sci USA 74:606, 1977.
41. Shay JW: Proc Nat Acad Sci USA 74:2461, 1977.

Journal of Supramolecular Structure 11:51−60 (1979)
Tumor Cell Surfaces and Malignancy 27−36

Endogenous Cyclic AMP Does Not Modulate Transport of Hexoses, Nucleosides, or Nucleobases in Chinese Hamster Ovary Cells

Robert M. Wohlhueter, Peter G.W. Plagemann, and J.R. Sheppard

Department of Microbiology (R.M.W., P.G.W.P.) and Genetics and Cell Biology (J.R.S.) and Dight Institute for Human Genetics (J.R.S.) University of Minnesota, Minneapolis, Minnesota 55455

In a previous study we have demonstrated that neither extracellular nor intracellular cyclic adenosine monophosphate (AMP) levels directly affect the uptake of nucleosides, nucleobases, or hexoses by various types of cultured mammalian cells. Uptake of these nutrients into cells, however, involves two processes operating in tandem: facilitated transport across the membrane and intracellular phosphorylation; and uptake rates generally reflect the rates of substrate phosphorylation rather than of transport. In the present study we have examined the question of whether substrate transport per se is regulated by intracellular cyclic AMP. Initially various cell lines, grown both in suspension and monolayer culture, were screened for their cyclic AMP response to prostaglandin E_1, isoproterenol, and inhibitors of cyclic AMP phosphodiesterase. Prostaglandin E_1 treatment of Chinese hamster ovary cells was selected as the system giving the largest and most consistent (50-fold to 100-fold) elevation of cyclic AMP. Rapid kinetic techniques were used to measure the transport of 3-O-methylglucose, thymidine, adenosine, hypoxanthine, and adenine in wild-type cells and in mutant sublines incapable of phosphorylating these substrates. In no case was an increase in intracellular cyclic AMP accompanied by a significant change in the rate of transport of these substrates, although prostaglandin E_1 slightly inhibited the transport of various substrates.

Key words: cyclic AMP; transport of nucleosides, nucleobases, and hexoses; Chinese hamster ovary cells.

Results of numerous studies have led to the view that hexose, nucleoside, and nucleobase transport in mammalian cells might be regulated in some manner by cyclic adenosine monophosphate (AMP). For example, the rapid increase in uridine uptake observed in density-inhibited or serum-starved, cultured mammalian cells consequent to mitogen stimulation was found to correlate with a decrease in intracellular cyclic AMP levels [1−7], and stimulation of cyclic AMP production by treatment of the cells with prostaglandin E_1 (PGE_1), theophylline, or dibutyryl cyclic AMP prevented the

0091-7419/79/1101-0051$02.00 © 1979 Alan R. Liss, Inc.

increase in uridine uptake caused by mitogens [1, 3] . Hexose uptake is also stimulated, although somewhat more slowly than uridine uptake, in mitogen-stimulated untransformed cultured cells [8] and lymphocytes [9, 10] , and the stimulation in lymphocytes is counteracted by increases in intracellular cyclic AMP concentration [10] . Furthermore, the insulin-stimulated glucose uptake by fat cells is accompanied by a decrease in intracellular cyclic AMP [11, 12] . There exists also an inverse correlation between changes in hexose uptake capacity and intracellular cyclic AMP levels when cells become transformed to tumor cells [8, 13, 14] .

In some studies incubation with high, exogenous concentrations of cyclic AMP or dibutyryl cyclic AMP were found to cause decreases in rates of uridine and thymidine uptake in Chinese hamster ovary (CHO) cells [15] , Balb 3T3 [3] , and neoplastic mast cells [16] , and of hypoxanthine uptake in Chinese hamster lung cells [17] ; and treatment of L cells with RO20-1274, an inhibitor of cyclic AMP phosphodiesterase, lowered the uridine uptake rate concomitant with an increase in cyclic AMP concentration [18] . But in other studies, such treatments increased uptake rates of thymidine and uridine in CV-1 monkey cells [19] and mouse L cells [18] , respectively, and of both substrates in human liver cells [20] .

Results of experiments measuring hexose uptake have been equally contradictory; incubation of untransformed and murine sarcoma virus-transformed Balb 3T3 cells [13, 21] and human glioma cells [22] with dibutyryl cyclic AMP plus theophylline has been reported to result in an increase of glucose uptake, whereas a similar treatment of polyoma virus-transformed 3T3 cells caused an inhibition of deoxyglucose uptake [23] . Incubation of 3T3 cells with adenosine also resulted in a decrease in 3-O-methylglucose uptake, and indirect evidence suggested that such effect might be related to an increase in intracellular cyclic AMP [24] .

The observed effects of extracellular cyclic AMP or dibutyryl cyclic AMP on substrate uptake rates, however, are probably secondary; they become apparent only after hours of incubation with cyclic nucleotides, whereas exposure of several lines of cultured mammalian cells to 1 mM dibutyryl cyclic AMP had no immediate effect on their uptake of uridine, thymidine, or deoxyglucose [25, 26] . Furthermore, we have previously shown that changes in intracellular cyclic AMP level induced in such cells by treatment with papaverine, PGE_1, or isoproterenol had no effect on the uptake of these substrates nor did it correlate with the inhibition of uridine, hypoxanthine, or deoxyglucose uptake caused by some of these substances [26] .

One complicating factor in all the studies summarized above is that they were conducted with cells in which the substrates were rapidly metabolized so that substrate uptake rather than transport through the membrane was measured. Uptake here is defined as the intracellular accumulation of radioactivity derived from extracellular, radioiabeled substrate. Uptake thus reflects the tandem operation of facilitated transport and intracellular phosphorylation plus subsequent metabolic conversion [27, 28] . Recent studies have shown that long-term (1–10 min) rates of uptake of nucleosides [20–32], nucleobases [33], and deoxyglucose [34] by various cell lines reflect mainly the rate of phosphorylation of these substrates rather than the rate of transport of the unmodified substrate through the plasma membrane (for review see Wohlhueter and Plagemann [35]). Our previous results [26] , therefore, did not unequivocally rule out an effect of cyclic AMP on the transport step per se. In the present study, we have examined this possibility by measuring the transport of nucleosides, nucleobases, and hexoses directly in cells incapable of metabolizing the substrates.

MATERIALS AND METHODS

Cell Culture

Sublines of CHO cells deficient in adenosine kinase (AK⁻), thymidine kinase (T6y-4), and hypoxanthine guanine phosphoribosyltransferase (VT-29, 6TG^r) were obtained from Dr. L. Siminovitch (University of Toronto) and a CHO line deficient in adenine phosphoribosyltransferase (DAP-12; Taylor et al [36]) from Dr. M. Taylor (Indiana University). These lines were all derived from proline auxotrophic clones of CHO cells (for convenience here designated "wild-type"). All lines of CHO cells, and lines of mouse lymphoma P388 cells, mouse L cells, and HeLa cells, were routinely propagated in suspension culture in Eagle's minimal essential medium for suspension culture supplemented with nonessential amino acids and 10% (v/v) heat-inactivated, fetal bovine serum as described previously [30, 31]. Cultures were incubated on a gyrotory shaker, except for cultures of more than 500 ml, which were incubated with magnetic stirring. Monolayer cultures in 25 cm³ Falcon flasks were established from suspension cultures and incubated in a CO_2 incubator. The growth medium was the same as used for suspension cultures, except that its base was Eagle's minimal medium for monolayer culture. Cells were enumerated with a Coulter counter. Cultures were routinely assayed for mycoplasma contamination by measuring the relative reates of incorporation of 5 μM [³H]uridine (40–80 cpm/pmole) and 5 μM [³H]uracil (40–80 cpm/pmole) into acid-insoluble material over a 30–60 min time period, similar to the method described by Schneider et al [37]. The incorporation of uracil was consistently very low in all cell lines used in this study and the ratio of uridine to uracil incorporation was > 500, indicating absence of mycoplasma.

Transport Studies

Cells were harvested from exponential phase suspension cultures by centrifugation at 400 g for 2 min and suspended to about $(1-3) \times 10^7$ cells per milliliter in basal medium 42 (BM42; Plagemann [38]) or glucose-free BM42B, as indicated in the appropriate experiments. The suspensions were supplemented where indicated with 60 or 120 μM PGE$_1$, incubated at 37° for 5 min, equilibrated at 25°, and then assayed for substrate transport. Substrate influx was measured against an intracellular concentration presumed to be effectively zero at zero time (the zero-trans protocol [27, 39]) using a rapid mixing/sampling technique which has been described in detail previously [27, 31]. Briefly, samples of 448 μl of suspension were mixed with 61 μl of a solution of labeled substrate at short intervals by means of a hand-operated dual syringe apparatus. The mixtures emerging from the mixing chamber were dispensed into 12 tubes mounted in an Eppendorf microcentrifuge. The tubes contained 100 μl of an oil mixture (final density = 1.034 g/ml). After the last sample had been mixed, the centrifuge was started, and within an estimated 2 sec, the cells had entered the oil phase, thus terminating transport. For sampling times in excess of 2 min, cell suspension and substrate solution were mixed in the same proportion provided by the mixing apparatus, and 509-μl samples were removed at appropriate times and centrifuged through oil. The culture fluid and oil were removed and the cell pellets were analyzed for radioactivity.

Total water space and extracellular water space in cell pellets obtained by centrifuging cells through the oil phase were determined in parallel runs in which substrate was replaced by [¹⁴C]carboxylinulin in ³H$_2$O [27]. All values for cell-associated radioactivity were corrected for radioactivity in the extracellular space of cell pellets,

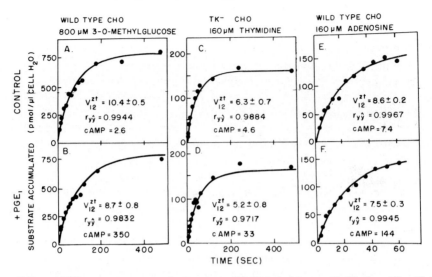

Fig. 1. Effect of PGE₁ pretreatment on the transport of 3-O-methylglucose (A, B), thymidine (C, D), and adenosine (E, F). Cells were harvested from exponential phase cultures of wild-type CHO (A, B, E, F) or thymidine kinase-deficient (TK⁻) CHO (C, D), and suspended to about 1.3×10^7 cells per milliliter in BM42B (C–F) or glucose-free BM42B (A, B). One portion of each suspension was supplemented with 120 μM PGE₁, and the treated (B, D, F) and untreated (A, C, E) suspensions were incubated at 37° for 5 min and then thermally equilibrated at 25°. In E and F both untreated and PGE₁-treated suspensions were also supplemented with 10 μM 2-deoxycoformycin during preincubation. Aliquots of the suspension were extracted for assay of intracellular cyclic AMP as described under Materials and Methods. Other aliquots of the suspension were assayed at 25° for transport of the appropriate substrates by the rapid kinetic technique; the substrate concentrations were 800 μM 3-O-methyl-[³H] D-glucose (190) cpm/μl); 160 μM [³H] thymidine (720 cpm/μl), or 240 μM [³H] adenosine (860 cpm/μl). Radioactivity per cell pellet was corrected for radioactivity trapped in extra-cellular water space and converted to pmoles/μl cell water ($S_{2,t}$) on the basis of the experimentally determined intracellular water space. The intracellular and extracellular water spaces in A and B, in C and D, and in E and F were 22.2 and 3.3, 8.4 and 3.2, and 10.9 and 5.3 μl/cell pellet, respectively. Equation 1 was fit to the time courses of substrate accumulation whereby all R parameters were constrained to equal each other and K was fixed at 5, 0.2, and 0.2 mM for 3-O-methylglucose, thymidine, and adenosine, respectively. The correlation coefficient ($r_{y,\,y}$) is indicated for each fit. v^{zt}_{12} values were calculated from K and the computed R parameters according to Equation 2.

and converted to pmoles per microliter cell water on the basis of the experimentally determined intracellular water space (Total water space − Inulin space/Cell pellet).

To evaluate transport rates an integrated rate equation (developed for zero-trans influx to conform to the simple carrier model of Eilam and Stein [39]) was fit by the method of least squares to time courses of accumulation of substrate to transmembrane equilibrium (for details see Refs. 28, 31):

$$S_{2,\,t} = S_1 \left[1 - \exp \left(- \frac{t + (R_{21} + R_{ee}S_1/K)S_{2,t}}{KR_{00} + R_{12}S_1 + R_{21}S_1 + S_1{}^2 R_{ee}/K} \right) \right] \qquad (1)$$

where $S_{2,t}$ = concentration of substrate inside the cell at time t ($S_{2,0} = 0$); S_1 = exogenous substrate concentration (and is taken as a constant); K = substrate carrier dissociation constant; and the R terms are resistant factors proportional to the time of a round of the carrier as defined by Eilam and Stein [39] and equal to the reciprocals of the corresponding maximum velocities. Equation 1 was fit to individual time courses of intracellular substrate accumulation at a single substrate concentration (see Fig. 1) with all R constants held equal (corresponding to a completely symmetrical carrier) and with K fixed (at 5 mM for 3-O-methylglucose, 200 μM for thymidine, 200 μM for adenosine, 1.5 mM for hypoxanthine, and 2 mM for adenine). These values of K were estimated in previous studies with CHO cells (summarized in Ref. 28 and unpublished observations).

Justification for the assumption of complete carrier symmetry is available as yet only for nucleoside transport in Novikoff rat hepatoma cells [31], but the reported zero-trans transport data for other cell lines, including CHO cells, support the view that carriers for nucleoside and nucleobase transport in cultured cells in general are symmetrical [28], ie, that transport is indifferent to direction and to whether the carrier is loaded or empty.

Initial velocities of zero-trans entry (v_{12}^{zt}) were calculated from K and the estimated R constant ($R_{12} = R_{ee} = R_{oo}$) according to the original zero-trans differential equation of Eilam and Stein (Eq. 18, Ref. 39) at $S_2 = 0$:

$$v_{12}^{zt} = \frac{KS_1}{K^2 R_{oo} + KR_{12}S_1} \tag{2}$$

Cyclic AMP Analyses

Samples of $(2-7) \times 10^7$ cells were collected by centrifugation, washed twice in phosphate buffered saline and extracted with 0.5–2 ml of a solution of cold ($0°$) 5% (w/v) trichloroacetic acid. The acid extracts were assayed for cyclic AMP by a modification of Gilman's method as described previously [14, 26] and for protein by the method of Lowry [40].

Chemicals

Radiochemicals were purchased as follows: 3-O-[^{3}H-methyl] methyl-D-glucose from ICN (Irvine, California); [^{3}H-methyl] thymidine and [G-^{3}H] hypoxanthine from Amersham/Searle (Arlington Heights, Illinois); [8-^{3}H] adenosine from Schwarz/Mann (Orangeburg, New York); and [^{14}C-carboxyl] carboxylinulin and ^{3}H$_2$O from New England Nuclear (Boston). Chemicals were obtained as follows: papaverine from Eastman Organic Chemicals (Rochester, New York) and isoproterenol and 1-methyl-3-isobutyl-xanthine from Sigma (St. Louis). PGE$_1$ was a gift from Dr. J. Pike, Upjohn Co. Other chemicals were reagent grade from standard suppliers.

RESULTS AND DISCUSSION

Suspensions of cells have a great advantage over monolayer cultures in studies on the facilitated transport of nucleosides, nucleobases, and hexoses in that the density of cells in suspension can be manipulated in such manner [$(2-5) \times 10^7$ cells per milliliter] that the intracellular H$_2$O space of the cells makes up at least 2% of the total water space of the suspension [27]. Thus, this proportion of total substrate added to the suspension will have accumulated intracellularly at equilibrium — a proportion that can be determined with reasonable accuracy. In contrast, in monolayer cultures at best only 0.2% of the total substrate can accumulate intracellularly in the absence of trapping

TABLE I. Effect of Various Treatments on the Intracellular Levels of Cyclic AMP in Various Cell Lines Propagated in Suspension or Monolayers

Culture	Treatment	Cyclic AMP (pmoles/mg protein) in			
		CHO	HeLa	P388	L
Suspension[a]	None	7.7	3.2	3.6	7.0[c]
	PGE$_1$	205.	8.7	8.1	ND[d]
	Papaverine	9.4	4.7	4.1	8.0
	Isoproterenol	9.4	3.1	4.8	ND
	MIX	6.1	ND	4.3	ND
	PGE$_1$ + MIX	267.	ND	8.0	ND
Monolayer[b]	None	27.	16	ND	13
	PGE$_1$	1,200.	9	ND	40
	Papaverine	38.	9	ND	23
	Isoproterenol	27.	9	ND	17

[a]Cells were collected from exponential phase cultures and suspended to $(0.5-3) \times 10^7$ cells per milliliter in serum-free BM42B containing, where indicated, 60 μM PGE$_1$, 200 μM papaverine, 100 μM isoproterenol, 0.5 mM 1-methyl-3-isobutylxanthine (MIX) or combinations thereof and incubated at 37° for 5 min. The cells from 4 ml of suspension were collected by centrifugation, washed twice in phosphate-buffered saline, and extracted with 0.5 ml cold 5% (w/v) trichloracetic acid. The acid extracts were analyzed for concentrations of cyclic AMP and protein as described in Materials and Methods.

[b]Cells were propagated in 25-cm^3 Falcon flasks and then analyzed as described above.

[c]Data from Sheppard and Plagemann [26].

[d]ND, not determined.

by phosphorylation. This low ratio of cell to total water hinders accurate estimates of intracellular substrate concentration. For these reasons it seemed preferable to use suspension cultures to assess the effect of endogenous cyclic AMP on substrate transport. Thus, the first prerequisite for these studies was to find cell lines in which cyclic AMP levels could be manipulated in some manner.

Previous studies have shown that the cyclic AMP levels of Novikoff rat hepatoma cells and mouse L cells propagated in suspension culture were unresponsive to treatment of the cells with PGE$_1$, isoproterenol, and various inhibitors of cyclic AMP phosphodiesterase [26]. We have now screened several other cell lines that can be grown in suspension culture for cyclic AMP response to such treatments (Table I). Treatment of CHO cells with PGE$_1$ was the only combination that elevated intracellular cyclic AMP levels by a factor of more than 2–3. In fact, in repeated experiments, the intracellular cyclic AMP level of wild-type CHO cells increased consistently between 20 and 100 times within 5 min of incubation with 60 or 120 μM PGE$_1$ (see also Table II). The elevated cyclic AMP levels persisted for at least 30 min in the presence of PGE$_1$ (data not shown). For comparative purposes we also determined the effect of the various treatments on intracellular cyclic AMP levels when the cells of the three lines that adhere to culture dishes were propagated in monolayer culture. In principle, the cell lines behaved the same whether propagated in suspension or monolayer culture, except that both the untreated and treated monolayer cultures possessed several times more cyclic AMP (expressed per milligram protein) than did the corresponding suspension cultures (Table I). A marked increase in cyclic AMP in response to PGE$_1$ has also been observed

TABLE II. Effect of PGE_1 Pretreatment on Cyclic AMP Concentrations and Initial Transport Velocities for Various Substrates in Wild-Type CHO Cells and Cells of Various Enzyme-Deficient Sublines Thereof*.

CHO cells	Substrate	μM	$v_{\frac{1}{2}}^{zt}$ (pmoles/μl cell $H_2O \cdot$sec)		[Cyclic AMP] (pmoles/mg protein)	
			Control	+PGE_1	Control	+PGE_1
Wild-type	3-O-methyl-	800	10.4 ± 0.5	8.7 ± 0.8	2.6	350
	glucose	800	10.8 ± 1.0	9.6 ± 0.8	4.0	226
		800	18.6 ± 1.1	12.8 ± 0.7	5.5	85
		800	16.4 ± 3.2	13.4 ± 2.1	3.1	179
TK$^-$	Thymidine	160	6.3 ± 0.7	5.2 ± 0.8	4.6	33
AK$^-$	Adenosine	80	6.1 ± 0.9	4.6 ± 0.7	6.1	39
		160	10.1 ± 0.6	8.3 ± 0.2	6.0	8.4
Wild-type	Adenosine	160	8.6 ± 0.2	7.5 ± 0.3	7.4	144
HGPRT$^-$	Hypoxanthine	160	3.2 ± 0.2	2.2 ± 0.2	ND[a]	ND
		320	4.7 ± 0.5	3.3 ± 0.3	4.7	5.4
APRT$^-$	Adenine	240	2.9 ± 0.3	2.4 ± 0.3	4.6	4.3
		240	5.3 ± 0.7	4.3 ± 0.6	4.6	5.9
Wild-type	Adenine	240	1.7 ± 0.2	1.2 ± 0.1	4.2	150
		480	8.2 ± 1.6	6.8 ± 1.0	3.3	148

*Values are from the experiments illustrated in Figure 1 and from other experiments conducted in the same manner. TK$^-$, AK$^-$, HGPRT$^-$, and APRT$^-$ are CHO sublines deficient in thymidine kinase, adenosine kinase, hypoxanthine/guanine phosphoribosyltransferase, and adenine phosphoribosyltransferase, respectively.

[a]ND, not determined.

in monolayer cultures of CHO cells by O'Neill and Hsie [41], and the adenylate cyclase of various types of hamster cells has been shown to be greatly stimulated by prostaglandins [42]. PGE_1 also causes an increase in cyclic AMP in 3T3 cells [1, 3, 26, 43] and human WI38 cells [44], but these cells cannot be propagated in suspension culture. The adenylate cyclase of L929 is greatly stimulated by PGE_1 [42, 46], but our line of L cells is unresponsive whether propagated in monolayers or suspension. The responses of 3T6 cells and some transformed 3T3 cells to prostaglandins, on the other hand, are minimal [26, 42, 45].

Figure 1 illustrates typical time courses of accumulation of 3-O-methyl-D-glucose, thymidine, and adenosine to transmembrane equilibrium in untreated and PGE_1-treated CHO cells in suspension. Table II summarizes the initial transport velocities for these substrates and for adenine and hypoxanthine in untreated and treated cells as well as the intracellular cyclic AMP concentrations observed in these cells at the time transport was measured.

The transport of each substrate was measured in cells unable to metabolize that substrate. 3-O-methylglucose is not phosphorylated in mammalian cells [47], so that its transport could be measured in wild-type cells without complication of metabolism. Transport of thymidine, hypoxanthine, adenosine, and adenine was measured in sublines of CHO cells deficient in thymidine kinase, hypoxanthine/guanine phosphoribosyltransferase, adenosine kinase, and adenine phosphoribosyltransferase, respectively, in which sublines no significant phosphorylation of the substrates was detected during

TABLE III. Direct Effect of PGE$_1$ on the Transport of Various Substrates in Wild-Type CHO Cells*

Substrate	μM	v_{12}^{zt} (pmoles/μl cell H$_2$O·sec)	
		Control	+PGE$_1$
3-O-Methylglucose	800	9.2 ± 1.9	7.4 ± 1.5
Adenosine	160	7.2 ± 0.2	6.7 ± 0.4
Thymidine	320	10.8 ± 0.5	8.8 ± 0.4
Hypoxanthine	320	5.1 ± 0.4	3.3 ± 0.2
Adenine	320	2.3 ± 0.1	2.4 ± 0.2

*Samples of a suspension of about 1.7 × 10^7 wild-type CHO cells per milliliter of BM42B (or of glucose-free BM42B for 3-O-methylglucose uptake measurements) were assayed for zero-trans accumulation of ^{3}H-labeled substrates at 25° by the rapid kinetic technique described in Materials and Methods and illustrated in Figure 1. For [^{3}H]adenosine transport measurements, the cells were preincubated with 10 μM 2-deoxycoformycin at 37° for 5 min and then at 25° for 2 min. Where indicated, PGE$_1$ was added simultaneously with substrate to a final concentration of 120μM. Radioactivity per cell pellet was corrected for substrate trapped in extracellular space (3.9 μl/pellet). The intracellular space was 12.1 μl/cell pellet. Equation 1 was fitted to the time courses of substrate accumulation comprised of 12–15 time points encompassing 2.5 sec to 2 min (see Fig. 1) with all R constants held constant and K fixed at 5, 0.2, 0.2, 1.5, and 2.5 mM for 3-O-methylglucose, adenosine, thymidine, hypoxanthine, and adenine, respectively. The correlation coefficients for the fits were all > 0.9.

4 min of incubation with the indicated concentrations of substrate (data not shown). It is noteworthy that sublines lacking either adenine- or hypoxanthine/guanine-phosphoribosyltransferase failed to respond to PGE$_1$ treatment. As yet we do not know what significance is to be attached to this observation. The two sublines in question were obtained by us from two different laboratories; whether the histories of the parental lines might contribute to the mutants' unresponsiveness is unclear.

In any case adenosine and adenine transport was also measured in our strain of wild-type CHO cells, which do respond to PGE$_1$. We have demonstrated previously that the initial time courses of accumulation of adenosine, adenine, and other nucleosides and nucleobases are about the same in wild-type cells as in cells lacking the respective enzymes responsible for their phosphorylation, provided the substrate concentration greatly exceeds the concentration that saturates the phosphorylating enzyme [28, 35].

Together, the results of Figure 1 and Table II indicate that the 10-fold to 100-fold increase in intracellular cyclic AMP concentration after PGE$_1$ treatment had little effect on the initial zero-trans transport velocities for the various substrates examined. Although the transport velocities were, in general, marginally lower in PGE$_1$-treated than in untreated cells, there is good reason to believe that this difference is not mediated by cyclic AMP, but is attributable to a direct effect of PGE$_1$ on the transport of these substrates: 1) A similar, slight decrease in transport v_{12}^{zt} was observed when PGE$_1$ was added simultaneously with substrate (Table III); 2) an inhibitory effect of PGE$_1$ was apparent in the hypoxanthine/guanine phosphoribosyltransferase-deficient cells, which do not respond to PGE$_1$ with elevated cyclic AMP levels; and 3) we have previously demonstrated that both PGE$_1$ and prostaglandin F$_{2\alpha}$ inhibit the uptake of nucleosides, hypoxanthine, deoxyglucose, and choline in Novikoff rat hepatoma cells, whose adenylate cyclase is also unresponsive to PGE$_1$ [48]. A recent report by Rozengurt et al [32] indicates that the involvement of cyclic AMP in uridine uptake by mitogen-stimulated 3T3 cells is distal to the transport step. An observed decrease in cyclic AMP correlated with an increase in the rate at which uridine was phosphorylated, while the rate of transport remained unchanged.

We conclude that the zero-trans transport of various substrates is not regulated by endogenous cyclic AMP, but that PGE_1 at concentrations of $60-120$ μM causes a slight direct inhibition of the transport of these substrates. That extracellular cyclic AMP and its dibutyryl derivative similarly have no effect on the transport of these substrates can be deduced from the lack of effect of these cyclic nucleotides at a concentration of 1 mM on the uptake of these nucleosides, nucleobases, and hexoses [26].

ACKNOWLEDGMENTS

This work was supported by US Public Health Service research grants GM24468, AM 23001, by a grant from the Leukemia Task Force, and by USPHS training grant CA 09138 (R.M.W.).

We thank John Erbe, Jill Myers, and Elizabeth Anton for excellent technical assistance, and Cheryl Thull for competently typing the manuscript.

REFERENCES

1. Rozengurt E, Jiminez De Azua L: Proc Natl Acad Sci USA 70:3609, 1973.
2. Kram R, Tomkins GM: Proc Natl Acad Sci USA 70:1659, 1973.
3. Kram R, Mamont P, Tomkins GM: Proc Natl Acad Sci USA 70:1432, 1973.
4. Jiminez de Azua L, Rozengurt E: Nature 251:624, 1974.
5. Jiminez de Azua L, Rozengurt E, Dulbecco R: Proc Natl Acad Sci USA 71:96, 1974.
6. Hare JD: Biochim Biophys Acta 282:401, 1972.
7. Hare JD: Biochim Biophys Acta 255:905, 1972.
8. Perdue JF: Chapter 4 in Nicolau C (ed): "Viral-Transformed Cell Membranes." New York: Academic, 1979.
9. Peters JH, Hausen P: Eur J Biochem 19:509, 1971.
10. Whitesell RR, Johnson RA, Tarpley H, Regen D: J Cell Biol 72:456, 1977.
11. Cuatrecasas P, Tell GPE: Proc Natl Acad Sci USA 70:485, 1973.
12. Taylor WM, Mak ML, Halperin ML: Proc Natl Acad Sci 73:4359, 1976.
13. Hatanaka M: Biochim Biophys Acta 355:77, 1974.
14. Sheppard JR: Nature 236:14, 1972.
15. Hauschka PV, Everhart LP, Rubin RW: Proc Natl Acad Sci USA 69:3542, 1972.
16. Lingwood CA, Thomas DB: J Cell Biol 61:359, 1974.
17. Alford BL, Barnes EM Jr: Arch Biochem Biophys 180:214, 1977.
18. Taylor-Papadimitriou J, Karmfyllis T, Eukarpidou A, Karamanlidou G: J Cell Sci 19:305, 1975.
19. Roller B, Hirai K, Defendi V: J Cell Physiol 83:163, 1974.
20. Ecker P: J Cell Sci 16:301, 1974.
21. Gazdar A, Hatanaka M, Herberman R, Russell E, Ikawa Y: Proc Soc Exp Biol Med 141:1044, 1972.
22. Walum E, Edström A: Exp Cell Res 100:111, 1976.
23. Grimes WJ, Schroeder JL: J Cell Biol 56:487, 1973.
24. Barnes DW, Brown VT, Colowick SP: J Cell Physiol 97:231, 1978.
25. Benedetto A, Casson EA: Biochim Biophys Acta 349:53, 1974.
26. Sheppard JR, Plagemann PGW: J Cell Physiol 85:163, 1975.
27. Wohlhueter RM, Marz R, Graff JC, Plagemann PGW: Methods Cell Biol 20:211, 1978.
28. Plagemann PGW, Wohlhueter RM: Curr Top Membr Transp (In press).
29. Marz R, Wohlhueter RM, Plagemann PGW: J Supramol Struct 6:433, 1977.
30. Plagemann PGW, Marz R, Wohlhueter RM: J Cell Physiol 97:49, 1978.
31. Wohlhueter RM, Marz R, Plagemann PGW: Biochim Biophys Acta 553:262, 1979.
32. Rozengurt E, Stein WD, Wigglesworth NM: Nature 267:442, 1977.
33. Marz R, Wohlhueter RM, Plagemann PGW: J Biol Chem 254:2329, 1979.

34. Graff JC, Wohlhueter RM, Plagemann PGW: J Cell Physiol 96:171, 1978.
35. Wohlhueter RM, Plagemann PGW: Int Rev Cytol (In press).
36. Taylor MW, Pipkorn JH, Tokito MK, Pozzatti RO Jr: Somatic Cell Gen 3:195, 1977.
37. Schneider EL, Stanbridge EF, Epstein CJ: Exp Cell Res 84:311, 1974.
38. Plagemann PGW: J Cell Physiol 77:213, 1971.
39. Eilam Y, Stein WD: Methods Membr Biol 2:283, 1974.
40. Lowry OH, Rosebrough NJ, Farr AL, Randall RJ: J Biol Chem 193:265, 1951.
41. O'Neill JP, Hsie AW: J Cyclic Nucleotide Res 4:169, 1978.
42. Perry CV, Johnson GS, Pastan I: J Biol Chem 246:5785, 1971.
43. Claesson HE, Lindgren JA, Hammarström S: Eur J Biochem 74:13, 1977.
44. Rindler MJ, Bashor MM, Spitzer N, Saier MH Jr: J Biol Chem 253:5431, 1978.
45. Samuelsson B, Grandström F, Green K, Hamberg M, Hammarström S: Ann Rev Biochem 44:669, 1975.
46. Magniello V, Vaughan M: Proc Natl Acad Sci USA 69:269, 1972.
47. Renner ED, Plagemann PGW, Bernlohr RW: J Biol Chem 247:5765, 1972.
48. Plagemann PGW, Sheppard JR: Biochem Biophys Res Commun 56:869, 1974.

Journal of Supramolecular Structure 11:61—67 (1979)
Tumor Cell Surfaces and Malignancy 37—43

Extracellular Lectin and Its Glycosaminoglycan Inhibitor in Chick Muscle Cultures

Howard Ceri, Paula J. Shadle, David Kobiler, and Samuel H. Barondes

Department of Psychiatry, Unviersity of California, San Diego, La Jolla, California 92093

Embryonic chick muscle contains two developmentally regulated lectins, which may be involved in cell interactions. These endogenous lectins are assayed as agglutinins of appropriate test erythrocytes. One of these, called lectin-2, interacts with specific glycosaminoglycans, especially heparin and dermatan sulfate. Lectin-2 is present at constant levels in both chick fibroblast and chick muscle cells throughout 14 days of culture but is released into the medium of cultured embryonic muscle after 7—8 days of culture, soon after myoblast fusion. Lectin-2 interacts strongly with a component of substrate-attached material in embryonic muscle cultures which is extractable from the culture dishes with alkali after the cells have been removed with ethylediaminetetraacetic acid. The active component in the substrate-attached material appears to be a glycosaminoglycan that is a more potent inhibitor of lectin-2 agglutination activity than any of the known glycosaminoglycans that we have tested. The active material is degraded by chondroitinase ABC but not by chondrotinase AC, hyaluronidase, or proteolytic enzymes and thus appears to be similar to dermatan sulfate. The results of these studies raise the possibility that lectin-2 functions by interacting with glycosaminoglycans, either associated with the cell surface or with the extracellular matrix.

Key words: lectin, glycosaminoglycan, extracellular material, cell matrix, cellular interactions, myoblast development

Specific surface interactions of developing cells with each other and with extracellular materials are believed to play an important role in tissue formation. While changes in cell surface components have been found during development, little is presently known about molecules which mediate specific cell interactions.

We have previously reported the presence of two developmentally regulated lectins in embryonic chick muscle that are candidates for a role in cellular interactions during development. The first (here referred to as lectin-1) has been purified by affinity chromatography [1, 2] and is assayed as an agglutinin of fixed trypsinized rabbit erythrocytes (here referred to as type I cells). Hemagglutination activity of this dimeric protein is inhibited by a number of sugars including lactose. Lectin-1 activity is low in extracts of pectoral muscle from 8-day-old chick embryos, rises to a maximum at about 16 days,

Received April 25, 1979; accepted May 15, 1979.

and then declines [3, 4]. The other lectin we have identified (here called lectin-2), also shows changes in activity in developing chick pectoral muscle [5] and is assayed as an agglutinin of modified erythrocytes (here called type II cells). These cells are type I cells that have been modified either by aging [5] or by alcohol washing [6]. Lectin-2 hemagglutination activity can be inhibited by low concentrations of several glycosaminoglycans [6]. It is also inhibited by several saccharides including N-acetyl-D-galactosamine [5, 6].

In the present report we show that lectin-2 is released into the medium of cultured chick embryo muscle cells after cell fusion has occurred. We also show marked inhibition of lectin-2 activity by a component of substrate-attached material (SAM) derived from cultured myoblasts. This inhibitor appears to be a glycosaminoglycan. Taken together our results suggest an extracellular function for lectin-2, perhaps a role in cell-matrix interactions.

MATERIALS AND METHODS

Cell Culture

Twelve-day chick embryo pectoral muscle was dissociated in 0.25% trypsin in Hanks' balanced salt solution and cultured on collagen surfaces at 4.5×10^4 cells per 1 cm^2 in Eagle's minimal essential medium supplemented with 10% fetal calf serum.

Lectin Extraction

Cell culture. Cells from 6–10 plates were lifted with phosphate-buffered saline (PBS) (0.075 M NaKPO$_4$, 0.075 M NaCl, pH 7.2) containing 2 mM ethylenediaminetetraacetic acid (EDTA). The cells were washed twice in PBS and homogenized in MEPBS (PBS containing 4 mM β-mercaptoethanol + 2 mM EDTA) containing 0.1 M lactose and 0.1 M N-acetyl-D-galactosamine.

Tissue. Lectin-1 and lectin-2 were extracted from 15-day chick embryo pectoral muscle in nine volumes of MEPBS containing 0.1 M lactose and 0.1 M N-acetyl-D-galactosamine [1, 5]. The extract was spun 1 h at 100,000g to remove debris and the supernatant was then centrifuged for 12 h at 100,000g [6]. The supernatant was found to contain all of the lectin-1 activity. The pellet was resuspended in 1 M NaCl + 4 mM β-mercaptoethanol and contained all of the lectin-2 activity [6].

Media. Media to be assayed for lectin activity were centrifuged at 1,000g for 10 min in a clinical centrifuge and used directly in hemagglutination assays.

Hemagglutination assays. Hemagglutination assays were done in microtiter V plates (Fisher Scientific) using serial twofold dilutions in MEPBS of extracts. Each well contained 0.025 ml lectin, 0.025 ml 0.15 M NaCl, 0.025 ml 1% bovine serum albumin in 0.15 M NaCl, and 0.025 ml of either 4% trypsinized glutaraldehyde-fixed rabbit red blood cells (type I cells [1]) or alcohol-washed trypsinized glutaraldehyde-fixed rabbit red blood cells (type II cells [6]) in PBS. Type I cells are specific for lectin-1 activity, while type II cells are specific for lectin-2 activity [6]. Substances to be tested for lectin inhibition were diluted in saline and replaced saline in the assay.

SAM Extraction

The media from 24- to 48-h myoblast cultures were removed and the cells lifted with PBS containing 2 mM EDTA followed by trituration [7]. Care was taken to remove all adherent cells. SAM was extracted in 0.1 N NaOH for 24 h at 37° [7], neutralized with PBS + 2 mM EDTA, and tested for inhibition of lectin-2 in hemagglutination assays. Each 100-mm culture plate yielded 4 ml of SAM extract containing 18 μg/ml of glucuronic acid, as determined by the orcinol method [8].

Glycosaminoglycan Extraction

Glycosaminoglycans (GAGs) were extracted from pectoral muscle of 15-day embryos by homogenization in three volumes of 0.4% NaCl, followed by centrifugation for 1 h at 100,000g. Subsequent purification was done by the method of Linker and Hovingh [9]. Briefly, the supernatant was precipitated with cetylpyridinium chloride and the precipitate, after washing with ethanol, was resuspended in buffer and digested with pronase. The

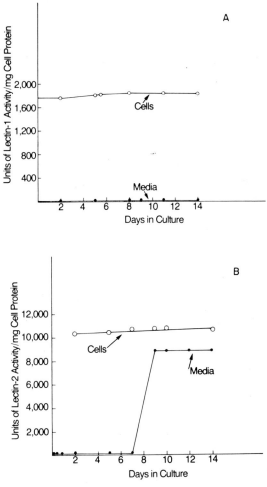

Fig. 1. Lectin-1 (A) and lectin-2 (B) activity in cell extracts and growth media of muscle cultures. Cultures were prepared and extracted as described in Methods. Lectin-1 activity was determined with type I cells and lectin-2 activity with type II cells as described in Methods. The units of lectin activity are the reciprocal of the titers (eg, a titer of 1:800 is referred to as 800 units). Each point is the average of duplicate values obtained from a single experiment. The overall results were confirmed in a replicate experiment.

TABLE I. Comparison of Characteristics of Lectin in Media From Muscle Cultures and Lectin-2

	Lectin-1	Lectin-2	Media
Agglutinates type I cells	+	0	0
Agglutinates type II cells	0	+	+
Inhibited by 10 mM lactose	+	0	0
Inhibited by 5 μg/ml heparin	0	+	+
Inhibited by extracts of SAM	0	+	+
Binds to p-aminophenyl lactoside column	+	0	0
Sedimented at 100,000g for 12 h	0	+	+

TABLE II. Comparative Potency of Extracts of SAM From Muscle Cultures, Muscle Tissue Extract, and Other Inhibitors of Lectin-2

	Concentration (μg/ml) that inhibits lectin-2 activity by 50%
Heparin	2.5
Dermatan sulfate	5.0
Heparan sulfate	12.5
Chondroitin-4-sulfate	>50
Chondroitin-6-sulfate	>50
Hyaluronic acid	>50
Muscle tissue extract	0.1[a]
NaOH extract of SAM	0.1[a]

[a]Specific activity determined by assuming that inhibitor is a glycosaminoglycan and that all uronic acid in these extracts is in active material.

GAGs were then precipitated with ethanol, dissolved in buffer, and tested for inhibitory activity in hemagglutination assays.

RESULTS

Extracellular Lectin-2 Activity

Extracts of embryonic chick skeletal muscle cultures had high levels of both lectin-1 and lectin-2 (Fig. 1A, B). Cells had a constant level of both lectin activities through 14 days in culture. During this period myoblast fusion and myotube formation took place.

The culture media showed no detectable lectin activity for seven days, followed by a dramatic rise of lectin-2 activity (Fig. 1B). Total extracellular lectin-2 activity in a given plate reached levels comparable to the lectin-2 activity that could be extracted from the cells on that plate. No lectin-1 activity was ever detected in the media (Fig. 1A). Mixing experiments in which purified lectin-1 was reacted with native or boiled media showed this was not due to the presence of an inhibitor in the culture media (data not shown).

The agglutinin found in the media was shown to meet functional criteria defining lectin-2 activity (Table I). It agglutinated type II but not type I erythrocytes; this agglutination was specifically blocked by heparin and extracts of SAM (see below) and not blocked by lactose. The activity failed to bind to a p-aminophenyl lactoside column, and sedimented in 12 h at 100,000g, as does lectin-2.

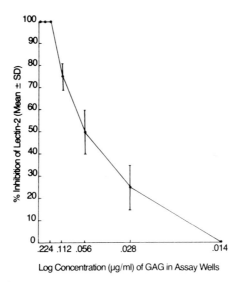

Fig. 2. Inhibition of lectin-2 activity by SAM from primary chick muscle cultures as a function of inhibitor concentration. SAM was extracted in 0.1 NaOH and neutralized with PBS, and serial dilutions were assayed for inhibition of lectin-2 activity. Glycosaminoglycans (GAG) content of the extracts was estimated by the orcionol method [8] assuming that 2.5 mg of GAG contains 1 mg of uronic acid.

SAM Inhibition of Lectin-2 Activity

Extracts prepared from SAM of myoblast cultures in 0.1 N NaOH and crude GAGs prepared from embryonic muscle tissue were extremely potent inhibitors of lectin-2 (Table II, Fig. 2). These substances had no detectable effect on lectin-1 activity. The potency of the extract of SAM as an inhibitor of lectin-2 is expressed in terms of GAG content of the extract, since we had previously found [6] that lectin-2 activity is sensitive to a group of iduronic acid-containg GAGs, including heparin, dermatan sulfate, and heparan sulfate, but not to other GAGs such as chondroitin sulfate or hyaluronic acid. As indicated in Table II, the extracted material from SAM or muscle tissue appears to be more potent than any of the standard GAGs. The specific activity of the GAG in these extracts may actually be much greater than would be estimated from uronic acid determination, since it is likely that, as with fibroblasts [10], there are several different GAGs in the SAM of muscle cultures and not all are active inhibitors.

The assumption that the inhibitor in the extracts is indeed a GAG is supported by a number of observations. First, the inhibitory activity of the extracts is resistant to prolonged digestion with trypsin or with pronase (Table III). It is also resistant to prolonged boiling, and can be precipitated by cetylpyridinium chloride (data not shown). Furthermore, the inhibitor is obviously highly anionic, since it binds tenaciously to a DEAE-cellulose column. In addition, the inhibitory activity in extracts of SAM can be completely destroyed by digestion with chondroitinase ABC (Table III). The same result was found with GAG preparations from embryonic muscle tissue. These results, coupled with studies of the effects of other enzymes, suggest that the inhibitor is similar to dermatan sulfate. This is suggested by the finding that the inhibitor is insensitive to testicular hyaluronidase, which digests hyaluronic acid and chondroitin sulfates, and is also insensitive to chondroitinase AC, which digests hyaluronic acid and chondroitin

TABLE III. Destruction of Inhibitory Activity of SAM by Chondroitinase ABC

	% Inhibition of lectin-2 agglutination activity
SAM	100
SAM + chondroitinase ABC	0
SAM + chondroitinase AC	100
SAM + hyaluronidase (testicular)	100
SAM + trypsin	100
SAM + pronase	100

SAM was incubated alone or with 2.5 units of chondroitinase ABC or AC (Sigma), or with 1 mg/ml of testicular hyaluronidase, trypsin, or pronase for 36 h at 37°C in PBS, pH 7.2 (pH 8 in the case of pronase). After incubation the samples treated with proteolytic enzymes were boiled for 5 min. Serial dilutions of all samples were then assayed for activity as lectin-2 inhibitors. SAM boiled or incubated alone for 36 h maintained full activity. Enzymes incubated alone had no effect on lectin-2 agglutination.

TABLE IV. Comparison of Lectin-2 and Fibronectin

Lectin-2	Fibronectin
Does not agglutinate formalinized sheep red blood cells	Agglutinates formalinized sheep red blood cells
EDTA-insensitive	EDTA blocks agglutination activity
β-mercaptoethanol preserves agglutination activity	β-mercaptoethanol dissociates to monomers with impaired binding
Does not bind to collagen[a]	Binds to collagen
Hemagglutination inhibited by N-acetyl-D-galactosamine but not N-acetyl-D-glucosamine	Hemagglutination not inhibited by N-acetyl-D-galactosamine; inhibited somewhat by D-galactosamine and D-glucosamine

Properties of fibronectin are documented in Yamada and Olden [11]. Properties of lectin-2 are based on Mir-Lechaire and Barondes [5] and Kobiler and Barondes [6], and on original observations made in the course of the present work.

[a]Lectin-2 was reacted with a collagen coated culture dish and the supernatant was assayed after incubation for 30 min. No activity was lost even when very dilute solutions of crude lectin were used.

sulfates (Table III). The only known glycosaminogylcan degraded by chondroitinase ABC but not by chondroitinase AC is dermatan sulfate.

Comparison of Lectin-2 and Fibronectin

Because fibronectin is also a known hemagglutinin that is present both on cell surfaces and in culture media of several cell types [11] and because it also interacts with heparin [12], it was necessary to discriminate between lectin-2 and fibronectin. The differences between lectin-2 and fibronectin, summarized in Table IV, indicate that they are distinct.

DISCUSSION

These results show that lectin-2 activity can be found in the medium of embryonic muscle culture, presumably owing to secretion by the muscle cells. This inference is based on our finding (data not shown) that there is no lectin-2 activity detectable in the medium of confluent or growing fibroblast cultures, although extracts of these cultures do contain lectin-2 activity. Presumably, then, the source of the lectin-2 in the medium of the muscle cultures is the muscle cells themselves, rather than fibroblasts in the cultures. Appearance of lectin-2 in the medium is not due to cell breakage, since the cultures show no visible deterioration and since another intracellular protein, lectin-1, was never found in the medium.Why lectin-2 appears in the medium, and only after substantial differentiation of the muscle cells, is presently unclear.

A possible extracellular function of lectin-2 is suggested by the finding that SAM from muscle cultures is rich in an inhibitor of this lectin. The inhibitor appears to be a glycosaminoglycan and the results suggest that the GAG binds to an active site on the lectin. It is notable that among the group of GAGs that act as inhibitors of lectin-2 some heparan sulfate is found associated with cell surfaces [13] and heparin binds to a cell surface protein [14]. One possible interpretation of these observations is that lectin-2 appears on the cell surface and plays a role in interactions of cells with GAGs either associated with other cells or bound within the extracellular matrix. An interaction of this complex with fibronectin might also occur. Appearance of free lectin-2 in the medium might result from an artifactual sloughing of this material but could also play some role in cellular attachment or detachment. Whatever the details, the observation that both lectin-2 and GAG that interacts with it are present outside muscle cells is suggestive of a functional interaction between these substances.

ACKNOWLEDGMENTS

This research was supported by grants from the McKnight Foundation and the US Public Health Service (MH 18282). H. Ceri was supported by a postdoctoral fellowship from the Medical Research Council of Canada, P. Shadle was supported by a National Science Foundation predoctoral fellowship, and D. Kobiler was supported, in part, by a Chaim Weizmann Fellowship. Dermatan sulfate, heparin, and heparan sulfate were the kind gift of Alfred Linker, University of Utah.

REFERENCES

1. Nowak T, Kobiler D, Roel LE, Barondes SH: J Biol Chem 252:6026, 1977.
2. Den H, Malinzak D, Rosenberg A: Biochem Biophys Res Commun 69:621, 1976.
3. Nowak T, Harwood PL, Barondes SH: Biochem Biophys Res Commun 68:650, 1976.
4. Kobiler D, Barondes SH: Develop Biol 60:326, 1977.
5. Mir-Lechaire FJ, Barondes SH: Nature 272:256, 1978.
6. Kobiler D, Barondes SH: FEBS Lett 101:257, 1979.
7. Culp LA, Rollins BJ, Baniel J, Hitri S: J Cell Biol 79:788, 1978.
8. Mejbaum R: J Physiol Chem 258:117, 1939.
9. Linker A, Hovingh P: Carbohydrate Res 29:41, 1973.
10. Rollins BJ, Culp LA: Biochemistry 18:141, 1979.
11. Yamada K, Olden K: Nature 275:179, 1978.
12. Ruoslahti E, Hayman EG: FEBS Lett 97:221, 1979.
13. Kraemer PM: Biochem Biophys Res Commun 78:1334, 1977.
14. Alimedia B, Busch C, Höök M: Thrombosis Res 12:773, 1978.

Journal of Supramolecular Structure 11:69–78 (1979)
Tumor Cell Surfaces and Malignancy 45–54

Cellular and Metabolic Specificity in the Interaction of Adhesion Proteins With Collagen and With Cells

H. K. Kleinman, A. T. Hewitt, J. C. Murray, L. A. Liotta, S. I. Rennard, J. P. Pennypacker, E. B. McGoodwin, G. R. Martin, and P. H. Fishman

Laboratory of Developmental Biology and Anomalies, National Institute of Dental Research (H.K.K., A.T.H., J.C.M., S.I.R., J.P.P., E.B.M., G.R.M.); Laboratory of Pathophysiology, National Cancer Institute (L.A.L.); and Developmental and Metabolic Neurology Branch, National Institute of Neurological and Communicative Disorders and Stroke (P.H.F.), National Institutes of Health, Bethesda, Maryland 20205

Fibronectin mediates the adhesion of fibroblasts to collagen substrates, binding first to the collagen and then to the cells. We report here that the interaction of the cells with the fibronectin-collagen complex is blocked by specific gangliosides, GD_{1a} and GT_1, and that the sugar moieties of these gangliosides contain the inhibitory activity. The gangliosides act by binding to fibronectin, suggesting that they may be the cell surface receptor for fibronectin.

Evidence is presented that other adhesion proteins or mechanisms of attachment exist for chondrocytes, epidermal cells, and transformed tumorigenic cells, since adhesion of these cells is not stimulated by fibronectin. Chondrocytes adhere via a serum factor that is more temperature-sensitive and less basic than fibronectin. Unlike that of fibroblasts chondrocyte adhesion is stimulated by low levels of gangliosides. Epidermal cells adhere preferentially to type IV (basement membrane) collagen but at a much slower rate than fibroblasts or chondrocytes. This suggests that these epidermal cells synthesize their own specific adhesion factor. Metastatic cells cultured from the T241 fibrosarcoma adhere rapidly to type IV collagen in the absence of fibronectin and do not synthesize significant amounts of collagen or fibronectin. Their growth, in contrast to that of normal fibroblasts, is unaffected by a specific inhibitor of collagen synthesis. These data indicate the importance of specific collagens and adhesion proteins in the adhesion of certain cells and suggest that a reduction in the synthesis of collagen and of fibronectin is related to some of the abnormalities observed in transformed cells.

Key words: cell adhesion, adhesion proteins, fibronectin, chondronectin, collagen substrates, gangliosides, cell surface

Received April 19, 1979; accepted May 21, 1979.

Fibroblasts use fibronectin, a large glycoprotein, to adhere to collagen substrates [1]. These cells synthesize their own fibronectin but under the usual culture conditions utilize the fibronectin present in serum to attach to collagen. The interaction follows a specific sequence of events starting with the binding of fibronectin to the collagen molecule [2]. The cells then bind to the fibronectin-collagen complex in a divalent cation-requiring, energy-dependent process [3]. The interaction of fibronectin with collagen is specific, and chromatography of fibronectin on collagen affinity columns is used to purify the protein in high yield from serum, tissue culture medium, or cell extracts [4, 5]. There appears to be a specific site within collagen to which fibronectin binds [6, 7]. Peptides from a similar locus on collagen types I, II, and III bind to fibronectin (Fig. 1). The binding site has been further located within a fragment of the α1(I) chain comprising residues 757–791. This sequence lacks carbohydrate and includes the bond cleaved by animal collagenase. The integrity of the collagenase-sensitive bond at residues 775–776 and of a chymotrypsin-sensitive bond at 779–780 are required for fibronectin binding [8]. The data suggest that a specific sequence of amino acids, perhaps containing a small number of residues, is the binding site for fibronectin on collagen. In addition, a specific binding site on fibronectin for collagen has been described [9, 10].

Here we report on the role of fibronectin and other serum proteins in the attachment of fibroblasts, chondrocytes, and epidermal cells to collagen. Further differences are noted in the attachment of cells from a metastatic fibrosarcoma. Finally, data are presented that are consistent with a role for certain complex gangliosides as the cell surface receptors for fibronectin.

MATERIALS AND METHODS

Materials

Collagen types I and IV were prepared from lathyritic rat skin [11] and a murine tumor [12], respectively, as previously described. Gangliosides were either obtained from Sigma Chemical Co. or Supelco, Inc., or were prepared as previously described [13].

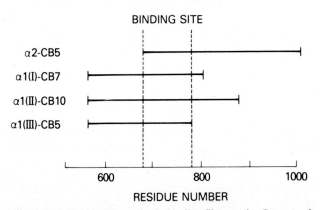

Fig. 1. Collagen cyanogen bromide peptides active in binding fibronectin. Cyanogen bromide peptides were prepared and isolated as already described and assayed for binding to fibronectin by either a radioimmunoassay or bioassay for activity in cell adhesion. Data on α2, α1 (I)-CB7, and α1 (II)-CB 10 from Dessau et al [7]; Data on α1 (I)-CB7 and α1 (II)-CB10 from Kleinman et al [6, 8]. Data on α1 (III)-CB5 from Kleinman and McGoodwin, unpublished observations.

Radioactive gangliosides were prepared as already described [14, 15]. Ceramides were obtained from Supelco, Inc., and oligosaccharides were obtained by ozonolysis of the ganglioside [16]. Cis-hydroxyproline was obtained from Sigma Chemical Co. Fibronectin was prepared by passing bovine serum (Colorado Serum Co.) over a denatured type I collagen Sepharose affinity column [4, 5] and eluting the bound fibronectin with 1 M KBr in 0.05 Tris containing 0.025 M 6-aminohexanoic acid, pH 5.3. The material that did not bind to the affinity column was considered to be fibronectin-free serum.

Cells

Chinese hamster ovary (CHO) cells were obtained from American Type Culture Collection. Chick sternal chondrocytes were obtained from day 14 embryonic chick sterna by dissociation with collagenase [17]. Epidermal cells were obtained from adult guinea pig epidermis by dissociation with trypsin [18]. Pulmonary metastatic tumor cells were selected in vivo from a pulmonary metastasis of the T241 fibrosarcoma [19].

Assay for Cell Adhesion

Collagen-coated bacteriologic plates [8] (35 mm) were preincubated for 1 h at 37° in 95% air, 5% CO_2 with Eagle's minimal essential medium (MEM) containing either serum, fibronectin, or fibronectin-free serum and 200 μg/ml of bovine serum albumin. The cells (usually 10^5) were then added for an additional incubation. The nonadherent cells were removed by gentle washing with 0.02 M phosphate-buffered saline (PBS). The attached cells were released with a solution of trypsin containing 0.1% ethylenediamine tetraacetic acid (EDTA) in PBS and were counted electronically.

Immunoprecipitation

Murine serum fibronectin (1 μg) was suspended in 1 ml MEM supplemented with albumin (20 μg) and was incubated with radioactive gangliosides for 60 min at 37° in 5% CO_2 (final pH 7.4). In some cases, the fibronectin was preincubated with denatured lathyritic rat skin collagen (2 μg) for 30 min at 37°. Rabbit antiserum (10 μl) against purified murine fibronectin was then added at a dilution of 1:5, a concentration previously shown capable of binding at least 5 μg of fibronectin. Samples were incubated for 2 h at 4°C. Samples were finally incubated with 100 μl of goat anti-rabbit immunoglobulin (1:4 dilution) (Miles Laboratories lot No. G105) at 4° overnight. No carrier was required and the blank was < 50 cpm. All incubations were performed in siliconized glass tubes. Samples were then spun over a sucrose cushion, dissolved in 0.5 ml of 0.5 N acetic acid, and counted.

RESULTS

Use of a Proline Analog to Distinguish Collagen-Dependent Cell Attachment

Studies by Kao and Prockop [20] have shown that cis-4-hydroxyproline prevents the growth of fibroblasts in culture. This compound is incorporated into peptide chains in place of proline and prevents the normal formation of trans-4-hydroxyproline in collagen. As a result, the collagen molecules do not form a triple helix and are not deposited into fibers [21]. Due to the known action of cis-hydroxyproline, the effect of this compound on the growth of fibroblasts is most likely due to its inhibition of the deposition of a collagen matrix. This proline analog can therefore be used to test whether collagen is necessary for the growth of cells in culture. In contrast to the previous observations on a tissue culture substrate where cell growth is inhibited in the presence of this analog, we found normal growth of fibroblasts on a collagen substrate in the presence of cis-4-hydroxyproline [22]. Thus, a collagen substrate is necessary for the growth of normal cells. However, the growth of cells from a metastatic tumor on tissue culture dishes was not altered by cis-4-hydroxyproline. These cells make little or no collagen or fibronectin (Table I) and attach preferentially to basement membrane collagen (Fig. 3). A low production of collagen is frequently observed with transformed cells [23], as is reduced production or surface retention [24] of fibronectin. The altered production of matrix components may be associated with cells that grow and spread abnormally.

Attachment Characteristics of Fibroblasts, Chondrocytes, Epidermal Cells, and Metastatic Tumorigenic Cells

As stated earlier, the attachment of trypsinized fibroblasts to collagen substrates is stimulated by serum and fibronectin (Fig. 2). The adherence of chondrocytes, epidermal cells and metastatic tumorigenic cells to collagen is not fibronectin-dependent (Figs. 2 and 3). Chondrocytes adhere well to type I collagen via a factor (presumably a protein) in the serum other than fibronectin (Fig. 2). This factor, which we have named chondronectin, is readily distinguished from fibronectin, since it is more temperature-sensitive than fibronectin ($t_{1/2} = 52°$ vs $t_{1/2} = 57°$ for 30 min), is separable from fibronectin by DEAE-cellulose column chromatography, and is produced by chondrocytes [25] in culture.

Epidermal cells adhere preferentially to type IV collagen, but their attachment is not stimulated by serum, fibronectin, or fibronectin-free serum (Fig. 3). These cells attach slowly to type IV collagen in comparison to fibroblasts or chondrocytes when incubated with serum [18]. Epidermal cells probably make their own specific attachment protein as indicated by their preferential binding to type IV collagen substrates and the extended time required for their attachment.

Cells from a fibrosarcoma (PMT-T241) were found to adhere preferentially to type IV collagen without the requirement for serum or fibronectin. Attachment under these conditions was rapid, suggesting that there was a preformed receptor on the cells. However, serum and fibronectin did stimulate the adhesion of these cells to type I collagen (Fig. 3). These observations indicate that these cells have the cell surface receptor for fibronectin but, in contrast to fibroblasts, do not synthesize significant amounts of fibronectin or of collagen (Table I).

TABLE I. Collagen and Fibronectin Synthesis and Cis-Hydroxyproline Sensitivity of Normal and Metastatic Cells

Cells	% Cells remaining after 5-day exposure to 25 μg/ml cis-hydroxyproline	% Collagenase-sensitive[a] ^{3}H-proline-labeled macromolecules	Fibronectin synthesis[b] (ng/cell/day)
Adult connective tissue cells	10	5.8	600
Pulmonary metastatic tumor cells	100[c]	None detected[d]	None detected

[a]Collagen determined by method of Peterkofsky and Diegelmann [32].
[b]Fibronectin determined by ELISA assay [33].
[c]Value indicates no difference in cell number between treated and untreated cultures.
[d]Chemical analyses could detect very low levels of hydroxyproline.

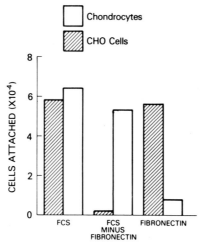

Fig. 2. Attachment properties of fibroblasts and chondrocytes on collagen type I in the presence of fetal calf serum (FCS), fibronectin, or serum minus fibronectin. Attachment assays were carried out as described in the Materials and Methods. Each point represents the mean of duplicate measurements, which did not differ by more than 10%.

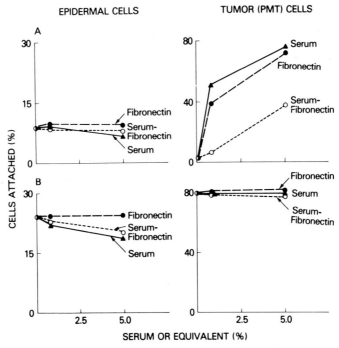

Fig. 3. Attachment properties of epidermal cells and metastatic tumor cells on collagen type I (A) and type IV (B) in the presence of increasing amounts of serum, fibronectin, or serum minus fibronectin. Attachment assays were carried out as described in Materials and Methods, except for the epidermal cells, which were allowed to attach for 18 h. Similar trends were observed with the epidermal cells after an incubation of 1.5 h, but the level of attachment was very low. The data on cell attachment are plotted as the amount of fibronectin present in that the percentage of serum indicated on the abscissa. Each point represents the mean of duplicate measurements, which did not differ by more than 10%.

Effect of Gangliosides on Cell Adhesion

The cell surface receptor(s) for fibronectin have not been identified. Because ganglioside synthesis [26] and fibronectin binding [27] are reduced in transformed cells, we have investigated the possible role of gangliosides in the interaction of fibronectin with the cell membrane. We studied the influence of a variety of gangliosides on CHO cell adhesion. As seen in Table II, GM_3, the simplest ganglioside tested, had no effect on cell adhesion and GM_2 and GM_1 were not as active in inhibiting cell adhesion as a mixture of gangliosides. GD_{1a} and GD_{1b} were more active, but GD_{1b}, which is an isomer of GD_{1a}, had less activity, suggesting the importance of the position of sialic acid. GT_1 was the most active ganglioside in inhibiting cell adhesion.

The activity of the gangliosides resided in the sugar portion since purified ceramides had no effect upon cell adhesion (Table II), while purified oligosaccharides from the ganglioside mixture retained some, but not all, of the activity. Since the position of sialic acid appeared important in the effect of gangliosides on cell adhesion, we next modified the sialic acid residues by mild periodate exposure. Oxidation of sialic acid residues from either mixed gangliosides or purified GD_{1a} reduced the activity significantly (Table II). Reduction of the oxidized products did not restore activity. The structure of the gangliosides as measured by thin-layer chromatography was not destroyed by the oxidation and reduction processes (not shown). In addition, free sugars, including sialic acid, glucose, galactose, N-acetyl glucosamine, and N-acetyl galactosamine, had no effect upon cell adhesion. These results suggest the specificity of the inhibition by gangliosides.

We next determined the mechanism by which the gangliosides were blocking cell adhesion. The ability of gangliosides to inhibit cell adhesion by blocking fibronectin binding to collagen or by blocking cell binding to the fibronectin-collagen complex was measured. Collagen-coated dishes were preincubated with gangliosides, rinsed to remove the unbound material, and then were used for the usual adhesion assays. Results from these experiments

TABLE II. Effect of Gangliosides and Their Components on CHO Cell Adhesion

Test compound	Amount required for 50% inhibition of cell adhesion (nmoles/100 μl)
Ganglioside mixture[a]	40
GM_3[b]	No activity
GM_2	89
GM_1	61
GD_{1b}	38
GD_{1a}	32
GT_1	$<<< 26$[c]
Periodate-treated ganglioside mixture	169
Periodate-treated and reduced ganglioside mixture	135
Periodate-treated and reduced GD_{1a}[d]	159
Oligosaccharides from ganglioside mixture	120
Ceramides[d]	$>>> 350$[e]

[a]Obtained from Sigma Chemical Co.
[b]Highly purified gangliosides.
[c]That level blocked cell adhesion 100%.
[d]Obtained from Supelco, Inc.
[e]That level had no effect upon cell adhesion.

demonstrated no inhibition of cell adhesion by gangliosides (Table IIIA). However, when the fibronectin-collagen complex was preincubated with gangliosides and then washed, cell adhesion was inhibited (Table IIIB). This suggests that gangliosides bind to the fibronectin-collagen complex. A direct demonstration of ganglioside binding to fibronectin was seen in preliminary studies in which radioactive gangliosides were mixed with fibronectin and antibodies against fibronectin were used to precipitate fibronectin and attached ganglioside. In these studies, we found that GD_{1a} bound better to fibronectin than did GM_1 (Table IV) in confirmation of the attachment data. The presence of collagen is not required for ganglioside binding. These studies indicate that gangliosides inhibit fibronectin-mediated cell adhesion by binding through their sugar residues to fibronectin.

The effect of gangliosides on chondrocyte cell adhesion was tested to determine how a cell whose adhesion is not mediated by fibronectin would respond to gangliosides. As seen in Figure 4, these cells responded differently. Chondrocyte adhesion was stimulated by low levels of gangliosides, and at higher concentrations cell adhesion returned to control levels. This confirms the cell specificity of the inhibition of gangliosides on fibronectin-mediated cell adhesiveness.

DISCUSSION

Many cells synthesize fibronectin in culture [27], and this protein is widely distributed in various anatomic sites [28]. However, cartilage [29] and various epithelial tissues do not appear to contain fibronectin. These observations correlate well with our survey of the attachment properties of various cells to collagen in vitro. Cells such as fibroblasts, hepatocytes, and periosteal cells produce fibronectin and use it to bind to collagen substrates [30]. Freshly isolated chondrocytes as well as cultured chondrocytes (unpublished observations) do not use fibronectin to attach to collagen [25]. Rather, they appear to use a different cell attachment factor, which we have named chondronectin. Chondrocytes, however, can synthesize fibronectin in culture [29], particularly when cultured with medium containing exogenous fibronectin. Fibronectin alters the morphology and biosynthetic activities of chondrocytes and appears to be a major factor accounting for their loss of chondrocyte

TABLE III. Mechanism of Ganglioside Inhibition of Fibronectin-Mediated Cell Adhesion

	A. Effect on fibronectin binding to collagen (cells $\times$ 10^4 attached: after fibronectin addition: % inhibition)[a]	B. Effect of cell binding to fibronectin-collagen complex (cells $\times$ 10^4 attached: % inhibition)[b]
No additions	18 (0)	24 (0)
Plus gangliosides	7 (61)	9 (62)
Plus gangliosides, then wash	18 (0)	10 (58)

Values represent mean of triplicate measurements that did not differ by more than 10%. In these experiments a quantity of ganglioside (0.58 μmole/ml) was used that is known to inhibit cell attachment by 60% in the presence of 0.2% serum or the equivalent amount of fibronectin.
[a]Collagen-coated dishes were incubated with a ganglioside mixture for one hour. Where indicated, the plates were rinsed several times, followed by the addition of serum or purified fibronectin and cell adhesion was measured as already described in Materials and Methods.
[b]Collagen-coated dishes, which had been preincubated with purified fibronectin for 1 h, were incubated with a ganglioside mixture for an additional hour. The plates were then washed several times where indicated and cell adhesion was measured as already described in Materials and Methods.

phenotype [31]. The behavior of other cells in culture may also be altered by the high levels of fibronectin present in serum. In addition to direct effects on the metabolism of cells, fibronectin may alter the population of cells retained in culture after passage of the cells.

Both quantitative and qualitative differences are noted in the attachment and binding of transformed cells to collagen. A line of highly metastatic mouse sarcoma cells (PMT)

TABLE IV. Measurement of Gangliosides Binding to Fibronectin by Immunoprecipitation of Labeled Gangliosides in the Presence of Fibronectin and Anti-fibronectin

	% Precipitated
A. ^{3}H-GM$_1$	
+ Fibronectin	16
+ Fibronectin + collagen	15
+ Collagen	3
B. ^{3}H-GD$_{1a}$	
+ Fibronectin	31
+ Fibronectin + collagen	30
+ Collagen	7

Immunoprecipitation of ^{3}H-ganglioside by anti-fibronectin: Each ganglioside was incubated with fibronectin, collagen, or both, followed by reaction with rabbit antifibronectin and precipitation by goat anti-rabbit IgG. Each value is the mean of two precipitations.

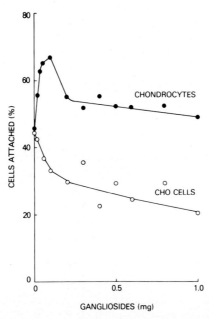

Fig. 4. Attachment of CHO cells and chondrocytes in the presence of increasing amounts of a ganglioside mixture. Collagen-coated dishes were incubated for 1 h with 1.5% fetal calf serum and the amount of ganglioside indicated. Then the cells were added and attachment was measured as described in Materials and Methods. The amount of serum employed is enough to support maximal attachment of CHO cells and 50% attachment of chondrocytes. The 50% attachment level of CHO cells is 0.2% serum. The gangliosides inhibit cell adhesion more at lower levels of serum. Each point represents the mean of duplicate measurements, which did not differ by more than 10%.

makes little or no fibronectin or collagen. In the presence of exogenous fibronectin, these cells can bind to a variety of collagen types. In the absence of fibronectin, PMT cells bind preferentially to type IV collagen. These differences may be related to the metastatic behavior of these cells. The lack of fibronectin and collagen may make these cells more peripatetic. The ability of these cells to bind to type IV collagen may allow circulating PMT cells to attach and penetrate endothelial basement membranes to initiate new growth. Other transformed but nonmetastatic cells produce less collagen and fibronectin than normal cells and do not show preferential binding to type IV collagen. Additionally, they retain less fibronectin on their surface [24]. These two changes appear to be related to the phenotypic changes associated with transformation.

As noted earlier, certain complex gangliosides have activities consistent with their role as cell surface binding sites for fibronectin. The studies reported here indicate that certain gangliosides, including GD_{1a} and GT_1, bind to fibronectin and block subsequent attachment of cells to the protein. The data also indicate that this activity resides in the oligosaccharide portion of the gangliosides and is dependent on intact sialic acid residues. Since the synthesis of these complex gangliosides is impaired in transformed cells [26], this could account for their reduced retention of fibronectin, and in turn could affect their malignant behavior.

ACKNOWLEDGMENTS

A. T. H. was supported by a National Institute of Health Postdoctoral Fellowship (Award #F-32DE05137).

REFERENCES

1. Pearlstein E: Nature 262:497, 1976.
2. Klebe RJ: Nature 250:248, 1974.
3. Klebe RJ: J Cell Physiol 86:231, 1975.
4. Hopper KE, Adelmann BC, Gentner G, Gay S: Immunology 30:249, 1976.
5. Engvall E, Ruoslahti E: Int J Cancer 20:1, 1977.
6. Kleinman HK, McGoodwin EB, Klebe RJ: Biochem Biophys Res Commun 72:426, 1976.
7. Dessau W, Adelmann BC, Timpl R, Martin GR: Biochem J 169:55, 1978.
8. Kleinman HK, McGoodwin EB, Martin GR, Klebe RJ, Fietzek PP, Woolley DE: J Biol Chem 253:5642, 1978.
9. Yamada KM, Kennedy DW: J Cell Biol 80:492, 1979.
10. Balian G, Click EM, Crouch E, Davidson JM, Bornstein P: J Biol Chem 254:1429, 1978.
11. Bornstein P, Piez KA: Biochemistry 5:3460, 1966.
12. Orkin RW, Gehron P, McGoodwin EB, Martin GR, Valentine T, Swarm R: J Exp Med 145:204, 1977.
13. Pacuszka T, Duffard RO, Nishimura RN, Brady RO, Fishman PH: J Biol Chem 253:5839, 1978.
14. Moss J, Fishman PH, Manganiello VC, Vaughan M, Brady RO: Proc Natl Acad Sci USA 73:1034, 1976.
15. Tallman JF, Fishman PH, Henneberry TC: Arch Biochem Biophys 182:556, 1977.
16. Fishman PH, Moss J, Osborne JO: Biochemistry 17:711, 1978.
17. Coon HG: Proc Natl Acad Sci USA 55:66, 1966.
18. Murray JC, Stingl G, Kleinman HK, Martin GR, Katz SI: J Cell Biol 80:197, 1979.
19. Liotta LA, Vembu D, Saini R, Boone C: Cancer Res 38:1231, 1978.
20. Kao WW, Prockop DJ: Nature 266:63, 1977.
21. Uitto J, Prockop DJ: Biochim Biophys Acta 336:234, 1974.
22. Liotta LA, Vembu D, Kleinman HK, Martin GR, Boone C: Nature 272:622, 1978.
23. Kamine J, Rubin H: J Cell Physiol 92:1, 1977.

24. Vaheri A, Mosher DF: Biochim Biophys Acta 516:1, 1978.
25. Hewitt AT, Kleinman HK, Pennypacker JP, Martin GR: J Cell Biol 79:151a, 1978.
26. Brady RO, Fishman PH: Biochim Biophys Acta 355:121, 1974.
27. Yamada KM, Olden K: Nature 275:179, 1978.
28. Stenman S, Vaheri A: J Exp Med 147:1054, 1978.
29. Dessau W, Sasse J, Timpl R, Jilek F, von der Mark K: J Cell Biol 79:342, 1978.
30. Kleinman HK, Murray JC, McGoodwin EB, Martin GR: J Invest Dermatol 71:9, 1978.
31. Pennypacker JP, Hassell JR, Yamada KM, Pratt RM: Exp Cell Res (In press).
32. Peterkofsky B, Diegelmann R: Biochemistry 10:988, 1971.
33. Schuurs A H WM, van Weemen BK: Clin Chim Acta 81:1, 1977.

Journal of Supramolecular Structure 11:79—93 (1979)
Tumor Cell Surfaces and Malignancy 55—69

Synergistic Stimulation of Early Events and DNA Synthesis by Phorbol Esters, Polypeptide Growth Factors, and Retinoids in Cultured Fibroblasts

Phillip Dicker and Enrique Rozengurt

Imperial Cancer Research Fund, Lincoln's Inn Fields, London WC2

12-O-Tetradecanoyl-phorbol-13-acetate (TPA), in the absence of serum, acts synergistically with a range of polypeptide growth factors to stimulate DNA synthesis in quiescent Swiss 3T3 cells. These growth factors include epidermal growth factor (EGF), insulin, and the peptide produced by BHK cells transformed by SV-40 virus (fibroblast-derived growth factor, FDGF). Retinoids also show mitogenic synergism with TPA or polypeptide growth factors. The spectrum of mitogenic synergisms displayed by TPA are similar to those of vasopressin, a pituitary peptide. However, TPA and vasopressin do not synergistically interact to stimulate DNA synthesis in quiescent 3T3 cells. This suggests that TPA and vasopressin act via an identical biochemical pathway. Several lines of evidence suggest rapid postreceptor convergence of the mitogenic mechanisms of action of the hormone and the tumor promotor. Thus, vasopressin and TPA both inhibit EGF binding to cellular receptors. Furthermore, TPA and vasopressin induce a similar array of early events in quiescent cells — most strikingly, identical stimulation of Rb^+ influx. Stimulation of ion flux is suggested as the possible convergence point of the pathway by which TPA and vasopressin act as mitogens.

Key words: Phorbol esters, retinoids, vasopressin, mitogens, uridine uptake, deoxyglucose uptake, ion fluxes

Normal, untransformed fibroblasts reduce their rate of entry into the S (DNA-synthesizing) phase of the cell cycle and accumulate in a highly viable state (called G_O, A, or R) under a large number of nonoptimal environmental conditions [1–4]. Under usual culture conditions, the limiting component is the concentration of serum present in the medium [5, 6]. Addition of serum to such quiescent cultures enhances the rates of protein and RNA synthesis and dramatically stimulates DNA synthesis and cell division. This large and reproducible transition of growth rate provides an experimental system for elucidating mechanisms of growth control.

Phorbol esters, a family of compounds with tumor-promoting activity, are strongly mitogenic to several types of quiescent cells in culture in the presence of limiting concentrations of serum [7]. The mitogenic potency is related to the potency of the phorbol ester as a tumor promoter in the two-stage system of skin carcinogenesis in mice [8]. 12-O-Tetradecanoyl-phorbol-13-acetate (TPA) is the most active tumor promotor and mitogen of the phorbol ester family.

Received March 18, 1979; accepted May 17, 1979.

0091-7419/79/1101-0079$02.90 © 1979 Alan R. Liss, Inc.

Recently we studied the mitogenic properties of TPA in quiescent cultures of fibroblastic cells. We found that the tumor promotor acts synergistically with other growth-promoting agents [9], rapidly stimulates an array of early metabolic changes, and causes a profound inhibition of the binding of radiolabeled epidermal growth factor (EGF) to cellular receptors [10]. The neurohypophyseal hormone vasopressin is also mitogenic for 3T3 cells [11]. We have found that many of its physiologic properties are similar to those of TPA. We propose that TPA modifies cell function by a mechanism similar to that of polypeptide hormones, like vasopressin.

INTERACTION OF TPA WITH DEFINED GROWTH FACTORS

Serum in the nutrient medium was shown to be an essential requirement for the mitogenic actions of TPA in cultures of mouse epidermal cells [12] and fibroblastic cells [7, 13]. The role of serum remained unresolved. We recently showed that TPA is mitogenic in the absence of serum if other growth factors are present [9]. Thus, quiescent cultures of Swiss 3T3 cells in the complete absence of serum are stimulated to undergo DNA synthesis by the addition of TPA together with either insulin, epidermal growth factor, or fibroblast-derived growth factor (FDGF), a polypeptide isolated from medium conditioned by BHK cells transformed by SV-40 virus [14] (Table I). The synergistic stimulation of DNA synthesis by TPA and defined growth factors can be demonstrated by measurements of total ^{3}H-Thymidine (^{3}H-TdR) incorporation into acid-insoluble material or by determination of the percentage of autoradiographically labeled nuclei incorporating ^{3}H-TdR (see Dicker and Rozengurt [9], and Table I).

The interaction between the tumor promotor and EGF or insulin is particularly striking, because neither of these substances produces a substantial stimulation of DNA synthesis by itself. In the presence of a fixed concentration of insulin, TPA stimulates DNA

TABLE I. Mitogenic Synergisms Between TPA and Growth Factors

		DNA synthesis			
		^{3}H-TdR incorporation[a]		Autoradiographically labeled nuclei[b]	
Additions	μg/ml	No TPA	100 ng/ml TPA	No TPA	100 ng/ml TPA
None		1	2	1	1
EGF	0.01	2	34	1	22
Insulin	1	2	95	1	70
FDGF	0.6	1	56	ND[c]	ND
FDGF	1.2	3	105	3	67
FDGF	2.4	46	97	ND	ND

[a]Cumulative ^{3}H-TdR incorporation, as measured in Rozengurt and Heppel [24], was determined over a 40-h exposure of quiescent cells to the additions indicated. Results are expressed as a percentage of incorporation produced by serum (10%) in the same experiment.
[b]Autoradiography was performed as in Rozengurt and Heppel [24] after a 40-h exposure of quiescent cells to ^{3}H-TdR and the additions indicated. Results are expressed as a percentage of the fraction of labeled nuclei produced by serum in the same experiment. Serum (10%) produced 80–90% autoradiographically labeled nuclei in these experiments.
[c]ND, not done.

synthesis in a dose-dependent manner (Fig. 1). The lowest concentration of TPA needed to show synergism consistently with 1 μg/ml insulin was 3 ng/ml. In contrast to the effect of TPA, phorbol itself, tested either in the absence or presence of insulin, was completely inactive in stimulating DNA synthesis. The close analogue, 4-O-methyl-12-O-tetradecanoyl-phorbol-13-acetate, was slightly mitogenic (18% of the maximal effect of TPA with insulin) at high concentrations (1 μg/ml) and in the presence of 1 μg/ml insulin. Phorbol is inactive as a tumor promotor while 4-O-methyl-12-O-tetradecanoyl-phorbol-13-acetate is a weak tumor promotor. Thus in our system the ability of phorbol esters to stimulate DNA synthesis in the presence of defined growth factors correlates well with the tumor-promoting potential of phorbol esters.

There is a striking synergistic interaction between growth-promoting polypeptides and TPA in stimulating quiescent cultures to recommence cell proliferation (Table II). In these experiments, the stimulating agents were added to medium containing depleted serum (see legend to Table II). Neither TPA nor insulin added to such cultures caused a substantial increase in growth, while together they caused a threefold increase in cell number. Similarly, although EGF and insulin together caused a threefold increase in cell number, the combination of the tumor promotor with both insulin and EGF resulted in a fivefold increase in cell number.

Hayashi and Sato [15] have demonstrated that several tumor epithelial cell lines grow in the absence of serum if growth factors are added to the medium. However, no fibroblastic cell retaining the ability to reversibly arrest in the G_0G_1 phase of the cell cycle has been reported to be able to proliferate in the absence of serum. Swiss 3T6 cells are fibroblastic cells that possess the reversible G_0G_1 arrest point [16]. Table III shows that 3T6

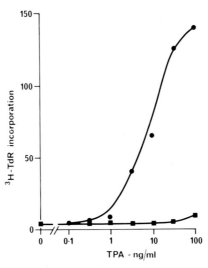

Fig. 1. Stimulation of ^{3}H-TdR incorporation by TPA and insulin into quiescent 3T3 cells. Cumulative ^{3}H-TdR incorporation (cpm $\times$ 10^{-3} per plate), measurement and conditions as in Rozengurt and Heppel [24], was determined over a 40-h exposure of quiescent cells to TPA in the absence (■) or presence (●) of 1 μg/ml insulin. Ten percent fetal bovine serum induced ^{3}H-TdR incorporation equal to 156 $\times$ 10^3 cpm per plate. As in all ^{3}H-TdR incorporations described in this review, quiescent cultures produced as in Rozengurt and Heppel [24] were washed twice in serum-free medium immediately prior to the experiment and experimental incubations were performed in a 1:1 mixture of Dulbecco's modified Eagle's medium (DMEM) and Waymouth medium.

TABLE II. TPA, EGF, and Insulin Stimulation of 3T3 Cell Proliferation

Addition	Cell number increase per 30-mm plate $\times 10^{-5}$ after 5 days	
	No TPA	200 ng/ml TPA
None	0	0.2
10 ng/ml EGF	0.5	1.5
1 μg/ml insulin	0.9	4.8
10 ng/ml EGF + 1 μg/ml insulin	3.9	8.8

Quiescent, confluent cultures of Swiss 3T3 cells were produced as in Rozengurt and Heppel [24]. Medium from parallel cultures was removed and one-third its volume of Waymouth's medium was added to replace low-molecular-weight nutrients that might have become depleted. TPA, insulin, and EGF were then added to give final concentrations as indicated. For each culture, two aliquots of cell suspension, produced by thorough trypsinization, were counted on a Coulter counter. Initial cell density was 2.3×10^5.

TABLE III. Proliferation of 3T6 Cells in Serum-Free Medium

Additions	Cells per 50-mm dish $\times 10^{-5}$
None	0.2
100 ng/ml TPA	2.0
1 μg/ml insulin	2.8
100 ng/ml TPA + 1 μg/ml insulin	10.8
0.5% fetal bovine serum	15.0

A 3T6 cell suspension was produced with crystalline trypsin, which was then neutralized with an excess of soya bean trypsin inhibitor. The cells were plated at 0.25×10^5 cells per 50-mm dish, in the absence of serum, in 1:1 Eagle's/Waymouth's plus 1.6 μM $FeSO_4$. The additions were made as above. Cultures were refed on days 4 and 8. On day 12 cultures were trypsinized and aliquots of the cell suspension were counted on a Coulter counter. The effect of 0.5% serum is shown for comparison.

cells can proliferate in serum-free medium if growth factors are present. Some proliferation of these cells occurs in the presence of insulin or TPA; however, a strikingly synergistic increase in proliferation occurs in the presence of both these factors. It should be noted that these experiments were performed with cells plated in the absence of serum (see footnote to Table III). Thus proliferation is indeed occurring in the complete absence of serum, and not owing to a residue left over from plating in serum.

The above results show that TPA apparently behaves as a growth factor in participating in complex synergistic interactions with growth-promoting polypeptides and, indeed, in stimulating cell proliferation. Thus, TPA may well be acting through the same type of mechanism as that used by peptide growth factors. This possibility receives further support in the next section, where we discuss a novel synergism between TPA, hormones, and a group of nonpeptide growth factors, the retinoids.

RETINOIDS AND TPA

Vitamin A and its derivatives have been reported to be inhibitors of cell proliferation [17] and also inducers of cell differentiation [18]. These properties are the reverse of TPA, which enhances cell proliferation and in many systems blocks cell differentiation [19]. Indeed retinoids have been shown to specifically reverse the effects of TPA, in several cell types. Thus retinoids block the mitogenic activity of TPA in lymphocytes [20] and the induction of ornithine decarboxylase produced by TPA in epithelial cells [21]. However, retinoic acid has been reported to minic TPA in increasing synthesis of plasminogen activator in chicken fibroblasts [22]. We therefore investigated the effects of retinoids on the stimulation of DNA synthesis produced by TPA, serum, or purified growth factors in 3T3 cells [23].

The combination of retinoic acid plus TPA synergistically produces 20–30% of the ^{3}H-TdR incorporation induced by saturating amounts of bovine serum (Table IV). Retinoic acid also drastically increases the amount of ^{3}H-TdR incorporation induced by EGF and TPA (Table IV and Fig. 2). Retinoic acid potentiates the mitogenic potency of TPA and EGF in a concentration-dependent manner. The minimal concentration of retinoic acid at which stimulation is consistently seen is 0.01 μM and maximal effects occur at about 1 μM. At 10 μM retinoic acid becomes strongly cytotoxic to 3T3 cells in the absence of serum.

Retinoic acid also exerts its stimulatory effects in the absence of TPA. Retinoic acid at 1 μM causes a considerable increase in ^{3}H-TdR incorporation induced by low concentrations of serum in cultures of quiescent Swiss 3T3 cells (Table IV). Likewise, retinoic acid markedly increases ^{3}H-TdR incorporation induced by low concentrations of FDGF (Table IV). TPA also enhances the mitogenic potency of FDGF (Table IV). In the presence of both TPA and retinoic acid, FDGF becomes a very potent mitogen at low concentrations. The enhancement of the potency of mitogens by retinoic acid was also found when the percentage of labeled nuclei incorporating ^{3}H-TdR was measured by autoradiography [23]. Retinol, retinal, and retinyl acetate all have stimulating effects on ^{3}H-TdR incorporation similar to those produced by retinoic acid (unpublished results).

Retinoic acid possesses growth-promoting activity when cell proliferation is monitored over a period of several days. Experiments performed in the presence of 2% serum

TABLE IV. Retinoic Acid Enhancement of the Mitogenic Potency of Growth Factors

Additions	^{3}H-TdR incorporation	
	No retinoic acid	Retinoic acid
None	1	1
TPA	1	25
EGF + TPA	18	68
Insulin + TPA	46	118
FDGF	3	40
FDGF + TPA	44	120
Fetal bovine serum	35	98

Concentrations of EGF, retinoic acid, insulin, TPA, fetal bovine serum, and FDGF were 0.01 μg/ml, 1 μM, 1 μg/ml, 0.1 μg/ml, 6% (v/v), and 1.2 μg/ml, respectively. ^{3}H-TdR incorporation was measured over 40 h as in Rozengurt and Heppel [24]. ^{3}H-TdR incorporation is expressed as a percentage of the incorporation induced by 10% fetal bovine serum.

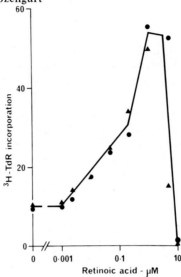

Fig. 2. Potentiation by retinoic acid of ³H-TdR incorporation induced by EGF and TPA or EGF and vasopressin in quiescent 3T3 cells. Cumulative ³H-TdR incorporation (cpm $\times$ 10⁻³ per plate) was determined over a 40-h exposure of cell cultures to retinoic acid with 10 ng/ml EGF and 100 ng/ml TPA (●) or with 10 ng/ml EGF and 10 ng/ml vasopressin (▲). Conditions and measurements were as in Rozengurt and Heppel [24]. EGF, TPA, vasopressin, or insulin alone induced incorporation of under 2×10^3 cpm per plate. Fetal bovine serum (10%) induced incorporation of 155×10^3 cpm per plate in this experiment.

in the medium (which does not support growth of Swiss 3T3 cells) demonstrate that retinoic acid causes a twofold to threefold increase in cell number. Furthermore, retinoic acid combined with either TPA, EGF, insulin, or FDGF synergistically caused a greater increase in cell number [23].

These results demonstrate that retinoids markedly enhance the mitogenic potency of a range of growth factors including TPA. Since high concentrations of FDGF [14] or the combination of insulin, EGF, and vasopressin [11] added in the absence of retinoids produce nearly maximal stimulation of DNA synthesis in Swiss 3T3 cells, retinoids are not required as essential nutrient molecules in this system. Their effects are probably due to a hormone-like, regulatory modulation of the mitogenic response. Intracellular retinoid-binding proteins have recently been isolated from many tissues, prompting the suggestion that these proteins mediate the biologic effects of retinoids, in a way similar to the role of steroid hormone receptors in responsive cells. Whatever the mechanism of action of retinoids, the fact that they potentiate the mitogenic activity of TPA as they do with other growth factors supports the notion that TPA performs its mitogenic actions via pathways like those used by other growth factors. Through which specific hormonal pathway does TPA exert its mitogenic effects? In the next section we produce strong evidence indicating that TPA activates the same mitogenic mechanisms as those stimulated by a defined peptide hormone, vasopressin.

SIMILARITIES IN THE MITOGENIC ACTIONS OF TPA AND VASOPRESSIN

Recent work from this laboratory has indicated that ionic fluxes may play a role in modulating the mitogenic response [24, 27]. These observations prompted us to test whether hormones or ionophores that stimulate ion fluxes are also able to regulate cell proliferation. We found that vasopressin, a neurohypophyseal nonapeptide that promotes Na^+ transport in several tissues, is a potent mitogen for Swiss 3T3 cells [11]. The hormone causes a shift of the dose response for the effect of serum on ^3H-TdR incorporation by quiescent cells. In the absence of added serum, the effect of vasopressin is greatly potentiated by insulin, EGF, and FDGF. Furthermore, we recently found that the mitogenic effect of vasopressin and EGF can be further enhanced by retinoic acid. Figure 2 shows the dose response of retinoic acid in the potentiation of EGF and vasopressin stimulation of ^3H-TdR incorporation in 3T3 cells. The dose response and extent of the enhancement by retinoic acid are similar to those seen in the presence of EGF and TPA (Fig. 2). Thus vasopressin appears to be able to replace TPA under these conditions. Nor is the equivalence of the mitogenic properties of vasopressin and TPA confined to the above situation. Table V illustrates that the phorbol ester and the nonapeptide produce identical stimulation of ^3H-TdR incorporation in the presence of several mitogens or combination of mitogens. Figure 3 shows that the time course of stimulation of ^3H-TdR incorporation caused by TPA and insulin is superimposeable with that caused by vasopressin and insulin. Further both vasopressin and TPA produce similar potentiation of the mitogenic potency of low concentrations of serum or FDGF (data not shown).

The similarities in the mitogenic properties of TPA and vasopressin suggest that these chemically diverse factors are stimulating DNA synthesis via identical pathways. If so, TPA and vasopressin should not synergistically increase each other's mitogenic activity. Results in Figure 4 demonstrate that this is indeed the case. TPA and vasopressin together cause no synergistic stimulation of DNA synthesis. That this is not because these molecules inter-

TABLE V. Similarity of Mitogenic Properties of TPA and Vasopressin

	^3H-TdR incorporation		
Additions	No addition	TPA	Vasopressin
None	1	2	1
EGF	1	14	10
EGF + retinoic acid	1	50	45
Insulin	1	60	58
Insulin + retinoic acid	2	105	93
EGF + insulin	21	93	98

Concentrations of EGF, retinoic acid, insulin, TPA, and vasopressin were 0.01 µg/ml, 1 µM, 1 µg/ml, 0.1 µg/ml, and 10 ng/ml, respectively. ^3H-TdR incorporation into acid-insoluble material was measured over 40 h as in Rozengurt and Heppel [24]. ^3H-TdR incorporation is expressed as a percentage of the incorporation induced by 10% fetal bovine serum.

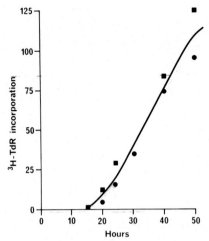

Fig. 3. Time course of ³H-TdR incorporation into quiescent 3T3 cells stimulated by TPA and insulin or vasopressin and insulin. Cumulative ³H-TdR incorporation (cpm × 10^{-3} per plate) was determined at various times after the addition of 100 ng/ml TPA and 1 μg/ml insulin (■) or 10 ng/ml vasopressin and 1 μg/ml insulin (●) to cell cultures. Conditions and ³H-TdR incorporation measurements were as in Rozengurt and Heppel [24]. Insulin, TPA, or vasopressin alone induced ³H-TdR incorporation of under 5 × 10^3 cpm per plate at 50 h. Fetal bovine serum (10%) induced incorporation of 239 × 10^3 cpm per plate at 50 h.

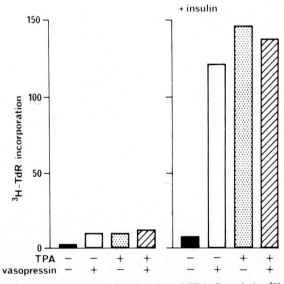

Fig. 4. Lack of mitogenic synergism between vasopressin and TPA. Cumulative ³H-TdR incorporation (cpm × 10^{-3} per plate) was measured over a 40-h exposure of cell cultures to various combinations at 100 ng/ml TPA, 10 ng/ml vasopressin, and 1 μg/ml insulin. Conditions and measurements were as in Rozengurt and Heppel [24]. Fetal bovine serum (10%) induced incorporation of 156 × 10^3 cpm per dish in this experiment.

fere with each other's action is shown by the fact that saturating levels of TPA and insulin produce the same amount of ^{3}H-TdR incorporation in the presence or absence of vasopressin. The findings shown in Figure 4 are in sharp contrast to the results obtained with other mitogenic molecules like FDGF, EGF, or insulin, which interact synergistically among themselves as well as with either TPA or vasopressin.

These results strongly indicate that TPA and vasopressin act via an identical pathway. This need not mean they act through the same initial receptor. Indeed the fact that TPA is mitogenic in 3T6 cells [9], whereas vasopressin is not active in these cells (unpublished data), suggests that this is not the case. Rather it seems that the series of events initiated by TPA or vasopressin binding to a cell converge at some postreceptor locus. An approach to defining the molecular nature of this common pathway is to investigate metabolic effects of TPA and vasopressin that occur much earlier than induction of DNA synthesis. Attempts in this direction are discussed in the following sections.

TPA STIMULATION OF EARLY EVENTS

When quiescent 3T3 cells are stimulated by serum or by defined growth factors, a complex array of biochemical changes occur [28]. These may be divided into primary, rapid, protein and RNA synthesis independent changes, and subsequent changes that are dependent on the synthesis of macromolecules [28]. The early events include stimulation of uridine and deoxyglucose uptake, increase in ion fluxes, and increase in the rate of glycolysis. If TPA exerts its mitogenic effects in a manner similar to other growth factors, it might be expected to trigger the same early events.

URIDINE UPTAKE

Quiescent 3T3 cells show a severalfold increase in the rate of uridine uptake when stimulated by serum [29, 30], EGF [31], insulin [31], or FDGF [14]. In the case of all these agents the stimulation occurs as follows: 1) After addition of the stimulant there is a lag of 5—15 min during which the rate of uridine uptake remains unchanged [14, 29, 31]; 2) after this lag period the rate of uridine uptake rapidly increases until the stimulated rate is reached, and then the rate of uridine uptake remains steady at its new elevated level [29, 31]; 3) the increase in uptake occurs primarily via an increase in the rate of phosphorylation and not in the rate of transport across the cell membrane [30, 31].

Figure 5 shows that TPA stimulates uridine uptake after a lag period of 10 min, followed by a rapid increase in the rate of uridine uptake. This kinetic conforms with uridine uptake stimulation induced by polypeptide growth factors.

To distinguish whether TPA stimulates transport of uridine across the membrane or its subsequent intracellular phosphorylation, the following experiments were performed. In both experiments cultures were stimulated with TPA for 40 min prior to the measurements of uptake. Figure 5 shows that the initial rate of entry of ^{3}H-uridine into TPA-stimulated cells does not differ from that of the controls. However, after 6—8 sec the rate of uptake in nonstimulated cultures levels off markedly. These results suggest that the initial rate of uridine *transport* is not substantially different in stimulated and nonstimulated cultures and that TPA stimulates the intracellular *trapping* of ^{3}H-uridine. To directly substantiate this conclusion, acid-soluble pools were separated chromatographically into charged and noncharged moieties (Table VI). Incubation with TPA considerably changes the composition of the acid-soluble pools in 3T3 cells; it increases the radioactivity re-

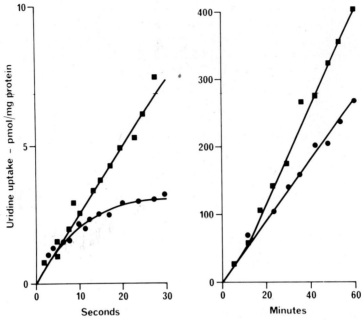

Fig. 5. TPA stimulation of uridine uptake. Left panel: Quiescent cultures of Swiss 3T3 cells were in-cubated with DMEM (●) or DMEM plus 100 ng/ml TPA (■) for 40 min. ³H-Uridine was then added at 10 μCi/ml, 28 Ci/mmole, for the times indicated. Cultures were then washed and ³H-uridine uptake measured as in Rozengurt et al [30]. Right panel: Quiescent cultures of Swiss 3T3 cells were exposed to 1 μCi/ml, 1 Ci/mmole ³H-uridine in DMEM (●) or DMEM plus 100 ng/ml TPA (■) at 0 min. At the times indicated cultures were washed and accumulative ³H-uridine uptake measured as in Rozengurt and Stein [29].

TABLE VI. ³H-Uridine Uptake Stimulated by TPA and Serum

Additions	% ³H-Uridine in phosphorylated pool after 6 sec	³H-Uridine uptake (pmoles/mg protein) 6 sec	³H-Uridine uptake (pmoles/mg protein) 10 min
None	58	1.2	41
100 ng/ml TPA	82	1.2	102
10% fetal bovine serum	88	1.3	125

Quiescent cultures of Swiss 3T3 cells, produced as in Methods, were exposed to DMEM plus the addi-tions indicated for 40 min. ³H-Uridine was then added at 1 μCi/ml, 1 Ci/mmole or 10 μCi/ml, 28 Ci/ mmole for 10 min and 6 sec uptake periods, respectively. Measurement of ³H-uridine uptake, and separation of phosphorylated and nonphosphorylated pools, was determined as described previously [31].

covered in the nucleoside phosphate pool from 58% of total counts in unstimulated cultures to 82% in cultures stimulated by TPA. Serum, which increases the radioactivity in the phos-phorylated pool to 88% of total counts, is shown for comparison. Clearly TPA stimulates the rate of conversion of ³H-uridine to phosphorylated nucleosides. Thus, TPA stimulates uridine uptake in quiescent 3T3 cells in the same fashion as other growth factors.

DEOXYGLUCOSE UPTAKE AND GLYCOLYSIS

When quiescent 3T3 cells are stimulated by serum, an increase in the rate of deoxyglucose uptake occurs in two distinct phases [14, 28, 32–34] : 1) In the first 30–60 min after serum addition the rate of deoxyglucose uptake increases severalfold, independently of protein synthesis; 2) by 6 h after serum stimulation the rate of deoxyglucose uptake dramatically increases to at least ten times that of quiescent cultures. This second phase of increase is inhibited by cycloheximide [32, 33].

The two-phase stimulation of deoxyglucose uptake by serum is demonstrated in Figure 6. The figure also demonstrates that either TPA or insulin alone causes an increase in the rate of deoxyglucose uptake after 45 min of incubation. They do not, however, cause a further increase after 6 h incubation. Thus TPA or insulin alone activates the first but not the second phase of the stimulation of deoxyglucose uptake. However, TPA and insulin added together do cause a second phase of stimulation of sugar uptake (Fig. 6). This finding suggests that ability to induce the cycloheximide-sensitive phase increase might be indicative of the mitogenic potential of a growth factor or combination of growth factors. Thus, neither TPA nor insulin alone causes substantial DNA synthesis when added to quiescent 3T3 cells, nor do they produce the second phase of deoxyglucose uptake stimu-

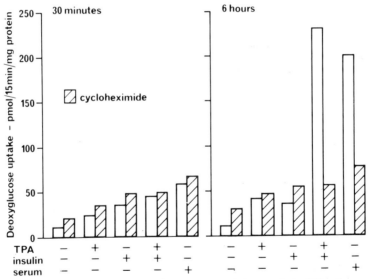

Fig. 6. TPA stimulation of deoxyglucose uptake. Left panel: Quiescent Swiss 3T3 cells were washed three times in DMEM minus glucose, then incubated with DMEM minus glucose in the presence (striped bars) or absence (plain bars) of 10 µg/ml cycloheximide plus the mitogens as indicated. After 30 min ³H-2-deoxyglucose was added at 1.25 µCi/ml, 2.5 µM and uptake measured as in De Asua and Rozengurt [32] during the subsequent 15 min. Right panel: Quiescent cultures of Swiss 3T3 cells were incubated in DMEM in the presence (striped bars) or absence (plain bars) of 10 µg/ml cycloheximide plus the mitogens as indicated. After 5.5 h the cultures were washed three times in DMEM minus glucose and exposed to DMEM minus glucose with (striped bars) or without (plain bars) 10 µg/ml cycloheximide plus the mitogens as indicated. After 30 min ³H-2-deoxyglucose was added at 1.25 µCi/ml, 2.5 µM and uptake was measured as in De Asua and Rozengurt [32] during the subsequent 15 min. For both panels concentrations of mitogens were 100 ng/ml, 1 µg/ml, 10% v/v for TPA, insulin, and fetal bovine serum, respectively. The serum was previously dialyzed against saline.

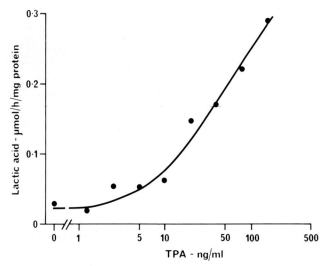

Fig. 7. TPA stimulation of lactic acid production. Quiescent cultures of 3T3 cells were exposed to TPA and cumulative lactic acid concentration in the medium was measured after 4 h. Conditions, medium, and assay for lactic acid production was as in Diamond et al [35].

lation. Serum, or TPA and insulin, induce both the second phase of deoxyglucose uptake and DNA synthesis.

Addition of serum or growth factors like EGF, insulin [35, 36], or FDGF (unpublished results) causes a stimulation of the glycolytic flux in quiescent 3T3 cells. Figure 7 shows that TPA also causes a concentration-dependent increase in glycolysis, as measured by the rate of lactic acid production. The stimulation of lactic acid production has been studied at high, saturating concentrations of extracellular glucose (25 mM), so the rate-limiting step in lactic acid production lies in the glycolytic pathway rather in the transport of glucose across the cell membrane [35]. TPA can synergistically increase lactic acid production still more in the presence of EGF [10].

Na$^+$, K$^+$ PUMP

One of the earliest changes produced subsequently to the addition of serum to quiescent cells is a stimulation of Rb$^+$ (a K$^+$ tracer) influx across the membrane [14, 24, 25, 27]. This increased flux represents an activation of the Na$^+$,K$^+$ pump, since it is inhibitable by ouabain. TPA similarly causes a rapid, ouabain-inhibitable increase in influx of Rb$^+$ when added to quiescent cells [37, 38].

Vasopressin, in general, induces an array of early events similar to those caused by TPA [27, 38, and unpublished results]. The similarity of their stimulation of Rb$^+$ uptake is most striking, especially considering that EGF and insulin show little enhancement of Rb$^+$ influx [24]. Both vasopressin and TPA produce an increase in the V$_{max}$ of ^{86}Rb uptake without altering the affinity of the uptake system for K$^+$ [38]. This again indicates a rapid, postreceptor convergence of the mitogenic mechanisms of action of TPA and vasopressin.

EFFECTS OF TPA ON EGF BINDING

The finding that TPA potentiated the mitogenic potency of various purified poly-peptides led us to test the effects of TPA on the binding of growth factors to cell surface receptors. We found, surprisingly, that TPA causes a potent, dose-dependent inhibition of ^{125}I-EGF binding [10]. TPA causes a tenfold decrease in the affinity of EGF receptors without a change in the number of receptors. We also produced evidence showing that TPA initially binds to a cell by a site other than the EGF receptor. That TPA exerts its mito-genic effects via a pathway not involving the EGF receptor is shown by the synergism of TPA and EGF in stimulation of DNA synthesis. EGF is able to initiate a biologic response when TPA inhibits its binding presumably because of the availability of "spare receptors" for the peptide. It is known that the maximal response to EGF can be obtained at concen-trations at which only a small fraction of EGF receptors are occupied.

The similarity of the mitogenic properties of TPA and vasopressin prompted the test-ing of the effects of vasopressin on EGF binding. Brown and Rozengurt [39] found that vasopressin inhibits EGF binding to Swiss 3T3 cells. The effect is specific since oxytocin, a peptide 10^3 times less potent than vasopressin in stimulating DNA synthesis, is also much less effective than vasopressin in inhibiting EGF binding. Thus TPA and vasopressin exert a similar effect on a membrane protein (the EGF receptor) soon after their addition to cell cultures. These findings provide further support to the idea that the pathways of action of these two mitogens converge very soon after they bind to 3T3 cells.

CONCLUSIONS

The biochemical mechanism of action of tumor promotors has aroused much interest. Knowledge of such mechanisms would indicate the best strategy for countering their ef-fects. The basis of the relationship between the mitogenic and tumor-promoting proper-ties of the phorbol esters is at present unknown. However, the two properties are not dis-sociable in the various members of the phorbol ester series. Thus elucidation of the means by which the esters exert their mitogenic effects should help in the understanding of their tumor-promoting properties.

We have shown that TPA, in the absence of serum, acts synergistically with a range of polypeptide growth factors to stimulate DNA synthesis in quiescent 3T3 cells. We also demonstrated a mitogenic synergism between TPA and a group of nonpeptide molecules, the retinoids. Likewise, the retinoids increased the mitogenic potency of polypeptide growth factors. These similarities suggested that TPA acted via mechanisms akin to those used by other growth factors. A similar conclusion has been reached by Weinstein and his co-workers [40, 41] on other grounds. They further advanced the possibility that, at least partly, the biologic effects of TPA could be mediated by the EGF receptor-effector trigger-ing system. This possibility seems unlikely, because EGF and TPA synergistically stimu-lated DNA synthesis in quiescent cells [9] and because TPA interacts with EGF receptors in a different manner from native EGF [10]. Thus, the important question is "Which specific hormonal path of action does TPA use to exert its mitogenic effect?" The answer appears to be that of vasopressin, since TPA and vasopressin have nearly identical patterns of mitogenic synergism with other factors, and they show no synergism with each other. This is clearly summarized in Table VII, which shows that 9 of 10 combinations between

TABLE VII. Mitogenic Interactions Between Various Growth Factors in Quiescent Swiss 3T3 Cells

Fixed concentration	Variable concentration					
	FDGF[a]	EGF	Insulin	Vasopressin	TPA	References
FDGF[a]		++	++	++	++	9, 11, 14
EGF	++		+	+	+	9, 11, 42
Insulin	++	+		++	++	9, 11, 14, 42
Vasopressin	++	+	++		0	11
TPA	++	+	++	0		9

Symbols: ++, Interaction of these factors induces ^{3}H-TdR incorporation of more than 40% of that caused by 10% fetal bovine serum; +, interaction of these factors induces ^{3}H-TdR incorporation of 10–40% of that caused by 10% fetal bovine serum; 0, no synergistic interaction.
[a]Concentrations of FDGF causing ^{3}H-TdR incorporation of less than 5% of that produced by 10% fetal bovine serum.

FDGF, EGF, insulin, vasopressin, and TPA act synergistically in stimulating DNA synthesis, while TPA and vasopressin do not potentiate the effect of each other.

We do not believe that TPA and vasopressin bind to the same cell surface receptor, because they show different cellular specificities in their biologic actions. Thus TPA and vasopressin seem initially to bind to different sites and their mitogenic train of events converge subsequently. That this convergence occurs soon after the initial binding is suggested by the ability of both TPA and vasopressin to rapidly inhibit EGF binding to its receptors. To further elucidate the nature of this convergence, we studied the stimulation of early events by TPA. The tumor promotor was shown to activate in quiescent cells a wide range of early events similar to those induced by other growth factors. Vasopressin also induces these early events. The stimulation of Rb$^+$ influx by TPA and vasopressin is strikingly similar. We conclude from the results given here that TPA's mechanism of action as a mitogen is of the same general nature as that of polypeptide growth factors. In particular the events that lead from vasopressin or TPA binding with a cell to their subsequent mitogenic effects seem to converge into the same pathway. Whether this convergence may have its basis in the identical stimulation of ion fluxes into quiescent cells by vasopressin and TPA is an important question that warrants further experimental work.

LITERATURE CITED

1. Smith JA, Martin L: Proc Natl Acad Sci USA 70:1263, 1973.
2. Pardee AB: Proc Natl Acad Sci USA 71:1286, 1974.
3. Pardee AB, Rozengurt E: In Fox CF (ed): "Biochemistry of Cell Walls and Membranes," 1975, vol 2, p 155.
4. Rozengurt E, Po CC: Nature 261:701, 1976.
5. Holley RW: Nature 258:487, 1975.
6. Rozengurt E: In Dumont JE, Brown BL, Marshall NJ (eds): "Eukaryotic Cell Function and Growth." New York: Plenum, 1976, p 711.
7. Sivak A: J Cell Physiol 80:167, 1972.
8. Yuspa SH et al: Nature 262:402, 1976.
9. Dicker P, Rozengurt E: Nature 276:723–726, 1978.
10. Brown KD, Dicker P, Rozengurt E: Biochem Biophys Res Commun 86:1073, 1979.
11. Rozengurt E, Legg A, Pettican P: Proc Natl Acad Sci USA 76:1284, 1979.

12. Yuspa SH, Licht U, Hennings H, Ben T, Patterson E, Slaga TJ: In Slaga TJ, Sivak A, Boutwell RKL (eds): "Mechanisms of Tumour Promotion and Co-carcinogenesis." New York: Raven, 1978, p 245.
13. Boynton AL, Whitfield JE, Isaacs RJ: J Cell Physiol 87:25, 1976.
14. Bourne H, Rozengurt E: Proc Natl Acad Sci USA 73:4555–4559, 1976.
15. Hayashi I, Sato G: Nature 259:132, 1976.
16. Mierzejewski K, Rozengurt E: Biochem Biophys Res Commun 73:271–278, 1976.
17. Lotan R, Nicolson GL: J Natl Cancer Inst 59:1717, 1977.
18. Strickland S, Mahdavi V: Cell 15:393, 1978.
19. Rovera G, O'Brien TG, Diamond L: Proc Natl Acad Sci USA 74:2894, 1977.
20. Kensler TW, Mueller GC: Cancer Res 38:771, 1978.
21. Verma AK, Rice HM, Shapas BG, Boutwell RK: Cancer Res 38:793, 1978.
22. Wilson EL, Reich E: Cell 15:385, 1978.
23. Dicker P, Rozengurt E: Biochem Biophys Res Commun (submitted for publication).
24. Rozengurt E, Heppel LA: Proc Natl Acad Sci USA 72:4492–4495, 1975.
25. Smith JB, Rozengurt E: J Cell Physiol 97:441–450, 1978.
26. Smith JB, Rozengurt E: Proc Natl Acad Sci USA 75:5560, 1978.
27. Rozengurt E, Mendoza S: Ann NY Acad Sci (In press).
28. Rozengurt E: In Hynes R (ed): "Surface Properties of Normal and Neoplastic Cells." Sussex, England: J. Wiley and Sons, 1979, p 322.
29. Rozengurt E, Stein WD: Biochim Biophys Acta 464:417, 1977.
30. Rozengurt E, Stein W, Wigglesworth N: Nature 267:442, 1977.
31. Rozengurt E, Mierzejewski K, Wigglesworth NM: J Cell Physiol 97:441, 1978.
32. De Asua GL, Rozengurt E: Nature 251:624, 1974.
33. Bradley WEC, Culp LA: Exp Cell Res 84:335, 1974.
34. Browenstein BL, Rozengurt E, De Asua GL, Stoker M: J Cell Physiol 85:579, 1975.
35. Diamond I, Legg A, Schneider JA, Rozengurt E: J Biol Chem 253:866–871, 1978.
36. Schneider JA, Diamond I, Rozengurt E: J Biol Chem 253:872, 1978.
37. Moroney J, Smith A, Tomli LD, Wenner CE: J Cell Physiol 95:287–294, 1978.
38. Mendoza S, Rozengurt E: Manuscript in preparation.
39. Brown K, Rozengurt E: Submitted for publication.
40. Lee L, Weinstein IB: Science 202:313, 1978.
41. Weinstein BI, Wigler M, Yamasaki H, Lee LS, Fisher PB, Mufson A: In Ruddon RW (ed): "Biological Markers of Neoplasia: Basic and Applied Aspects." Amsterdam: Elsevier/North-Holland, 1978, p 451.
42. Mierzejewski K, Rozengurt E: Biochem Biophys Res Commun 83:874, 1978.

Journal of Supramolecular Structure 11:95–104 (1979)
Tumor Cell Surfaces and Malignancy 71–80

Cell Surface Fibronectin and Oncogenic Transformation

Richard O. Hynes, Antonia T. Destree, Margaret E. Perkins, and Denisa D. Wagner

Department of Biology, Center for Cancer Research, Massachusetts Institute of Technology, Cambridge, Massachusetts 02139

Fibronectin is a large glycoprotein at the cell surface of many different cell types; a related protein is present in plasma. Fibronectin is a dimer of 230,000-dalton subunits and also occurs in larger aggregates; it forms fibrillar networks at the cell surface, between cells and substrata and between adjacent cells, and it is not a typical membrane protein. Cell surface fibronectin is reduced in amount or absent on transformed cells and in many cases its loss correlates with acquisition of tumorigenicity and, in particular, metastatic ability. Exceptions to the correlations with transformation and tumorigenicity exist. Loss of fibronectin and the resulting reduced adhesion appear to be involved in pleiotropic alterations in cell behavior and may be responsible for several aspects of the transformed phenotype in vitro. Fibronectin interacts with other macromolecules (collagen/gelatin, fibrin/fibrinogen, proteoglycans) and is apparently connected to microfilaments inside the cell.

Key words: fibronectin structure and properties, cytoskeleton, cell surface proteins, fibronectin distribution, fibronectin interactions, transformation

Since the initial report in 1973 that a large protein was lost from the surfaces of virally transformed cells [1], there has been a large amount of work that has by and large confirmed the generality of this observation. This surface protein is now generally known as fibronectin. Some of the probable implications of the loss of fibronectin for the transformed phenotype in vitro are becoming clear, and several analyses have attempted to clarify possible relationships with the malignant phenotype in vivo. In this article, we shall briefly review the current state of this area of research. No attempt will be made to be exhaustive, but we will rather summarize the main points that are established and attempt to identify the outstanding questions that require further research. Several detailed reviews of the subject have been published and these may be consulted for more complete bibliographies [2–4].

Received April 30, 1979; accepted May 7, 1979.

DISTRIBUTION OF FIBRONECTINS

Although cell surface fibronectin was first described in fibroblasts, it has subsequently been detected on many other cell types in culture (Table I). Analysis of tissue sections by immunofluorescence or immunoelectron microscopy has also identified cross-reacting material in many locations in vivo [22–24]. The discovery [33] that cell surface fibronectin – variously known as LETS protein, CSP, SF-antigen, galactoprotein a or Z – is immunologically related to a plasma and serum protein known as cold-insoluble globulin (CIg), leads to recognition of an even wider distribution of proteins of this type. These proteins are known collectively as fibronectins. Although they are cross-reactive immunologically, exact identity has not been shown. In fact, it seems clear that the cell surface form identified on cultured cells, which is rather insoluble [34, 35], differs somewhat from the soluble plasma form. The cellular source of the plasma form has not been identified. The possibility of cell type-specific differences among fibronectins has not been studied in any detail, and there has been little biochemical analysis of the antigenically related material detected in tissue sections.

The major in vivo locations of fibronectins are in soft connective tissue stroma, associated with basement membranes, and in body fluids such as plasma and cerebrospinal and amniotic fluids (Table I). In tissue culture, fibronectin has been most extensively studied on fibroblasts, of which it is a major surface protein, consistent with the connective tissue location in vivo. Other major producers in culture are myoblasts, endothelial cells, and amniotic cells (Table I), and several other cell types have been reported to produce fibronectin, usually at lower levels [15–21]. Some apparent discrepancies exist between the in vivo and in vitro distributions. Neural tissues, both neuronal and glial, appear to lack fibronectin in vivo, but some glial cells have been reported to make it in vitro. Similarly, cartilage in vivo is free of fibronectin [31], and while differentiated chondrocytes in culture also lack fibronectin, predifferentiated or dedifferentiated chondrocytes do synthesize it [31, 32]. Hormonal regulation of fibronectin production has been demonstrated [36, 37] and cells regulate their levels in response to growth conditions [38, 39]. Clearly, therefore, the levels produced by a given cell type can be modulated.

STRUCTURE OF FIBRONECTIN

Fibronectins, both cell surface and plasma forms, are large glycoproteins with subunit molecular weights of 230,000 ± 20,000, and are about 5–7% carbohydrate. Most or all the carbohydrate side chains appear to be of the complex asparagine-linked type [40, 41]. The carbohydrate contents of fibronectin chains appear to vary [14, 42]. Fibronectins are in fact dimers of the basic subunits held together by disulfide bonds [26, 27, 34, 35, 42–44]. The interchain disulfide bonds are located very close to one end [42, 45], probably the C terminal [46, 47]. On the cell surface, but not in plasma, fibronectin also occurs as high-molecular-weight aggregates whose integrity depends on disulfide bonds [43, 44]. Disulfide-bonded aggregates could arise through reaction of the single free sulfhydryl group present on each subunit of fibronectin [42]. Within fibronectin, there appear to be globular domains joined by flexible regions, as determined by physical methods [48, 49]. Different domains can be separated by partial proteolytic digestion [42]. These separable fragments differ in composition. There is a small (25,000–30,000 daltons), highly disulfide-bonded but carbohydrate-free region and a larger (200,000 daltons) fragment that is relatively poor in cystine, but contains most of the carbohydrate and the free sulfhydryl [42]. The 200,000-dalton fragment can be further fragmented to yield a fragment of

30,000–40,000 daltons that contains the site by which fibronectin binds to gelatin [50–52] and a different fragment, which binds to heparin [53, 54], is also probably located in the 200,000-dalton region.

PROPERTIES OF CELL SURFACE FIBRONECTIN

Cell surface fibronectin is arranged in fibrillar arrays that can be detected by immuno-fluorescence or immunoelectron microscopy (Fig. 1). The pattern of the fibrils varies for different cells and, for a given cell type, depends on culture conditions, especially cell density. Isolated cells have fibronectin predominantly beneath them, between the cell and the substratum [39]. Cells in contact often have fibronectin between them, and dense cultures have elaborate fibrillar networks around and above the cells (Fig. 1). Fibronectin is most prevalent in dense or growth-arrested cultures; growing cells have less, and mitotic cells have very little [38, 39].

Cell surface fibronectin is relatively immobile and does not readily form patches and caps, as do certain integral membrane proteins [39, 55, 56]. The fibrils can be left behind on the substratum when cells are detached [39] and although some crude plasma membrane preparations contain fibronectin, it is possible to separate fibronectin from plasma membrane vesicles and it can be isolated in a nonmembranous cell surface fraction probably corresponding with the cell surface coat [57, 58].

All of these results suggest that fibronectin is not a typical membrane protein but should be considered rather as a constituent of the surface coat, glycocalyx, or extracellular matrix. Consistent with this idea is the difficulty of solubilizing fibronectin from cell surfaces. This cannot be accomplished by nonionic detergents, high- or low-salt, or chelating agents, but requires chaotropic reagents [34]. Release from cell surfaces is also promoted by reducing agents, a phenomenon that is consistent with the extensive disulfide bonding [43]. The fibrillar matrix of fibronectin is readily removed by proteolytic enzymes.

TABLE I. Distribution of Fibronectins

	Representative references
In vitro – Cell surface and secreted	
Fibroblasts – primary cultures and established lines	1, 2, 5–8
Myoblasts – primary cultures and established lines	9, 10
Endothelial cells	11–13
Amniotic cells	14
Some glial cells	15
Some epithelial cells	16–18
Teratocarcinoma embryoid bodies	19–21
In vivo	
Basement membranes	22–24
Soft connective tissue stroma	22–24
Plasma 300 μg/ml (serum has less)	25–27
Amniotic fluid	14, 28
Cerebrospinal fluid	29
Absent from:	
Preimplantation embryos (mouse)	20, 24
Neural tissue (neuronal and glial)	30
Cartilage and differentiated chondrocytes	31, 32

FIBRONECTIN AND TRANSFORMATION

In most cases, transformation of cells by DNA or RNA tumor viruses leads to loss of fibronectin from the cell surface, although some exceptions do occur. If the viruses are temperature-sensitive for transformation, then the loss of fibronectin is temperature-sensitive. Chemical and spontaneous transformants have been less extensively studied, but in many cases they also showed reduced levels of cell surface fibronectin. Transformants of fibroblasts, myoblasts [9], glial cells [15], and epithelial cells [16] have all been reported to lose fibronectin. Thus, there is a good, albeit not universal, correlation between loss of fibronectin and in vitro transformation of several cell types by a variety of transforming agents (see reviews in references 2–4).

The exact degree of parallelism between in vitro transformation and tumorigenicity and malignancy in vivo remains uncertain. Several studies have investigated the relationship between loss of fibronectin and in vivo aspects of the tumor phenotype. In a series of adenovirus-transformed rat cells, there was a good correlation with tumorigenicity [59]. In other series of cells, the correlation was less good [60, 61]. In these studies, the correlation was between in vitro expression of fibronectin and hyperplasia in vivo. More recent studies using immunofluorescence analysis of tumor sections have shown a much better correlation between in vivo expression of fibronectin and tumorigenicity [62]. It appears that some transformed cells that do not express fibronectin in vivo can turn on expression in vitro. This is reminiscent of the behavior of some normal cells discussed earlier. In any event, it now seems likely that some of the lack of correlation between in vitro expression of fibronectin and in vivo tumorigenicity may arise from cells that are in vitro false-positive for fibronectin. Also several studies have suggested that the best correlation is between loss of fibronectin and acquisition of metastatic capability, rather than with hyperplasia [62–64]. It remains to be seen how well these correlations will stand up to further experimental tests but, at present, the correlations are good enough to suggest that fibronectin plays a significant role in some aspect(s) of in vitro transformation and in vivo malignancy.

In order to investigate directly its role in the determination of various parameters of the transformed phenotype in vitro, purified fibronectin has been added to cultures of transformed cells. This causes increased adhesion, flattening, and elongation of cells and the cells align with each other in patterns characteristic of normal cells [65, 66]. The cells show reduced numbers of microvilli and surface ruffles [67] and show increased organization of microfilaments into bundles [66, 68]. In contrast with these effects on adhesion and morphology, fibronectin has no effect on growth in monolayers [65] or in agar (I. U. Ali, unpublished data) nor on cyclic AMP levels[65] or the rates of nutrient transport [66, 69].

The simplest interpretation of the pleiotropic effects of fibronectin on transformed cells is that the primary effect is to increase adhesion to the substratum and that the other properties follow from this. This is outlined in Figure 2. Thus, increased adhesion would lead to cell flattening on the substratum; this would lead in turn to reduction in surface microvilli and ruffles, since the surface membrane in these structures would be utilized in the increase in overall surface area associated with spreading. Several workers have proposed that contact inhibition of movement [70, 71] can best be explained as a reflection of inhibition of underlapping consequent upon effective cell-substratum adhesion [72–74]. Increasing the adhesion by adding fibronectin would therefore be expected to lead to reduced underlapping and thus to contact inhibition of movement and alignment of the cells. It has been argued that the effects of fibronectin on microfilament organization can also be ascribed merely to adhesion [68]. However, other explanations are also possible

[66] and, in light of recent results to be discussed later, it appears that the effects of fibronectin on the cytoskeleton are more complex and also involve direct interactions (see next section).

Thus, a plausible hypothesis is that the pleiotropic effects of fibronectin on the behavior of cells arise from an increase in cell-substratum adhesion. The corollary of this hypothesis is that reduction of fibronectin levels by transformation could lead to reduced cell-substratum adhesion and consequently to alterations in the parameters discussed above, all of which alterations are characteristics of the transformed phenotype.

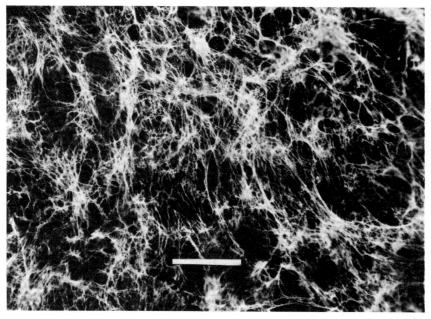

Fig. 1. Fibrillar network of fibronectin on confluent culture of NIL.8 hamster fibroblastic cells. Cells were grown to confluence, fixed, and stained with antibody to fibronectin. Magnification: bar represents 50 μ.

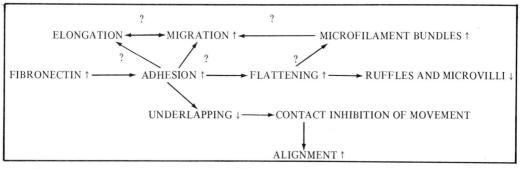

Fig. 2. Diagrammatic representation of the effects of fibronectin on transformed cells. Fibronectin has been shown to produce all of the effects shown: The diagram predicts likely interrelationships among the effects. Hence, increased adhesion is thought to lead to cell flattening and thus to reduced numbers of ruffles and microvilli. Question marks indicate questionable interrelationships such as a simple induction of microfilament bundles by cell flattening (see text) or the possible relationships among adhesion, migration, and cell elongation, which are not clearly understood.

The reasons for the reduced levels of fibronectin that occur on transformation remain incompletely understood. Reduced rates of biosynthesis provide a partial explanation [75, 76] but increased turnover [5, 8, 75] and decreased ability to bind fibronectin [47, 77] also contribute. The possibility that transformation-induced proteolytic enzymes, in particular plasminogen activator, might be responsible for removal of fibronectin has been examined. It is clear that plasminogen is not required [78–80] and that extensive cleavage of fibronectin into the characteristic proteolytic fragments discussed earlier does not occur [80]. However, subtle cleavage of fibronectin or cleavage of a molecule necessary for its binding to cells by proteolytic enzymes not requiring plasminogen remain possibilities.

FIBRONECTIN AND THE CYTOSKELETON

Since alterations in fibronectin and alterations in the organization of the cytoskeleton, in particular of microfilament bundles, both occur on transformation, it seemed possible that the two might be related. This idea was strengthened by the effects of fibronectin readdition on the arrangement of microfilament bundles [66, 68] and by the observation that cytochalasin B, a drug that disassembles cytoplasmic microfilaments, leads to release of fibronectin from the cell surface [39, 81]. Double-label immunofluorescence analyses showed that there was definite correspondence between the fibrillar arrays of fibronectin and actin in cells under a variety of conditions [82] (Fig. 3), and recent electron microscopic analysis has confirmed this [83]. These results suggest a transmembrane connection between fibronectin and microfilaments. Analogous investigations have failed to detect any relationship between fibronectin and microtubules or intermediate filaments [39, 81, 82].

Hence, it appears that the influence of exogenously added fibronectin on microfilaments is likely to be more direct than a simple effect on cell spreading. The patterns of fibronectin are consistent with an involvement in adhesion plaques at the base of the cell. These plaques are sites of attachment of microfilament bundles to the plasma membrane [84, 85].

Since neither actin nor fibronectin appears to be an integral membrane protein, there must be intervening proteins connecting the two. It is therefore of some interest to investigate the molecules with which fibronectin interacts.

INTERACTIONS OF FIBRONECTIN

Plasma fibronectin is known to interact with fibrin and can even be cross-linked to it by factor XIII transglutaminase [27]. Numerous studies have shown that fibronectins interact with collagen, especially when it is denatured to gelatin. In fact, affinity chromatography on gelatin-Sepharose is now the major step in purification of fibronectin [86]. Codistribution of fibronectin and collagen at the cell surface has been reported [87]. Fibronectin can be cross-linked by chemical cross-linked by chemical cross-linkers to sulfated proteoglycans [77], which suggests that it is also in close proximity with them at the cell surface. Fragments of fibronectin with specific affinities for gelatin and glycosaminoglycans have been isolated [50–53]. It therefore seems clear from a variety of lines of evidence that fibronectin can interact through specific binding sites with extracellular macromolecules (collagen, proteoglycans, fibrin). It is also known that fibronectin at the cell surface forms high-molecular-weight aggregates that dissociate on reduction of disulfide bonds [43, 44]. Disulfide bond formation either with itself or with other cell surface molecules is apparently essential for fibronectin to bind to or be retained at the surface [42, 88].

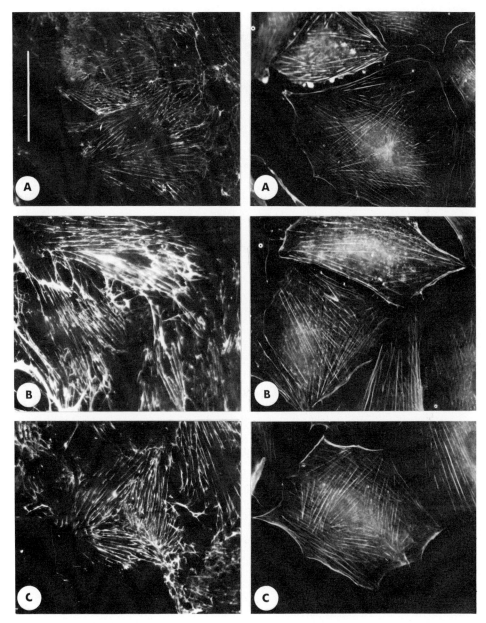

Fig. 3. Double-label immunofluorescence of actin (right) and fibronectin (left). NIL.8 cells were growth-arrested by culture in 0.3% serum, fixed, permeabilized with acetone, and double-stained. Note the correspondences between arrays of actin inside cells and arrays of fibronectin between cells and substratum. Lack of complete identity shows that the antisera do not cross-react. Bar represents 50 μ.

Knowledge of these interactions does not yet provide any insight into the means by which fibronectin might interact with the cytoskeleton, since the latter interaction presumably involves integral membrane proteins. The recent observations that fibronectin may interact with certain gangliosides [89] may be the first indication of interactions with the plasma membrane. It is clear that much research remains to be done in this area, since discovery of the means by which fibronectin binds to the cell surface may lead to an understanding of a) its transmembrane effects, b) the reasons for reduced binding and retention of fibronectin by transformed cells and, therefore, the reasons behind the loss of fibronectin that is associated with transformation and that leads to pleiotropic alterations in cellular phenotype.

CONCLUSIONS

It is now clear that loss of cell surface fibronectin is a frequent correlate of oncogenic transformation. Studies on the relevance of this loss for the behavior of cells in vitro suggest that fibronectin is involved in cell-substratum adhesion and thus has effects on various aspects of morphology and motility that are related to adhesion. The relevance to in vivo parameters is less clear, although many results suggest a correlation with tumorigenicity and most recently with metastasis. The in vitro data that suggest a role for fibronectin in adhesion would be consistent with a role in invasion and metastasis, both of which probably involve alterations in adhesion. One could make plausible arguments extrapolating the in vitro results to the in vivo situation. However, at this point it remains uncertain exactly what role loss of fibronectin plays in vivo, and this will no doubt be a major area of future research.

The many binding affinities shown by fibronectin present an interesting problem in protein chemistry. How are all these binding sites arranged within the large glycoprotein? Their functional relevance has also to be analyzed. One of the more interesting interactions of fibronectin is with microfilaments. The molecular basis of this transmembrane interaction is completely unknown and offers an attractive, if difficult, problem for investigation.

The reasons for loss of fibronectin on transformation also need further analysis. Insights may well arise from analyses of the interactions of fibronectin. There is also the question of regulation of rates of biosynthesis both on transformation and in normal cells that can modulate their rates of synthesis over large ranges.

Fibronectins have provided a fertile area for research over the past five or six years and seem likely to do so for a few years more.

ACKNOWLEDGMENTS

This research was supported by grants from the US Public Health Service, the National Cancer Institute (PO1 CA10451 to S.E. Luria and RO1 CA17007 to R.O. Hynes) and from the American Cancer Society (VC258). R.O.H. was the recipient of a National Institutes & Health Research Career Development Award and M.E.P. of a Damon Runyon Postdoctoral Fellowship.

REFERENCES

1. Hynes RO: Proc Natl Acad Sci USA 70:3170, 1973.
2. Hynes RO: Biochim Biophys Acta Rev Cancer 458:73, 1976.
3. Yamada KM, Olden K: Nature 275:179, 1978.

4. Vaheri A, Mosher DF: Biochim Biophys Acta Rev 516:1, 1978.
5. Robbins PW, Wickus GG, Branton PE, Gaffney BJ, Hirschberg CB, Fuchs P, Blumberg PM: Cold Spring Harbor Symp Quant Biol 39:1173, 1974.
6. Yamada KM, Weston JA: Proc Natl Acad Sci USA 71:3492, 1974.
7. Gahmberg CG, Kiehn D, Hakomori S: Nature 248:413, 1974.
8. Hynes RO, Wyke JA: Virology 64:492, 1975.
9. Hynes RO, Martin GS, Critchley DR, Shearer M, Epstein CJ: Dev Biol 48:35, 1976.
10. Chen LB: Cell 10:393, 1977.
11. Jaffe EA, Mosher DF: J Exp Med 147:1779, 1978.
12. Macarak EJ, Kirby E, Kirk T, Kefalides NA: Proc Natl Acad Sci USA 75:2621, 1978.
13. Birdwell CR, Gospodarowicz D, Nicolson GL: Proc Natl Acad Sci USA 75:3273, 1978.
14. Crouch E, Balian G, Holbrook K, Duksin D, Bornstein P: J Cell Biol 78:701, 1979.
15. Vaheri A, Ruoslahti E, Wastermark B, Ponten J: J Exp Med 143:64, 1976.
16. Chen LB, Maitland N, Gallimore PH, McDougall JK: Exp Cell Res 106:39, 1977.
17. Quaroni A, Isselbacher KJ, Ruoslahti E: Proc Natl Acad Sci USA 75:5548, 1978.
18. Smith HS, Riggs JL, Mosesson, MW: Cancer Res (In press).
19. Wartiovaara J, Leivo I, Virtanen I, Vaheri A, Graham CF: Nature 272:355, 1978.
20. Zetter BR, Martin GR: Proc Natl Acad Sci USA 75:2324, 1978.
21. Wolfe J, Mautner V, Hogan B, Tilly R: Exp Cell Res 118:63, 1979.
22. Linder E, Vaheri A, Ruoslahti E, Wartiovaara J: J Exp Med 142:41, 1975.
23. Stenman S, Vaheri A: J Exp Med 147:1054, 1978.
24. Wartiovaara J, Leivo I, Vaheri A: Dev Biol 69:247, 1979.
25. Mosesson MW, Umfleet RA: J Biol Chem 245:5728, 1970.
26. Mosesson MW, Chen AB, Huseby RM: Biochim Biophys Acta 386:509, 1975.
27. Mosher DF: J Biol Chem 250:6614, 1975.
28. Chen AB, Mosesson MW, Solish GT: Am J Obstet Gynecol 125:958, 1976.
29. Kuusela P, Vaheri A, Palo J, Ruoslahti E: J Lab Clin Med 92:595, 1978.
30. Schachner M, Schoonmaker G, Hynes RO: Brain Res 158:149, 1978.
31. Dessau W, Sasse J, Timpl R, Jilek F, Von Der Mark K: J Cell Biol 79:342, 1978.
32. Hassell JR, Pennypacker JP, Yamada KM, Pratt RM: Ann NY Acad Sci 312:406, 1978.
33. Ruoslahti E, Vaheri A: J Exp Med 141:497, 1975.
34. Hynes RO, Destree AT, Mautner VM: In Marchesi VT (ed): "Membranes and Neoplasia," New York: Alan R. Liss, Inc., 1976, p 189.
35. Yamada KM, Schlessinger DH, Kennedy DW, Pastan I: Biochemistry 16:5552, 1977.
36. Chen LB, Gudor RC, Sun TT, Chen AB, Mosesson MW: Science 197:776, 1977.
37. Furcht LT, Mosher DF, Wendelschafer-Crabb G, Woodbridge PA, Foidart JM: Nature 277:393, 1979.
38. Hynes RO, Bye JM: Cell 3:113, 1974.
39. Mautner V, Hynes RO: J Cell Biol 75:743, 1977.
40. Carter WG, Hakomori S: Biochemistry 18:730, 1979.
41. Olden K, Pratt RM, Yamada KM: Cell 13:461, 1978.
42. Wagner DD, Hynes RO: J Biol Chem (In press).
43. Hynes RO, Destree AT: Proc Natl Acad Sci USA 74:2855, 1977.
44. Keski-Oja J, Mosher DF, Vaheri A: Biochem Biophys Res Commun 74:699, 1977.
45. Jilek F, Hormann H: Hoppe-Seyler's Z Physiol Chem 358:133, 1977.
46. Iwanaga S, Suzuki K, Hashimoto S: Ann NY Acad Sci 312:56, 1978.
47. Hynes RO, Ali IU, Destree AT, Mautner V, Perkins ME, Senger DR, Wagner DD, Smith KK: Ann NY Acad Sci 312:317, 1978.
48. Alexander SS, Colonna G, Yamada KM, Pastan I, Edelhoch H: J Biol Chem 253:5820, 1978.
49. Alexander SS, Colonna G, Edelhoch H: J Biol Chem 254:1501, 1979.
50. Balian G, Click EM, Crouch E, Davidson JM, Bornstein P: J Biol Chem 254:1429, 1979.
51. Hahn LHE, Yamada KM: Proc Natl Acad Sci USA 76:1160, 1979.
52. Ruoslahti E, Hayman E, Kuusela P, Shively JE, Engvall E: J Biol Chem (In press).
53. Yamada KM, Hahn LHE, Olden K: Proceedings of 1979 ICN–UCLA Symposium on "Tumor Cell Surfaces and Malignancy," New York: Alan R. Liss, Inc. (In press).
54. Stathakis NE, Mosesson MW: J Clin Invest 60:855, 1977.
55. Schlessinger J, Barak LS, Hammes GG, Yamada KM, Pastan I, Webb WL, Elson EL: Proc Natl Acad Sci USA 74:2909, 1977.

56. Yamada KM: J Cell Biol 78:520, 1978.
57. Graham JM, Hynes RO, Davidson EA, Bainton DF: Cell 4:353, 1975.
58. Graham JM, Hynes RO, Rowlatt C, Sandall JK: Ann NY Acad Sci 312:221, 1978.
59. Chen LB, Gallimore PH, McDougall JK: Proc Natl Acad Sci USA 73:3570, 1976.
60. Marciani DJ, Lyons LB, Thompson EB: Cancer Res 36:2937, 1976.
61. Der CJ, Stanbridge EJ: Cell 51:1241, 1978.
62. Chen LB, Summerhayes I, Segal R, Walsh ML, Hsieh P, Silagi S: Proceedings of 1979 ICN-UCLA Symposium on "Tumor Cell Surfaces and Malignancy," New York: Alan R. Liss, Inc. (In press).
63. Chen LB, Burridge K, Murray A, Walsh ML, Copple CD, Bushnell A, McDougall JK, Gallimore PH: Ann NY Acad Sci 312:366, 1978.
64. Smith HS, Riggs JL, Mosesson MW: Cancer Res (In press).
65. Yamada KM, Yamada SS, Pastan I: Proc Natl Acad Sci USA 73:1217, 1976.
66. Ali IU, Mautner VM, Lanza RP, Hynes RO: Cell 11:115, 1977.
67. Yamada KM, Ohanian SH, Pastan I: Cell 9:241, 1976.
68. Willingham MC, Yamada KM, Yamada SS, Pouyssegur J, Pastan I: Cell 10:375, 1977.
69. Yamada KM, Pastan I: J Cell Physiol 89:827, 1976.
70. Abercrombie M, Heaysman J: Exp Cell Res 6:293, 1954.
71. Abercrombie M: In Vitro 6:128, 1970.
72. Harris A: Exp Cell Res 77:285, 1973.
73. Bell PB: J Cell Biol 74:963, 1977.
74. Trinkaus JP, Betchaku T, Krulikowski LS Exp Cell Res 64:291, 1971.
75. Olden K, Yamada KM: Cell 11:957, 1977.
76. Hynes RO, Destree AT, Mautner VM, Ali IU: J Supramol Struct 7:397, 1977.
77. Perkins ME, Ji TH, Hynes RO: Cell 16:941, 1979.
78. Hynes RO, Wyke JA, Bye JM, Humphryes KC, Pearlstein ES: In Reich E, Shaw E, Rifkin DB (eds): "Proteases and Biological Control." Cold Spring Harbor, New York: Cold Spring Harbor Laboratories, 1975, p 931.
79. Hynes RO, Pearlstein ES: J Supramol Struct 4:1, 1976.
80. Mahdavi V, Hynes RO: Biochim Biophys Acta 542:191, 1978.
81. Ali IU, Hynes RO: Biochim Biophys Acta 471:16, 1977.
82. Hynes RO, Destree AT: Cell 15:875, 1978.
83. Singer II: Cell 16:675, 1979.
84. Abercrombie M, Heaysman JEM, Pegrum SM: Exp Cell Res 67:359, 1971.
85. Abercrombie M, Dunn GA: Exp Cell Res 92:57, 1975.
86. Engvall E, Ruoslahti E: Int J Cancer 20:1, 1977.
87. Vaheri A, Kurkinen M, Lehto VP, Linder E, Timpl R: Proc Natl Acad Sci USA 75:4944, 1978.
88. Ali IU, Hynes RO: Biochim Biophys Acta 510:140, 1978.
89. Kleinman HK, Hewitt AT, Pennypacker JP, McGoodwin EB, Martin GR, Fishman PH: J Supramol Struct 11:69, 1979.

Journal of Supramolecular Structure 11:105–111 (1979)
Tumor Cell Surfaces and Malignancy 81–91

Tumor Metastases and Cell-Mediated Immunity in a Model System in DBA/2 Mice. VIII. Expression and Shedding of Fcγ Receptors on Metastatic Tumor Cell Variants

Volker Schirrmacher and Wolfgang Jacobs

Institut für Immunologie und Genetik am Deutschen Krebsforschungszentrum, Im Neuenheimer Feld 280, D-6900 Heidelberg, Federal Republic of Germany

The expression of receptors for the Fc portion of IgG immunoglobin molecules was studied on tumor cell lines with high and low metastatic capacity. Two tumor cell lines from DBA/2 mice that had high metastatic activity, ESb and MDAY-D2, contained a high percentage of Fc receptor positive cells, as detected in a rosette assay with IgG antibody-coated erythrocytes (EA). In contrast, the low metastatic parental line Eb, from which ESb was derived, contained only a low percentage of EA-rosette-forming cells. ESb ascites tumor cells adapted to tissue culture in the presence of 2-mercaptoethanol (2ME) had a high expression of Fc receptors, whereas a cell line adapted to tissue culture in the absence of 2ME had a low expression of Fc receptors.

"Soluble" Fc receptors were detectable by their ability to bind to EA and to cause blocking of rosette formation. They were found to be present in fluids from tumor-bearing animals, such as serum and cell-free ascites. Even animals with an ascites tumor of the low-metastatic line Eb contained "soluble" Fc receptors.

The results are discussed with regard to their possible significance for tumor metastasis.

Key words: tumor metastases, Fc receptor, shedding, tumor variants

Properties of tumor cells that may be important for tumor cell dissemination and formation of metastasis are investigated in a syngeneic tumor model system in DBA/2 mice. The system consists of a methylcholanthrene-induced lymphoma (Eb) with low metastatic potential and a spontaneous variant thereof (ESb) with high metastatic capability. An unrelated methylcholanthrene-induced tumor (MDAY-D2) with pronounced metastasizing capacity is included for comparison. The major characteristics of these tumor cells have already been described [1–4] and are summarized in Table I. We showed

Received May 18, 1979; accepted June 25, 1979

TABLE I. Properties of the Tumor Cells of the Model System: Summary

	Eb	ESb	MDAY-D2
Strain of origin	DBA/2	DBA/2	DBA/2
Induction	MC,1955[a]	from Eb, 1968	see [15]
Tumorigenicity (TD_{50}, SC)	10^3-10^4	$<10^1$	$<10^1$
Metastasizing capacity	+	++++	++++
Invasiveness in vitro	±	+++	+++
Immunogenicity	++++	+	ND
Histiocytes at primary tumor	+++	±	+
Cell surface morphology: microvilli	+	++	++
Cell surface antigens			
H-2	K^d, D^d	K^d, D^d	K^d, D^d (NO K^k)
THY 1.2	+	+	−
Ig	−	−	−
Cell surface dynamics[b]			
Shedding	+	+++	ND
Modulation	+	+++	ND

[a]MC = methylcholanthrene ; ND = not done
[b]Of H-2 antigens.

that ESb and MDAY-D2 but not Eb tumor cells had the capacity to adhere to and invade syngeneic normal mouse tissue in vitro [1, 5]. Furthermore, ESb tumor cells had more microvilli [1] and showed increased shedding of histocompatibility antigens [6]. The local primary tumors of the two metastatic lines were less infiltrated by host-derived macrophage-like cells than those of the tumor Eb [1]

In previous studies [4, 7] we have also defined the tumor antigens of the tumor lines Eb and ESb. The results are summarized in Table II. Tumor protection experiments revealed the presence of tumor-associated transplantation antigens (TATA) on both Eb and ESb tumor cells. TATAs of Eb and ESb were distinct and non-cross-reactive. Two antigens, one (1) characteristic for Eb and cross-reacting with a radion-induced BALB/c lymphoma, RLδl, the other (2) characteristic for ESb and not cross-reacting with a number of unrelated tumor cells could be defined in this way. Similar antigens were characterized by means of tumor-specific syngeneic cytotoxic T lymphocytes (CTL). The similarity of the specificity patterns of protective antitumor immunity in vivo and of cytolytic T cells in vitro suggests that the latter can recognize TATAs and may thus play an important role in the establishment of protective immunity.

In the present study we report on the expression of receptors for the Fc portion of IgG immunoglobulin molecules — so-called Fcγ receptors. Fc receptors are expressed on a number of different cells such as B cells, activated T cells, macrophages, mast cells, monocytes, and various malignant cell populations. Fcγ receptors have a high affinity for the Fc portion of IgG molecules and only low affinity for Fc portions of IgM. They only weakly interact with free antibody but show a strong binding to antigen-antibody complexes, aggregated IgG, or cell-bound IgG antibody. These receptors play an essential role in antibody-dependent cell-mediated cytotoxicity. Recently a suppressive activity of Fc receptors expressed on activated T cells has also been reported [8].

We will show that both the metastatic cell lines ESb and MDAY-D2 contained a high percentage of cells with Fc receptors, as measured by the EA rosette assay, whereas the nonmetastatic line Eb had only very few of these rosetting cells. Furthermore, we will report that cell-free Fc receptors can be detected in the serum and ascites fluid from tumor-bearing animals.

TABLE II. Definition of Tumor Antigens in the Model System Eb/ESb

	Eb	ESb	MDAY-D2	P-815	SL2	RLδ1	RBL-5
I. TATA[a]							
1	+	–	–	–	–	+	–
2	–	+	–	–	–	–	–
II. T_K target[b]							
1	+	–	–	–	–	+	–
2	–	+	–	–	–	–	–

[a]TATA = tumor-associated transplantation antigen.
[b]Target antigens of syngeneic tumor-specific killer T cells.

MATERIALS AND METHODS

EA-Rosette Assay

Antibody-coated erythrocytes (EA) were prepared as follows: A 1% suspension of washed sheep erythrocytes (SRCB) was incubated for 30 min at room temperature with a subagglutinating amount of a rabbit IgG anti-sheep erythrocyte antibody (R-antiSRCB). The coated erythrocytes were washed twice in PBS. Tumor cells for the rosette assay were taken either from tissue culture as described [4] or from the ascites of tumor-bearing animals. In the latter situation the cells were preincubated at a density of 5×10^6/ml in Falcon flasks in a horizontal position for 30 min at 37°C to keep the tumor cells from contaminating host-derived adhering cells (macrophages and B lymphocytes). This procedure was performed twice. The rosette assay between tumor cells and the EA suspension was performed in small plastic tubes (F.A. Greiner, Nürtingen) as follows: 50 μl PBS, 50 μl of the tumor test cells (6×10^6/ml) and 50 μl of the 1% EA suspension was added, mixed, and centrifuged for 3 min at 150g in a WIFUG-table centrifuge. The pellet was carefully resuspended and assessed for content of rosettes in a counting chamber by assaying about 200–400 cells per sample. The tumor cells that formed rosettes were usually covered with 3–10 erythrocytes per cell. Uncoated erythrocytes were not bound by the tumor cells.

Blocking of Rosette Formation With Fc Receptor Containing Test Fluid

An EA-rosette-blocking assay was established to test for "soluble" Fc receptors in the supernatant of tumor cell cultures or in the ascites fluid or serum from tumor-bearing animals. These fluids were spun for 10 min in a Beckman airfuge and 50 μl of the EA cell pellet was incubated with 50 μl of the test solution for 45 min at room temperature. After two washings these preincubated EA cells were assayed with the tumor cells for rosette formation, as described above. The following controls were included: uncoated erythrocytes as a negative control, serum from normal animals instead of tumor-bearing animals, and EA cells that were not preincubated with test solutions (positive control). Normal DBA/2 spleen cells served as a positive control in all rosette assays.

All other materials and methods have been described elsewhere [1–4].

RESULTS

Expression of Fcγ Receptors on Metastatic and Nonmetastatic Tumor Cell Lines

The ability of the three tumor lines of our model system to form EA-rosettes with sheep red blood cells (SRBC) coated with decreasing amounts of a rabbit anti-SRBC serum was tested. The results are shown in Figures 1 and 2 and Table III. Whereas only 6–8% of

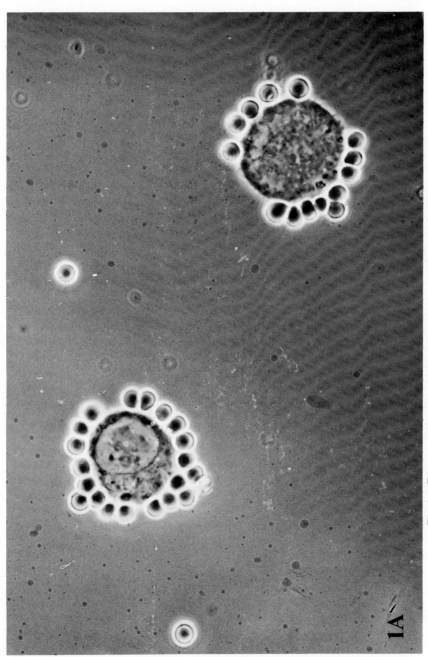

Fig. 1A. EA-rosettes formed by the tumor line MDAY-D2 [magnification, × 3,150].

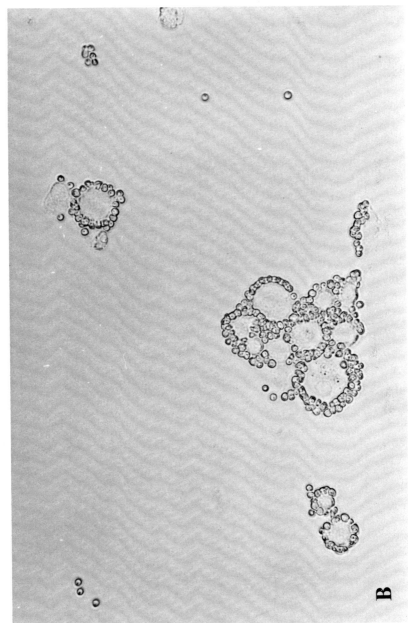

Fig. 1B. EA-rosettes formed by the tumor line ESb [magnification, × 2,000].

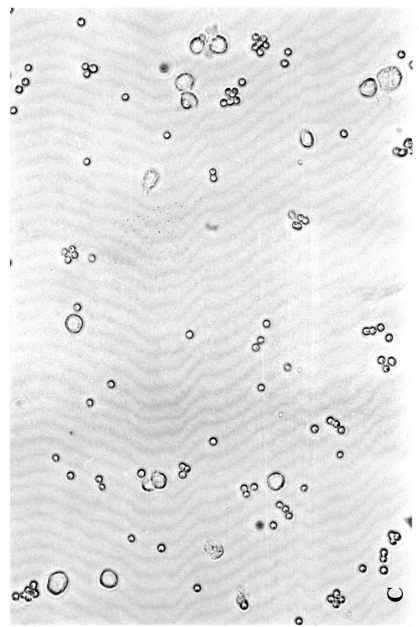

Fig. 1C. Negative results for rosette formation were obtained with the majority of cells from tumor Eb [magnification, × 1,250].

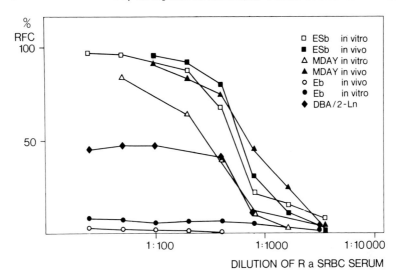

Fig. 2. Dependency of EA-rosette formation on the dilution of antiserum used for coating the red cells. The different cell types studied are indicated; MDAY = MDAY-D2; DBA/2-Ln = normal spleen cells from DBA/2.

TABLE III. RFC$_{50}$ Titer of Tumor Cell Lines and of Normal Spleen Cells

Cell type	% EA-RFC (maximal)	RFC$_{50}$ titer[a]	% RFC with non-coated SRBC
Eb in vitro	6	1:500	1
Eb in vivo	8	1:500	1
ESb in vitro	95	1:520	0
ESb in vivo	97	1:620	2
MDAY-D2 in vitro	87	1:360	1
MDAY-D2 in vivo	95	1:720	1
DBA/2 spleen cells	46	1:550	0

[a]Highest R anti-SRBC dilution giving 50% of the maximal % EA-RFC.

the nonmetastatic parental line Eb formed rosettes, more than 90% of the cells of the two metastatic tumor lines formed rosettes with the antibody-coated erythrocytes. Typical examples of the microscopic pictures are given in Figure 1.

The R-anti-SRBC serum used had a log$_2$ haemagglutination titer of 10, which was mercaptoethanol-resistant and thus consisted mostly of IgG antibody. Under the conditions of the rosette assay no agglutination occurred at antiserum dilutions higher than 1:50. The highest antibody dilution at which 50% of the maximal numbers of rosettes were formed (RFC$_{50}$ titer) was determined from Figure 1, and the results are represented in Table III. Normal spleen cells from DBA/2 mice were tested for comparison. They formed up to 46% EA-rosettes and had an RFC$_{50}$ titer of 1:550. The RFC$_{50}$ titer of ESb tumor lines from tissue culture or from in vivo and of MDAY-D2 from in vivo were similar or somewhat higher. The only cells with a lower RFC$_{50}$ titer than normal cells were MDAY-D2 tumor cells from tissue culture.

Because of this difference in the expression of Fc receptors between tumor cells from in vivo and from tissue culture, we studied the stability of this marker on tumor cells passaged for various periods in tissue culture. MDAY-D2 ascites tumor cells after depletion of adherent cells formed EA rosettes up to 95%. After several passages of these cells in tissue culture this maximal number of EA-RFC decreased to lower than 50%. When ESb ascites tumor cells were treated similarly the percentage EA-RFC remained rather constant under tissue culture conditions, provided the medium contained 5×10^{-5} M 2-mercaptoethanol (2-ME). When 2-ME was omitted from the tissue culture medium, it was difficult to maintain viable ESb tumor cells in vitro. One particular tumor line, ESb_G, however, was established under these 2-ME-free tissue culture conditions. The number of EA-RFC of this line was much lower than that of the line cultured in the presence of 2-ME. In the first passage numbers it was around 20% and decreased to 10%. When the line ESb_G from tissue culture passage number 7 was inoculated back into DBA/2 mice intraperitoneally, the ascites tumor cells harvested 12 days later, after adsorption of adherent cells, were again more than 90% positive in the rosette assay (Table IV).

The ability of various other tumor lines of different histologic type and origin to form EA rosettes was also tested. The results obtained with tumor cells adapted to tissue culture are presented in Table V. The ability of various lymphoma lines to form EA-rosettes was found to vary from 3% (RBL-5) to 20% (SL2), 60% (ULMC, AKR-A) and 90% (LSTRA, SBR-1). No correlation was found with the tumor type or strain of origin.

Blocking of EA Rosette Formation by Preincubation of EA With Fc Receptor Containing Test Fluids

The possibility that the rosette-forming tumor cell lines not only express Fc receptors on the cell surface but actively shed this material into the environment similar to H-2 antigens [6] was studied. The presence of Fc receptors in ascites fluids or in the serum from tumor-bearing animals was investigated by testing these fluids for their ability to block the rosette formation between EA and the tumor cells. The antibody-coated erythrocytes were preincubated with the test fluids, then washed twice, and tested for their ability to bind to ESb tumor cells. The results from several experiments are summarized in Table VI. Pretreatment of EA with normal mouse serum had no blocking effect, whereas pretreatment with serum from ESb, MDAY-D2, or Eb tumor-bearing animals caused about 90% blocking

TABLE IV. Expression of Fc Receptors on Tumor Cells Passaged in Tissue Culture or in Vivo

Tumor cell	In vivo[a]	In vitro[b]					In vitro → In vivo[c]
		% EA-RFC					
PT		1	2	4	7	10	
ESb	97	92	91	89	84	84	84
ESb_G	97	23	23	ND	11	ND	93
MDAY-D2	95	94	94	ND	53	43	ND

[a]Washed ascites tumor cells after depletion of adherent cells.

[b]Tumor cells adapted to suspension tissue culture; the numbers of passage in tissue culture (PT) are indicated; ESb and MDAY-D2 were cultured in medium with 5×10^{-5} M 2-ME. The line ESb_G was adapted to tissue culture in medium without 2-ME: the viability at PT 1 was only 45%.

[c]Tissue culture cells from PT 7 were inoculated intraperitoneally into DBA/2♀ mice; results shown are from day 12 ascites tumor cells.

TABLE V. EA-Rosette Formation by Various Low Metastatic Tumor Cells Adapted to Tissue Culture

Tumor line	Type[a]	Strain of origin	% EA-RFC
SL2	L	DBA/2	20
P-815	M	DBA/2	80
ULMC	L	BALB/c	62
Meth. A	S	BALB/c	5
LSTRA	L	BALB/c	94
RBL-5	L	C57bl/6	3
AKR-A	L	AKR	61
SBR-1	L	B10.BR	92
Normal spleen cells	–	DBA/2	46

[a]L = lymphoma; S = sarcoma; M = mastocytoma.

TABLE VI. Blocking of Rosette-Formation Between EA and ESb Tumor Cells by Preincubation of EA With Fc Receptor Containing Test Fluids

| Serum | Preincubation of EA[a] | | | % EA-RFC[b] | % Blocking |
	Ascites Fluid	Fresh	Frozen		
–	–	–	–	90	–
NMS	–	+	–	90	0
NMS	–	–	+	90	0
ESb (day 6)	–	+	–	11	88
ESb (day 5)	–	–	+	92	0
MDAY-D2 (day 9)	–	+	–	9	90
MDAY-D2 (day 8)	–	–	+	77	14
Eb (day 5)	–	+	–	10	89
Eb (day 5)	–	–	+	78	13
–	ESb (day 6)	+	–	15	83
–	ESb (day 6)	–	+	83	8
–	MDAY-D2 (day 9)	+	–	26	71
–	MDAY-D2 (day 8)	–	+	91	0
–	Eb (day 5)	+	–	40	56
–	Eb (day 5)	–	+	91	0

[a]EA were prepared by coating SRBC with 1:200 diluted RaSRBC; 50 μl EA pellet was preincubated at room temperature for 45 min with 50 μl test fluid (serum or ascites); after two washings these EA preparations were used for the test; test fluids were not heat-inactivated and were used either fresh or after storage at –20°C. (day 6) indicates day 6 after tumor inoculation.

[b]% Rosettes formed with ESb ascites tumor cells after depletion of adherent cells.

in this assay. Similar results were obtained with ascites fluids from tumor-bearing animals. Here the Eb ascites fluid was less inhibitory than the fluids from ESb or MDAY-D2 ascites. It is noteworthy that the test fluids had to be fresh. If they were frozen and thawed most of the blocking activity was destroyed.

DISCUSSION

Membranes of mammalian cells possess various recognition units that enable them to react to various environmental stimuli. A good example is the receptors for hormones and growth factors on malignant cells which can have a profound influence on tumor growth and dissemination [9, 10]. Here we describe the expression of another type of receptor on tumor cells: the Fc receptor which is specific for immunoglobulin molecules bound in an antigen-antibody complex form. The biological significance of Fc receptors, which are present on a variety of normal and malignant cells is not clear but has been a matter of consideration in recent years [11–14].

Using an EA-rosette assay for the detection of Fc receptors, we found that the metastatic tumor variant ESb was positive, whereas the nonmetastatic parental line Eb was mostly negative. Similarly, the metastatic tumor line MDAY-D2 was found to be EA-rosette-positive, whereas the nonmetastatic original line MDAY was negative, as described recently by Kerbel et al [15]. Of course, more tumor lines with and without metastatic properties need to be investigated to test for general significance of these findings.

As shown in Table V, the ability to form EA-rosettes is not restricted to high metastatic tumor cells. A variety of low metastatic tumors, all deprived of contaminating host cells by adaptation to tissue culture, contained a high percentage of EA-RFC. The presence of Fc receptors on tumor cells is thus certainly not a property that enables them to metastasize. However, it is possible that tumor cell variants possessing Fc receptors have an advantage for metastasis formation over Fc receptor negative cells and might thus be selected out.

The EA-rosette assay is in our hands a convenient quick assay to distinguish the two tumor lines Eb and ESb. As shown from the results in Table IV, the expression of Fc receptors on ESb ascites tumor cells remained rather stable when the cells were passaged in tissue culture. Eb ascites tumor cells passaged in tissue culture also remained at the low level of 5–8% of EA-positive cells (Table III). An exception was the cell line ESb_G, which represented an ESb line adapted to tissue culture in the absence of 2-mercaptoethanol, a condition where Eb cells grow easily but where most of the ESb cells die. The observed shift in the expression of Fc receptors on the ESb_G line from high to low and back from low to high when the cells were grown again in vivo could represent a phenotypic variation influenced by the different environment. Since such shifts did not occur with the other two lines, we favor an alternative explanation; namely, that the shifts indicate the outgrowth of either Eb-like or ESb-like cells from a heterogeneous cell population under in vivo or in vitro culture conditions.

The differences observed in the EA-rosette assay between Eb and ESb tumor cells could mean either a qualitative or a quantitative difference in the expression of Fc receptors on these cells. Anderson and Grey [16] have shown that L5178 lymphoma cells, which are equivalent to Eb, carry receptors for aggregated IgG. Using an autoradiographic binding assay employing ^{125}I-labeled aggregated IgG2B, the grain counts of various cell types were as follows: 40–50 grains/cell/day for P815 mastocytoma cells and macrophages, 20–30 for allogeneically activated thymocytes, 2–3 for splenocytes, 1 for L5178 lymphoma cells, and 0.6 for positive thymocytes. Neauport-Sautes and Fridman [17] showed that an immunoglobulin-binding factor (IBF) was produced by internally labeled L1578-Y thymoma cells. After precipitation with antigen-antibody complexes the factor, a glycoprotein, was shown to consist of a major unit of 40,000 daltons and a minor unit of 20,000 daltons. Frade and Kourilsky [18] also used the T cell lymphoma L5178-Y to extract a glycoprotein having Fc receptor properties. Studies with lactoperoxidase-catalyzed surface-iodination [19] suggest that the Fc receptor from several different cell sources contains a polypeptide chain with a mol wt of about 120,000, which is highly susceptible to proteolytic degradation after cell lysis. These studies suggest that the negative results obtained with Eb cells (L5178-YE) in the EA-rosette assay are not due to an absence of Fc receptors on these cells. They rather suggest a lower sensitivity of the rosette assay as compared with the above-described Fc receptor detection assays. If this is the case, then our results would indicate a quantitative rather than a qualitative difference in the expression of Fc receptors on Eb and ESb cells. The metastatic tumor variant has probably a higher density of Fc receptors than the parental line.

This conclusion seems to be supported by the blocking experiments performed with ascites fluid and serum from tumor-bearing animals. Here, even the fluids from Eb tumor-bearing animals had blocking activity, indicating the presence of cell-free Fc receptors. No quantitative experiments have yet been performed to test for differences in the amount of blocking activity in the fluids from animals bearing metastatic or nonmetastatic tumor cell lines. Also the exact nature of the blocking activity needs to be demonstrated. The instability of the blocking activity to freezing and thawing is in accord with the assumption that it is cell-free Fc receptor material, since this was shown before to be sensitive to this treatment [17].

In connection with metastasis the acquisition of Fc receptors by tumor cells might have selective advantage for one of several reasons: 1) it would enable the cells to bind immune complexes; these could have a stimulatory effect on tumor growth [20], cause masking of tumor-specific antigens, and/or lead to changes in the tumor cell traffic, with enhanced sequestration in the liver [21], 2) the release of "soluble" Fc receptors into body fluids might have important implications in the regulation of immune responsiveness; for instance, suppressive activity of IBF produced by L5178-Y on the humoral immune response in vitro has recently been demonstrated [17].

REFERENCES

1. Schirrmacher V, Shantz G, Clauer K, Komitowski D, Zimmermann H–P, Lohmann-Matthes ML: Int J Cancer 23:233, 1979.
2. Schirrmacher V, Shantz G: In Müller-Ruchholtz W, Müller-Hermelink HK (eds): "Function and Structure of the Immune System." New York: Plenum Press, 1979, pp 769–775.
3. Shantz G, Schirrmacher V: In Quastel MR (ed): "Cell Biology and Immunology of Leukocyte Function." New York: Academic Press, 1979, pp 725–736.
4. Schirrmacher V, Bosslet K, Shantz G, Clauer K, Hübsch D: Int J Cancer 23:245, 1979.
5. Lohmann-Matthes ML, Schleich A, Shantz G, Schirrmacher V: J.N.C.I., submitted.
6. Davey GC, Currie GA, Alexander P: Br J Cancer 33:9, 1976.
7. Bosslet K, Schirrmacher V, Shantz G: Int J Cancer 24, Sept. issue, 1979.
8. Gisler RH, Fridman WH: J Exp Med 142:507, 1975.
9. Lippmann M: In Heusen IC et al (eds): "Trends in Research and Treatment." Breast Cancer, New York: Raven Press, 1976, pp 111–139.
10. McGuire WL, Raynaud J-P, Baulieu E-E (eds): "Progesterone Receptors in Normal and Neoplastic Tissues. Progress in Cancer Research and Therapy." New York: Raven Press, vol. 4, 1977.
11. Kerbel RS, Davies AJS: Cell 3:105, 1974.
12. Ramasamy R, Munro A, Milstein C: Nature 249:573, 1974.
13. Rubin B, Hertel-Wulff B: Scand J Immunol 4:451, 1975.
14. Halloran P, Schirrmacher V: In Cinader B (ed): "Immunology of Receptors." New York: Marcel Dekker, 1977, pp 201–219.
15. Kerbel RS, Twiddy RR, Robertson DM: Int J Cancer 22:583, 1978.
16. Anderson CL, Grey HM: J Exp Med 139:1175, 1974.
17. Neauport-Sautes C, Fridman WH: J Immunol 119:1269, 1977.
18. Frade R, Kourilsky FM: Eur J Immunol 7:663, 1977.
19. Bourgois A, Abney ER, Parkhouse RME: Eur J Immunol 7:691, 1977.
20. Shearer WT, Philipott GW, Parker CW: Science 182:1357, 1973.
21. Stutman O: Transplant Rev 5:969, 1973.

Journal of Supramolecular Structure 11:147–166 (1979)
Tumor Cell Surfaces and Malignancy 93–112

Properties of Epithelial Cells Cultured From Human Carcinomas and Nonmalignant Tissues

Helene S. Smith, Adeline J. Hackett, John L. Riggs, Michael W. Mosesson, Judie R. Walton, and Martha R. Stampfer

Donner Research Laboratory, University of California, Berkeley, California 94720, and Peralta Cancer Research Institute, Oakland, California 94625 (H.S.S., A.J.H., M.R.S.); California State Department of Health Services, Berkeley, California 94720 (J.L.R.); Department of Medicine, Downstate Medical Center, State University of New York, Brooklyn, New York 11203 (M.W.M); and Lawrence Livermore Laboratory, University of California, Livermore, California 94550 (J.R.W.)

Human epithelial cell cultures were examined for expression of plasminogen activator and fibronectin matrix. All of the cells examined showed ultrastructural evidence suggesting their epithelial origin, including microvilli and specialized junctions. The nonmalignant cells were also negative for endothelial cell markers (ie, they lacked factor VIII antigen, a nonthrombogenic surface and Weibel-Palade bodies). The nonmalignant lines all produced large amounts of plasminogen activator, whereas the tumor-derived lines showed a gradation of activities, ranging from lines having as much activity as the nonmalignant lines to lines having little or no activity above background. For both normal and malignant cells, addition of dexamethesone only slightly decreased the levels of plasminogen activator. By immunofluorescence microscopy, normal bladder and fetal intestine epithelial cells showed fibronectin in a globular and fibrillar matrix. In contrast, normal mammary epithelial cells had a much diminished amount of fibronectin with a punctate distribution.

Key words: carcinoma and nonmalignant cells, fibronectin, human epithelial cells, plasminogen activator

Transformation by various agents (ie, chemicals, viruses) or spontaneously has been associated with various in vitro changes, including increased production of plasminogen activator [1–3], loss of fibronectin containing surface matrix [4], abnormal morphology [5], decreased serum requirements [6], acquisition of colony-forming ability on contact-inhibited monolayers [7], increased plating efficiency on plastic, infinite life in culture [8], and acquisition of the ability to produce tumors when inoculated into immunosuppressed mice [9]. Depending on the cell type and/or the trans-

Received April 23, 1979; accepted May 24, 1979.

forming agent, the properties among this list of alterations that are relevant may differ. For example, many of the properties found to correlate with fibroblast transformation such as refractility, piling up of cells, decreased serum requirement, and increased activation of plasminogen, did not apply to chemically induced transformation of rat liver epithelial cells [10]. Two other properties relevant to fibroblast transformation — ie, agglutination by concanavallin A and karyotypic changes — also did not correlate with epithelial cell transformation [11]. In recent studies, plating efficiency on plastic correlated with tumorigenicity for rat tracheal epithelial cells [12] but not for mouse epidermal cells [13]. Anchorage independence appears to be an important marker for epithelial cell transformation [10, 12–14] and for various fibroblast systems [15–17]; however, there seems to be little correlation between growth in agar and transformation for adeno-virus transformed cells [18]. Loss of a fibronectin-containing surface matrix is associated with fibroblast transformation in most [4] but not all [19] systems.

Except for human gliomas [20], there is very little information available on which any of the above criteria are applicable for human malignancies. Despite the fact that approximately 90% of human malignancies are carcinomas, ie cancers of epithelial cell origin, there have been almost no systematic comparisons of the in vitro properties of human epithelial cell lines derived from nonmalignant specimens and specimens representing various stages of malignant progression. The major difficulty has been that currently used media favor outgrowth from the normal stromal components; hence most of the epithelial lines* that have been developed [see reference 22 for a summary] represent the rare variant capable of overgrowing normal fibroblasts. Thus, it is not surprising that Marshall et al [23], when examining human carcinomas of bladder and colon origin, found that all 5 of the lines examined had lost topo-inhibition and grew on contact-inhibited fibroblasts.

We have approached the problem of determining which in vitro parameters correlate with malignancy in humans by developing cell lines of various human carcinomas and nonmalignant epithelial tissues and then comparing their properties [24–27]. The cell lines were cultured by techniques that we developed to remove contaminating fibroblasts; hence these lines, which have not been subjected to the selective pressure of overgrowing normal fibroblasts, may represent types of epithelial cells not previously studied in vitro. Among the lines that grew well enough to be extensively characterized were at least a few lines representing stages of malignant progression, including specimens of metastatic vs primary carcinoma origin as well as lines derived from nonmalignant tissue. In addition, there has been a recent report on techniques to routinely culture normal human mammary epithelium for at least one to two subcultures [29]. In this paper we describe some of our studies to characterize these cultures for various transformation parameters.

MATERIALS AND METHODS

Cell Culture

Epithelial cell lines. All of the cell lines used (listed in Table I) were obtained from the Cell Culture Laboratory, Naval Supply Center (Oakland, CA). The growth medium used was Dulbecco's modification of Eagle's minimum essential medium (#H21HG; GIBCO

---

*Nomenclature used conforms with that of Fedoroff [21]: A "cell line" arises from a primary culture at the first subculture, whereas an "established cell line" is one that has demonstrated the potential to be subcultured indefinitely.

TABLE I. Summary of Source and Nuclear Morphology of Human Epithelial Cell Lines

Cell source (designation)[a]	Nuclear ultrastructure[b]	Morphology[c]
Derived from nonmalignant tissue		
Fetal intestine (74Int)	Smooth contour lacking invaginations,	Normal
Fetal intestine (677Int)	uniform nuclear envelope, dispersed	Normal
Fetal intestine (680Int)	chromatin, few if any nuclear	Normal
Adult bladder (767B1)	bodies or perichromatin granules	Normal
Derived from primary carcinomas		
Colon (675T)	Tortuous contour with extensive	Abnormal
Colon (785T)	invaginations, irregular nuclear	Abnormal
Breast (578)[d]	envelope, condensed chromatin, many	Very abnormal
Transitional cell (761T)	nuclear bodies and perichromatin granules	Abnormal
Derived from metastatic carcinomas		
Stomach to muscle (746T)	Indistinguishable from primary	Very abnormal
Pancreas to lymph node (766T)	carcinoma lines	Very abnormal
Adenocarcinoma to sacrum (696T)		Very abnormal
Adenocarcinoma to hip (700T)		Very abnormal
Breast to pleura (MCF7)[e]		Very abnormal

[a]Unless otherwise indicated, lines are described in references 24, 26–28.
[b]Summarized from reference 28.
[c]Summarized from reference 24.
[d]Described in reference 25.
[e]Described in reference 40.

Grand Island, NY) containing 4.5 gm glucose/liter and supplemented with 10% fetal calf serum and 10 μg/ml insulin (Calbiochem, San Diego, CA).

Primary mammary cell cultures. Primary cultures of breast epithelial cells were prepared as described elsewhere in detail [29] from specimens of reduction mammoplasties. The specimen was washed in Ham's F-12 medium containing 5% fetal calf serum and antibiotics. Skin tissue and any grossly damaged tissue were cut off. The remaining tissue was gently lacerated with opposed scalpels, areas of lobulated fat were removed and placed directly into Ham's medium containing 5% fetal calf serum, antibiotics, 200 units/ml of collagenase (Sigma, St. Louis, MO), and 100 units/ml of hyaluronidase (Sigma, St. Louis, MO). The tissue was incubated at $37°$C at room temperature with gentle rotation with fresh enzyme solution being added every 12–24 h, until by light microscopy the mammary organoids (ducts, ductules, and lobules) were without association with stromal elements. The organoids were separated from single cells by filtration through a polyester cloth filter of 95 μm pore (Pekap, Tetko, Inc., Monterey Park, CA), washed off the filter, and plated in tissue cultures vessels in a mixture of Ham's F-12 medium and Dulbecco's modified Eagle's medium (1:1) plus 5% fetal calf serum, mixed with conditioned medium from several human epithelial cell lines, and containing insulin (5 μg/ml), hydrocortisone (5 μg/ml), 17β-estradiol, and 5-dihydrotestosterone (10^{-9} M), triiodothyronine (5 $\times$ 10^{-8} M), epidermal growth factor (5 ng/ml), and antibiotics. Cells were subcultured by exposure to STV (calcium and magnesium free saline, 0.05% trypsin, 0.02% versine).

Electron Microscopy

Cells were glutaraldehyde fixed in situ (2.5% glutaraldehyde in 0.1 M cacodylate buffer pH 7.3), post-fixed with 1% buffered osmium tetroxide followed by 2% ethanolic uranyl acetate. The specimens were dehydrated in graded ethanol and embedded with Epon. After polymerization, cells were sectioned parallel to the substrate surface with a diamond knife, were mounted on grids, examined, and photographed with a Philips EMZ01 electron microscope operated at an accelerating voltage of 50 V.

Immunofluorescence Studies

Cells were trypsinized and plated onto coverslips at approximately 10^5 cells per 60 mm diameter dish. When the cells reached confluence the coverslips were rinsed with phosphate-buffered saline, fixed in cold acetone, air dried, and kept frozen until assayed.

The indirect fluorescent antibody procedure used in this study has been described [30]. Briefly, dilutions of the antisera were reacted with the fixed cells on coverslips for approximately 1 h at $37°C$ in a moist chamber. The coverslips were then washed with phosphate-buffered saline (PBS) and reacted with goat anti-rabbit globulin that had been conjugated with fluorescein isothiocyanate [31] for an additional hour at $37°C$. The coverslips were washed again and mounted in Elvanol mounting medium on a microscope slide.

Antibody to plasma fibronectin was prepared in rabbits as previously described [32]. The specificity of the antiserum for tissue and plasma forms of fibronectin has been well established [33–35]. Rabbit antiserum to human factor VIII antigen was obtained from Berring Diagnostics (Calbiochem Co.).

Plasminogen Activator

Multi-well linbro dishes coated with ^{125}I-labeled fibrinogen were prepared as described [36]. Each well was incubated with 2.0 ml of medium containing 10% fetal calf serum plus 0.5 NIH units of thrombin for 24 h and then washed once with TD buffer (0.024 M Tris, ph 7.4; 0.14 M NaCl; 0.05 M KCL; 0.0037 M Na_2HPO_4). Unless otherwise indicated, cells that had been trypsinized 4 to 5 days prior to the experiment and that were nearly, but not completely, confluent were trypsinized, and 10^5 cells were added to each well in 2.0 ml of medium. The cells were initially allowed to settle for 5 h in medium containing 2.5% fetal calf serum; subsequently they were incubated with medium containing 2.5% dog serum; since fetal calf serum has been found to possess high levels of plasmin inhibitors. Plasminogen-free dog serum was prepared as described elsewhere [3]. For each of these experiments, one human embryo lung fibroblast line, HeLu, which was positive for plasminogen activator, and one human embryo skin fibroblast line, HeSk, which did not produce plasminogen activator [37, 38], were assayed as controls.

For studies using dexamethasone, cells were grown for 3 days prior to the experiment and maintained throughout the assay in the indicated concentration of dexamethasone, which was added to the medium from a $5 \times 10^{-5}M$ stock solution in ethanol. The culture receiving no dexamethasone was treated in an identical manner with an equivalent volume of ethanol. To perform the assay, cells were replaced on ^{125}I-fibrin-coated dishes in medium containing 2.5% fetal calf serum plus dexamethasone or ethanol.

Binding Of Platelets

Platelets prepared from 60–120 ml human whole blood according to the procedure described by Tollefsen [39] were generously provided by Drs. D. Gospodarowicz and I. Vlodafsky (University of California, San Francisco, CA). To observe platelet binding,

2×10^8 platelets were added to confluent cultures of cells in 35 mm culture dishes containing 1 ml of Dulbecco's modified Eagle's medium with 0.25% bovine serum albumin and incubated for 30 minutes at $37°C$ in a humidified CO_2 incubator. Following incubation, the cultures were washed 10 times with the same medium and viewed under phase microscopy.

RESULTS

Description Of The Cell Lines

The source of the cell lines used in this study and a summary of their morphologies and nuclear ultrastructures are shown in Table I. The lines derived from nonmalignant tissue were uniform in morphology and ultrastructure and could readily be distinguished from those lines derived from malignant tissues, which were morphologically [24] and ultrastructurally [28] abnormal.

The lines derived from both normal and malignant tissues showed ultrastructural evidence suggesting their epithelial origin, including microvilli and specialized junctions [41]. Microvilli were plentiful on the free surfaces of the cells in areas where the cells did not closely oppose each other (Fig. 1A). Desmosome-like structures and specialized junctions were also characteristic of these cultures. Figure 1B illustrates adjacent cell membranes lying approximately parallel to each other, occasionally bridged by desmosome attachments (small arrows). In this preparation, the desmosomes appear as dense plaques with short filaments on their cytoplasmic faces. In the middle of this picture, one of the cells has a persistent hemidesmosome (large arrow). Although the membranes are somewhat retracted from each other at this site, flocculent material is just visible in the intervening space. Tight junctions were also readily distinguishable in the cell lines. Figure 2 illustrates a tight junction lined by short fibrils that protrude perpendicularly from the junction into the cytoplasm of the opposing cells (inset). An electron-dense material fills the 100 Å space that separates cells in this region.

Since all of the lines showed the cuboidal morphology [24], specialized cell-attachments, and microvilli typical of epithelium, it is likely that they were not derived from normal stromal fibroblasts; however, somewhat similar structures have been reported for vascular endothelium [42]. All of the lines derived from malignant tissues also showed extensive morphologic and ultrastructural abnormalities; therefore, it is not likely that they were derived from normal vascular tissue. However, the possibility remained that the lines derived from nonmalignant tissue were vascular in origin. Although endothelial-specific organelles (Weibel-Palade bodies) were never observed in the electron microscope, recent studies suggest that bona fide endothelial cells need not have this marker [43]. To exclude the possibility that the lines derived from nonmalignant tissue were endothelial in origin, three lines (767B1, 74Int, and 680Int) were tested for an endothelial cell marker, antihemophilic factor (factor VIII antigen), by immunofluorescence microscopy. In contrast to human umbilical vein endothelial cells, which were positive in the assay (Fig. 3A), all three cell lines were negative as illustrated for fetal intestine line 74Int (Fig. 3B). Normal endothelial cells in culture also have a nonthrombogenic cell surface and do not bind platelets. Therefore, we have examined the same three nonmalignant lines (767B1, 74Int, and 680Int) for their ability to bind washed human platelets. As illustrated in Figure 4A, cultured normal bovine endothelial cells did not bind platelets. The few platelets remaining after washing the culture adhered only to the plastic surface accessible at intercellular junctions and not to the cellular membranes. In contrast all three lines (74Int, 680Int, and 767B1) tested for bound

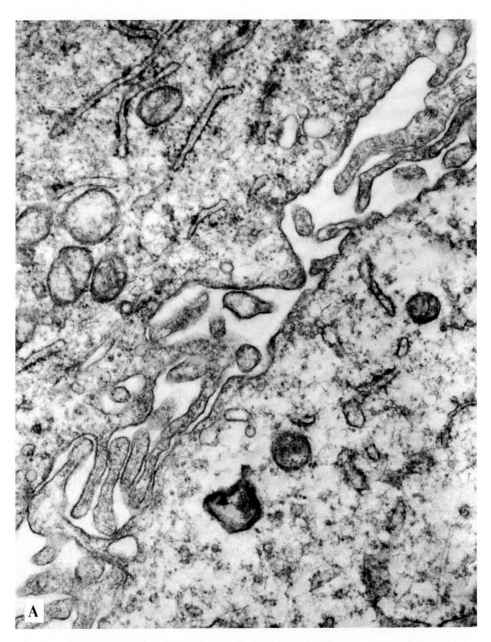

Fig. 1. Ultrastructure of epithelial cells. Fetal intestine line (680Int), passage 16. A) Microvilli; bar = 0.2 μ; B) desmosomes (small arrow) and persistent hemidesmosome (large arrow); bar = 0.5 μ.

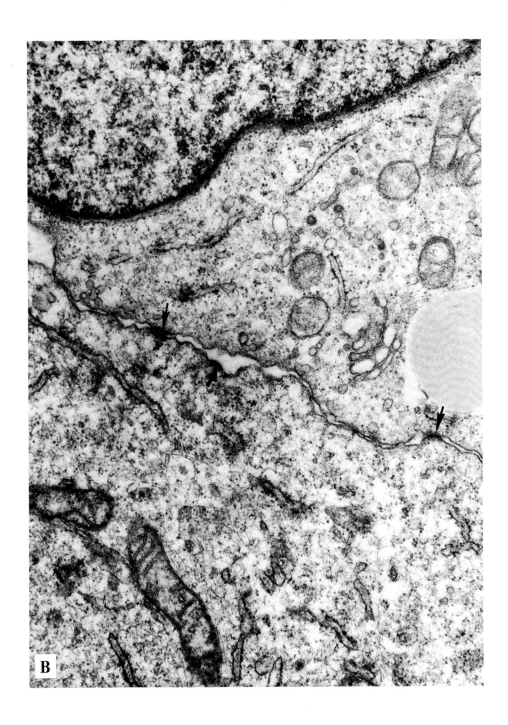

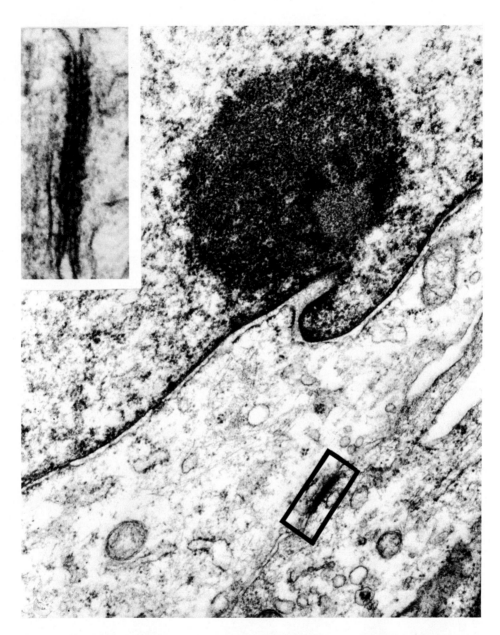

Fig. 2. Ultrastructure of epithelial cells. Fetal intestine line (680Int), passage 16. Figure illustrates a tight junction (arrow); bar = 0.2 μ. Inset shows tight junction at high magnification; bar = 0.1 μ.

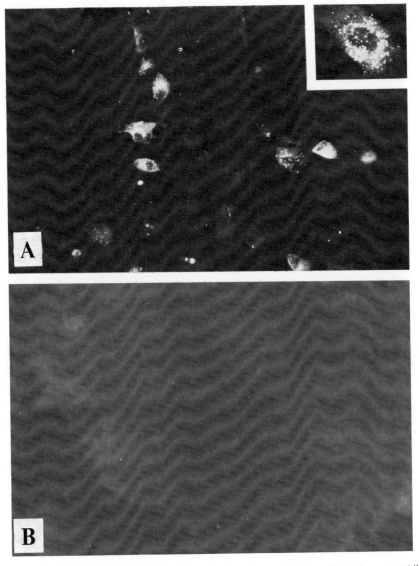

Fig. 3. Expression of antihemophilic factor (factor VIII antigen). A) Subconfluent human umbilical vein endothelial cells with approximately 20% of the cells showing bright fluorescence. Inset shows higher magnification of positive cell with discrete punctate pattern of fluorescence. B) Confluent monolayer of fetal intestine cells (74Int), with no positive cells.

platelets. Both lines derived from fetal intestine caused the platelets to coalesce into large aggregates (Fig. 4B) while the line derived from adult bladder (767B1) bound the platelets singly and did not cause platelet aggregation (data not shown).

Characterization Of The Cells For Properties Associated With Transformation

All of the epithelial lines derived from nonmalignant tissue showed extensive aibility to activate plasminogen. Figure 5 illustrates a typical experiment showing extensive solubili-

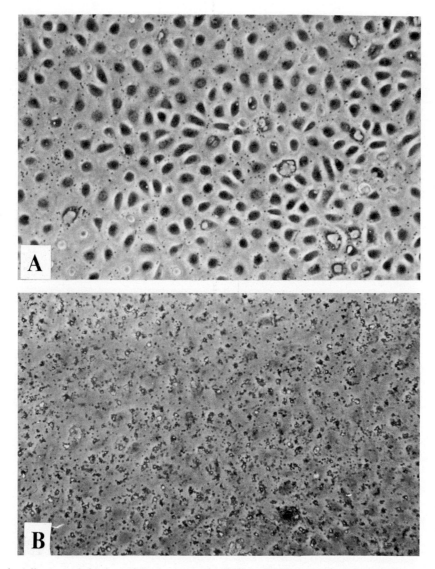

Fig. 4. Adherence of platelets. A) Bovine aorta endothelial cells; Note few platelets adhering only at intercellular junctions. B) Fetal intestine cells (74Int). Note extensive adherence and aggregation of platelets.

zation of ^{125}I-fibrin by an epithelial line derived from normal adult bladder. This activity was plasminogen dependent since it was absent when plasminogen was removed from the medium.

The carcinoma-derived lines varied in their production of plasminogen activator. Figure 6 illustrates the extremes of activity observed among the carcinoma-derived lines. The transitional cell carcinoma line, 761T, showed even more activity than the positive control line, HeLu, whereas the metastatic carcinoma line, 696T, showed little if any activity above background. In the experiment illustrated in Figure 2, the positive control,

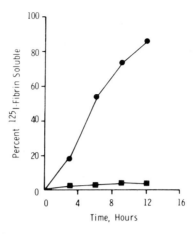

Fig. 5. Fibrinolytic activity of an epithelial cell line derived from nonmalignant adult bladder (767B1). Cells at passage 13 were plated on ^{125}I-fibrin-coated dishes in medium containing 2.5% plasminogen-free dog serum. After 12 hours, the assay was initiated by replacing the original medium with fresh medium containing either 2.5% dog serum (●——●), or 2.5% plasminogen-free (■——■) dog serum.

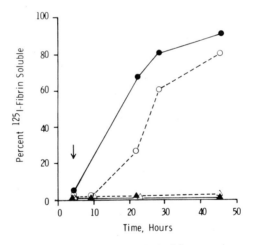

Fig. 6. Fibrinolytic activities of epithelial cell lines derived from carcinomas. Cells were plated on ^{125}I-fibrin-coated dishes in medium containing 2.5% fetal calf serum. Arrow indicates time of shift to medium containing 2.5% dog serum. Transitional cell carcinoma (761T), passage 24, ●——● ; metastatic carcinoma (696T), passages 21 ▲——▲ ; control human embryo lung (HeLu), --○--○; control human embryo skin (HeSk), △--△--.

HeLu, showed a lag before any activity was detected. Similar lags were also observed for some of the carcinoma lines; the length of these lags varied from one experiment to another. Table II illustrates the data gathered from typical experiments on each cell line. The data are presented as time required for 20% solubilization of the ^{125}I-fibrin; hence, the longer the time, the lower the amount of plasminogen activator produced. All of the lines derived from nonmalignant tissues produced large amounts of plasminogen activator, even at the earliest passage tested, passage 5. The tumor-derived lines varied in activity;

TABLE II. Plasminogen Activator in Human Epithelial Cells

Source of cells (designation, passage)	Time for 20% solubilization of ^{125}I-fibrin
Derived from nonmalignant tissue	
Fetal intestine (74Int, 19)	3
Fetal intestine (677Int, 6)	5
Fetal intestine (680Int, 5)	6
Adult bladder (767B1, 13)	3
Derived from primary carcinomas	
Colon (675T, 11)	5
Colon (785T, 6)	5
Breast (578T, 13)	75[a]
(578T, 40)	27
Trans. cell (761T, 22)	5
Derived from metastatic carcinoma	
Stomach to muscle (746T, 15)	19
Pancreas to lymph node (766, 15)	9
Adenocarcinoma to sacrum (696T, 20)	BKG
(696T, 50)	11
Adenocarcinoma to hip (700T, 16)	13
(700T, 50)	18

[a]Extrapolated from last data point at 42 hours.

6 cell lines had as much activity as the nonmalignant lines; 1 carcinoma-derived line was negative, and 2 lines produced intermediate amounts of plasminogen activator. There was no consistent difference in growth rate between the lines with low or high levels of plasminogen activator. In some cases an increase in plasminogen activator was observed at higher passages. The metastatic carcinoma line, 696T, which showed little activity at passage 15, showed extensive activity at passage 50. The breast carcinoma-derived line, 578T, also produced more plasminogen activator at passage 40 than at passage 13. The time for 20% solubilization of ^{125}I-fibrin at passage 40 was 27 hours, in contrast to an extrapolated 75 hours at passage 13. Another metastatic line, 700T, produced similar levels of plasminogen activator from passage 16 to passage 50. None of the other cell lines were tested beyond passage 25.

Several studies have shown that the plasminogen activators produced by certain nonmalignant cells can be suppressed by corticosteroids [37, 44]. To determine whether corticosteroids could inhibit the plasminogen activator activity found in these epithelial cells, an adult normal epithelial cell line (767B1), a normal fetal line (680Int), and a colon carcinoma line (675T) were incubated for 3 days in various concentrations of dexamethasone prior to assaying for plasminogen activator. A slight diminution in the amount of fibrinolysis was observed in the presence of 10^{-6} M dexamethasone; however, the response was similar for all 3 lines. No further decrease was found when 3×10^{-6} M dexamethasone was used (data not shown).

For most of the lines, including the control lines, HeLu and HeSK, the fibrinolytic activity did not vary when monkey serum rather than dog serum was used as the source of plasminogen. The metastatic stomach carcinoma line, 746T, was unique in that the fibrinolytic activity in dog serum was consistently higher than in monkey serum. Two other lines (578T and 696T) that had little detectable fibrinolytic activity in dog serum did show some activity when monkey serum was used as the source of plasminogen.

The same cell lines have been characterized for a number of other properties associated with transformation, including growth on contact-inhibited monolayers and in methocel, tumorigenicity in immunosuppressed mice [27], and loss of an external fibronectin containing matrix (H.S. Smith, J.R. Riggs, M.W. Mossesson, Production of Fibronectin by Human Epithelial Cells in Culture, Cancer Research, in press). A summary of these results is presented in Table III. For the growth properties, cell lines derived from normal tissue were negative, whereas the carcinoma-derived lines varied in their expression, with some lines being more abnormal than others. In most cases, the lines derived from metastatic lesions had more abnormal properties than did those derived from primary carcinomas. The metastatic adenocarcinoma line, 696T, was a notable exception. At low passages the line was negative for growth on monolayers, in methocel, and in mice. After extensive subculture, the cells gained the ability to grow on monolayers but were still negative for growth in methocel or in immunosuppressed mice. These same cells also increased production of plasminogen activator as a function of passage (Table II). The altered properties at high passage were not the result of an inadvertent contamination of the culture with a different cell line since both high and low passage cells contained identifying marker chromosomes upon giemsa banding (personal communication, Dr. W. Nelson-Rees, Cell Culture Laboratory, Naval Supply Center, Oakland CA). In most cases where cells grew both on monolayers and in methocel, the efficiency of plating was much higher on the monolayers than in the methocel. The highest plating efficiency observed in methocel was only 2.5%.

All of the lines derived from normal tissue as well as primary carcinomas were positive for a fibronectin matrix by immunofluorescence microscopy. In contrast, cell lines from metastatic carcinomas showed little if any fibronectin, including low passages of metastatic adenocarcinoma (line 696T), which showed no other abnormal growth properties. The 696T line also altered in expression of fibronectin as a function of passage; a small amount of fibronectin in an extracellular matrix was observed after extensive subculture.

Further Studies On Fibronectin Synthesis By Human Mammary Epithelial Cells

Recently, Stampfer et al [29] developed a conditioned media that reproducibly supports extensive growth of human mammary epithelial cells in primary and secondary culture. These cells have been shown to have typical epithelial-type specialized junctions and microvilli [29]; in addition, they bind antibodies raised against the human milk fat globule, a property specific to human mammary epithelium (J. A. Peterson, J. C. Bartholomew, M. Stampfer, R. L. Ceriani. Quantitative Changes in Expression of Human Mammary Epithelial Antigens in Breast Cancer as Measured by Flow Cytometry, data to be published). Within these epithelial cultures is also a small proportion of cells with a morphological appearance suggestive of myoepithelium. In addition, with the separation techniques described by Stampfer et al [29], pure cultures of fibroblastic stromal cells can be obtained from the same specimens. We have examined cultures of these various cell types from two reduction mammoplasty specimens for presence of fibronectin by immunofluorescence

TABLE III. Summary of Various Growth Properties of Human Epithelial Cell Lines

Source of cells (designation, passage)	Efficiency of plating (%) [a,b]			Tumorigenicity [b,c]	Fibronectin matrix [d]
	Epithelial cell monolayers	Fibroblast monolayers	Large colonies in methocel		
Derived from nonmalignant tissue					
Fetal intestine (74Int, 12–15)	<0.01	<0.01	<0.005	-	+
Fetal intestine (677Int, 7–9)	<0.01	<0.01	<0.005	-	+
Fetal intestine (680Int, 12–13)	<0.02	<0.02	<0.005	-	+
Adult bladder (767B1, 10–17)	<0.02	<0.02	<0.005	-	+
Derived from primary carcinoma					
Colon (675T, 8–10)	2.6[e]	<0.02	<0.005	-	+
Colon (785T, 9–17)	0.06[e]	<0.02	<0.005	[f]	+
Breast (578T, 10–28)	50	48	0.03		+
Trans. cell (761T, 18–22)	<0.02	<0.02	<0.005	-	+
Derived from metastatic carcinomas					
Stomach to muscle (746T, 11–14)	46	36	0.05	+	-
Pancreas to lymph node (766T, 15–16)	5.4	3.4	1.0	+	-
Adenocarcinoma to sacrum (696T, 16)	<0.05	<0.05	<0.005	-	+[g]
(696T, 50–52)	57	70	<0.005	-	
Adenocarcinoma to hip (700T, 9–15)	12	33	0.04	+	-
(700T, 50)	25	90	2.5	NT	NT

a Efficiency of plating = (number of colonies formed/number of cells plated) multiplied by 100.
b Summarized from reference 27.
c Mice immunosuppressed with antithymocyte serum.
d Summarized from Smith, Riggs and Mosesson (Cancer Research, in press).
e Visible microscopically only.
f These cells have been reported to produce tumors in congenitally athymic-asplenic (lasat) mice [45].
g Very scanty, dust-like pattern.

microscopy. In contrast to normal human fetal intestine cells, which produce a fluorescent pattern consisting of globular material attached to long fibrous-like structures (Fig. 7a), the normal mammary epithelial cells show a diminished, punctate and dust-like pattern (Fig. 7B) in both primary and secondary cultures. In contrast, both the putative myoepithelial cells (Fig. 7C) and the fibroblasts (Fig. 7D) distribute the fibronectin as an extensive fibrillar lacy network.

DISCUSSION

We have attempted to define how some of the properties associated with in vitro transformation apply to human carcinoma induction. Figure 8 diagrams the progression to malignancy of a typical mammary duct, illustrating the in vivo situation [46, 47], for which we would like to develop a model in culture. In the normal duct (Fig. 8A) a uniform layer of epithelial cells with a regular and normal morphology is separated from the blood vessels and stroma by a basement membrane. As these cells progress to an atypical, premalignant state, they lose growth control and proliferate extensively; morphologically, the atypical cells can become as irregular and pleomorphic as frank carcinoma cells (Fig. 8B). The notable difference between this extreme atypia (sometimes described as "carcinoma in situ") and frank carcinoma is the relationship of the epithelial cells to the basement membrane. In contrast to the premalignant state, where the normal relationship of the various cellular components is maintained, the carcinoma cells invade the basement membrane and grow in the surrounding stromal matrix (Fig. 8C). This progression from normality to carcinoma can follow alternate paths of development; it can occur by either gradual or abrupt changes, and it continues beyond the stage of primary carcinoma to metastases.

Associated with each step in malignant progression, there must be changes in cellular physiology which could potentially be measured in vitro. According to the principles of malignant progression defined in vivo [46, 47], a particular change might appear early on some pathways to malignancy and late on others, whereas another change may be present and important for some pathway to malignancy but not all pathways. Ideally, there may be properties that always and only appear when cells become malignant, but this alternative may not necessarily be true. Finally, there may be "enhancing" properties, which are themselves not necessarily responsible for the malignant phenotype but which confer on malignant cells an increased growth advantage.

We have approached the problem of determining which in vitro parameters correlate with malignancy in humans by culturing cells from tissues representing various stages of malignant progression. Although all of the lines cultured from malignant tissue were morphologically [24, 26] and ultrastructurally [28] abnormal (in contrast to those derived from nonmalignant tissues, which appeared normal), we cannot say for certain that all of the tumor-derived cells are capable of invasive growth. Because of the nature of malignant progression, the frank carcinoma is comprised of a heterogeneous population, only some cells of which may be invasive. Although a metastatic lesion is likely to be enriched for more invasive cells, it also may be heterogeneous, possibly having arisen from a clump of primary tumor cells only some of which are capable of initiating growth at the metastatic site. Once proliferation has been initiated by these more aggressive cells, the noninvasive cells may again commence proliferation.

Because of the central role that invasion of the basement membrane plays in carcinoma induction, we examined the lines for synthesis of fibronectin, a protein found associated with basement membranes as well as connective tissue in various normal human tissues

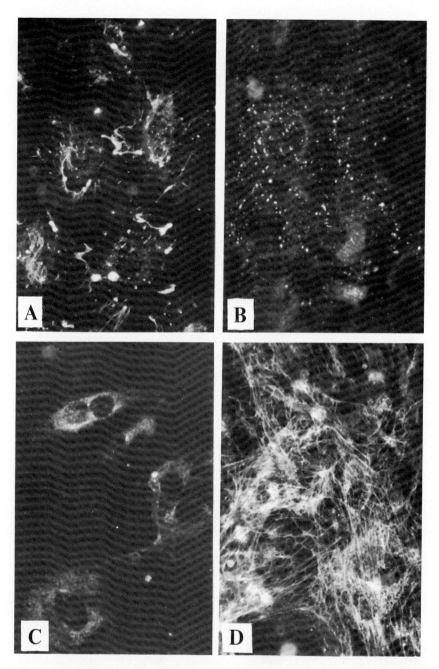

Fig. 7. Expression of fibronectin by various human cells in culture. A) Normal fetal intestine line 680Int showing globular and fibrillar pattern. B) Normal mammary epithelial cells H48RE in primary culture showing punctate and dust-like pattern. C) Putative myoepithelial cell in same epithelial culture as B), showing extensive fibrillar matrix. D) Normal fibroblasts in secondary culture from same patient as B), showing extensive fibrillar matrix.

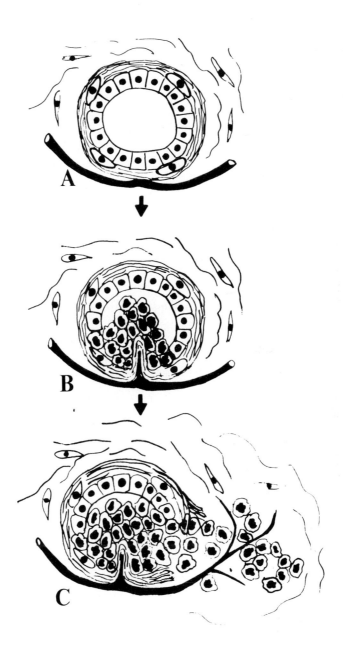

Fig. 8. Diagram of progression to malignancy of a typical mammary duct. A) Normal mammary duct. Note uniform polar epithelial cells and myoepithelial cells surrounding the lumen separated by basement membrane from the blood vessels and stroma. B) Atypical hyperplasia. Note the abnormal pleomorphic cells and intact basement membrane. C) Frank carcinoma. Note the disruption of basement membrane and invasion of epithelial cells into stromal area.

[48]. Absence of fibronectin in an external cellular matrix has been associated with transformation in many [4] but not all [19] systems. We have found that all the cell lines derived from metastatic tissues were negative for fibronectin, whereas those derived from nonmalignant tissues of primary carcinomas all produced fibronectin in an extracellular matrix. These observations suggest that absence of a fibronectin matrix in vitro may be a marker of invasive growth for human epithelial cells. However, this conclusion must be considered only tentative. When we extended these studies to primary and secondary cultures of normal mammary cells, we found that they produced a much diminished amount of fibronectin with a punctate and dusty cellular distribution rather than the extensive matrix produced by the nonmalignant lines derived from adult bladder and fetal intestine. These differences may be related to the fact that mammary ducts contain, in addition to the epithelial cells, myoepithelial cells, which may be involved in basement membrane synthesis. That putative cultured myoepithelial cells produced an extensive fibronectin matrix supports this hypothesis. In contrast, there are no myoepithelial cells in either bladder or intestine; therefore, the epithelial cells may be responsible for basement membrane synthesis in these organs. These observations point out the need to distinguish organ-specific properties from tumor-specific properties. Therefore, it will be important to compare the in vitro properties of cells cultured from specimens representing different stages of malignant progression in a single organ system.

How do the various other properties associated with in vitro transformation fit into the scheme of malignant progression? For properties such as growth on contact-inhibited monolayers, in methocel, or in immunosuppressed mice, the nonmalignant lines were negative, whereas the carcinoma-derived lines varied in expression, with some lines being more abnormal than others. The lines derived from metastatic lesions tended to have more abnormal properties than those derived from primary carcinomas, with the exception of one metastatic line, 696T, which was negative in these assays. Inasmuch as the tumor-derived lines were not consistantly positive in the assays tested, these in vitro parameters probably do not represent changes essential to the malignant state. The fact that the nonmalignant lines were negative for these properties suggests that the markers are somehow related to malignancy even if they are not essential. Therefore, with the reservation that many more studies are needed, we suggest that such properties may be "enhancing" and confer on malignant cells an increased growth advantage.

Finally, increased production of the protease, plasminogen activator, has been associated with transformation in many [1–3, 36–38, 49] but not all systems [10, 19, 50, 51]. For example epithelial cells derived from normal rat liver produced extensive amounts of plasminogen activator [10, 51]. Among the human epithelial lines that we studied, the level of plasminogen activator in culture also did not correlate with malignancy. The control nonmalignant epithelial cell lines all produced large amounts of plasminogen activator, whereas the tumor-derived lines showed a gradation of activities, ranging from lines having as much activity as the nonmalignant cells to lines having little or no activity above background. Since some of the nonmalignant lines were derived from fetal tissue, expression of plasminogen activator might be related to their fetal origin. However, nonmalignant adult bladder also produced extensive plasminogen activator, which suggests that adult human epithelial cells, like rat liver epithelial cells, produce plasminogen activator.

ACKNOWLEDGMENTS

We wish to thank Dr. Daniel B. Rifkin (New York University) for providing the ^{125}I-labeled fibrinogen-coated plates for the plasminogen activator studies, and also Drs. Dennis

Gospodarowicz and Israel Vlodafsky (University of California Medical Center, San Francisco, CA) for providing us with freshly prepared platelets and normal endothelial cell cultures.

We also wish to acknowledge the excellent technical assistance of Mr. Sylvester and Ms. A. Pang. This work was supported by National Cancer Institute contract CP70510, NIH Program project grant HL-17419, American Cancer Society grant DPT-72A and US Department of Energy Contract W-7405-ENG-48.

REFERENCES

1. Unkeless J, Tobia A, Ossowski L, Quigley J, Rifkin D, Reich E: J Exp Med 137:85, 1973.
2. Ossowski L, Unkeless J, Tobia A, Quigley J, Rifkin D, and Reich E: J Exp Med 137:112, 1973.
3. Quigley J, Ossowski L, Reich E: J Biol Chem 249:4306, 1974.
4. Hynes RO: Biochem Biophys Acta 458:73, 1976.
5. Handleman SL, Sanford KK, Tarone RE, Parshao R: In Vitro 13:526, 1977.
6. Smith H, Scher C, Todaro G: Virology 44:359, 1971.
7. Aaronson SA, Todaro GJ, Freeman AE: Exp Cell Res 61:1, 1970.
8. Ponten J: Biochem Biophys Acta 458:398, 1976.
9. Aaronson S, Todaro G: Science 162:1024, 1968.
10. Montesano R, Drevon C, Kuroki T, Saint Vincent L, Handleman S, Sanford KK, DeFeo D, Weinstein IB: J Natl Cancer Inst 59:1651, 1977.
11. Katsuta H, Takaoka T: In Nakahara W, Takayama S, Sugemura T, Odashima S (eds):"Topics in Chemical Carcinogenesis." Tokyo: University of Tokyo Press, 1972, p 389.
12. Marchok AC, Rhoton JC, Nettesheim P: Cancer Res 38:2030,1978.
13. Colburn NH, Vorder Bruegge WF, Bates JR, Gray RH, Rossen JD, Kelsey WH, Shemada T: Cancer Res 38:624, 1978.
14. Berkey JJ, Zolotar L: In Vitro 13:63,1977.
15. Shin S, Freedman FH, Risser R, Pollock R: Proc Natl Acad Sci USA 72:4435, 1975.
16. Tucker RW, Sanford KK, Handleman SL, Jones GM: Cancer Res 37:1571, 1977.
17. Barrett JC, Ts'o POP: Proc Natl Acad Sci USA 75:3761, 1978.
18. Gallimore PH, McDougall JK, Chen LB: Cell 10:667, 1977.
19. Pearlstein E, Hynes RO, Franks LM, Hemmings VJ: Cancer Res 36:1475, 1976.
20. Ponten J: In Fogh J (ed): "Human Tumor Cells In Vitro." New York: Plenum Press, 1975, p 175.
21. Federoff S: J Natl Cancer Inst 38:607, 1967.
22. Fogh J, Trempe G: In Fogh, J (ed): "Human Tumor Cells In Vitro". New York Plenum Press, 1975, p 115.
23. Marshall CJ, Franks LM, Carbonell AW: J Natl Cancer Inst 59:1743, 1977.
24. Owens R, Smith HS, Nelson-Rees W, Springer EL: J Natl Cancer Inst 56:843, 1976.
25. Hackett A, Smith HS, Springer EL, Owens R, Nelson-Rees WA, Riggs JL, Gardner MB: J Natl Cancer Inst 58:1795, 1977.
26. Smith HS, Owens R, Nelson-Rees W, Springer EL, Dollbaum C, Hackett A: In Nieburgs HE (ed): "Prevention and Detection of Cancer," Vol 2. New York: Marcel Dekker, 1978, p 1465.
27. Smith HS: J Natl Cancer Inst 62:225, 1979.
28. Smith HS, Springer EL, Hackett AJ: Cancer Res 39:332, 1979.
29. Stampfer MR, Hollowes R, Hackett AJ: In Vitro (in press).
30. Riggs JL. McAllister RM. Lennette EH: J Gen Virol 25:21, 1974.
31. Riggs JL, Seiwald RJ, Burckhalter JH, Downs CM, Metcalf TG: Am J Pathol 34:1081, 1958.
32. Mosesson MW, Umfleet RA: J Biol Chem 245:5728, 1970.
33. Chen AB, Amrani DL, Mosesson MW, Biochem Biophys Acta 493:310, 1977.
34. Chen AB, Mosesson MW: Anal Biochem 79:144, 1977.
35. Cooper HA, Wagner RH, Mosesson MW: J Lab Clin Med 84:258, 1974.
36. Rifkin D, Pollack R: J Cell Biol 73:47, 1977.
37. Rifkin D, Loeb J, Moore G, Reich E: J Exp Med 139:1317, 1974.
38. Rifkin D, Pollack R: In Ribbons D, Brew K (eds):"Proteolysis and Physiological Regulation." New York:Academic Press, 1976, p 263.
39. Tollefsen DM, Feagler JR, Majerus PW: J Biol Chem 249:2646, 1974.
40. Soule HD, Vazquez J, Long A, Albert S, Brennan M: J Natl Cancer Inst 51:1409, 1973.

41. Franks LM, Wilson PD: Int Rev Cytol 48:55, 1977
42. Haudenschild CC, Cotran RS, Gimbrone MA, Folkman J: J Ultrastruct Res 50:22, 1975.
43. Gospodarowicz D, Moran J, Braun D, Birdwell C: Proc Natl Acad Sci USA 73:4120, 1976.
44. Vassali J, Hamilton J, Reich E: Cell 8:271, 1976.
45. Gershwin ME, Ikeda RM, Erickson K, Owens R: J Natl Cancer Inst 61:245, 1978.
46. Foulds L: "Neoplastic Development," Vol I. New York: Academic Press, 1969.
47. Foulds L: "Neoplastic Development," Vol II. New York: Academic Press, 1975.
48. Stenman S, Vaheri AJ: J Exp Med 145:1054, 1978.
49. Barrett JC, Crawford BD, Grady DL, Hester LD, Jones PA, Benedict WF, Ts'o POP: Cancer 37:3815, 1977.
50. Chibber BA, Niles RM, Prehn L, Sorof S: Biochem Biophys Res Commun 65:806, 1975.
51. San RHC, Rice JM, Williams GM: Cancer Lett 3:243, 1977.

Journal of Supramolecular Structure 11:167–174 (1979)
Tumor Cell Surfaces and Malignancy 113–120

The Detection, Immunofluorescent Localization, and Thrombin Induced Release of Human Platelet-Associated Fibronectin Antigen

Mark H. Ginsberg, Richard G. Painter, Charles Birdwell, and Edward F. Plow, with the technical assistance of Jane Forsyth

Research Institute of Scripps Clinic, La Jolla, California 92037

Platelets are cells which develop adhesive properties following stimulation. Since fibronectin (fn) mediates adhesive properties of several cells, we sought evidence for platelet associated fn. Lysates of suspensions of washed human platelets containing ≤ 50 ng soluble fn/10^9 cells contained 2.85 μg fn antigen per 10^9 cells. The platelet fn antigen competition curve showed a similar slope to the curve for purified plasma fn suggesting antigenic identity. Immunofluorescent staining for fn was minimal in intact cells suggesting that the majority of fn antigen is intracellular. In permeable platelets, fluorescent staining for fn was seen in a punctate distribution suggesting a granule localization. Stimulation of platelet secretion by thrombin released platelet fn antigen. Suramin, a drug which inhibits platelet secretion, inhibited fn release. The apparent secretion of platelet fn, taken with the immunofluorescent data, support the localization of a portion of platelet fn antigen in a storage granule.

Key words: cellular adhesion, platelets, fibronectin, hemostasis

Platelets are anucleate cells which circulate freely in blood. Following stimulation by agents such as collagen or thrombin, platelets adhere to surfaces, to each other, to collagen or fibrin. Thus these cells represent potential models for the study of cellular adhesion. The fibronectins (fn) such as cold insoluble globulin [1] and the large external transformation-sensitive protein [2] are a group of glycoproteins found in plasma and on the surfaces of certain cells [3,4]. These proteins have now been implicated in a number of cellular activities, including the adhesion of cells to one another or to substrata [3,4]. This adhesion promoting property may be mediated by the affinity of fn for collagen [5] and fibrin [6]. The presence of fn antigen in platelets was suggested by Mosesson and Umfleet [6], raising the possibility that platelet fn may be involved in the adhesive properties of platelets.

In this article, we described studies which confirm [7, 8] the presence of fn antigen in platelets and which provide evidence supporting the intracellular localization of at least a portion of it in storage granules.

Received April 20, 1979; accepted June 18, 1979.

MATERIALS AND METHODS

Plasma fn

Plasma fn was purified by passage of 2 ml plasma/ml over gelatin sepharose beads as described by Engvall and Ruoslahti [5]. Bound fn was eluted with 1 M NaBr, pH 5.3. Homogeneity of fn was verified by polyacrylamide gel electrophoresis in the presence of β mercaptoethanol and sodium dodecyl sulfate (SDS PAGE) in which greater than 95% of Coomassie blue stained material was associated with a closely spaced doublet of apparent M_r=230,000. The fn produced contained $\leq$0.2 μg Factor VIII antigen/mg by crossed immunoelectrophoresis (kindly performed by Dr. T.S. Zimmerman, Scripps Clinic).

Anti-fn

Anti-fn was prepared by immunization of rabbits or goats with 1 mg subcutaneous doses of fn in complete Freund's adjuvant on a bimonthly schedule. The anti-fn produced was absorbed by passage through a gelatin-sepharose column and a sepharose column to which plasma depleted of fn was coupled. Fn antibodies were affinity purified on fn-sepharose (5 mg fn/ml beads). Following application of the antiserum and thorough washing, affinity purified anti-fn was eluted. F(ab')2 fragments were prepared by digestion of 7.5 mg purified antibody with 200 μg of pepsin at pH 4.0 for 18 hr at 37°C followed by extensive dialysis. Control F(ab')2 fragments were prepared from the IgG fraction isolated by DEAE-cellulose chromatography of preimmunization bleedings. Digestion of >97% of the IgG to F(ab')2 fragments was observed by SDS-PAGE.

Radioimmunoassay

Fn was radiolabeled with ^{125}I to a specific activity of 0.5-1 μCi/μg, and the double antibody radioimmunoassay was developed similar to those previously described by this laboratory [8, 9]. Assays were performed in plastic, siliconized tubes at 22°C with ^{125}I-fn at 15 ng/ml in a buffer system of 0.025 M NaCl, 0.04 M sodium borate, pH 8.3 containing 1% heat-inactivated normal rabbit serum and 1 mM EDTA. The precipitability of the ligand in 10% trichloracetic acid was usually >90% and non-specific precipitation by second antibody was <5%. ^{125}I fibrinogen was not bound in this assay and purified Factor VIII antigen at 1 unit/ml (7.5 μg/ml) produced no inhibition of fn binding. The radioimmunoassay for platelet factor 4 was performed by previously described methods [10].

Platelets

Platelet-rich plasma was prepared as described [11] and the platelets pelleted by centrifugation at 1,000 × g for 20 min and resuspended in modified Tyrode's buffer [12]. The suspension was then gel filtered [13] on sepharose 2B in modified Tyrode's. ^{125}I-fn, added to the platelet-rich plasma, was not detected in the isolated platelet fraction; and, on this basis, a contribution of $\leq$200 ng fn/10^9 platelets due to plasma contamination was estimated. For extraction, platelets were pelleted at 1,000 × g for 10 min and 0.5% triton-X 100 (J.T. Baker Chemical Co., Phillipsburg, NJ) added. After 30 min at 22°C, the mixture was centrifuged and the supernatant analysed. In experiments in which release was measured, platelets were prelabeled either with ^{3}H serotonin or ^{14}C serotonin + ^{51}Cr as previously described [12]. Varying quantities of purified human thrombin (a generous gift of Dr. John Fenton) were added and the mixture incubated at 37°C for 30 min. Reactions were stopped by addition of 0.5% (final concentration) formaldehyde, the platelets centrifuged at 2,000

X g for 20 min and supernatants taken for measurement of radioactivity, platelet factor 4 and fn. Percent release of any constituent was defined as

$$\frac{Cx(u) - Cx(b)}{Cx(+) - Cx(b)} \times 100$$

Where Cx = concentration in thrombin treated supernatant (u) or buffer treated (b) supernatant Cx(+) = concentration in 0.5% triton X-100 lysate.

Immunofluorescence

Immunofluorescent staining was performed on 2% formaldehyde fixed platelets on polylysine-coated circular glass cover slips. The cells were treated for 3 min with 0.1% triton X-100 to render them permeable to antibody or were permitted to remain intact. They were then incubated for 20 min with either goat F(ab')2 anti-fn or nonimmune-F(ab')2. The cells were rinsed with PBS and stained for 20 min with rhodamine-labeled rabbit F(ab')2 anti-goat immunoglobin (Cappel Lab, Cochranville, PA). The platelets were viewed with a Zeiss Universal microscope equipped with an HBO 50W mercury lamp and an IVFI epifluorescence condenser with a BP 546 excitation filter, a KT 580 chromatic splitter and an LP 590 barrier filter.

RESULTS

Detection of Platelet fn Antigen

In order to determine whether platelets contain fn antigen, washed human platelets were lysed in Triton X-100 and assayed for fn in radioimmunoassay. When platelets, isolated by differential centrifugation and gel filtration, were pelleted by centrifugation, ≤50 ng/ml, fn was detected in the supernatant by radioimmunoassay indicating a minimal carryover of soluble plasma fn. In contrast, fn antigen was detected in the 0.5% Triton extract of the washed platelets (Triton alone was without effect in this assay). As shown in Figure 1 the platelet lysate produced complete competitive inhibition of similar slope to the purified fn indicating apparent antigenic identity between the platelet and purified plasma fn. Analysis of platelet extracts from 12 adult donors showed an average fn level of 2.85 ± 1.24 (S.D.) $\mu g/10^9$ platelets. A plasma fn level of 270 ± 176 μg was obtained from 8 donors similar to reported levels [14]. The yield of detected platelet fn antigen was not increased by increasing the Triton X concentration up to 10-fold nor by addition of 1% 2-mercaptoethanol nor 6M Urea. Thus, at 0.5% Triton X-100 extraction of platelet fn antigen appears complete.

Immunofluorescent Localization of Platelet fn Antigen

The above experiments established the presence of cell-associated fn antigen in platelet suspension. To determine whether the antigen was platelet derived and to assess its accessibility in the resting cell, indirect immunofluorescent staining was performed using F(ab')2 fragments of immunochemically purified goat anti-fn and rhodamine labeled F(ab')2 fragments of rabbit anti-goat Ig. As shown in Figure 2, resting, intact platelets showed only a light, variable, surface speckled staining. When these cells were made permeable to the immunofluorescent reagents, either by detergent treatment (as shown) or by freezing and thawing, staining was markedly enhanced and was present in the punctate pattern with multiple discrete foci per cell. Thus, the detected fn antigen was platelet-associated and the bulk of antigen was inaccessible to immunofluorescent reagents in intact cells.

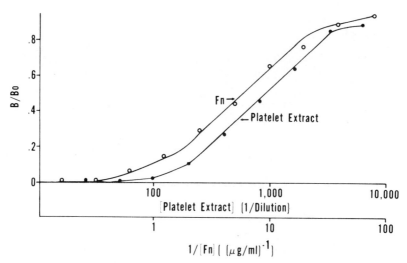

Fig. 1. Inhibition of binding fn – anti-fn by purified plasma fn or platelet extract. Various dilutions of platelet extract or purified plasma fn were assayed using the fn radioimmunoassay described in Materials and Methods. B = fraction of ^{125}I-labeled fn bound in the presence of competing antigen. Bo = fraction bound in the absence of competing antigen. (●————●) platelet extract, (○————○) plasma fn.

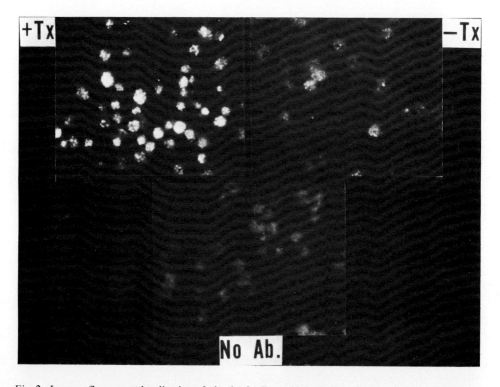

Fig. 2. Immunofluorescent localization of platelet fn. Formaldehyde fixed human platelets either intact (–Tx) or permeabilized with 0.1% Triton X-100 (+Tx) were stained with goat F(ab')2 anti-fn followed by rhodaminated rabbit anti goat Ig. Prebleed F(ab')2 staining of triton permeabilized platelets (no Ab) is shown below, blocking controls and prebleed staining of intact cells had a similar appearance.

Thrombin-Induced Secretion of Platelet fn Antigen

The immunofluorescent experiments described above are consistent with an intracellular location for a major portion of platelet fn. One possibility for such location would be in a storage granule. To test this, the effect of thrombin, a protease which releases the contents of platelet storage granules, was examined. As shown in Figure 3, thrombin stimulated release of platelet fn into the supernatant fluid. Serotonin, a dense body constituent [15] and platelet factor 4, a probable alpha-granule constituent [16], were virtually all released by thrombin. In contrast, consistently less than half of Triton X extractable fn was released by thrombin. To insure that thrombin was not inducing destruction of platelet fn antigen, thus accounting for incomplete release, the thrombin-treated platelets were lysed in Triton X-100 and assayed for fn antigen. As shown in Table I, sufficient fn remained in the thrombin treated platelet pellet to account for the fn not released into the supernatant. Thus, thrombin induced only a partial release of platelet fn antigen. In experiments in which ^{51}Cr loss was assayed, less than 1% occurred, indicating that fn release was a selective (ie non-lytic) phenomenon.

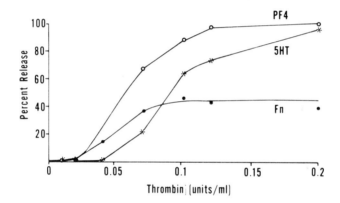

Fig. 3. Thrombin induced release of platelet fn antigen: 100 μl of solutions of various concentrations of thrombin were mixed with 400 μl of platelets and the mixture incubated at 37°C for 30 min. Reactions were stopped and percent release determined as described in Materials and Methods. (o———o) platelet factor 4, (☆———☆) serotonin, (●———●) fibronectin. Means of duplicate determinations.

TABLE I. Recovery of fn Antigen From Thrombin Stimulated Platelets

Source	Fibronectin content (μg/ml)
Thrombin stimulated supernatant	2.83 ± 0.2
Thrombin stimulated pellet	6.23 ± 2.6
Total fn in resting platelets	8.98 ± 0.8

100 μl of thrombin, 12.5 units/ml, were added to 400 μl of platelet suspension and the mixture incubated at 37°C for 30 min. The platelets were sedimented by centrifugation, and the supernatant removed and assayed for fn antigen (Thrombin stimulated supernatant). 500 μl of a 0.15 m NaCl solution containing 0.5% Triton X-100 were added to the pellet and the resulting mixture assayed for fn antigen (Thrombin stimulated pellet). To determine the total fn, 400 μl of resting platelets were added to 100 μl 2.5% Triton X-100 and the resultant lysate assayed for fn.

The above experiments indicated that thrombin released a portion of platelet fn antigen into the supernatant. This raised the possibility that thrombin proteolytically cleaved platelet surface fn (or an fn receptor) in a manner analagous to trypsin induced release of fn from fibroblast cultures. To test this possibility, the release of platelet fn in the presence of an inhibitor of platelet secretion was assayed. As shown in Table II, 2.5×10^{-4} M Suramin abolished thrombin induced serotonin [17] and platelet factor 4 secretion. Fibronectin release was inhibited as well. Up to 5×10^{-4} M Suramin did not inhibit thrombin-induced clotting of plasma, verifying that the thrombin was proteolytically active in the presence of the concentrations of Suramin used.

DISCUSSION

The data provided in this report indicate that washed human platelets contain detergent extractable fn-related antigen. The bulk of platelet fn antigen was inaccessible to immunofluorescent reagents in resting intact platelets. When the cells were made permeable, fn antigen stained in a punctate intracellular distribution. When platelet secretion was triggered by thrombin, platelet fn antigen was partially released and fn release was inhibited by an inhibitor of platelet secretion. Taken together with the immunofluorescent localization – the apparent secretion of platelet fn antigen supports the localization of at least a portion of it in storage granules.

The presence of an average of 2.85 μg fn antigen per 10^9 platelets was detected by radioimmunoassay of a platelet lysate. The possibility that this represents contaminating soluble plasma fn appears to be ruled out for three reasons: 1) When radiolabeled plasma fn was added to the platelet rich plasma prior to washing, less than 200 ng/10^9 platelets of plasma fn was detected in the resulting suspension of washed platelets; 2) When the suspension of washed platelets was centrifuged, less than 50 ng fn antigen/10^9 platelets was detected in the platelet free supernatant; 3) Platelet associated fn antigen was demonstrated by immunofluorescence. The slopes of the inhibition curves for platelet and plasma fn antigens were similar, suggesting that the platelet antigen is immunochemically and structurally related to the plasma antigen. Whether the 2 proteins are indeed identical cannot be ascertained from the data presented here. The level of platelet fn antigen reported here is similar to the value (3.44 μg/10^9 platelets) recently reported by Zucker et al [18] in an electroimmunoassay. Since 10^9 platelets represents approximately one milligram of platelet protein, fn related antigen then represents approximately 0.3% of platelet protein.

TABLE II. Effect of Suramin on Release of Platelet fn

	Percent Release		
Treatment	Fn	PF4	Serotonin
Thrombin	28.3	71.1	78.3
Thrombin + 2.5×10^{-4} M Suramin	0	0	0.8

100 μl thrombin (5 units/ml) plus 100 μl Suramin (2.5×10^{-3} M) or Tyrode's solution were added to plastic tubes followed by 800 μl of platelet suspension. Following incubation at 37°C for 30 min, 1 ml of 1% formaldehyde was added, the mixture centrifuged and percent release of each constituent determined as described in Materials and Methods.

Immunofluorescent examination of intact platelets revealed only a variable, very light speckled surface staining. This staining was specific in that it was absent from pre-bleed and blocking controls. When the platelets were made permeable, staining for fn antigen was markedly enhanced. This suggests that most of the fn antigen is in the interior of resting platelets rather than on the surface. This is corroborated by the results of Hynes et al [19] who reported that they were unable to stain intact platelets for fn. Since they used whole antiserum rather than F(ab')2 fragments of affinity purified antibody, and stained in the presence of plasma proteins, it is possible that the anticipated high background may have obscured the minor degree of staining which we observed. Furthermore, Phillips and Agin [20] did not report radiolabeling of proteins the size of fn on the surface of resting platelets. Thus, based on immunofluorescence and cell surface labeling studies there is little detectable fn on the surface of resting platelets.

The punctate pattern of fn immunofluorescent staining in permeable resting platelets was highly similar to the pattern observed for a probable alpha granule constituent, platelet factor 4 [21]. In addition, we confirmed [18] that, like platelet storage granule constituents, fn antigen is released from thrombin-stimulated platelets. Release was selective and was inhibited by an inhibitor of platelet secretion, indicating that fn release may occur by secretion. Taken together with the immunofluorescent results, these data indicate that a portion of platelet fn is present in an intracellular storage granule. This possibility is supported by subcellular fractionation studies [18] in which platelet associated fn was reported to be present in alpha granule rich fractions.

Resting platelets are discrete and are non-adherent as judged by their ability to circulate freely in blood. Following stimulation platelets may adhere to each other, to collagen, to surfaces, or to fibrin. The data presented here indicate that the bulk of platelet fn antigen is intracellular, and may be released upon thrombin stimulation, possibly from storage granules. How releasable or nonreleasable platelet fn might participate in the generation of platelet adhesiveness is then an important question for future investigation.

ACKNOWLEDGMENTS

The authors gratefully acknowledge the expert secretarial assistance of Ms. Monica Bartlett, the artwork of Ms. Betsy Cargo, and photography of Mr. Gerry Sandford. The authors also acknowledge Dr. Marjorie Zucker for making available a manuscript in press.

This research was supported in part by grants HL 16411, AI 7007, and CA-23929 and is publication #1777 of Scripps Clinic and Research Foundation. Mark H. Ginsberg is the recipient of Clinical Investigator Award #AM00393. Richard G. Painter is the recipient of RCDA #AM00437. Charles Birdwell and Edward Plow are recipients of Established Investigatorships of the American Heart Association.

REFERENCES

1. Morrison P, Edsall R, Miller SG: J Am Chem Soc 70:3103, 1948.
2. Hynes RO, Bye JM: Cell 3:113, 1974.
3. Yamada KM, Olden K: Nature (Lond) 275:179, 1978.
4. Vaheri A, Mosher DF: Biochim Biophys Acta 516:1, 1978.
5. Engvall E, Ruoslahti E: Int J Cancer 20:1, 1977.
6. Mosesson MW, Umfleet RA: J Biol Chem 245:5728, 1970.
7. Bensusan H, Koh T, Henry K et al: Proc Natl Acad Sci USA 75:5864, 1978.

8. Plow EF, Birdwell C, Ginsberg MH: J Clin Invest 63:540, 1979.
9. Plow EF, Hougie C, Edgington TS: J Immunol 107:1495, 1971.
10. Ginsberg MH, Hoskins R, Sigrist P, Painter RG: J Biol Chem. In press.
11. Ginsberg MH, Henson PM: J Exp Med 147:207, 1978.
12. Ginsberg MH, Kozin F, O'Malley M, McCarty DJ: J Clin Invest 60:999, 1977.
13. Tangen O, Berman HJ, Marfey P: Thromb Diath Haemorrh 25:268, 1971.
14. Mosher DF, Williams E: J Lab Clin Med 91:729, 1978.
15. Henson PM, Ginsberg MH, Morrison DC in Poste G, Nicolson G (eds): "Membrane Fusion." New York: Elsevier, No. Holland, 1978, p. 411.
16. Niewiarowski S: Thromb Haemostasis 38:924, 1977.
17. Pollard HB, Goldman KT, Pazoles C, Shulman NR: Proc Natl Acad Sci USA 74:5295, 1977.
18. Zucker MB, Mosesson MW, Broekman MJ, Kaplan KL: Blood 54:8, 1979
19. Hynes RO, Ali IU, Destree AT, Mautner V, Perkins ME, Senger DR, Wagner DD, Smith KK: Ann NY Acad Sci 312:317, 1977.
20. Phillips DR, Agin PP: Biochim Biophys Acta 352:218, 1974.
21. Ginsberg MH, Taylor L, Painter RG: Submitted for publication.

Journal of Supramolecular Structure 11:175—187 (1979)
Tumor Cell Surfaces and Malignancy 121—133

Growth Control by Cell to Cell Contact

Richard Bunge, Luis Glaser, Michael Lieberman, Dan Raben, James Salzer,
Brock Whittenberger, and Thomas Woolsey

*Departments of Biological Chemistry and Anatomy and Neurobiology, Division of Biology
and Biomedical Sciences, Washington University School of Medicine, St. Louis, Missouri
63110.*

Control of cell growth by cell to cell contact is reviewed with particular emphasis on two systems — contact inhibition of growth observed with Swiss 3T3 cells and the mitogenic stimulation of Schwann cells by dorsal root ganglia neurites. In both cases the biological effect can be reproduced by the addition of surface membranes to the corresponding cells. In the case of contact inhibition of 3T3 cells, biological activity appears to correlate with membrane binding to the cells. An octylglucoside extract of 3T3 plasma membranes retains the biological activity (growth inhibition) of the original membranes.

Key words: growth control, 3T3 cells, Schwann cells, neurites, plasma membranes

While the purpose of this review is to discuss recent advances in the study of the effect of cell to cell contact on growth control, the subject can be put into the general context of specific cell to cell adhesion. The problem has been examined in a number of systems, of which the best studied are dissociated embryonic cells in which it has been demonstrated that specific cell to cell adhesion can occur [for review, see references 1—4]. These results imply that there are molecules present on the cell surface that can interact with the surface of other cells (either homologous or heterologous) and result in cell to cell adhesion. Such adhesion is believed to be important in terms of normal development, but in a number of instances it is also likely that specific cell to cell adhesion will have an effect on the physiological properties of the cells; that is, a cell in contact with certain other cells may behave in a different manner or respond in a different way to external stimuli than a cell that is growing in relative isolation. The problem with a number of the approaches that have been used to study cell to cell adhesion is that it is very difficult to distinguish biologically meaningful cell to cell adhesion — that is, adhesion between cells, which has a developmental or physiological consequence, in contrast to intercellular adhesion, which happens to represent a laboratory curiosity in the sense that two normally unrelated cell types fortuitously have ligands on the cell surface that can interact. Therefore, it is of great interest to study cell interactions in which there are physiological consequences of cell adhesion. This review concentrates on two such examples and mentions a few others that have been less well investigated but may represent fruitful areas for further investigation.

Received March 18, 1979; accepted June 18, 1979.

0091-7419/79/1102-0175$02.60 © 1979 Alan R. Liss, Inc.

The two systems that will be discussed in detail are 1) contact inhibition of growth, a situation in which contact between 3T3 cells is followed by cessation of growth (in this situation a negative growth signal is generated) [3, 5–8], and 2) contact stimulation of growth, a situation in which contact between the surface of a neurite and a Schwann cell induces cell division in the Schwann cells (in this case a positive growth signal is generated) [9–11].

CONTACT INHIBITION OF GROWTH

The subject of contact inhibition of growth is an old one and a one that has been debated for a number of years. The specific question that has been asked is whether the cessation of growth observed at confluence with a number of "normal" fibroblastic cell lines at high cell density is due to a contact phenomenon or represents the failure of nutrients or other mitogenic factors in the medium to reach the cell surface. The latter could result either because the factors are depleted from the medium [12] or because a diffusion boundary layer exists near the cell surface [13, 14].

Classical experiments by Dulbecco [7] have shown that if a nongrowing confluent monolayer of cells is wounded, new cells will grow into the wound area, indicating that depletion of growth factors or other nutrients from the bulk medium was not responsible for contact inhibition of growth. A slightly different way of looking at such experiments is shown in Figure 1. The conclusion drawn from this experiment is essentially the same as that in the original Dulbecco experiments as well as similar experiments by Holley and Kiernan [15]; ie, that 3T3 cells at confluence do not grow, in spite of the fact that they are in a medium that can support the growth of sparse cells.

The question has been raised, however, as to whether growth is limited because of an inability of mitogenic factors to reach the cell surface at a rate rapid enough to have an effect on the cells, since the cells generally degrade or utilize mitogenic factors [13, 14]. A test of this proposal has been carried out by increasing the viscosity of the medium. This should result in a further reduction of cell growth if diffusion limitation of growth exists [16]. Since neither the rate nor the extent of cell growth was altered by changes in viscosity, it appears unlikely that growth under these conditions with Swiss 3T3 cells is diffusion limited.* A similar conclusion by a different approach was reached by Thrash and Cunningham [17], who showed that cell density as well as medium components can limit the density of Swiss and Balb 3T3 cells. We can, therefore, assume that among the signals for growth that a cell is capable of receiving there are both positive signals, such as those brought about by the binding of known mitogens to the cell surface, and negative signals, which are derived in the particular case that is under discussion by contact with other cells. Contact could therefore be considered in the same light as the interaction of hormones with a surface receptor. These interactions between cells ultimately produce an intracellular signal which at the present time has not been defined, and which is responsible for the cessation of growth.

Not all cultured "normal" fibroblastic cells exhibit the same extent of growth control as do 3T3 cells, and for some lines this property is only apparent in low concentrations of serum [3]. One of the simplest ways in which cell to cell contact could inhibit cell growth

---

*Some reinterpretation of these observations has been presented in the "Matters Arising" section of Nature (274:722, 1978) by H. G. Maroudas, B. Whittenberger and L. Glaser, as well as a different interpretation by R. W. Holley and J. H. Baldwin in Nature (278:283, 1979).

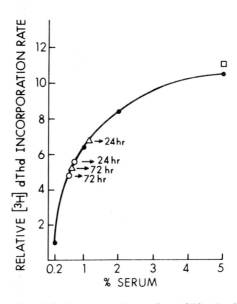

Fig. 1. Depletion of mitogenic activity from serum by confluent 3T3 cells. Cells were plated in both Linbro multi-well dishes (2 cm² per well, 1.2×10^3 cells per well) and Falcon 35 mm dishes (6×10^4 cells per dish) in DME/10% calf serum/L-[³⁵S]-methionine (1 μCi/ml). Medium was also plated on empty 35 mm dishes as a control. Seventy-two hours after plating, the medium in the Linbro dishes was changed to DME/0.2% calf serum/L-[⁻³⁵S]-methionine (1 μCi/ml) (0.6 ml per well). Prior to the addition of the low serum medium the wells were rinsed twice with DME to remove residual serum. In addition, the medium in all the 35 mm dishes (including the dishes with no cells) was changed to DME/10% serum utilizing two different serum lots (this will generate 72-hour depleted medium). Forty-eight hours later the medium in one-half of the 35 mm dishes was changed (DME/10% calf serum, 2 serum lots) to generate 24-hour depleted medium. Twenty-four hours later the medium was removed from the 35 mm dishes (5 sets of samples: serum lots 1 and 2, both 24- and 72-hour depleted, and the medium over empty plastic for 72 h), brought to 1 μCi/ml in L-[³⁵S]-methionine (stock at 1,000 μCi/ml), and added to the starved cells in the Linbro dishes (1.0 ml/well). In addition, medium containing 0.2%, 1.0%, 2.0%, or 5.0% serum was also added to starved cells. The dishes were pulsed with [³H]-dThd (6.7 Ci/ mmole) from 21 to 25 hours after the medium change, and the data were collected and analyzed by the double-label technique previously described [37]. Symbols: •, standard curve determinations; △, serum lot 32060 (K.C. Biological); ○, serum lot 328074 (K.C. Biological); □, medium incubated over empty plastic. The cells from which the depleted medium was taken were assayed for DNA synthesis and had 10% the rate of a sparse culture for the 24-hour depleted medium (both serum lots) and 2% the rate of a sparse culture for the 72-hour depleted medium (both serum lots). Similar results have been obtained in independent experiments by autoradiography. The data show that incubation of medium with confluent cells results in only a partial depletion of mitogenic activity for sparse cells.

would be if cell contact changed either the number of receptors for mitogens and/or the ability of these receptors to function. The concentration of receptors for mitogenic factors in confluent density-inhibited cells has only been investigated in a limited number of cases. The concentration is generally similar to or higher than that observed in sparse cells [for example, see references 8, 18]. In BSC-1 cells, the level of receptor for epidermal growth factor decreases tenfold at confluence, perhaps as a consequence of cell to cell contact (our interpretation) [19].

If growth is in part controlled by the interaction of molecules present at the cell surface, then it is possible to consider that a plasma membrane fraction of such cells when added to sparse cells (ie, subconfluent cells, which do not have extensive cell to cell contact with other cells), may result in the cessation of growth if the cells recognize membranes in the same manner as they recognize other cells.

The probability that such an experiment would actually succeed was greatly increased by the fact that, in a number of cases where specific cell adhesion had been examined, it was known that plasma membranes retain the ability to bind to cells with the same or similar specificity as the cells from which they were derived [see for example references 20, 21]. In addition, a limited number of experiments suggested that the developmental patterns of slime molds could be altered by the addition of homologous plasma membranes [22, 23]. In previous experiments in which adhesion of plasma membranes to cells was measured, it was concluded that only one of the two complementary cell surface adhesive molecules remained functional in isolated plasma membranes [20]. It is not known whether this is a general phenomenon, but the proposed experiments require that this component be the one that elicits a response in the target cell.

An extensive series of studies has therefore been carried out in order to determine whether a plasma membrane fraction derived from 3T3 cells can, in fact, induce the cessation of growth of a sparse culture of the same cells. The system is clearly one that needs to be approached with caution, because cessation of growth, which is the parameter to be measured, could be due to a variety of "toxic effects" that would not be related to contact inhibition of growth.

Plasma membranes from 3T3 cells when added to sparse cells lead to the cessation of growth in a time and concentration dependent manner. This effect is not due to general toxicity since the same membranes do not have an effect on SV40 transformed 3T3 cells. The effect is reversible, in that removal of the membranes by trypsinization followed by replating of the cells results in reinitiation of growth. Control experiments have shown that the membranes do not act by removing essential nutrients from the bulk medium which would be a trivial cause for the cessation of cell growth [24].

The cells that are arrested by the addition of membranes are arrested early in the G_1 phase of growth, a situation identical to that which obtains during contact at high cell density. The kinetics by which membranes interact with cells are such that in each cell cycle, even at saturating membrane concentrations, only a maximum of 40–50% of the cells are arrested. The remainder of the cells go through an additional cell cycle, and if membranes are still present about 40–50% of these cells will now be arrested in G_1. This leads to a model of growth control which suggests that during each cell cycle, presumably early in G_1, the sensitivity of the cells to contact to other cells (or in this case membranes), is reset at different levels. If this sensitivity is below some threshold value, the cells can be arrested by addition of membranes or, presumably, by contact with other cells. If this signal is set above some threshold value, then the cells can continue through the cell cycle. In the next cell cycle this sensitivity will again be randomized, and some cells will become sensitive to contact inhibition [25]. Previous experiments by Martz and Steinberg [26], in which the growth of 3T3 cells in contact with other cells was followed by cinematography, would be in agreement with this type of model, as would recent experiments on growth control by nutrient starvation [27]. In the experiments by Martz and Steinberg, cells with extensive contact with other cells were observed after cell division. About 50% of such cells divided again within 24 hours, whereas the other 50% failed to divide during the maximum time period of observation (72 hours).

Membranes prepared from erythrocytes are not active in inhibiting the growth of 3T3 cells, and membranes prepared from SV40 transformed 3T3 cells show less activity than those prepared from 3T3 cells. Thus, one would conclude that SV40 transformed 3T3 cells, which do not show density-dependent inhibition of growth, have lost the ability to respond to contact with other cells but can still generate a signal by contact with normal cells. The relevant molecules are still present in the plasma membrane of SV3T3 cells, although apparently at a somewhat lower concentration than in the 3T3 cells.

Addition of membranes to cells will also reduce the rate of uptake of α-aminoisobutyric acid and uridine [28], an effect which resembles that observed at high cell density [for review see references 3, 29, 30]. On the other hand, addition of membranes has no effect on the rate of uptake of 2-deoxyglucose or inorganic phosphate by sparse 3T3 cells, and thus these two parameters seem to be dissociable from the cessation of growth seen at high density [28] — ie, contact inhibition of growth. These data are complementary to those obtained by Cunningham and co-workers, which also suggested that transport of glucose and inorganic phosphate was not directly related to growth control [29], and to the finding of Lever that contact did not alter the ability of membrane vesicles to transport glucose [31]. A summary of these data is shown in Figure 2A. (It should be noted that the use of membranes for such experiments has a number of advantages, since the cell density in the presence of membranes is low and any effects due to nutrient depletion by high cell density are therefore minimized.) SV40 transformed 3T3 cells show a weak response to the addition of membranes, in that the uptake rate of α-aminoisobutyric acid and uridine is decreased, but there is no effect on cell growth or on the rate of uptake of 2-deoxyglucose. Whether this response represents a decreased ability of these cells to respond to the same stimuli as 3T3 cells or a nonspecific effect is not known. At membrane concentrations that give maximal inhibition of uptake of 3T3 cells there is very little effect on the uptake rate of α-aminoisobutyric acid and uridine by SV3T3 cells, but at high concentrations of membranes

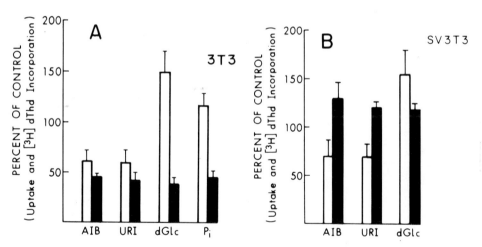

Fig. 2. Effect of 3T3 plasma membranes on solute transport. A. The bar graph summarizes a large number of experiments in which the rate of solute uptake was measured after 48 h of incubation of Swiss 3T3 cells with saturating levels of membranes (16 to 20 phosphodiesterase units per 35 mm dish) [28]. Open bars indicate rate of solute uptake; closed bars, the corresponding rate of DNA synthesis. B. Similar data obtained for SV3T3 cells (for details see text). The data shown are for 20 PDE units (alkaline phosphodiesterase [24]) per 35 mm dish. Maximal inhibition of solute uptake by 3T3 cells occurs at 4 PDE units/dish, a level at which SV3T3 cells show a very low response. Thus solute uptake (α-aminoisobutyric acid and uridine) is at least five times more sensitive to membrane addition in 3T3 cells than in SV3T3 cells. Abbreviations: AIB, α-aminoisobutyric acid; URI, uridine; dGlc, 2-deoxy-D-glucose; Pi, inorganic phosphate.

the inhibition can be as large as that observed with 3T3 cells (Fig. 2B). The data in Figure 2B were obtained at 20 phosphodiesterase units of membranes per 35 mm dish, whereas the maximum effect of membranes on transport with 3T3 cells is obtained at 4 phosphodiesterase units/35 mm dish, at which level there is very little effect on the rate of nutrient uptake by SV3T3 cells. The effect on nutrient uptake by SV3T3 cells is unlikely to be due to steric effects, since the rate of 2-deoxyglucose appears not to be affected and monosaccharides and amino acids are molecules of roughly equivalent size.

We have devised a technique for measuring the binding of membranes to cells on a dish by the use of ^{125}I-labeled plasma membranes, which retain the ability to block cell

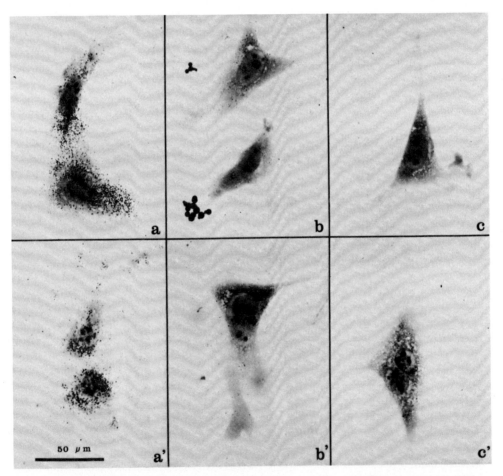

Fig. 3. Binding of ^{125}I-labeled plasma membranes to 3T3 cells. Plasma membranes were labeled with ^{125}I by the glucose oxidase lactoperoxidase method, and added to cells in Linbro wells at concentrations of 6 PDE units/dish (a, b, c) or 2 PDE units/dish (a', b', c'). After 48 h the medium was removed, the cells fixed with glutaraldehyde and dipped in emulsion. a,a', 5% serum; b,b', 25% serum; c,c', 5% serum with heat-inactivated membranes. The levels of DNA synthesis as a percent of control were: a, 41%; a', 51%; b, 77%; b', 93%; c, 110%; c', 124%. High serum reduces, or heat inactivation of membranes abolishes, both biological activity and binding of membranes to cells. Cells have been lightly stained with Giemsa. Note that panels b,b' and c,c' have very few grains compared to a and a' and that an increase in membrane concentration (panel a compared to a') increases the labeling of cells.

growth. By autoradiography it is possible to determine the amount of ^{125}I present on the cells as well as that present on plastic. The conclusions from a number of experiments, although still somewhat preliminary, suggest the following: 1) The plasma membranes from 3T3 cells will bind to the cells on the dish, but only a small fraction (less than 2% of added counts) is internalized. 2) Membranes that have been inactivated by heat treatment do not bind and do not block cell growth. 3) High concentrations of serum that compete with the biological activity of the membranes, in the sense that higher concentrations of membranes are needed to produce the same biological activity in the presence of high serum as in low serum, prevent the binding of membranes to the cells (Fig. 3), and 4) At the moment there appears to be a rough correlation between the amount of membrane bound and biological activity. Additional experiments, especially experiments with defined mitogens, will have to be carried out to determine whether, in fact, serum acts in part by preventing the interaction of membranes with cells and, by implication, the interaction of cells with each other. Should this possibility turn out to be correct, it would be a very exciting phenomenon and could be considered analogous to down regulation of hormonal receptors. In this case mitogens would decrease the affinity of receptors on the cell surface that can bind to other cells or membranes, thereby decreasing the effect of cell to cell contact.

It should be pointed out that experiments by Peterson et al [32] have shown that membranes will prevent the mitogenic stimulation of 3T3 cells by the defined mitogen epidermal growth factor using membranes prepared from a 3T3 mutant, which lacks epidermal growth factor receptors. Thus the blockage of the effect of epidermal growth factor cannot simply be due to trapping of this hormone by the membranes. Membranes appear to act in part by down regulating the receptors for epidermal growth factor at the cell surface, and it is attractive to speculate that the converse may also be true — that certain mitogens might decrease the concentration of the cell surface receptors that mediate the binding to other cells. This observation is not without precedence in that several growth factors, notably nerve growth factor and epidermal growth factor, have been shown to alter the adhesive properties of cells [33–35].

As summarized in Table I, all the data obtained to date suggest that the interaction of isolated plasma membranes with cells parallels the biological effects observed at high cell density. It therefore seemed reasonable to proceed to attempt to solubilize the membrane component or components responsible for this action, and this has been accomplished by the use of the detergent octylglucoside [36]. As shown in Figure 4 and Table II [37], the extract basically appears to act in the same way as the membranes, and efforts to purify the components present in this extract are in progress. We conclude from these data that contact inhibition of growth mediated by molecules on the cell surface is one of the important signals that regulates cell growth under culture conditions. Only if the appropriate mole-

TABLE I. Characteristics of Growth Inhibition of 3T3 Cells by Plasma Membranes

1) Concentration is time dependent and reversible.
2) Maximally 50% of cells are arrested in each cell cycle.
3) Cells are arrested in G_1 at a restriction point probably identical to that observed in low serum (G_0).
4) Membranes induce decrease in rate of uptake of α-aminoisobutyric acid and uridine but not of Pi and glucose.
5) The membranes compete with mitogenic factors and serum.
6) Membranes bind to cells and are not extensively internalized.
7) Membrane activity and membrane binding to cells is prevented by mild heat treatment.

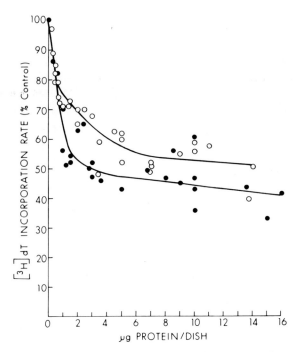

Fig. 4. Effect of an octylglucoside extract of membranes on DNA synthesis. Sparse 3T3 cells were incubated with the indicated concentrations of membranes (●) or an octylglucoside extract of membranes (○) for 24 hours, after which the rate of thymidine incorporation into DNA was measured during a 2-hour pulse with [³H]-dThd as described. Eight separate experiments are included in this figure [37].

TABLE II. Biological Activity of Octylglucoside Extract of 3T3 Plasma Membranes

1) Inhibits DNA synthesis in 3T3 cells in a concentration-dependent manner to a maximum of 50%.
2) Inhibition is reversible.
3) Inhibition of 50% is due to a steady state of cells becoming inhibited and escaping from inhibition.
4) Inhibition can be blocked by high concentrations of serum and other mitogens.
5) Inhibitory activity is heat labile.

cules are purified and their interaction with the cell surface is defined will we be able to get past the current descriptive phase of these investigations. It is important to point out again that the inhibition of growth by contact is *only one* of the signals that control cell growth and that under different conditions cell growth can be controlled by the availability of nutrients or mitogens, as has been discussed in detail by Thrash and Cunningham [17]. This distinction is important to keep in mind when assessing a number of observations in the literature.

Recently a cell surface component [38, 39] has been described which is obtained by urea extraction of cells and which also blocks growth of 3T3 cells. The reversibility of this effect is not known, and the precise portion of the cell cycle in which these cells are arrested has not yet been determined. This surface component is inactivated by incubating cells with UDP-GlcNAc. When we incubate 3T3 cells with UDP-GlcNAc and then isolate from these cells a plasma membrane enriched fraction or an octylglucoside extract of these

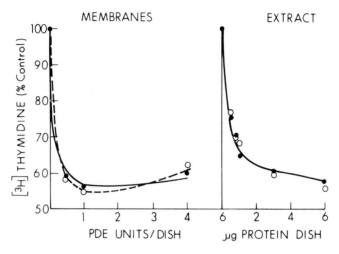

Fig. 5. Effect of UDP-GlcNAc on inhibitory components present in 3T3 membranes. Swiss 3T3 cells were grown to confluence in 1,585 cm² roller bottles. To 2 roller bottles at confluence was added enough sterile UDP-GlcNAc in culture medium to bring the final concentration to 0.5 mM. Controls received an equivalent quantity of medium with no nucleotide addition. After 5 hours a plasma membrane fraction was prepared from these cells and an aliquot of the membrane fraction was extracted with octylglucoside. The enrichment of these membrane fractions for phosphodiesterase was identical in control membranes and those prepared from UDP-GlcNAc-treated cells. Panel A shows the ability of these membranes to inhibit DNA synthesis in 3T3 cells after 24 hours of incubation with cells, and panel B shows similar data for the octylglucoside extract. ●, Control membranes or extract; ○, membranes or extract from cells incubated with UDP-GlcNAc. Note that the membranes and extracts prepared from cells incubated with UDP-GlcNAc give results identical to those observed with control samples.

membranes, their activity is identical to that of control membranes (Fig. 5). Thus the molecules present in the plasma membrane fraction that reversibly inhibit cell growth appear to be different from those obtained by urea extraction.

GROWTH CONTROL OF SCHWANN CELLS

In 1976 Wood and Bunge [9, 10] developed methods for the preparation of dorsal root ganglia from 16-day-old rat embryos free of fibroblasts and containing only neurons and Schwann cells. When these ganglia were maintained in culture these investigators could show that the neurons extended neurites and that Schwann cells would proliferate to ensheath these neurites. When the ganglion somata were removed and the neurites were allowed to degenerate the Schwann cells remained quiescent. Addition of a ganglion (which itself was devoid of any Schwann cells because of a prior treatment with antimitotic agents) to such a culture of quiescent Schwann cells restored their ability to grow and, after a period of several weeks, myelin was formed in relation to the axons growing from the ganglia. It was suggested that this growth control of Schwann cells might be related to contact with the neurites.

We have, therefore, carried out experiments whose design and principle is similar to that used for 3T3 cells [11]. Quiescent Schwann cells, which on 24-hour labeling with [³H]-thymidine show less than one nucleus in 200 labeled with thymidine, were incubated for two days with a membrane fraction prepared from dorsal root ganglia neurites (Fig. 6).

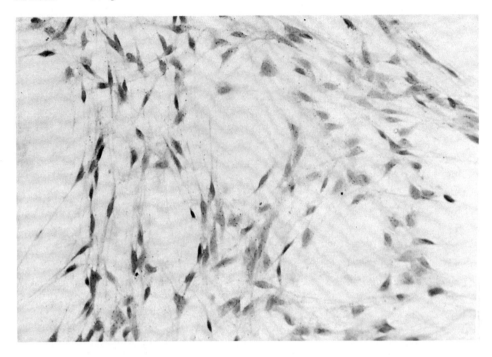

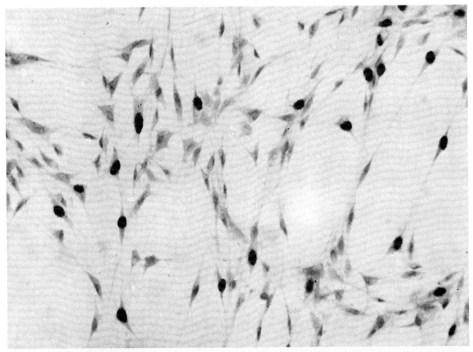

Fig. 6. Mitogenic effect of neurite membranes on Schwann cells. Quiescent Schwann cells [10, 11] were incubated for two successive 24-hour periods with neurite membranes and labeled with [³H]-thymidine for the second 24-hour period followed by autoradiography. Top panel: control cells not incubated with neurites. Bottom panel: cells incubated with neurites. Note presence of labeled nuclei in bottom panel and their absence in top panel. (Labeled nuclei appear black due to high grain density toluidine blue stain; magnification, × 300.)

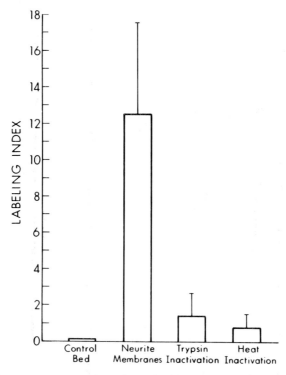

Fig. 7. Effect of various treatments on mitogenic activity of neurite membranes. The bar graph summarizes a series of experiments in which quiescent Schwann cells were incubated either with neurite membranes or with neurite membranes prepared from dorsal root ganglia pretreated with trypsin (0.05% at 34° for 30 or 60 min) before removal of the ganglia and preparation of the neurite membranes. Trypsin was inhibited with trypsin inhibitor at the end of the incubation. Heat-inactivated membranes were prepared by heating neurite membranes at 60° for 10 min. Note that pretreatment of intact ganglion before isolation of neurite membranes abolishes biological activity. Incubation with membranes was for 48 h — in the last 24 hours, in the presence of 1 μC/ml of [³H]-thymidine. Labeling index is the percent of labeled nuclei. Note the very large stimulation of [³H]-thymidine incorporation by Schwann cells incubated with neurite membranes.

Under these conditions, 20% and sometimes up to 30% of the cells can be labeled with thymidine during a 24-hour incubation. Thus the membrane fraction appears to be mitogenic for Schwann cells. A series of control experiments has shown that the relevant ligand appears to be on the surface of the neurite since it is inactivated by a short treatment with external trypsin (Fig. 7) and appears to be absent from the cytoplasmic fraction of the neurites.

This system is one that lacks some of the drawbacks of the 3T3 system discussed previously — namely, the effect of membranes on cells is a positive one; that is, heterologous cell to cell contact stimulates the Schwann cells to enter into S phase. The detection of this positive signal by itself directly excludes any toxic effect that the membranes might have on cells. The system is one that is of considerable biological interest and is highly specific. The membranes prepared from neurites cannot be replaced by a number of mitogenic compounds or with plasma membranes fractions obtained from a variety of other neuronal and non-neuronal cells in tissue culture. The isolation of the neurite membrane components responsible for this effect will require the development of a source of this mitogenic material other than the primary cultures now in use, since they yield insufficient material for successful biochemical characterization of the components.

Schwann cells have also been prepared from sciatic nerve by Raff and coworkers [40–42] and a Schwann cell-containing fraction has been prepared from chick sympathetic ganglia [43, 44]. These Schwann cell preparations show several different properties from the ones that have been used in the experiments summarized above; most notably, they grow, although slowly, in the absence of any neurites or neurite membranes. Their relation to the cells that have been prepared by the method of Wood is not entirely clear. Both cell types will respond to cholera toxin as a mitogen, although cells prepared by the method of Wood do so only weakly. The Schwann cell-enriched fraction of Hanson and Partlow [44] is stimulated to grow by a neuronal homogenate, and the Schwann cells prepared by Raff et al respond to pituitary extracts [40]. It remains for the future to ascertain the relation between these various types of Schwann cells. It should be clear, however, that the response to a surface mitogenic signal derived from neurites and that to an apparently soluble component present in pituitary extracts are not necessarily mutually exclusive phenomena.

Schwann cells can be defined by morphology, antigenicity, presence of S-100, and, most stringently, the ability to myelinate appropriate axons. Not all the available preparations of Schwann cells in culture have been subjected to all the above tests, and cells prepared by different procedures may differ, either because they are derived from different cell populations or because their properties have altered as a result of culture conditions.

GENERAL CONCLUSION

At this time the principal conclusion from this work is that cell to cell contact can have physiological consequences for cells and these can be mimicked by suitably prepared surface membrane fractions. This is clearly only the first step in the elucidation of the chemical components present in membranes responsible for these effects. Systems that respond in this way have clear advantages over systems in which cell to cell adhesion is simply examined as an adhesive phenomenon, not the least of which is that the biological effect represents an amplification of the binding signal that facilitates the assay for specific binding. There are a number of systems more or less well defined in the literature in which it is possible that cell to cell contact also results in biological response such as induction of specific proteins. Two specific examples that come to mind are the induction of S-100 protein at high cell densities, as first described by Pfeiffer et al [45, 46], and another, more recent description of induction of enzymes and transmitter synthesis in pheochromocytoma PC12 [47]. Both of these systems should be amenable to the types of investigation that have been described for 3T3 cells and for Schwann cells. Different systems that appear less amenable to chemical investigation are the formation of junctions between cells, observed in a number of systems, where the formation of the junction clearly must follow cell contact, but where the formation of the junction requires the presence of two living cells [for some recent examples, see references 48–51].

We have not attempted to present in this brief review a comprehensive list of references. A more detailed set of references to work in this field can be found in published papers as well as in two recent comprehensive reviews [41, 52].

ACKNOWLEDGMENTS

This work was supported by grants from NIH, GM 18405, EY 01255 and NSF PCM 77-15972. M. L. is supported by a fellowship from the Damon Runyon-Walter Winchell Fund (DR6-168-F); D. R. by grant GM 07067; J. S. and B. W. by grant GM 02016; M. L. by Damon Runyon Fellowship DRG-168-F. Authors have been listed in alphabetical order.

REFERENCES

1. Shur BD, Roth S: Biochim Biophys Acta 415:473–512, 1975.
2. Marchase RB, Vosbeck K, Roth S: Biochim Biophys Acta 457:385–416, 1976.
3. Pardee AB, Dubrow R, Hamlin J, Kletzien R: Ann Rev Biochem 47:715–750, 1970.
4. Frazier WA, Glaser L: Ann Rev Biochem 48:491–523, 1979.
5. Todaro GJ, Green H, Goldberg BD: Proc Natl Acad Sci USA 51:66–73, 1963.
6. Stoker MGP, Rubin H: Nature 215:171–172, 1967.
7. Dulbecco R: Nature 227:802–806, 1970.
8. Westermark B: Proc Natl Acad Sci USA 74:1619–1621, 1977.
9. Wood PM, Bunge RP: Nature 254:662–664, 1975.
10. Wood PM: Brain Res 115:361–375, 1976.
11. Salzer J, Glaser L, Bunge RM: (in preparation).
12. Holley R, Kiernan J: Proc Natl Acad Sci USA 60:300–304, 1968.
13. Stoker MGP: Nature 246:200–203, 1973.
14. Stoker M, Piggott D: Cell 3:207–215, 1974.
15. Holley RW, Kiernan JA: In Wolstenholme GEW, Knight J (eds): Ciba Found Symp: "Growth Control in Cell Cultures." London: Churchill-Livingstone, 1971, pp 3–15.
16. Whittenberger B, Glaser L: Nature 272:821–823, 1978.
17. Thrash CR, Cunningham DD: J Cell Physiol 86:301–310, 1975.
18. Thomopoulus P, Roth J, Lovelace E, Pastan I: Cell 8:417–423, 1976.
19. Holley RW, Armour R, Baldwin JH, Brown KD, Yeh YC: Proc Natl Acad Sci USA 74:5046–5050, 1977.
20. Santala R, Gottlieb DI, Littman D, Glaser L: J Biol Chem 252:7625–7634, 1977.
21. Obrink B, Kuhlenschmidt MS, Roseman S: Proc Natl Acad Sci USA 74:1077–1081, 1977.
22. McMahon D, Hoffman S, Fry W, West C: In McMahon D, et al (eds): "Developmental Biology Pattern Formation, Gene Regulation." Palo Alto, California: W. H. Benjamin, 1975, pp 60–75.
23. Tuchman J, Smart JE, Lodisch HF: Dev Biol 51:77–85, 1976.
24. Whittenberger B, Glaser L: Proc Natl Acad Sci USA 74:2251–2255, 1977.
25. Whittenberger B, Raben D, Glaser L: J Supramol Struct 10:307–327, 1979.
26. Martz E, Steinberg MS: J Cell Physiol 79:189–210, 1972.
27. Riddle VGH, Rossow PW, Pardee DB: J Cell Biol 79:11a, 1978.
28. Lieberman MA, Raben D, Whittenberger B, Glaser L: J Biol Chem 254:6357–6361, 1979.
29. Barsh GS, Cunningham DD: J Supramol Struct 7:61–77, 1977.
30. Parnes JR, Isselbacher KJ: Prog Exp Tumor Res 22:79–122, 1978.
31. Lever JE: J Cell Physiol 89:779–787, 1976.
32. Peterson SW, Vale R, Das M, Fox CF: J Supramol Struct Suppl 2:126, 1978.
33. Merrell R, Pulliam MW, Randono L, Boyd LF, Bradshaw RA, Glaser L: Proc Natl Acad Sci USA 72:4270–4274, 1975.
34. Schubert D, Whitlock C: Proc Natl Acad Sci USA 74:4055–4058, 1977.
35. Aharonov A, Vladovsky I, Preiss RM, Fox CF, Herschman HR: J Cell Physiol 95:195–202, 1978.
36. Baron C, Thompson TE: Biochim Biophys Acta 382:276–285, 1975.
37. Whittenberger B, Raben D, Lieberman MA, Glaser L: Proc Natl Acad Sci USA 75:5457–5461, 1978.
38. Natraj CV, Datta P: Proc Natl Acad Sci USA 75:3859–3862, 1978.
39. Natraj CV, Datta P: Proc Natl Acad Sci USA 75:6115–6119, 1978.
40. Brockes JP, Fields KF, Raff MC: Nature 266:364–366, 1977.
41. Raff MC, Smith AH, Brockes JF: Nature 273:672–673, 1978.
42. Raff MC, Abney E, Brockes JP, Smith AH: Cell 15:813–822, 1978.
43. McCarthy KD, Partlow LM: Brain Res 114:415–426, 1976.
44. Hanson GR, Partlow LM: Brain Res 159:195–210, 1978.
45. Pfeiffer GE, Herschman HR, Lightbody J, Sato G: J Cell Physiol 75:329–340, 1970.
46. Labourdette S, Mahony JB, Brown IR, Marks A: Eur J Biochem 81:591–597, 1977.
47. Lucas CA, Edgar D, Thoenen H: Exp Cell Res (in press).
48. Pitts JA, Burk RR: Nature 269:762–764, 1977.
49. Griepp EB, Peacock JH, Bernfield MR, Revel JP: Exp Cell Res 113:273–282, 1978.
50. Lawrence TS, Beers WH, Gilula NB: Nature 272:501–506, 1978.
51. Lowenstein WR, Kanno Y, Socolar SJ: Nature 279:133–136, 1978.
52. Glaser L: Rev Physiol Biochem Pharmacol 83:89–122, 1978.

Journal of Supramolecular Structure 11:189—195 (1979)
Tumor Cell Surfaces and Malignancy 135—141

Mitotic Factors From Mammalian Cells: A Preliminary Characterization

Prasad S. Sunkara, David A. Wright, and Potu N. Rao

Departments of Developmental Therapeutics (P.S.S. and P.N.R.) and Biology (D.A.W.), The University of Texas System Cancer Center, M.D. Anderson Hospital and Tumor Institute, Houston, Texas 77030

The objective of this study was the preliminary characterization of the factors from mitotic HeLa cells that can induce meiotic maturation in Xenopus laevis oocytes. We found that this factor is a heat-labile, Ca^{2+}-sensitive, nondialyzable protein with a sedimentation value of 4-5S. Furthermore, no new protein synthesis was found to be required for this mitotic factor to induce maturation in the amphibian oocytes. These data suggest that the factors involved in the breakdown of nuclear membrane and the condensation of chromosomes that are associated with three different phenomena, mitosis, meiosis, and premature chromosome condensation, are very similar in different animal species.

Key words: mitotic factors, oocyte maturation

In amphibians, meiotic maturation of ovarian oocytes involves the breakdown of the germinal vesicle (nucleus), chromosome condensation, and progression through the first meiotic division. This maturation process can be induced either by incubating fully grown oocytes with progesterone or by normal ovulation in vivo [1—5]. Since maturation is not induced when progesterone is injected into the oocyte [6, 7], the existence of a cytoplasmic factor, produced in the oocyte in response to progesterone treatment, has been postulated. Indeed, when cytoplasmic extracts from matured oocytes are injected into immature oocytes they induce maturation [7—9]. Recent reports suggest that maturation-promoting activity (MPA) is present not only in maturing oocytes but also in early cleavage stages of amphibian embryos undergoing synchronous cell division [10]. The MPA appears to fluctuate during the division cycle of the embryonic cells and reaches a peak during mitosis [10]. The factor from the mature oocytes was found to be a heat-labile protein that is magnesium-dependent and calcium-sensitive and exists in three different molecular sizes [9].

Received April 27, 1979; accepted June 29, 1979.

Recently we have shown that extracts of mitotic HeLa cells can induce germinal vesicle breakdown (GVBD) and chromosome condensation in amphibian oocytes, indicating that these factors have no species barriers [11]. Further, we observed a cyclical change in the levels of MPA during the HeLa cell cycle. The MPA was not present in either G_1 or S phase cells. The mitotic factors accumulated slowly in the beginning of G_2 but proceeded at a progressively rapid rate during late G_2 and reached a threshold at the G_2-mitotic transition when the nuclear membrane breaks down and chromatin condenses into chromosomes. The present study is an attempt at preliminary characterization of the mitotic factors from HeLa cells that induce maturation in amphibian oocytes.

MATERIALS AND METHODS

Cells and Cell Synchrony

HeLa cells were grown as spinner cultures at $37°C$ in Eagle's minimal essential medium (MEM) supplemented with nonessential amino acids, heat-inactivated fetal calf serum (10%), sodium pyruvate, glutamine, and penicillin-streptomycin mixture [12]. These cells have a cell cycle time of 22 hours consisting of 10.5 hr of pre-DNA synthetic (G_1) period, 7 hours of of DNA synthetic period, 3.5 hr of post-DNA synthetic (G_2) period and 1.0 hour of mitosis. To obtain mitotic populations, HeLa cells were first partially synchronized by a single TdR block, and then they were incubated at $37°C$ for about 10 hr in a chamber filled with N_2O at a pressure of 80 lb/in^2 (5.36 atm). The rounded and loosely attached mitotic cells were selectively detached by gentle pipetting, which yielded a population with a mitotic index of 98% [13].

Preparation of HeLa Cell Extracts

Extracts of mitotic cells were prepared by suspending cells at a concentration of 20 $\times 10^6$ cells/ml of extraction medium containing 0.2M NaCl, 0.25M sucrose, 0.01M $MgSO_4$, 0.002M EGTA, and 0.01M Na_2HPO_4/NaH_2PO_4, pH 6.5 [9, 11]. In some experiments Ca^{2+}, Mg^{2+}, and EGTA-free buffer was used. Cell extracts were obtained by hand homogenization using a Teflon pestle/glass homogenizer (20 strokes) at $4°C$. The homogenate was centrifuged at 30,000 $\times$ g for 30 min in a refrigerated Sorvall RC5 centrifuge at $4°C$. The supernatants thus obtained were used for the assay of MPA in Xenopus laevis oocytes. Protein concentration in the extracts was determined by the method of Bradford [14] using bovine serum albumin as the standard.

Preparation of Xenopus Oocytes

Oocytes were obtained by surgically removing a portion of the ovaries from X. laevis females. With a small incision that can be closed by a few stitches, multiple harvests of oocytes can be obtained from the same animal. All operations on oocytes were conducted using amphibian Ringer's solution supplemented with $MgCl_2 \cdot 6H_2O$ (0.12 grams/liter). Oocytes were manually dissected from their follicles after pretreatment of the ovarian fragments with collagenase (1 mg/ml) [3].

Assay for Maturation Promoting Activity

Cell extracts were assayed by injecting 65 nl into each oocyte. Injected oocytes were inspected for GVBD after 1 to 3 hr. Germinal vesicle breakdown was detected by a depigmentation of an area of the animal hemisphere [3]. Presence or absence of the germinal vesicle was also determined by dissection of the oocyte. Some oocytes were fixed in Smith's fluid, dehydrated with amylacetate [15], embedded in paraffin, sectioned at 7 μ and stained with Feulgen and fast green [16].

Sucrose Gradient Density Centrifugation

5-ml linear 5–20% sucrose gradients in 10 mM phosphate buffer (pH 6.5) containing 0.002M EGTA were prepared in polyallomer centrifuge tubes. The 100,000 × g supernatants obtained from mitotic cell extracts (0.4 ml) were layered on the gradients and centrifuged at 85,000 × g for 17 hr in a Beckman SW 50.1 rotor at 4°C. The gradients were fractionated into 0.25-ml aliquots using an ISCO microfractionater. Each fraction was used to assay for MPA and protein content. These fractions were also assayed for the presence of mannose phosphate isomerase, malate dehydrogenase, 6 phosphogluconate dehydrogenase, lactate dehydrogenase, and malic enzyme [17], present in HeLa cell extracts, as internal standards for determining the sedimentation profile.

RESULTS

Throughout this study either whole or subfractions of the mitotic extracts were assayed for their MPA as indicated by GVBD and chromosome condensation in Xenopus oocytes. The results of this study indicate that maturation could be induced in 100% of the oocytes injected with the mitotic extracts. In some of the oocytes we could clearly see the first polar body (Fig. 1).

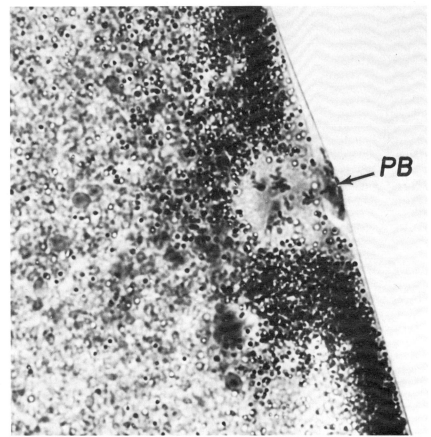

Fig. 1. Germinal vesicle breakdown and chromosome condensation in Xenopus laevis oocyte 4 hr after injection with HeLa cell mitotic extract (65 nl containing a total of 221 ng protein). Oocyte fixed in Smiths fluid; sections stained with Feulgen-fast green. Magnification approximately 1,320×. Note the presence of first polar body (PB) between plasma membrane of the egg and the vitelline membrane. The condensed chromosomes of the oocyte are located on the spindle of the arrested second meiotic division in the region relatively clear of pigment granules.

Nature of Mitotic Factors

Incubation of freshly prepared mitotic extracts (7 mg/ml) with RNase (1.5 units/ml) at 25°C for 1 hr had no effect on the MPA (Table I). However, a similar treatment with protease (subtilopeptidase-A from B. subtilis)(0.2 units/ml) reduced this activity to 18% as compared to 100% in untreated extract. Neither RNase nor protease at the concentrations tested showed any toxic effects on the oocytes. These enzymes per se were unable to induce GVBD.

Effect of Cycloheximide on Maturation Promoting Activity of Mitotic Factors

Oocytes were incubated for 1 hr in Ringer's solution containing cycloheximide at a concentration (20 μg/ml) known to inhibit protein synthesis in amphibian oocytes [18]. These oocytes were then injected with mitotic extracts (7 mg/ml) and further incubated for 2 hr with cycloheximide (20 μg/ml). The data shown in Table II indicate that the MPA induced by the mitotic factors is not dependent on new protein synthesis.

Effect of Ca^{2+} and Mg^{2+} on Maturation Promoting Activity of the Mitotic Factors

The MPA of the mitotic factors, which was highly sensitive to Ca^{2+} (1 mM), was unaffected by Mg^{2+} even at relatively high concentrations (10 mM) (Table III).

TABLE I. Effect of RNase and Protease Treatments on the Maturation Promoting Activity of Mitotic Cell Extracts

Substance injected	No. of oocytes injected	No. showing GVBD	% GVBD
Mitotic extracts	11	11	100
RNase (1.5 units/ml) alone	11	0	0
Mitotic extracts treated with RNase (1.5 units/ml)	5	5	100
Protease (0.2 units/ml) alone	11	0	0
Mitotic extracts treated with protease (0.2 units/ml)	11	2	18

Freshly prepared mitotic extracts (7 mg of protein/ml) were incubated with either RNase or protease at 25°C for 1 hr. At the end of incubation, 65 nl of the treated extracts were injected into each oocyte.

TABLE II. Maturation Promoting Activity of Mitotic Cell Extracts in Cycloheximide-Treated Oocytes

Treatment	No. of oocytes	No. showing GVBD	% GVBD
Injected with mitotic extract	11	11	100
Incubated with cycloheximide (20 μg/ml) alone	8	0	0
Mitotic extracts injected into cycloheximide-treated oocytes	12	12	100

Oocytes were incubated with cycloheximide (20 μg/ml) for 1 hr prior to injection. After injection of the mitotic extract, oocytes were further inucbated with cycloheximide for another 1.75 hr at which time they were scored for GVBD.

Heat-Sensitivity of the Mitotic Factors

Incubation of the mitotic extract at 40°C for 10 min had no significant effect on its MPA (Table IV). However, a 10-min incubation at 50°C or higher resulted in a rapid loss of this activity as evidenced by the decrease in the frequency of GVBD. Extracts incubated at 60° and 100°C did show some precipitate upon centrifugation. On the other hand heat treatment of the extract at 50°C did not give any precipitate upon centrifugation but showed a rapid loss of activity ruling out the possibility of mitotic factor being entrapped in the precipitated material.

Effect of Dialysis and pH of the Extraction Medium on the Activity of the Mitotic Factors

The MPA of the mitotic extracts was not affected by dialysing it against extraction medium of different pH's (Table V). However, the activity of the extract was lost when dialized against extraction medium with a pH of 8.0.

TABLE III. Effect of Ca^{2+} and Mg^{2+} on Maturation Promoting Activity of Mitotic Cell Extracts

Oocytes injected with	No. of oocytes injected	No. of oocytes showing GVBD	% GVBD
Ca^{2+} and Mg^{2+} - free buffer (CMF buffer)	7	0	0
Mitotic extract in CMF buffer	9	8	89
Mitotic extract in CMF buffer +1 mM Mg^{2+}	8	7	88
Mitotic extract in CMF buffer +2.5 mM Mg^{2+}	8	8	100
Mitotic extract in CMF +10 mM Mg^{2+}	13	13	100
Mitotic extract in CMF buffer +1 mM Ca^{2+}	10	0	0

A total volume of 65 nl of extracts made from 20×10^6 cells/ml (7 mg of protein/ml) was injected into each oocyte.

TABLE IV. Effect of Temperature on the Maturation Promoting Activity of Mitotic Cell Extracts

Temperature	No. of oocytes injected	No. of oocytes showing GVBD	% GVBD
0°C	10	9	90
40°C	12	10	83
50°C	12	1	8.3
60°C	6	0	0
100°C	6	0	0

Freshly prepared mitotic extracts were incubated at different temperatures for 10 min. At the end of incubation, extracts were centrifuged at $30,000 \times g$ at 4°C to remove the precipitate. A total volume of 65 nl of the supernatant was injected into each oocyte.

Preliminary Characterization of the Mitotic Factors

In order to determine the molecular size of the factors that possess the MPA, the mitotic extract was centrifuged on linear sucrose density gradients (5–20%) and the various fractions collected were assayed for activity. Activity was observed in a single distinct peak (Fig. 2). The sedimentation value of this fraction was estimated to be about 4-5S.

TABLE V. Effect of pH of the Extraction Medium on the Maturation Promoting Activity of Mitotic Cell Extracts

pH of dialysis buffer	No. of oocytes injected	No. showing GVBD	% GVBD
Undialyzed	10	10	100
6.5	10	10	100
7.0	10	10	100
7.5	10	10	100
8.0	10	1	10

Mitotic extracts were dialyzed overnight against buffers of different pH and 65 nl of the dialyzed extracts were injected into each oocyte. The oocytes were examined for GVBD at 1.75 hr after the injection.

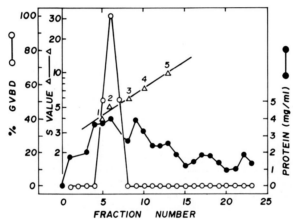

Fig. 2. Separation of mitotic factors on sucrose gradients. Mitotic extract (0.4 ml; 15 mg/ml) was layered on 5 ml linear sucrose gradient (5–20%) and spun at 85,000 X g for 17 hr in a Beckman SW50-1 rotor. The fractions were collected from the top by a fraction collector. Each of these fractions was assayed for maturation promoting activity and for the presence of (1) mannose phosphate isomerase (3.9S), (2) malate dehydrogenase (5S), (3) 6 phosphogluconate dehydrogenase (6S), (4) lactate dehydrogenase (7.3S), and (5) malic enzyme (10S) as internal standards.

DISCUSSION

The results of this study suggest that the factors from mitotic HeLa cells that can induce GVBD and chromosome condensation in Xenopus oocytes are heat-labile, nondialyzable and Ca^{2+}-sensitive proteins. It was also found that synthesis of new proteins was not required for the induction of maturation by the mitotic factors. Furthermore, the MPA appears to reside in a protein of a single molecular size of 4-5S.

The characteristics of the mitotic factors from HeLa cells appear to be similar to those of the maturation promoting factors isolated from the cytoplasms of mature amphibian oocytes, which were also found to be heat-labile and Ca^{2+}-sensitive proteins [9]. Unlike the mitotic factor that has a single molecular size (4-5S), the factor from the oocytes have three different forms, 4S, 15S and 32S [9].

The present study further confirms our earlier observation [11] that factors involved in the breakdown of the nuclear membrane and the condensation of chromosomes, which are associated with three different phenomena, mitotis, meiosis, and premature chromosome condensation, appear to be very similar if not identical in different animal species. Whether this particular factor (4-5S protein) from the mitotic cells, which induces maturation in amphibian oocytes, can also induce premature chromosome condensation in mammalian cells remains to be tested.

ACKNOWLEDGMENTS

We thank Dr. C.G. Shasrabuddhe for his help with the sucrose gradients. This investigation was supported by grants CA-11520, CA-14528, CA-23878 from the National Cancer Institute and GM-23252 from the Institute of General Medical Sciences, DHEW.

REFERENCES

1. Masui Y: J Exp Zool 166:365, 1967.
2. Subtelny S, Smith LD, Ecker RE: J Exp Zool 168:39, 1968.
3. Merriam RW: J Exp Zool 180:421, 1972.
4. Wasserman WJ, Masui Y: Biol Reprod 11:133, 1974.
5. Dettlaff T, Nikitina LA, Stoeva OG: J Embryol Exp Morphol 12:851, 1964.
6. Masui Y, Markert CL: J Exp Zool 177:129, 1971.
7. Smith LD, Ecker RE: Dev Biol 25:233, 1971.
8. Drury KC, Schorderet-Slatkine S: Cell 4:269, 1975.
9. Wasserman WJ, Masui Y: Science 191:1266, 1976.
10. Wasserman WJ, Smith LD: J Cell Biol R 15, 1978.
11. Sunkara PS, Wright DA, Rao PN: Proc Natl Acad Sci USA 76:2799, 1979.
12. Rao PN, Engelberg J: Science 148:1092, 1965.
13. Rao PN: Science 160:774, 1968.
14. Bradford MM: Ann Biochem 72:248, 1976.
15. Drury HF: Stain Technol 16:21, 1941.
16. Subtelny S, Bradt C: J Morphol 112:45, 1963.
17. Sicilaino MJ, Shaw CR: In Smith I (ed): "Chromatographic and Electrophoretic Techniques." London: Heinemann, Volar, pp 185–209, 1976.
18. Wasserman W, Masui Y: Exp Cell Res 91:381, 1975.

Journal of Supramolecular Structure 11:197–205 (1979)
Tumor Cell Surfaces and Malignancy 143–151

Pyrimidine Biosynthesis in Normal and Transformed Cells

Mayo Uziel and James Selkirk

Biology Division, Oak Ridge National Laboratory, Oak Ridge, Tennessee 37830

We have developed procedures for sensitive measurement of specific radio-activities of pyrimidine nucleosides excreted from cells in culture. The changes in the observed values reflect dilution of the added isotope through de novo biosynthesis of nonradioactive pyrimidine nucleosides or by shifting and equilibration of other nucleotide pools into the free uridine pool. It is thus possible to monitor uridine biosynthesis occurring in intact cells without destroying or disrupting the cell population. On comparing a series of normal and transformed lines, we have observed several growth-dependent patterns of change in specific activity and levels of uridine excretion and the temporal appearance of these changes.

Hamster embyro fibroblasts slows pyrimidine biosynthesis at mid-growth while the hamster cell line V79 continues to dilute the pyrimidine pool at about 7% of the rate observed during exponential growth at confluence. Both cells exhibit Urd excretion beginning at one-half maximal growth.

Passageable normal rat liver cells (IARC-20) also show a cessation of pyrimidine biosynthesis with a prior increase in uridine excretion. Two chemically transformed lines IARC-28 and IARC-19 derived from IARC-20 show different patterns. IARC-19 begins uridine excretion in early log growth and the specific activity continues to decrease at about 2% of the rate observed during exponential growth at confluence. The IARC-28 cells also begin excretion in early log growth but pyrimidine biosynthesis stops at about midlog. This method may prove to be an additional aid in recognizing and differentiating transformed cells in culture that do not exhibit the transformed phenotype.

Key words: pyrimidine biosynthesis, V79, IARC19, IARC20, IARC28, biomarker, pleiotropy, confluence, rat liver epithelial cells

We have recently discovered uridine and cytidine to be normal excretion products of cells in culture and the excretion process is regulated so that the maximal rate of excretion occurs as the cells enter G_1/G_0 [1]. The excretion of uracil and deoxynucleosides is also known to occur in fibroblast cultures, especially with mutants blocked in a utilization step [2]. It would appear that the processes leading to the normal excretion of these compounds is related to the balance of salvage and de novo synthetic pathways.

Received April 23, 1979; accepted July 2, 1979.

The balance between salvage and de novo biosynthetic pathways in growing cells is regulated by several phenomena including the concentration of base or nucleoside in the medium [3, 4]. For example, the presence of Urd in culture of HTC cells can introduce a repression of Urd synthesis that requires new RNA and protein synthesis for derepression [3]. On the other hand, studies of key enzymes in the biosynthetic pathway of normal and transformed cells have shown certain key enzymes to increase in malignantly transformed cells [5]. Pyrimidine biosynthesis is one of these pleiotropic manifestations along with increased utilization of UDP and its derivatives and decreased rates of catabolism of uracil and thymine [5].

The normal presence of nucleosides in the medium provides a unique opportunity to continuously monitor biosynthesis and excretion of uridine. Using recently developed techniques for affinity chromatography and sensitive analysis of nucleosides in culture, we have examined sets of fibroblastic and epithelial cells to see if we could detect the transformation dependent pleiotropic effects on pyrimidine biosynthesis and salvage.

MATERIALS AND METHODS

Growth of Cells

Syrian hamster embryo fibroblasts obtained from Charles River Farms were grown in DMEM supplemented with 0.45% glucose and 10% FCS in 8.5% CO_2 at 37°C and 98% R.H. [1]. The cells grew synchronously in tertiary subculture when confluent secondary cells (seeded at 2×10^6 cells per 100 mm dish and grown for 72 hrs) were suspended at 200,000 per ml in the medium and 10 ml added to each 100 mm plate. The V79, IARC-20, IARC-19, and IARC-28 lines were grown in William's medium according to Montesano [6]. See the figure legends for plating data. Cells were counted with a hemocytometer or a cytofluorograph. These cell lines were routinely checked for PPLO and found negative.

Radioactive Labeling

Either 2-[^{14}C]Urd (58 μCi/μmol, Schwartz/Mann) or 6-[^{3}H]Urd (20 ci/mmol, New England Nuclear) were used as the radioactive tracers. The label was diluted in fresh medium so that 1 ml of medium contained the correct amount of tracer. This was added to the cells 7 hrs after seeding. See figure legends for the amount of radioactivity added.

All samples were counted by adding 3 ml of scintillation fluid to 0.2 ml of aqueous sample. All samples were counted in a Beckman LS250 for 10 minutes.

Uridine Isolation and Analysis

Two ml of medium was processed as described in [7]. The nucleoside, adsorbed to 2 ml of the affinity column were collected by elution with 30 ml acetic acid and then lyophilized. The residue was dissolved in about 1 ml of water and transferred to conical test tubes and lyophilized again. The residue was dissolved in 0.2 ml of the initial chromatographic solvent (1.5% v/v acetonitrile 0.03 M NH_4 phosphate pH 5.1). The analyses were done with a Water's C18 ODS μBondpak column at a flow rate of 0.67 ml/min at room temperature [1]. The fractions (0.22 ml) 11 to 60 were counted for radioactivity. The solvent was changed to 20% acetonitrile at 15 min to cleanse the column and returned to the original solvent at 35 min for reequilibration. Uridine eluted at 12.3 min (8.25 ml) with this system.

The amount of uridine was measured by comparison of the peak height to standards. We routinely analyze at least 250 pmoles based on absorbancy measurements and usually

1,000 pmoles so the outer range of precision is ± 10%. The error range is very close to the symbol size on the exponential plot. The sensitivity of the assay is 25 pmoles for a peak height of 0.0008 A at 254 nm. The absorbance (A) was measured continuously with an LDC monitor (1 cm light path 8 μl cell volume) using a recorder span of 0.08 or 0.02 depending on the amount of uridine in the sample.

RESULTS

Pyrimidine Metabolism in Hamster Cells

Figure 1 shows the excretion properties of synchronized III° HEF grown to confluence and then stimulated to grow again by replacement of the culture fluid with fresh medium. The specific activity of uridine in the medium decreases exponentially as it equilibrates with the endogenous pools and newly synthesized uridine. At 46 hr, the cell number is 1/2 the cell number at confluence and the specific activity of the excreted uridine becomes constant. The excretion of uridine appears to have begun earlier, between 30 and 40 hr post seeding as the cells were in G_2 phase. At 72 hr the medium was replaced and a burst of cell growth occurred accompanied by an additional decrease in uridine specific activity due to additional biosynthesis of uridine. The specific activity becomes constant after the additional growth. The number of cells increase by 41% and the specific activity decreased from the level before changing the medium. The endogenous uridine in the medium contributes less than 5% to this change. The rate of isotope dilution decreases from 4 per hr in exponential growth to zero in the G_1/G_0 state.

Figure 2 illustrates the change in uridine concentration and specific activity in cultures of V79. The excretion process begins during exponential growth approximately two generations before the cells reach a maximum number. The cells continuously take up the external uridine during early log growth until a minimum is reached at about 40 hr after seeding. The specific activity continues to decrease throughout the incubation period at a rate of 3 per hr during exponential growth to 0.5 per hr at about 1/2 maximal growth to 0.1 per hr when growth ends.

Pyrimidine Metabolism in Liver Epithelial Cells

Montesano [6] has observed these cells to be morphologically indistinguishable from the normal phenotype and will not overgrow at confluence. These IARC cells, however, show metabolic differences between the normal and transformed phenotype. IARC-20, a passageable epithelial cell line derived from normal rat liver grows to confluence with uridine excretion beginning at about 1/2 maximum cell number (Fig. 3) as with the hamster embryo fibroblasts. In contrast to the HEF, the specific activity becomes constant at a time closer to confluence. The rate of isotope dilution goes from a value of 15 in early log to zero at confluence.

IARC-19, a malignantly transformed line, shows density inhibited growth and the culture appearance is very similar to the IARC-20 line (Fig. 4). The excretion of uridine however begins about 3 generation times prior to confluence and the specific activity continues to decrease from a rate of 4 per hr during exponential growth to a value of 0.06 per hr at maximum cell number.

IARC-20 also shows early changes in excretion (about 4 generation times before confluence) (Fig. 5) but the specific activity change becomes zero at about 1/2 maximum growth. The appearance of the culture is again not strikingly different than the normal cell population.

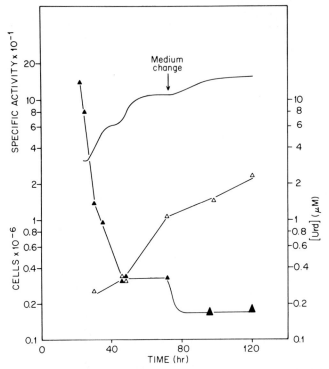

Fig. 1. Metabolism of uridine in synchronous growing hamster embryo fibroblasts. The cells were plated at 200,000 per ml from dilute suspension of 3-day-old, confluent, II° hamster embryo fibroblasts. After 7 hr the medium was replaced with fresh medium, 0.02 μCi/ml Urd was added to 0.4 μM and left for continuous labeling. At the times indicated duplicate cell counts were made in the cytofluorograph; the medium was collected and analyzed for uridine concentration and specific activity. Cell counts ———; uridine concentration — △ —; uridine specific activity — ▲ —. The medium was changed at 72 hr.

DISCUSSION

We have presented two examples of phenotypic variation of pyrimidine biosynthesis and excretion when comparing morphologically similar normal and transformed cell lines of fibroblasts and epithelial cells that do not exhibit overgrowth. There was no predictable form to the variation except that there was a difference in one or both properties when comparing the normal and transformed lines. V79 is a rapidly growing fibroblastic line obtained from normal hamster lung that can produce tumors in nude mice [E. Huberman, personal communication]. The putative normal counterpart is the 3rd subculture of hamster embryo fibroblasts. Of the parameters measured, only the specific activity change differs between these fibroblastic cells and that continues to decrease in the V79 cells. Considering the net synthesis of RNA that occurred, the time period, and the rate of isotope dilution in the culture, the continued decrease can arise only from a continued de novo synthesis of uridine.

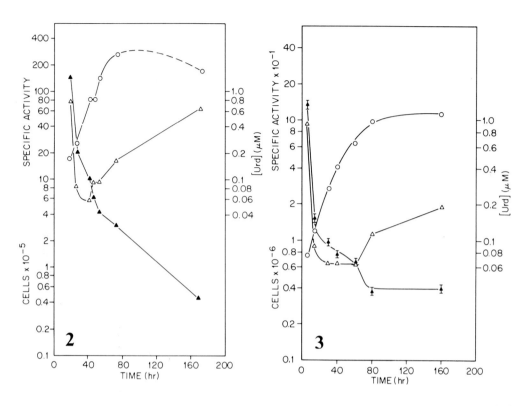

Fig. 2. Pyrimidine metabolism in V79 cells. Freshly confluent cells were collected with trypsin and seeded at 2×10^6 cells per 100 mm dish. After 7 hr the medium was replaced with fresh medium containing 0.1 μCi/ml of 0.1 μM uridine. At the indicated times the medium was collected and the cells counted. The culture fluid was analyzed for uridine concentration and specific activity. Uridine concentration —— △ ——; uridine specific activity —— ▲ ——; and cell count —— ○ ——.

Fig. 3. Pyrimidine metabolism in IARC-20 cells. Freshly confluent cells were collected with trypsin and seeded at 1×10^5 cells per 100 mm dish. After 7 hr the medium was replaced with fresh medium containing 0.1 μCi/ml of 0.1 μM uridine. At the indicated times the medium was collected and the cells counted. The culture fluid was analyzed for uridine concentration and specific activity. Uridine concentration —— △ ——; uridine specific activity —— ▲ ——; and cell count —— ○ ——.

The malignantly transformed IARC lines show a more complex set of changes. IARC-19 differs from the normal IARC-20 cells in two ways: continued de novo synthesis at confluence while the control specific activity becomes constant and, a much earlier appearance of the excretion process; 20% of maximum cell growth compared to 70% of maximum cell growth in IARC-20. IARC-28 shows a difference only in the early appearance of uridine excretion at 10% maximum cell growth. At confluence de novo synthesis ends as with IARC-20. Because of potential phenotype variations it is probably better to compare cells from a common parental line. For example, the liver-derived normal epithelial line ends biosynthesis near confluence rather than at 1/2 maximum growth.

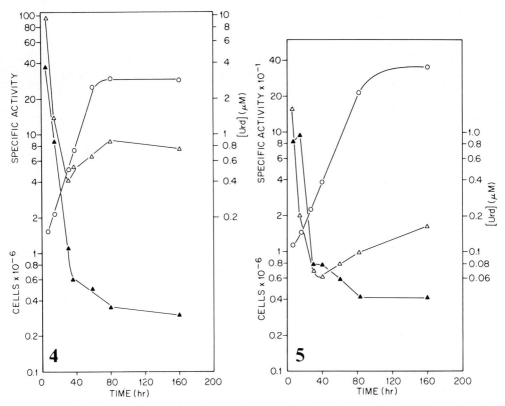

Fig. 4. Pyrimidine metabolism in IARC-19 cells. Freshly confluent cells were collected with trypsin and seeded at 1×10^5 cells per 100 mm dish. After 7 hr the medium was replaced with fresh medium containing 0.1 μCi/ml of 0.1 μM uridine. At the indicated times the medium was collected and the cells counted. The culture fluid was analyzed for uridine concentration and specific activity. Uridine concentration — $\triangle$ —; uridine specific activity — $\blacktriangle$ —; and cell count — $\circ$ —.

Fig. 5. Pyrimidine metabolism in IARC-28 cells. Freshly confluent cells were collected with trypsin and seeded at 1×10^5 cells per 100 mm dish. After 7 hr the medium was replaced with fresh medium containing 0.1 μCi/ml of 0.1 μM uridine. At the indicated times the medium was collected and the cells counted. The culture fluid was analyzed for uridine concentration and specific activity. Uridine concentration — $\triangle$ —; uridine specific activity — $\blacktriangle$ —; and cell count — $\circ$ —.

The above comparisons are useful at this time primarily to illustrate that different metabolic phenotypes can be observed independent of morphological growth characteristics. The value of this system as a marker for malignant transformation will depend on many more examples where the normal and transformed cells are derived from the same cell population also under well-controlled conditions of growth.

The prospects for this type of data to become a biomarker for carcinogenesis are based on Weber's extensive studies of malignancy-linked biochemical processes [5]. Pyrimidine biosynthesis is one of several metabolic systems that expresses a class I biochemical imbalance, ie, malignancy linked. The pleiotropic mainfestations of the biochemical imbalance include increased rates of de novo synthesis of UMP and deoxynucleotides coupled with a decreased level of catabolic enzymes. This environment in the malignant cell would be expected to minimize loss of Urd from the cell and increase the biosynthetic capacity to form pyrimidine nucleotides. Our observations are consistent with this model however, we have observed the changes in concentration and time of appearance of uridine in the medium not to be predictable based on the normal or transformed phenotype. The fibroblasts excrete almost 10 times more uridine than the liver epithelial cells at comparable growth states (see uridine concentration at confluence Figs. 1–5) while the level of excretion from the transformed cells can be the same or different than the normal counterpart (Figs. 3–5). The time when excretion begins can vary from 10% to 50% of maximum cell number. The absence of predictable change reflects the complexity of the overall metabolic balance for each cell type and the lack of specific knowledge concerning the events regulating excretion.

The excretion and specific activity changes reflect different aspects of the metabolic pathways described in Fig. 6. The amount of Urd in the medium will depend on several kinetic processes: 1) the balance of influx and efflux; 2) the rate of intracellular Urd formation; and/or 3) the appearance of new enzyme systems that would favor release of Urd from the cell. Thus, compartmentalization could contribute to the rate of Urd excretion, and to the observed specific activity. Whether or not the excretion process per se can alter observed specific activities will depend on both the size and specific activity of the presumed compartment. The fact that the different cell populations show a variable time for appearance of the excretion products would suggest that the excretion process and de novo synthesis are not necessarily coordinately linked.

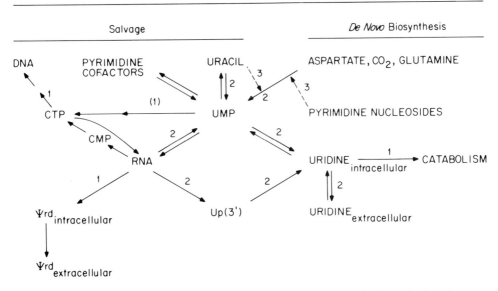

DILUTION OF ISOTOPE IN CULTURE RESULTS IN VARIABLE SPECIFIC ACTIVITIES DEPENDING ON THE PRESENCE OF ACTIVE PATHWAYS, POOL EQUILIBRATION TIME AND CONCENTRATION OF ENDOGENOUS COMPOUNDS

Fig. 6. Summary of uridine metabolism. The several sources of salvage and the biosynthetic pathways are illustrated. The dotted lines indicate regulatory blocks and the putative inducer. The numbers refer to the utilization of uridine. 1. Irreversible loss of uridine through conversion. The parenthesis indicates the process may not be complete. 2. Sources of metabolism dependent isotope dilution. 3. Regulation of biosynthesis.

The specific activity measurement is a function of the several variables illustrated in Fig. 7. These are kinetic factors, reflecting the rate of equilibration of the various pools, and quantitative limits, determined by the total amount of the endogenous pools (which are generally low due to overall cell growth of a factor of 10 or more), the amount of catabolism to non-Urd derivatives and the increase in Urd by de novo synthesis. The initial specific activity will be determined by the input label plus any endogenous Urd (Fig. 7). The subsequent changes will reflect equilibration with RNA breakdown products, uridylate derivatives, and endogenous uracil derived from ribo- and deoxy-ribonucleosides. The ultimate value for the specific activity of uridine will then be determined by the size of the endogenous pool, compartmentalization, the amount of de novo synthesis and irreversible losses of Urd through modification (eg, to pseudo-uridine) and other metabolic end products if these processes are not continuous through the cell cycle. The specific activity can thus become constant under one of the two conditions, compensating input of a high specific activity compartment and de novo synthesis — an unlikely prospect considering the time factors — or a cessation of de novo biosynthesis. However, in those times when the specific activity is changing there is little doubt that compartment shifts are occurring as well as dilution by de novo synthesis. The latter is known to occur in the hamster embryo fibroblasts (Uziel and Selkirk, unpublished results), in addition, the amount of the enzymes for de novo biosynthesis of pyrimidines has been observed to reach a maximum during S and then falls to a very low values at mitosis in 3T3 and HTC cells [4] which is consistent with the observed end to de novo synthesis at confluence in the hamster embryo fibroblasts and the liver cell lines.

Several parameters associated with uridine excretion have been shown to vary on comparaing normal and transformed cell populations. These include the changes in concentration of uridine in the medium, the specific activity changes and the temporal relationship of these measurements to the cell cycle and growth stage. The correlation of these events to the appearance of a new homeostatis in the transformed cells is still speculative; however, de novo biosynthesis can be monitored by measuring the specific activity of extracellular uridine. The prediction of the direction and extent of change in specific activity is not yet possible without prior specific knowledge on the levels key enzymes. On the other hand, with the use of selected substrates such as orotic acid, the empirical observations may be used to describe the intracellular state of some of the key enzymes. This latter approach may provide a basis for nondestructive (cell) assessment of transformation-dependent change in homeostatis.

$$\text{SPECIFIC ACTIVITY:} \quad \frac{C_i \text{ (URIDINE)}}{\left[\text{Moles (Urd}_{\text{LABEL}} + \text{Urd}_{\text{ENDOGENOUS (MEDIUM)}} + \text{Urd}_{\text{(SALVAGE)}} + \text{Urd}_{\text{(DE NOVO BIOSYNTHETIC)}}\right]}$$

VARIABLES: A) RATE OF BIOSYNTHESIS; RATE OF RNA TURNOVER

B) CATABOLISM WILL BECOME A VARIABLE IF THE BREAKDOWN IS COMPARTMENTALIZED.

Fig. 7. Specific activity measurements. The calculation of specific activity depends on four major compartments. Two are invariant, the original label and endogenous uridine. One is variant with a fixed limit, the pool of uridine derivatives initially present in the cells. And one compartment is variant depending upon the regulatory processes operating on de novo biosynthesis.

ACKNOWLEDGMENTS

We thank K. Dearstone and A.J. Bandy for their technical assistance. The V79 cells were obtained from E. Huberman of the Biology Division, ORNL. We thank R. Montesano for the several IARC cell lines.

Research sponsored by the Office of Health and Environmental Research, U.S. Department of Energy (Contract No. 40-740-78), under contract W-7405-eng-26 with the Union Carbide Corporation and the Environmental Protection Agency (Contract No. 79-D-XO533).

REFERENCES

1. Uziel M, Selkirk JK: J Cell Physiol 99:217, 1979.
2. Chan TS, Meuth M, Green H: J Cell Physiol 83:263, 1974.
3. Hoogenrad NJ, Lee DC: J Biol Chem 249:2763, 1974.
4. Mitchell AD, Hoogenrad NJ: Exp Cell Res 93:105, 1975.
5. Weber G, Prajda N, Williams JC: In Davis W, Maltoni C (eds): "Advance in Tumor Prevention, Detection and Characterization, Vol 3." 1976.
6. Montesano R, Vincent LS, Drevon C, Tomatis L: Int J Cancer 16:550, 1975.
7. Uziel M, Smith LH, Taylor S: Clin Chem 22:1451, 1976.

Journal of Supramolecular Structure 11:207–216 (1979)
Tumor Cell Surfaces and Malignancy 153–162

Growth of Kidney Epithelial Cells in Hormone-Supplemented, Serum-Free Medium

Mary Taub and Gordon H. Sato

Department of Biology, University of California, San Diego, La Jolla, California 92093

Madin Darby canine kidney cells can grow in synthetic medium supplemented with 5 factors – insulin, transferrin, prostaglandin E_1, hydrocortisone and tri-iodothyronine – as a serum substitute. These 5 factors permit growth for one month in the absence of serum, and a growth rate equivalent to that observed in serum-supplemented medium. Dibutyryl cAMP substitutes for prostaglandin E_1 in the medium, suggesting that increased growth of Maden Darby canine kidney cells results from increased intracellular cAMP. Potential applications of the serum-free medium are discussed. The medium permits the selective growth of primary epithelial cell cultures in the absence of fibroblast over-growth, and a defined analysis of the mechanisms by which hormones regulate hemicyst formation.

Key words: renal epithelium, primary cultures, prostaglandins, mammalian cell growth

Hormones are important regulators of kidney epithelial cell growth and function in vivo. They play an important role in regulating transepithelial solute transport by renal tubule cells [1], and have been implicated in regulating kidney growth during development [1, 2] and in response to injury [2]. However, studies concerning the mechanisms by which hormones affect these processes have been difficult because of the complex structure of the kidney.

Cultured kidney epithelial cells provide convenient systems to study hormonal regulation of kidney functions. The Madin Darby canine kidney cell line (MDCK) for example, functions in culture like tubular epithelial cells [3–5]. At confluency MDCK cells form multicellular hemicysts (groups of cells slightly raised from the tissue culture dish surface) [3]; hemicyst formation has been attributed to the transport of salt and water from the mucosal surface of the cells (facing the culture medium) through the serosal surface of the cells (facing the dish surface) [4]. The tubule segment from which MDCK cells are derived was not identified. However, the MDCK cell line responds to

Received April 25, 1979; accepted July 6, 1979.

arginine vasopressin by producing cAMP [6]. The latter response is distinctive of distal tubule cells.

Other kidney epithelial cell lines are also available, which form hemicysts, including monkey kidney (LLC-MK$_2$) and bovine kidney (MDBK) cells [8]. However, the available lines are relatively "leaky" epithelia [4, 5], as the transepithelial potential generated by such cells is low [4, 5]. As a consequence the utility of such cell lines for studies concerning transepithelial solute flux is limited. Thus the development of additional culture systems of kidney epithelial cells, and hormone-supplemented, serum-free media may prove to be an important tool towards these ends.

Previously, serum in tissue culture medium has impeded studies concerning the regulation of animal cell growth and differentiated function in vitro by hormones. However, Sato and coworkers have demonstrated that serum can be replaced as a growth requiring supplement by specific hormones and accessory factors, which differ according to cell type [9–11]. This paper reports the long-term growth of MDCK cells in a serum-free culture medium supplemented with insulin, transferrin, PGE$_1$, hydrocortisone, and triiodothyronine (T$_3$). These 5 components are the minimal number required to attain the growth rate observed in serum-supplemented medium [12]. The utilization of the medium to support the growth of primary kidney epithelial cell cultures, as well as established kidney lines has been demonstrated. The medium should also prove useful to study regulation of vectorial solute transport processes in cultured kidney cells.

MATERIALS AND METHODS

Cells and Maintenance

The canine kidney epithelial cell line MDCK [3] was obtained from Dr. John Holland at the University of California at San Diego. Stock cultures were routinely incubated in a humidified 5% CO$_2$/95% air mixture at 37°C; the growth medium for stock cultures was a 50:50 mixture of Dulbecco's Modified Eagle's Medium (DME) and Ham's F12 Medium supplemented with 5% horse serum and 2.5% fetal calf serum. Serum-free growth experiments were also conducted using a 50:50 mixture of DME and F12(SF-DME/F12) based upon the observation that the growth rate of MDCK cells in serum-free DME/F12 supplemented with 5 μg/ml insulin and 5 μg/ml transferrin was maximal when using this combination of the two media. All media were supplemented with 10 mM N-2-hydroxypiperazine-N'-2-ethane-sulfonic acid (HEPES), sodium bicarbonate at 1.1 mg/ml, 92 IU/ml penicillin, 200 μg/ml streptomycin, 25 μg/ml ampicillin, and 10^{-8}M selenium. Triple-distilled water was used for medium preparation.

To initiate primary kidney cultures, the kidneys from 10-day-old mice (Balb/c) were minced into 1 mm diameter pieces. Kidney cell suspensions were prepared from the mince following the method of Leffert and Paul [13] with the modification that the cells were incubated in a 0.3% EDTA, 0.1% trypsin solution containing 1 mg/ml collagenase (Worthington) and 0.1% soybean trypsin inhibitor. Prior to use, cells were pelleted by centrifugation and resuspended in SF-DME/F12.

Cell Growth and Plating Efficiency

Logarithmically growing MDCK cells were trypsinized using a 0.3% EDTA, 0.1% trypsin solution. The cells were then treated with an equal volume of 0.1% soybean trypsin inhibitor, pelleted by centrifugation, and resuspended in SF-DME/F12. After repeating this procedure, the cells were inoculated into tissue culture dishes containing medium. After an appropriate incubation period, the cells were trypsinized and counted with a Coulter counter. The dosage response to added factors was assayed by measuring cell number after a 4-day incubation period. Unless otherwise mentioned, the determinations of cell number were made in triplicate.

To determine the plating efficiency of MDCK cells, 500 cells were inoculated into 60 mm dishes containing 4 ml of medium (determinations were in triplicate); one week later colonies were fixed with formalin, stained with 0.5% crystal violet, and counted.

Materials

Hormones, including prostaglandins (J. Pike, Upjohn Co.), epidermal growth factor (EGF) and fibroblast growth factor (FGF) (Collaborative Research), purified human transferrin (original source Behring diagnostics, obtained from R. W. Holley, Salk Institute), purified bovine insulin (original source Eli Lilly, obtained from J. Lever, Salk Institute), and selenium (R. Ham, University of Colorado) were gifts. Dibutyryl cAMP, isobutyl methylxanthine (IBMX), bovine insulin, human transferrin, triiodothyronine and hydrocortisone were obtained from Sigma Co.

RESULTS

Growth of MDCK Cells in a Hormone-Supplemented, Serum-Free Medium

MDCK cells grew at 1.5 doublings per day in SF-DME/F12 supplemented with 10% fetal calf serum (Fig. 1). When serum was deleted from the medium the growth rate was

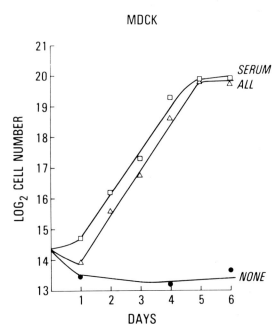

Fig. 1. The effect of medium supplementation of MDCK cell growth. MDCK cells were inoculated at 2.5×10^4 cells/dish into 60 mm dishes containing SF-DME/F12 supplemented with a) 10% fetal calf serum △; b) PGE_1, 25 ng/ml; T_3, 5×10^{-12}M; hydrocortisone, 5×10^{-8}M; insulin 5 μg/ml; transferrin, 5 μg/ml □; or no additional factors ●.

less than 0.4 doublings per day. However, MDCK cells grew at 1.5 doublings per day when SF-DME/F12 was supplemented with PGE_1, hydrocortisone, triiodothyronine, insulin and transferrin (Medium K-1) in the absence of serum (Fig. 1). The ability of Medium K-1 (SF-DME/F12 supplemented with the 5 components) to support clone formation, and the long-term growth of MDCK cells was also studied. The plating efficiency of MDCK cells in Medium K-1 was 70% of that observed in the serum-supplemented medium, and MDCK cells also successfully grew over a 5-week test period (through 4 passages) in Medium K-1.

The optimal concentrations of the hormones in Medium K-1 were determined by assaying the effect of hormone concentration on MDCK cell growth (Table I). With the exception of insulin, all hormones caused maximal growth stimulation at physiological concentrations (Table I). The effects of different prostaglandins on growth were similarly compared between 1 and 1,000 ng/ml [12]. PGE_2 caused equivalent growth stimulation to PGE_1 while $PGF_2\alpha$ and PGA_1 did not have significant growth stimulatory effects.

The relative effects of the individual components in Medium K-1 on cell growth were compared by means of a hormone deletion study (Fig. 2). Omission of either PGE_1 or transferrin from Medium K-1 was more deleterious to cell growth (growth was inhibited by over 50%) than the omission of hydrocortisone, T_3 or insulin; the growth inhibition resulting from the removal of T_3 was observed only after a 6-day time interval. These observations indicate that PGE_1 and transferrin are the most critical of the 5 factors for MDCK cell growth in serum-free medium. However, no growth stimulation was observed when SF-DME/F12 was supplemented with only one of these factors. Increased growth was observed, however, when SF-DME/F12 was supplemented with 2 components, either transferrin and PGE_1, or transferrin and insulin (Table II).

The Mechanism of Action of PGE_1

As PGE_1 a) is one of the most critical components in Medium K-1 for growth, and b) specifically stimulates growth of MDCK cells, rather than the other cell types studied [8], the mechanism by which PGE_1 enhances MDCK cell growth was of interest. The possibility that PGE_1 stimulates growth as a result of its stimulatory effects on cAMP production was also examined with respect to its effects on cell growth in SF-DME/F12 sup-

TABLE I. Concentration Optima of Supplements in Medium K-1

Medium supplement	Optimal concentration range	Concentration in Medium K-1
Insulin	$5-10\ \mu g/ml$	$5\ \mu g/ml$
Transferrin	$5-20\ \mu g/ml$	$5\ \mu g/ml$
PGE_1	$25-1,000\ ng/ml$	$25\ ng/ml$
T_3	$5 \times 10^{-12}M$	$5 \times 10^{-12}M$
Hydrocortisone	$5 \times 10^{-9}-10^{-7}M$	$5 \times 10^{-8}M$

The dependence of MDCK cell growth on hormone concentration was determined as follows. The optimal dosage of each factor was determined in the presence of the other 4 factors (insulin, 5 $\mu g/ml$; transferrin, 5 $\mu g/ml$; T_3, $5 \times 10^{-12}M$; hydrocortisone, $5 \times 10^{-8}M$; PGE_1, 25 ng/ml), with the exception that the T_3 optima were determined in the absence of hydrocortisone. Determinations were made in triplicate after 4 days. The effect of each hormone on cell growth was expressed as the percentage of the control cell number (the cell number in 35 mm dishes lacking the hormone being studied) as described in Taub et al [12].

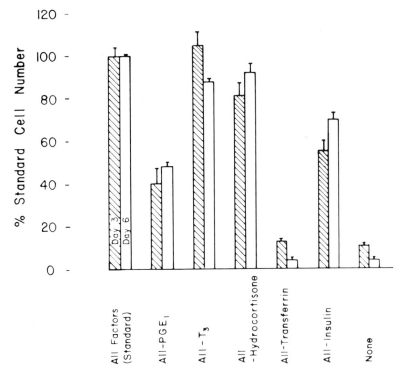

Fig. 2. The effect of deletion of a factor from hormone-supplemented medium on MDCK cell growth. MDCK cells were inoculated at 5×10^4/dish into 60 mm dishes containing a) SF-DME/F12 and 5 factors (PGE_1, 25 ng/ml; T_3, 5×10^{-12}M; hydrocortisone, 5×10^{-8}M; transferrin, 5 μg/ml; insulin, 5 μg/ml); b) SF-DME/F12 and 4 of the above factors or c) SF-DME/F12 (alone). Cell number was assayed in triplicate on days 3 and 6. In Medium K-1 the cell number was 1.1×10^6 on day 3 and 3.7×10^6 on day 6.

TABLE II. Synergistic Effects of Medium Supplements on Cell Growth

Medium supplement	Percentage standard cell number
None	2 ± 0
Insulin	2 ± 0
PGE_1	2 ± 0
T_3	1 ± 0
Transferrin	2 ± 0
Hydrocortisone (HC)	1 ± 0
Transferrin, PGE_1	22 ± 6
Transferrin, insulin	29 ± 6
Insulin, PGE_1	3 ± 0
Insulin, transferrin, PGE_1	82 ± 7
Insulin, transferrin, PGE_1, HC, T_3 (Std)	100 ± 7

MDCK cells were inoculated into dishes containing SF-DME/F12 supplemented with different combinations of the 5 factors in Medium K-1 (insulin, 5 μg/ml; transferrin, 5 μg/ml; T_3, 5×10^{-12}M; hydrocortisone, 5×10^{-8}M; PGE_1, 25 ng/ml). Growth was assayed in dishes in triplicate after 4 days, and was compared to the cell number in Medium K-1 (Standard).

TABLE III. Effect of Hormones on Hemicyst Formation

Added components	Hemicysts/field	Percentage of monolayer as hemicyst
Insulin, transferrin (Standard)	0	0
Standard + PGE$_1$	2.7 ± 2.1	8 ± 5
Standard + PGE$_1$ + hydrocortisone	10.4 ± 3.4	32 ± 10
Standard + PGE$_1$ + T$_3$	6.0 ± 3.8	18 ± 9
Standard + T$_3$	0	0
10% Fetal calf serum	1.3 ± 1.3	12 ± 31

MDCK cells were grown to confluency in SF-DME/F12 supplemented with the components indicated above (insulin, 5 μg/ml; transferrin, 5 μg/ml; PGE$_1$, 25 ng/ml; hydrocortisone, 5 × 10^{-8}M; T$_3$, 5 × 10^{-12}). The average number of hemicysts per field was estimated by counting 10 microscope fields at 100× magnification using a Nikon microscope. The hemicyst size was estimated from the diameter hemicysts, determined using a Nikon microscope grid, and compared to the total field size, also using the grid. The above estimations permitted a calculation of the percentage of monolayer of hemicyst.

plemented with insulin (5 μg/ml), and transferrin (5 μg/ml). Dibutyryl cAMP (0.5 mM) was not only growth stimulatory to MDCK cells, but also substituted for PGE$_1$ in Medium K-1, permitting optimal growth to occur. At a similar concentration sodium butyrate had no effect on growth. Three other factors which affect cAMP metabolism in MDCK cells were also studied. While isobutyl methylxanthine (0.5 mM) (a phosphodiesterase inhibitor) and glucagon (5 μg/ml) were also growth stimulatory, arginine vasopressin had no significant growth-enhancing effect.

Applicability of Serum-Free Medium to Examine Regulation of Hemicyst Formation

In serum-supplemented medium confluent monolayers of MDCK cells form domes or hemicysts, a process which depends upon the vectorial transport of salt and water across the monolayer. MDCK cells maintained in Medium K-1 not only were similar morphologically to cells in serum-supplemented medium, but also formed hemicysts.

The effect of the 5 components in Medium K-1 on hemicyst formation was examined (Table III). No hemicysts were observed in monolayers grown to confluency in SF-DME/F12 containing only insulin and transferrin. However, when SF-DME/F12 was supplemented with PGE$_1$ in addition to insulin and transferrin, hemicyst formation was apparent. The addition of hydrocortisone further increased the frequency of hemicysts, and this effect of hydrocortisone was observed only when PGE$_1$ was present.

Applicability of Medium K-1 for Growth of Primary Kidney Cultures

The simultaneous growth of both fibroblasts and epithelial cells in primary kidney cultures has complicated studies of tubular transport functions. The possibility that Medium K-1 would permit the selective growth of epithelial cells in primary kidney cultures was examined.

When baby mouse kidney cells were inoculated at 5 × 10^3 cells/cm^2 into either Medium K-1 or SF-DME/F12 supplemented with 10% fetal calf serum, 25% of the cells attached, and grew exponentially (0.6 doublings per day). Microscope examinations indicated that initially over 99% of the attached cells were epithelial in morphology under both culture conditions. However, in serum-supplemented medium after 5 days 13% of the cells were fibroblasts and after 11 days the majority of the cell population was fibroblastic (Fig.

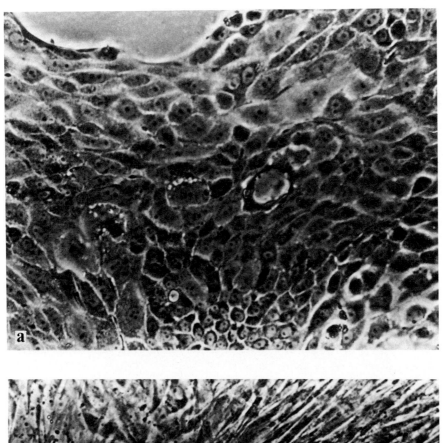

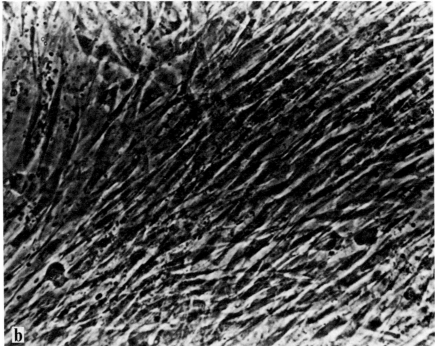

Fig. 3. Primary baby mouse kidney cultures. Baby mouse kidney cells were distributed at 10^4 cells/ 35 mm dish into dishes containing either a) Medium K-1 or b) SF-DME/F12 supplemented with 10% fetal calf serum. Eleven days later the cells were photographed. The suspension of baby mouse kidney cells was prepared as described in Materials and Methods.

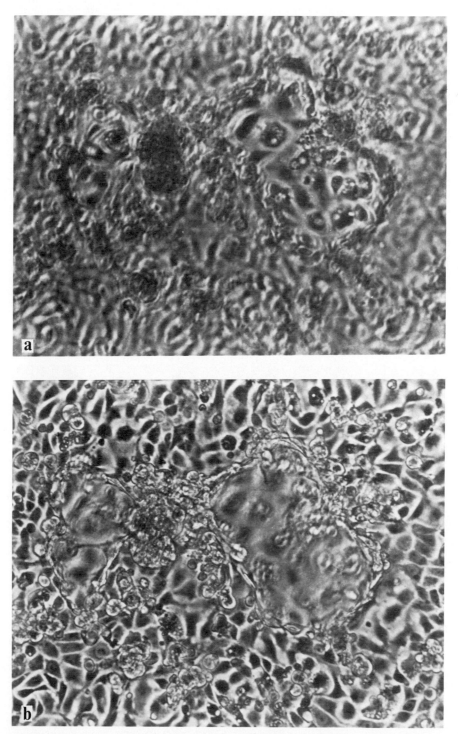

Fig. 4. Hemicyst formation by primary cultures. Baby mouse kidney cells were distributed at $5 \times 10^4/$ 35 mm dish into Medium K-1. Hemicyst formation was observed in confluent cultures.

TABLE IV. Growth of Kidney Cell Lines in Medium K-1

Cell type		Growth rate (doublings/day)	
		SF-DME/F12	
Cell line	Species of origin	+ FCS	Medium K-1
LLC-MK$_2$ (7)	Monkey	1.6	1.6
MDBK (8)	Bovine	0.8	1.0
BSC-1	Monkey	0.7	0.4
NRK (15)	Rat	1.3	0.1
RAG (16)	Rat	1.6	1.2
MDCK (3)	Canine	1.5	1.5

Cells were inoculated at 2.5×10^4/60 mm dish into dishes containing SF-DME/F12 supplemented with 10% fetal calf serum. The next day the medium was removed by aspiration, the cells were washed three times with SF-DME/F12, and then incubated with Medium K-1 or SF-DME/F12 supplemented with 10% fetal calf serum. The growth rate was estimated from daily cell counts in duplicate dishes over a 5-day period.

3b). During this time interval no equivalent fibroblast overgrowth was observed in Medium K-1 (Fig. 3a). Although hemicyst formation was observed in primary cultures maintained in Medium K-1 (Fig. 4), it is particularly interesting that no such hemicysts were observed in SF-DME/F12 supplemented with 10% fetal calf serum.

The observation that baby mouse kidney cells grew in Medium K-1 (a dog kidney medium) suggested that Medium K-1 could be used for the maintenance of kidney epithelial cells derived from a number of animal species. Indeed, primary cultures of human fetal, baby rabbit and adult wolf kidney cells were all maintained in Medium K-1 in the absence of fibroblast overgrowth.

However, these observations do not indicate whether all types of epithelial cells in mammalian kidneys can grow in Medium K-1. To test this possibility, the effect of Medium K-1 on the growth of a number of kidney epithelial cell lines was examined. Table IV illustrates that 4 of the 6 kidney cell lines tested grew at equivalent rates in Medium K-1 and SF-DME/F12 supplemented with 10% fetal calf serum after a serum preincubation overnight. However, the BSC-1 cell line grew at only 57% of the rate observed in serum-supplemented medium.

DISCUSSION

When SF-DME/F12 was supplemented with insulin, transferrin, PGE$_1$, T$_3$ and hydrocortisone (Medium K-1), the kidney epithelial cell line MDCK was maintained one month in the absence of serum. MDCK cells proliferated at equivalent rates in Medium K-1 and in SF-DME/F12 supplemented with 10% fetal calf serum.

Although the addition of each of these 5 components was necessary to obtain optimal growth of MDCK cells, the deletion of either PGE$_1$ or transferrin from Medium K-1 had the most severe inhibitory effects on growth, as compared to the deletion of any other factor. Of interest in regard to the PGE$_1$ requirement is the observation that prostaglandins are produced in large quantities by the renal medulla [17]. Thus in vivo prostaglandins may regulate renal growth as well as systemic blood pressure [17].

These studies introduce the possibility that cAMP mediates the growth-stimulatory effects of PGE$_1$ on MDCK cells. Dibutyryl cAMP could substitute for PGE$_1$ in the medium;

moreover, other factors which affect cAMP production in MDCK cells, including PGE_2, glucagon, and isobutyl methylxanthine also enhanced growth [12], with the exception of arginine vasopressin. However, increased intracellular cAMP may still be correlated with growth, if arginine vasopressin affects a distinct compartment of intracellular cAMP, as compared to the other factors. The proposed correlation between increased intracellular cAMP levels and growth in MDCK cells is contrasted with the correlation between decreased intracellular cAMP levels and growth previously made in fibroblast cultures [18].

The extent to which Medium K-1 can be applied to cultured kidney cells has been examined. The studies indicate that the hormone-supplemented medium has little species specificity, as kidney epithelial cells from mouse, monkey, and man were maintained in Medium K-1. Second, in primary kidney cultures the hormone-supplemented medium permitted the selective growth of the epithelial cells, rather than the fibroblasts. Thus, the problem of fibroblast overgrowth which occurs in serum-supplemented medium can be avoided. Finally, Medium K-1 is apparently not universally applicable for all epithelial cells in the kidney. Only one of the two monkey kidney epithelial lines tested grew at equivalent rates in Medium K-1 and serum-supplemented medium. Conceivably, alternative media may be developed for the selective growth of different types of kidney epithelial cells in primary cultures. The availability of such hormone-supplemented media should make primary kidney cultures a more powerful tool for studies concerning kidney function.

ACKNOWLEDGMENTS

The investigators thank Dr. Jane Bottenstein for critical reading of the manuscript. The work was supported by NIH-GM 17019, NIH-CA 19731, NIH-GM 17702, and NSF PCM 76-80785 to G.S. M.T. was supported by an NIH postdoctoral fellowship (NIH 1 F32 CA05917-01).

REFERENCES

1. Katz A, Lindheimer MD: Ann Rev Physiol 39:97, 1977.
2. Reiter RJ: In Nowinski WW, Goss RS (eds): "Compensatory Renal Hypertrophy." New York: Academic Press, p 183, 1969.
3. Leighton JL, Estes W, Mansukhani S, Brada Z: Cancer 26:7022, 1970.
4. Misfeldt DS, Hamamoto SJ, Pitelka DR: Proc Natl Acad Sci USA 73:1212, 1976.
5. Cereiijido M, Robbins ES, Dolan WJ, Rotundo CA, Sabatini DD: J Cell Biol 77:853, 1978.
6. Rindler MJ, Chuman L, Schaeffer L, Saier MH: J Cell Biol (In press).
7. Hull RN, Cherry WR, Johnson IS: Anat Rec 124:450, 1956.
8. Madin SH, Darby NB: Proc Soc Exp Biol Med 122:931, 1966.
9. Sato GH, Reid L: In Rickenberg HV (ed): "Biochemistry and Mode of Action of Hormones II." Baltimore: University Park Press, Vol 20:215, 1978.
10. Hayashi I, Sato G: Nature 259:132, 1976.
11. Sato GH: In Litwak G (ed): "Biochemical Action of Hormones." New York: Academic Press, Vol III:391, 1975.
12. Taub M, Chuman L, Saier MH, Sato G: Proc Natl Acad Sci USA (In press).
13. Leffert HL, Paul D: J Cell Biol 52:559, 1972.
14. Hopps HE, Bernheim BC, Nisalak A, Hin Tjio S, Smadell SE: J Immunol 91:416, 1963.
15. Duc-Ngugen H, Rosenblum EN, Zeigel RF: J Bacteriol 92:1133, 1966.
16. Klebe RS, Chen T, Ruddle FH: J Cell Biol 45:74, 1970.
17. Lee JB, Attalah AA: In Kurtzmann NA, Martinez-Maldonado M (eds): "Pathophysiology of the Kidney." Springfield: Charles C. Thomas, 1977.
18. Pastan IH, Johnson GS, Anderson WD: Ann Rev Biochem 44:491, 1975.

Journal of Supramolecular Structure 11:217–225 (1979)
Tumor Cell Surfaces and Malignancy 163–171

Human Fibrosarcoma Cells Produce Fibronectin-Releasing Peptides

Jorma Keski-Oja, Hans Marquardt, Joseph E. De Larco, and George J. Todaro

Laboratory of Viral Carcinogenesis, National Cancer Institute, National Institutes of Health, Bethesda, Maryland 20205

A sensitive radioimmunoassay, specific for human fibronectin, was used to measure the ability of certain biologically active polypeptides to release fibronectin from cultured human lung fibroblasts into their culture media. Concentrated, serum-free culture supernatant from a human fibrosarcoma cell line was fractionated by gel filtration chromatography in the presence of acetic acid. Various polypeptides with molecular weights between 46,000 and 6,000 were tested for their ability to release fibronectin from cells. The column fraction, containing polypeptides with an apparent molecular weight of 10,000, exhibited the ability to rapidly release fibronectin from target cells. The activity could be inhibited by phenylmethyl sulphonylfluoride. Several other hormonal factors, tested in parallel with the column fractions, failed to show this effect. The 10,000 dalton molecular weight polypeptides may represent a family of cellular gene products responsible for maintenance of low levels of surface associated fibronectin in fibrosarcoma cells and thus be related to their infiltrating properties by preventing the formation of the extra-cellular matrix.

Key words: fibrosarcoma culture media, gel permeation chromatography, fibronectin-radioimmuno-assay, fibronectin-releasing peptides

Transformed cells frequently show a characteristic loss of cell surface-associated fibronectin [1–3]. Certain biochemically known agents can induce the release of fibronectin from cells. Several proteases release fibronectin from the cell surfaces [4–6], also human thrombin from human fibroblasts [7]. On the other hand, fibronectin is released from cells in apparently intact form by either urea [8] or cytochalasin B, a microfilament disrupting agent [9, 10]. Certain tumor promoters, namely, the biologically active phorbol esters, are also capable of inducing a rapid release of fibronectin from cells [11] but thus far no cell-derived factors have been identified.

Abbreviations: EGF, epidermal growth factor; SGFs, sarcoma growth factors; MSA, multiplication stimulating activity; SDS, sodium dodecyl sulphate; K, 10^3 (in molecular weights); BSA, bovine serum albumin; PBS, phosphate buffered saline; PMSF, phenylmethyl sulphonyfluoride; FCS, fetal calf serum.

Received April 27, 1979; accepted July 2, 1979.

Transformed cells and tumor cell lines produce factors assumed to be important for their altered growth properties. The production of certain growth factors may explain the molecular background and mechanisms needed for the invasive properties of different types of tumors [12]. Established lines of human fibrosarcomas have been used to study the altered properties of malignant cells. An established human fibrosarcoma cell line (8387) [13] has been shown to produce a family of polypeptides with multiplication stimulating activity (MSA) [14]. This fibrosarcoma line grows in soft agar, is tumorigenic in nude mice [13] and has low levels of surface-associated fibronectin [our unpublished observation]. Fibrosarcoma cells also produce increased amounts of plasminogen activators [15, 16], and express reduced amounts of surface-associated fibronectin [1, 2]. Very little, however, is known about the mechanisms of fibronectin release from transformed cells. The tissue invasiveness of malignant cells may, at least to some extent, be a result of their ability to pervade fibronectin-containing structures that are probably important in the formation of the extracellular matrix. In this report we describe how fibroblast-associated fibronectin can be released from the cells by a partially purified, 10,000 molecular weight polypeptide(s) that is apparently of proteolytic character, obtained from the serum-free culture media of the established human fibrosarcoma line (8387).

MATERIALS AND METHODS

Isolation of Peptides From Human Fibrosarcoma Culture Media

Supernatant fluids from a human fibrosarcoma cell line (8387) were collected using serum-free Waymouth's medium. The low molecular weight peptides were partially purified from the supernatants by a method that utilizes the natural affinity of these peptides for a high molecular weight binding protein [17, 18]. The medium was ultrafiltered at neutral pH using a high flow Amicon hollow fiber apparatus (50,000 dalton exclusion) and the retentate was acidified to pH 2.3 to dissociate the peptides from their binding protein. Chromatography was carried out on a Bio-Gel P-100 column which was eluted with 1M acetic acid. Five different pooled column fractions with molecular weights varying between 46,000 and 6,000 were used for assays (see below).

Radioimmunoassay for Fibronectin

A specific antibody to human plasma fibronectin was raised by immunizing rabbits. The immunizing antigen was purified by gelatin-Sepharose affinity chromatography and DEAE-cellulose chromatography, as described previously [11, 19]. Antifibronectin antiserum produced in rabbits, was adsorbed with 2 volumes of fetal calf serum (37°C for two hours and 4°C for 18 hours) and clarified by centrifugation. This adsorption removed all cross-reacting antibodies against bovine fibronectin and medium containing 10% FCS caused no inhibition in the binding. Plasma from mouse and rat or tissue culture media from cell lines of heterologous species failed to compete in the assay. This radioimmunoassay using preadsorbed immune sera and ^{125}I-labeled human plasma fibronectin is thus specific for human fibronectin [7, 11].

Purified human fibronectin was iodinated by using 2 μg chloramine-T for 10 μg of protein in 0.4 M phosphate buffer (pH 7.6). The reaction was carried out for one minute at room temperature and then quenched with a saturated solution of tyrosine. Iodinated protein was recovered in the void volume of a Bio-Gel P-60 column. Competition radioimmunoassay was performed by a double antibody precipitation method [7, 11]. In brief, the appropriate dilution of rabbit antifibronectin was chosen for the precipitation of $\sim$50% of input radiolabeled fibronectin. The antisera was first incubated with serial dilutions of un-labeled competing test antigen samples at 37°C for 2 hours. Approximately 20,000 dpm of ^{125}I-fibronectin was then added and incubated for an additional 2 hours at 37°C. The immune complex was incubated at 37°C for 1 hour and 4°C for 3 hours with sheep anti-rabbit immunoglobulin as the second antibody. The immune precipitate was washed 3 times with cold PBS. The amount of ^{125}I-fibronectin in the precipitate was directly measured in a gamma counter.

A solution of fibronectin in 0.5% BSA served as standard. It was necessary to divide the standard and freeze in small aliquots to prevent the loss of the antigenic activity which occurs with repeated freezing and thawing [20]. The competition curves were linear between 4–40 ng of fibronectin and the variation between two identical samples tested in parallel was less than 5% [11].

Cell Cultures and the Assay for Fibronectin Release

Diploid human embryo lung fibroblasts (CCL-137) were obtained from the American Type Culture Collection, Rockville, Maryland. Cells were grown on plastic tissue culture dishes (Falcon Industries, Oxnard, California) at 37°C in Eagle's basal medium supplemented with 10% fetal calf serum, 100 IU/ml penicillin, and 50 μg/ml streptomycin. Cells were between passages 13 and 19. Upon reaching confluency, 3–6 days after subculture the growth medium was removed and the cells were washed thrice with the binding buffer (Dulbecco's modification of Eagle's media plus 50 mM N,N-bis-(2 hydroxyethyl)-2-aminoethanesulphonic acid and 1 mg/ml of BSA, pH 6.8). The experiments were carried out in binding buffer. After the cultures were incubated at 37°C for the time described, the medium was collected and clarified by centrifugation at 300 × g for 10 minutes and their fibronectin concentrations were determined by radioimmunoassays. The attached cells were washed 3 times with cold PBS and extracted with 500 μl of urea-Triton solution (1% Triton X-100, 6 M urea, 1 mM PMSF). The protein concentrations of the cell extracts were determined [21].

Labeling of Cells With ^{35}S-Methionine

Cultures of human lung fibroblasts were washed three times with methionine-free media and then labeled with 30 μCi/ml of ^{35}S-methionine (103 μCi/mmol, The Radiochemical Centre, Amersham, England) in methionine-free media for 4 hours. The labeling was terminated by washing the cells with media containing excess of unlabeled methionine. The cultures were then incubated in the binding buffer as shown. Upon termination of the incubation the media of the cells were collected, clarified by centrifugation (300 × g), and the polypeptides were precipitated with cold trichloracetic acid (10% final concentration) and analyzed in SDS-polyacrylamide gels.

SDS-Polyacrylamide Gel Electrophoresis

SDS-Polyacrylamide gels were prepared according to previously published methods [22, 23]. Purified plasma fibronectin (subunit molecular weight 220,000), phosphorylase b (molecular weight 94,000), bovine serum albumin (molecular weight 68,000) ovalbumin (molecular weight 45,000) carbonic anhydrase (molecular weight 29,000), myoglobin (molecular weight 17,200) and bromphenol blue were used as markers for molecular weight and mobility.

RESULTS

The Release of Fibronectin by Fibrosarcoma Derived Polypeptides

Five different pooled column fractions, isolated by gel filtration as described, were analyzed for their ability to release fibronectin from confluent cultures of human lung fibroblasts. The mobilities of the major protein bands of the pooled fractions were between 46,000 and 6,000 daltons in SDS-polyacrylamide gel electrophoresis. Equal amounts of protein were added to the serum-free media of the cells. The column fraction that contained polypeptides with an apparent molecular weight of 10,000, contained an activity that released fibronectin from the cells into their serum-free media. (Table I). Cultured fibroblasts produced and released a basal level of fibronectin into their media, and the amounts of fibronectin released from cultures treated with the other column fractions did not differ significantly from this control value.

When the 10K-peptide pool was analyzed in SDS-polyacrylamide gels, it contained a major protein band with apparent molecular weight of 10,300 and a minor band of 9,300 (Fig. 1). So far, attempts to purify these individual peptides have been unsuccessful.

To study how much of the 10K-fraction was needed to bring about the release, we used different concentrations as shown in Figure 2. Microgram quantities of the fraction were necessary suggesting either a low specific activity or that only a fraction of the total protein is active. The release of fibronectin is time dependent (Fig. 3). An increase in the fibronectin content in the media of the cells treated with 10K-peptides was seen within 30 minutes after the onset.

Analysis of the Released Molecules

To analyze the sizes of the cellular molecules released to the medium, cells were labeled with radioactive methionine and then incubated with the 10K fraction polypeptides ($10 \mu g$/ml) for 4 hours. The released polypeptides were precipitated with trichloracetic acid and analyzed by SDS-polyacrylamide gel electrophoresis followed by autoradiography (Fig. 4). The polypeptide patterns were apparently identical. The released radiolabeled polypeptides that comigrated with the subunits of purified human plasma fibronectin and with the 220,000 molecular weight polypeptides secreted from

TABLE I. Fibronectin-Releasing Ability of Different Pooled Column Fractions*

Pool No.	Apparent mol wt.	Total fibronectin released to media (μg)	Difference between treated and control plates (μg)
1	46K–24K	1.0	0
2	14K–13K	0.8	0
3	12K	0.8	0
4	10K	5.1	4.1
5	6K	1.1	0.1
–	control	1.0	0

*Averages of duplicate dishes.
Human lung fibroblasts were cultivated on 60 mm diameter dishes and upon confluency washed 3 times with binding buffer before assay. The cells were then incubated for 4 hours in 2.5 ml of binding buffer with different pooled column fractions (5 μg/ml final concentration). The fibronectin concentrations of the media were determined by radioimmunoassays. The protein concentrations of the cultures were $422 \pm 37 \mu g$. The molecular weights given represent the mobilities of the major protein bands of the pools in SDS-polyacrylamide gels.

untreated cells, did not show signs of major proteolytic cleavages, as is seen in the case of trypsin treated cells [6], suggesting that only a minor part of fibronectin was cleaved during the treatment of the cells with 10K-peptides.

Effects of Some Hormonal Factors on the Release of Fibronectin

We analyzed the 10,000 molecular weight polypeptides produced by an established human lung carcinoma cell line (9812) as a control, as well as several known hormonal factors. None of them caused the release of fibronectin from the treated cells (Table II). The effects of some proteinase inhibitors were studied in parallel. If phenylmethyl sulphonylfluoride was present with the 10K-peptide(s), it was able to inhibit the fibronectin releasing activity of this material. Phenylmethyl sulphonylfluoride blocked the fibronectin-releasing activity of this 10K-peptide(s) at the concentration of 10 μg/ml, suggesting that the activity present in this fraction is of proteolytic character, possibly a serine protease. The activity was also inhibited by leupeptin (10 μg/ml) and soybean trypsin inhibitor (40 μg/ml).

DISCUSSION

We have shown in this study that human fibrosarcoma cells produce an activity that can release fibronectin from cultured human fibrobalsts. This protein is a small acid-stable peptide with an apparent molecular weight of 10,000 and it acts as a protease. The size of the fibronectin molecules found in the media of the cells treated with these 10K-

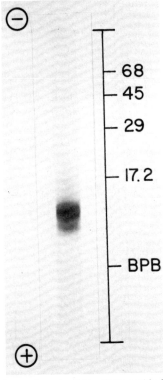

Fig. 1. SDS-polyacrylamide gel electrophoresis of the 10K-peptide fraction. A lyophilized aliquot of the column fraction was incubated in 10% SDS and 5% mercaptoethanol at +100°C for 3 minutes and analyzed in a 10% SDS-polyacrylamide gel and stained with coomassie blue. Molecular weight and mobility markers ($\times 10^3$) were bovine serum albumin, ovalbumin, carbonic anhydrase, myoglobin and bromphenol blue (BPB).

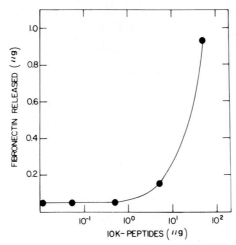

Fig. 2. The dependence of fibronectin release to increasing concentrations of the 10K-peptides (averages of duplicate dishes). Confluent cultures of human lung fibroblasts were exposed to increasing concentrations of 10K-peptides in serum-free media for 2 hours. Prior to the experiment the cultures were incubated in serum-free media for 12 hours. The supernatants were clarified by centrifugation and their fibronectin concentrations were determined by radioimmunoassays. The protein concentrations of the cultures were 206 ± 15 μg. Abscissa: the concentration of 10K-peptides (μg); Ordinate: fibronectin released into the media (μg).

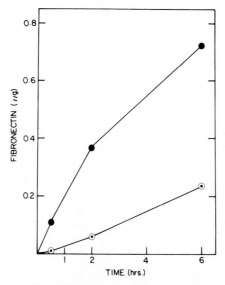

Fig. 3. Time course of fibronectin release by 10K-peptides (averages of duplicate dishes). Human lung fibroblasts were cultivated on 35 mm diameter plastic petri dishes. Confluent cultures were washed twice with binding buffer and incubated in binding buffer for 12 hours before the assay. The cultures were then washed 3 times and incubated in 1 ml of binding buffer with (●——●) or without (○——○) the 10K-peptides (5 μg/ml) the times indicated and the fibronectin concentrations of the media were determined by radioimmunoassay. The protein concentrations of the cultures were 294 ± 19 μg. Abscissa: total fibronectin released (μg); Ordinate: time (hours).

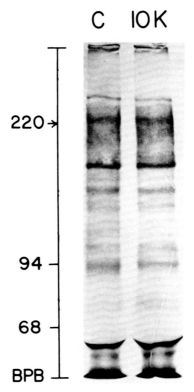

Fig. 4. SDS-polyacrylamide gel electrophoresis of the polypeptides released from cultured fibroblasts by 10K-peptides. Cultures of human lung fibroblasts were labeled with ^{35}S-methionine (50 μCi/ml) for 4 hours. The cells were then washed with serum-free media containing excess of unlabeled methionine and incubated in serum-free media plus 10K-peptides (5 μg/ml) for 3 hours. The polypeptides of the supernatants were precipitated with trichloracetic acid (10% final concentration), washed with acetone, and analyzed in a 5% gel slab with spacer. The gel was then subjected to autoradiography shown here. C: supernatant from control cells; 10K: supernatant from cells treated with 10K-peptides. An arrow indicates the position of purified plasma fibronectin run in parallel with the samples. Molecular weights of the marker proteins ($\times 10^3$) are given.

TABLE II. Effects of Some Hormonal Factors on the Fibronectin Production of Cultured Human Fibroblasts

Factor	Fibronectin in media (μg)
None	0.8
EGF (2 ng/ml)	0.6
Insulin (5 μg/ml)	0.8
Dexamethasone (50 ng/ml)	0.9
SGFs (20 μg/ml)	0.7
Rat 10K-MSA-Peptides (100 ng/ml)	0.7
10K-peptides from lung carcinoma cells (5 μg/ml)	0.8
10K-peptides (5 μg/ml)	3.3
10K-peptides (5 μg/ml) + PMSF (10 μg/ml)	0.7

Dense cultures of human lung fibroblast (60 mm diameter dishes) were washed with binding buffer and exposed to the hormones described in 3 ml of binding buffer for 3 hours. The fibronectin concentrations of the media were determined by radioimmunoassays. The protein concentrations of the cultures were 373 ± 17 μg.

peptides was apparently unaltered, suggesting that there may be a specific site close to the plasma membrane where the peptides act.

Virus-transformed and tumor-derived cell lines produce growth factors assumed to be important for their altered growth behavior [12, 17]. The sarcoma-derived peptide fractions described contain growth stimulating activities [14, 18]. Therefore, it was of value to try to correlate whether the release of fibronectin is linked to the MSA-like stimulation of growth. We tested sarcoma growth factors [24], rat MSA-peptides of the molecular weight of 10,000 [25], insulin, and epidermal growth factor in an analogous study. The 10,000 molecular weight fraction with growth promoting properties [Todaro et al, unpublished observations] from the supernatants of human lung carcinoma cells (9812), was used as a control. None of these peptides were able to cause a rapid release of fibronectin from cultured human fibroblasts into their media. Murine sarcoma growth factors, although able to reversibly transform murine cells [24], did not release fibronectin from human fibroblasts. We did not, however, test them in murine cell cultures, where they might be effective. The fibronectin-releasing activity produced by the fibrosarcoma cells is apparently unrelated to the growth promoting (MSA) peptides, but is a small molecular weight peptide that is copurified together with 10,000 molecular weight MSA-peptides. We have not succeeded in purifying these activities apart from each other thus far. It is not known whether the 10K-peptide(s) is also produced by other cell lines. This will be studied later after the further purification of the peptide(s).

The 10K-peptides may be related to plasminogen activators that are produced by transformed cells [15, 16]; however, the reported molecular weights of plasminogen activators produced by cultured fibroblasts are between 85,000–36,000 [26] which would suggest this activity is distinct from these factors. The ability of the 10K-peptide(s) to activate plasminogen has not been studied thus far. The role of plasminogen activators in the release of fibronectin is not clear. Removal of plasminogen from transformed cells does not restore their cell surface fibronectin [27]. Several proteases including trypsin [6, 28] and thrombin [7] release fibronectin from cells. Thrombin apparently attacks a specific site close to the membrane and releases fibronectin molecules that are apparently unaltered in size [7], whereas trypsin causes a significant cleavage [6, 28]. Transformed cells produce and release fibronectin into their media without detectable difference in size when compared to fibronectins produced by normal cells [29]. This does not exclude the possibility of the cleavage of a short polypeptide. Thus, fibronectins produced by transformed cells might have different affinities to the cellular skeletal actin-containing structures proposed to serve as inserting structures for cell surface fibronectin [30–32].

The 10K-peptide(s) described here is the first cell-derived factor found to release fibronectin. This peptide(s) may help sarcoma cells in destroying the extracellular matrix that contains fibronectin [33–36] and thus they may somehow be related to the infiltrating properties of fibrosarcoma cells.

ACKNOWLEDGMENTS

We thank Ms. Estelle Harvey and Ms. Linda Toler for their fine assistance and Ms. Ellen Fleming for secretarial help. This research was supported by the Virus-Cancer Program of the National Institutes of Health.

REFERENCES

1. Hynes RO: Biochim Biophys Acta 458:73, 1976.
2. Vaheri A, Mosher DF: Biochim Biophys Acta 516:1, 1978.
3. Yamada KM, Olden K: Nature 275, 179, 1978.
4. Blumberg PM, Robbins PW: Cell 6:137, 1975.
5. Zetter BR, Chen LB, Buchanan JM: Cell 7:407, 1976.
6. Keski-Oja J, Vaheri A, Ruoslahti E: Int J Cancer 17:261, 1976.
7. Mosher DF, Vaheri A: Exp Cell Res 112:323, 1978.
8. Yamada KM, Weston JA: Proc Natl Acad Sci USA 71:3492, 1974.
9. Ali IU, Hynes RO: Biochim Biophys Acta 471:16, 1977.
10. Kurkinen M, Vaheri A, Wartiovaara J: Exp Cell Res 111:127, 1978.
11. Keski-Oja J, Shoyab M, De Larco JE, Todaro GJ: Int J Cancer 24:222, 1979.
12. Todaro GJ, De Larco JE: Cancer Res 38:4147, 1970.
13. Aaronson S, Todaro GJ, Freeman A: Exp Cell Res 61:1, 1970.
14. De Larco JE, Todaro GJ: Nature 272:365, 1978.
15. Unkeless JC, Tobia A, Ossowski L, Quigley JP, Rifkin DB, Reich E: J Exp Med 137:85, 1973.
16. Ossowski L, Unkeless JC, Tobia A, Quigeley JP, Rifkin DB, Reich E: J Exp Med 137:112, 1973.
17. Todaro GJ, De Larco JE, Marquardt H, Bryant ML, Sherwin SA, Sliski AH: Cold Spring Harbor Symp Quant Biol, vol. 6 (In press) 1979.
18. Marquardt H, De Larco JE, Todaro GJ: (Manuscript in preparation) 1979.
19. Engvall E, Ruoslahti E: Int J Cancer 20:1, 1977.
20. Alexander SS, Colonna G Jr, Yamada KM, Pastan I, Edelhoch H: J Biol Chem 253:5820, 1978.
21. Lowry OH, Rosebrough NJ, Farr AL, Randall RJ: J Biol Chem 193:265, 1951.
22. Laemmli UK: Nature 277:680, 1970.
23. Weber K, Osborn M: J Biol Chem 244:4406, 1969.
24. De Larco JE, Todaro GJ: Proc Natl Acad Sci USA 75:4001, 1978.
25. Dulak NC, Temin HM: J Cell Physiol 81:153, 1973.
26. Vetterlein D, Young PL, Bell TE, Roblin R: J Biol Chem 254:575, 1979.
27. Pearlstein E, Hynes RO, Franks LM, Hemmings VJ: Cancer Res 36:1775, 1976.
28. Hynes RO: Proc Natl Acad Sci USA 70:3170, 1973.
29. Vaheri A, Ruoslahti E: J Exp Med 142:530, 1975.
30. Hynes RO, Destree AT: Cell 15:875, 1978.
31. Singer II: Cell 16:675, 1979.
32. Keski-Oja J, Sen A, Todaro GJ: J Cell Biol (abstract, in press) 1979.
33. Vaheri A, Kurkinen M, Lehto V-P, Linder E, Timpl R: Proc Natl Acad Sci USA 75:4944, 1978.
34. Chen LB, Murray A, Segal RA, Bushnell A, Walsh ML: Cell 14:377, 1978.
35. Furcht LT, Mosher DF, Wendelschafer-Crabb G: Cell 13:268, 1978.
36. Hedman K, Kurkinen M, Alitalo K, Vaheri A, Johansson S, Höök M: J Cell Biol 81:83, 1979.

Journal of Supramolecular Structure 11:227—235 (1979)
Tumor Cell Surfaces and Malignancy 173—181

Inhibition of Blood Coagulation Factor XIII$_a$-Mediated Cross-Linking Between Fibronectin and Collagen by Polyamines

Deane F. Mosher, Peter E. Schad, and Hynda K. Kleinman

Department of Medicine, University of Wisconsin, Madison, Wisconsin 53706 (D.F.M., P.E.S.) and Laboratory of Developmental Biology and Anomalies, National Institute of Dental Research, Bethesda, Maryland 20014 (H.K.K.)

Soluble fibronectin is found in body fluids and media of cultured adherent cells. Insoluble fibronectin is found in tissue stroma and in extracellular matrices of cultured cells. Fibronectin is a substrate for factor XIII$_a$ (plasma transglutaminase) and can be cross-linked to collagen and to the α chain of fibrin. We have used sodium dodecyl sulfate-polyacrylamide gel electrophoresis to investigate the possibility that factor XIII$_a$-mediated cross-linking is influenced by polyamines. Spermidine inhibited cross-linking between fibronectin and type I collagen, isolated α1 (I) collagen chains, or iodinated cyanogen bromide fragment 7 of α1 (I) chains (^{125}I-α1 (I)-CB7). Half-maximal inhibition of cross-linking between ^{125}I-α1 (I)-CB7 and fibronectin was observed when 0.1 mM spermine or spermidine was present. Spermidine, 0.7 mM, partially inhibited cross-linking between fibronectin and the α chain of fibrin but failed to inhibit cross-linking between the fibrin monomers of a fibrin clot. Spermidine also failed to inhibit cross-linking between fibronectin molecules when aggregation of fibronectin was induced with dithiothreitol. In contrast, 0.7 mM monodansylcadaverine inhibited fibronectin-collagen, fibronectin-fibrin, fibronectin-fibronectin, and fibrin-fibrin cross-linking. Spermidine or spermine, 0.7 mM, enhanced the cross-linking between molecules of partially amidinated fibronectin, suggesting that N^{1,8}-(di-γ-glutamyl)-polyamine cross-linkages were formed. Spermidine and spermine failed to enhance cross-linking between monomers of amidinated fibrin. These results indicate that physiologic concentrations of polyamines specifically disturb transglutaminase-catalyzed cross-linking between fibronectin and collagen.

Key words: fibronectin, factor XIII, transglutaminase, collagen, polyamine, ϵ(γ-glutamyl)-lysine

Received April 25, 1979; accepted July 8, 1979.

Fibronectin is a glycopretein found in extracellular fluids, and connective tissues and associated with basement membranes (reviewed in Vaheri and Mosher [1] and Yamada and Olden [2]) and is present in the extracellular fibrillar matrix of substrate-attached cells in culture [3–6]. Collagen binds to fibronectin [7–10] and is a second component of the matrix [11, 12]. A specific region of the type I collagen $\alpha1$ (I) chain, which is generated by cyanogen bromide cleavage and designated $\alpha1$ (I)-CB7, comprises residues 552–822 and contains the principal binding site for fibronectin [9, 10].

Transglutaminases are a class of calcium ion-dependent enzymes that catalyze an acyl transfer reaction in which γ-carboxamide groups of peptide-bound glutaminyl residues are acyl donors and a variety of primary amines, including the -ϵ-amino groups of peptide-bound lysyl residues, are acyl acceptors. By this reaction, transglutaminases catalyze the formation of ϵ-(γ-glutamyl)-lysine linkages between proteins. As recently reviewed by Folk and Finlayson, transglutaminases are widely distributed and are throught to catalyse biologically important cross-linking of fibrin, hair proteins, keratin, and proteins of seminal fluid [13]. Fibronectin is a substrate for transglutaminases of plasma [14, 15] and liver [16] and can be cross-linked to itself [14, 16], fibrin [14, 17, 18], and collagen [19]. Fibronectin in the extracellular fibrillar matrix of cultured fibroblasts can be extensively cross-linked by exogenous plasma transglutaminase [20].

Polyamines are widely distributed and are thought to play important roles in cell proliferation and other biologic processes (reviewed in Tabor and Tabor [21] and Jänne et al [22]). These compounds can serve as acyl acceptors for liver [23, 24] and plasma [24] transglutaminase. Polyamines also dissociated fibronectin from gelatin [25]. In the present paper, we report that polyamines specifically inhibit transglutaminase-catalyzed cross-linking between collagen and fibronectin.

METHODS

Materials

Bolton Hunter reagent (1,500 Ci/mmole) was from New England Nuclear, Coomassie brilliant blue R-250 was from BioRad Laboratories, spermine and spermidine were from Sigma Chemicals, and human thrombin was a generous gift from Dr. John Fenton II, New York State Department of Health.

Purification of Proteins and Protein Fragments

Human fibrinogen, human factor XIII, human plasma fibronectin, lathyritic rat type I collagen, calf skin type III collagen, and cyanogen bromide peptides of $\alpha1$ (I) chains of calf skin type I collagen were prepared as described elsewhere [19].

Radiolabeling of $\alpha1$ (I)-CB7

Cyanogen bromide fragment 7 of bovine $\alpha1$ (I) chains [$\alpha1$ (I)-CB7] was reacted with Bolton Hunter reagent as described elsewhere [19]. Approximately 10^{-2} moles of ^{125}I-reagent was incorporated per mole of $\alpha1$ (I)-CB7.

Amidination of Proteins

Fibronectin and fibrinogen in 20 mM sodium borate, 0.15 M sodium chloride, pH 8.3, were incubated for 2 h at $0°$ with 0.33 M and 0.28 M ethyl acetimidate, respectively. Unreacted reagent was removed by extensive dialysis. Approximately 84% of the lysyl residues in fibronectin and 99% of the lysyl residues in fibrinogen were modified, as assessed by spectroscopy after reaction of the modified proteins with trinitrobenzene sulfonate [26].

Cross-Linking Reactions

Factor XIII_a-mediated cross-linking was performed in 10 mM Tris, 140 mM sodium chloride, pH 7.4 (Tris-buffered saline), containing the indicated amount of calcium chloride. Concentrated stock solutions of the polyamines were made in Tris-buffered saline and titrated to pH 7.4 prior to addition. Proteins to be added were in Tris-buffered saline, with the exception of type I and type III collagen. Prior to being added to the incubations, the collagens were either in 5 mM acetic acid or in 10 mM Tris, 400 mM sodium chloride, pH 7.4. Solutions of Tris and sodium chloride were added along with the collagens in order to make the final ionic strengths and hydrogen ion concentrations constant. The incubations were terminated by addition of an equal volume of 2% sodium dodecyl sulfate, 2% β-mercaptoethanol, followed by heating for 3 min at $95°C$.

Sodium Dodecyl Sulfate-Polyacrylamide Gel Electrophoresis

Polyacrylamide gel electrophoresis in sodium dodecyl sulfate was performed in cylindrical gels or discontinuous slab gels as described previously [19]. After staining with Coomassie brilliant blue R-250, collagen bands were metachromatic [27] and could be identified by their red color. Slabs containing ^{125}I-proteins were dried and analyzed by autoradiography. Inhibition of cross-linking by polyamines was quantitated by analysis of densitometry tracings of autoradiograms:

% Inhibition = 100 − 100X

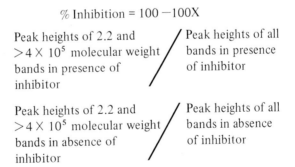

RESULTS

Fibronectin could be cross-linked to isolated α1 (I) collagen chains at $22°$ or $37°$ and to native type I collagen at $37°$ (Fig. 1). Complexes with apparent molecular weights of 3.3, 5.0, and $> 10 \times 10^5$ were formed. These complexes were not formed if factor XIII, thrombin, calcium ion, fibronectin, or collagen was omitted from the reaction mixture [19]. Inclusion of 1 mM spermidine in the reaction mixture completely inhibited formation of the complexes (Fig. 1).

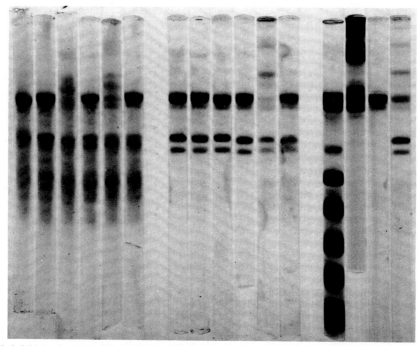

Fig. 1. Inhibition by spermidine of factor XIII$_a$-mediated cross-linking between fibronectin and α1 (I) collagen chains or fibronectin and type I collagen. The reduced products of 13 different incubations were analyzed by sodium dodecyl sulfate-polyacrylamide gel electrophoresis through 4% cylindrical gels. All incubations contained fibronectin, 270 μg/ml; factor XIII, 25 μg/ml; thrombin 1 unit/ml; and 10 mM calcium ion. Incubations 1–6 contained α1 (I) collagen chains, 1 mg/ml; incubations 7–12 contained type I collagen, 400 μg/ml. Even-numbered incubations contained 1 mM spermidine. Incubations were for 2 h at the following temperatures: incubations 1, 2, 7, and 8 at 0°; incubations 3, 4, 9, and 10 at 22°; and incubations 5, 6, 11, and 12 at 37°. Gel 13 contains the following reduced molecular-weight markers: fibronectin, 2.0 × 10^5; phosphorylase, 9.3 × 10^4; albumin, 6.8 × 10^4; ovalbumin, 4.3 × 10^4; chymotrypsinogen, 2.45 × 10^4; and hemoglobin, 1.65 × 10^4. Gel 14 contains nonreduced fibronectin; the major band has a nominal molecular weight of 4.0 × 10^5. Gel 15 contains the products of an incubation in which fibronectin and cross-linking reagents but no collagen were present. Gel 16 contains products of the same incubation as gel 11; the incubation was sampled at 5 min rather than 2 h.

Fibronectin also could be cross-linked to ^{125}I-α1(I)-CB7, which is known to contain a binding site for fibronectin [9, 10] (Fig. 2). Cross-linking was not observed if factor XIII, thrombin, calcium ion, or fibronectin was omitted from the reaction mixture. Cross-linking was partially inhibited by 1–100 μM spermine or spermidine (Fig. 2) and completely inhibited by 1 mM spermine or spermidine (data not shown). Half-inhibition was observed when these polyamines were present at concentrations of approximately 100 μM.

Spermidine, 0.7 mM, inhibited fibronectin-collagen and fibronectin-fibrin but not fibronectin-fibronectin and fibrin-fibrin cross-linking (Fig. 3). As shown in gels 1–4, fibronectin can be cross-linked to itself in the presence of dithiothreitol [14] to form dimers of 4.0 × 10^5 MW and higher-molecular-weight oligomers. Formation of oligomers and loss of staining from the 2.0 × 10^5 MW monomer band were inhibited by monodansylcadaverine but not by spermidine. As shown in gels 5–8 of Figure 3, both spermidine and monodansyl-cadaverine inhibited the cross-linking of fibronectin and α1 (I) collagen chains. Gels 9–12

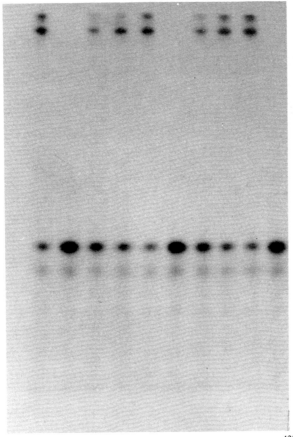

Fig. 2. Inhibition of factor XIII$_a$-mediated cross-linking between fibronectin and ^{125}I-α1 (I)-CB7 of α1 (I) collagen chains by spermine and spermidine. The reduced products of ten different incubations were analyzed by sodium dodecyl sulfate-polyacrylamide gel electrophoresis through a 3% /8% discontinuous slab gel. The slab was analyzed by autoradiography. All incubations contained fibronectin, 270 μg/ml, and ^{125}I-α1 (I)-CB7, 3 μg/ml. Incubations 1, 3–5, and 7–9 contained 10 mM calcium ion; factor XIII, 25 μg/ml; and thrombin, 1 unit/ml. Incubations 3, 4, and 5 contained 100 μM, 10 μM, and 1 μM spermine, respectively; incubations 7, 8, and 9 contained 100 μM, 10 μM, and 1 μM spermidine, respectively. Incubations 2, 6, and 10 contained 10 mM ethylenediaminetetraacetic acid (EDTA) instead of calcium and no factor XIII or thrombin. Incubations were for 2 h at 37°C. Approximately 5 × 10^3 CPM were added to each slot of the gel. Apparent molecular weights of the non-cross-linked ^{125}I-α1 (I)-CB7 bands (narrow arrows) are 3.3 × 10^4 and 2.9 × 10^4; apparent molecular weights of cross-linked ^{125}I-α1(I)-CB7 (broad arrows) are 2.2 and > 4.0 × 10^5.

of Figure 3 show that formation of 2.6 and 3.0 × 10^5 MW complexes, which consist of fibronectin and the α chains of fibrin [14, 18], and loss of staining from the band representing fibronectin monomer were partially inhibited by spermidine and more completely inhibited by monodansylcadaverine. Gels 9–16 show that formation of the cross-linked 9.3 × 10^4 MW dimer of the γ-chains of fibrin, loss of staining from the 4.7 × 10^4 MW γ-chain band, formation of the various cross-linked multimers of the α chains of fibrin, and loss of staining from the 7.2 × 10^4 MW α-chain band were inhibited by monodansylcadaverine but not by spermidine.

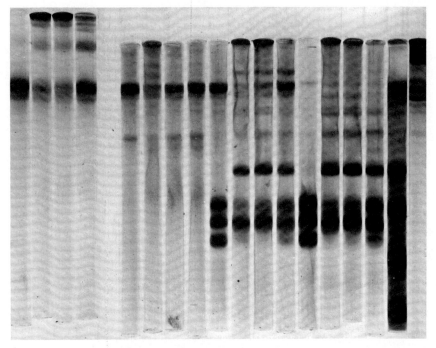

Fig. 3. Inhibition of factor XIII$_a$-mediated fibronectin-collagen and fibronectin-fibrin but not fibronectin-fibronectin or fibrin-fibrin cross-linking by spermidine. The reduced products of 16 different incubations
were analyzed by sodium dodecyl sulfate-polyacrylamide gel electrophoresis through 4% (gel 1–4)
or 5% (gels 5–18) cylindrical gels. Incubations 1–4 contained fibronectin, 710 μg/ml, and 10 mM dithiothreitol; incubations 5–8 contained fibronectin, 270 μg/ml, and isolated α1 (I) collagen chains, 250
μg/ml; incubations 9–12 contained fibronectin, 270 μg/ml, and fibrinogen, 730 μg/ml; and incubations
13–16 contained fibrinogen, 1.4 mg/ml. Incubations 2–4, 6–8, 10–12, and 14–16 contained factor
XIII, 25 μg/ml; thrombin, 1 unit/ml; and 10 mM calcium ion. Incubations 1, 5, 9, and 13 contained 10
mM EDTA instead of calcium ion and no factor XIII or thrombin. Incubations 3, 7, 11, and 15 contained 0.67 mM spermidine; incubations 4, 8, 12, and 16 contained 0.63 mM monodansylcadaverine.
Incubations 1–8 were for 2 h at 37°C; incubations 9–16 were for 2 h at 0°. Gels 17 and 18 contained
reduced size markers and nonreduced fibronectin, respectively (see Fig. 1). Fibronectin-fibrin cross-
linking was studied at 0° rather than 37° because fibrin α-chain polymer formation is less marked at the
lower temperature [14].

Spermidine could enhance cross-linking between peptide chains by means of a transfer reaction between the carboxamide group of a glutaminyl residue in each chain and both
primary amino groups of the polyamine [24]. To examine this possibility, we followed
the lead of Schrode and Folk [24] and attempted to cross-link amidinated fibronectin
and fibrin in the presence and absence of polyamines (Fig. 4). Modification of lysyl residues in fibrinogen was virtually complete, yielding a product that could not be cross-
linked (Fig. 4, slot 7). Lysyl residues in fibronectin were not completely modified and the
amidinated fibronectin could be partially cross-linked in the presence of dithiothreitol
(Fig. 4, slot 2). Spermine or spermidine enhanced cross-linking of amidinated fibronectin (Fig. 4, slots 3 and 4) but not of amidinated fibrin (Fig. 4, slots 8 and 9). Spermine
or spermidine enhanced cross-linking between amidinated fibronectin and amidinated
fibrin (Fig. 4, slots 13 and 14).

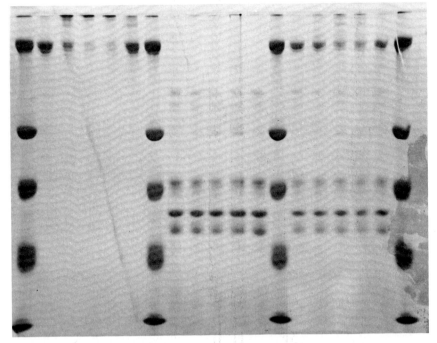

Fig. 4. Effects of spermidine, spermine, and monodansylcadaverine on factor XIII$_a$-mediated cross-linking of amidinated fibronectin and fibrin. The reduced products of 15 different incubations were analyzed by sodium dodecyl sulfate-polyacrylamide gel electrophoresis through a 3%/8% slab gel. Incubations contained factor XIII, 25 μg/ml; thrombin, 1 unit/ml; and 10 mM calcium ion. Incubations 1–5 contained amidinated fibronectin, 720 μg/ml, and 10 mM dithiothreitol. Incubations 6–10 contained amidinated fibrinogen, 1.2 mg/ml. Incubations 11–15 contained amidinated fibronectin, 310 μg/ml, and amidinated fibrinogen, 610 μg/ml. Incubations 1, 6, and 11 contained 10 mM EDTA instead of calcium ion. Incubations 3, 8, and 13 contained 0.67 mM spermidine; incubations 4, 9, and 14 contained 0.67 mM spermine; and incubations 5, 10, and 15 contained 0.63 mM monodansylcadaverine. Incubations 1–5 were at 37°C for 2 h. Incubations 6–15 were at 0° for 2 h. Molecular-weight markers (see Fig. 1) were analyzed on every sixth slot.

DISCUSSION

Vuento and Vaheri demonstrated that polyamines bind to fibronectin during gel filtration and can be used to dissociate fibronectin from insolubilized gelatin [25]. The present experiments demonstrate that polyamines inhibit factor XIII$_a$-mediated cross-linking between fibronectin and collagen. The same concentrations of polyamines had little effect on factor XIII$_a$-mediated cross-linking among fibrin molecules and enhanced factor XIII$_a$-mediated cross-linking among molecules of amidinated fibronectin. Cross-linking of amidinated fibronectin presumably is enhanced by formation of $N^{1,n}$-(di-γ-glutamyl)-polyamine cross-linkages, as described by Schrode and Folk [24]. Monodansylcadaverine, which is the best-known inhibitor of factor XIII$_a$-mediated fibrin-fibrin cross-linking [28, 29], also inhibited fibronectin-fibrin, fibronectin-fibronectin, and fibronectin-collagen cross-linking. The results suggest that polyamines specifically interact with the fibronec-tinyl-factor XIII$_a$ acyl-enzyme intermediate [30–32] and compete with lysyl residues of collagen as acyl acceptors in factor XIII_a -mediated cross-linking. In contrast, monodansyl-cadaverine apparently reacts with both the fibrinyl-factor XIII_a and fibronectinyl-factor XIII_a acyl-enzyme intermediates and is a more general inhibitor of factors XIII_a -mediated cross-linking.

Previous studies suggest that fibrin and collagen compete for the same binding site on fibronectin. Loss of fibronectin into the fibrin clot is less when denatured collagen is present during clotting [7], and $\alpha 1$ (I)-CB7 inhibits cross-linking of the α chain of fibrin to fibronectin [19]. Conversely, fibrinogen inhibits the binding of fibronectin to denatured collagen [7], and fibrin inhibits the cross-linking of ^{125}I-$\alpha 1$ (I)-CB7 to fibronectin [19]. In our experiments, polyamines had a dual effect on fibronectin-fibrin cross-linking. Spermidine and spermine enhanced cross-linking of amidinated fibronectin and amidinated fibrin (Fig. 4), presumably by being incorporated into $N^{1, n}$-(di-γ-glutamyl)-polyamine cross-linkages. However, spermidine partially inhibited cross-linking between unmodified fibronectin and unmodified fibrin (Fig. 3). The α chain of fibrin contains glutaminyl residues which are susceptible to the action of factor XIII_a [13], whereas we have been unable to demonstrate susceptible glutaminyl residues in collagen (unpublished results). We suspect that polyamines compete as acyl acceptors in factor XIII_a-mediated cross-linking between fibronectin and fibrin just as between fibronectin and collagen. However, the competition may be partially masked when assayed by polyacrylamide gel electrophoresis because of formation of $N^{1, n}$-(di-γ-glutamyl)-polyamine cross-linkages between reactive glutaminyl residues in fibronectin and reactive glutaminyl residues in fibrin.

Further experiments are needed to determine the significance of the present findings. The concentrations of polyamines and their biosynthetic enzymes increase when enkaryotic cells proliferate [21, 22]. Both tissue transglutaminases and the plasma enzyme are widely distributed [13]. One can think of a number of ways in which the formation of the extracellular fibronectin-collagen matrix could be influenced by polyamines. For instance, transglutaminase-catalyzed incorporation of a polyamine into fibronectin might make fibronectin incapable of associating with collagen. Conversely, polyamines could disrupt noncovalent associations between fibronectin and collagen [25], but not cross-linked fibronectin-collagen complexes. To test such hypotheses, it will be necessary to characterize the biochemistry of the fibronectin-collagen and fibronectin-polyamine interactions in more detail and to correlate biochemical studies with events which take place in cultures of proliferating cells and in proliferating tissues.

ACKNOWLEDGMENTS

This work was supported by the National Institutes of Health (HL 21644) and the University of Wisconsin Graduate School. It was done during the tenure of an Established Investigatorship from the American Heart Association and its Wisconsin Affiliate to Deane F. Mosher.

REFERENCES

1. Vaheri A, Mosher DF: Biochim Biophys Acta 516:1, 1978.
2. Yamada KM, Olden K: Nature 275:179, 1978.
3. Furcht LT, Mosher DF, Wendelschafer-Crabb G: Cell 13:262, 1978.
4. Hedman K, Vaheri A, Wartiovaara J: J Cell Biol 76:748, 1978.
5. Chen LB, Murray A, Segal RA, Bushnell A, Walsh ML: Cell 14:377, 1978.
6. Crouch E, Balian G, Holbrook K, Duksin D, Bornstein P: J Cell Biol 78:701, 1978.

7. Engvall E, Ruoslahti E, Miller EJ: J Exp Med 147:1584, 1978.
8. Jilke F, Hörmann H: Hoppe-Seyler's Z Physiol Chem 359:247, 1978.
9. Dessau W, Adelmann BC, Timpl R, Martin GR: Biochem J 169:55. 1978.
10. Kleinman HK, McGoodwin EB, Martin GR, Klebe RJ, Fietzek PP, Woolley DE: J Biol Chem 753: 5642, 1978.
11. Bornstein P, Ash JF: Proc Natl Acad Sci USA 74:2480, 1977.
12. Vaheri A, Kurkinen M, Lehto V-P, Linder E, Timpl R: Proc Natl Acad Sci USA 75:4944, 1978.
13. Folk JE, Finlayson JS: Adv Protein Chem 31:1, 1977.
14. Mosher DF: J Biol Chem 250:6614, 1975.
15. Jilek F, Hörmann H: Hoppe-Seyler's Z Physiol Chem 358:1165, 1977.
16. Birckbichler PJ, Patterson MK, Jr: Ann NY Acad Sci 312:354, 1978.
17. Mosher DF: J Biol Chem 251:1639, 1976.
18. Iwanaga S, Suzuki K, Hashimoto S: Ann NY Acad Sci 312:56, 1978.
19. Mosher DF, Schad PE, Kleinman HK: J Clin Invest 64:781, 1979.
20. Keski-Oja J, Mosher DF, Vaheri A: Cell 9:29, 1976.
21. Tabor CW, Tabor H: Ann Rev Biochem 45:285, 1976.
22. Jänne J, Pösö H, Raina A: Biochim Biophys Acta 473:241, 1978.
23. Clarke DD, Mycek MJ, Neidle A, Waelsch H: Arch Biochem Biophys 126:44, 1959.
24. Schrode J, Folk JE: J Biol Chem 253:4837, 1978.
25. Vuento M, Vaheri A: Biochem J 175:333, 1978.
26. Wofsy L, Singer SJ: Biochemistry 2:104, 1963.
27. Micko S, Schlaepfer WW: Anal Biochem 88:566, 1978.
28. Lorand L, Rule NG, Ong HH, Furlanetto R, Jacobsen A, Downey J,Örner N, Bruner-Lorand J: Biochemistry 7:1214, 1968.
29. Nilsson JLG, Stenberg P, Ljunggren C, Hoffman K-J, Lunden R, Eriksson O, Lorand L: Ann NY Acad Sci 202:286, 1972.
30. Pincus JH, Waelsch H: Arch Biochem Biophys 126:44, 1968.
31. Curtis CG, Stenberg P, Brown KL, Baron A, Chen C, Gary A, Simpson I, Lorand L: Biochemistry 13:3257, 1974.
32. Gross M, Whetzel NH, Folk JE: J Biol Chem 252:3752, 1977.

Journal of Supramolecular Structure 11:237–250 (1979)
Tumor Cell Surfaces and Malignancy 183–196

Influence of Buffer Ions and Divalent Cations on Coated Vesicle Disassembly and Reassembly

Michael P. Woodward and Thomas F. Roth

Department of Biological Sciences, University of Maryland Baltimore County, Catonsville, Maryland 21228

Disruption of the coat of coated vesicles is accompanied by the release of clathrin and other proteins in soluble form. The ability of solubilized coated vesicle proteins to reassemble into empty coats is influenced by Mg^{2+}, Tris ion concentration, pH, and ionic strength. The proteins solubilized by 2 M urea spontaneously reassemble into empty coats following dialysis into isolation buffer (0.1 M MES–1 mM EGTA–1 mM $MgCl_2$–0.02% NaN_3, pH 6.8). Such reassembled coats have sedimentation properties similar to untreated coated vesicles. Clathrin is the predominant protein of reassembled coats; most of the other proteins present in native coated vesicles are absent. We have found that Mg^{2+} is important in the coat assembly reaction. At pH 8 in 0.01 M or 0.1 M Tris, coats dissociate; however, 10 mM $MgCl_2$ prevents dissociation. If the coats are first dissociated at pH 8 and then the $MgCl_2$ is raised to 10 mM, reassembly occurs. These results suggest that Mg^{2+} stabilizes the coat lattice and promotes reassembly. This hypothesis is supported by our observations that increasing Mg^{2+} (10 μM–10 mM) increases reassembly whereas chelation of Mg^{2+} by (EGTA) inhibits reassembly. Coats reassembled in low-Tris (0.01 M, pH 8) supernatants containing 10 mM $MgCl_2$ do not sediment, but upon dialysis into isolation buffer (pH 6.8), these coats become sedimentable. Nonsedimentable coats are noted also either when partially purified clathrin (peak I from Sepharose CL4B columns) is dialyzed into low-ionic-strength buffer or when peaks I and II are dialyzed into isolation buffer. Such nonsedimentable coats may represent intermediates in the assembly reaction which have normal morphology but lack some of the physical properties of native coats. We present a model suggesting that tightly intertwined antiparallel clathrin dimers form the edges of the coat lattice.

Key words: coated vesicles, coat dissembly, coat reassembly, coat dissociation, clathrin

Abbreviations used: SDS, sodium dodecyl sulfate; PAGE, polyacrylamide gel electrophoresis; EGTA, ethyleneglycoltetraacetic acid; MES, 2-(N-morpholino)ethanesulfonic acid.

Received May 21, 1979; accepted July 13, 1979.

Morphologic evidence has suggested that coated vesicles are the intracellular organelles responsible for receptor-mediated protein transport [1–3] and neuronal membrane recycling [4, 5]. Until recently, however, little was known concerning the structure and biochemical composition of coated vesicles. Pioneering structural studies by Kanaseki and Kadota [6] and Kadota and Kadota [7] have revealed that the coat consists of a lattice of interlocked hexagons and pentagons. The most striking image is that resulting from the assembly of 20 hexagons and 12 pentagons to form a spherical lattice. An elegant study by Crowther et al [8] supported these observations and demonstrated that there were other possible arrangements of hexagons and pentagons. Woods et al [9] made similar observations on coated vesicles from porcine brain and chicken oocyte. In addition they found that larger assemblies occurred in chicken oocytes [9]. A common observation of all of the preceding studies is that the coat lattice consists of rod-shaped particles which assemble into interlocked hexagons and pentagons. Ockleford [10] has proposed, on the basis of observations of coated vesicles in human placentas, that the sides of the hexagons and pentagons are composed of ridges of protein rather than rods.

Concurrent with these morphologic studies were investigations of the protein composition of purified coated vesicle preparations. Pearse [11] observed that porcine brain-coated vesicle preparations contained a single major protein (mol wt = 180,000 daltons), which she estimated made up greater than 80% of the total protein. Subsequently, she found that this protein, clathrin, was common to coated vesicles from a variety of sources [12]. Blitz et al [13] found that in addition to clathrin two other proteins were consistently found in significant amounts of brain coated vesicle preparations. Woods et al [9] also observed similar proteins in chicken oocyte and porcine brain coated vesicle preparations. Woodward and Roth [14] quantitated the amount of protein in the various bands observed in SDS gel electrophoretic patterns of porcine brain-coated vesicle preparations and found that clathrin, a 125,000-dalton protein, and a 55,000-dalton protein occurred with a mole ratio of approximately 2:1:2.

Pearse [11, 12] and Blitz et al [13] have argued that chlathrin is the sole structural protein of the coat lattice, since it is the major band on SDS gels. In support of this Blitz et al [13] found that clathrin was the major protein solubilized by 2 M urea. Partial confirmation of this hypothesis has come from studies by Woodward and Roth [14], Kartenbeck [15], Schook et al [16], and Keen et al [17], who have found that coats can reassemble spontaneously in solutions of solubilized coated vesicle proteins under appropriate conditions. However, it is still not certain that clathrin is the sole structural protein of the lattice or that it can catalyze its own self assembly. In this report we present further studies of the role of clathrin in coat structure.

METHODS

Isolation Procedure

Coated vesicles were prepared as described by Woodward and Roth [14]. Isolation buffer contained 0.1 M MES–1 mM $MgCl_2$–1 mM EGTA–0.2% NaN_3 (pH 6.8). The purity of the preparations was monitored by electron microscopy of negatively stained samples or thin section images as described previously [14].

Electrophoresis Methods

SDS-polyacrylamide gel electrophoresis was performed using 10% slab gels according to Laemmli [18]. Gels were simultaneously fixed and stained in 30% isopropanol–10% acetic acid–0.05%. Coomassie blue R250 and destained in 10% isopropanol–10% acetic acid.

Protein Concentration

Protein concentrations were estimated from the amount of tryptophan fluorescence at 340 nm. Bovine serum albumin was used to construct a standard curve.

Centrifuation Procedures

Sucrose density grandient centrifugation. Coated vesicle preparations were analyzed on 10–30% (w/w) linear sucrose density gradients using a SW40 rotor. The gradients were centrifuged for 2 h at 57,000 g at 4°C. They were fractionated by upward displacement with 50% sucrose. Fractions were monitored by absorbance at 280 nm, electron microscopy, and SDS-polyacrylamide gel electrophoresis.

Airfuge centrifugation. Samples were centrifuged at room temperature for 20 min at 107,000 g in a Beckman Airfuge to separate reassembled coats from soluble proteins.

Sepharose CL4B chromatography. Coated vesicle proteins solubilized with 0.5 M Tris-isolation buffer (pH 7.0) [17] were chromatographed at room temperature on a Sepharose CL4B column (1.5 X 100 cm) in 0.5 M Tris-isolation buffer (pH 7.0) at 10 ml/h.

RESULTS

Purified coated vesicle preparations consisting of empty coats and coated vesicles contain many proteins [14]. We sought to determine which of these proteins are structural elements of the coat lattice by investigating in vitro reassembled coats.

Protein Composition and Structure of Reassembled Coats

Although a variety of reagents disrupt coat morphology and promote the release of clathrin, as well as other proteins [14], we observe only small differences between the resultant SDS-polyacrylamide gel patterns. Coated vesicles dissociated in 2 M urea, 0.25 M $MgCl_2$, or 10 mM Tris (pH 8) reassemble as empty coats after dialysis of the soluble proteins into isolation buffer [14]. These coats exhibit sizes and symmetries similar to those seen in undissociated coated vesicles [14]. In particular, empty coats with six-fold rotational symmetry are frequently observed (Fig. 1a). Isolated hexagons or pentagons, which could be intermediates in the reassembly reaction, are not evident. In high magnification, high-resolution images of negatively stained coats, the edges of the lattice often appear to have a helical substructure. This aspect of coat morphology is enhanced in Markham-rotated images (Fig. 1a).

To determine if reassembled coats have sedimentation properties similar to control coats, we purified reassembled coats on 10–30% (w/w) linear sucrose density gradients. Comparison of the sedimentation profile of empty coats reassembled from 2 M urea supernatants with that of undissociated preparations suggests that the two preparations have identical sedimentation characteristics (Fig. 2a). Both reassembled and untreated coats exhibited broad profiles on these gradients, the peak fractions having a sedimentation coefficient of approximately 200S. Coats were observed only at sucrose concentrations greater than 15% (w/w). The width of the peaks does not appear to be due to aggregation or association of the coats, since negatively stained images of the fractions did not contain clusters of coats. Rather, the broad sedimentation profile may be due to the size heterogeneity of the preparations.

Gradient fractions containing reassembled coats (lanes 7–14, Fig. 2b) appear to consist predominantly of clathrin when analyzed on SDS-polyacrylamide gels. The group of bands in the region of 90,000–125,000 daltons and 55,000 daltons, present in untreated preparations (lanes 6–14, Fig. 2c), are present in very much reduced amounts in

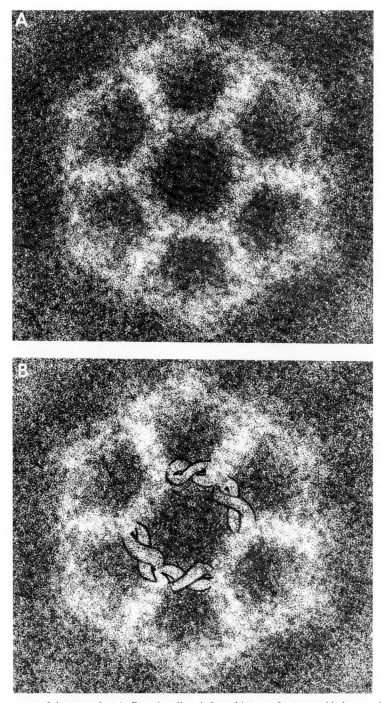

Fig. 1. Structure of the coat edge. A: Rotationally reinforced image of a reassembled coat with six-fold symmetry. We frequently observe such coats in both untreated and reassembled preparations. The lattice edges appear to be composed of intertwined rods. Negatively stained with uranyl acetate. × 1,200,000. B: To aid in visualizing the substructure of the lattice edges in A we have outlined the rods comprising several of the edges.

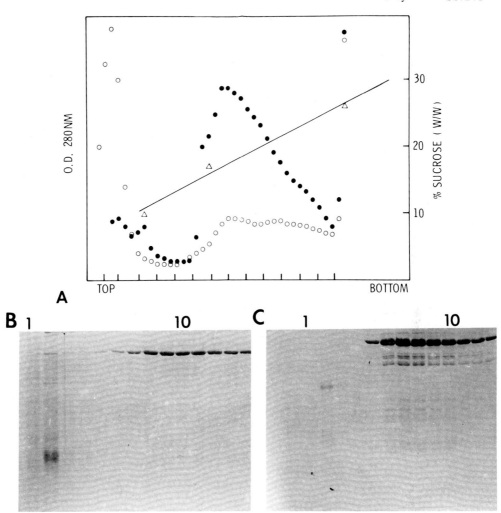

Fig. 2. A: Sedimentation profiles of reassembled coats (○) and untreated coated vesicles preparations (●). Aliquots of reassembled and native preparations were centrifuged in parallel on 10–30% (w/w) linear sucrose density gradients. Coats were observed between 15% and 26% (w/w) sucrose on both gradients. Most of the minor proteins remained at the top of the reassembled coat gradients, whereas they cosedimented with the native coats. The gradients were centrifuged for 2 h at 57,000g in a Beckman SW40 rotor. The hash marks on the abscissa indicate fractions analyzed by SDS-poly-acrylmaide gel electrophoresis. B, C: Comparison of the proteins present in reassembled coats (B) and native preparations (C). Fractions of the reassembled and untreated gradients were analyzed by SDS-polyacylamide gel electrophoresis. Reassembled coats (lanes 7–14) appear to have fewer proteins than untreated coated vesicle preparations (lanes 6–14). In particular, the relative amounts of the 125,000-dalton proteins and 55,000-dalton proteins are markedly diminished in reassembled coats. Most of the minor bands (lanes 1 and 2) do not cosediment with reassembled coats.

reassembled coats. Many of the minor proteins present in the 2 M urea supernatant remain at the top of the gradient (lanes 1 and 2, Fig. 2b), whereas the majority of the clathrin is found in reassembled coats. These results suggest that clathrin is the predominant structural element of the coat.

MgCl$_2$ and Tris Effects on Reassembly

In some preliminary experiments using preparations dissociated at pH $>$ 7.5 we observed that the MgCl$_2$ and Tris concentration of the dissociating buffer profoundly affected the reassembly equilibrium. Coated vesicles dissociated in low Tris (10 mM Tris-10 μM MgCl$_2$ – 1 mM EGTA, pH 8) or high Tris (100 mM Tris–10 μM MgCl$_2$ –1 mM EGTA, pH 8.3) reassembled when dialyzed into isolation buffer (pH 6.5) containing 10 μM MgCl$_2$. However, if 10 mM MgCl$_2$ was present in the dissociating buffer, no dissociation was observed, which suggests to us that MgCl$_2$ stabilizes the coat and might promote reassembly. This possibility was tested by examination of the effect MgCl$_2$ has on reassembly at pH 8 or 8.3 and during dialysis into isolation buffer (pH 6.8).

Effect of MgCl$_2$ on Reassembly in 100 mM Tris (pH 8.3)

Reassembled coats form in preparations dissociated in high Tris at pH 8.3 if the MgCl$_2$ concentration is raised to 10 mM (Table I). The substantial increase in the amount of protein which sediments in the presence of 10 mM MgCl$_2$ (Table I) suggests that these coats sediment like native coats. At concentrations of MgCl$_2$ less than 10 mM, no coats are observed in the electron microscope and the majority of protein does not sediment, indicating that reassembly has not occurred. The material which does sediment at less than 10 mM MgCl$_2$ consists of vesicles and protein aggregates.

Since these results at pH 8.3 support the hypothesis that Mg^{2+} promoted reassembly, we next examined if increasing the MgCl$_2$ concentration shifted the reassembly equilibrium toward the assembled state at pH 6.8. After preparations dissociated in high Tris are dialyzed against isolation buffer (pH 6.8) containing 10 μM to 10 mM MgCl$_2$, reassembled coats, but not filamentous aggregates, are observed in the electron microscope. Interestingly, as the concentration of MgCl$_2$ is increased, more protein sediments, which suggests that more reassembly occurs as the concentration of MgCl$_2$ is raised (Table II).

Effect of MgCl$_2$ on Reassembly of 100 mM Tris (pH 8.3) Supernatants

We previously observed [14] that vesicle and aggregate free supernatants obtained following dissociation of coated vesicles with 2 M urea reassembled when dialyzed into isolation buffer at pH 6.8. This indicated that the 2 M urea supernatants contained all the proteins necessary for reassembly. Since supernatants from coated vesicles dissociated from both high and low Tris contained essentially the same proteins as 2 M urea supernatants as judged by SDS PAGE, we predicted they would also reassemble. However, when the high-Tris supernatants were tested for reassembly at pH 8 and 8.3, or following dialysis into isolation buffer at pH 6.8, no reassembly was observed (Table III). Raising the MgCl$_2$ concentration to 10mM did not result in reassembly as it did in noncentrifuged preparations (see Table II).

Effect of MgCl$_2$ on Reassembly of 10 mM Tris Supernatants

In contrast to the results of the previous experiment, reassembly did take place when the supernatants from coated vesicles dissociated in low Tris, instead of high Tris, were dialyzed against isolation buffer (pH 6.8) (Table IV). Coats reassemble at pH 8 (low Tris), in the presence of 10 mM MgCl$_2$, but these coats do not sediment under conditions which pellet control preparations. However, dialysis of each supernatant into isolation buffer (pH 6.8) containing 10 μM to 10 mM MgCl$_2$ resulted in the formation of coats which did sediment (Table IV). Despite the fact that the coats which reassembled at pH 8 (10 mM MgCl$_2$) did not sediment, they appear morphologically identical to those which did sediment at pH 6.8.

TABLE I. Effect of [MgCl$_2$] on Reassembly in 100 mM Tris (pH 8.3)

[MgCl$_2$]:	10 μM	100 μM	1 mM	10 mM	20 mM
Preparation I					
Coats present	–	–	–	+	+
% Protein sedimentable	26	35	31	75	nd
Preparation 2					
Coats present	–	–	–	+	
% Protein sedimentable	37	38	43	69	

Coated vesicles were dissociated with 100 mM Tris pH 8.3. (The buffer also contained either 100 mM MES – 10 μM MgCl$_2$ – 1 mM EGTA or 10 M MgCl$_2$ – 1 mM EGTA.) Following dissociation aliquots were adjusted to 10 μM, 100 μM, 1 mM, 10 mM, or 20 mM MgCl$_2$ and then assayed by electron microscopy for the presence of coats and by centrifugation for sedimentable particles.

TABLE II. Effect of [MgCl$_2$] on Reassembly of Preparations Dissociated in 100 mM Tris (pH 8.3) and Then Dialyzed Into Isolation Buffer (pH 6.8)

[MgCl$_2$]:	10 μM	100 μM	1 mM	10 mM
Coats present	+	+	+	+
% Protein sedimentable	62	74	70	80

Coated vesicles were dissociated with 100 mM Tris (pH 8.3) as in Table I. Separate portions of the preparations were adjusted to 10 M, 100 μM, 1 mM, or 10 mM MgCl$_2$, dialyzed into isolation buffer at pH 6.8 containing the same MgCl$_2$ concentration, and then assayed for the presence of coats by electron microscopy and by centrifugation for sedimentable particles.

TABLE III. Effect of [MgCl$_2$] on Reassembly of 100 mM Tris (pH 8.3) Supernatants Dialyzed Into Isolation Buffer (pH 6.8)

[MgCl$_2$]:	10 μM	100 μM	1 mM
Coats present	–	–	–

Coated vesicles were dissociated by dialysis into 100 mM Tris (pH 8.3) containing 10 μM, 100 μM, or 1 mM MgCl$_2$. The dissociated preparations were centrifuged to remove vesicles and aggregates (Beckman Airfuge for 20 min, 107,000 g), then dialyzed into isolation buffer (pH 6.8) containing the same MgCl$_2$ concentrations, and assayed for the presence of coats by electron microscopy.

TABLE IV. Effect of [MgCl$_2$] on Reassembly of 10 mM Tris (pH 8) Supernatants

[MgCl$_2$]:	10 μM	100 μM	1 mM	10 mM
Coats present (pH 8)	–	–	–	+[a]
% Protein sedimentable	8	8	13	18
Coats present (pH 6.8)	+	+	+	+

A coated vesicle preparation was dissociated by dialysis into 10 mM Tris – 10μM MgCl$_2$ – 1 mM EGTA (pH 8) and then centrifuged for 20 min at 107,000g in a Beckman Airfuge to remove vesicles and aggregates. Separate portions of the supernatant were brought to 10 μM, 100 μM, 1 mM or 10 mM MgCl$_2$ and assayed by negative staining for the presence of coats and by centrifugation for sedimentable particles. Then the aliquots were dialyzed into isolation buffer (pH 6.8) at the same MgCl$_2$ concentrations and assayed for the presence of coats by electron microscopy.

[a]Normal-looking coats were present but were nonsedimentable.

Effect of EGTA on Reassembly

If $MgCl_2$ promotes coat reassembly, it should be possible to inhibit its effect through the use of chelating agents. This possibility was tested by dialyzing preparations dissociated in 100 mM Tris–10 μM $MgCl_2$ (pH 8.3) into isolation buffer at pH 6.8 containing 100 μM to 10 mM EGTA (Table V). Although reassembly was observed at all concentrations of EGTA tested, less protein sedimented with increasing EGTA concentration. These results suggest that EGTA inhibited coat assembly and are consistent with our hypothesis that $MgCl_2$ promotes reassembly.

The divalent cation induction of coat reassembly appears to be specific for $MgCl_2$. For, when 10 mM $CaCl_2$, $MnCl_2$, $ZnCl_2$, or $FeCl_2$ was added to preparations dissociated in 10 mM or 100 mM Tris at pH 8, large aggregates of protein formed. Such aggregates were often in the form of filamentous bundles. Lower concentrations of these ions were not tested.

Effect of [Tris] on Reassembly

The ability of the 10 mM but not the 100 mM Tris supernatants to reassemble suggested that the physical properties of one or more proteins necessary for assembly may have been altered. To determine whether this inhibition was due to Tris or to increased ionic strength, a preparation was dissociated with low Tris and centrifuged, and portions of the supernatant were adjusted to low Tris, high Tris, or high NaCl (Table VI).

The presence of 1 mM $MgCl_2$ did not promote reassembly in any of the fractions at pH 8.0 (Table VI), and little protein sedimented upon centrifugation of the treated supernatants (Table VI). However, upon dialysis to pH 6.8 in isolation buffer, coats reassembled from both low Tris and 10 mM Tris–100 mM NaCl supernatants, but no coats were observed in the high-Tris supernatant (Table VI). This suggests that the effects on reassembly we observed were due to the Tris molecule rather than higher ionic strength.

Fractionation of Coated Vesicle Proteins

Our experiments with 2 M urea and low-Tris supernatants show that the proteins necessary for reassembly can be released in soluble form. However, these supernatants may well contain more proteins than those needed for reassembly. In order to determine which proteins are required for reassembly or are part of the coat lattice, we attempted to fractionate the 2M urea and low-Tris supernatants by chromatography on Agarose A-5M, but found that the columns did not separate the proteins (data not shown). This suggested to us that neither 2M urea nor low Tris completely disrupts the protein-protein interactions of the lattice. However, we were able to separate some of the coated vesicle proteins by chromatography on Sepharose CL-4B columns equilibrated with 0.5 M Tris-isolation buffer (pH 7) using the method of Keen et al [17].

Both we and Keen et al [17] find that unfractionated 0.5 M Tris supernatants reassemble when dialyzed into isolation buffer. However, unlike Keen et al [17] we found that such reassembled coats did sediment like control coats, whereas they observed that the coats did not sediment on sucrose gradients. The source of this difference is unknown to us.

Chromatography on Sepharose CL4B columns separates the proteins into two major peaks (Fig. 3a). Both we and Keen et al [17] find that the faster-eluting peak (peak I) contains clathrin and that peak II contains several proteins including the 95,000-

TABLE V. Effect of [EGTA] on Reassembly of Preparations Dissociated in 100 mM Tris (pH 8.3) and Then Dialyzed Into Isolation Buffer (pH 6.8)

[EGTA]:	100 μM	1 mM	10 mM
Coats present	+	+	+
% Protein sedimentable	72	68	46

Coated vesicles were dissociated in 100 mM Tris (pH 8.3) and then separate aliquots were dialyzed into isolation buffer containing 100 μM, 1 mM, or 10 mM EGTA at pH 6.8. Following dialysis the solutions were assayed for the presence of coats by electron microscopy and centrifugation for sedimentable particles.

TABLE VI. Effect of [Tris] on Reassembly

	10 mM Tris	100 mM Tris	10 mM Tris–100 mM NaCl
Coats present (pH 8)	–	–	–
% Protein sedimentable	13	16	nd
Coats present following dialysis to pH 6.8	+	–	+

A coated vesicle preparation was dissociated by dialysis into 10 mM Tris–10 μM MgCl$_2$–1 mM EGTA (pH 8) and then centrifuged 20 min at 107,000g to remove vesicles and aggregates. Separate portions of the supernatant were adjusted to 10 mM Tris–1 mM MgCl$_2$, 100 mM Tris–1 mM MgCl$_2$, or 10 mM Tris–100 mM NaCl–1 mM MgCl$_2$. These aliquots were assayed for the presence of coats by electron microscopy and for sedimentable particles by centrifugation in a Beckman Airfuge (20 min at 107,000g). The resultant supernatants were dialyzed into isolation buffer and then assayed for the presence of coats.

and 125,000-dalton proteins. However, unlike Keen et al [17] we find that peak I also contains two proteins with molecular weights near 30,000 daltons (Fig. 3b) in addition to clathrin.

We find, as did Keen et al [17], that neither peak I nor peak II alone reassembled when dialyzed into isolation buffer at pH 6.5, but that an equal mixture of peaks I and II did reassemble when dialyzed into isolation buffer (pH 6.5). However, the coats formed do not sediment. Peak I alone did reassemble when dialyzed against 10 mM MES–1 mM EDTA–1 mM CaCl$_2$ (pH 6.5), but it too did not sediment. Thus it appears that the ability of the proteins of peak I to reassemble is influenced by ionic strength and accessory proteins. That these coats did not sediment suggests that other factors necessary for coat stabilization were absent.

DISCUSSION

Pure preparations of coated vesicles contain a plethora of proteins which, after being solubilized by a variety of treatments, can reassemble into intact coats. This ability to reassemble has provided us with a major tool for examining which proteins are involved in coat structure, which proteins are important in regulating reassembly, and what ionic conditions are necessary for reassembly.

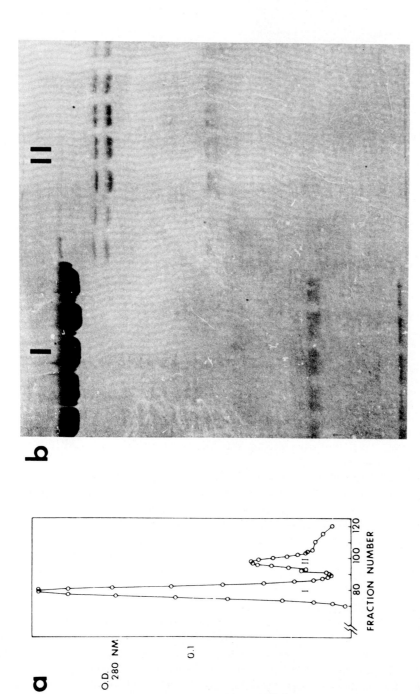

Fig. 3. Separation of coated vesicle proteins by chromatography on Sepharose CL4B. a: Elution profile of 0.5 M Tris-isolation buffer (pH 7.0) supernatants on Sepharose CL4B. Coated vesicle proteins solubilized by treatment with 0.5 M Tris-isolation buffer (pH 7.0) were chromatographed on a Sepharose CL4B column equilibrated with 0.5 M Tris-isolation buffer; b: SDS-polyacrylamide gel patterns of peaks I and II. Aliquots of peaks I and II were analyzed by SDS-polyacrylamide gel electrophoresis. Peak I consists primarily of clathrin. Peak II contains the 125,000-dalton proteins and the 55,000-dalton protein.

Proteins Involved in the Coat Lattice

We find that treatment of coated vesicles with 2 M urea, low Tris (10 mM, pH 8), and 0.5 M Tris-isolation buffer (pH 7) yields soluble protein preparations which reassemble into sedimentable coats when dialyzed against isolation buffer. These coats appear to have a morphology and size distribution similar to untreated preparations when examined in the electron microscope. Similar observations on the morphology of reassembled coats have been made by other investigators [15–17].

Reassembled coats, untreated coats, and coated vesicles have similar sedimentation properties on linear sucrose density gradients; however, their protein compositions are not identical. Coats reassembled from 2 M urea supernatants appear to consist predominantly of clathrin; however, other proteins are present. This observation tends to support the contention of others [11, 12, 15–17] that clathrin is the sole lattice protein. However, our observation that clathrin and the two 30,000-dalton proteins of peak I from Sepharose CL4B can reassemble into coats with normal morphology does not support the hypothesis that clathrin is the sole protein comprising the rods of the coat lattice. That the coats reassembled from peak I did not sediment was unfortunate, since it prevented our determining whether the two 30,000-dalton proteins cosedimented with reassembled coats. However, the two 30,000-dalton proteins are present in the reassembled coats following gradient purification of coats reassembled from 2 M urea supernatants. These observations strongly suggest that the two 30,000-dalton proteins are involved in the coat lattice. More detailed tests of this hypothesis are being presented in a separate communication [19].

MgCl$_2$ Effects on Reassembly

It is becoming increasingly clear from our work and that of others [16, 17] that the factors involved in promoting coat assembly are quite complex. Our results indicate that Mg^{2+} may be important in modulating the dissociation-reassembly equilibrium, since preparations dissociated in high or low Tris (pH 8) spontaneously reassemble at pH 8 in the presence of 10 mM MgCl$_2$, whereas lower concentrations of MgCl$_2$ are ineffective. The transition from no coats to coats occurs abruptly, which suggests that the process is cooperative and virtually all or none if sufficient Mg^{2+} is present. The apparent absence of partial coats is also consistent with this suggestion. When preparations dissociated with Tris (pH 8) are dialyzed into isolation buffer containing increasing concentrations of MgCl$_2$, more clathrin appears to reassemble into coats. This suggests that Mg^{2+} shifts the equilibrium toward reassembly and that it may stabilize the coat lattice. Such a role for Mg^{2+} is supported by our observation that increased chelation of Mg^{2+} increases the amount of nonsedimentable protein under reassembly conditions, and the observation of Schook et al [16] that chelation of Mg^{2+} with 6 mM EDTA or 5–10 mM adenosine triphosphate (ATP) interferes with reassembly.

The cation requirement appears to be specific for Mg^{2+}, since in our hands replacement of Mg^{2+} by 10 mM CaCl$_2$, FeCl$_2$, ZnCl$_2$, or MnCl$_2$ promotes the formation of filaments rather than coats. This is contrary to the report by Schook et al [16] that coats reassemble when partially purified clathrin preparations are dialyzed against isolation buffer (pH 6.8) containing 50–100 mM CaCl$_2$; however, the lower concentrations we used were not tested. Keen et al [17] observed that partially purified clathrin requires Ca^{2+} to reassemble but that this requirement is abolished if a hypothesized reassembly promotor protein(s) is present. Such apparent abolishment of the Ca^{2+} requirement suggests that the reassembly reaction is influenced by the presence of accessory proteins. Thus the varied effects of Ca^{2+} and Mg^{2+} observed by several workers may be due to differences in the protein composition of their preparations.

Tris Effects on Reassembly

The procedures used to prepare soluble coated vesicle proteins appear to affect the ability of such proteins to reassemble. Supernatants from preparations dissociated with low Tris (0.01 M, pH 8), 2 M urea, 0.25 M $MgCl_2$ [14], or 0.5 M Tris-isolation buffer (pH 7.0) reassemble when dialyzed against isolation buffer. In contrast, high-Tris (0.1 M, pH 8) supernatants do not reassemble when dialyzed against isolation buffer under the same conditions. That this effect is due to Tris and not to ionic strength is supported by our observation that replacement of Tris with NaCl results in supernatants from which coats will reassemble when dialyzed into isolation buffer. Whether Tris alters the properties of the soluble proteins sufficiently to either promote the sedimentation of an accessory protein necessary for reassembly or perturb protein-protein interactions necessary for reassembly is as yet unclear.

Reassembly Intermediates

In our studies of reassembly we have observed complete coats, but neither partial coats nor isolated hexagonal or pentagonal arrays were observed. This suggested that the reassembly reaction was essentially all or none; however, there is evidence which suggests that intermediate states do exist. When 10 mM $MgCl_2$ is present in low-Tris (10 mM, pH 8) supernatants, morphologically normal but nonsedimentable coats are observed. Following dialysis into isolation buffer (pH 6.8), these coats become sedimentable. Another instance in which nonsedimentable coats are observed occurs following dialysis of either partially purified clathrin (peak I from Sepharose CL4B columns) into low-ionic-strength buffer or peaks I and II into isolation buffer. Our hypothesis of reassembly intermediates is also supported by the work of Keen et al [17], who found that under certain ionic conditions coats reassemble but do not sediment. The existence of these intermediate states, which have normal morphology but are nonsedimentable, provides us with a tool for exploring how such factors as pH, divalent cations, ionic strength, and accessory proteins mediate and stabilize coat assembly. By determining how such factors effect the formation of intermediates in vitro, we hope to gain new insights as to how the reaction proceeds inside the cell.

Coat Structure

Kanaseki and Kadota [6] and Crowther et al [8] propose that the coat lattice consists of rods assembled into a spherical network of interlocking hexagons and pentagons. Crowther et al [8] postulated that the rods are comprised by clathrin dimers. However, no evidence was presented to show substructure in the rods. Our observations of Markham-rotated high-magnification images of both native and reassembled coats show a substructure in the rods consistent with a lattice edge made up of tightly intertwined molecules (Fig. 1).

Since the rods comprising the lattice are approximately 65Å in diameter and 165Å long [14], there is sufficient volume for a maximum of 4.5×10^5 daltons of protein based upon a partial specific volume of 0.735 cm^3/g. Thus there is enough volume for a clathrin dimer but not a trimer in each rod. Therefore, we propose that the rods are composed of intertwined antiparallel dimers of clathrin (Fig. 4). In this model, unlike that of

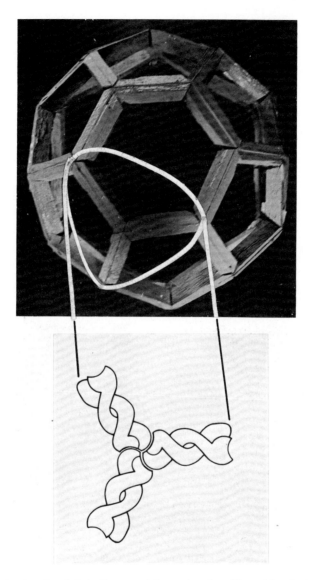

Fig. 4. Proposed structure for clathrin dimers and the coat vertices. We envision the lattice edge as consisting of an intertwined antiparallel clathrin dimer. Thus at each vertex six clathrin molecules interact. The head of one dimer interacts with the tail of an adjacent dimer. The proposed vertex structure is shown in relation to the entire coat lattice. The lattice structure shown is consistent with the six-fold symmetrical images we observe and is similar to that proposed by Crowther et al [8].

Crowther et al [8], a lattice vertex would involve three clathrin dimers in which the head of one dimer would interact with the tail of an adjacent dimer. In this organization only one class of clathrin-clathrin recognition sites is needed.

ACKNOWLEDGMENTS

This work was supported by grants HD 11519 and HD 09549 from The National Institutes of Health. This work is submitted as partial fulfillment of the requirements for the PhD by Michael P. Woodward.

The authors are grateful to Drs. P. G. Sokolove and C. D. Linden for many helpful discussions.

REFERENCES

1. Roth TF, Porter KR: J Cell Biol 20:313, 1964.
2. Roth TF, Cutting SA, Atlas SB: J Supramol Struct 4:527, 1976.
3. Anderson RGW, Goldstein SL, Brown MS: Proc Natl Acad Sci 73:2434, 1976.
4. Heuser JE, Reese TS: J Cell Biol 57:315, 1973.
5. Douglas WW, Nagasawa J, Schultz RA: Nature 232:340, 1971.
6. Kanaseki T, Kadota K: J Cell Biol 42:202, 1969.
7. Kadota K, Kadota T: J Cell Biol 58:135, 1973.
8. Crowther RA, Finch ST, Pearse BMF: J Mol Biol 103:785, 1976.
9. Woods JW, Woodward MP, Roth TF: J Cell Sci 30:87, 1978.
10. Ockleford CD: J Cell Sci 21:83, 1976.
11. Pearse BMF: J Mol Biol 97:93, 1975.
12. Pearse BMF: Proc Natl Acad Sci 73:1255, 1976.
13. Blitz AL, Fine RE, Toselli PA: J Cell Biol 75:135, 1977.
14. Woodward MP, Roth RF: Proc Natl Acad Sci 75:135, 1978.
15. Kartenbeck J: Cell Biol Inter Rep 2:457, 1978.
16. Schook W, Puszkin S, Bloom W, Ores C, Kochwa S: Proc Natl Acad Sci 76:116, 1979.
17. Keen JH, Willingham MC, Pastan IH: Cell 16:303, 1979.
18. Laemmli UK: Nature 222:680, 1970.
19. Linden CD, Woodward MP, Roth TF: In preparation.

Journal of Supramolecular Structure 11:251—258 (1979)
Tumor Cell Surfaces and Malignancy 197—204

Isolation and Characterization of a Variant of B16-Mouse Melanoma Resistant to MSH Growth Inhibition

Richard M. Niles and Mary P. Logue

Boston University School of Medicine, Division of Surgery, Department of Biochemistry, Boston, Massachusetts 02118

A variant of B-16 F_1 mouse melanoma was selected for its ability to survive and replicate in the presence of melanocyte-stimulating hormone (MSH). Although the variant (MR-4) was completely resistant to growth inhibition by MSH, cyclic AMP was still able to block cell replication. Tyrosinase activity in MR-4 cells was considerably lower than in B-16 F_1 cells. MSH induced a twofold to threefold increase in tyrosinase activity in both cell types, but the absolute activity in MR-4 remained significantly less than in the parental cells. MR-4 cells were also found to have a markedly depressed cyclic AMP-dependent protein kinase activity relative to B-16 F_1 cells. The protein kinase from both cell types was stimulated by cyclic AMP, but the level of MR-4 kinase activity at maximal cyclic AMP concentrations remained considerably lower than B-16 F_1 kinase activity under the same conditions. In both cell types adenylate cyclase activity was markedly stimulated by MSH. When equal numbers of viable F_1 and MR-4 cells were injected subcutaneously into C57/B1 mice, the MR-4 cells formed tumors earlier and killed the host sooner than the parental F_1 cells. We conclude that the biochemical alteration which allows MR-4 cells to replicate in the presence of MSH is a low level of tyrosinase activity, which in turn may be the result of low cyclic AMP-dependent protein kinase activity.

Key words: tumorigenicity, cyclic AMP-dependent protein kinase, tyrosinase MSH-growth-resistant variant, mouse melanoma

Melanocyte-stimulating hormone (MSH) can inhibit the growth of cultured melanoma cells [1, 2]. It is not clear whether this growth inhibition is due to the ability of MSH to increase intracellular cyclic AMP levels [3, 4] or due to the accumulation of cytotoxic intermediates of melanin biosynthesis [5]. Analogs of cyclic AMP have been demonstrated to alter melanoma cell morphology [2], inhibit cell replication [6], and stimulate melanogenesis [7]. The relationship between MSH and cyclic AMP and the effects they have on cultured melanoma cells has been the subject of intensive study and debate.

Received March 29, 1979; accepted July 13, 1979.

We have previously reported that B-16 mouse melanoma metastatic variants differ markedly in control of melanogenesis [8] and regulation of cyclic AMP metabolism [9]. In an attempt to determine the relationship among melanogenesis, cyclic AMP metabolism, and metastatic potential we isolated variants of B-16 F_1 (low metastatic potential) mouse melanoma cells which were resistant to growth inhibition by MSH. We report here some of the properties of these resistant cells and their biochemical alterations which enable them to replicate in the presence of MSH.

MATERIALS AND METHODS

Isolation of Cells Resistant to MSH Growth Inhibition

B-16 F_1 (low metastatic potential) mouse melanoma cells were obtained through the courtesy of Dr. I. J. Fidler, Frederick Cancer Research Laboratories, Frederick, Maryland. Stock cultures of these cells were routinely maintained in minimal essential medium (MEM) containing Earle's salts, nonessential amino acids, vitamin solution, L-glutamine (2 mM), sodium pyruvate (1 mM), 50 μg/ml streptomycin sulfate, 50 units/ml penicillin G + 10% heat-inactivated fetal bovine serum (Gibco), adjusted to a final pH of 7.4 and were grown in a 37°C, 95% air–5% CO_2 humidified incubator.

Unfortunately we were not successful in achieving a one-step selection procedure for the isolation of resistant cells. Therefore a sequential two-step procedure was followed. We seeded 1×10^5 B-16 F_1 cells into T-25 flasks. One day later, the medium was aspirated and the flasks were refed with medium containing 0.2 μg/ml MSH. After 7 days in this medium (refeeding every other day) the surviving cells were seeded into another T-25 and grown in the presence of 2 μg/ml MSH for 7 days. After this time the cells were prepared for cloning by the seeding of 100 viable cells onto 60-mm dishes with medium containing 2 μg/ml MSH. After allowance of 2 weeks for colony development ten individual clones were isolated using stainless steel cloning cylinders.

Cell Growth Measurements

Various clones or parental cells were seeded at 1.0×10^5/60-mm dish. One day later cells were refed with either unsupplemented medium or medium containing 0.2 μg/ml MSH. In some experiments 0.5 mM 8-bromocyclic AMP (8BrA) + 0.2 mM 1-methyl-3-isobutyl-xanthine (MIX) was also added to the culture medium. At 24, 48, and 72 hours after addition of these compounds, triplicate plates were processed for cell counts with a model B Coulter Counter.

Tyrosinase Assay

Parental or variant cells were seeded at $(0.4–3.0) \times 10^5$/100-mm dish. One day after seeding all plates were refed with complete medium $\pm$ 0.2 μg/ml MSH. Twenty-four hours after this refeeding tyrosinase was measured as described previously [8].

Protein Kinase Assay

Kinase activity was measured by the assay of Corbin et al [10]. Mouse melanoma parental and variant cells were grown to confluence on 100-mm culture dishes. We prepared cells for assay by washing the monolayer three times with 4 ml of 0.05 M phosphate buffer (pH 6.8), scraping the cells from the dishes ($\sim$4 $\times$ 10^6/dish) with a rubber policeman, and sonicating the resultant suspension (1.5 ml) for 30 seconds at setting #3 in a model WI85 sonifer (Heat Systems, Plainview, New York). The reaction mixture consisted of 0.05 M phosphate buffer (pH 6.8), 0.2 mM γ-^{32}P ATP (180 cpm/pmole), 0.5 mg histone (type II-

A) ± various concentrations of cyclic AMP, and 20 μl of cell homogenate. Following a 10-minute incubation at 30°C, 50 μl of the reaction mixture was pipetted onto Whatman 3-MM filter paper disks (2.3-mm diameter; Whatman, Inc., Clifton, New Jersey). The disks were dropped into ice-cold 10% trichloroacetic acid (TCA) and washed in sequence with 10% TCA, 95% ethanol, and ether. After drying, the filters were placed in scintillation vials containing Aquasol (New England Nuclear, Boston, Massachusetts) and counted. All experimental samples were corrected for endogenous phosphorylation, ie, the amount of phosphorylation in the absence of histone or the absence of cyclic AMP.

Cyclic AMP Measurements

Parental and variant mouse melanoma cells were prepared and assayed for the ability of MSH to increase intracellular cyclic AMP levels by previously described techniques [9], with the exception that 35-mm dishes were employed and cell densities at the time of stimulation were much lower than previously reported.

Assay of Tumor Growth

Viable cells (1×10^5) of F_1 and variant lines were injected subcutaneously into C57/Bl mice — ten mice for each cell type. Mice were checked every other day for appearance of tumors and the time at which tumors became palpable was recorded. Tumor development in each individual mouse was then followed and the time required to kill the host was noted.

RESULTS

Following isolation of clones from the parental B-16 F_1 cells, they were tested for growth in the absence and presence of MSH. Only 4 of 10 clones showed significant resistance to MSH-induced growth inhibition. One clone (#4) was completely unaffected by MSH even after 72 h of treatment. This particular clone was utilized for further investigation and was given the designation B-16-F_1-MR-4.

F_1 and MR-4 cells were tested for growth in the presence of MSH or 8-BrcA + MIX (Fig. 1). F_1 cells were found to be growth-inhibited by both MSH and 8-BrcA + MIX, although the cyclic AMP analog was more effective. The MR-4 clone differed from F_1 in several aspects. First, the growth rate of untreated MR-4 cells was greater than control F_1 cells. Second, MR-4 cells treated with MSH were not growth-inhibited, while MR-4 cells treated with the cyclic AMP analog were significantly inhibited at all time points. In summary, F_1 was growth-inhibited by both MSH and cyclic AMP, the latter being more effective; MR-4 had a higher replication rate than F_1, was completely resistant to inhibition by MSH, but was susceptible to inhibition by exogenously supplied cyclic AMP.

We suspected that one reason why MR-4 was resistant to MSH-induced growth inhibition was an alteration in tyrosinase, the key enzyme in melanin biosynthesis, since Pawelek et al [2] found that variants of S91 mouse molanoma cells resistant to MSH growth inhibition invariably had altered tyrosinase activities. Therefore, we measured tyrosinase activity in F_1 and MR-4 cells that had been incubated in the absence or presence of MSH for 24 h. Under our assay conditions, the enzyme activity from both cell lines was linear with respect to time and protein concentration. The data (Table I) clearly show that there was a marked reduction of MR-4 basal tyrosinase activity, ie, the activity present in the absence of MSH. Also, MSH was able to stimulate tyrosinase activity approximately threefold in F_1, while only a twofold stimulation was achieved in MR-4, and the absolute levels of hormonally induced tyrosinase activity were six times less in MR-4 than in F_1.

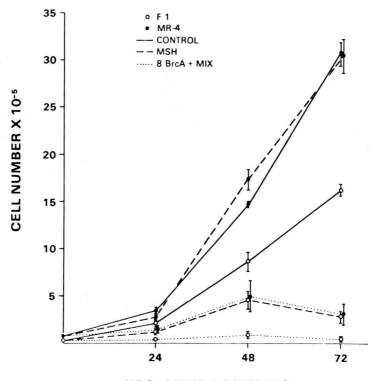

HRS. AFTER REFEEDING

Fig. 1. Growth of F_1 and MR-4 cells in the absence or presence of MSH or 8-bromocyclic AMP + 1-methyl-3-isobutylxanthine. Cells were seeded at 1×10^5/60-mm culture dish. One day later the cells were refed with complete medium $\pm$ 0.2 μg/ml MSH, or $\pm$ 5 $\times$ 10^{-4} M 8-bromocyclic AMP + 2 $\times$ 10^{-4} M 1-methyl-3-isobutylxanthine. At 24, 48, and 72 h after refeeding, plates were processed for cell counts. The data are represented as the mean $\pm$ SEM (bars above and below the data points) of triplicate plates.

Since we had shown that MR-4 cells were still inhibited by the exogenous addition of cyclic AMP, there existed the possibility that MSH failed to inhibit growth because of receptor-adenylate cyclase dysfunctions and hence insufficient production of intracellular cyclic AMP. Therefore we measured the ability of MSH to increase cyclic AMP levels in intact F_1 and MR-4 cells.

The data in Table II clearly show that at any time point measured MR-4 cells produced more cyclic AMP in response to MSH than did F_1 cells. Therefore it is unlikely that the failure of MR-4 cells to be inhibited by MSH is due to a defect in the MSH-receptor-adenylate cyclase complex.

Since it appears that the only mechanism through which cyclic AMP exerts its physiologic actions is the activation of cyclic AMP-dependent protein kinase, we decided to examine the possibility that changes in protein kinase activity might be responsible for MR-4 resistance to MSH. Both F_1 and MR-4 were assayed for protein kinase activity using histone as the phosphate acceptor and using various concentrations of cyclic AMP to stimulate the enzyme. Our assay conditions resulted in linearity with respect to time and protein concentration for the kinases from each cell line. It is apparent from the data (Table III and Fig. 2) that the protein kinase activity of MR-4 differs substantially from that of F_1. The specific activity of the MR-4 kinase under all four assay conditions (Table III)

TABLE I. Tyrosinase Activity in F_1 and MR-4 Cells

Cell type	Specific activity
F_1	8.6
F_1 + 0.2 μg/ml MSH	26.5
MR-4	2.0
MR-4 + 0.2 μg/ml MSH	4.1

Cells were prepared and assayed for tyrosinase activity as described in Materials and Methods. Specific activity is defined as nanomoles of tyrosine hydroxylated per 10^6 cells per hour. Cell densities at the time of the experiment were as follows: F_1 control, 3.4×10^6; MR-4 control, 4.8×10^6; F_1-MSH, 2.4×10^6; MR-4-MSH, 4.4×10^6. The experiment was repeated two additional times with similar results.

TABLE II. Effect of MSH on Cyclic AMP Levels in Intact F_1 and MR-4 Cells

Cell type	Incubation time (min)	Picomoles cyclic AMP/10^5 cells
F_1	5	161 ± 24
	15	393 ± 36
	30	326 ± 12
	60	302 ± 49
MR-4	5	729 ± 72
	15	1,698 ± 37
	30	814 ± 182
	60	443 ± 52

Cells were prepared for hormone stimulation and cyclic AMP was extracted and quantitated as described in Materials and Methods. MSH was present at a concentration of 0.2 μg/ml. Control levels of cyclic AMP at all time points were 0.7 ± 0.2 pm/10^5 cells (F_1) and 1.2 ± 0.3 pm/10^5 cells (MR-4). The data are represented as the mean ± SEM of triplicate plates, each assayed in duplicate in the radioimmunoassay determination for cyclic AMP levels.

TABLE III. Protein Kinase Activity in F_1 and MR-4 Cells

	Picomoles ^{32}P transferred to histone/10^6 cells	
Reaction mixture	F_1	MR-4
–cyclic AMP, –histone	92.0	40.6
+cyclic AMP, –histone	160.7	48.6
–cyclic AMP, +histone	305.1	60.4
+cyclic AMP, +histone	635.2	127.4

Cells were prepared and assayed for protein kinase activity as described in Materials and Methods. The concentration of cyclic AMP used in this experiment was 2 μM. The entire experiment was repeated three additional times with similar results. Cell numbers at the time of the experiment were 2.8×10^5 (F_1) and 4.0×10^5 (MR-4).

was markedly depressed relative to F_1. Also the MR-4 protein kinase was almost maximally stimulated by low concentrations of cyclic AMP (10^{-8} M), while a similar enzyme preparation from F_1 required 10^{-6} M cyclic AMP to be maximally stimulated. At the point of optimal stimulation of protein kinase in both cell lines, the specific activity of F_1 was still 2.8 times higher than the specific activity of MR-4 (Fig. 2).

We next compared the biologic activity (tumor formation) of F_1 and MR-4 cells. When an equal number of viable cells were injected subcutaneously into C57/B1 mice, it was observed that the MR-4 cells formed palpable tumors earlier (an average of 5 days vs 13 days) and killed their host sooner (an average of 14 days vs 22 days after appearance of tumor) than did F_1 cells (Table IV).

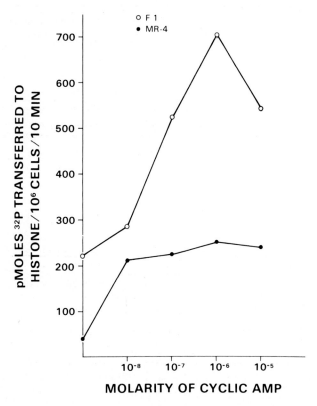

Fig. 2. Protein kinase activity in F_1 and MR-4 cell homogenates as a function of cyclic AMP concentration. Cells were prepared and assayed for protein kinase activity as described in Materials and Methods. Specific activity is expressed as picomoles of ^{32}P transferred from γ-^{32}P ATP to histone per 10^6 cells. Cell densities at the time of assay were 6.3×10^6 (F_1) and 6.1×10^6 (MR-4). The experiment was repeated three additional times with similar results. The initial points on the y axis represent the enzyme activity in the absence of any added cyclic AMP.

TABLE IV. Tumorogenicity of F_1 and MR-4 Cells

Cell type	Latency period (days)		Survival time (days)	
	Range	Ave	Range	Ave
F_1	9–18	13	12–28	22
MR-4	4–6	5	10–18	14

The protocol for assaying tumorogenicity is described in Materials and Methods. Latency period is the length of time before the appearance of a palpable mass. Survival time is defined as the period of time the mouse survived following the appearance of the tumor. There were ten mice in each treatment group.

DISCUSSION

The results presented in this communication suggest that the biochemical alterations which allow MR-4 cells to grow in the presence of MSH are markedly lower levels of tyrosinase and cyclic AMP-dependent protein kinase activities. Pawelek et al [2] have also found depressed tyrosinase activity in two mutants of Cloudman S91 melanoma cells selected for their ability to replicate in the presence of MSH. However, in contrast to their results, we found that MR-4 cells were markedly inhibited by the exogenous addition of 8BrcA to the culture media. Also unlike our MR-4 cells, the Cloudman S91 melanoma mutants did not have depressed cyclic AMP-dependent protein kinase activity.

The mechanism whereby MSH inhibits cell replication has been the subject of controversy. Some feel that the cytostatic action of MSH is due to its ability to increase intracellular cyclic AMP, high levels of which have been demonstrated to be a negative regulator of growth in many types of cultured cells [11–13]. Other investigators believe that MSH indirectly inhibits growth by its stimulation of melanin biosynthesis, the intermediates of which are known to be cytotoxic [5, 14–16]. On the basis of our results we would argue that both groups are partially correct. It is obvious that the markedly lower tyrosinase activity in MR-4 even in the presence of MSH leads to a much lower rate of melanin production and hence a noncytotoxic level of intermediates. In fact when parental F_1 cells are grown on tyrosine-free medium MSH no longer inhibits cell proliferation (data not shown). On the other hand, although MR-4 cells are resistant to MSH, they are still growth-inhibited by cyclic AMP, although not to the same extent as F_1 cells. This may be the result of a *persistent* activation of protein kinase, leading to an imbalance of phosphorylation-dephosphorylation reactions which may be necessary for replication. Alternatively the cyclic AMP may be metabolized to a cytotoxic product by the cells, although this possibility was not likely in our experiments since the potent phosphodiesterase inhibitor MIX was included in the incubation mixture.

The mechanism responsible for depressed protein kinase activity in MR-4 cells is currently under investigation. Among the possibilities are decreased synthesis of holoenzyme, increased turnover of holoenzymes, increased production of regulatory subunits or decreased production of catalytic subunits, and increased production of protein kinase inhibitors. It should be noted that kinase activity in MR-4 was depressed relative to that in F_1 under all four assay conditions (no cAMP, no histone; +cAMP, −histone; −cAMP, +histone; and +cAMP, +histone). From these data it could be argued that the alteration affects the holoenzyme rather than one or the other subunits.

There is convincing evidence that cyclic AMP is the intracellular mediator of MSH-induced tyrosinase activity and hence melanogenesis [3, 4, 7, 17]. Since the only known mechanism through which cyclic AMP exerts its physiologic response is the activation of protein kinase [18, 19], it is presumed that phosphorylation of specific proteins is the mechanism through which MSH increases tyrosinase activity [20, 21]. In light of the biochemical alterations we have demonstrated in MR-4, namely, depressed tyrosinase and protein kinase activity, it is tempting to speculate that in the B-16 mouse melanoma system *total* tyrosinase activity, ie, the activity present in either the absence or presence of MSH, is regulated by cyclic AMP-dependent protein kinase. This hypothesis is strengthened by our recent observations that another variant of F_1 selected for enhanced pulmonary metastatic potential in vivo (B-16-F_{10}) has markedly depressed tyrosinase activity relative to F_1 [8] and also has significantly lower protein kinase activity (Niles and Logue, unpublished observations). This hypothesis could be tested by obtaining a variant of F_1 which had completely defective or absent protein kinase. Such cells should have no detectable levels of tyrosinase activity and hence would be amelanotic melanomas.

The mechanism whereby MR-4 cells accumulate more cyclic AMP in response to MSH than do F_1 cells is currently under investigation. However, it is interesting to note that Bourne et al [19] found that mutants of S49 lymphoma cells resistant to dibutyryl cyclic AMP accumulated significantly more cyclic AMP in response to catecholamines, prostaglandins, and cholera toxin than did wild-type cells.

Our original objective in obtaining F_1 variants resistant to MSH-induced growth inhibition was to obtain cells with altered cyclic AMP metabolism. Using this approach, we hope to determine what role the altered cyclic AMP metabolism we have previously observed for F_{10} cells [8, 9] plays in their enhanced metastatic potential. The data we have acquired concerning the biologic behavior of MR-4 indicate that they have increased malignant potential relative to F_1 cells. It is possible that the ability of the MR-4 cells to resist MSH-induced growth inhibition and hence grow more rapidly than F_1 in vitro may account for their greater rate of growth in vivo. In cooperation with Dr. I. J. Fidler of the Frederick Cancer Research Center, a comparative study of the pulmonary metastatic potential of F_1 and MR-4 is currently in progress. Thus it appears that the selective alteration of a few biochemical parameters can result in a progression of malignancy.

ACKNOWLEDGMENTS

We wish to express our appreciation to Dr. I. J. Fidler, Frederick Cancer Research Laboratories, Frederick, Maryland, for supplying us with the parental B-16-F_1 cell line and to Ramona Boylan for typing and editing this manuscript. This work was supported in part by grant CA 18913 from the National Cancer Institute.

REFERENCES

1. Wong G, Pawelek J: Nature New Biol 241:213, 1973.
2. Pawelek J, Sansone M, Koch N, Christie G, Halaban R, Hendee J, Lerner AB, Varga JM: Proc Natl Acad Sci USA 72:951, 1975.
3. Pawelek J, Wong G, Sansone M, Morowitz J: Yale J Biol Med 46:337, 1973.
4. Kreiner PW, Gold CJ, Keirns JJ, Brock WA, Bitensky MW: Yale J Biol Med 46:583, 1973.
5. Graham DG, Tiffany SM, Vogel FS: J Invest Dermatol 70:113, 1978.
6. Dipasquale A, McGuire J: J Cell Physiol 93:395, 1977.
7. Johnson GS, Pastan J: Nature New Biol 237:267, 1972.
8. Niles RM, Makarski J: J Natl Cancer Inst 61:523, 1978.
9. Niles RM, Makarski J: J Cell Physiol 96:355, 1978.
10. Corbin JD, Keely SL, Park CR: J Biol Chem 250:218, 1975.
11. Sheppard JR: Proc Natl Acad Sci USA 68:1316, 1971.
12. Johnson GS, Friedman RM, Pastan IH: Proc Natl Acad Sci USA 68:425, 1971.
13. Pastan IH, Johnson GS, Anderson WB: Annu Rev Biochem 44:491, 1975.
14. Lerner AB: Am J Med 51:141, 1971.
15. Halaban R, Lerner AB: Exp Cell Res 108:111, 1977.
16. Halaban R, Lerner AB: Exp Cell Res 108:119, 1977.
17. Kreider JW, Wade DR, Rosenthal M, Densley T: J Natl Cancer Inst 54:1457, 1975.
18. Kuo JF, Greengard P: Proc Natl Acad Sci USA 64:1349, 1969.
19. Bourne HR, Coffino P, Tompkins GM: J Cell Physiol 85:611, 1975.
20. Wong G, Pawelek J: Nature 255:644, 1975.
21. Korner A, Pawelek J: Nature 267:444, 1977.

Journal of Supramolecular Structure 11:259–267 (1979)
Tumor Cell Surfaces and Malignancy 205–213

Mechanisms of Thrombin-Stimulated Cell Division

Dennis D. Cunningham, Kevin C. Glenn, Joffre B. Baker, Robert L. Simmer, and David A. Low

Department of Microbiology, College of Medicine, University of California, Irvine, California 92717

Addition of highly purified thrombin to cultures of several kinds of nondividing fibroblasts brings about cell division. This stimulation occurs in serum-free medium, permitting studies on its mechanism under chemically defined conditions. Previous studies have shown that action of thrombin at the cell surface is sufficient to cause cell division and that the proteolytic activity of thrombin is required for its mitogenic effect. These results prompted experiments which showed that there is a cell surface receptor for thrombin and that thrombin must bind to its receptor and cleave it to stimulate cell division. Some of the thrombin that binds to its receptors becomes attached to them by a linkage that appears to be covalent. However, it is presently unknown whether this direct thrombin receptor complex plays a role in the stimulation.

These results raise a number of questions that should be explored in future studies. They also provide a foundation on which to build hypotheses about tentative molecular mechanisms that might be involved in the stimulation. Knowledge that thrombin must cleave its receptor to bring about cell division suggests two alternative mechanisms for stimulation by proteolysis. In one the receptor is a negative effector which prevents cell division when it is intact, but not after it has been cleaved. Alternatively, a fragment of the receptor could be a positive effector. In this mechanism, proteolysis by thrombin would produce a specific receptor fragment which brings about cell proliferation. If every protease which cleaves the receptor also stimulates cell division, the receptor is probably a negative effector. In contrast, if certain proteases cleave the receptor but do not stimulate the cells, a fragment of the receptor is likely a positive effector. With negative regulation by the receptor, the controlling events would occur before proteolysis of it, and it might be possible to find putative regulatory molecules by identification of nearest neighbors of the receptor. This should be possible by using bifunctional crosslinking reagents. If a fragment of the thrombin receptor turns out to be a positive effector, it should be possible to identify and study fragments by analyzing the metabolic fate of the receptor. Techniques are now available for this kind of analysis and it should also be possible to determine whether receptor fragments remain in the membrane or whether they are translocated to specific sites within the cell. A

Received May 30, 1979; accepted July 25, 1979.

critical question to be asked is which of these events and interactions involving the thrombin receptor are necessary for stimulation of cell division. It now appears that the best way to answer this question is to examine these events in a large number of cloned cell populations that are responsive or unresponsive to the mitogenic action of thrombin. If a thrombin-mediated event occurs in all responsive clones but is altered or absent in some unresponsive clones, it is probably necessary for stimulation of cell division.

Key words: cell surface receptors, proteolysis of receptors, positive or negative regulation

Recent studies have shown that thrombin is an effective mitogen for several kinds of cultured fibroblasts. Addition of it to nondividing cultures of chick embryo (CE), mouse embryo (ME), or human foreskin (HF) cells causes about one round of cell division. Under optimal conditions, this treatment leads to a 60–80% increase in cell number with CE and ME cells and about a 40% increase with HF cells [1–3].

Investigations on the mechanism of thrombin-stimulated cell division have been aided by several properties of the system. First, cell division can be brought about by adding highly purified thrombin to serum-free cultures. Although factors normally present in the animal are absent, this system permits experiments to be conducted under chemically defined conditions. Second, the proteolytic activity of thrombin is required for its mitogenic action [2, 4], indicating that proteolysis is a primary event in the stimulation. Third, it has been possible to derive cells that are unresponsive to the mitogenic action of thrombin from responsive populations of cells [3]. By studying thrombin-mediated events in both responsive and unresponsive populations, it should be possible to determine which events are necessary for thrombin-stimulated cell division and which are not [5]. Finally, thrombin action at the cell surface is sufficient to bring about cell division [6]. Knowledge of this property of the system has facilitated studies on it by identifying a limited part of the cell on which to focus initial experiments.

In the first section of this article we will briefly summarize and discuss studies to date on thrombin-stimulated cell division, emphasizing results which have provided clues about molecular events involved. This will provide a framework for the second section where we will extrapolate to more detailed molecular mechanisms which are necessarily hypothetical at this time. Here, the emphasis will be on models and mechanisms which are amenable to experimental evaluation. We have recently published a summary of our work on thrombin-stimulated cell division which contains supporting experimental data [7].

REVIEW OF THROMBIN-STIMULATED CELL DIVISION

Action of Thrombin at the Cell Surface is Sufficient to Stimulate

We decided that the first goal in probing the mechanism of the stimulation should be identification of the cellular site(s) where the primary interactions with thrombin take place. The first specific question was whether thrombin could stimulate by acting at the cell surface or whether it had to be internalized. This question has been asked previously for other polypeptide growth factors and hormones, but the answers have not been conclusive. Early studies with polypeptides linked to Sepharose beads indicated that action at the cell surface was sufficient to elicit a biological response [8–11]. However, subsequent experiments showed that there was sufficient release of polypeptides from these

Sepharose beads [12–15] (sometimes in a "superactive" form [16]) to question this conclusion. It has also been questioned on the basis of extensive uptake of polypeptide factors by cultured cells [17–19], and demonstrations of receptors for insulin [20] and nerve growth factor [21, 22] in the nucleus.

We approached this question for thrombin by linking it to carboxylate-modified polystyrene beads via a peptide bond using a water-soluble carbodiimide reagent [6]. These thrombin beads stimulated division of cells; however, beads with nonmitogenic proteins like bovine serum albumin or ovalbumin similarly linked to them did not cause the cells to divide. The critical question, of course, was whether the stimulation by thrombin beads could be accounted for by release of thrombin from the beads. Carefully controlled experiments employing ^{125}I-thrombin linked to polystyrene beads demonstrated that there was not sufficient release either into the medium or directly into cells to account for any of the cell division caused by the thrombin beads. This permitted us to conclude that action of thrombin at the cell surface was sufficient to stimulate cells to divide [6]. Analogous experiments with trypsin, another protease that is mitogenic for CE cells, demonstrated that it also can produce cell division by action at the cell surface [23].

Binding of Thrombin to Its Cell Surface Receptors is Necessary for Stimulation

The above results indicated that it would be fruitful to examine the cell surface for specific interactions with thrombin. Binding studies with ^{125}I-thrombin, in the absence and presence of a large excess of unlabeled thrombin, showed that ME, HF, and CE cells bind thrombin specifically, indicating the presence of receptors for thrombin [24, 25]. The fraction of total binding that was specific was greater for ME cells than CE or HF cells so we have conducted most of our binding experiments with ME cells. The receptors on ME cells appear to be unique for thrombin, since neither insulin nor epidermal growth factor (EGF) compete significantly for the binding of ^{125}I-thrombin. The thrombin receptor is actually on the cell surface, since about 80% of ^{125}I-thrombin specifically bound under steady state conditions can be removed by brief treatments with trypsin which do not disrupt cells. Scatchard analyses of ^{125}I-thrombin binding data are linear over a broad range of thrombin concentrations, indicating a single affinity class of receptors [24].

The conclusion that thrombin must bind to its receptors on ME cells to stimulate cell division came from experiments in which small amounts of calf serum were added along with thrombin. Addition of calf serum to a final concentration of 0.1% markedly inhibited stimulation of ME cell division by thrombin. This low concentration of serum markedly inhibited the binding of thrombin to its cell surface receptors, but it did not inhibit either the proteolytic activity of thrombin or its nonspecific association with the cells. Scatchard analyses of ^{125}I-thrombin binding data in the presence and absence of serum showed that the inhibition by serum resulted from a masking of thrombin receptors on cells and not from binding of ^{125}I-thrombin by serum components [24].

Photoaffinity Labeling of the Thrombin Receptor

The indication, noted above, that there was a single affinity class of thrombin receptors suggested the possibility that they could be identified as a discrete molecular species by photoaffinity labeling techniques. By employing procedures developed by Fox and his collaborators to radiolabel the EGF receptors on mouse 3T3 cells [26, 27], we labeled the thrombin receptors on ME [28] and CE [5] cells with ^{125}I-thrombin conjugated to a photoreactive reagent. These experiments revealed that there was significant labeling of what appeared to be only a single component or receptor on the cell surface. The apparent molecular weight of the receptor was about 50,000 for ME cells, and 43,000 for CE cells. The absolute values of these molecular weights must be interpreted with caution since the receptors might be glycoproteins. Nevertheless, the ability to identify the labeled thrombin-receptor complex on gels has enabled us to make some interesting conclusions.

Thrombin Must Cleave Its Receptors to Stimulate Cell Division

A question that is very basic to the mechanism of stimulation by thrombin is whether its proteolytic activity is required for mitogenic action. It appears that proteolysis is indeed necessary, since thrombin that has been inactivated with either diisopropyl-fluorophosphate (DFP) or phenyl methyl sulfonyl fluoride (PMSF) is no longer mitogenic even though these inactivated thrombins bind to cells like active thrombin [4]. This requirement for proteolysis prompted us to search for cell surface components whose cleavage by thrombin was necessary for stimulation of cell division. We did this by looking for cell surface components that were cleaved by thrombin on CE cells that were responsive to its mitogenic action, but which were not cleaved or were absent on CE cells that did not divide after thrombin treatment [5]. Cleavage of cell surface proteins was monitored by labeling cell surface components of control and thrombin-treated cells with $^{125}I^-$ by lactoperoxidase-catalyzed iodination. These studies revealed a cell surface component of 43,000 daltons (43k) that was removed by thrombin from the responsive cells. An apparently identical component was present on four separately isolated populations of unresponsive cells, but it was not removed by mitogenic treatments with thrombin. Thus, removal of it appears necessary for thrombin-stimulated cell division. It is noteworthy that 43k was not removed from responsive cells by DFP-inactivated thrombin. This shows that proteolysis by thrombin and not a cellular protease was responsible for its removal. It was also not removed during serum stimulation, demonstrating that its removal was not simply a consequence of initiating cell division [5].

As noted above, the photoaffinity labeling experiments showed that the molecular weight of the thrombin receptor on CE cells was 43,000. Because of the identity of their apparent molecular weights, it appears that 43k, identified by labeling with $^{125}I^-$ and lactoperoxidase, is the thrombin receptor. It should be pointed out that there has been some variability in the migration on sodium dodecyl sulfate (SDS) polyacrylamide gels of the thrombin receptor complex of CE cells from experiment to experiment, depending on the condition used to solubilize the cells. However, there was a corresponding variation in the migration of ^{125}I-thrombin so the estimated molecular weight of the thrombin receptor remains at about 43,000. Thus, the studies to date indicate that thrombin must cleave its receptor to stimulate cell division although this conclusion is based on measurements of molecular weight that necessarily involve some uncertainty. It is noteworthy that the unresponsive cells still specifically bound ^{125}I-thrombin, consistent with the observation that 43k was still present on their cell surface. Thus, their inability to divide after thrombin treatment can be attributed to an absence of cleavage of their receptors rather than an inability of the receptors to bind thrombin.

Direct Linkage of Thrombin to Its Cell Surface Receptors

Another event has been identified which is a consequence of interaction between thrombin and its cellular receptors. When ^{125}I-thrombin is incubated with HF, ME, or

CE cells in the absence of any crosslinking reagent, a significant amount of the thrombin that is specifically bound becomes directly linked to its receptors [29, 30]. For HF cells, this amount is over 50%; it is about 1–10% for ME and CE cells. This linkage appears to be covalent since it survives boiling in 3% SDS and 1.0% 2-mercaptoethanol.

It is noteworthy that the linkage can be disrupted by incubation at pH 12 or treatment with hydroxylamine [30]. This suggests that the linkage between thrombin and its receptors involves an acyl group, analogous to the linkage that occurs between thrombin and antithrombin III [31, 32]. This ester linkage is formed between an arginine carboxyl group of antithrombin III, and the hydroxyl group of the active site serine of thrombin, representing a stable intermediate of a proteolytic event [31]. In this case, the released peptide fragment has a molecular weight of about 6,000 since the apparent molecular weight of the thrombin-antithrombin III complex under reducing conditions is about 90,000, while that of antithrombin III is about 63,000, and thrombin is about 33,000 [33]. Our preliminary experiments are consistent with the possibility that formation of the direct thrombin receptor complex is analogous to formation of the thrombin-antithrombin III complex, and that only a small peptide from the receptor is released upon complex formation. Clearly, there are many questions about the thrombin receptor complex that remain to be answered. If it turns out to be a stable intermediate of a proteolytic reaction, like the thrombin-antithrombin III complex, it will be important to investigate any relationship it might have to the cleavage of the thrombin receptor identified by experiments discussed in the preceding section [5].

POSSIBLE MECHANISMS FOR THROMBIN-STIMULATED CELL DIVISION

The above results suggest some likely models or mechanisms for the stimulation by thrombin. They also raise a number of questions that should be addressed in future studies. There are many possibilities, and in this section we will discuss some testable alternatives that are providing direction to our experiments.

Purification of the Thrombin Receptor

Many studies on the mechanism by which the receptor participates in stimulation of cell division would be greatly facilitated by a purified receptor and antibodies to it. For example, availability of a purified receptor would permit a direct test of whether the receptor is identical to the 43,000 dalton cell surface component identified by iodination with $^{125}I^-$ and lactoperoxidase. We are currently developing several purification procedures. One of these involves incubating cells with ^{125}I-thrombin and purifying the directly linked ^{125}I-thrombin receptor complex. With this method, the assay during purification simply involves measurements of ^{125}I-radioactivity, and the receptor can be liberated from the ^{125}I-thrombin receptor complex after purification by treatment with hydroxylamine or pH 12 as noted above. Our preliminary experiments indicate that human placenta will be useful for this purification since it forms a large amount of the ^{125}I-thrombin receptor complex upon incubation with ^{125}I-thrombin. We have found that the complex binds to heparin with a high affinity, and this has provided the basis for an effective affinity purification step. In addition, the ^{125}I-thrombin receptor complex can be precipitated by antibodies to thrombin, and this should facilitate the development of a second affinity purification step. Combined with standard fractionation techniques, these highly selective purifications should enable us to extensively purify the thrombin receptor complex, and thus the receptor.

We are also developing procedures to directly purify the receptor itself. Our experiments have shown that it binds with high affinity to heparin, and this should make it possible to develop an affinity purification step as with the thrombin receptor complex. It will be interesting to compare the directly purified receptor with the receptor that is liberated by hydroxylamine or pH 12 treatment from the purified ^{125}I-thrombin receptor complex. As noted earlier, formation of this complex probably involves removal of a small fragment from the receptor. It will be possible to study this problem directly when both receptor preparations have been purified.

The Thrombin Receptor as a Positive or Negative Effector

The conclusion that thrombin must cleave its receptor to stimulate cell division suggests two alternative mechanisms by which proteolysis could trigger cell division. One possibility is that the thrombin receptor is a negative effector which in its intact state participates in the development of a negative signal to prevent cell division. The other possibility is that cleavage of the receptor by thrombin produces a specific receptor fragment which is a positive effector and signals the cell to divide. It should be possible to distinguish between these two possibilities by examining the ability of a number of different proteases to stimulate cell division and cleave the thrombin receptor. If every protease which cleaves the receptor also stimulates the cell to divide, it would appear that the receptor functions as a negative effector. On the other hand, if there are proteases which cleave the receptor but do not stimulate cell division, it is likely that proteolysis of the receptor by thrombin produces a specific positive fragment which is central to the development of the mitogenic signal.

It is noteworthy that thrombin must be present continuously in the medium to produce maximal cell division, even though a one hour exposure to it removes its receptors from the cell surface [5]. However, the receptors are replaced within three hours after changing to thrombin-free medium [5]. Therefore, if the thrombin receptor is a negative effector, it must be removed continuously to allow maximal cell division; replacement of it would stop events leading to cell proliferation. On the other hand, if a specific fragment of the receptor is a positive effector, the above results predict it would have a short half-life. As evidence becomes available for either alternative, it will be important to develop approaches to test these predictions.

Approaches for Studying Negative Regulation by the Receptor

There are several possible mechanisms which could account for negative regulation where the thrombin receptor prevents cell division when it is intact but not after it has been cleaved by any one of several proteases. For example, the intact receptor might interact with and inhibit a membrane enzyme necessary for production of a product that is rate limiting for cell division; cleavage of the receptor would prevent inhibition of enzymatic activity and lead to stimulation of cell division. Alternatively, the intact receptor, but not a cleaved receptor, might bind a cytoplasmic agent which permits or causes cell division when free but not when bound to the receptor. Such an agent could be a component of the structural or contractile apparatus, an ion, or a specific positive regulatory molecule. There are, of course, many possibilities. The important point is that with negative regulation by the thrombin receptor, the key controlling events would occur before proteolysis of it. Thus, if the experiments in the preceding section indicate that the receptor is a negative effector, it would be furitful to identify cellular components that are bound to the thrombin receptor and to determine if proteolysis of the receptor affects this association. Protein-nearest neighbors of the receptor could be identified by previously developed techniques employing a reversible bifunctional imidoester cross-linking reagent, immunoadsorption with antibodies to thrombin, and two-dimensional diagonal electrophoresis [34–36]. This approach would facilitate identification of putative regulatory components that are bound to the thrombin receptor in its intact state but not after proteolytic cleavage of it.

Approaches for Studying Positive Regulation by the Receptor

If certain proteases can cleave the thrombin receptor without producing cell division, it is likely that stimulation by thrombin involves production of a specific receptor fragment which is a positive effector. In view of the very limited and specific proteolysis by thrombin of protein substrates [37], such a mechanism is certainly feasible.

From our present perspective, it appears that positive regulation by a fragment of the receptor would be easier to explore than negative regulation by the intact receptor. This is largely because a first step in examining positive regulation would be a study of the metabolic fate of the receptor, and it is now possible to propose feasible approaches for this. One avenue has been provided by model studies on the EGF receptor involving linkage of ^{125}I-EGF to its receptors by a photoactivable cross-linking reagent [26, 27]. Since the crosslinked ^{125}I-EGF receptor complex was the only labeled component in the cells, it was possible to examine the cellular processing of it during continued incubation of the cells [27]. We have used analogous techniques to label the thrombin receptor on ME [28] and CE [5] cells with ^{125}I-thrombin conjugated to a photoactivable crosslinking reagent, and this should permit analysis of the metabolic fate of the thrombin receptor.

As noted above, we recently found that ^{125}I-thrombin in the absence of a cross-linking reagent becomes directly linked to its cellular receptors [29, 30]. By following the fate of this linked component during continued incubation of cells, it should be possible to evaluate the metabolic fate of the spontaneously-formed direct thrombin receptor complex. In these studies, it will be important to determine if linkage of ^{125}I-thrombin to its receptor might alter subsequent processing of it. Only a fraction of the receptors that bind thrombin become crosslinked to it, and the subsequent metabolic fate of linked and unlinked receptors might be different. However, studies on the EGF receptor have shown that the same discrete fragments are produced after EGF binding whether or not EGF is crosslinked to the receptor. This conclusion came from experiments showing that the fragments derived from the EGF receptor were the same whether the linkage with the photoactivable crosslinking reagent was brought about before or after processing of the receptor [27]. In addition, when cells are incubated with ^{125}I-EGF, some of the specifically bound ^{125}I-EGF becomes directly linked to its receptors as does thrombin [29, 38]. Upon continued incubation, this complex is processed to fragments that are identical in size to the fragments identified with the photoactivable derivative of ^{125}I-EGF [38].

Preliminary experiments suggest that a portion of the direct ^{125}I-thrombin receptor complex is removed upon continued incubation of cells. After this incubation and treatment at pH 12 to disrupt the linkage between ^{125}I-thrombin and its receptor, the ^{125}I-radioactivity migrated with intact thrombin, indicating that a part of the receptor rather than a part of the thrombin had been removed from the thrombin receptor complex. Since the thrombin remained intact during the metabolism of the thrombin receptor complex, it should be possible to immunoprecipitate the metabolized thrombin receptor complex from NP40-solubilized extracts of ^{35}S-methionine-labeled cells using antibodies to thrombin. Treatment of the immunoprecipitate at pH 12 should then release the ^{35}S-labeled receptor fragment from the metabolized thrombin receptor complex. This labeled fragment would be useful for many studies.

Determination of Which Events Are Necessary for Thrombin-Stimulated Cell Division

Since thrombin must bind to its cellular receptor and cleave it to stimulate cell division [5, 24], a first step in analyzing the mechanism of thrombin stimulation is to identify and define molecular changes in the thrombin receptor after thrombin binds to it. Then, it is important to evaluate which of these events are necessary for the stimulation and which are not.

An approach which we are refining is to examine these events in cells that are responsive and ones which are unresponsive to the mitogenic action of thrombin [3, 5]. Thrombin-mediated events which occur in all of the responsive populations but which do not occur or are altered in some of the unresponsive populations are probably necessary for the stimulation. We have conducted some of our experiments on uncloned populations of responsive and unresponsive CE cells [5]. We are now developing procedures to select and clone cells that are responsive or unresponsive to thrombin so it will be possible to conduct experiments on homogenous populations of cells. Since these experiments necessarily require cells that are capable of undergoing a large number of population doublings in culture, we are focusing attention on established cell lines. Preliminary experiments indicate that a line of Chinese hamster lung cells will be well suited for these studies. The above approach should enable us to address important issues. For example, a central question now is whether formation of the direct thrombin receptor complex is necessary for thrombin-stimulated cell division. There are indications that it might not be necessary since ME and CE cells are more sensitive to the mitogenic action of thrombin than HF cells, yet formation of the direct thrombin receptor complex is much more extensive with HF cells [30]. On the other hand, certain results suggest a correlation between formation of the complex and stimulation by thrombin. The important point here is that the clearest means for resolving this issue will be examination of thrombin receptor complex formation in a large number of cloned responsive and unresponsive cells.

The approaches discussed in this section might enable us to define a metabolic pathway for the thrombin receptor that is involved in the control of cell proliferation. If these studies identify receptor fragments that are necessary for stimulation, it would be important to extend the above techniques and examine the fate of these fragments. Some might be further metabolized to species that are also necessary for stimulation. An active fragment could bring about its biological effects in the membrane of the cell surface or endocytosed vesicles, or it could be released from the membrane and produce its effects by interacting with a soluble cell component or with the nucleus or another cellular organelle. Thus, it would be important to examine the fate of these receptor fragments in terms of their location in the cell after continued incubation. This information probably could be obtained by EM autoradiography if the fate of the receptor were studied by following the fate of the ^{125}I-thrombin receptor complex. Then, responsive and unresponsive clones could be used to determine whether certain associations of receptor fragments with cellular components are necessary for thrombin-stimulated cell division.

ACKNOWLEDGMENTS

We thank Dr. John W. Fenton II for gifts of highly purified human thrombin [39] and for helpful discussions. This work was supported by grant CA 12306 from the National Cancer Institute. D.D.C. was supported by Research Career Development Award CA 00171 from the National Cancer Institute. K.C.G. and D.A.L. were supported by NIH Predoctoral Training Grants GM 07311 and GM 07134, respectively.

REFERENCES

1. Chen LB, Buchanan JM: Proc Natl Acad Sci USA 72:131, 1975.
2. Pohjanpelto P: J Cell Physiol 91:387, 1977.
3. Carney DH, Glenn KC, Cunningham DD: J Cell Physiol 95:13, 1978.
4. Glenn KC, Carney DH, Cunningham DD, Fenton JW II (manuscript in preparation).
5. Glenn KC, Cunningham DD: Nature 278:711, 1979.
6. Carney DH, Cunningham DD: Cell 14:811, 1978.
7. Cunningham DD, Carney DH, Glenn KC: In Ross R, Sato G (eds): "Hormones and Cell Culture." New York: Cold Spring Harbor Press, Vol 6, 1979, p 199.
8. Cuatrecasas P: Proc Natl Acad Sci USA 63:450, 1969.
9. Blatt LM, Kimm KH: J Biol Chem 246:4895, 1971.
10. Anderson J, Melchers F: Proc Natl Acad Sci USA 70:416, 1972.
11. Frazier WA, Boyd LF, Bradshaw RA: Proc Natl Acad Sci USA 70:2931, 1973.
12. Davidson MB, Van Herle AJ, Gerschenson LE: Endocrinology 93:1442, 1973.
13. Garwin JL, Gelehrter TD: Arch Biochem Biophys 164:52, 1974.
14. Bolander FF, Fellows RE: Biochem 14:2938, 1975.
15. Kolb JH, Renner R, Hepp KD, Weiss L, Wieland OH: Proc Natl Acad Sci USA 74:248, 1975.
16. Topper YJ, Oka T, Vonderhaar BK, Wilcheck M: J Cell Physiol 89:647, 1976.
17. Zetter BR, Chen LB, Buchanan JM: Proc Natl Acad Sci USA 74:596, 1977.
18. Martin BM, Quigley JP; J Cell Physiol 96:155, 1978.
19. Neville DM, Chang TM: In Kleinzeller A, Bronner F (eds): "Current Topics in Membranes and Transport." New York: Academic Press, 1978, p 65.
20. Goldfine ID, Smith GJ, Wong KY, Jones AL: Proc Natl Acad Sci USA 74:1368, 1977.
21. Andres RY, Jeng I, Bradshaw RA: Proc Natl Acad Sci USA 74:2785, 1977.
22. Yankner BA, Shooter EM: Proc Natl Acad Sci USA 76:1269, 1979.
23. Carney DH, Cunningham DD: Nature 268:602, 1977.
24. Carney DH, Cunningham DD: Cell 15:1341, 1978.
25. Perdue JF, Lubenskyi W, Kivity E, Susanto I: J Cell Biol 79:CS235, 1978.
26. Das M, Miyakawa T, Fox CF, Pruss RM, Aharohov A, Hershcman H: Proc Natl Acad Sci USA 74:2790, 1977.
27. Das M, Fox CF: Proc Natl Acad Sci USA 75:2644, 1978.
28. Carney DH, Glenn KC, Cunningham DD, Das M, Fox CF, Fenton JW II, J Biol Chem 254:6244, 1979.
29. Baker JB, Simmer RL, Glenn KC, Cunningham DD: Nature 278:743, 1979.
30. Simmer RL, Baker JB, Cunningham DD: (submitted, J Surpamol Struct).
31. Rosenberg RD, Damus PS: J Biol Chem 248:6490, 1973.
32. Owen WG: Biochim Biophys Acta 405:380, 1975.
33. Chandra S, Bang NU: In Lundblad RL, Fenton JW II, Mann KG (eds): "Chemistry and Biology of Thrombin." Ann Arbor: Ann Arbor Science, 1977, p 421.
34. Wang K, Richards FM: J Biol Chem 249:8005, 1974.
35. Ruoho A, Bartlett PA, Dutton A, Singer SJ: Biochim Biophys Res Commun 63:417, 1975.
36. Takemoto LJ, Miyakawa T, Fox CF: In Revel J, Henning U, Fox CF (eds): "Cell Shape and Surface Architecture." New York: Alan R Liss, p 605.
37. Blombach B, Hessel B, Hogg D, Claesson G: In Lundblad RL, Fenton JW II, Mann KG (eds): "Chemistry and Biology of Thrombin." Ann Arbor: Ann Arbor Science, 1977, p 275.
38. Linsley PS, Blifield C, Wrann M, Fox CF: Nature 278:745, 1979.
39. Fenton JW II, Fasco MJ, Stackrow AB, Aronson DL, Young AM, Finlayson JS: J Biol Chem 252:3587, 1977.

Journal of Supramolecular Structure 11:269–281 (1979)
Tumor Cell Surfaces and Malignancy 215–227

Fibronectin Associated With the Glial Component of Embryonic Brain Cell Cultures

Clifford J. Kavinsky and Beatrice B. Garber

Department of Biology, University of Chicago, Chicago, Illinois 60637

In a basic approach to investigations of neuronal–glial interactions during both normal brain development and its pathogenesis, embryonic brain cell populations were fractionated into purified neuronal and glial components. Using separation procedures based on differential adhesion and cytotoxicity, the isolated neuronal and glial phenotypes could be identified by distinct morphological and biochemical characteristics, including the visualization of glial fibrillary acid protein (GFA) within glial cells in immunohistochemical assays with monospecific anti-GFA serum.

When unfractionated cerebrum cells dissociated from 10-day chick or 14-day mouse embryos were plated as monolayers and cultured for 1–14 days, monospecific antiserum against fibronectin (LETS glycoprotein) was found to react with many, but not all, of the cells as revealed by indirect immunofluorescence microscopy. The isolated neuronal and glial components of these populations were used to determine whether the appearance of membrane-associated fibronectin was characteristic of one cell type or the other, or both, and if neuronal–glial cell interaction was required for its expression. It was found that the surfaces of glial cells, completely isolated from neurons, showed an intense fluorescent reaction to the anti-fibronectin serum. In contrast, the purified neuronal cultures showed no fluorescence with either the anti-GFA or anti-fibronectin sera. These results demonstrate fibronectin as a cell surface protein associated primarily with glial cells and independent of neuronal–glial cell interaction for its expression. Furthermore, the results indicate that the fibronectin observed on glial cell surfaces in these cultures is produced endogenously and is not due to the preferential binding of fibronectin present in the culture medium. The role of fibronectin as an adhesive molecule in neuronal–glial interactions is discussed.

Key words: fibronectin, cell fractionation, glial fibrillary acidic protein, immunofluorescent labeling, neuronal–glial cell interactions, brain cell culture.

The role of the cell surface in mediating many important cellular functions such as intercellular adhesion [1], motility [2], growth control [3], and selective transport [4] has stimulated widespread interest in identifying function-related membrane macromolecules both in normal and in pathological tissues, with special emphasis on neoplasia [5–7].

Received May 3, 1979; accepted July 16, 1979.

Although such studies have been useful in characterizing membrane constitutents of a wide variety of cell types, progress concerning cells derived from the central nervous system has been hampered by the inherent complexities encountered when working with brain tissues, particularly with respect to the heterogeneity of cell types and the paucity of reliable bio-chemical markers for their identification. Despite these difficulties, a 54,000 dalton poly-peptide originally obtained in purified form from multiple sclerosis plaques of human brain tissue [8,9], and more recently from normal human brain [10], has been revealed to be expressed exclusively by neuroglia, particularly the astrocytic components [9], and to be correlated with cytoplasmic 100 Å filaments [11]. Due to an abundance of dicarboxylic amino acids this protein has been termed the glial fibrillary acidic protein (GFA) and is used as a diagnostic indicator for glial cells.

Recently, much attention has been focused on a high molecular weight (220,000 dalton) glycoprotein that has been shown to be a prominent cell surface component of many cell types grown in vitro, including fibroblasts [12–16], epithelial cells [17], myoblasts [18–20], and vascular endothelial cells [21–23]. Furthermore, this substance, now referred to as fibronectin, has been demonstrated to be a constitutent of plasma and serum, present in high concentration, and antigenically identical to the cold-insoluble globulin (CIg) reported by Mosseson [24–27]. The ubiquitous nature of fibronectin exhibited in vitro reflects its presence in a wide variety of embryonic and adult tissues examined in situ [28–30], where it is found primarily in association with basement membrane and connective tissue [31,32]. Examination of cells following neoplastic transformation reveals a marked reduction or complete absence of fibronectin [33–36]. This loss of fibronectin is a result of decreased biosynthetic activity [37] and has been correlated with the tumorigenic capabilities of cells in a series of adenovirus-transformed rat cell lines [38]. Fibronectin has been postulated to play a role in cell adhesion [39,40] and to influence cell morphology [41–43] and motility [44]. If such is the case, then expression of this glycoprotein by cellular elements of the brain during neurogenesis may be of importance in understanding the many complex cell migrations and interactions that occur during development of the central nervous system and in elucidating the alterations in cell behavior associated with neoplasia.

To approach the question of cell surface fibronectin expression in the developing brain, we have examined monolayer cultures of embryonic cerebral cells by indirect immunofluorescent assays using antisera directed against purified fibronectin. The use of methodologies developed in this laboratory for the preparation of homogeneous populations of neurons or glia suitable for extended culture and histochemical analysis permitted the localization of fibronectin with respect to particular cell types. We have obtained evidence, reported here, that developing glial cells, whose identity is verified by immunofluorescence assays with anti-GFA serum, produce cell-surface-associated fibro-nectin. In contrast, fibronectin is not detectable in pure neuronal cultures. The implica-tions of glial fibronectin for neuronal adhesion and migration during normal development and also in neoplasia are considered in the discussion.

METHODS

Preparation of Cell Cultures

Using sterile techniques, cerebral lobes from 10-day chick or 14-day mouse embryos were dissociated into single cell suspensions according to standard procedures developed by Garber and Moscona [45]. Embryos were staged using previously established guidelines [46,47]. The tissues were freed of meninges, cut into 2mm^3 pieces, incubated in calcium-

magnesium-free Tyrode's solution (CMF) at 37°C for 20 min, and then enzymatically dissociated in 0.1% trypsin (Grand Island Biological) at 37°C for 35–40 min under a 5% CO_2 –
95% air atmosphere. After 3 washes in CMF, culture medium was added and the tissues
were dispersed into single cell suspensions by flushing them repeatedly through a fine-bore
pipette. Aliquots ($3-6 \times 10^6$ cells/dish) were dispensed into 35 mm Falcon tissue culture
dishes containing 3 ml of culture medium (Eagle's basal medium, supplemented with 3.8
mg/ml d-glucose, 15% fetal bovine serum, 1% l-glutamine, and 1% penicillin-streptomycin
solution, 50 units each/ml).

Homogeneous glial cultures were prepared by taking advantage of the ability of glial
cells to adhere to the underlying substratum at a faster rate than neurons [48]. Selected
brain cell suspensions were plated for 10 min, then the supernatant medium containing the
unattached neurons was removed, and fresh medium was added. A glial-enriched culture was
obtained from the plated cells. Residual neuronal contaminants were effectively removed
by subculturing the glial cultures after they reached confluence. The neurons' restricted
capacity to reattach in secondary culture, plus the glial cells' continued mitotic activity resulted in over 95% purity in secondary glial cultures.

The supernatant medium from the initial plating of the cell suspension was used to
prepare homogeneous neuronal cultures. Following a second 15-min preparative plating to
remove carry-over glial contaminants, a neuron-enriched fraction was obtained by plating
the cells remaining in this second supernatant. Two 24-h treatments of 10^{-4} M cytosine-d-
arabinoside (ARA-c, Sigma) proved to be effective in removing residual glial cells from these
enriched neuronal cultures. The neuronal populations thus obtained were determined to
have over 97% purity. The identification of neurons and glia was made on the basis of
morphological criteria, tritated thymidine assays for mitotic activity, and histochemical
assays for acetylcholinesterase and butyrylcholinesterase [49].

Pretreatment of culture dishes with poly-l-lysine (5 μg/ml; Sigma, mol wt 340,000)
markedly facilitated the attachment of cells to the plastic surface [50] and was used routinely for both the sequential plating steps and the final purified preparations.

Early passage fibroblasts, prepared from 18-day mouse embryos according to previously published protocols [51] were grown in 100 mm Falcon tissue culture dishes containing
10 ml growth medium (Dulbecco's modified Eagle's medium supplemented with 10% fetal
bovine serum and 1% penicillin-streptomycin solution). Upon reaching confluence, cells
were subcultured using 0.25% trypsin and seeded at densities of 10^6 cells/100 mm plate.

Purification of Fibronectin From Fetal Bovine Serum

Fibronectin was purified from human plasma and fetal bovine serum (FBS) by affinity chromatography according to previously published methods [52,53]. Briefly, chromatography was carried out at room temperature using BrCN-activated Sepharose 4B (Pharmacia) coupled to gelatin (Sigma, type I). Purification was carried out by first passing 40 ml
of plasma or serum through a Sepharose 2B column to remove minor contaminants having
affinity for the Sepharose. The voided material was subsequently passed through the gelatin-
sepharose column. The fibronectin was eluted off the column as a single peak with 4 M urea
(Schwarz/Mann) in 0.05 M tris buffer, pH 7.5, and then dialyzed extensively against the
same buffer at 4°C. Passing the unabsorbed fraction through a second gelatin-Sepharose
column did not increase the yield of fibronectin. Eluting the column with 8 M urea also
had no effect on total yield. Protein determinations conducted according to the method
of Lowry [54], using bovine serum albumin standards, revealed FBS to contain approximately
62.5 μg/ml of fibronectin. This value, however, was observed to be variable, changing signi-

ficantly with different lots of FBS. Analyses of the various fractions in a sodium dodecyl sulfate-polyacrylamide gel electrophoresis system, using 7.5% slab gels according to the method of Laemmli [55], revealed that the fibronectin band present in the starting material was not detectable in the void volume of the gelatin-Sepharose column, and that reduced samples of the affinity purified material migrated as a single band with an apparent molecular weight of approximately 220,000 daltons. Adjacent wells containing purified preparations isolated from human plasma and cell surface fibronectin extracted from intact cultures of chick embryo fibroblasts [43] revealed that the human and bovine plasma fibronectins comigrated while the cell surface fibronectin was displaced slightly toward the cathode.

Analyses of samples by gel double-diffusion in agarose using rabbit serum containing antibodies to human plasma fibrotectin gave strong reactions with both the human plasma and FBS starting materials and the affinity-purified preparations while yielding no detectable precipitin bands against the voided material of the gelatin-Sepharose column. These observations, taken together with the results obtained by electrophoretic analysis, established that the purification protocol did, in fact, remove all fibronectin from the starting material and that the purified material obtained was fibronectin.

The FBS from which the bovine fibronectin had been removed was subsequently reconstituted to its original protein concentration by Amicon filtration, dialyzed extensively against Tyrode's solution, Millipore filtered, and used in the preparation of cell growth medium.

Antisera

Rabbit serum that contained antibodies to the fibronectin of human plasma was prepared by injecting highly purified fibronectin. The serum fraction was immunoabsorbed with the supernatant of Cohn fraction I. The resulting high titer antiserum was monospecific, as determined both by immunoelectrophoresis and by direct binding of fibronectin antibodies to the appropriate band on polyacrylamide gels [56]. This antiserum was generously supplied by Dr. Lan Bo Chen. The interspecies cross-reactivity of antisera prepared against purified fibronectin has been reported elsewhere [57]. Twenty μl of this antiserum was absorbed with 100 μg of purified plasma fibronectin. Following centrifugation, the supernatant was tested for residual immunoreactivity in immunofluorescence assays.

Antisera against GFA, kindly supplied by Dr. Doris Dahl, was obtained by injections of purified GFA (isolated from human spinal cord) into rabbits. Immunoelectrophoresis of the resulting antiserum gave evidence of its monospecificity [10].

Immunofluorescence

For examination of cell surface-associated fibronectin, cell monolayers plated on poly-l-lysine-coated glass coverslips (12 mm, Kimble) were extensively washed in Hank's balanced salt solution (HBSS) with bicarbonate buffer, pH 7.4, and placed in a humidified chamber. Ten μl of fibronectin antiserum prepared from rabbits injected with human plasma fibronectin, diluted 1:80 with HBSS, was layered on the coverslips and incubated for 30 min at 37°C. After washing in HBSS, the coverslips were then layered with 10 μl of fluorescein isothiocyanate-conjugated (FITC) IgG antibody from goat anti-rabbit serum (Cappel), diluted 1:20 with HBSS. After a second 30 min incubation at 37°C, coverslips were again washed in HBSS and were subsequently fixed in 2% paraformaldehyde in phosphate-buffered saline (PBS) for 30 min. Following fixation, the coverslips were washed in PBS and mounted on microscope slides with Elvanol. Parallel samples of unfixed cells were similarly prepared.

Control samples consisting of 1) cells incubated with normal rabbit serum in place of the specific antibody, 2) preparations in which the anti-fibronectin serum was omitted, and 3) coverslips exposed to normal goat serum prior to labeling with the FITC-conjugated antibody were also prepared. Fluorescence was observed using a Zeiss fluorescence microscope equipped with epi-illumination.

For intracellular visualization of GFA, coverslip preparations were fixed in formyl alcohol (9 parts 95% ethanol:1 part 37% formalin) for 20 min at 4°C. Cold acetone (½ volume) was then added for 15 min, followed by a 30 min exposure to 100% acetone at 4°C. After extensive washing and treatment with Tween 80 detergent (Sigma, 3% aqueous solution) for 1 min at 20°C, the cells were again washed and subsequently labeled in the manner described above, using rabbit anti-human GFA serum, diluted 1:50 with PBS. Appropriate controls were carried out, as described above for the anti-fibronectin serum.

RESULTS

Morphology of Whole Cerebrum Cell Cultures

Following dissociation of cerebral tissue from chick or mouse embryos, the resulting cell suspension, when examined under phase-contrast microscopy, revealed single, phase-dark cells, many of which had prominent nucleoli. These cells could be grouped into two general size classes: $10-15 \mu$, and $3-7 \mu$ in diameter. These observations were consistent with those reported by Varon and Raiborn [48], who used analogous cell systems. On the basis of evidence presented here and in previously published studies using identical or similar cell models [58–62], it appeared that the larger rounded cells were neuronal in origin, and that the smaller proliferative cells were glial precursors. By 72 hours, the small, nonaggregated cells (glioblasts) took on a flattened, spread-out appearance typical of epithelial morphology and exhibited irregular contours and many cytoplasmic granulations. These cells proliferated rapidly and achieved confluence by 7 days in culture.

During this period the neurons had increased in size and retained their rounded cell bodies, each with a clear nucleus and prominent nucleolus. The neuronal cells, mostly bipolar in appearance, aggregated into clusters. These aggregates invariably rested upon the underlying glial monolayer, suggesting a perferential affinity for the glial cells, or their exudates, as substrates rather than for the culture dish surface (Fig. 1A). Cell processes, first observed extending from neuronal aggregates after 24 h, fasciculated into fiber bundles, some of which were over 3 mm long after 7 days in culture. These nerve fibers formed an intricate meshwork which interconnected with other neuronal aggregates within the culture. Neuronal perikarya were found moving along the newly formed fascicles and the underlying glial monolayer.

Separation of Neuronal and Glial Cell Types

Separated homogeneous populations of glial cells and neurons were prepared from dissociated cerebral cell suspensions by exploiting a combination of differential adhesiveness to the culture dish during the initial plating and differential cytotoxic responses to the nucleoside analogue, cytosine-d-arabinoside, as described in Methods. Along with inhibition of DNA polymerase activity, ARA-c produced selective toxic effects on the actively dividing glial components, while apparently having no effect on neurons, which are postmitotic at this gestational age [58,63]. Examination of purified neuronal cultures after treatment with ARA-c revealed an absence of glial elements, while the neuronal aggregates and interconnecting fiber tracts remained intact (Fig. 1B). Poly-l-lysine pretreatment of neuron-

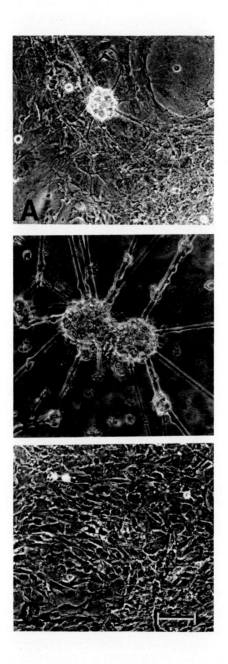

Fig. 1. Ten-day chick embryonic cerebral monolayer cultures, phase-contrast. (A) Mixed culture of neurons and glia after 7 days in culture. (B) Homogeneous neuronal culture after 7 days in culture. (C) Homogeneous glial culture after 7 days in culture (bar = 90μ; magnification, $\times$ 150).

al cultures was critical for attachment of neuronal elements to the surface of the culture dish, since the glial cells, which normally form the neuronal substratum, were absent.

Initial glial cultures obtained by rapid plating, although substantially enriched for glial cells, contained varying numbers of neuronal contaminants, which were effectively removed by subculture after the glia reached confluence. Phase microscopic examination of purified glial cultures obtained in this way revealed cells with an exclusively epithelial morphology (Fig. 1C).

Expression of GFA by Epithelial Components

Comparative immunofluorescent analysis of fractionated mouse monolayer cultures using rabbit serum containing antibodies to human GFA, revealed the presence of GFA in the epithelial glial cell fraction, and its absence in the neuronal fraction. Parallel preparations of glial cells treated with normal rabbit serum yielded no detectable specific fluorescence (Fig. 2C,D). Furthermore, mouse embryo fibroblasts similarly prepared were also GFA-negative (Fig. 2E,F). At early states of culture, only 5—10% of the glial cells expressed this protein; however, after 14 days in culture essentially 100% of the cells in the glial cultures were GFA-positive. The antigen was distributed within the cytoplasm as filamentous arrays, which were randomly oriented within the somatic portion of the cell. GFA protein within the filopodia consistently had a polarized configuration oriented parallel to the long axis of the process (Fig. 2A,B). These results confirmed the classification of these epithelial cells as glial by immunochemical criteria and demonstrated that differentiation of these cells progresses in vitro.

Distribution of Fibronectin

With antiserum directed against fibronectin, indirect immunofluorescent staining of embryonic chick and mouse cerebral cells in monolayer cultures containing both neurons and glia revealed that fibronectin, or a closely related molecule, was associated with the cell surface of many, but not all, of the cells. That fibronectin antiserum was reacting with an antigen of cellular origin, and not a serum contaminant, was established by growing the cells in culture medium containing serum from which the fibronectin had previously been removed (see Methods). Cells fixed in 2% paraformaldehyde following antibody labeling had immunofluorescent staining patterns identical to those of parallel live preparations. Protocols in which the cells were fixed before labeling, however, consistently introduced a low level of diffuse background fluorescence not evident in post-fixed or live preparations. Cells prepared in the manner described in Methods served to establish the localization of fibronectin at the external cell surface. Prior absorption of the fibronectin antiserum with purified human plasma fibronectin abolished all detectable specific fluorescence. Similarly, cells treated with pre-immune rabbit serum or FITC-conjugated goat anti-rabbit serum alone yielded no specific fluorescence.

Upon further examination, it was found that fibronectin expressed in heterogeneous cultures of cerebral cell populations could be detected as early as 24 h in culture. More significantly, fibronectin was localized to cells with a flattened epithelial morphology, indicative of glial origins. Moreover, the rounded neuronal elements did not express the antigen. Immunofluorescent examination of homogeneous glial cell cultures demonstrated that the glial cells were the source of fibronectin expression demonstrated earlier in the whole cerebral cell monolayers. In isolated glial cell cultures fibronectin increased in a strictly density-dependent manner. In sparse cultures there was little detectable fibronectin on the surface of the glial cells. However, it was noted that the fibronectin present in these cultures was

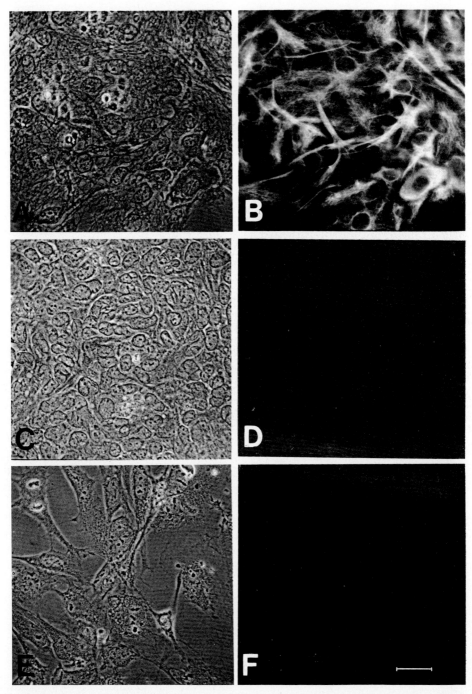

Fig. 2. Homogeneous glial monolayer after 14 days in culture, (A) viewed with phase-contrast; (B) corresponding field showing indirect immunofluorescent visualization of intracellular GFA; (C) parallel homogeneous glial preparation viewed under phase contrast; (D) corresponding field showing indirect immunofluorescent reaction with normal rabbit serum; (E) mouse embryo fibroblasts after 14 days in culture viewed under phase-contrast; (F) corresponding field labeled with GFA antiserum (bar = 10μ; magnification, $\times$ 400).

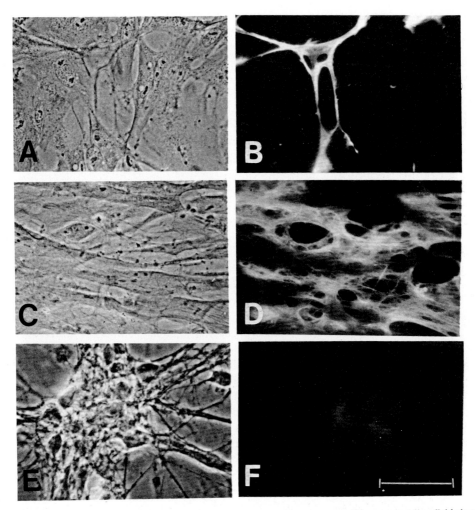

Fig. 3. (A) Purified glial cell fraction after 72 h in culture, phase-contrast; (B) corresponding field show-ing indirect immunofluorescent distribution of cell surface fibronectin; (C) homogeneous population of confluent glial cells after 7 days in culture, phase-contrast; (D) corresponding immunofluorescent stain-ing of fibronectin. Note dense fibrillar-like network associated with cell processes; (E) purified neuronal monolayer culture after 7 days, phase-contrast; (F) corresponding field after staining with antifibronectin serum (bar = 30μ; magnification, $\times$ 400).

localized on filopodial-like processes (see Fig. 3A,B). With progressive proliferation, the cells became increasingly dense, and after 7–10 days reached confluence. Concomitantly, the fibronectin level increased and was observable as a dense matrix closely associated with the surface of the culture dish (Fig. 3C,D).

Glial cells grown in serum from which the fibronectin had been removed by affinity chromatography showed no alteration in their ability to attach and spread on the under-lying substratum, nor in the pattern of fibronectin-specific fluorescence observed. While this result does not ensure that serum fibronectin will not bind to the cells in culture, it does indicate that most of the specific fluorescence observed is not attributable to serum-derived protein.

In contrast to the intense fluorescence seen in glial cell cultures with the anti-fibro-nectin serum, immunofluorescent examination of corresponding pure neuronal cultures demonstrated that the neurons were devoid of fibronectin (Fig. 3E,F). Thus, fibronectin is expressed by the glial component of developing cerebral cell populations and serves as a diagnostic marker of this cell type in vitro.

DISCUSSION

The results presented above suggest that fibronectin, a well-characterized cell surface glycoprotein, may provide a useful biochemical marker for developing glial cells grown in vitro. This is consistent with the recent demonstration of fibronectin in cultures of normal adult human glial cells [64]. While immunological data demonstrate that there are antigenic determinants shared by fibronectin and cell surface components on young glial cells, these tests do not permit direct identification of the cell surface antigen as fibronectin. However, the disposition, topographical arrangement, and general properties of the glial antigen — ie, density dependence and fibrillar appearance — are consistent with those expected for fibronectin.

Expression of fibronectin by glial cells, and its absence in neuronal elements, may represent a significant cell surface property governing neuronal—glial interactions during neurogenesis. In view of the ubiquitous nature of fibronectin, it is quite unlikely that it participates in the establishment of highly specific intercellular contacts. However, a general adhesive role for fibronectin cannot be ruled out. It is possible that this substance, expressed by immature glia during development, may serve to bring cellular elements into close opposition to one another in a nonspecific manner. Subsequently, adherent cells may further interact with one another in accordance with the histogenetic program. Similar mechanisms may be involved in facilitating the migrations of newly born neuronal cells to their final positions in the cephalic wall. This notion is not without precedent, since such a role for radial glia has been previously put forward by Rakic [65,66].

We have shown that neuronal cells in the absence of glia and of glial-associated fibro-nectin retain properties for mutual adhesion and aggregate to form tightly coherent cell clusters under these conditions. However, in the presence of glia, neurons tend to adhere to the glial substrate and to move away from their neuronal neighbors. Such neuronal—glial cell interactions, observed earlier in explant cultures [67,68] and monolayer cultures [60], suggest that fibronectin may play a role as an adhesive molecule, enabling neurons to extend pseudopodial outgrowths along a glial framework. In the case of freely moving neurons, this could result in the directed migration and translocation of neurons along predetermined pathways; in the case of anchored neurons, the elongation of axonal or dendritic processes could result in the alignment of cortical elements or the establishment of fibrous tracts.

The proposal that such a mechanism is operative in the intact embryo is, of course, contingent upon demonstrating fibronectin in brain tissues developing in situ. Recent obser-vations by Schachner et al [69], using immunofluorescent assays, have indicated that fibro-nectin can be seen neither in intact adult nor embryonic tissues. However, these results may be due to the dynamic state of fibronectin in vivo — eg, a rapid turnover of fibronectin on glial cell surfaces in vivo or its appearance in a less polymerized form than that exhibited in monolayer cell cultures. Further analysis of the dichotomous expression and behavior of this molecule in vivo and in vitro seems warranted, and investigations are in progress to address this question by more sensitive methods for detection of fibronectin in brain tissues both in situ and in 3-dimensional aggregates reconstituted in vitro.

Since the neoplastic counterparts of normal fibronectin-producing cells have generally been shown to be devoid of fibronectin [12,64], it is of interest to note that cerebral glial-derived cells of the C_6 astrocytoma line do not express fibronectin [70]. When dissociated C_6 astrocytoma cells were plated on a confluent sheet of embryonic glial cells, it was found that they failed to adhere to normal glia and, instead, penetrated between the normal glial cell junctions [71]. The astrocytoma cells then migrated underneath the normal glial sheet attaching preferentially to the culture dish surface. The possibility that neoplastic alterations of glial cell surface properties operative in tissue invasiveness may also involve fibronectin raises provocative questions. Not only may the absence of fibronectin on astrocytoma cells prevent cell–cell contacts and tissue relationships with normal glial cells, but, in addition, proteolytic activity by the neoplastic glial cells may also destroy the preexisting fibronectin mediated cell–cell and cell–substrate adhesiveness that preserves the integrity of the normal tissue.

In conclusion, the demonstration of fibronectin associated with the glial component of embryonic brain tissue may be related to the neuromesenchymal function of glia in neurogenesis, particularly in terms of the stromal support it provides for developing neuronal networks.

ACKNOWLEDGMENTS

We would like to thank Dr. Lan Bo Chen and Dr. Doris Dahl for providing anti-fibronectin and anti-GFA sera. Appreciation is also extended to Dr. Ken Yamada for his contribution of purified cell-extracted fibronectin. We are also grateful to Marion Sullivan for her secretarial assistance during the preparation of the manuscript.

This work was supported by NIH grants CA 19265, NS 10714, and GM 07151.

REFERENCES

1. Moscona AA: In Moscona AA (ed): "The Cell Surface and Development." New York: John Wiley & Sons, 1974, pp 67–100.
2. Abercrombie M, Heaysman JEM, Pegrum SM:Exp Cell Res 67:359–367, 1971.
3. Sefton BM, Rubin H: Nature 227:843, 1970.
4. Bretscher MS, Raff MC: Nature 258:43–49, 1975.
5. Hynes RO:Biochim Biophys Acta 458:73–108, 1976.
6. Nicolson GL:Biochim Biophys Acta 457:57–108, 1976.
7. Nicolson GL:Biochim Biophys Acta 458:1–72, 1976.
8. Uyeda CT, Eng LF, Bignami A: Brain Res 37:81–89, 1972.
9. Bignami A, Dahl D: J Comp Neurol 153:27–38, 1974.
10. Dahl D, Bignami A: Brain Res 116:150–157, 1976.
11. Schachner M, Smith C, Schoonmaker G: Dev Neurosci 1:1–14, 1978.
12. Critchley DR, Wyke JA, Hynes RO:Biochim Biophys Acta 436:335–352, 1976.
13. Hogg NM:Proc Natl Acad Sci USA 71:489–492, 1974.

14. Graham JM, Hynes RO, Davidson EA, Brainton DE: Cell 4:353–365, 1975.
15. Hynes RO, Humphreyes KD: J Cell Biol 62:438–448, 1974.
16. Wartiovaara J, Linder E, Ruoslahti E, Vaheri A: J Exp Med 140:1622–1633, 1974.
17. Chen LB, Maithland N, Gallimore PH, McDougall JK: J Exp Cell Res 106:39–46, 1977.
18. Hynes RO, Martin GS, Shearer M, Critchley DR, Epstein CJ: Dev Biol 48:35–46, 1976.
19. Chen LB: Cell 10:393–400, 1977.
20. Furcht LT, Mosher DF, Wendelschafer-Crabb G:Cell 13:263–271, 1978.
21. Birdwell GR, Gospodarowicz D, Nicolson GL: Proc Natl Acad Sci USA 75:3275–3277, 1978.
22. Macarak EJ, Kirby E, Kirk T, Kefalides NA: Proc Natl Acad Sci USA 75:2621–2625, 1978.
23. Jaffe EA, Mosher DF: Ann NY Acad Sci 312:122–131, 1978.
24. Ruoslahti E, Vaheri A, Kuusela P, Linder E: Biochim Biophys Acta 322:352–358, 1973.
25. Ruoslahti E, Vaheri A: J Exp Med 141:499–501, 1975.
26. Mosseson MW, Umfleet RA: J Biol Chem 245:5728–5736, 1970.
27. Yamada KM, Olden K: Nature 275:179–184, 1978.
28. Wartiovaara J, Leivo I, Virtanen I, Vaheri A, Graham CF: Ann NY Acad Sci 312:132–141, 1978.
29. Wartiovaara J, Leivo I, Vaheri A: Dev Biol 69:247–257, 1979.
30. Linder E, Vaheri A, Ruoslahti E, Wartiovaara J: J Exp Med 142:41–49, 1975.
31. Linder E, Stenman S, Lehto VP, Vaheri A: Ann NY Acad Sci 312:151–159, 1978.
32. Bray BA: Ann NY Acad Sci 312:142–150, 1978.
33. Hynes RO, Wyke JA: Virology 64:492–504, 1975.
34. Hynes RO: Proc Natl Acad Sci USA 70:3170–3174, 1973.
35. Stone KR, Smith RE, Joklik WK: Virology 58:86–100, 1974.
36. Hynes RO, Ali IU, Destree AT, Mautner V, Perkins ME, Senger DR, Wagner DD, Smith KK, Pastan I: Ann NY Acad Sci 312:256–277, 1978.
37. Olden K, Yamada KM: Cell 11:957–969, 1977.
38. Chen LB, Gallimore PH, McDougall JK: Proc Natl Acad Sci USA 73:3570–3574, 1976.
39. Yamada KM, Yamada SS, Pastan I: Proc Natl Acad Sci USA 72:3158–3162, 1975.
40. Hynes RO, Destree AF: Cell 15:875–886, 1978.
41. Yamada KM, Yamada SS, Pastan I: Proc Natl Acad Sci USA 73:1217–1221, 1976.
42. Chen LB, Murray A, Segal RA, Bushnell A, Walsh ML: Cell 14:377–391, 1978.
43. Yamada KM, Olden K, Pastan I: Ann NY Acad Sci 312:256–277, 1978.
44. Ali IU, Hynes RO: Cell 14:439–446, 1978.
45. Garber BB, Moscona AA: Dev Biol 27:217–234, 1972.
46. Gruneberg H: Heredity 34:89–92, 1943.
47. Hamburger V, Hamilton HL: J Morphol 88:49–92, 1951.
48. Varon S, Raiborn C: Brain Res 12:180–199, 1969.
49. Stanley S, Garber BB, Wong YC: (in preparation).
50. Yavin E, Yavin Z: J Cell Biol 62:540–546, 1974.
51. Rein A, Rubin H: Exp Cell Res 49:666–678, 1968.
52. Engvall E, Ruoslahti E: Int J Cancer 20:1–5, 1977.
53. Ruoslahti E, Engvall E: Ann NY Acad Sci 312:178–191, 1978.
54. Lowry OH: J Biol Chem 193:265, 1951.
55. Laemmli UK: Nature 227:680–685, 1970.
56. Burridge K: Proc Natl Acad Sci USA 73:4457–4561, 1976.
57. Kuusela P, Ruoslahti E, Engvall E, Vaheri A: Immunochemistry 13:639–642, 1976.
58. Tsai HM: Ph.D. Dissertation. University of Chicago, 1977.
59. Peterson GR, Webster GW, Shuster L: Dev Biol 34:867–870, 1975.
60. Wong YC, Garber BB:Proc 9th Int Cong Elec Mic 3:602, 1978.
61. Crain SM, Peterson ER: Science 188:275–278, 1975.
62. Dichter MA: Brain Res 149:279–293, 1978.
63. Fischbach GD: Dev Biol 28:407–429, 1972.
64. Vaheri A, Ruoslahti E, Westermark B, Ponten J: J Exp Med 143:64–72, 1976.
65. Rakic P: Brain Res 33:471–476, 1972.
66. Rakic P: J Comp Neurol 145:61–68, 1972.

67. Peterson ER, Crain SM, Murray MR: Z Zellforsch 66:130–145, 1965.
68. Guillery RW, Sobkowicz HM, Scott GL: J Comp Neurol 140:1–34, 1978.
69. Schachner M, Schoonmaker G, Hynes RO: Brain Res 158:149–158, 1978.
70. Kavinsky CJ, Garber BB: J Cell Biol 79:99, 1978.
71. Wong YC, Garber BB: Proc 9th Int Cong Elec Mic 2:308–309, 1978.

Journal of Supramolecular Structure 11:349–359 (1979)
Tumor Cell Surfaces and Malignancy 229–239

The Serum-Free Growth of Balb/c 3T3 Cells in Medium Supplemented With Bovine Colostrum

M. Klagsbrun and J. Neumann

Departments of Surgery and Biological Chemistry, Children's Hospital Medical Center and Harvard Medical School, Boston, Massachusetts 02115

Bovine milk contains growth promoting factors that stimulate DNA synthesis and cell division in confluent monolayers of quiescent Balb/c 3T3 cells. The growth factor activity was highest in colostrum obtained within 24 hours after birth of a calf. Samples of milk obtained 32 hours and 60 hours after birth were 20% and 1% as active respectively as was a sample obtained 8 hours after birth in stimulating DNA synthesis. No activity was detectable 3 days after birth or thereafter. A similar temporal dependence was found in sheep's milk. Bovine colostrum obtained on the day of a calf's birth can be substituted for serum and will support the growth of sparse Balb/c 3T3 cells to confluence. In Dulbecco's modified Eagle's medium (DMEM) supplemented with 2.5% (vol/vol) bovine colostrum, the number of Balb/c 3T3 cells in a dish increased 35-fold, from 2.0×10^4 cells to 7×10^5 cells. The generation time was approximately 38 hours. Proliferation of cells was characterized by formation of clusters of confluent Balb/c 3T3 cells which were smaller in size and more tightly packed than were Balb/c 3T3 cells grown to confluence in serum. No proliferation was detected in DMEM supplemented with milk obtained 10 days after birth of a calf or in DMEM supplemented with bovine serum albumen.

Key words: colostrum, milk, serum, growth factors, mitogens, DNA synthesis, proliferation, 3T3 cells, serum-free growth

In a previous report, we have demonstrated that human breast milk stimulates DNA synthesis and cell division in confluent monolayers of quiescent Balb/c 3T3 cells [1]. The mitogenic activity of the human milk is due to the presence of growth promoting factors that are polypeptides with molecular weights between 14,000 and 18,000 and isoelectric points between 4.4 and 4.7.

Received April 27, 1979; accepted July 2, 1979.

Balb/c 3T3 cells were established as a cell culture line by Aaronson and Todaro [2]. Since then, these cells have been used extensively to study growth control in cell culture [3–5]. Balb/c 3T3 cells are routinely grown in medium supplemented with serum. It is believed that serum contains growth promoting factors that are necessary in order for these cells to proliferate. The factors in serum necessary for the growth of 3T3 cells are thought to be potent mitogenic substances that are derived from platelets [6–8]. The presence of growth factors in milk raises the possibility that the serum requirement of Balb/c 3T3 cells may be replaced with milk. Initial attempts in this laboratory to grow these cells in human milk were unsuccessful. However, it was observed that human colostrum was a better source of growth factor activity than was human milk obtained from the same woman later in her lactation period. Since human colostrum was not readily available for large scale cell culture experiments, bovine colostrum was tried instead.

In this report, we demonstrate that bovine colostrum will stimulate DNA synthesis and cell division in confluent Balb/c 3T3 cells. In addition, these cells, when plated sparsely, will grow to confluence in a medium in which serum has been replaced by colostrum. Successful growth in the absence of serum is only possible using colostrum obtained within 24 hours after birth of a calf. Milk obtained later in the lactation period is inactive.

MATERIALS AND METHODS

Source of Milk

Bovine milk was kindly provided by Dr. Edward Kingsbury of the Department of Veterinary and Animal Sciences at the University of Massachusetts (Amherst, Massachusetts). The milk was obtained from Holstein and Jersey cows and was frozen immediately after milking. The concentration of protein in milk was determined by the method of Lowry [9].

Preparation of Milk for Cell Culture

Frozen milk samples were thawed and spun in a RC-5 superspeed Sorvall centrifuge at $12,000 \times$ g for 30 minutes. The fat which floated on top of the spun milk was removed and discarded. Cellular debris and other sediment at the bottom of the centrifuge tube was also discarded. Milk samples were sterilized by filtration through Nalgene filter units. The presence in milk of casein micelles [10] and other particles makes filtration of milk at concentrations of 10% (vol/vol) or greater difficult. Samples of milk at concentrations of 10% (vol/vol) or less were sterilized by diluting milk into medium, prefiltering with 0.80 micron Nalgene filter units and then by filtering with 0.45 micron Nalgene filter units.

Cells and Cell Culture

Mouse Balb/c 3T3 embryo cells (clone A31) were obtained from Dr. C. D. Scher (Sidney Farber Cancer Center, Boston, Massachusetts). The cells were grown at $37°C$ in Dulbecco's modified Eagle's medium (DMEM, Gibco, Grand Island, New York) containing 4.5 gm of glucose per liter, penicillin (50 U/ml) and streptomycin (50 μg/ml), and supplemented with either calf serum (Colorado Serum Co., Denver, Colorado) or bovine milk prepared as described above.

Proliferation of Sparse Cells

The kinetics of Balb/c 3T3 cell proliferation were measured using the following protocol; Balb/c 3T3 cells were detached by incubation with 0.1% (vol/vol) trypsin and 0.02% EDTA (Gibco) in phosphate buffered saline lacking calcium and magnesium. The cells were resuspended in DMEM at a concentration of 10^4 cells/ml and 1 ml of cells was plated into each well of a 24-well microtiter plate (16 mm diameter, Costar, Cambridge, Massachusetts). Approximately 4 hours after plating, the DMEM containing unattached cells was removed and the number of attached cells was counted. The plating efficiency under these conditions was about 20 to 40%. The attached cells were then fed with unsupplemented DMEM or with DMEM supplemented with either milk or with serum. On every third or fourth day, duplicate wells were counted and the rest of the cells were refed with fresh medium. The number of cells in a well was measured by detachment of cells with trypsin and counting in a Coulter Model ZF electronic particle counter (Coulter Electronics).

DNA Synthesis and Cell Division in Confluent Cells

The preparation of confluent Balb/c 3T3 cells in a 96-well microtiter plate (Falcon); the measurement of DNA synthesis by scintillation counting and by autoradiography, and the measurement of cell division by detachment with trypsin followed by counting in a Coulter counter, have been described previously [1, 11].

Photography

Balb/c 3T3 cells were photographed under phase and after fixation and staining. Cells were fixed and stained using the following steps; washing with 0.15 M NaCl, addition of cold methanol for 5 minutes, addition of 10% buffered formalin phosphate for 5 minutes, a rinse with cold H_2O and addition of toluidene blue (0.1% in H_2O) for 1 minute. Photographs were taken using a Nikon Model MS inverted phase microscope with a Wild Heerbrugg Model MK4 camera attachment.

RESULTS

Stimulation of DNA Synthesis by Milk

Samples of milk were obtained from cows within 24 hours after birth of a calf (day 1) and at regular intervals thereafter up to a period of 2 weeks. The milk samples were tested for the ability to stimulate DNA synthesis in quiescent confluent Balb/c 3T3 cells. The stimulatory activity in relation to the time elapsed since birth of a calf, of milk samples obtained from 3 cows is shown in Figure 1. In each case, milk obtained on the day of birth, that is the colostrum, was the most active in stimulating DNA synthesis in the Balb/c 3T3 cells. A concentration of 1% (vol/vol) bovine colostrum was sufficient to label every nucleus in the Balb/c 3T3 population. The stimulatory activity of the bovine milk declined very rapidly after the day of birth. A milk sample obtained 32 hours after birth was only 20% as active in stimulating DNA synthesis as was a sample obtained 8 hours after birth when measured at a final concentration of 1% (vol/vol). On the third day postpartum (60 hours) and thereafter no stimulatory activity could be detected. The decline in stimulatory activity was not due solely to the drop in the protein concentration of milk. While the protein concentration of milk obtained 60 hours after

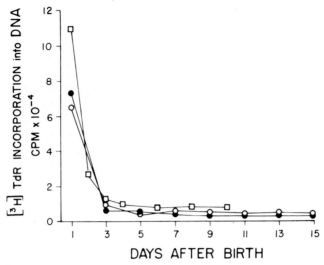

Fig. 1. Stimulation of DNA synthesis in Balb/c 3T3 cells by bovine milk obtained at various times after birth of a calf. Quiescent monolayers of confluent Balb/c 3T3 cells were prepared by plating approximately 10^4 cells into each 0.3 cm^2 well of a 96-place microtiter plate. The cells were maintained in Dulbecco's modified Eagle's medium (DMEM) supplemented with 10% calf serum for 7 to 10 days in order to deplete the serum of growth promoting factors. Milk was obtained from 3 different cows on the day a calf was born (day 1) and at regular intervals thereafter. The milk samples were added to the confluent monolayers of quiescent Balb/c 3T3 cells without any medium change along with (^{3}H) TdR (6.7 Ci/mmol, 4 μCi/ml) and incubated for a period of 40–48 hours. The cells were fixed with methanol and TCA and DNA synthesis was measured by scintillation counting. The final concentration of milk in each microtiter well was 1.0% (vol/vol). The background incorporation of the quiescent cells was 3,000 cpm while 20% (vol/vol) calf serum stimulated the incorporation of approximately 80,000 cpm.

birth was about 20% of that obtained 8 hours after birth, the stimulatory activity of the former was less than 1% that of the latter. A similar pattern was observed with sheep's milk. Sheep colostrum obtained on the day of a lamb's birth stimulated DNA synthesis but milk obtained 2 days later did not (Fig. 2).

Confluent monolayers of Balb/c 3T3 cells can be stimulated to synthesize DNA by addition of fresh bovine serum [12]. The stimulatory activity of bovine colostrum and bovine serum were compared (Fig. 3). Bovine colostrum at a concentration of 0.25% (vol/vol) was as active as bovine serum at a concentration of 2.5% (vol/vol). Maximum stimulation of Balb/c 3T3 cells was obtained with 1% (vol/vol) colostrum and 10% (vol/vol) serum. Therefore colostrum was about ten times as active as serum on a per volume basis in stimulating DNA synthesis in confluent Balb/c 3T3 cells. The protein concentration of bovine colostrum is about 200–250 mg/ml and that of bovine serum is about 70–100 mg/ml. Thus the specific activity of colostrum is 3–5 times greater than that of serum.

Stimulation of Cell Division by Milk

Colostrum obtained on the day of birth of a calf induced cell division in confluent quiescent Balb/c 3T3 cells as well as DNA synthesis (Fig. 4). The stimulation of cell division by the colostrum was concentration-dependent. A concentration of 0.8% (vol/

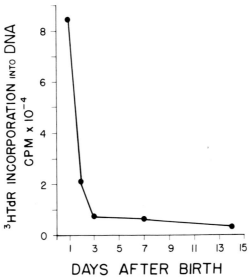

Fig. 2. Stimulation of DNA synthesis by sheep's milk obtained at various times after birth of a lamb. Milk was obtained from a sheep on the day of a lamb's birth and at regular intervals thereafter. Samples of milk at a final concentration of 1.0% (vol/vol) were added along with (^{3}H) TdR to confluent monolayers of quiescent Balb/c 3T3 cells and DNA synthesis was measured as described in Figure 1.

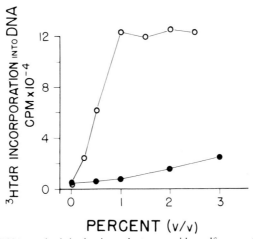

Fig. 3. Stimulation of DNA synthesis by bovine colostrum and by calf serum. Confluent monolayers of Balb/c 3T3 cells were incubated with various concentrations of bovine colostrum obtained on the day of the birth of a calf (O−O) and with various cocentrations of calf serum (●−●) along with (^{3}H) TdR. DNA synthesis was measured as described in Figure 1.

vol) milk induced an approximate 6-fold increase in cell number in a period of 6 days. By comparison, milk obtained from the same cow 10 days after birth of the calf was inactive in stimulating cell division.

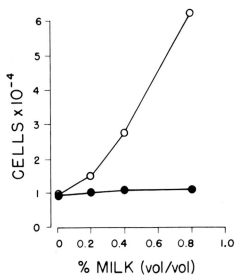

Fig. 4. Stimulation of cell division by bovine milk. Confluent monolayers of quiescent Balb/c 3T3 cells were incubated for 6 days with various concentrations of colostrum obtained on the day of the birth of a calf (O–O) and milk obtained 10 days after birth of a calf (●–●). The final concentration of milk used were 0, 0.2, 0.4, and 0.8% (vol/vol). The cells were refed on day 3 of the experiment. On day 6 of the experiment, the cells were detached from the microtiter wells by incubation with 0.1% (wt/vol) trypsin and counted in a Coulter counter.

The Proliferation of 3T3 Cells in Medium Supplemented With Milk Instead of Serum

Bovine colostrum, like serum, contains factors that stimulate DNA synthesis and cell division in Balb/c 3T3 cells. The presence of these factors suggests that Balb/c 3T3 cells may proliferate in a medium which has been supplemented with bovine colostrum instead of serum. To test this possibility, Balb/c 3T3 cells were trypsinized, plated sparsely in unsupplemented DMEM and, after attachement, were grown in DMEM supplemented with either bovine colostrum obtained on the day of birth of a calf, or in DMEM supplemented with bovine serum. The optimal concentration of bovine colostrum needed for growth of Balb/c 3T3 cells was found to be between 1.0 and 2.5% (vol/vol). At higher concentrations, the cells, while remaining viable, became less adhesive and detached from the dish. The optimal serum concentration was 10% (vol/vol). There was no growth of Balb/c 3T3 cells in DMEM supplemented with milk obtained 10 days after birth, in DMEM supplemented with bovine serum albumen (5 mg/ml), or in unsupplemented DMEM. The growth curves of Balb/c 3T3 cells grown in DMEM supplemented with 2.5% (vol/vol) colostrum, 2.5% (vol/vol) serum and 10% (vol/vol) serum are shown in Figure 5. In 10% (vol/vol) serum, there was immediate exponential growth with a generation time of about 28 hours. The cell number increased 100-fold before a maximum saturation density was obtained 8 days after plating. In 2.5% (vol/vol) serum, after a lag period of about 3 days, the cells grew with a generation time of about 28 hours, increased in number by 50-fold, and reached a maximum saturation density in 10 days which was about one half that of cells grown in 10% (vol/vol) serum. It has been shown previously that the final saturation density of Balb/c 3T3 cells is directly proportional to the amount of serum in the culture medium [13]. In 2.5% (vol/vol) colostrum, after a 3-day lag period,

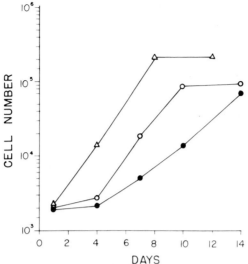

Fig. 5. The growth of Balb/c 3T3 in DMEM supplemented with either bovine colostrum or calf serum. Balb/c 3T3 cells were plated sparsely in DMEM at a density of approximately 5×10^3 cells/cm^2 and those cells that attached were grown in the appropriate medium according to the protocol described in Materials and Methods. Every third or fourth day cells in duplicate wells were trypsinized and counted while all remaining cells were refed with the approproate medium. DMEM + 10% serum (△–△); DMEM + 2.5% serum (○–○); DMEM + 2.5% bovine colostrum (●–●).

the cells proliferated, but grew more slowly than was the case in serum. The generation time in colostrum was about 38 hours and the increase in cell number was about 35-fold in 14 days. The density of Balb/c 3T3 cells in a well the day after plating is shown in Figure 6A. The density of cells after 12 days' growth in 2.5% (vol/vol) colostrum and in 10% (vol/vol) serum is shown in Figure 6B and Figure 6C, respectively.

Patterns of Cell Growth in Colostrum and in Serum

The pattern of Balb/c 3T3 cell growth in colostrum was different than in serum. Cells in serum grew uniformly throughout the dish, and eventually formed a monolayer that covered the total available surface. On the other hand, the cells in colostrum grew in clusters leaving gaps in the dish. The confluent cells in the clusters were smaller and more densely packed (Fig. 6B) than were the confluent cells grown in 10% (vol/vol) serum (Fig. 6C). After reaching a high cell density, the clusters often lost their ability to adhere to the plastic substrate, and rolled up to form aggregates which detached from the dish. Figure 7 shows a mass of aggregated cells after detachment. The lower saturation density and apparent longer generation time of Balb/c 3T3 cells grown in colostrum was due in part to the loss of cells into the medium during growth. In a few experiments when cell loss due to lack of adhesion was small, Balb/c 3T3 cells grew in colostrum with a generation time equivalent to that found in serum, approximately 28 hours.

Characterization of Bovine Milk

Initial characterization of the factors in bovine milk necessary for the growth of cells in the absence of serum indicated the following: 1) the factors are resistant to the conditions of pasteurization. Milk heated to 61°C for 2 hours and then cooled quickly

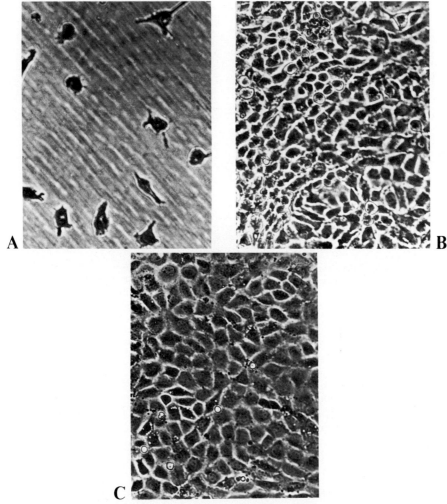

Fig. 6. Photomicrographs of Balb/c 3T3 cells grown in DMEM + colostrum or in DMEM + serum. The Balb/c 3T3 cells grown as described in Figure 5 were photographed at 1 day and 12 days after plating. A, DMEM + 2.5% colostrum 1 day after plating. B, DMEM + 2.5% colostrum 12 days after plating. C, DMEM + 10% serum 12 days after plating. The cells in 6A were photographed after fixation and staining. The cells in 6B and 6C were photographed under phase.

on ice was fully active in supporting cell growth; 2) defatted, skimmed milk is as active as whole milk, suggesting that the growth stimulating activity of bovine colostrum resides in milk protein rather than in milk fat; 3) adjustment of the pH of milk to 4.6 by addition of HC1 results in the precipitation of casein. The supernatant fraction remaining after removal of precipitated casein by centrifugation retained the ability to stimulate DNA synthesis in quiescent Balb/c 3T3 cells. This fraction, often referred to as whey, also contained the immunoglobulins and albumens of milk.

DISCUSSION

Bovine milk can be substituted for serum in order to grow sparse Balb/c 3T3 cells to confluence. However, only milk obtained within 24 hours after birth of a calf, that is the colostrum, will support cell growth. Milk obtained later in the lactation period is in-

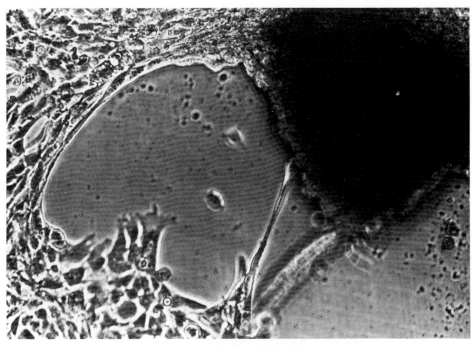

Fig. 7. Photomicrograph of an aggregate of Balb/c 3T3 cells formed during growth in colostrum. Balb/c 3T3 cells were grown in DMEM + 2.5% colostrum. After 15 days in culture, some areas of the dish were found to contain cellular aggregates. An aggregate of cells (top right) is shown coming off the dish leaving a gap in the center. The cells were photographed under phase.

active despite the presence of substantial amounts of protein, lipid, carbohydrate and other nutrients. It is not clear why the milk obtained later is inactive. Perhaps the cow synthesizes mitogenic substances just prior to, or at the time of birth. The mitogens would appear in the first milk but would be diluted out in milk obtained subsequently. Alternatively, the growth promoting factors may be inactivated, or inhibitors of growth factors may appear as the lactation period progresses.

A temporal dependence of growth factor activity is also found in sheep and human milk. The growth factor activity of milk is determined by measuring the stimulation of DNA synthesis in quiescent Balb/c 3T3 cells [1]. In both the cow and the sheep, the level of DNA synthesis that is stimulated by milk obtained 1 day and 2 days after birth is only 20% and 1% respectively of the level stimulated by milk obtained on the day of birth. The decline in growth factor activity with the passage of time is not as dramatic in human milk as it is in animal milk. Preliminary results obtained with the milk of 5 women indicates that a loss of growth factor activity of up to 80% occurs in the first 20 days after birth. However, the growth factor activity of human milk never disappears completely and is detectable even 3 months after birth of the infant.

The growth patterns of Balb/c 3T3 cells in serum and in colostrum are different. Cells at the optimal serum concentration of 10%, grow uniformly throughout the dish, become confluent and adhere very tightly to the plastic substratum. In contrast, at the optimal colostrum concentration of 2.5%, cell growth is characterized by the formation of clusters of cells and of empty gaps on the dish. The cells in the clusters are smaller and packed more densely than are cells grown in 10% serum (Fig. 6). In addition, the cells grown in colostrum are less adhesive than those grown in serum. Eventually clusters of cells roll up to form large aggregates that detach from the dish (Fig. 7). The lowered adhesion to the plastic substratum of colostrum-grown cells compared to serum-grown cells might be related to different levels of adhesion promoting factors such as fibronectin [14]. The loss of cells from the dish makes it difficult to obtain an accurate generation time for the growth of Balb/c 3T3 cells in colostrum. However, under optimal conditions the generation time of cells grown in colostrum is equivalent to that of cells grown in serum, approximately 28 hours.

Both colostrum and serum will support the growth of Balb/c 3T3 cells. However, the growth promoting factors in colostrum and in serum are probably not the same. The growth factors in serum required to make Balb/c 3T3 competent for growth are derived from platelets [6–8]. The human platelet-derived growth factors are cationic polypeptides with isoelectric points between 9.7 and 10,2 [15, 16]. In contrast, the growth factors in human and bovine milk that stimulate the growth of Balb/c 3T3 cells are anionic polypepties with isolelectric points between 4.4 and 5.0. We have found no evidence to date for the presence of cationic growth factors in milk. In addition, we have shown that the activity of the human milk growth factor is resistant to disulfide bond reduction by sulfhydryl reducing agents such as 2-mercaptoethanol and dithiothreitol [1]. These reagents inactivate the human platelet-derived growth factor irreversibly [15, 16].

The use of colostrum to supplement culture medium provides a new approach to cell culture. Previously, it has been thought that Balb/c 3T3 cells require some blood-derived fraction such as serum or a combination of platelet-poor plasma and platelet-derived growth factor for proliferation. However, it is now apparent that other sources of growth factor activity besides blood can be used for the growth of these cells. We have found that other cell types such as epithelial cells and myoblasts will proliferate in colostrum-supplemented medium. Thus, the growth of cells in colostrum may be a general phenomenon. The use of colostrum in cell culture may provide several benefits. For example, it may be possible to grow cells in colostrum that are difficult to grow in serum. In addition, serum often contains virus, hormones and other molecules which may be undesirable in certain cultures such as those used to prepare vaccines. The use of colostrum would be a feasible alternative that might minimize some of the problems that are associated with growth in serum.

ACKNOWLEDGMENTS

I would like to thank Dr. J. Kadish, Dr. B. Zetter, Dr. D Tapper, S. Smith, G. Emanuel and R. Rybach for their contributions to this study. This work was supported by grant RO1-CA21763 from the National Cancer Institute.

REFERENCES

1. Klagsbrun M: Proc Natl Acad Sci USA 75:5057, 1978.
2. Aaronson SA, Todaro GJ: Science 162:1024, 1968.
3. Holley RW, Kiernan JA: Proc Natl Acad Sci USA 60:300, 1968.
4. Dulbecco R: Nature 227:802, 1970.
5. Holley RW: Nature 258:487, 1975.
6. Kohler N, Lipton A: Exp Cell Res 87:297, 1974.
7. Pledger WJ, Stiles CD, Antoniades HN, Scher CD: Proc Natl Acad Sci USA 74:4481, 1977.
8. Vogel A, Raines E, Kariya B, Rivest J, Ross R: Proc Natl Acad Sci USA 75:2810, 1978.
9. Lowry OH, Rosebrough NJ, Farr AL, Randall RJ: J Biol Chem 193:265, 1951.

10, Jenness R: In Larson B, Smith VR (eds): "Lactation." New York: Academic Press, 1974, Vol III, pp 3–107.
11. Klagsbrun M, Langer R, Levenson R, Smith S, Lillehei C: Exp Cell Res 105:99, 1977.
12. Todaro GJ, Lazar GK, Green H: J Cell Comp Physiol 66:325, 1965.
13. Todaro GJ, Matsuya Y, Bloom S, Robbins A, Green H: In Defendi V, Stoker M (eds): "Growth Regulating Substances for Animal Cells in Culture." Philadelphia: Wistar Institute Press, 1967, pp 87–98.
14. Hynes RO, Ali IU, Destree AT, Mutner V, Perkins ME, Singer DR, Wagner DD, Smith KK: Ann NY Acad Sci 312:317, 1978.
15. Ross R, Vogel A: Cell 14:203, 1978.
16. Antoniades HN, Scher CD, Stiles CD: Proc Natl Acad Sci USA, In press, 1979.

Journal of Supramolecular Structure 11:361–370 (1979)
Tumor Cell Surfaces and Malignancy 241–250

Stimulation of Human Vascular Endothelial Cell Growth by a Platelet-Derived Growth Factor and Thrombin

Bruce R. Zetter and Harry N. Antoniades

*Department of Surgery, Children's Hospital Medical Center, and Department of
Medical Microbiology and Molecular Genetics, Harvard Medical School, Boston,
Massachusetts 02115 (B.R.Z.), and Center for Blood Research and the Department
of Nutrition, Harvard University School of Public Health, Boston, Massachusetts 02115
(H.N.A.)*

Repair of a vascular wound is mediated by migration and subsequent replication of the endothelial cells that form the inner lining of blood vessels. We
have measured the growth response of human umbilical vein endothelial cells
(HuE) to two polypeptides that are transiently produced in high concentrations at the site of a wound; the platelet-derived growth factor (PDGF) and
the protease thrombin. When 10^4 HuE cells are seeded as a dense island (2-mm
diameter) in the center of a 16-mm tissue culture well in medium containing
20% human serum derived from platelet-poor plasma (PDS), no increase in cell
number or colony size is observed. With the addition of 0.5 ng/ml partially
purified PDGF, colony size increases and the number of cells after 8 days is
4.8×10^4. When human thrombin (1 μg/ml) is added along with the PDGF, the
cell number rises to 9.2×10^4. Thrombin alone stimulates no increase in cell
number. Although partially purified PDGF stimulates endothelial cells maintained in PDS as well as those maintained in whole blood serum (WBS), pure
PDGF is active only when assayed in medium that contains WBS and is supplemented with thrombin. These results suggest the existence of a second class of
platelet-derived factors that enable HuE cells to respond to the mitogenic activity of the purified platelet mitogen and thrombin.

Key words: endothelial cells, platelet-derived growth factor, thrombin, wound healing

The endothelial cells that form the inner lining of blood vessels have an extremely
low turnover rate and rarely undergo mitosis in the normal adult vasculature in vivo [1–3].
These cells do, however, proliferate during the healing process that follows a vascular injury [4–6]. In tissue culture, endothelial cells also exhibit a stringent growth control in
which cells in a confluent monolayer fail to proliferate in response to serum growth factors unless gaps or wounds are first made in the monolayer [7–9].

Received April 25, 1979; accepted July 16, 1979.

In recent years, considerable progress has been made in identifying mitogens present in the circulation that can stimulate division of cells in culture [10–12]. Two classes of polypeptides have been identified that can be expected to be produced in high concentration at a wound site and that might be relevant to the endothelial cell proliferation that occurs in wound healing. The first class of these polypeptides is the growth factors released from platelet granules during platelet activation. Such platelet-derived growth factors have been found to induce proliferation of several different cell types including smooth muscle cells [13, 14], human and mouse fibroblasts [15–22], glial cells [23, 24], and mammary tumor cells [25]. Recently, a polypeptide growth factor derived from human platelets has been purified to homogeneity [26]. The platelet-derived growth factor (PDGF) is a heat-stable polypeptide with an isoelectric point of 9.8 and a molecular weight of approximately 13,000 as judged by analytical SDS-polyacrylamide gel electrophoresis. The properties of PDGF are identical to those of the serum-derived growth factor previously isolated from whole human serum [19].

The second polypeptide of potential interest for vascular wound healing is thrombin, a highly specific protease that is produced in high concentration at a wound site as a result of coagulation [27]. Thrombin has been found to directly stimulate cell division or to potentiate the mitogenic response of cells to other growth factors in systems as diverse as the chick embryo fibroblast [28–31], mouse splenocyte [32], mouse, rabbit, and human fibroblast [33–36], and human but not bovine endothelial cells [37, 38]. In the studies described herein, we have investigated the possibility that thrombin and platelet-derived growth factors might act *together* to simulate endothelial cell proliferation. Our results support this conclusion.

METHODS

Purification of Platelet-Derived Growth Factors

The platelet-derived growth factor (PDGF) was purified according to previously published techniques [26]. In the present report, experiments described as being performed with "partially purified" PDGF employed material prepared by heat treatment of washed human platelets followed by ion-exchange chromatography, gel filtration in 1 M acetic acid, and isoelectric focusing, whereas experiments performed with "purified" PDGF employed material that had been further fractionated using preparative SDS-polyacrylamide gel electrophoresis [26]. Using Balb/c 3T3 cells as an assay, the pure PDGF was estimated to have a specific activity of about 5×10^6 units per milligram protein. One unit is defined as the amount of PDGF capable of inducing DNA synthesis in 50% of a population of quiescent Balb/c 3T3 (clone A31) cells.

Preparation of Whole Blood Serum and Plasma-Derived Serum

Human whole blood serum (WBS) and serum derived from platelet-poor plasma (PDS) were prepared according to the method of Ross et al [22] with the omission of the final chromatography of PDS on CM-Sephadex. PDS preparations were discarded if they were found to induce proliferation when added at a concentration of 20% (v/v) to sparse cultures of Balb/c 3T3 cells.

Maintenance of Human Vascular Endothelial Cells in Tissue Culture

Primary cultures of human umbilical vein endothelial cells were isolated in the laboratory of Dr. M. Gimbrone (Harvard Medical School) according to established procedures [39]. Cultures were discarded if they contained any smooth muscle colonies as detected by morphology or by the presence of thrombogenic cells to which exogenously added platelets would adhere [40]. Cells were trypsinized and split at a ratio of 1:5 into gelatin-coated Falcon T25 tissue culture flasks. To prepare the gelatin-coated substratum, the flasks were flooded with 5 ml of 1% (w/v) Difco gelatin in calcium- and magnesium-free phosphate-buffered saline. The flasks were allowed to stand at $4°C$ over night. Just before use, the gelatin was warmed to room temperature and aspirated, and the dishes were washed twice with medium. The culture medium was HEPES-buffered medium 199 (H199, Microbiological Associates) supplemented with 25 μg/ml endothelial cell growth supplement (ECGS, Collaborative Research), 250 ng/ml fibroblast growth factor (courtesy of Dr. D. Gospodarowicz, University of California, San Francisco), and 1 μg/ml human alpha-thrombin (generously provided by Dr. J. Fenton, Albany). After ten passages, the cultures were discarded and new primary cultures isolated.

Cell Growth Assays

All growth assays were carried out in gelatin-coated Falcon 24-well culture dishes. For studies on sparse cultures, 10^4 cells were dispersed randomly into each well. For studies on outgrowth from dense cultures, 10^4 cells were seeded as a dense island in the center of each well according to the method of Folkman and Butterfield (manuscript submitted for publication). In this method, the wells are first partially filled with 0.7 ml of agar solution (1% Difco agar in medium 199 with 10% human serum or PDS) which is allowed to harden in the well. With a cork borer, a 2-mm hole is punched into the agar in the center of each 16-mm well. Then 10^4 cells are seeded into each hole in a total volume of 10 μl and allowed to settle for 10 min before the entire well is flooded with 0.5 ml H199 medium containing 20% PDS and incubated over night at $37°C$. Each well now contains a 2-mm colony of 10^4 cells still surrounded by an agar plug. When the agar plug is removed by means of a sterile curved spatula, the small, dense colony can grow out to fill the entire 16-mm well. After removal of the agar plug, the wells are refilled with 0.8 ml of fresh medium containing either PDS or WBS and the growth factor to be assayed. Fresh medium and fresh growth factors are added every 2 days until the conclusion of the experiment, at which time the cells are removed with 0.25% trypsin and counted on a Coulter Zf particle counter.

RESULTS

Platelet-Derived Growth Factors Stimulate Endothelial Cell Proliferation

When partially purified human PDGF is added to cultures of human umbilical vein endothelial cells that have been seeded as dense islands with room to outgrow onto the culture dish, cell proliferation is stimulated (Fig. 1). The amount of cell proliferation stimulated by PDGF increases as the concentration of either PDS or whole blood serum is in-

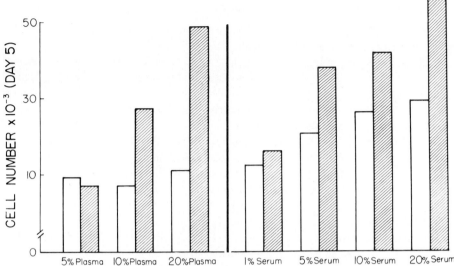

Fig. 1. Response of human umbilical vein endothelial (HuE) cells to PDGF. HuE cells (10^4) were seeded as a dense 2-mm island in the center of a 12-mm tissue culture well in medium containing 5% PDS. After 18 h, the medium was replaced with fresh medium containing either plasma (PDS, left panel) or whole blood serum (WBS, right panel) at the concentrations indicated. Shaded columns represent cultures supplemented with 5 ng/ml partially purified PDGF prepared as described in Methods.

creased. In some experiments, WBS alone stimulated a small increase in cell number. For example, in Figure 1, cell number can be seen to increase from 1×10^4 to 1.9×10^4 after 3 days in WBS alone. When experiments are carried out over longer time periods, WBS is found to stimulate proliferation only transiently over a period of 2–3 days (Fig. 2), and in many experiments no increase at all is seen in the presence of WBS alone. Stimulation by PDGF, on the other hand, was consistently observed in every experiment performed.

Thrombin Potentiates PDGF-Induced Endothelial Cell Proliferation

We have previously demonstrated that although thrombin cannot by itself stimulate endothelial cell proliferation, it can potentiate the growth response to other mitogens [33, 37, 38]. As shown in Figure 2, thrombin potentiates the PDGF-induced proliferation of human endothelial cells. When 10^4 cells were seeded as a dense island in medium H199 supplemented with 20% human WBS, only a small increase in cell number was observed within 8 days in the presence or absence of 1 μg/ml purified human thrombin. In the presence of 5 ng/ml partially purified PDGF, the cell number after 8 days was 4.2×10^4. However, with the addition of PDGF and thrombin, the cell number after 8 days was 9.2×10^4. The pattern of the growth curve indicates that although the initial growth rate is the same for cells growing in PDGF as for those growing in PDGF plus thrombin, the presence of thrombin allows the cells to continue dividing at this rate for a longer period of time. Since the experiment is terminated before the expanding colony totally fills the dish, the increase in cell number observed is not simply the result of a higher saturation density in PDGF plus thrombin.

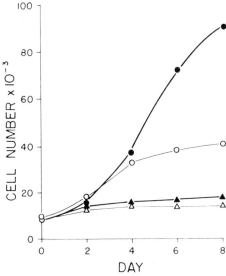

Fig. 2. Response of HuE cells to PDGF and thrombin. HuE cells were seeded as described in the legend to Figure 1, and maintained in medium containing 20% WBS alone (△—△), or supplemented with either 2 μg/ml human thrombin (▲—▲), 5 ng/ml partial purified PDGF (○—○), or 5 ng/ml partially purified PDGF plus 1 μg/ml human thrombin (●—●). Fresh medium and growth factors were added every 2 days.

Diminished Response of Sparse Endothelial Cell Cultures

The experiments described above employed a protocol in which 10^4 cells were seeded in a 2-mm circle in the center of a 16-mm well so that the increase in cell number observed represents outgrowth from the dense island of cells. In contrast, when the same number of cells are dispersed as a sparse culture in the same well, the cells display a diminished responsiveness to the mitogenic activity of PDGF and thrombin (Table I). After 6 days, the cell number in cultures supplemented with 5 ng/ml partially purified PDGF and 1 μg/ml thrombin is 62,428 if the cells were seeded as a dense island, but only 14,107 in cultures where 10,000 cells had been seeded sparsely. The sparse cells fail to proliferate even when plated in wells previously filled with an agar plug. It is of interest that as the cells proliferate in the dense culture, they tend to maintain contact with the other cells in the island rather than migrating away from the island and then dividing. This results in a circle of growing cells that increases in diameter daily.

Response to Increasing Concentration of Partially Purified PDGF

Figure 3 shows the proliferative response of human endothelial cells to increasing concentration of partially purified PDGF in the presence or absence of 1 μg/ml human thrombin. This material stimulates endothelial cell proliferation whether the experiment is carried out in PDS (left panel) or in WBS (right panel) and the response is stimulated by thrombin in both cases. It is important to note that the dose response to PDGF or to PDGF plus thrombin is described by a bell-shaped curve. High concentrations of PDGF are inhibitory to endothelial cell proliferation.

TABLE I. Effect of Cell Density on Endothelial Cell Response to PDGF and Thrombin*

	10^4 Cells sparsely seeded	10^4 Cells seeded as dense island
Control	$8,423^a \pm 162$	$9,686 \pm 274$
+ 1 μg/ml thrombin	$7,760 \pm 384$	$12,402 \pm 270$
+ 5 ng/ml PDGF	$11,212 \pm 566$	$29,566 \pm 946$
+ 5 ng/ml PDGF + 1 μg/ml thrombin	$14,107 \pm 322$	$62,428 \pm 1,242$

*All values represent the mean of three samples.
[a]Cell numbers after 6 days.

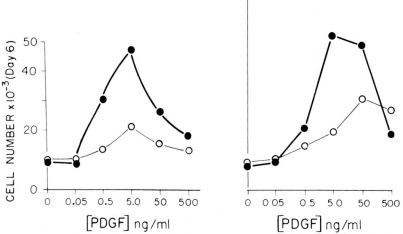

Fig. 3. Dose response of HuE cells to partially purified PDGF. HuE cells, seeded as dense islands, were treated with increasing concentrations of partially purified PDGF (o–o), or partially purified PDGF plus 1 μg/ml thrombin (•–•) in medium supplemented with either 20% PDS (left panel) or 20% WBS (right panel). Fresh medium and factors were added every 2 days.

Response to Increasing Concentration of Purified PDGF

The response of endothelial cells to the purified mitogen (Fig. 4) is surprisingly different from that of the partially purified material. Purified PDGF stimulates human endothelial cell proliferation only when assayed in whole blood serum supplemented with 1 μg/ml of pure human thrombin. It has no effect on endothelial cell proliferation when assayed in platelet-poor PDS. The maximal response is observed with 0.5 ng/ml of the pure mitogen in WBS supplemented with thrombin. Higher concentrations are again inhibitory to cell growth. These results differ from the situation with mouse fibroblasts [26], in which the pure factor has been shown to be mitogenic when assayed in medium containing platelet-poor plasma.

DISCUSSION

The mitogenic activity of factors secreted by platelets is now well documented [12–25]. Since these factors are secreted during the platelet activation that occurs during wound healing, it is not surprising that cells such as fibroblasts and vascular smooth muscle cells

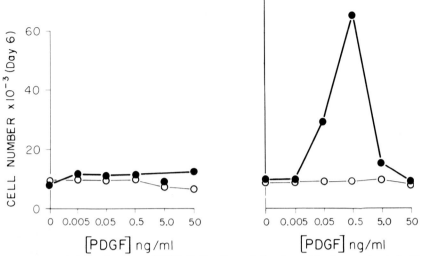

Fig. 4. Response of HuE cells to pure PDGF. HuE cells, seeded as dense islands, were treated with increasing concentrations of pure PDGF (○–○) or pure PDGF plus 1 μg/ml thrombin (●–●) in medium supplemented with either 20% human PDS (left panel) or 20% human WBS (right panel). Fresh medium and factors were added every 2 days.

that regenerate during wound healing are among those that respond to PDGF as a mitogen in vitro. The endothelial cells that line the inner surfaces of blood vessels are also required to regenerate after a vascular wound is made, yet the literature regarding the effect of PDGF on endothelial cell proliferation is not conclusive. Although endothelial cell proliferation in vitro has been reported to be stimulated by the inclusion of whole platelets in the growth medium [41, 42], platelet extracts and partially purified platelet factor preparations have not previously been found to be active [43–45].

We now report that under certain experimental conditions, human umbilical vein endothelial cells are stimulated to divide by human platelet-derived growth factors and that this stimulation is markedly enhanced by addition of the protease thrombin to the cultures. Thrombin alone is not mitogenic for these cells. Our results indicate that endothelial cells will respond to PDGF and thrombin if the cells are plated onto gelatin-coated dishes in the form of a small, dense island of cells that has room to outgrow into a comparatively large area. On the other hand, the same number of cells seeded sparsely onto the same size culture dish will not respond to the growth factors. This suggests that endothelial cell proliferation may be influenced by factors such as cell density, cell–cell contact, or other forms of metabolic cooperation that are more likely to occur when the cells are seeded as a dense island. It should be noted that in veins and arteries in vivo, endothelial cells are virtually never found at sparse densities and that the repair of a vascular wound generally involves outgrowth from a dense cell population proximal to the wound. Outgrowth from a dense culture of endothelial cells may, therefore, be more relevant to physiologic conditions than growth from sparse cultures. This type of growth control may be more relevant for endothelial cells than for other cell types that grow in different configurations in vivo.

Since whole blood serum contains material secreted by platelets during clotting, WBS contains PDGF and this may account for the initial observation made by several groups that fibroblasts and smooth-muscle cells will proliferate in WBS, but not in platelet-poor plasma or plasma-derived serum [13, 15, 18, 21]. Since our results demonstrate that PDGF can stimulate endothelial cell proliferation even when the cells are maintained in 20% WBS, we conclude that this concentration of WBS contains an amount of PDGF that is subsaturating for endothelial cell growth. It is conceivable, however, that the amount of PDGF produced locally by a platelet aggregate in vivo may be higher than that present in WBS.

An intriguing possibility raised by these results is that platelets may produce more than one factor that affects endothelial cell proliferation. The evidence for this is that pure PDGF is mitogenic for endothelial cells only when assayed in WBS. In PDS, pure PDGF is inactive. Since WBS contains other platelet-derived material in addition to subsaturating levels of PDGF, these other platelet-derived factors may be conditioning factors essential for endothelial cell proliferation. Since pure PDGF stimulates 3T3 cell proliferation in platelet-poor plasma [26], these other factors must not be essential for the growth of fibroblasts. Further evidence of possible secondary platelet-derived growth factors is provided by the observation that *partially purified* preparations of PDGF will support endothelial cell growth in PDS whereas *pure* PDGF will not. One explanation for this observation is that the partially purified PDGF contains the secondary factors necessary for endothelial cell proliferation that are absent in PDS but present in WBS. Thrombin itself is not likely to be an active component of the partially pure PDGF, since this material undergoes a heat treatment that renders thrombin inactive [26].

In summary, maximal stimulation of human endothelial cell proliferation is observed when cells are seeded as a dense island with room to outgrow on a gelatin-coated substratum and incubated in medium supplemented with human WBS, human PDGF, and human alpha-thrombin. A failure to observe an effect of PDGF on endothelial cell proliferation might, therefore, occur if the cells are seeded at sparse population density, if thrombin is omitted from the reaction mixture, or if the various components of the system (cells, serum, thrombin, and platelet factor) are not all derived from the same species.

Whereas thrombin and platelet-derived growth factors are both produced in high concentration at the site of a vascular wound, we would propose a model for wound healing in which blood clotting and cell proliferation are mechanistically interrelated (Fig. 5). The platelet adhesion and aggregation that occur during wound healing play an important role in the closure of the wound by the platelet plug. At the same time, platelet-derived growth factors are released which will stimulate proliferation of vascular endothelial cells as well as smooth-muscle cells [13]. Thrombin is formed during the coagulation cascade that occurs in response to vascular injury. Thrombin plays a crucial role in clot formation by converting soluble fibrinogen to a polymeric fibrin clot. At the same time, thrombin will potentiate the response of endothelial cells to the mitogenic properties of the platelet-derived growth factors. In a recent report, Pohjanpelto has demonstrated a synergistic effect of thrombin and platelet extract on the growth of human fibroblasts [46]. Further work will be necessary to determine if the combination of PDGF and thrombin may indeed be relevant to the proliferation of other cell types that regenerate after injury, including the fibroblasts of vascular adventitia and vascular smooth-muscle cells.

ACKNOWLEDGMENTS

We wish to thank Dr. J. Buchanan for stimulating us to undertake these studies and Dr. J. Folkman for advice and support. We also thank Dr. M. Gimbrone for providing primary cultures of human umbilical vein endothelial cells, Dr. J. Fenton for his generous

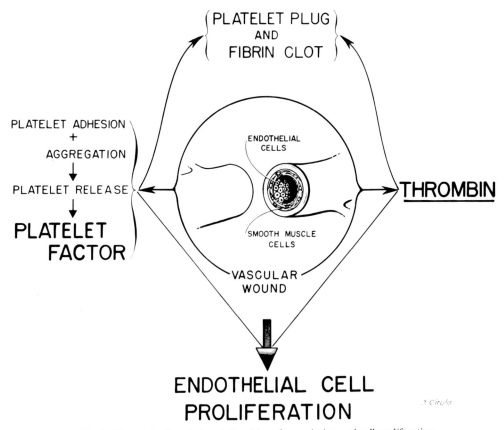

Fig. 5. Wound healing: Interrelationships of coagulation and cell proliferation.

gift of pure human alpha-thrombin, and Drs. C. Scher, C. Stiles, and M. Simons for their helpful advice, as well as M. J. Canavan for her editorial assistance. This work was supported by grant Nos. 5R01CA14019 and CA15388 from the National Institutes of Health.

REFERENCES

1. Engerman RL, Pfaffenbach D, Davis MD: Lab Invest 17:738, 1967.
2. Spaet TH, Lejnieks I: Proc Soc Exp Biol Med 125:1197, 1967.
3. Schwartz SM, Benditt EP: Circ Res 41:248, 1977.
4. Poole JCF, Sanders AG, Florey HW: J Pathol Bacteriol 75:133, 1958.
5. Cliff WJ: Trans Roy Soc London, Ser B 246:395, 1963.
6. Schoefl GI: Ann NY Acad Sci 116:789, 1964.
7. Haudenschild CC, Zahniser D, Folkman J, Klagsbrun M: Exp Cell Res 98:175, 1976.
8. Sholley MM, Gimbrone MA, Cotran RS: Lab Invest 36:18, 1977.
9. Wall RT, Harker LA, Striker GE: Lab Invest 38:523, 1978.
10. Gospodarowicz D, Moran JS: Ann Rev Biochem 45:531, 1976.
11. Ross R, Sato GH (eds): "Cold Spring Harbor Conference on Cell Proliferation." Cold Spring Harbor, New York: Cold Spring Harbor Press, 1978, vol 6.
12. Chen LB: In Tooze J (ed): "The Transformed Cell." Cold Spring Harbor, New York: Cold Spring Harbor Press (In press).
13. Ross R, Glomset J, Kariya B, Harker L: Proc Natl Acad Sci USA 71:1207, 1974.
14. Rutherford RB, Ross R: J Cell Biol 193:1094, 1976.

15. Balk SD: Proc Natl Acad Sci USA 68:271, 1971.
16. Kohler N, Lipton A: Exp Cell Res 87:297, 1974.
17. Antoniades HN, Stathakos D, Scher CD: Proc Natl Acad Sci USA 72:2603, 1975.
18. Scher CD, Stathakos D, Antoniades HN: Nature 247:279, 1974.
19. Antoniades HN, Scher CD: Proc Natl Acad Sci USA 74: 1973, 1977.
20. Pledger WJ, Stiles CD, Antoniades HN, Scher CD: Proc Natl Acad Sci USA 74:4481, 1977.
21. Vogel A, Raines E, Kariya B, Rivest MJ, Ross R: Proc Natl Acad Sci USA 75:2810, 1978.
22. Ross R, Nist C, Kariya B, Rivest MJ, Raines E, Callis J: J Cell Physiol 97:497, 1978.
23. Busch C, Wasteson A, Westermark B: Throm Res 8:493, 1976.
24. Heldin CH, Wasteson A, Westermark B: Exp Cell Res 98:175, 1977.
25. Eastment CT, Sirbasku DA: J Cell Physiol 97:17, 1978.
26. Antoniades HN, Scher CD, Stiles CD: Proc Natl Acad Sci USA 76:1809, 1979.
27. Lundblad RL, Fenton JW, Mann KG (eds): "Chemistry and Biology of Thrombin." Ann Arbor, Michigan: Ann Arbor Press, 1977.
28. Chen LB, Buchanan JM: Proc Natl Acad Sci USA 72:131, 1975.
29. Carney DH, Cunningham DD: Cell 14:811, 1978.
30. Zetter BR, Chen LB, Buchanan JM: Proc Natl Acad Sci USA 74:596, 1977.
31. Martin BM, Quigley JM: J Cell Physiol 96:155, 1978.
32. Chen LB, Teng NNH, Buchanan JM: Exp Cell Res 101:41, 1976.
33. Zetter BR, Sun TT, Chen LB, Buchanan JM: J Cell Physiol 92:233, 1977.
34. Pohjanpelto P: J Cell Physiol 91:387, 1977.
35. Pohjanpelto P: J Cell Physiol 95:189, 1978.
36. Carney DH, Glenn KC, Cunningham DD: J Cell Physiol 95:13, 1978.
37. Zetter BR, Gospodarowicz D: In Lundblad RL, Fenton JW, Mann KG (eds): "Chemistry and Biology of Thrombin." Ann Arbor, Michigan: Ann Arbor Press, 1977, p 551.
38. Gospodarowicz D, Brown KD, Birdwell CR, Zetter BR: J Cell Biol 77:774, 1978.
39. Gimbrone MA, Cotran RS, Folkman J: J Cell Biol 60:673, 1974.
40. Zetter BR, Johnson LK, Shuman MA, Gospodarowicz D: Cell 14:501, 1978.
41. Saba SR, Mason RG: Thromb Res 7:807, 1975.
42. D'Amore P, Shepro D: J Cell Physiol 92:177, 1977.
43. Thorgeirsson G, Robertson AL: Atherosclerosis 30:67, 1978.
44. Wall RT, Harker LA, Quadracci LJ, Striker GE: J Cell Physiol 96:203, 1978.
45. Davies PF, Ross R: J Cell Biol 79:663, 1978.
46. Pohjanpelto P: Thromb Res 14:353, 1979.

Journal of Supramolecular Structure 11:371–390 (1979)
Tumor Cell Surfaces and Malignancy 251–270

Isolation and Immunological Characterization of an Iron-Regulated, Transformation-Sensitive Cell Surface Protein of Normal Rat Kidney Cells

J. A. Fernandez-Pol

Radioimmunoassay Laboratory, VA Medical Center and the Department of Medicine, Division of Nuclear Medicine, St. Louis University, St. Louis, Missouri 63125

We have analyzed the surface proteins of cultured normal rat kidney (NRK) cells and virus-transformed NRK cells subjected to iron deprivation. Such a treatment specifically induces two transformation-sensitive plasma membrane-associated glycoproteins with a subunit molecular weight of 160,000 (160 K) and 130,000 (130 K) daltons in NRK cells. In these cells the 160 K glycoprotein is readily available to lactoperoxidase-mediated iodination, and the 130 K is apparently inaccessible to iodination. Major differences were revealed when iodinated membrane proteins of normal and virus-transformed cells subjected to iron deprivation were compared. In Kirsten sarcoma virus-transformed NRK cells the 160 K glycoprotein was weakly labeled. In two clones of simian virus 40-transformed NRK cells the 160 K glycoprotein was weakly labeled or not at all. The 130 K glycoprotein was inaccessible to iodination in all the virus-transformed cell lines.

The 160 K and 130 K glycoproteins were isolated from plasma membranes of NRK cells using preparative SDS gel electrophoresis. Antibodies generated against these glycoproteins stained the external surfaces of NRK cells and induced antigen redistribution. Evidence presented suggests that 160 K and 130 K are plasma membrane-associated procollagen molecules. A possible interaction of these proteins with transferrin is also described. The data suggest that these proteins may have an important role in the sequence of events leading to transformation

Key words: viral transformation, iron starvation, membrane proteins, procollagen

Iron has been previously implicated in the control of cell growth in cultured cells [1–4]. Though its main effects have been determined, the molecular aspects of the suggested control function remains undefined. This element is important in a number of metabolic processes. It is essential in DNA synthesis as a cofactor of the enzyme ribonucleotide reductase. It is also required in collagen synthesis at the level of proline and

Abbreviations: NRK, normal rat kidney; SV, simian virus 40; K, Kirsten sarcoma virus; DME, Dulbecco-Vogts modified Eagle's medium; PAGE, polyacrylamide gel electrophoresis; SDS, sodium dodecyl sulfate; PMSF, phenyl methylsulfonylfluoride; PBS, phosphate-buffered saline.

Received March 18, 1979; accepted July 2, 1979.

lysine hydroxylation. Experimental evidence that iron deprivation affects both of these processes in cultured cells has been presented [5, 6].

We have previously demonstrated that NRK cells express two membrane-associated glycoproteins in response to iron deprivation [7]. These membrane glycoproteins are of interest because their synthesis can be experimentally regulated by the cellular concentration of iron and because they can exist associated with the plasma membrane in two molecular forms, partially glycosylated and fully glycosylated [7]. These two proteins are decreased when cells are transformed by oncogenic viruses, and their decrease might correlate with the development of the transformed phenotype [7].

In this study, we have labeled external cell proteins by a lactoperoxidase-catalyzed iodination procedure to explore further the nature and location of the membrane glycoproteins with subunit molecular weight 160 K and 130 K induced by iron depletion. Evidence presented here suggests that 160 K and 130 K are procollagen molecules that are associated with the plasma membrane. Isolation, immunological characterization, and preliminary data that suggest a possible interaction of these proteins with transferrin are also presented.

METHODS

Cell Culture

Cells were grown in Dulbecco-Vogt modified Eagle's medium containing 10% (vol/vol) calf serum (Colorado Serum Company) as previously described [8]. NRK-B Cl 8, K-NRK Cl 32, SV-NRK P8C12T7, and SV-NRK-B Cl 2 were kindly supplied by Dr. R. Ting (Biotech Research, Inc.). Unless otherwise indicated subconfluent cells were used in this study.

It has been shown that desferrioxamine, a highly specific iron-chelating agent, selectively deprives iron from the cells [1, 7]. Thus to investigate the effects of iron deprivation on membrane protein patterns in normal and transformed cells, cultures were grown with or without desferrioxamine (325–396 μg/ml), and the membranes were analyzed after set incubation periods.

Cell Surface Labeling

Monolayer cultures were surface labeled as described by Hynes [9]. The growth medium was removed and the cells were washed three times with PBS (pH 7.2). The cells in a 100-mm dish were labeled in 2 ml PBS containing glucose (5 mM), lactoperoxidase (40 μg) (Calbiochem), glucose oxidase (0.2 U) (Calbiochem or Worthington), and 100 μCi carrier-free Na-^{125}I (New England Nuclear). After 10 min incubation at room temperature, labeling was terminated by addition of PBI (phosphate-buffered saline in which NaCl was replaced by NaI). The PBI contained 2 mM PMSF to inhibit proteases. The medium was removed and the cells were washed twice with PBS containing 2 mM PMSF. The cells were then scraped from the dish into Earle's BSS containing 10% sucrose, and the membranes were isolated as described below. In some experiments, the cells were labeled in suspension after removal from the dishes by scraping. All washings and fractionation buffers contained 2 mM PMSF.

Protease Treatment of the Cells

Subconfluent cells were treated as described in [10]. Collagenase treatment of the cells was carried out only in the presence of 2 mM N-ethylmaleimide and 1 mM PMSF. Purified collagenase and trypsin were obtained from Worthington Biochemical Corporation.

Metabolic Labeling of Cells

The cultures were metabolically labeled with radioactive precursors, [14C]-glucosamine, [14C]-galactose, [14C]-glucose, [14C]-mannose, and [14C]-proline by culturing in complete DME medium. Pulse labeling of the cells with [35S] methionine (644-1270 μCi/mmole) was performed as indicated elsewhere [7].

Preparation of Transferrin

Purified human (Boheringer) or bovine (Calbiochem) transferrin were stored at 4°C in the iron-free form. The transferrins were converted to the iron-saturated form and titrated [11] by addition of $Fe(ClO_4)_2$ in the presence of 20 mM $NaHCO_3$ and 1 mM nitrilotriacetate (NTA). After iron saturation of transferrin, possible contaminating NTA was removed by Sephadex G-25 column chromatography. Transferrin peak (void volume) was lyophilized and purity of the preparation (greater than 98%) was determined by SDS electrophoresis.

Surface Labeling of Cells in the Presence of Transferrin

After 14 h of growth in the presence or absence of desferrioxamine (325–350 μg/ml), 90% iron-saturated differric transferrin in 200 μl iron-free DME medium (Custom made, Microbiological Associates) containing 0.1% bovine serum albumin (Chelex-100 treated, Bio Rad; Nutritional Biochemicals) was added to the cultures. Final transferrin concentration in growth media was 20 μM. The cells were incubated in the tissue culture incubator for 30 min. This incubation period was chosen because preliminary experiments showed maximal cellular binding of ^{125}I transferrin at this time (unpublished). A set of control cultures were identically treated, but transferrin was omitted from the preparation. Then the cells were surface labeled by the lactoperoxidase iodination procedure, and the plasma cell membranes were analyzed by SDS-PAGE.

Membrane Isolation and Analysis of Membrane Proteins by Polyacrylamide Gel Electrophoresis

The plasma membranes were isolated by the method of Brunette and Till [12] as modified by Stone et al [13]. SDS gel electrophoresis was performed following the basic procedure of Laemmli [14]. When radioactive proteins were analyzed, autoradiographs were obtained by exposing dried gels to Kodak RP Royal "X-Omat" film. The amount of protein or radioactivity in each band was estimated by measuring the areas under the peaks by a Digitizer (Elographic, Tennessee). Protein standard for molecular weight estimation were myosin (200 K), phosphorylase B (94 K), β-galactosidase (130 K), bovine serum albumin (68 K) and ovalbumin (43 K) (Bio Rad Laboratories).

Isolation of 160 K and 130 K from NRK Cells

The glycoproteins were isolated and partially purifed using plasma membranes from confluent NRK-B cells grown in 102 dishes 150 mm in diameter. After 72 h of growth in normal medium the cells were treated with 390 μg/ml of desferrioxamine for 11 h. Then the cells were collected and the plasma membranes were isolated. After boiling for 3 min and reduction with dithiothreitol (0.1 M), the preparations were electrophoresed on 5% to 12% exponential gradient preparative slab gels. Two narrow slices were cut near the edges of the fixed (50% trichloroacetic acid) gels and stained with Coommassie blue to locate the 160 K and 130 K glycoproteins. These glycoproteins were the major stained proteins in that molecular weight region. The stained strips were aligned with the fixed gels, and the protein bands were cut from the gels. The gel was triturated at 0–4°C with a Dounce homogenizer, and the protein was eluted with three extractions at 37°C in 4 ml of 5 mM ammonium bicarbonate, 0.05% SDS, and 0.5 mM PMSF. This procedure yielded approximately 1,300 μg of 160 K and 1,200 μg of 130 K with a purity greater than 95% as estimated by reelectrophoresis and Coomassie blue staining. The protein preparations were lyophilized and resuspended in 1.5 ml PBS.

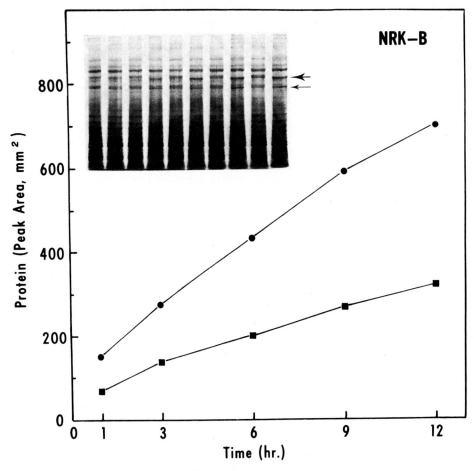

Fig. 1A. Selective effects of iron deprivation on plasma membrane profiles of NRK cells. Cells were plated at 1×10^6 per 100-mm dish. Forty-eight hours later, the medium was replaced. Dishes were divided into two sets: One set contained normal medium (control); the other set contained added desferrioxamine (350 μg/ml). At regular intervals after the initiation of the treatment, cells were collected and plasma membrane proteins were analyzed in exponential 5% to 12% acrylamide gels; polypeptide membranes that contained 100 μg of protein was applied to each lane. Protein bands were stained with Coomassie brilliant blue and were quantitated with an electronic planimeter and expressed as peak area. Inset: Duplicate lines correspond to control and desferrioxamine treated cells for each of the indicated times. Large and small arrows indicate 160 K and 130 K, respectively. Symbols: ●, 160 K; ■, 130 K.

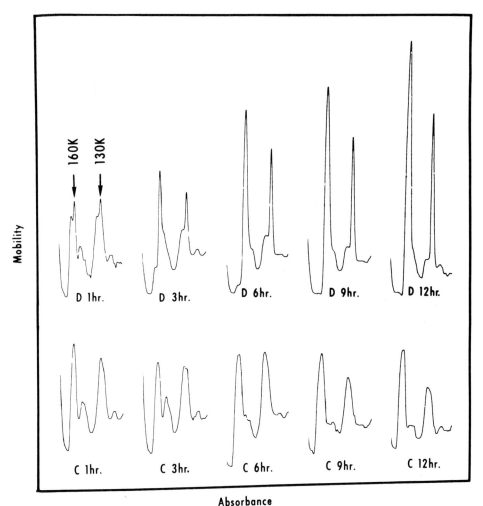

Absorbance

Fig. 1B. Selective effects of iron deprivation on plasma membrane protein profiles of NRK cells (continued). Densitometric scans of Coomassie blue stained gels of the regions of interest of control [C] and desferrioxamine treated cells [D] are shown.

Production of Anti 160 K and 130 K Antiserum

Rabbits were immunized three times at 2-week intervals intradermally at multiple sites with 80 μg of the protein preparations in 0.5 ml of PBS emulsified with 1 ml of Freund's complete (first injection) or incomplete (last two injections) adjuvant. Seven days after the last injection the rabbits were bled. Gamma globulins were obtained from the serum by three precipitations with 40% ammonium sulfate at 4°C. The pellet was dissolved in Ca^{++}, Mg^{++}-free PBS and was dialyzed extensively against the same buffer. Dialysis was stopped when dialysate was negative for sulfates [15].

Immunoreactivity in Polyacrylamide Gels

The membrane proteins were separated by SDS-PAGE as indicated above. The reactivity of the antiserum with membrane proteins was determined as described elsewhere [16].

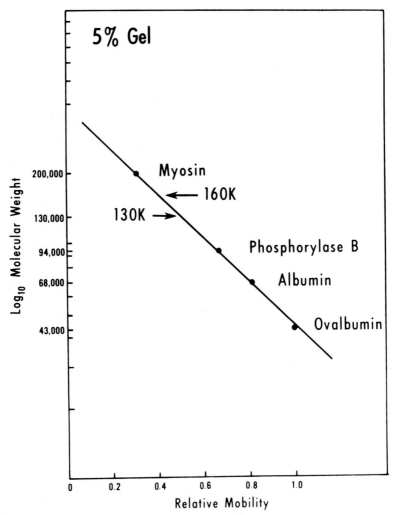

Fig. 1C. Selective effects of iron deprivation on plasma membrane protein profiles of NRK cells (continued). Molecular weight versus mobility plot of standard proteins separated in 5% SDS polyacrylamide gels. Positions of 160 K and 130 K are indicated.

Immunofluroscense Localization

NRK cells ($1-4 \times 10^4$ cells) were grown on coverslips (ethanol sterilized) in 35 mm culture dishes for 36 to 72 h. Then, new media with or without desferrioxamine (350 μg/ml) were added. After 3 h of incubation the cells were washed twice with PBS at 37°C and fixed in PBS containing 4% formaldehyde and 5% (wt vol) sucrose at room temperature for 30 min [17]. The cultures were then rinsed 4 times with PBS. A set of cultures was used without further treatment while another set was treated with acetone to permit intracellular staining [18]. After incubation of the cells with the antisera (1:50 dilution in 1 ml) for 60 min, the cells were rinsed with PBS and they were exposed to the IgG fraction of goat anti-rabbit IgG coupled to fluorescein (Miles Laboratories) for 60 min. After rinsing with PBS the cells were mounted in phosphate-buffered glycerol. Cells were examined with a Zeiss microscope equipped with fluorescence optics. For studies of antigen distribution, cultured cells were exposed to gamma globulin fractions (1 mg/ml) added to the culture medium. The cells were incubated for 1-3 h at 37°C, rinsed with PBS, fixed, and stained as described above.

Electron Microscopy

After incubation of the glycoproteins and/or transferrin in PBS containing 1 mM $CaCl_2$ and $MgCl_2$ at $37°C$ for 15 min, supernatant samples and pellets collected by centrifugation were prepared for electron microscopy as indicated elsewhere [19]. After negative staining with 1% uranyl acetate, the specimens were examined in a Philips 200 transmission electron microscope.

Other Procedures

Aliquots of the solubilized plasma membrane preparation were used for determination of protein [20], total radioactivity, and trichloroacetic acid-precipitable radioactivity. Metal-free water was used in the preparation of all transferrin solutions. Cells were counted with a Coulter counter. Protein was measured by the method of Lowry et al [21] or Bio Rad. Ouchterlony analyses were performed as indicated elsewhere [15]. Areas were estimated by a standard computer program developed at this laboratory. Unless otherwise noted, all the measurements were carried out in triplicate, and the results reported here were reproduced in four separate experiments each.

RESULTS

Relationship of the 163 K and 160 K Glycoproteins

We have evaluated this relationship by comparison of plasma membrane protein patterns of NRK cells grown in the presence or absence of desferrioxamine (Figs. 1A and B). The 5% to 12% exponential gel shown in Figure 1 demonstrates that the mobility of 163 K of NRK cells starved for iron is altered to a lower apparent molecular weight, 160 K. In the case of 132 K and 130 K a similar phenomenon was observed. Thus, when the cells were grown under conditions of iron deprivation, 163 K and 132 K ceased to be synthesized, and 160 K and 130 K were synthesized in their place. Further details of the relationship between iron depletion and kinetics of accumulation of 160 K and 130 K will be published elsewhere [7].

The 160 K and 130 K molecular weights used in the description of our data correspond to the lowest apparent molecular weight determined in a 5% gel (Fig. 1C) in cells treated with desferrioxamine for 24 h. The apparent molecular weight of the iron-regulated proteins after 6 h of treatment was about 170 K and 140 K, as determined in a 5% to 12% exponential acrylamide gel.

These glycoproteins were efficiently labeled with [14C]-glucosamine and to a much lower specific activity with radioactive [14C]-glucose, [14C]-galactose, and [14C]-mannose. They were also metabolically labeled with [35S] methionine and [14C]-proline. The amount of glycosylation particularly with [14C]-galactose appeared to be dependent on the presence or absence of iron. Further details of these results are reported elsewhere [7].

Characterization of 160 K and 130 K Glycoproteins Induced by Iron Deprivation in NRK Cells

Cell surface proteins were iodinated by the lactoperoxidase-catalyzed iodination procedure which apparently labels cell surface proteins but not internal proteins [9]. Iodination of the surface of NRK cells subjected to iron deprivation labeled a protein of apparent molecular weight of 160 K daltons (Fig. 2). In control cells, 160 K was absent, and a relatively broad band of 163 K was found in its place. Thus, iron deprivation resulted in the expression of a cell surface protein, 160 K. No significant changes in

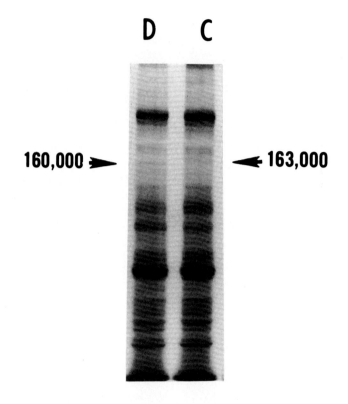

Fig. 2. Effect of iron starvation on surface proteins of plasma membrane of NRK cells. Cells were labeled in monolayer by the glucose oxidase lactoperoxidase-catalyzed iodination procedure [9]. The plasma membranes were isolated and analyzed in exponential 5% to 12% acrylamide gels. Plasma membrane samples applied to each lane contained equal quantities of cell membrane protein (100 μg). D. Iodination pattern of NRK cells grown in the presence of desferrioxamine. Cells were plated at 1×10^6 cells per 100-mm dish. Forty-eight hours later, new medium containing desferrioxamine (325 μg/ml) was added. Following 14 h of treatment, cells were iodinated. In this autoradiogram, a sharp protein band with a molecular weight of 160,000, is iodinated. C. Control, untreated cells, shows 163 K glycoprotein.

mobility were seen in other membrane-associated proteins of cells subjected to iron deprivation, though decreases in the labeling of some proteins were observed (Fig. 2). To ascertain whether 160 K was firmly bound to the cell membranes or loosely attached, the cells were incubated and washed extensively with PBS at 37°C. After this procedure, the ^{125}I-labeled 160 K was not decreased. Thus, 160 K appears to be firmly associated with the plasma membrane. The intensity of the iodinated band of 160 K daltons was enriched in plasma membrane preparations. The 160 K glycoprotein was iodinated in isolated membrane preparations. No evidence was found that the 130 K glycoprotein detected by Coomassie blue staining (Fig. 1) or [^{35}S] methionine labeling comigrates with a 130 K lactoperoxidase-labeled glycoprotein. The 130 K glycoprotein could not be significantly iodinated in isolated cell membranes. These data suggest that 130 K glycoprotein induced by iron deprivation is not accessible to iodinization. However, the possibility that iodination may have altered the mobility of 130 K detected by metabolic labeling to a protein of slightly lower molecular weight has not been ruled out.

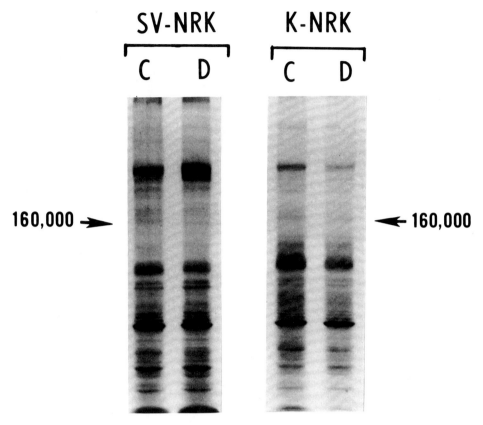

Fig. 3. Iodination of cell surface proteins of SV-NRK-B C12 and K-NRK cells subjected to iron deprivation. Cells were treated as indicated in Figure 2. C. Control, untreated cells; D. desferrioxamine treated cells.

Further experiments suggested that 160 K protein is exposed at the outer cell surface since trypsinization of the cells removed most of the label associated with 160 K. The 160 K glycoprotein, metabolically labeled with [^{35}S] methionine, was readily degraded by treatment with trypsin (1 μg/ml of trypsin at 37°C for 3 h). However, tryptic digestion with a decreased quantity of trypsin (0.1 μg/ml) did not remove all the label associated with 160 K. The 130 K glycoprotein could be partially removed by 1 μg/ml of trypsin. Treatment of the cell surface with highly purified collagenase (10 units/ml for 3 hr at 37°C) effectively removed 160 K and 130 K. The 160 K and 130 K bands comigrated with authentic proline-labeled procollagen. These data suggest that 160 K and 130 K are related to the procollagen.

Surface Labeling of Transformed Cells Subjected to Iron Deprivation

We have examined transformed cell lines for differences in the distribution of cell surface proteins after 12 h or 16 h of iron deprivation. Figure 3 shows that the plasma membrane polypeptide patterns of K-NRK cells grown in the presence or absence of desferrioxamine were not significantly different, with the exception of one band of apparent molecular weight close to 160 K daltons. This band is weakly labeled in com-

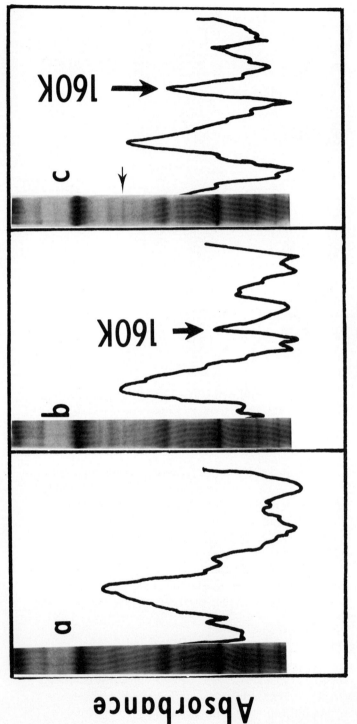

Mobility

Fig. 4. Iodination of cell surface proteins of NRK cells subjected to iron deprivation after exposure to added transferrin. Cells were plated at 1×10^6 per 100-mm dish. Forty-eight hours later, the medium was removed and new medium with or without desferrioxamine (325 μg/ml) was added. After 14 h, transferrin was added to the cultures (final concentration, 20 μM) and cultures were incubated at 37°C for 30 min. A set of control cultures were identically treated but without transferrin. Then the cells were iodinated by the lactoperoxidase procedure. Plasma membranes were prepared from 5 to 8 dishes for each condition, normalized for equal protein (100 μg), and analyzed by SDS electrophoresis in 5% to 12% exponential acrylamide gels. Autoradiograms of (a) control, untreated cells, (b) desferrioxamine-treated cells plus 20 μM transferrin, (c) desferrioxamine treated cells, no additions. Note that the labeled protein at 160,000 mol wt is present in both (b) and (c) preparations but the relative activity is different. Prior exposure of the cells to transferrin decreases the specific activity of the 160 K species. Densitometric scans of autoradiogram of the regions of interest are shown.

parison to 160 K in NRK cells (Fig. 2). Thus, 160 K is a surface protein in K-NRK cells but apparently is less accessible to iodination, or the quantities on the cell surface are reduced in comparison to the untransformed counterpart. As shown in Figure 3, when SV-NRK-B C12 cell cultures were grown in the presence of desferrioxamine, 160 K showed weak labeling. In another clone of SV-NRK cells, 160 K could not be detected (not shown). The difference between these two clones in membrane polypeptide distribution and response to iron deprivation indicates clonal variation. These findings are in accordance with results obtained by metabolic labeling of transformed cells [7]. 130 K could not be detected in any transformed cell line. The data suggest that 160 K and 163 K are surface proteins whose surface expression is modified by iron and is altered by viral oncogenic transformation.

Possible Interaction of 160 K with Transferrin in Cultured NRK Cells

Intact NRK cells, grown in the presence or absence of desferrioxamine, were loaded with exogenous differic transferrin prior to the lactoperioxidase iodination procedure. In the autoradiographs, 163 K and 160 K were evident in control and treated cells, respectively (Fig. 4). Note that the labeled 160 K band is very sharp and easily seen in the autoradiographs of cells unexposed to exogenously added transferrin (Fig. 4c). In contrast, this component is significantly reduced in cells preloaded with transferrin (Fig. 4b). Although in our hands, lactoperoxidase iodination is a semiquantitative procedure, we decided to estimate the loss of label in the surface polypeptide bands of cells exposed to transferrin prior to iodination. As can be observed in Figure 4b, a significant decrease of about 55% in the iodination of the 160 K band after prior incubation with transferrin was detected.

TABLE I. Estimated Inhibition of Lactoperoxidase Iodination of 160 K and 163 K Proteins by Transferrin in NRK Cells

Protein	% Inhibition	
	Human transferrin	Bovine transferrin
160 K (induced)	62	79
163 K (control)	45	73

Cells were plated at 1×10^6 per 100-mm dish. Forty-eight hours later, the medium was removed and new medium with or without desferrioxamine (325 µg/ml) was added. After 14 h, transferrin was added to the cultures (final concentration, 20 µM) and cultures were incubated at 37°C for 30 min. A set of control cultures was identically treated but without transferrin. Then the cells were iodinated by the lactoperoxidase procedure. Plasma membranes were prepared from 5 to 8 dishes for each condition, normalized for equal protein, and analyzed by SDS electrophoresis in 5% to 12% acrylamide gradient. Autoradiograph bands were quantitated and expressed as peak area. The percent inhibition was calculated by dividing the decrease in area of iron-regulated proteins in transferrin-treated cultures by the area of iron-regulated proteins in cells unexposed to transferrin. The data are expressed as an average of three experiments and, for bovine transferrin, as an average of two experiments. For details, see text.

The loss of radioactivity, however, was never complete. No other major differences were noted. Experiments with bovine transferrin showed that this protein also partially prevented the labeling of 163 K and 160 K of NRK cells (Table I). Thus, human or bovine transferrin, with certain selectivity, partially inhibits the iodination of these bands. The experiments described above were also performed with K-NRK and SV-NRK cells to ascertain whether differences in the pattern of 160 K labeling or other membrane proteins would be found in these cells. There was a significant difference in the labeling of 160 K in K-NRK cells with or without prior incubation with transferrin in three separate experiments (65% inhibition). Other membrane proteins remained unchanged. No significant differences were observed between protein bands of SV-NRK cells exposed or unexposed to transferrin prior to iodination. No significant changes in other membrane proteins were found when the membrane proteins of transformed cells were analyzed in exponential 7% to 16% gels.

Isolation of 160 K and 130 K Glycoproteins from NRK Cells

The partial purification procedure of 160 K and 130 K glycoproteins involved plasma membrane preparation followed by preparative SDS-PAGE. We estimated by Coomassie blue staining that 160 K and 130 K represent about 3% and 1%, respectively, of total proteins of the membrane preparation. One major band was present upon re-electrophoresis on analytical SDS-PAGE in each of the cases. The isolated glycoproteins migrated within the same molecular weight as the original proteins and showed minimal ($< 2\%$) or undetectable contamination by other cell proteins of different molecular weights, as determined by Coomassie blue staining of SDS-PAGE. The isolated 160 K and 130 K proteins apparently correspond to proteins originally identified by metabolic labeling, since the 160 K and 130 K membrane proteins detected by Coomassie blue staining and the 160 K and 130 K proteins metabolically labeled comigrate [7]. Thus, because the 160 K and 130 K proteins are well separated by SDS-PAGE from other proteins, the isolation procedure apparently afforded a relatively homogenous preparation of the glycoproteins with minimal contamination by other proteins of different molecular weight. These preparations appeared to be of suffcient purity to justify further physical-chemical and immunological characterization.

Possible Interaction of 160 K With Transferrin as Revealed by Electron Microscopy

An interaction of possible biological relevance between 160 K and transferrin was suggested by the lactoperoxidase study. These observations prompted us to investigate the possible interaction of 160 K, 130 K, and transferrin under a variety of experimental conditions by transmission electron microscopy after negative staining. When 160 K (0.03 μg/ul), 130 K (0.03 μg/ul), or transferrin (0.1 μg/ul) (< 5 or 90% iron-saturated) were incubated at 37°C in PBS containing 1 mM Ca^{++} and Mg^{++}, a random distribution of protein particles was observed (not shown). In a few instances molecular aggregates were seen in 160 K preparations, which did not show a tendency to be organized. When 160 K was incubated with 5% iron-saturated transferrin striated aggregates were visible in the preparations (Fig. 5a). The incubation of 160 K with 90% iron-saturated transferrin was found to produce extensive aggregates showing striations, but apparently to a lower extent (not shown). The incubation of 160 K, 130 K, and transferrin resulted in the formation of globular protein aggregates that appear to coprecipitate (or copolymerize) with filaments in certain organized fashion (Fig. 5b). In none of the control conditions, which consisted in all other possible combinations of 160 K, 130 K, and transferrin were these structures observed.

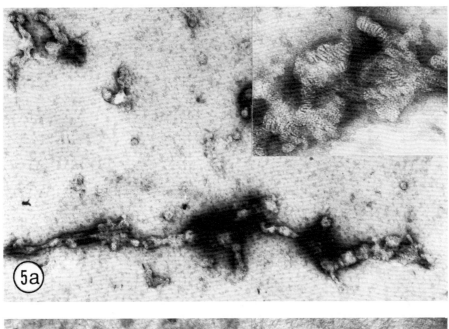

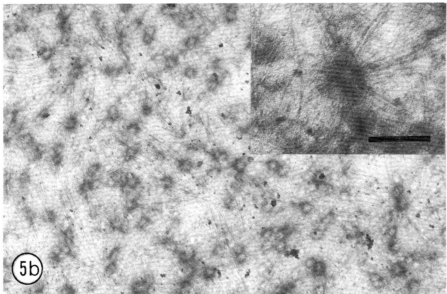

Fig. 5. Electron micrographs of 160 K, 130 K, and transferrin. The 160 K glycoprotein from NRK cells can assume different supramolecular structures depending on the presence or absence of transferrin and/or 130 K glycoprotein. The proteins were incubated in PBS (pH 7.4) containing 1 mM $CaCl_2$ and $MgCl_2$ at 37°C for 30 min. The supernatant of the reaction was applied to carbon-coated specimen grids and negatively stained with 1% uranyl acetate as described by Huxley [19]. Preparations were observed in a Philips 200 transmission electron microscope. (a) Irregulary striated aggregates are the most prevalent structure observed in the preparations of 160 K and 5% iron-saturated transferrin (magnification, × 54,538). Inset: Corresponds to right lower field (magnification, × 176,800). (b) Reticular networks and protein aggregates are observed in preparations of 160 K, 130 K, and 5% iron-saturated transferrin (magnification, × 55,566). Inset: Shows detail of a structure in close association with filaments (magnification, × 176,800), bar measures 1,000 Å.

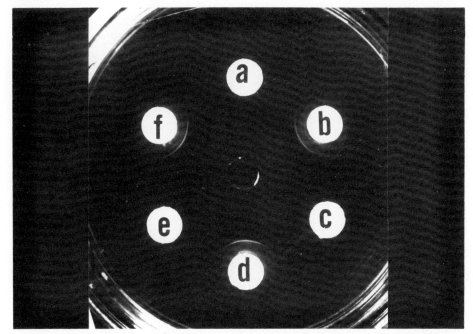

Fig. 6. Immunodiffusion of isolated 130 K glycoprotein in center well against preimmune (diluted 1:12) (wells a, c, and e) and immune (diluted 1:1,000) (wells b, d, and f) from a rabbit injected three times with 130 K protein as described in Methods.

Immunological Specificity of the Antiserum to the 160 K Glycoprotein

The antiserum to the 160 K glycoprotein reacted with 160 K, producing a single sharp precipitin band as determined by Ouchterlony analysis. The anti-160 K antibody did not react with 130 K or with a plasma membrane preparation obtained identically as described above but from which 160 K and 130 K were omitted. The reaction of 160 K with anti-160 K antisera apparently was specific since preimmune serum did not significantly react with 160 K. Additional evidence of specificity of anti-160 K antisera was provided by the method of Olden and Yamada [16]. With this procedure, the antiserum to the 160 K glycoprotein reacted only with one protein in an SDS-PAGE of total membrane proteins, as estimated by a significant densitometric increase (50% over controls), which comigrates with the 160 K glycoprotein. The reaction apparently was specific, since nonimmune sera did not react with any proteins in control gels. Anti-130 K

Fig. 7. A. Immunological localization of 160 K in NRK cells. Cells were plated on coverslips at 2×10^4 per 35-mm dish. Forty-eight hours later, the medium was replaced. Cells were grown for 3 h in the presence of 350 μg/ml desferrioxamine. The cells were then fixed in formaldehyde and stained by indirect immunofluorescence with anti-160 K antibody (diluted 1:50) as described in Methods. Cells photographed with the microscope focused on lower surfaces. (B, C, D, E). Antibody induced redistribution of 160 K in NRK cells. Density of plating was 1×10^4 (B, C), 4×10^4 (D), and 2×10^4 (E, F) cells per 35-mm dish. Forty-eight hours later the medium was replaced and the cells were cultured in the presence of 350 μg/ml desferrioxamine for 3 h. The cells were then cultures for 1 h (B), 2 h (C, D, E), or 3 h (F) with 1 mg/ml anti-160 K globulin, then fixed and stained. (B, D, E): NRK cells photographed with the microscope focused on mid-portions of the cells; (C, F): Microscope focused on upper surfaces of cells (fluorescence micrographs; magnification, $\times$ 500).

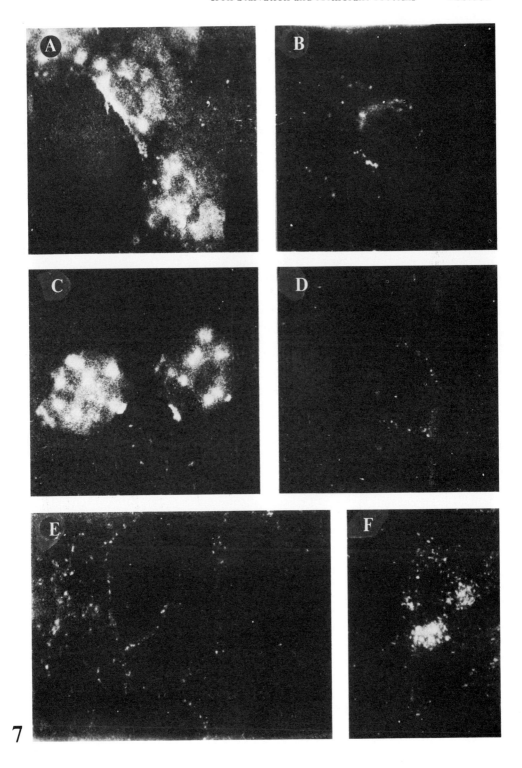

7

reacted with 130 K and cross-reacted with 160 K, indicating that 130 K and 160 K glyco-proteins share common antigenic determinants. The reaction of 130 K with anti-130 K antibodies appeared to be specific, since preimmune serum did not significantly react with 130 K (Fig. 6). The 130 K antiserum did not significantly react with other proteins of the membrane preparations. The antiserum to 130 K is therefore not entirely specific, where-as the anti-160 K is directed against the 160 K cell surface glycoprotein.

Immunofluorescence Localization and Antigen Redistribution

NRK cells were fixed, exposed to antibody against 160 K, and stained using in-direct immunofluorescence. Figure 7A shows that 160 K was found on the cell surface of subconfluent NRK cells in a diffuse pattern. Focal points of increased staining appeared to correspond to cell attachment areas and blebs. By cell density analysis we were able to demonstrate spatial transitions in the nature of 160 K antigen since con-fluent cells showed staining located preferentially in the intercellular spaces (not shown). Immunofluorescence data showed surface staining in both control and treated cells, in-dicating either that 160 K is present in controls or, more likely, that anti-160 K cross-reacts with 163 K. When the interior of NRK cells was rendered accessible to the anti-body by altering the plasma membrane with acetone, the antibody stained both the cell surface and the perinuclear cytoplasm of subconfluent cells (not shown). In confluent cells, however, the cell surface but not the cytoplasm was stained. The 160 K glycoprotein of NRK cells could be redistributed by exposure of cultured cells to the anti-160 K anti-body (Fig. 7B). In subconfluent cultures of NRK cells rearrangements of surface antigens occurred after incubation for 1–3 h in the presence of anti-160K added to the culture medium (Fig. 7C). The 160 K antigen concentration and spatial distribution appeared to be dependent upon cell density, since confluent cells showed significant staining and antigen redistribution in peripheral areas of the cell (Figs. 7D and E). The apparent in-tensity or frequency of staining of the cell surfaces of iron-deprived and control cells was compared. The cell surface fluorescence of the desferrioxamine-treated cells appeared to be increased in comparison to untreated cells (not shown). The difference in the staining of the two types of conditions was consistent and evident both in dorsal and equatorial sections of the cell surface. Areas of concentration of antibody were seen in about 30% of the cells after 3 h of incubation with anti-160 K antiserum (Fig. 7F). Redistribution of antigens with nonimmune rabbit gamma globulins was negative. These antibody-induced redistributions indicate that the 160 K glycoprotein is exposed at the cell surface and is mobile in the plane of the membrane. Similar results were obtained with antiserum against 130 K (data not shown). Since the anti-130 K antiserum cross-reacts with 160 K glycoprotein, these results with 130 K are difficult to interpret. Thus, further work will be necessary to define more precisely the nature of the association of 130 K to cell mem-branes. Results of these experiments suggest that the 160 K or a related antigen is present in controls, that antigen concentration is related to cell density, and that iron depletion appeared to significantly alter the antigen abundance.

DISCUSSION

In the present study we have shown that cultured cells express different surface protein patterns as a result of iron deprivation. Under such conditions an exterior plasma membrane-associated protein, 160 K of NRK cells, was detected in small concentrations or not at all on virus-transformed derivatives. Additionally, the data suggest that the ex-pression of 160 K to the cell exterior may be experimentally regulated by intracellular iron concentrations. Because lactoperoxidase-catalyzed iodination involves the possibility of cell penetration by [125]I [22], the possibility arose that the results observed with 160 K might be artifactual. That this was not the case was suggested by the facts that antibodies against 160 K localized on the cell surface, that the protein is enriched in membrane preparations, and that it is sensitive to trypsinization. The 130 K polypeptide was apparently not accessible to iodination in both untransformed and transformed cells. This suggests that it is either not located at the surface or contains no iodinizable groups, or its configuration is such that the residues are not available to iodination. Experiments with virus-transformed cells suggested that changes in iodinization of 160 K manifested by absent or weak iodination may be related to transformation. The loss or decrease concentrations of a number of membrane proteins have been noted before and may be a direct result of the expression of viral genetic information [23].

Treatment of the cell surface with purified collagenase removed 160 K and 130 K, suggesting that these molecules are related to procollagen. Experimental work has established a critical role for iron in the synthesis of collagen [6, 24]. The biosynthesis of collagen occurs in a series of sequential steps [24–26]. Iron has been shown to be required for the hydroxylation of both proline and lysine in procollagen. It has been shown that in connective tissue treated with an iron chelator such as 2,2′-dipyridyl, proline and lysine are incorporated into procollagen but there is no synthesis of hydroxyproline or hydroxylysine [24, 26]. It has been recently demonstrated that fibroblast cultures treated with desferrioxamine show inhibition of DNA synthesis and reduced collagen formation, with an apparent increase in the amounts of collagen produced with reduced doses of the agent [27]. The present findings support the view that desferrioxamine effects on membrane-associated proteins involve collagen synthesis and inhibition of proline and lysine hydroxylase activity. This in turn would result in the accumulation in the cell and also on the cell membrane of under-hydroxylated collagen precursors. Furthermore, the protein would be under-glycosylated since the incorporation of galactose and glucose, which attach to the hydroxylysine residues, would be prevented [24]. Thus, the present data and other results [7] suggest that the under-glycosylated 160 K and 130 K seen in our preparations are under-hydroxylated procollagen molecules. It has been shown that procollagen is retained by the cells in the endoplasmic reticulum when treated with 2,2′-dipyridyl [28]. This suggests that procollagen should not be susceptible to iodination unless a fraction of the molecules are associated with the cell membrane and are exposed to the extracellular space. Under our conditions, it appears that 160 K is exposed to the extracellular space. Our data are in accordance with current ideas about cell surface architecture of collagen [29] and also with the evidence reported that collagen is membrane bound and that it is patched and capped by anti-collagen sera in human fibroblasts [30]. Thus, the data suggest that 160 K is related to procollagen, is associated with the cell membrane, and is exposed to the external environment.

The significance and mechanisms of the decreased or absent 160 K on the surfaces of transformed cells as determined by surface iodination remain to be determined. Several possible explanations exist for this finding: It could be due to reduced synthesis, increased degradation, or enhanced release of the glycoprotein. Recent work has shown decreased cellular messenger RNA coding for various high molecular weight proteins in transformed cells [31]. The results presented in a subsequent paper [7] allow one to consider the first model since the proteins appear in the surface of transformed cells at reduced rates, in comparison to normal cells, as demonstrated by metabolic labeling. Since 160 K and 130 K are most likely related to procollagen, our data are in accordance with the observation that collagen synthesis is altered in cultured fibroblasts after transformation by some oncogenic viruses [32, 33], chemicals [32], and the potent tumor promoter phorbol 12-myristate 13-acetate [34]. Thus, the decreased accumulation of 160 K and 130 K may be due to the inability of virus-transformed NRK cells to synthesize sufficient quantities of these proteins. The present findings also imply that the concentration of these proteins in or on the plasma membrane may be of certain importance to growth arrest [7] and morphological changes [7, 27] induced by iron deprivation. Thus, our data provide evidence of biochemical concomitants of morphological and growth changes which are altered by transformation.

A point of particular interest is the function of 160 K and 130 K associated with the cell membranes and the apparent inhibition of iodination of 160 K glycoprotein by transferrin. They may simply have the well-known structural role as precursors of collagen [26]. However, other possibilities may also be considered. One obvious possible role for 160 K or a subset of this protein is that it is a component of the transferrin receptor, because it is a cell surface protein, and because one might expect that the receptor complex for transferrin is regulated by iron availability. That the transferrin receptor in some cells may be susceptible of detection by lactoperoxidase iodination appears to be likely for several reasons discussed elsewhere [35]. Furthermore, Witt and Woodworth have recently shown that the iodination of a putative 190 K transferrin receptor of reticulocyte is partially inhibited by its association with transferrin, presumably because the interaction of transferrin and its receptor shields some of the tyrosine residues from attack by the lactoperoxidase molecule [35]. Using this approach it was possible to demonstrate a differential decrease in the iodination of the 160 K protein in the membranes of intact NRK cells that have been preloaded with differic transferrin in those unexposed to transferrin. However, an alternative explanation for these findings is that transferrin interacts with 160 K and the complex transferrin-160 K is internalized [36], with a subsequent reduction in the number of molecules of 160 K available for iodination. Electron microscopy evidence provided further support for the idea that transferrin, 160 K, and 130 K interact in certain fashion. This finding may not be suprising since precursors of collagen or collagen itself have been shown to interact with glycoproteins [37], to produce specific mono- or polymorphic arrangements [37, 38], and to bind Fe^{3+} [39]. Furthermore, it is known that collagen molecules may be precipitated in a variety of different polymorphic forms; which polymorph occurs is determined mainly by the conditions of precipitation [38]. Taken together, these few data and published reports indicate in vivo and in vitro interactions that may or may not be entirely specific but that may be of possible physiological relevance. The molecular events described in this paper may represent an early step in the transferrin-cell interaction, which is followed by binding of transferrin to the receptor. Further extensive study is necessary to confirm the speculation concerning specificity and physiological implications of this interaction.

In conclusion, the present findings show that, upon iron starvation, normal and some transformed cells display a new cell surface glycoprotein, related to procollagen, which can be shown to interact with transferrin. Our results on the latter point are only suggestive, and only when the proteins are isolated in pure form can definite knowledge of these interactions be obtained. Finally, the results presented in this paper yield additional insight into interactions between surface proteins, growth media proteins, and iron, which could facilitate the detailed understanding of factors controlling cell shape and growth in vitro.

NOTE ADDED IN PROOF

Specific antibodies against procollagen propeptides, generously provided by Dr. Kao, showed similar staining characteristics as the anti-160 K antibodies.

ACKNOWLEDGMENTS

The author thanks K. Baer, P. Hamilton, M. Still, and D. Klos for expert technical assistance, and James Daly for establishing the computer programs necessary to evaluate denistometric scans. Valuable secretarial assistance was provided by J. Becker and J. Barrett. The technical assistance in electron microscopy of Ray Narconis and Jesse Urhahn is acknowledged. I thank Dr. Winston Whei-Yang Kao, Ophthalmology Research Lab, Eye & Ear Hospital, Pittsburgh, Pennsylvania, for kindly providing us with antibodies against procollagen propeptides.

This study was supported by VA MRISS 657/2620-01 and NIH PHS RR05388-17.

REFERENCES

1. Robbins E, Fant J, Norton W: Proc Natl Acad Sci USA 69:3708, 1972.
2. Messmer TO: Exp Cell Res 77:404, 1973.
3. Rudland PS, Durbin H, Clingan D, Jimenez de Asua L: Biochem Biophys Res Commun 75:556, 1977.
4. Fernandez-Pol JA: Cell 14:489, 1978.
5. Hoffbrand AV, Ganeshaguru K, Hooton JWL, Tattersall MHN: Br J Hematol 33:517, 1976.
6. Prockop DJ: Fed Proc 30:984, 1971.
7. Fernandez-Pol JA: In prepration.
8. Fernandez-Pol JA, Bono VH, Johnson GS: Proc Natl Acad Sci USA 74:2889, 1977.
9. Hynes RO: Proc Natl Acad Sci USA 70:3170, 1973.
10. Carter WG, Hakomori S: J Biol Chem 253:2867, 1978.
11. Graham G, Bates GW: J Lab Clin Med 88:477, 1976.
12. Brunette DM, Till JE: J Membr Biol 5:215, 1971.
13. Stone KR, Smith RE, Joklik WK: Virology 68:86, 1974.
14. Laemmli UK: Nature 227:690, 1970.
15. Garvey JS, Cremer NE, Sussdorf DH: "Methods in Immunology." Williamsport, Massachusetts: WA Benjamin, Inc., 1977, p 218; 313.
16. Olden K, Yamada KM: Anal Biochem 78:483, 1977.
17. Pouyssegur J, Yamada KM: Cell 13:139, 1978.
18. Pollack R, Rifkin D: Cell 6:495, 1975.
19. Huxley HE: J Mol Biol 7:281, 1963.
20. Peterson GL: Anal Biochem 83:346, 1977.
21. Lowry OH, Rosebrough NJ, Farr AL, Randall RJ: J Biol Chem 193:265, 1951.
22. Morrison M: In Fleischer, Packer L (eds): "Methods in Enzymology," Vol XXXII. New York: Academic Press, 1974, p 103.
23. Hynes RO: Biochim Biophys Acta 458:73, 1976.
24. Prockop DJ, Berg RA, Kivirikko KI, Uitto J: In Ramachandra GN, Reddi AH (eds): "Biochemistry of Collagen." New York: Plenum Press, 1976, p 163.
25. Bornstein P: Ann Rev Biochem 43:567, 1974.
26. Fessler JH, Fessler LI: Ann Rev Biochem 47:129, 1978.
27. Hunt J, Richards RJ, Harwood R, Jacobs A: Br J Hematol 41:69, 1979.
28. Uitto J, Hoffman HP, Prockop DJ: Science 190:1202, 1975.
29. Bornstein P, Duksin D, Balian G, Davidson JM, Crouch E: J NY Acad Sci 312:93, 1978.
30. Faulk WP, Conochie LB, Temple A, Papamichail M: Nature 256:123, 1975.
31. Adams SL, Sobel ME, Howard BH, Olden K, Yamada KM, de Crombrugghe BD, Pastan I: Proc Natl Acad Sci USA 74:3399, 1977.

32. Hata RI, Peterkofsky B: Proc Natl Acad Sci USA 74:2933, 1977.
33. Kamine J, Rubin H: J Cell Physiol 92:1, 1977.
34. Delclos KB, Blumberg PM: Cancer Res 39:1667, 1979.
35. Witt DP, Woodworth RC: Biochemistry 17:3913, 1978.
36. Silverstein SC, Steinman RM, Cohan ZA: Ann Rev Biochem 46:669, 1977.
37. Eisen AZ, Gross J: In Fitzpatrick TB et al (eds): "Dermatology in General Medicine." New York: McGraw-Hill, 1971, p 147.
38. Miller A: In Ramachamdran GN, Reddi AH (eds): "Biochemistry of Collagen." New York: Plenum Press, 1976, p 85.
39. Rosmus J, Vanick O, Marl J, Deyl Z: Experientia 23:898, 1967.

Journal of Supramolecular Structure 11:391–399 (1979)
Tumor Cell Surfaces and Malignancy 271–279

Carbohydrate Structure of the Major Glycopeptide From Human Cold-Insoluble Globulin

Susan J. Fisher and Roger A. Laine

Department of Biochemistry, University of Kentucky College of Medicine, Lexington, Kentucky, 40536

Cold-insoluble globulin (CIg) is a member of a group of circulating and cell-associated, high-molecular-weight glycoproteins termed fibronectins. CIg was isolated from human plasma by affinity chromatography on gelatin-Sepharose. SDS-polyacrylamide gel electrophoresis of the purified glycoprotein gave a double band that migrated near myosin. The CIg glycopeptides were released by pronase digestion and isolated by chromatography on Sephadex G-50. Affinity chromatography of the major G-50 peak on Con A-Sepharose resulted in two fractions: one-third of the glycopeptides were unbound and two-thirds were weakly bound (WB). Sugar composition analysis of the unbound glycopeptides by GLC of the trimethylsilyl methyl glycosides gave the following molar ratios: sialic acid, 2.5; galactose, 3.0; N-acetylglucosamine, 4.9; and mannose, 3.0. Sugar composition analysis of the WB glycopeptides gave the following molar ratios: sialic acid, 1.7; galactose, 2.0; N-acetylglucosamine, 4.1; and mannose, 3.0. The WB CIg glycopeptides cochromatographed on Sephadex G-50 with WB transferrin glycopeptides giving an estimated molecular weight of 2,800. After degradation with neuraminidase alone or sequentially with β-galactosidase the CIg and transferrin glycopeptides again cochromatographed. Methylation linkage analysis of the intact and the partially degraded glycopeptides indicated that the carbohydrate structure of the major human CIg glycopeptide resembles that of the major glycopeptide from transferrin.

Key words: cold-insoluble globulin, carbohydrate structure, human plasma

Cold-insoluble globulin (CIg) is a component of plasma and a member of a group of high-molecular-weight glycoproteins which are known collectively as fibronectins [1]. The

The costs of publication of this article were defrayed in part by the payment of page charges. This article must therefore be marked "advertisement" in accordance with 18 USC section 1734 solely to indicate this fact.

Abbreviations used: CIg, cold-insoluble globulin; LETS, large, external, transformation-sensitive; WB, weakly bound; SDS, sodium dodecyl sulfate; Con A, concanavalin A; PAS, periodic acid-Schiff; SFA, surface fibroblast antigen; CSP, cell surface protein.

Received May 10, 1979; accepted July 16, 1979.

cellular forms have been variously referred to as LETS [2], galactoprotein a [3, 4], SFA [5], CSP [6], and Zeta [7], while the circulating form, CIg, has been shown to be very similar to another serum protein, opsonic, α_2 SB glycoprotein [8].

The cell-associated and circulating fibronectins confer, to varying degrees, several adhesive properties to cultured cells. Comparison of the biologic activities of the two forms from chicken and from man have shown that they have identical activities with regard to mediating cell attachment to collagen and cell spreading on culture substrata. However, the cellular glycoproteins are 50 times more reactive in restoring normal morphology to transformed cells and 150 times more reactive in hemagglutination [9].

It appears that the two forms, while sharing many structural similarities, may also exhibit some differences. Attempts to produce a monospecific antiserum which does not cross-react with both forms have thus far not been reported successful [10, 11]. In addition, fibronectins from both sources have been reported to have similar isoelectric points and to produce similar CnBr cleavage products [12]. However, in some gel electrophoresis systems, the plasma and cellular forms have been shown to behave differently. The circulating fibronectins migrate as a doublet, while the cellular glycoproteins form a more slowly migrating, single, diffuse band [9, 13, 14].

It is unknown whether these differences will be accounted for by variations in the amino acid and/or the carbohydrate composition of the cellular and the plasma glycoproteins. In the first part of a study designed to compare the carbohydrate structure of glycopeptides isolated from human plasma and cell-associated fibronectins, we have determined the chemical structure of the major glycopeptide from CIg.

MATERIALS AND METHODS

CIg was isolated from fresh human serum by affinity chromatography according to the method of Engvall and Ruoslahti [15]. Whole blood (600 ml) was obtained and allowed to clot for 1 h at room temperature (25°C). Subsequent steps in the CIg isolation were carried out at 4°C. The blood was centrifuged for 15 min at 1,000g and the resulting serum was fractionated on a gelatin-Sepharose column containing 10 mg gelatin (Knox) per milliliter Sepharose. The column was washed with ten volumes of phosphate-buffered saline, pH 7.2, containing 0.01 M sodium citrate and the bound material was eluted with 200 ml of 1 M sodium iodide, dialyzed overnight against distilled water, and lyophilized. The product was assayed for protein according to the method of Lowry et al [16] and for homogeneity by SDS-polyacrylamide gel electrophoresis on 7.5% gels [17] in the presence of 2-mercaptoethanol with CIg complexed to fibrinogen (A. B. Kabi Company, Stockholm) as a standard. The gels were stained for protein with Coomassie blue [18] or for carbohydrate with PAS [19].

CIg, transferrin (human, Calbiochem), and fetuin (type III, Sigma Chemical Company) were digested with pronase and the solubilized glycopeptides were isolated by chromatography on a 30 × 1.5-cm Sephadex G-50 column. Columns were eluted with 0.1 M pyridine acetate buffer, pH 5.0. Fractions (1 ml) were collected and assayed for hexose by the method of Dubois et al [20]. An aliquot of the CIg, transferrin, and fetuin glycopeptides was N-acetylated with [³H]-acetic anhydride [21], mixed with the corresponding unlabeled glycopeptides and subjected to further fractionation on Con A-Sepharose [22]. The sugar composition of the unbound and WB CIg glycopeptides was determined after methanolysis by gas-liquid chromatography of the trimethylsilyl methyl glycosides [23, 24] on a Perkin-Elmer gas chromatograph, model 3920, equipped with a flame ionization detector and a 1.9-meter × 2-mm column of 3% OV-101 on 100–120 Supelcoport (Supelco., Inc.,

Bellefonte, Pennsylvania). Carrier gas was nitrogen at 45 ml/min. Peaks were integrated with a Spectra-physics "Minigrator." Amino acid analysis of the CIg glycopeptides was performed on a modified Technicon Amino Acid Analyzer by Dr. S. K. Chan, University of Kentucky.

The CIg and transferrin glycopeptides which were weakly bound to Con A-Sepharose were partially degraded with neuraminidase (type V, Sigma Chemical Company) alone or sequentially with a β-galactosidase and β-N-acetylhexosaminidase isolated from jack bean meal [25, 26] (gifts of Dr. Y.-T. Li, Tulane University, New Orleans). The resulting glyco-peptides were chromatographed on a 30 × 1.5-cm Sephadex G-50 column. Fractions (1 ml) were collected and assayed for radioactivity. Fractions containing either the intact or par-tially degraded glycopeptides were pooled and linkage positions were determined by meth-ylation analysis [Björndal et al, 27, 28] as modified by Järnefelt et al [29]. Instrumental conditions for the mass spectrometer were as follows: Finnigan model 3300-6110 with chemical ionization using methane at 1 torr and source temperature of 60°C; transfer lines were kept at 250°C. Other source parameters were as follows: collector, 34.2 V; electron multiplier, 1,950 V; emission current, 60 mA; ionizing electron energy, 150 eV; ion energy,

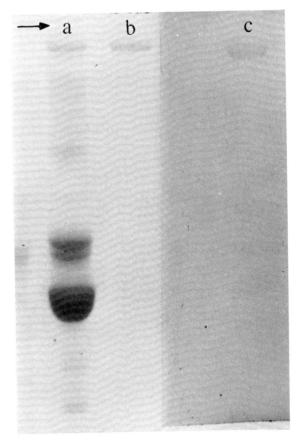

Fig. 1. SDS-polyacrylamide gel electrophoresis (arrow indicates origin) a: 10 μg CIg complexed with fibrinogen; b: 10 μg purified CIg stained for protein with Coomassie blue; c: 25 μg purified CIg stained for carbohydrate with PAS.

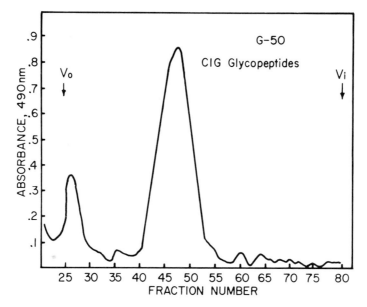

Fig. 2. Sephadex G-50 chromatography of CIg glycopeptides. Fractions 40–55 were pooled for further analysis. Vo = void volume; Vi = inclusion volume.

22.3 V; extractor, 25.6 V. Data acquisition was in the mass fragmentography mode using m/e 264 for terminal hexoses, m/e 292 for monosubstituted hexoses, m/e 320 for branched hexoses, and m/e 393 for monosubstituted amino sugars (MH-60 ions). Mass chromatograms for these ions were summed and a composite chromatogram plotted. All possible ions resulting from common sugars were searched.

RESULTS

SDS-polyacrylamide gel electrophoresis of the eluate from the gelatin-Sepharose column gave a high-molecular-weight band which appears as a diffuse doublet under close scrutiny but photographs as a single band as stained with Coomassie blue or PAS and which migrated with a CIg standard (Fig. 1). No other bands could be visualized by either method of staining. Chromatography of the total pronase-solubilized CIg glycopeptides on Sephadex G-50 (Fig. 2) gave a small peak at the void volume which could not be degraded by further protease treatment and a broad major peak corresponding to an approximate molecular weight of 2,800. The small void peak has not been further characterized.

Fractionation of the labeled transferrin, fetuin, and the major G-50 peak of the CIg glycopeptides by affinity chromatography on Con A-Sepharose (Fig. 3) yielded the following patterns. From fetuin, the glycopeptides (panel A) eluted entirely in the unbound fraction [30, 31]. From transferrin, one-fourth of the glycopeptides eluted in the unbound fraction and three-fourths in the weakly bound (WB) fraction. The transferrin glycopeptides which were not bound to the affinity column are probably of the "fetuin," triantennary type [32]. Fractionation of the major G-50 peak of the CIg glycopeptides on Con A-Sepharose (panel C) gave a pattern which closely resembled that obtained for the transferrin glycopeptides. One-third of the CIg glycopeptides passed through the col-

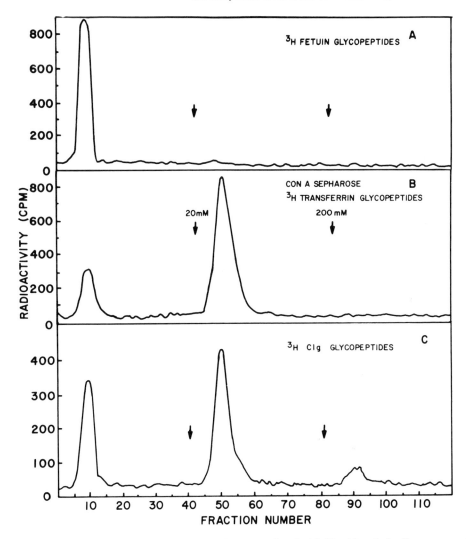

Fig. 3. Con A-Sepharose chromatography. Fractions were eluted with 20 mM methyl α-D-mannopyrano-side and 200 mM methyl α-D-mannopyranoside.

umn and two-thirds were weakly bound, indicating that the single peak obtained on Sephadex G-50 (Fig. 2) could be a mixture of the biantennary and the triantennary glycopeptides.

The major fraction of CIg glycopeptides, weakly bound to Con A-Sepharose, was isolated for initial structural characterization. Based on three mannose residues, the molar ratios of galactose, N-acetylglucosamine, and N-acetylneuraminic acid were found to be 3.0, 4.9, and 2.5, respectively, for the unbound fraction and 2.0, 4.1, and 1.7 for the WB glycopeptides. Since the average chain contains three mannose residues and asparagine, the CIg glycopeptides probably have an N-glycosyl-linked core structure. The transferrin biantennary glycopeptides which were weakly bound to the affinity column and which cochromatographed on Sephadex G-50 with the WB CIg glycopeptides (Fig. 4, panels A

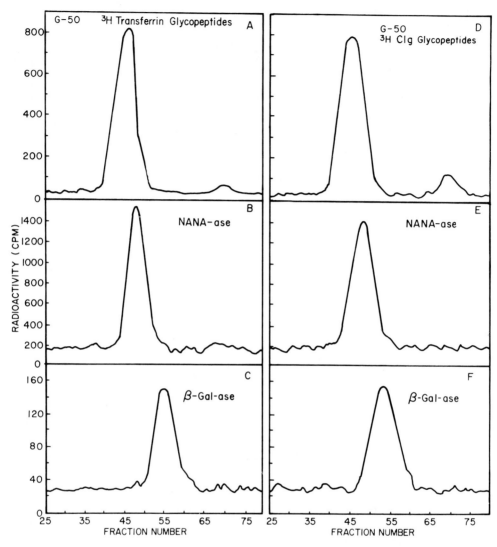

Fig. 4. Sephadex G-50 chromatography of intact and partially degraded WB transferrin (A–C) and CIg (D–F) glycopeptides. NANA-ase = neuraminidase degraded; β-Gal-ase = sequential degradation with neuraminidase and β-galactosidase.

and D), served as a standard compound for the remaining experiments. After partial degradation with neuraminidase the WB CIg and transferrin glycopeptides cochromatographed (Fig. 4, panels B and E) but with reduced apparent molecular weights, corresponding to the loss of two sialic acid residues. Subsequently to treatment with β-galactosidase the WB glycopeptides again cochromatographed (Fig. 4, panels C and F) with correspondingly lower molecular weights.

Comparison of the methylation analysis of the WB CIg and transferrin glycopeptides showed the linkage and the position of corresponding residues to be identical, both in the intact and in the partially degraded glycopeptides. Intact transferrin (Fig. 5, panel

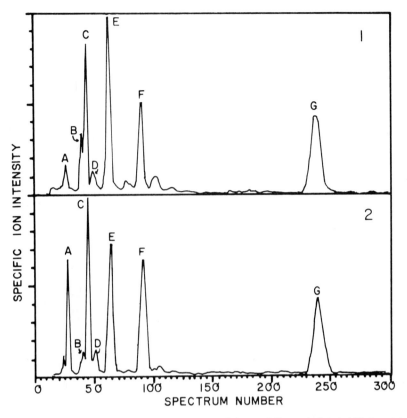

Fig. 5. Reconstructed multiple ion gas chromatogram of the partially methylated alditol acetates of the WB transferrin (panel 1) and CIg (panel 2) glycopeptides. Graphs are composite tracings of the following MH-60 ions: m/e 264 = terminal hexose; 292 = internal hexose; 320 = disubstituted hexose; 393 = mono-substituted amino hexose. A peak consisting of phthalate plasticizer at scan number 210, which gave signal at m/e 393, has been omitted. A = terminal hexose; B = 3-galactose; C = 2-mannose; D = 4-glucose; E = 6-galactose; F = 3,6-mannose; G = 4-N-acetylglucosamine.

TABLE I. Summary of Methylation Linkage Analysis of Sequentially Degraded Biantennary CIg and Transferrin Glycopeptides

Treatment	Branched residues	Internal residues	Terminal residues
NANA-ase	3,6-Mannose	2-Mannose, 4-Glucosamine	Galactose
NANA-ase, β-Gal-ase	3,6-Mannose	2-Mannose, 4-Glucosamine	Glucosamine
NANA-ase, β-Gal-ase, β-Hex-ase	3,6-Mannose	4-Glucosamine	Mannose

NANA-ase = neuraminidase; β-Gal-ase = β-galactosidase; β-Hex-ase = β-hexosaminidase.

1) and CIg glycopeptides (Fig. 5, panel 2) contained 3,6-substituted mannose, 2-mannose, 6-galactose, 4-glucosamine, and minor amounts of terminal- and 3-galactose. Methylation linkage analysis of the partially degraded glycopeptides is summarized in Table I. Following neuraminidase treatment there was a decrease in internal galactose and a concomitant increase in terminal galactose. After sequential degradation with neuraminidase and β-galactosidase the galactose residues were sharply reduced and half the glucosamine appeared in the terminal position. The terminal glucosamine residues were removed by degradation with β-hexosaminidase, after which approximately two-thirds of the mannose residues appeared in the terminal position. A trace amount of 4-glucose (less than 0.1 mole/3 mannose residues) was present in all WB transferrin and CIg preparations.

DISCUSSION

Two major classes of CIg glycopeptides were distinguished by affinity chromatography on Con A-Sepharose. 1) Two-thirds of the CIg glycopeptides were weakly bound (WB) to the lectin column. Consistent with the previously established structural requirements for Con A binding [31], the WB CIg glycopeptides contained three mannose residues, two of which were 2-linked. The structure of this glycopeptide was shown to be identical to that previously determined for the major biantennary transferrin glycopeptide [32] which also binds weakly to Con A [30]. Except for the presence of a small amount of terminal and 3-galactose residues, indicating that some of the WB CIg chains are either unsialylated or sialylated on the 3 position of galactose, other structural heterogeneity was not detected in this fraction. 2) A smaller portion (one-third) of the CIg glycopeptides passed through the Con A-Sepharose. Methylation analysis of this fraction (data not shown) indicated that the unbound CIg glycopeptides contain both 3,6- and 2,4-linked mannose, as does the fetuin triantennary glycopeptide [33]. It is probable that the 2,4-linked mannose residues, which prevent fetuin glycopeptides from binding to Con A [30, 31], also give rise to the unbound CIg fraction. The possibility that this fraction is a mixture of tri- and tetraantennary glycopeptides has not been excluded.

In close agreement with earlier observations [34, 35], human CIg was found to have a carbohydrate content of approximately 4%. From the Con A binding data each subunit of CIg, of molecular mass 210,000, may contain an average of two biantennary and one triantennary carbohydrate chains, which give a combined molecular mass of 7,277, corresponding to a carbohydrate content of 3.5%. The small void peak obtained from chromatography of the glycopeptides on Sephadex G-50 may constitute the remaining 0.5% of the calculated CIg carbohydrate content of 4%. Although the carbohydrate composition of human CIg corresponds to previously published results [36], neither type of chain contains 4-linked galactose or 4-linked mannose, which were recently reported by Wrann [36] to be components of human CIg. Galactosamine and fucose, which were shown by Carter and Hakomori to be components of LETS glycopeptides isolated from hamster embryo fibroblasts [37], were not detected in the human preparation. Stoichiometric amounts of glucose, reported in LETS glycopeptides from chick embryo fibroblasts [38], were not present in the CIg glycopeptides.

Since the carbohydrate structures of CIg resemble those carried by many other proteins, it seems likely that the specialized functions which have been proposed for this glycoprotein do not reside in the carbohydrate portion of the molecule. Instead, glycosylation may in this case be related to a more generalized function such as stabilization of the molecule against proteolytic digestion [39], maintenance of protein solubility, or clearance from the plasma [40].

ACKNOWLEDGMENTS

This work was supported by grant GM 23902 and Postdoctoral Fellowship HD 05687 (S.F.) from the National Institutes of Health.

We wish to thank Dr. S. K. Chan for performing the amino acid analysis, Dr. Y.-T. Li for generous gifts of β-galactosidase and β-hexosaminidase, and Diane Wiginton for expert technical assistance. We are grateful to Chris Cirulli for his participation in this project and to Professors S. K. Chan, Robert L. Lester, and Johan Järnefelt for many helpful discussions.

REFERENCES

1. Kuusela P, Ruoslahti E, Engvall E, Vaheri A: Immunochemistry 13:639, 1976.
2. Hynes RO, Bye JM: Cell 3:113, 1974.
3. Gahmberg CG, Hakomori S: Proc Natl Acad Sci USA 70:3329, 1973.
4. Gahmberg CG, Kiehn D, Hakomori S: Nature 248:413, 1974.
5. Ruoslahti E, Vaheri A, Kuusela P, Linder E: Biochim Biophys Acta 322:352, 1973.
6. Yamada KM, Weston JA: Proc Natl Acad Sci USA 71:3492, 1974.
7. Robbins PW, Wickus GG, Branton PE, Gaffney BJ, Hirschberg CB, Fuchs P, Blumberg PM: Cold Spring Harb Symp Quant Biol 39:1173, 1974.
8. Blumenstock FA, Saba TM, Weber P, Laffin R: J Biol Chem 253:4287, 1978.
9. Yamada KM, Kennedy DW: J Cell Biol 80:492, 1979.
10. Ruoslahti E, Vaheri A: J Exp Med 141:497, 1975.
11. Burridge K: Proc Natl Acad Sci USA 73:4457, 1976.
12. Vuento M, Wrann M, Ruoslahti E: FEBS Lett 82:227, 1977.
13. Crouch E, Balian G, Holbrook K, Duskin D, Bornstein P: J Cell Biol 78:701, 1978.
14. Keski-Oja J, Mosher DF, Vaheri A: Biochem Biophys Res Commun 74:699, 1977.
15. Engvall E, Ruoslahti E: Int J Cancer 20:1, 1977.
16. Lowry OH, Rosebrough NJ, Farr AL, Randall RJ: J Biol Chem 193:265, 1951.
17. Laemmli UK: Nature 277:680, 1970.
18. Segrest JP, Jackson RL: Methods Enzymol 28(Part B):54, 1972.
19. Carlson RW, Wada GH, Sussman HH: J Biol Chem 251:4139, 1976.
20. Dubois M, Gilles KA, Hamilton JK, Rebers PA, Smith F: Anal Chem 28:350, 1956.
21. Roseman S, Ludowieg J: J Am Chem Soc 76:301, 1954.
22. Krusius T: FEBS Lett 66:86, 1976.
23. Sweeley CC, Walker B: Anal Biochem 36:1461, 1964.
24. Bhatti T, Chambers RE, Clamp JR: Biochim Biophys Acta 222:339, 1970.
25. Li S-C, Mazzotta MY, Chien S-F, Li Y-T: J Biol Chem 250:6786, 1975.
26. Li S-C, Li Y-T: J Biol Chem 245:5153, 1970.
27. Björndal H, Lindberg B, Svensson S: Carbohydrate Res 5:433, 1967.
28. Björndal H, Lindberg B, Pilotti Ä, Svensson S: Carbohydrate Res 15:339, 1970.
29. Järnefelt J, Rush J, Li Y-T, Laine RA: J Biol Chem 253:8006, 1978.
30. Krusius T, Finne J, Rauvala H: FEBS Lett 71:117, 1976.
31. Baenziger J, Fiete D: J Biol Chem 254:2400, 1979.
32. Spik G, Bayard B, Fournet G, Strecker S, Bouquelet S, Montreuil J: FEBS Lett 50:296, 1975.
33. Baenziger J, Fiete D: J Biol Chem 254:789, 1979.
34. Mosesson MW, Chen AB, Huseby RM: Biochim Biophys Acta 386:509, 1975.
35. Vuento M, Wrann M, Ruoslahti E: FEBS Lett 82:227, 1977.
36. Wrann M: Biochem Biophys Res Commun 84:269, 1978.
37. Carter WG, Hakomori S: Biochemistry 18:730, 1979.
38. Yamada KM, Schlesinger DH, Kennedy DW, Pastan I: Biochemistry 16:5552, 1977.
39. Olden K, Pratt RM, Yamada KM: Cell 13:461, 1978.
40. Ashwell G, Morell AG: Adv Enzymol 41:99, 1974.

Journal of Supramolecular Structure 11:401–427 (1979)
Tumor Cell Surfaces and Malignancy 281–307

Fibronectin and Proteoglycans as Determinants of Cell-Substratum Adhesion

Lloyd A. Culp, Ben A. Murray, and Barrett J. Rollins

Department of Microbiology, Case Western Reserve University, Cleveland, Ohio 44106

When normal or SV40-transformed Balb/c 3T3 cells are treated with the
Ca^{++}-specific chelator EGTA, they round up and pull away from their footpad
adhesion sites to the serum-coated tissue culture substrate, as shown by scanning electron microscope studies. Elastic membranous retraction fibers break
upon culture agitation, leaving adhesion sites as substrate-attached material
(SAM) (Cells leave "footprints" of substrate adhesion sites during movement
by a very similar process.) SAM contains 1–2% of the cell's total protein and
phospholipid content and 5–10% of its glucosamine-radiolabeled polysaccharide,
most of which is glycosaminoglycan (GAG). By one- and two-dimensional
sodium dodecyl sulfate-polyacrylamide gel electrophoresis, there is considerable
enrichment in SAM for specific GAGs; for the glycoprotein fibronectin; and
for the cytoskeletal proteins actin, myosin, and the subunit protein of the
10 nm-diameter filaments. Fibrillar fibronectin of cellular origin and substratum-
bound fibronectin of serum origin (cold-insoluble globulin, CIg) have been
visualized by immunofluorescence microscopy. The GAG composition in SAM
has been examined under different cellular growth and attachment conditions.
Heparan sulfate content correlates with glycopeptide content (derived from
glycoprotein). Newly attaching cells deposit SAM with principally heparan
sulfate and fibronectin and little of the other GAGs. Hyaluronate and chron-
droitin proteoglycans are *coordinately* deposited in SAM as cells begin spreading and movement over the substrate. Cells attaching to serum-coated or CIg-
coated substrates deposited SAM with identical compositions. The proteoglycan
nature of the GAGs in SAM has been examined, as well as the ability of proteoglycans to form two classes of reversibly dissociable "supramolecular
complexes" — one class with heparan sulfate and glycopeptide-containing
material and the second with hyaluronate-chondroitin complexes. Enzymatic
digestion of "intact" SAM with trypsin or testicular hyaluronidase indicates
that (1) only a small portion of long-term radiolabeled fibronectin and cytoskeletal protein is bound to the substrate via hyaluronate or chondroitin
classes of GAG; (2) most of the fibronectin, cytoskeletal protein and heparan

Abbreviations: EGTA, ethylenebis (oxyethylenenitrilo) tetra acetic acid; SAM, substrate-attached
material; SDS, sodium dodecyl sulfate; PAGE, polyacrylamide gel electrophoresis; BSA, bovine serum
albumin; GAG, glycosaminoglycan; GAP, glycosaminoglycan-associated protein; CIg, cold-insoluble
globulin; TPCK, L-1-tosylamide-2-phenylethylchloromethyl ketone; PMSF, phenylmethylsulfonyl
fluoride; PBS, phosphate-buffered saline.

Received April 9, 1979; accepted July 6, 1979.

sulfate coordinately resist solubilization; and (3) newly synthesized fibronectin, which is metabolically labile in SAM, is linked to SAM by hyaluronate- and/or chondroitin-dependent binding. All of our studies indicate that heparan sulfate is a direct mediator of adhesion of cells to the substrate, possibly by binding to both cell-surface fibronectin and substrate-bound CIg in the serum coating; hyaluronate-chondroitin complexes in SAM appear to be most important in motility of cells by binding and labilizing fibronectin at the periphery of footpad adhesions, with subsequent cytoskeletal disorganization.

Key words: fibronectin, glycosaminoglycans, proteoglycans, adhesion, substrate-attached material cytoskeleton, immunofluorescence, heparan sulfate

Adhesive interactions between cells and between cells and noncellular matrix materials appear to be involved in a number of interesting and important biological processes, including normal and abnormal morphogenesis and malignant invasion. Many workers have studied the biological properties of these adhesive interactions and have demonstrated both quantitative and qualitative differences in adhesion that may be biologically important, but the underlying molecular mechanisms have been difficult to unravel [1].

Recently, fibronectin, a large protein found on the surface of many vertebrate cells [2, 3] and in vertebrate plasma, where it is known as cold-insoluble globulin (CIg) [3], has been shown to be involved in the normal adhesion of some avian and mammalian cell types to extracellular substrata [1]. For many cell types, fibronectin must be adsorbed to the substratum for normal cell attachment and spreading to occur [4], and addition of exogenous fibronectin causes many poorly adherent transformed cell lines, which are depleted of surface fibronectin, to spread out and adhere more tightly to the substratum [3]. The mechanism(s) by which fibronectin brings about these effects is unknown, but the known affinity of fibronectin for fibrous matrix materials such as collagens [5, 6] and heparin [7] raises the possibility that fibronectin may directly mediate in some fashion an adhesive interaction involving cells, fibrillar components, and fibronectin (cellular and/or substratum-bound). This possibility is strengthened by the demonstration that anti-whole-cell antibodies or concanavalin A, when bound to culture dishes, can mediate BHK cell attachment and spreading, which is morphologically and kinetically similar to that seen when dish-bound fibronectin is employed [8].

Clearly, it would be easier to study such molecular interactions in adhesion if the adhesive cell surface sites could be at least partially purified away from the rest of the cell. Such a preparation can be generated from a variety of cell types by treatment with the calcium-specific chelator EGTA [9]. The cells round up and retract away from their substrate adhesion sites; the retraction fibers connecting the cells to the adherent material eventually break, leaving the adhesion sites and associated material still firmly bound to the dish [10]. In the past few years we and our colleagues have examined the cellular origins and biochemical composition of this substrate-attached material (SAM) in some detail [1, 9–21]. More recently, we have begun experiments to examine the structural and functional interrelationships between the various components of SAM [15; Rollins and Culp, in preparation]. Although our results are not yet conclusive, they suggest that fibronectin in SAM is specifically associated with certain classes of glycosaminoglycans and proteoglycans. These interactions, then, may be part of the molecular mechanism of cell-substratum adhesion.

GROSS COMPOSITION OF SUBSTRATE-ATTACHED MATERIAL

Initial studies in our laboratory showed that SAM contains 1–2% of the cell's total protein content (as detected by incorporation of radiolabeled leucine) and 5–10% of the cell's polysaccharide (as detected by incorporation of radiolabeled glucosamine) [21]. There is little or no detectable nucleic acid, showing that SAM does not simply consist of a small number of cells that are resistant to detachment. Most of the polysaccharide represents glycosaminoglycans (GAGs) [12, 16], which drew our attention to these long-chain polysaccharides as possible mediators of adhesion. More recently Cathcart and Culp [14] have shown that SAM also contains 1–2% of the cell's phospholipid. These results, together with scanning electron microscopic studies discussed below, suggested that SAM represents discrete regions of the cell surface specialized for adhesion. Further work in our laboratory has been designed to test this hypothesis and to dissect further the structure and function of the components of SAM.

SAM REPRESENTS CELL-SUBSTRATUM ADHESION SITES

If biochemical studies of SAM are to have any relevance to cell-substratum adhesion, it is essential to show that SAM does not represent material that is secreted by the cells into the medium during growth or EGTA-mediated detachment and that then binds secondarily to the substratum. Contamination of SAM by whole cells is routinely less than 0.01%. Autoradiographic experiments with SAM metabolically labeled with ^{3}H-leucine or ^{3}H-glucosamine show that most of the incorporated label is found specifically located in areas to which cells were formerly attached and not in areas of the substratum that were free of cells [17]. Fibronectin shows a similarly restricted distribution when visualized by indirect immunofluorescence (see below). Furthermore, deposition of radiolabeled SAM onto the substratum ceases when the cells have completely covered the substratum, although the amount of radiolabeled macromolecular material shed into the medium continues to increase [19]. At least some of this material should have access to the substratum, since antibody is able to penetrate under the cells (see below).

There is considerable evidence that SAM represents the areas by which the cells are tightly bound to the tissue culture substratum, probably through the mediation of a tightly adsorbed layer of serum proteins. Micromanipulation experiments indicate that many cell types adhere to the substratum at multiple focal adhesive plaques [22]. SAM is indeed tightly adherent to the dish; the material is largely resistant to extraction with a wide variety of nonionic detergents, chaotropic agents, and salts [Cathcart and Culp, in preparation]. Of all the treatments tested, only extraction with 0.2% sodium dodecyl sulfate quantitatively solubilizes both protein and polysaccharide. Extraction with 0.5% sodium deoxychloate, 5 M urea, or 0.5% nonionic detergent (Triton X-100, Nonidet P-40, or Tween 40) solubilized 40% or less of either material. Sodium dodecyl sulfate-polyacrylamide gel electrophoresis (SDS-PAGE) patterns of solubilized and resistant material after these treatments were generally very similar, one exception being that part of the actin in SAM could be selectively extracted by nonionic detergent or by ATP plus KCl [Cathcart and Culp, in preparation]. Thus, the great majority of proteins and polysaccharides in SAM are *coordinately* released or retained, arguing that these materials are indeed structurally associated in SAM. High-resolution autoradiography [17] and immunofluorescent staining of fibronectin (see below) reveal that SAM components are distributed in localized pools under the cell. Material of similar morphology can be visualized by scanning electron micro-

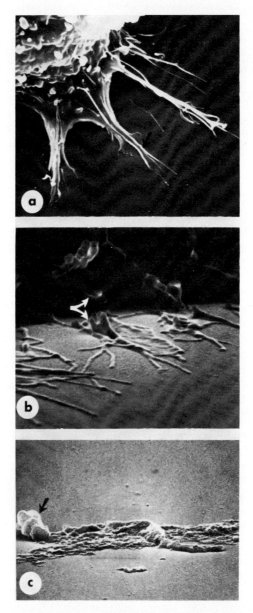

Fig. 1. Cellular origin of substrate-attached material. Swiss 3T3 cells were detached by EGTA treatment after growth to confluence and then allowed to reattach to fresh glass substrate in medium containing 10% serum. Specimens were processed for scanning electron microscopic observation by fixation in buffered glutaraldehyde, dehydration with graded alcohols and freon, and critical-point drying. Samples were sputter-coated with gold-palladium before SEM analysis. (a) A cell 2 h after attachment, showing well-developed footpads at the arrows (original magnification, $\times$ 6,500; 20° tilt); (b) a cell detaching after 10 min of treatment in 0.5 mM EGTA in PBS with gentle shaking, showing shearing of the labile retraction fiber (at the arrows) that connects the cell body to the footpad (original magnification, $\times$ 13,500; 80° tilt); (c) morphology of SAM after removal of cells that had been grown for 24 h, showing the remnant of the retraction fiber at the arrow (original magnification, $\times$ 13,500; 80° tilt). (Reprinted from Culp et al [20], with permission of the publisher.)

scopy of SAM (Fig. 1) [10, 20] and of material left behind after mechanical removal of cells [23–26]. When cells are examined microscopically during the detachment process, they are seen to round up and retract away from this firmly bound material (Fig. 1) [10, 20]. Finally, SAM differs in protein [11, 27], phospholipid [14], and polysaccharide [12] composition from whole cell or enriched surface membrane preparations, suggesting that it represents a specialized region of the cell surface. For example, SAM, whole cell preparations, and enriched membrane fractions prepared by two different methods all have the same classes of phospholipids present, but SAM is enriched for phosphatidylserine and has a higher ratio of phosphatidylethanolamine to phosphatidylcholine than do other preparations [14].

Proteins of SAM

The protein composition of SAM has been investigated by sodium dodecyl sulfate-polyacrylamide gel electrophoresis (SDS-PAGE) of the SDS-extracted radiolabeled material (Fig. 2). A number of species are enriched with respect to solubilized whole membranes. In particular, fibronectin (C_0), myosin (C_a), and actin (C_2) can be identified. By analogy with other systems [30–33], C_1 represents the subunit protein of one or more types of 10 nm "intermediate" filaments. SAM contains, at most, trace amounts of collagen [13], so collagen does not appear to be involved in cell-substratum adhesion in this system.

To resolve further the biochemical complexity of the proteins in SAM and to assist in further identifying the unknown components, we turned to the high-resolution two-dimensional electrophoresis system described by O'Farrell [34]. Proteins are isoelectrically focused in a cylindrical gel in the first dimension, followed by sizing analysis on a slab SDS-PAGE gel in the second dimension.

When substrate-attached proteins were analyzed on two-dimensional gels, a minor radioactive cellular protein, identified as "α" in Figure 3, co-electrophoresed with porcine skeletal α-actinin [28]. The concentrations of this α-actinin-like protein in SAM were very low compared to the amounts of actin and myosin. A minor band in the SAM of these cells, which migrates more slowly than the C_b band, has recently been shown to bind mono-specific antibody to α-actinin [J. Schollmeyer, personal communication]. The presence of α-actinin in substrate adhesion sites is of considerable interest, since this protein may be the internal membrane attachment site for actin-containing microfilaments in gut epithelial microvilli [29]. Also, the immunofluorescent distribution of α-actinin in spreading rat embryo cells exhibits a condensed focal pattern similar to the pattern observed with anti-actin [30], and some of these condensed foci may be cell-substrate adhesion sites. Other evidence will be required to determine if this protein acts as the internal membrane binding component for the actin-containing microfilaments in these adhesion sites; however, the very small quantity of this protein in SAM may argue against a major anchorage role for this protein.

The C_b band in Figure 2 is resolved into two components on two-dimensional gels — the major component, C_{b1}, and the minor component, C_{b2}, in Figure 3. Neither of these components appears to be glycosylated, since precursor radioactive glucosamine cannot be incorporated into the C_b bands [11]. Fibronectin (C_0) displays considerable micro-heterogeneity in the isoelectric focusing direction, some of which may be derived from the fact that it is a sialylated glycoprotein [27]. This microheterogeneity is probably not due to a monomer-dimer equilibrium via disulfide crosslinkage [35], since isoelectric focusing was performed with samples in 5% mercaptoethanol.

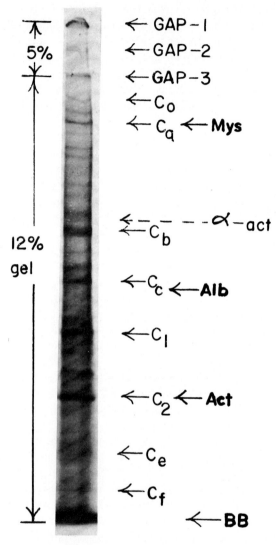

Fig. 2. Slab SDS-PAGE analysis of leucine-radiolabeled SVT2 substrate-attached material. As described previously [11], ^{14}C-leucine-radiolabeled SVT2 SAM was prepared after growth of cells for 48 h in radioactive medium, and the SAM was harvested by SDS extraction after EGTA-mediated detachment of cells. 20,000 cpm of SAM in sample buffer were electrophoresed in a 12% ORTEC slab gel at 40 mA/gel. The gel was then dried and autoradiographed for 8 weeks. Marker proteins of rabbit skeletal muscle myosin (Mys), rabbit skeletal muscle actin (Act), bovine serum albumin (Alb), and porcine skeletal muscle α-actinin (α-act) were electrophoresed on the same gel and detected by staining with Coomassie blue. The nomenclature for cellular proteins (C) in SAM has been described previously [11, 20, 21], and the following components have been identified: GAP, glycosaminoglycan-associated protein; C_o, fibronectin; C_a, myosin; C_2, actin.

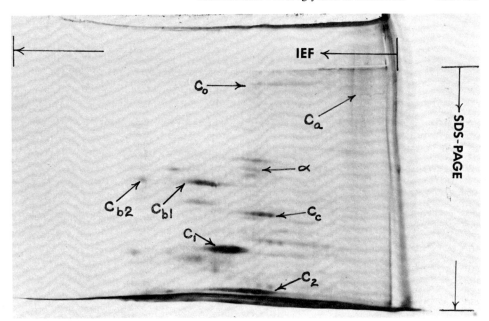

Fig. 3. Two-dimensional electrophoresis of the larger proteins in SAM. Isoelectric focusing was performed in 2 mm diameter (12 cm length) cylindrical gels as described by O'Farrell [34] using a mixture of 1.6% pH 5–7 ampholines and 0.4% pH 3–10 ampholines. These gels were frozen at $-20°C$ until they were used for SDS-PAGE. Slab SDS-PAGE gels for the second dimension were poured in the following order: a 12% or 20% ORTEC separating gel as described previously [11], depending on the size range of proteins being analyzed; then a 2 cm length 5% ORTEC stacking gel; finally a 0.5 cm length 2% agarose gel (containing 0.075 M Tris sulfate, pH 8.4) into which was embedded the isoelectric-focused cylindrical gel. A thin layer of sample buffer was applied at the surface of the agarose gel. Electrophoresis was performed as described by O'Farrell for nonequilibrated samples at 40 mA/gel. After electrophoresis, the slab gels were dried and autoradiographed for 1–4 months. 25,000 cpm of ^{14}C-leucine-radiolabeled SVT2 SAM was isoelectrically focused (IEF) in a cylindrical gel in the first dimension. Then this gel was mounted in an agarose overlay and electrophoresed into an SDS-PAGE gel (12% ORTEC gel) as the second dimension. Basic proteins are distributed on the right side and acidic proteins on the left side of the gel. Two micrograms each of carrier rabbit skeletal muscle actin and porcine skeletal muscle α-actinin were also present in the sample and were detected by Coomassie staining – the former co-electrophoresed with radioactive component C_2 and the latter with the radioactive spot marked α. The gel was dried, and radioactive components were detected by autoradiography as shown here.

The prominent C_1 protein (mol wt 55,000), which is completely lacking in tryptophan residues and which has been shown not to be tubulin [11], migrates in these O'Farrell gels identically to the "52K" protein identified by Brown et al [31] as the subunit protein of the 10 nm-diameter, non-actin containing filaments of fibroblasts. This protein, as well as actin (C_2), is observed in SAM in similar relative concentrations from both normal and virus-transformed cells under many different growth conditions ($C_1 : C_2 = 0.5–0.6$), suggesting that both classes of filaments are tightly associated in the substrate adhesion site of cells in a well-defined molar ratio [1, 11, 20, 21]. However, the immature adhesion sites of newly attaching, EGTA-subcultured 3T3 or SVT2 cells contain much higher levels of C_1 relative to actin or myosin ($C_1 : C_2 = 1.5–2.0$) [11, 20, 21]. This suggests that these filaments play an important role in reorganization of cell surface material at these adhesion sites.

Previous evidence [11, 20, 21] has demonstrated that the C_2 band is actin. When SAM preparations are electrophoresed on O'Farrell gels using 20% slab SDS-PAGE gels to improve the resolution of low molecular weight proteins, the actin band (C_2) can be resolved into two equivalent pools (Fig. 4) with different isoelectric points corresponding to the beta and gamma forms of actin observed in non-muscle cells [36, 37]. The relative amounts of the beta and gamma forms of actin were similar in SAM and whole cell extracts. It thus appears that the EGTA-resistant, adhesion-site-bound actin is not an enrichment of either class of actin and reflects the actin composition of the whole cell.

Fibronectin in SAM

Since fibronectin has been implicated in cell-substratum adhesion [3, 4], we decided to investigate the topographic distribution of this protein in SAM. Taking advantage of the immunological cross-reactivity between fibronectins of different species [38] and the easy purification of plasma fibronectin by affinity chromatography on immobilized gelatin [5, 6], we prepared, purified, and characterized monospecific goat and rabbit antibodies against human plasma fibronectin (cold-insoluble globulin; CIg) [Murray and Culp, in preparation]. The specificity of the antibodies was verified by double diffusion analysis (Ouchterlony) and crossed-immunoelectrophoresis [39]. With the immunoperoxidase-staining technique for SDS-PAGE of Olden and Yamada [40], these antibodies specifically stain a band in SAM that comigrates with authentic fibronectin (data not shown).

We first used indirect immunofluorescence analysis of formaldehyde-fixed cultures to examine fibronectin distribution before the cells were removed. The results were similar to the patterns observed by others in other cell types [3, 41, 42] (Fig. 5). Cell-associated fibronectin-specific fluorescence was visible as a pattern of supracellular fibers; the pattern grew much more extensive and more intricate as the cultures grew denser. In the sparser cultures fibrillar fluorescence often coincided with the boundary between two cells, but

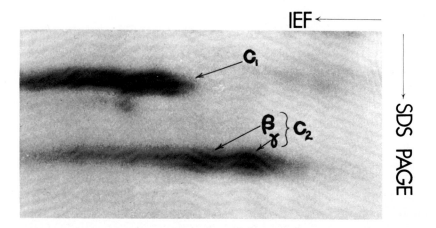

Fig. 4. Two-dimensional electrophoresis of the smaller proteins in SAM. ^{14}C-leucine-radiolabeled SVT2 SAM was electrophoresed as described in Figure 3, except a 20% ORTEC slab SDS-PAGE gel was used to improve the resolution of smaller proteins. Only a portion of the autoradiogram is shown. Rabbit skeletal muscle actin (2 μg added as carrier) co-electrophoresed with the C_2 radioactive component in SAM, which has previously been shown to be actin by a number of criteria [11, 21].

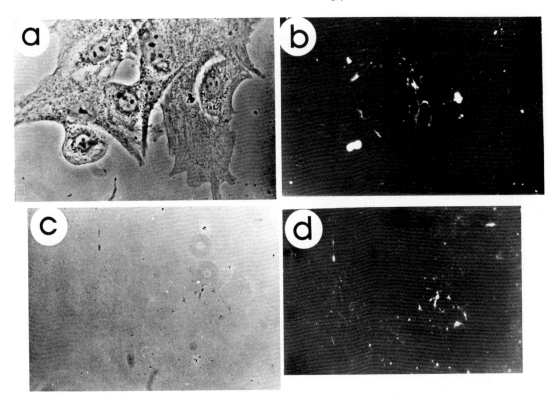

Fig. 5. Immunofluorescence analysis of Balb/c 3T3 cells and SAM. Balb/c 3T3 cells were grown on 11 × 22 cm glass coverslips as described previously [18]. At 24 h after seeding, the cells were washed three times with phosphate-buffered saline containing 1 mM each CaCl$_2$ and MgCl$_2$ and fixed for 20 min in the same buffer containing 3.7% formaldehyde. After three 5-min washes in buffer lacking formaldehyde, cells were stained for 30 min at room temperature with 4 μg/ml affinity-purified rabbit antibody directed against purified human plasma fibronectin [Murray and Culp, in preparation]. After three more washes, the coverslips were further stained with fluorescein-labeled goat antibody to rabbit immunoglobulin (Miles Laboratories, 1/64 dilution), washed, and mounted in a barbital-buffered saline solution at pH 9. For SAM preparations, cells were released from coverslips by treatment with 0.5 mM EGTA in buffer lacking divalent cations [9] followed by gentle pipetting. The coverslips were then washed and fixed (using buffer lacking divalent cations) and processed as above. Samples were examined on a Leitz Ortholux microscope equipped with phase-contrast optics and epifluorescence illumination at an original magnification of 400 ×. (a) 3T3 cells visualized by phase-contrast optics; (b) fluorescence image of the same field; (c) 3T3 SAM visualized by phase-contrast optics; (d) fluorescence image of the same field.

this correspondence was lost as the cultures grew denser. By differential focusing we could also see fluorescent fibers *underneath* the cells, suggesting that the antibody was able to penetrate between the cell and substratum; this has not been observed in all other systems [41]. This staining probably did not arise by penetration of the antibodies *through* the cell, since diffuse intracellular staining was seen only in preparations in which the integrity of the membrane had been impaired by extraction with 0.5% Triton X-100 for 5 min. The fibrillar staining was also seen with antibodies that had been absorbed with insolubilized bovine CIg, so this presumably represents fibronectin synthesized by the cells. In contrast, a continuous layer of fluorescence was visualized bound to the substratum; this staining *was* abolished by the above absorption, and so it probably represents bovine CIg adsorbed to the substratum from the calf serum in the tissue culture medium. In sparse cultures, this substratum-bound fluorescence frequently was reduced or absent directly beneath and around cells and in "tracks" leading up to cells; these tracks resembled in their appearance the "phagokinetic tracks" seen by Albrecht-Buehler [43]. We do not yet know whether this decreased fluorescence is a result of the loss of substrate-bound CIg or of the masking of CIg antigenic determinants by some other material.

We found many similar features when we examined SAM by immunofluorescence (Fig. 5). There was considerable fibrillar and punctate fluorescence localized to areas of the approximate size and shape of single cells or small groups of cells. The continuous substratum fluorescence with dark "tracks" was also seen. As with the cell cultures, only the fibrillar and punctate fluorescence was stained with antibodies previously adsorbed with bovine CIg to prevent reactivity of the antibody with substratum-adsorbed serum proteins. This does not rule out the possibility that *some* of the fibrillar and punctate fluorescence may represent bovine CIg absorbed from the medium. It is interesting that the amount of fibronectin-specific fluorescence of any kind (continuous, fibrillar, or punctate) decreases drastically in SAM generated from very dense cultures grown on glass coverslips; this decrease is *not* observed on plastic coverslips (data not shown). A similar finding was briefly noted by Mautner and Hynes [41] for NIL cells. This observation is being further investigated.

Serum Components in SAM

Material synthesized by cells in SAM can be detected by incorporation of appropriately radiolabeled precursors. In addition, SAM also contains adsorbed serum proteins. At least twelve such components can be detected by SDS-PAGE analysis [11; Haas and Culp, in preparation], including bovine serum albumin (BSA). However, BSA alone will not support normal cell attachment and spreading when adsorbed to a substratum. Grinnell and others have shown that purified plasma fibronectin (CIg), when adsorbed to the substratum, will mediate normal attachment and spreading of BHK cells [4]; we have confirmed this result for Balb/c 3T3 and SVT2 cells [Murray, Haas and Culp, in preparation). It has been reported for one cell line that serum deprived of CIg by passage over immobilized gelatin is deficient in normal cell spreading [44]. As discussed earlier, CIg adsorbed from the medium can be detected by immunofluorescence, but by SDS-PAGE analysis CIg seems to be a minor component of the proteins adsorbed to the substratum [Haas and Culp, in preparation].

Since substratum-bound CIg probably represents the primary site of interaction between cellular adhesive material and the substratum, SAM produced on substrata coated with purified CIg should resemble SAM produced in the usual manner on serum-coated substrata. SDS-PAGE analysis shows that this is, in fact, the case [Murray and Culp, in preparation]. SAM from cells attaching on CIg-coated substrata contains as much cellular fibronectin as SAM from cells attaching to serum-coated substrata. This suggests that CIg in the serum layer cannot functionally substitute for cell surface fibronectin. This interpretation is supported by the finding that cell-surface fibronectin and high molecular weight proteoglycans are the major iodinatable cell-surface components incorporated into new adhesion sites when cells are prelabled with ^{131}I by the lactoperoxidase technique, removed with EGTA, and allowed to reattach onto a fresh substratum before preparing SAM; in contrast, the released cells themselves contain many iodinated species by SDS-PAGE [Cathcart and Culp, in preparation]. Even though these cells retain surface-iodinated fibronectin, they still require substratum-bound CIg for normal attachment and spreading.

Furthermore, when cells are removed by trypsin treatment under conditions that remove all surface-associated fibronectin and are allowed to attach to fresh substrata, the SAM that is laid down contains normal amounts of metabolically labeled (cell-derived) fibronectin [Buniel and Culp, unpublished results] ; this presumably derives from intracellular or newly synthesized fibronectin.

Interestingly, the *quantity* of ^{3}H-glucosamine-polysaccharide retained when pre-labeled SVT2 cells are allowed to reattach to a substratum for 1 h before they are removed is considerably greater when the substratum was precoated with purified CIg rather than with serum. SVT2 cells on CIg-coated substrata also spread more extensively than they do on the serum-coated substrata.

Glycosaminoglycans in SAM

A role for complex carbohydrates in cell adhesion has been postulated on the basis of evidence from a wide variety of studies [reviewed in reference 1]. The molecular structure of these carbohydrates is unclear, but much attention has been focused on glycoproteins, and, in particular, on fibronectin, as described earlier [3, 11, 21, 46–49]. Considerable attention also has been paid to cell surface glycosaminoglycans (GAGs), but most of these experiments have yielded only indirect evidence for an adhesive role for GAGs.

A promising line of investigation was begun when it was discovered that SAM is highly enriched for GAGs when compared to the rest of the cell [11, 16, 52]. Initially, only hyaluronic acid was chemically identified in SAM [16]. Metabolic radiolabeling with $^{35}SO_4$, however, revealed the presence of sulfated GAG [16, 52], and when glucosamine- or sulfate-radiolabeled SAM was analysed by SDS-PAGE, nearly all of the radioactivity was found in three high molecular weight GAG-associated bands [11].

The GAGs in SAM have since been examined in greater detail and have been compared with the GAGs in the rest of the cell [12]. We hoped that a specific redistribution of the GAGs in SAM would suggest their functional role(s) in adhesion. Table I shows the distribution of radioactivity among the various GAGs and glycopeptide in the cell-associated, EGTA-soluble, and substrate-attached material of 3T3 cells after exposure to ^{3}H-glucosamine for 72 h. Both EGTA-soluble material and SAM are relatively enriched for GAG.

The distribution of specific GAGs in this preparation from 3T3 cells (and SVT2 cells, not shown) reveals several patterns. Essentially, the relative amounts of chondroitin 4-sulfate and unsulfated chondroitin rise in SAM as compared to cell-associated material, whereas the relative amount of dermatan sulfate falls. These rises and falls are reproducible. Also, the rise and fall in the relative amount of heparan sulfate in the various fractions tends to be paralleled by the changes in amount of glycopeptide in the same fractions.

Thus it is apparent that GAGs are redistributed in cellular adhesion sites. This does not in itself demonstrate functionality for the GAGs, and so we compared SAM from cells adherent for only 1 h (before they begin to spread) to SAM from cells adherent for 72 h (during which time they move several cell diameters [53], leaving a SAM enriched for footprints). Table II shows the distribution of radioactivity in polysaccharides from these preparations in 3T3 cells. Results for SVT2 cells were similar. The most striking result is the enrichment for heparan sulfate in newly formed footpads. It is almost three times the amount seen in footprint-enriched SAM. This parallels the large rise in radiolabeled glyco-peptide content in SAM from these reattaching cells. That these changes are occurring *specifically* at the footpad is indicated by the similarity between the *cell-associated* GAG distributions in long-term radiolabeled and reattaching cells.

In summary, newly formed adhesion sites are highly enriched for heparan sulfate and

TABLE I. Distribution of Long-Term Radiolabeled Polysaccharides in 3T3 Cells*

Polysaccharide[a]	% Radioactivity[b]			
	Cell-associated	EGTA-soluble	Cell+ EGTA[c]	Substrate-attached
Glycopeptide	73.6	36.0	72.7	27.9
GAG	26.4	64.0	27.3	72.1
Total	100.0	100.0	100.0	100.0
HS	48.8	22.2	48.2	26.3
6S	0.8	1.1	0.8	2.3
4S	5.7	8.3	5.8	22.4
DS	24.0	11.7	23.7	2.7
OS	3.1	18.0	3.5	23.6
HA	17.6	38.7	18.0	22.7
Total	100.0	100.0	100.0	100.0

*Analytical procedures have been described by Rollins and Culp [12]. Briefly, cultures of 3T3 cells were labeled for 72 h with ^{3}H-glucosamine, following which the cells were detached by EGTA treatment. Substrate-attached polysaccharide is material resistant to EGTA-mediated release; cell-associated polysaccharide is material that is found in the washed pellet after a low-speed centrifugation; and EGTA-soluble polysaccharide is material that remains in the supernatant after the low-speed centrifugation. Polysaccharides were isolated by ethanol precipitation of Pronase-digested fractions. Hyaluronic acid, dermatan sulfate, and the chondroitins were identified and quantitated by paper chromatography of chondroitinase AC and chondroitinase ABC digests. Heparan sulfate and glycopeptide were identified and quantitated by Sepharose CL-6B chromatography of chondroitinase ABC digests; heparan sulfate was measured as material sensitive to nitrous acid degradation.

[a]HS, heparan sulfate; 6S, chondroitin 6-sulfate; 4S, chondroitin 4-sulfate; DS, dermatan sulfate; OS, unsulfated chondroitin; HA, hyaluronic acid.

[b]Glycopeptide and GAG are shown as the percentage of total polysaccharide radioactivity, whereas the individual GAGs are shown as the percentage of total GAG radioactivity.

[c]The precentage of radioactivity in the (cell + EGTA) fractions contained in a specific polysaccharide was determined as follows:

$$\% \text{ radioactivity} = \frac{(\text{cpm of specific polysaccharide in cell-associated and EGTA-soluble material})}{(\text{cpm of total polysaccharide in cell-associated and EGTA-soluble material})} \times 100$$

depleted of hyaluronic acid and the chondroitins, as compared to the rest of the cell. As the adhesion sites mature — ie, as the cells begin to spread — there is a progressive accumulation of unsulfated chondroitin and hyaluronic acid in a fairly constant proportion. This accumulation occurs *coordinately* and *specifically* at the adhesion site, suggesting that the chondroitins and hyaluronic acid may be somehow associated with each other. This situation is reminiscent of the hyaluronate-chondroitin proteoglycan complexes in cartilage [54–56].

Proteoglycans in SAM

Most glycosaminoglycans are found as parts of large proteoglycans [56, 57]. We devised techniques to analyze intact GAG-containing molecules from SAM. The effect of

TABLE II. Distribution of Radiolabeled Polysaccharides in SAM From Long-term Radiolabeled and Reattaching Cells*

Cellular fraction	Polysaccharide[a]	% Radioactivity[b]	
		Long-term	Reattaching
Cell-associated	Glycopeptide	73.6	59.7
	GAG	26.4	40.3
	Total	100.0	100.0
	HS	48.8	56.8
	6S	0.8	2.5
	4S	5.7	4.3
	DS	24.0	17.7
	OS	3.1	2.5
	HA	17.6	16.2
	Total	100.0	100.0
SAM	Glycopeptide	27.9	66.6
	GAG	72.1	33.4
	Total	100.0	100.0
	HS	26.3	80.2
	6S	2.3	1.6
	4S	22.4	8.0
	DS	2.7	0.9
	OS	23.6	4.8
	HA	22.7	4.5
	Total	100.0	100.0

*3T3 cells were grown in the presence of ^{3}H-glucosamine for 72 h as described in Table I (long-term), and the polysaccharides were analyzed for radioactivity. Alternatively, long-term radiolabeled cells were removed from dishes with EGTA, washed in cold PBS, and replated in fresh dishes. After 1 h SAM polysaccharides were analyzed as usual (reattaching).
[a]HS, heparan sulfate; 6S, chondroitin 6-sulfate; 4S, chondroitin 4-sulfate; DS, dermatan sulfate; OS, unsulfated chondroitin; HA, hyaluronic acid.
[b]Glycopeptide and GAG are shown as the percentage of total polysaccharide radioactivity, whereas the individual GAGs are shown as the percentage of total GAG radioactivity.

proteolytic treatment of these species was then assessed in an attempt to demonstrate the existence of proteoglycans [Rollins and Culp, in preparation].

The carbohydrate-containing species of SAM were initially separated by molecular sieve chromatography on Sepharose CL-2B in an SDS buffer. The resulting profile from a preparation doubly labeled with ^{35}SO$_4$ and ^{3}H-glucosamine is shown in Figure 6. Three classes of glucosamine-labeled material were resolved, of which two (areas II and III) were sulfated. The profile was not altered by omission of protease inhibitors or by reduction and alkylation of SAM before analysis. Similar results were seen with SAM from 3T3 or SVT2 cells.

SAM was also electrophoresed in SDS buffer on 1.5–10% concave logarithmic poly-acrylamide gels containing 1% agarose for structural support (Fig. 7A). The three areas separated by electrophoresis correspond to the three areas of SAM separable by gel chromatography (Fig. 7B–D). The material of highest apparent molecular weight migrates as a relatively sharp band and is not labeled with ^{35}SO$_4$ or ^{14}C-leucine (data not shown).

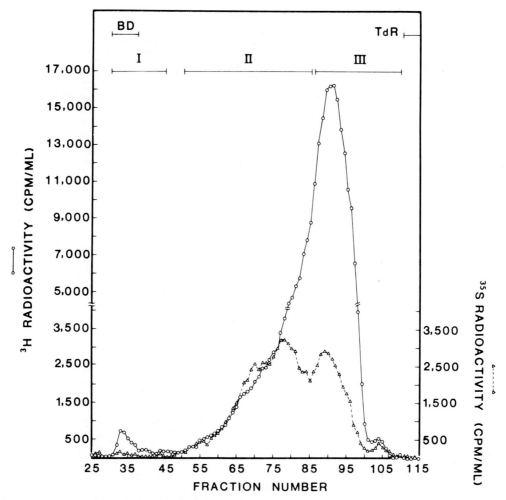

Fig. 6. SDS chromatography on Sepharose CL-2B of SAM from long-term ^{3}H-glucosamine, [35]SO$_4$ radiolabeled SVT2 cells. SVT2 cells were grown for 72 h in the presence of ^{3}H-glucosamine and Na$_2$[35]SO$_4$ and then removed with EGTA (containing PMSF). The SAM was extracted with SDS (also containing PMSF) and, after vacuum dialysis, it was chromatographed on a column of Sepharose CL-2B (1 × 120 cm, eluted with 120 mM Tris-HCl (pH 7.4), 0.2% SDS) [Rollins and Culp, Biochemistry, in press].

The other two ^{14}C-glucosamine-labeled areas are diffuse and the areas are not well separated. Both are labeled by [35]SO$_4$ and ^{14}C-leucine. Similar patterns were seen for SVT2 cell SAM.

    In order to identify the proteoglycans in SAM, the areas of radioactivity shown in Figure 6 were analyzed for carbohydrates before and after Pronase digestion. Such analysis has shown that the material in area I of Figure 6 is entirely composed of hyaluronic acid, the eluted position of which does not change after Pronase digestion. Area II is composed of the other GAGs, along with some glycopeptide. Digestion of this material with Pronase showed that all of the chondroitin species and some 50% of the heparan sulfate species are structurally attached to protein as defined by a change in column elution position after Pronase digestion. Analysis of area III, which contained the rest of the GAG along with

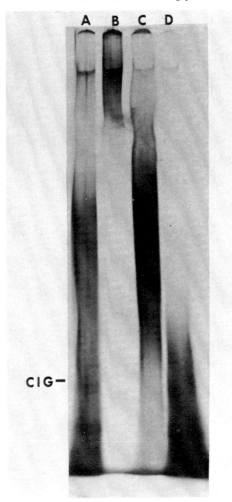

Fig. 7. SDS-PAGE on gradient gels of chromatographically fractionated SAM from long-term radio-labeled 3T3 cells. An aliquot of SDS-extracted SAM from long-term ^{14}C-glucosamine radiolabeled 3T3 cells was electrophoresed on a 1.5–10% concave logarithmic polyacrylamide gel containing 1% agarose. Another aliquot was chromatographed on Sepharose CL-2B as described in the legend to Figure 6. The indicated areas in Figure 6 were collected and electrophoresed on the same gel as the unfractionated SAM: well B, area I; well C, area II; well D, area III. The position of human CIg after electrophoresis is indicated [Rollins and Culp, Biochemistry, in press].

much glycopeptide, yielded essentially similar results. Table III (based on unpublished data of Rollins and Culp) summarizes the proteoglycan species thus far identified in SAM on the basis of their apparent hydrodynamic sizes before and after Pronase digestion.

Association of SAM Proteoglycans

In order to assess the ability of SAM proteoglycans to interact with each other, or with other components in SAM, we adapted some techniques used in cartilage research [56, 58, 59] for use with SAM (Fig. 8) [Rollins and Culp, in preparation]. When a 4.0 M guanidine hydrochloride extract of long-term ^{3}H-glucosamine/[35]SO$_4$ radiolabeled SAM is

TABLE III. Proteoglycan and GAG Species in SAM*

Radiolabeling conditions	Species[a]	Comments
Long-term	HA	No detectable protein, largest apparent molecular weight
	4S-6S-OS	Larger molecular weight proteoglycan, present in large amounts
	4S-OS	Smaller molecular weight proteoglycan, present in small amounts
	HS	Proteoglycan
	DS	Proteoglycan
Reattaching	HA	No detectable protein
	6S-OS	Largest proteoglycan in reattaching cell SAM
	4S-OS	Smaller molecular weight proteoglycan
	HS	Proteoglycan
	DS	Probably not in proteoglycan form

*These species are tentatively identified by their behavior on gel chromatography before and after Pronase digestion (see text).
[a]HS, heparan sulfate; 6S, chondroitin 6-sulfate; 4S, chondroitin 4-sulfate; DS, dermatan sulfate; OS, unsulfated chondroitin; HA, hyaluronic acid. Species are named by the carbohydrate components they contain.

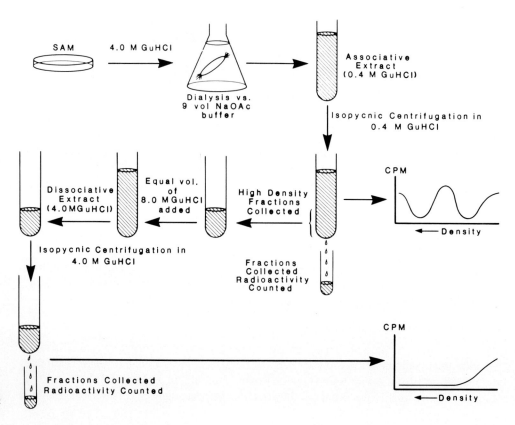

dialyzed to associative conditions (0.4 M guanidine hydrochloride) and centrifuged to equilibrium in a cesium chloride gradient, the profile of Figure 9A results. There are two major peaks of radioactivity at densities greater than 1.580 g/ml. The denser peak, at the bottom of the gradient, has a much higher ratio of ^{35}S to ^{3}H radioactivity than does the peak of intermediate density. There is also a small area of ^{35}S and ^{3}H radioactivity at the top of the gradient.

When the material banding at densities greater than 1.580 g/ml (fractions 1–8, Fig. 9A) is brought to dissociative conditions (4.0 M guanidine hydrochloride) and again centrifuged to equilibrium in cesium chloride, the radioactivity is distributed as shown in Figure 9B. Although small amounts of ^{35}S and ^{3}H radioactivity are at the bottom of the gradient, over 80% of the ^{3}H and 75% of the ^{35}S radioactivity bands at densities less than 1.580 g/ml. This material can be dialyzed to 0.4 M guanidine hydrochloride and recentrifuged to give the same pattern as fractions 1–8 in Figure 9A (data not shown). Thus the carbohydrates in SAM are capable of undergoing a reversible association into highly negatively charged aggregates.

The material at the bottom of the gradient (fractions 1 and 2, Fig. 9A), comprising only 6% of the total radioactivity, is over 80% GAG. Of this GAG, about 40% is heparan sulfate, and the rest is chondroitinase ABC–digestible material. The band of intermediate density (fractions 3–9) is over 80% heparan sulfate and comprises 31% of the total radioactivity. There is also a small amount of other GAG and glycopeptide in this fraction. Thus the high-density material is qualitatively different from the intermediate-density material (both by analysis here and by ^{35}S:^{3}H ratios in Figure 9A), but both areas are capable of being disaggregated by 4.0 M guanidine hydrochloride. The least dense fractions (10–12), with 14% of the total radioactivity, have nearly equal amounts of heparan sulfate and glycopeptide and are slightly depleted of glycopeptide.

The material sticking to the centrifuge tube (routinely 48% of the total radioactivity) is highly enriched for chondroitinase-digestible GAG. A smaller amount of glycopeptide and even less heparan sulfate also stick to the tube. No radioactivity was found adherent to any of the other surfaces used in these experiments (eg, dialysis tubing).

In order to assess the role of intact protein in the observed aggregation phenomenon, SAM was tested for its ability to aggregate after extensive protease digestion. A typical associative sedimentation equilibrium analysis of long-term radiolabeled SVT2 cell SAM is shown in Figure 10A. Fractions 1–9 were combined and digested for 24 h with Pronase in the presence or absence of SDS. This material was extensively dialyzed, then made 0.4 M in guanidine hydrochloride and centrifuged under these associative conditions. This treatment had little effect on the aggregation of the intermediate-density material

---

Fig. 8. Isopycnic centrifugation of SAM under associative and dissociative conditions. Radiolabeled cells were removed from dishes with EGTA, and the SAM remaining on the dishes was extracted with 4.0 M guanidine hydrochloride in 0.054 M sodium acetate (pH 5.8) at 4°C for 48 h. The extract was dialysed against 9 vol 0.05 M sodium acetate to reduce the concentration of guanidine hydrochloride to 0.4 M. These are defined as associative conditions [56]. The associative extract was brought to a loading density of 1.63 g/ml cesium chloride and centrifuged in a Beckman 50 Ti rotor at 34,000 rpm at 18°C for 48 h. After centrifugation, 1 ml fractions were collected by piercing the bottom of the centrifuge tube, and the density and radioactivity of each sample was determined. The lower two-thirds of the associative gradient was brought to dissociative conditions (4.0 M guanidine hydrochloride), cesium chloride was added to a density of 1.54 g/ml, and centrifugation and analysis of the gradient were performed as described for the associative gradients.

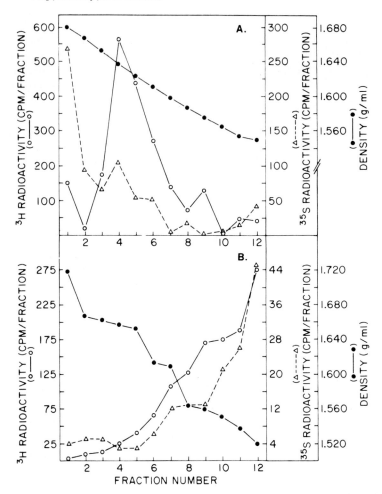

Fig. 9. Associative and dissociative isopycnic centrifugation of SAM from long-term ^{3}H-glucosamine, ^{35}SO$_4$ radiolabeled 3T3 cells. SAM from long-term ^{3}H-glucosamine/^{35}SO$_4$ radiolabeled 3T3 cells was extracted with 4.0 M guanidine hydrochloride, concentrated, and dialyzed to 0.4 M guanidine hydrochloride as described in Figure 8. Cesium chloride was added to this extract to a density of 1.63 g/ml and the mixture was centrifuged to equilibrium (A). Fractions 1–8 from A. were combined and made 4.0 M in guanidine hydrochloride. Cesium chloride was added to a density of 1.54 g/ml, and the mixture was centrifuged to equilibrium (B). Approximately 1 ml fractions were collected from the bottoms of the centrifuge tubes and the density (–●–●–), ^{3}H (–○–○–), and ^{35}S (–△–△–) radioactivity of each fraction were determined as described in Figure 8 [Rollins and Culp, Biochemistry, in press].

(fractions 3–7) but altered the appearance of the densest aggregate (fractions 1–2) (see Fig. 10B). This effect, although slight, was observed reproducibly in several experiments.

In cartilage [56], hyaluronic acid is a multivalent ligand, binding several proteoglycan subunits along its length. To assess the possible multivalency of hyaluronic acid in SAM, an aliquot of combined fractions 1–9 in Figure 10A was dissociated by adding an equal volume of 8.0 M guanidine hydrochloride. To this dissociated mixture was added 100 μg of HA-80, a hyaluronidase digestion product from hyaluronic acid consisting of approximately 80 repeating units. The size of this oligomer (a maximum of 0.003% of the size of

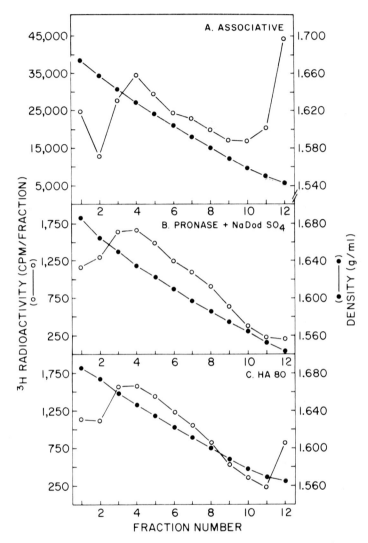

Fig. 10. Effect of Pronase digestion and HA80 on the behavior in isopycnic centrifugation of SAM from long-term ^{3}H-glucosamine radiolabeled SVT2 cells. SAM from long-term ^{3}H-glucosamine radiolabeled SVT2 cells was extracted with 4.0 M guanidine hydrochloride, dialyzed to associative conditions, and centrifuged to equilibrium in cesium chloride (A). Fractions 1–9 of this associative gradient were digested with Pronase and recentrifuged under associative conditions to give a profile indistinguishable from that seen in fractions 1–9 in A. This material was divided into two aliquots. One aliquot was made 0.2% in SDS and redigested with Pronase. This digest was dialyzed and recentrifuged (B). The other aliquot was made 4.0 M in guanidine hydrochloride, 100 μg HA80 were added, and the mixture was then dialyzed back to 0.4 M guanidine hydrochloride and recentrifuged (C). Fractions were collected and their densities (–●–●–) and content of ^{3}H radioactivity (–○–○–) were measured as described in Figure 8 [Rollins and Culp, Biochemistry, in press].

most of the hyaluronic acid in SAM) corresponds to the distance between attached proteoglycan subunits in the cartilage aggregate [56].

The dissociative mixture was kept at 4°C for 24 h, then dialyzed against 9 volumes of buffer to bring it back to associative conditions. This mixture was centrifuged as usual, and the result is shown in Figure 10C. A little less than 10% of the total radioactivity was found in the least dense fraction of the gradient, indicating a competitive effect of the HA-80 on aggregate formation. This effect was observed reproducibly in several experiments. This suggests that the HA-80 may have competed against cartilage-like aggregate formation in the higher density area of the gradient.

In cartilage, it has been elegantly shown that the formation of the protein–polysaccharide complex is due to interaction of the core protein of the chondroitin-keratin proteoglycan subunit with hyaluronic acid (an interaction further stabilized by another glycoprotein) [56–58]. All of the elements of the cartilage aggregate system (except the glycoprotein link) have been shown to be present in these lower gradient fractions of guanidine-extracted SAM. Furthermore, the addition of HA-80 to presumably aggregated material leads to the displacement of some of the formerly aggregated material from the densest gradient fractions. These results suggest, but by no means demonstrate, that a small proportion of the macromolecular aggregates in SAM may resemble cartilage proteoglycan aggregates. We are now examining this possibility by further experimentation.

The majority of complex formation in SAM, however, seems to be somewhat independent of the presence of intact protein. The behavior of the intermediate density fractions of SAM in isopycnic centrifugation is not altered by Pronase digestion either in the absence or the presence of SDS. The other major difference from the cartilage system is the striking enrichment for heparan sulfate in this intermediate-density material. Over 82% of all the carbohydrate in the fractions of density between 1.600 g/ml and 1.660 g/ml is heparan sulfate. The fact that 4.0 M guanidine hydrochloride can force nearly all of this material to band at densities less than 1.600 g/ml suggests that SAM contains polysaccharides that have the potential to form aggregates consisting mostly of heparan sulfate. Whether the heparan sulfate is combining with itself and/or other components to form these aggregates cannot be determined from these experiments.

The existence of aggregates in the high-density fractions of these associative gradients has not been rigorously demonstrated by this work. There are, however, precedents specifically involving heparin derivatives. Macromolecular heparin from rat skin [60] and native heparin from rat peritoneal mast cells [61] have been shown to be large molecular weight proteoglycans (1.1×10^6 mol wt and 750,000 mol wt, respectively) which are resistant to protease digestion (including Pronase) but are degraded to free carbohydrate chains by alkali and can be shown to contain xylose and serine. Thus the heparan sulfate in SAM could be engaging in protein-mediated interactions with itself or other components, and yet this protein would remain insensitive to protease treatment.

Alternatively, the observed aggregation phenomenon could be due to carbohydrate–carbohydrate interaction. If these interactions are mediated by hydrogen bonds, or if they depend in some way on specific conformations of the polysaccharides (some of which are known to be hydrogen bond-directed [57]), then guanidine hydrochloride should be able to disrupt the interactions by its ability to disrupt hydrogen bonding.

That SAM is not identical to cartilage is not surprising. The suggested interactions involving the heparan sulfate of SAM are, however, unique since, until now, no tissue system has been described in which "macromolecular" heparan sulfate of heparan sulfate proteoglycans are known to play a role. Whether this phenomenon is functionally related to the enrichment for heparan sulfate in the early adhesion site is unknown.

Protein—Polysaccharide Interrelationships in SAM

To examine further the structural and functional relationships between the various components of SAM, we have carried out digestion experiments with trypsin and hyaluronidase [15]. Trypsinization of SAM with purified TPCK-trypsin at low concentrations (1–10 μg/ml) for 15 min releases 70–80% of the ^{3}H-glucosamine-labeled polysaccharide but only 35–45% of the ^{3}H-leucine-labeled protein. Previous work has shown that most of the ^{3}H-glucosamine-labeled material in SAM is glycosaminoglycan [16]. These results were typical of both 48-hour-labeled (long-term) and 2-hour-labeled (short-term) SAM. Chemical analysis revealed that trypsinization selectively solubilizes hyaluronate and the chondroitins, whereas heparan sulfate is quite resistant to solubilization. Also, heparan sulfate in SAM is not exchangeable with exogenously added heparin [Culp, unpublished data], in contrast to the exchangeability observed for heparan sulfate on other regions of the cell surface [45].

SDS-PAGE analysis of the trypsin-resistant material from these cultures (Fig. 11) revealed that only a few leucine-labeled bands are selectively labile to trypsin treatment. The large GAP-1 band is lost selectively from both long-term and short-term preparations, even at very low trypsin concentrations (1 μg/ml); this band is associated chiefly with the chondroitins [15].

Fibronectin in SAM is not selectively labile to trypsin in long-term radiolabeled preparations, in contrast to the fibronectin found on other regions of the cell surface [2]; however, the metabolically labile, pulse-radiolabeled (short-term) fibronectin in this adhesive material is selectively labile to digestion. Consistent with this, the fibrillar pattern of immunofluorescence of fibronectin in SAM, which would be expected to reflect the properties chiefly of the more abundant, long-term radiolabeled fibronectin, is resistant to trypsin digestion under the conditions used here [Murray and Culp, unpublished data]. These results suggest that most of the fibronectin in SAM is contained within a highly resistant adhesive structure rich in heparan sulfate; however, *newly synthesized* fibronectin is present in a much more labile structure, along with hyaluronate and the chondroitins. Upon chasing pulse-radiolabeled cells with cold leucine before preparing SAM, some but not all of this fibronectin becomes incorporated into the resistant material [12, 15], again demonstrating the process of maturation that the adhesion sites undergo. However, these experiments could not address the question of the nature of the interaction between the fibronectin and the respective glycosaminoglycans, if any, since there are many other proteins in SAM whose digestion might disrupt a labile structure, releasing glycosaminoglycans and fibronectin.

We then turned to digestion with testicular hyaluronidase, which will digest hyaluronic acid and the chondroitins but not heparan sulfate. Hyaluronidase solubilized about half of the labeled polysaccharide in long-term or short-term labeled SAM, consistent with the glycosaminoglycan content of these preparations, but digested only 10–15% of the polysaccharide from reattaching-cell SAM, consistent with the high heparan sulfate content of this material. Hyaluronidase treatment released only about 10–15% of the labeled protein from long-term radiolabeled preparations, about 5% from short-term preparations, and almost none from reattachment preparations. Protein patterns on SDS-PAGE of resistant and soluble material from long-term labeled SAM are very similar to each other and to the

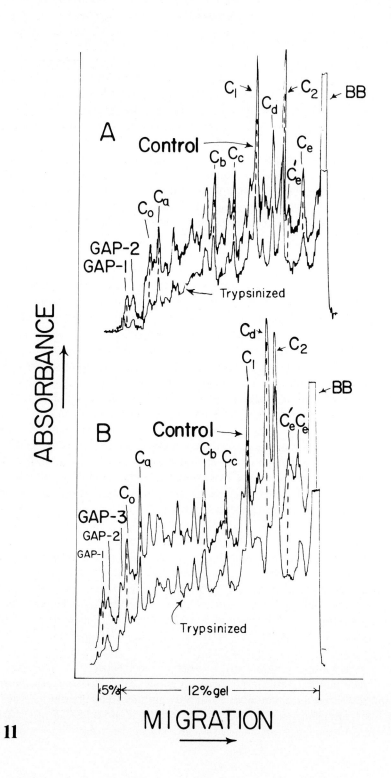

11

pattern of undigested material, with perhaps a slight enrichment in the C_0 band (fibronectin) in the released material. This may reflect a small amount of newly synthesized fibronectin in long-term labeled material (see below). Only small quantities (10% or less) of heparan sulfate, fibronectin, and cytoskeletal protein were solubilized under conditions which solubilized greater than 90% of the hyaluronate and the chondroitins [15]. Furthermore, immunofluorescence microscopy also showed that the (long-term) fibronectin in SAM is resistant to hyaluronidase digestion [Murray and Culp, unpublished data]. Interestingly, in short-term labeled material, the C_0 band was specifically and completely released by hyaluronidase digestion, and no radiolabeled cytoskeletal protein was released under these conditions.

Thus newly synthesized fibronectin is bound to SAM by a hyaluronidase-sensitive structure, perhaps in a cartilage-like proteoglycan, as discussed above. Unfortunately, because of the difficulty of obtaining heparan-sulfate-digesting enzymes of sufficient specificity and purity, we have not yet been able to carry out a similar analysis for the hyaluronidase-resistant heparan-sulfate-containing material.

A Model for Cell-Substratum Adhesion

The foregoing data and discussion suggest a tentative model of adhesion and a description of the molecular events occurring within the adhesion site (Fig. 12). During the early adhesive interaction with the substrate (< 1 h), no cell spreading has occurred, and the dependence of this interaction on metabolic activity or cytoskeletal function is minimal [18]. It is also during this period that SAM is strikingly enriched for heparan sulfate. The fact that heparin binds strongly and specifically to CIg [7] suggests that this initial adhesive interaction may involve cell-surface heparan sulfate acting as a cross-link between the cell-surface fibronectin [11, 62], and substrate-bound CIg (Fig. 12A). This correlates with all of the experimental indications to date that the cell-adhesion and spreading factor found in serum is CIg, as discussed earlier.

Over 72 h an accumulation of certain proteoglycan species occurs specifically in the adhesion site. There is a relative increase in the proportion of hyaluronic acid and of proteoglycans containing the galactosaminoglycans (dermatan sulfate and the chondroitins). (For concreteness, the proteoglycans in the model of Figure 12 are depicted as complexes analogous to the proteoglycans found in cartilage [56, 57], but as discussed earlier, this form of organization is by no means established for the SAM proteoglycans.) This accumulation could be the chemical reflection of the physiological maturation that the footpad undergoes as it loosens its connections with the cell body to become a footprint [1, 63]. The mechanism whereby such an accumulation of polysaccharide might weaken the foot-

---

Fig. 11. SDS-PAGE analyses of trypsin-treated SAM. SAM was prepared from SVT2 cultures grown for 48 h (A) or 2 h (B) in radioactive leucine-containing medium. Control preparations received no trypsin, whereas trypsinized preparations were treated with 5 μg/ml for 15 min at 37°C. Trypsin activity was destroyed with soybean trypsin inhibitor and PMSF and SAMs were isolated for SDS-PAGE analyses as described elsewhere [11, 15]. 10,000 cpm of SAM of control (48 h), control (2 h), and trypsinized (2 h) samples were electrophoresed in adjacent wells of a slab gel, whereas only 6,000 cpm of the trypsinized (48 h) sample was used; the gel was fluorographed. Various proteins are identified in the legend to Figure 2 or in the text. Treatment with trypsin concentrations varying between 0.25 and 10 μg/ml generated the pattern differences shown here (reprinted from reference 15 with permission of the publisher).

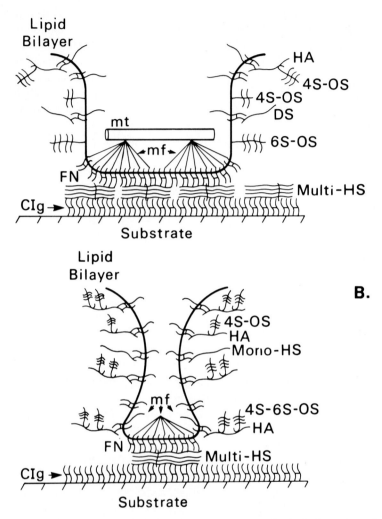

Fig. 12. Model of cell-substrate adhesion. Identifiable components of a single footpad are shown in the newly formed adhesion site of reattaching cells (A) and in the fully matured adhesion site just before the cell breaks its connection with the footpad (B). See text for details. Multi-HS, macromolecular or proteoglycan heparin sulfate multivalent for fibronectin; mono-HS, heparin sulfate chains monovalent for fibronection; FN, fibronectin; CIg, cold-insoluble globulin; 6S-OS, undersulfated chondroitin 6-sulfate proteoglycan; 4S-OS, undersulfated chondroitin 4-sulfate proteoglycan; 4S-6S-OS, incompletely sulfated chondroitin 4-sulfate and chondroitin 6-sulfate proteoglycan; DS, dermatan sulfate; HA, hyaluronic acid; mf, microfilaments; mt, microtubule.

pad remains obscure, but a suggested model is shown in Figure 12B. If hyaluronic acid and the galactosaminoglycan-containing proteoglycans are monovalent in their interaction with fibronectin, then during their accumulation in the adhesion site, they may be able to compete with multivalent heparan sulfate for binding to fibronectin. Monovalent heparan sulfate chains could act in the same manner. If fibronectin is connected in some wasy to the cell's cytoskeletal apparatus [41], such a competition could lead to a localized destabilization of this apparatus and subsequent pinching off of the footpad.

There are several examples of systems in which stimuli for cell growth, movement, and detachment are correlated with hyaluronic acid accumulation, consistent with the proposed model [64, 65]. Conversely, cessation of growth and movement has been observed to be accompanied by a decrease in hyaluronic acid production [66, 67]. Furthermore, Kraemer and his colleagues have isolated CHO cell variants in which the strength of cell-substratum adhesion is inversely correlated with the capacity to synthesize hyaluronic acid [68–70]. One subline is resistant to detachment from the substratum and synthesizes little or no hyaluronic acid, as well as reduced amounts of other complex carbohydrates at the cell periphery [68, 69]. Conversely, an easily detached variant has three times more detectable label in surface hyaluronic acid than does the parent cell [69]. Furthermore, in the parent CHO cell, an anchorage-dependent Chinese hamster cell line, the synthesis and deposition of hyaluronic acid into cell surface material is stimulated by cell attachment to and growth on a solid substratum [70]. All of these results are consistent with the negative modulatory role of hyaluronic acid (and some proteoglycans) in physiologically mature footpads proposed in our model.

In this model, then, the differences in adhesive strength between nontransformed and transformed cells could be explained in two ways. One possibility is that the adhesion sites of transformed cells accumulate more hyaluronic acid, galactosaminoglycan, and monovalent heparan sulfate, or less fibronectin, than do the adhesion sites of nontransformed cells. This would lead to a greater degree of cytoskeletal depolymerization and greater ease of detachment of transformed cells. However, we found no such differences between SAM prepared from transformed and nontransformed cell lines.

The other possibility is a defect in cytoskeletal organization or attachment to the membrane [71, 72]. Immunofluorescence and electron micrographic studies suggest that the cytoskeleton is, indeed, less well organized in transformed cells than in nontransformed cells [73–75]. Thus the material in SAM that actually effects adhesion of the cell surface to the substrate might be expected to be conserved in both normal and transformed cells, since both cell types are adhesive. Such conservation was, in fact, observed.

We believe that our model provides a reasonable interpretation for the available experimental evidence on cell-substratum adhesion, but many points clearly remain to be established. In particular, we are examining the physical and biochemical interactions between fibronectin and the proteoglycans and glycosaminoglycans in SAM, and we are examining more closely the roles of cell-surface-bound and substratum-bound fibronectin in the structure and function of SAM. Such studies should clarify the actual relationships between the various macromolecular components of SAM and may pave the way for a detailed molecular description of the cell-substratum adhesion site.

ACKNOWLEDGMENTS

We thank Josefina Buniel, Sara Hitri, and Riva Ansbacher for technical assistance, Dr. Martha Cathcart and Dr. Robert Haas for data and discussions, and Dr. Judy Schollmeyer for supplying results prior to publication. Dr. Richard Robson generously supplied samples of porcine skeletal muscle and chicken gizzard α-actinins. This work was supported in part by American Cancer Society research grant BC-217, National Cancer Institute research grant CA13513, and National Institute of Arthritis Metabolic and Digestive Diseases research grant AM 25646. Dr. Lloyd A. Culp was a Career Development Awardee of the

National Cancer Institute (CA70709). Ben A. Murray and Barrett J. Rollins were supported by U.S. Public Health Service Training grants GM 07225 and GM 07250, respectively.

NOTE ADDED IN PROOF

We now have additional evidence for fibronectin:proteoglycan binding in adhesion sites by examining the ability of GAGs isolated from substrate-attached material to bind to CIG-Sepharose columns. Most of the heparan sulfate in SAM binds very well to CIG, whereas the unsulfated and sulfated chondroitins do not bind [J. Laterra and L. Culp, unpublished data] . This supports the conclusion that multivalent heparan proteoglycans are direct mediators of the adhesive bond (Fig. 12).

REFERENCES

1. Culp LA: Curr Topics Memb Transport 11:327, 1978.
2. Hynes RO: Biochim Biophys Acta 458:73, 1976.
3. Yamada KM, Olden K: Nature 275:179, 1978.
4. Grinnell F: Int Rev Cytol 53:65, 1978.
5. Engvall E, Ruoslahti E: Int J Cancer 20:1, 1977.
6. Ruoslahti E, Vuento M, Engvall E: Biochim Biophys Acta 534:210, 1978.
7. Stathakis NE, Mosesson MW: J Clin Invest 60:855, 1977.
8. Grinnell F, Hays DG: Exp Cell Res 116:275, 1978.
9. Culp LA, Black PH: Biochemistry 11:2161, 1972.
10. Rosen JJ, Culp LA: Exp Cell Res 107:139, 1977.
11. Culp LA: Biochemistry 15:4094, 1976.
12. Rollins BJ, Culp LA: Biochemistry 18:141, 1979.
13. Culp LA, Bensusan H: Nature 273:680, 1978.
14. Cathcart MK, Culp LA: Biochemistry 18:1167, 1979.
15. Culp LA, Rollins BJ, Buniel J, Hitri S: J Cell Biol 79:788, 1978.
16. Terry AH, Culp LA: Biochemistry 13:414, 1974.
17. Culp LA: Exp Cell Res 92:467, 1975.
18. Mapstone TB, Culp LA: J Cell Sci 20:479, 1976.
19. Culp LA, Terry AH, Buniel JF: Biochemistry 14:406, 1975.
20. Culp LA, Buniel JF, Rosen JJ: In Harmon RE (ed): "Cell Surface Carbodydrate Chemistry." New York: Academic Press, 1978, p 205.
21. Culp LA: J Supramol Struct 5:239, 1976.
22. Harris AK: Dev Biol 35:97, 1973.
23. Revel JP, Hoch P, Ho D: Exp Cell Res 84:207, 1974.
24. Revel JP, Wolken K: Exp Cell Res 78:1, 1973.
25. Badley RA, Lloyd CW, Woods A, Carruthers L, Allcock C, Rees DA: Exp Cell Res 117:231, 1978.
26. Whur P, Koppel H, Urquhart CM, Williams DC: J Cell Sci 24:265, 1977.
27. Vessey AR, Culp LA: Virology 86:556, 1978.
28. Suzuki A, Goll DE, Singh I, Allen RE, Robson RM, Stromer MH: J Biol Chem 251:6860, 1976.
29. Mooseker MA, Tilney LG: J Cell Biol 67:725, 1975.
30. Lazarides E: J Cell Biol 68:202, 1976.
31. Brown S, Levinson W, Spudich JA: J Supramol Struct 5:119, 1976.
32. Starger JM, Goldman RD: Proc Natl Acad Sci USA 74:2422, 1977.
33. Hynes RO, Destree AT: Cell 13:151, 1978.
34. O'Farrell PH: J Biol Chem 250:4007, 1975.
35. Hynes RO, Destree A: Proc Natl Acad Sci USA 74:2855, 1977.
36. Whalen RG, Butler-Browne GS, Gros F: Proc Natl Acad Sci USA 73:2018, 1976.
37. Garrels JI, Gibson W: Cell 9:793, 1976.
38. Kuusela P, Ruoslahti E, Engvall E, Vaheri A: Immunochemistry 13:639, 1976.
39. Axelsen NH, Krøll J, Weeke B (eds): Scand J Immunol 2 (Suppl 1), 1973.

40. Olden K, Yamada KM: Anal Biochem 78:483, 1977.
41. Mautner V, Hynes RO: J Cell Biol 75:743, 1978.
42. Hedman K, Vaheri A, Wartiovaara J: J Cell Biol 76:748, 1978.
43. Albrecht-Buehler G: Cell 11:395, 1977.
44. Thom D, Powell AJ, Badley RA, Woods A, Smith CG, Rees DA: Ann NY Acad Sci 312:453, 1978.
45. Kraemer PM: Biochem Biophys Res Commun 78:1334, 1977.
46. Klebe RJ: Nature 250:248, 1974.
47. Pearlstein E: Nature 262:497, 1976.
48. Hynes RO, Destree AT, Mautner VM, Ali IU: J Supramol Struct 7:397, 1977.
49. Vaheri A, Kurkinen M, Lehto V-P, Linder E, Timpl R: Proc Natl Acad Sci USA 75:4944, 1978.
50. Pessac B, Defendi V: Science 175:898, 1972.
51. Underhill C, Dorfman A: Exp Cell Res 117:155, 1978.
52. Roblin R, Albert SO, Gelb NA, Black PH: Biochemistry 14:347, 1975.
53. Gail MH, Boone CW: Exp Cell Res 70:33, 1972.
54. Hardingham TE, Muir HE: Biochim Biophys Acta 279:401, 1972.
55. Hascall VC, Heinegård D: J Biol Chem 249:4232, 1974.
56. Hascall VC: J Supramol Struct 7:101, 1977.
57. Lindahl U, Höök M: Ann Rev Biochem 47:385, 1978.
58. Sajdera SW, Hascall VC: J Biol Chem 244:77, 1969.
59. Hascall VC, Sajdera SW: J Biol Chem 244:2384, 1969.
60. Horner AA: J Biol Chem 246:231, 1971.
61. Yurt RW, Leid RW Jr, Austen KF, Silbert JE: J Biol Chem 252:518, 1977.
62. Kleinman HK, McGoodwin EB, Klebe RJ: Biochem Biophys Res Commun 72:426, 1976.
63. Chen W-T: J Cell Biol 75:416a, 1977.
64. Tomida M, Koyama H, Ono T: J Cell Physiol 86:121, 1975.
65. Lembach KJ: J Cell Physiol 89:277, 1976.
66. Morris CC: Ann NY Acad Sci 86:179, 1960.
67. Tomida M, Koyama H, Ono T: Biochim Biophys Acta 338:352, 1974.
68. Atherly AG, Barnhart BJ, Kraemer PM: J Cell Physiol 90:375, 1977.
69. Barnhart BJ, Cox SH, Kraemer PM: (in preparation).
70. Kraemer PM, Barnhart BJ: Exp Cell Res 114:153, 1978.
71. Rees DA, Lloyd CW, Thom D: Nature 267:124, 1977.
72. Edelman GM: Science 192:218, 1976.
73. Willingham MC, Yamada KM, Yamada SS, Pouysségur J, Pastan I: Cell 10:375, 1977.
74. McNutt NS, Culp LA, Black PH: J Cell Biol 50:691, 1971.
75. McNutt NS, Culp LA, Black PH: J Cell Biol 56:412, 1973.

Journal of Supramolecular Structure 11:467–476 (1979)
Tumor Cell Surfaces and Malignancy 309–318

Growth Rate and Chromosome Number of Tumor Cell Lines With Different Metastatic Potential

Maria A. Cifone, Margaret L. Kripke, and Isaiah J. Fidler

Cancer Biology Program, NCI Frederick Cancer Research Center, Frederick, Maryland 21701

We investigated whether the metastatic potential of various tumor cell lines was related to chromosome counts or to rate of growth in vitro or in vivo. Clones of known metastatic potential derived from a C3H⁻ fibrosarcoma induced by UV radiation (UV-2237) and from C57BL/6 B16 melanoma were tested for these characteristics. No correlation was found between the growth rate of these clones in monolayer culture or at a subcutaneous site and their ability to produce metastases. The cells from clones of UV-2237 were mainly in the diploid range with only one exception, and the B16 clones were all hyperploid. Thus, there was also no correlation between malignant behavior of the clones and gross changes in chromosome number.

Key words: metastatic potential, growth rates, chromosome number and range

Clinical and morphologic observations of human neoplasia have suggested that tumors may progress from benign to malignant behavior over a period of time [1–4]. The progression of evolution of a tumor has been attributed to the emergence of new variant cells that have a selective advantage for growth in vivo. It has been suggested that such variants have an increased growth rate and that they also have an abnormal number of chromosomes [5–8]. In general, benign (noninvasive, nonmetastasizing) tumors are thought to be well-differentiated and to grow slowly; mitotic figures are infrequent, and those present are usually normal. In contrast, malignant (metastasizing) tumors are usually undifferentiated and consist of a large number of dividing cells. These dividing cells may have many abnormal chromosomes and higher chromosome numbers, and they may exhibit varying degrees of anaplasia [4].

Despite numerous observations, it is still unclear whether an increased growth rate or change in chromosome number are requisite for the progression of tumors from a benign to a malignant state. This issue cannot be resolved by morphologic examination of clinical specimens, nor can studies be performed on a variety of tumors of different histologic types and of possible different etiologies obtained from different donors. Instead, studies must be performed on neoplastic cell lines isolated from a single neoplasm

Received March 18, 1979; accepted July 26, 1979.

that have defined biologic behavior in vivo. Recent cloning studies demonstrated that two murine neoplasms, the C57BL/6 B16 melanoma [9] and a C3H⁻ fibrosarcoma induced by ultraviolet (UV) radiation [10] are heterogeneous and contain subpopulations of cells with differing capacities for metastasis. These clones breed true upon recloning. The availability of these clones, which vary in their metastatic behavior in vivo, affords us an opportunity to investigate which properties of cloned tumor cell populations are associated with metastasis. In these experiments we wished to determine whether the metastatic potential of a variety of tumor cell clones was associated with an abnormal chromosome number and/or with a rapid growth rate, as measured in animals or in cell cultures.

MATERIALS AND METHODS

Animals

Specific-pathogen-free C57BL/6 and C3H/HeN (MTV⁻) (C3H⁻) mice were obtained from the Animal Production Area of the Frederick Cancer Research Center. Within a single experiment all mice were age- and sex-matched.

Cell Cultures

The B16 melanoma, which arose in a C57BL/6 mouse, was established in culture as described previously [11, 12]. In the present studies we used in vitro cloned lines derived from our B16 parent culture [9]. The UV-2237 is a fibrosarcoma that was induced by chronic UV irradiation of a female C3H− mouse. The tumor was established in culture from the first in vivo passage in immunosuppressed syngeneic mice, and cells of the sixth in vitro passage were cloned as previously reported. All cell lines were grown as monolayers on plastic flasks in MEM Autopow medium (Flow Laboratories, Rockville, Maryland) supplemented with 10% fetal calf serum (FCS), glutamine, nonessential amino acids and vitamins designated as complete minimum essential medium (CMEM) (Grand Island Biological Co., Grand Island, New York). The cultures were maintained at 37°C in a humidified incubator in an atmosphere containing 5% CO_2. All cell lines were examined and found free of Mycoplasma [13] and the following murine viruses: reovirus type 3, pneumonia virus of mice, K virus, Theiler's virus, Sendai virus, minute virus of mice, mouse adenovirus, mouse hepatitis virus, lymphocytic choriomeningitis virus, ectromelia virus, and lactate dehydrogenase virus (Microbiological Associates, Walkersville, Maryland). In order to assure reproducibility between in vivo and in vitro assays the cultures were tested within 2 weeks after recovery from frozen stocks.

The tumor cells were harvested from subconfluent cultures (50–70% confluent) by rinsing the monolayers with 0.25% trypsin–0.02% versene solution. After 1 min, the flasks were tapped sharply to dislodge the monolayers, and the cells were washed in CMEM with 10% FCS. The cells were resuspended in Hanks's balanced salt solution (HBSS) for counting and injection. Only suspensions containing single cells of > 90% viability were used for injection.

Experimental Pulmonary Metastasis

Unanesthetized mice were inoculated IV via the tail vein with 0.2 ml of 5×10^4 (B16) or 1×10^5 (UV-2237) viable single tumor cells suspended in HBSS. All mice were killed 18 days after tumor cell injection, and their lungs were removed, rinsed in water, and fixed in formalin (B16) or Bouin's fixative (UV-2237). The number of lung tumor colonies was determined by counting surface metastases under a dissecting microscope,

since most experimental metastases in mice are located at the surface of the lung [14].
Metastases were counted in a blind fashion by two observers.

In Vitro Growth Rate Determinations

Cell lines were plated at a density of 10^4 cells per 60-mm plastic petri dish (Falcon Plastics, Oxnard, California). Duplicate cultures were trypsinized, and the number of cells per dish was determined every 24 h for 5 days with a Coulter Counter (Coulter Electronics, Inc., Hialeah, Florida).

Tumor Growth in Vivo

C3H$^-$ mice (8 weeks old) were injected subcutaneously with 10^6 cells of the UV-2237 fibrosarcoma clones (5 mice per group). The tumors were measured with a caliper once a week in three diameters, and the average tumor diameter was determined for each animal.

Chromosome Analysis

Tumor cells were plated at 10^6 per 100-mm plastic petri dish, and 24–36 h later the cultures were incubated with 1 μg/ml Colcemid (Calbiochem, La Jolla, California). At the end of 2 h at 37°C, the cells were trypsinized (0.25% trypsin–0.02% EDTA), centrifuged, and resuspended in 0.075 M KCl for 45 min. Samples were fixed three times in methanol-acetic acid (3:1) and then resuspended in this fixative. The fixed cells were dropped onto slides. Chromosome counts from at least 100 cells were made on each cell line. The differences in chromosome numbers were analyzed by Student's t test, the Mann-Whitney U test, and the Median test.

RESULTS

Tumor Growth Rate vs Metastatic Potential

Clones of the B16 melanoma were classified as having low, intermediate, or high metastatic potential. These categories were based on the number of macroscopic tumor colonies present in the lungs of syngeneic mice injected IV 18 days earlier with 5×10^4 tumor cells. The clones of low metastatic potential (clone numbers 16, 15, and 12) produced less than a median of seven lung colonies in groups of ten recipients, the intermediate parent B16 line gave 40 lung colonies, and the highly metastatic clone (number 9) produced more than 500 tumor colonies per recipient (Table I).

Clones of the UV-2237 fibrosarcoma were also classified as having low, intermediate, or high metastatic potential based on the number of tumor colonies present in the lungs of mice injected IV 18 days earlier with 1×10^5 tumor cells. In this tumor system the formation of lung metastases correlates with the formation of extrapulmonary metastases and with the formation of spontaneous metastases from subcutaneously growing tumors [10]. The clones of low metastatic potential (numbers 15 and 38) produced less than a median of two lung colonies in groups of ten recipients. The highly metastatic clones (numbers 39 and 25) produced more than 135 tumor colonies per recipient. Intermediate clones form a continuous series between clones which are obviously "low" and those which are obviously "high."

In spite of the wide variation of metastatic behavior of the B16 or UV-2237 clones, the doubling times of these cell lines in monolayer culture did not differ significantly from each other (Tables II, III). For UV-2237 clones, the doubling times ranged from 17 to 24 h, and there was no positive correlation between short doubling time and high metastatic potential (Table III).

TABLE I. Quantitative Lung Colony Assay With B16 Melanoma or UV-2237 Fibrosarcoma Clones

Syngeneic[a] recipients	Tumor source	Median number (range) of pulmonary metastases
C57BL/6	B16 parent[b]	40.5 (8–131)
	Clone 15	5 (2– 20)
	Clone 16	3.5 (0– 15)
	Clone 12	6 (0– 34)
	Clone 9	>500
C3H–	UV-2237 parent[c]	160.5 (17–300)
	Clone 38	2 (0– 8)
	Clone 15	1 (0– 9)
	Clone 42	5 (0– 39)
	Clone 43	9.5 (0– 78)
	Clone 26	25.5 (4–212)
	Clone 39	135 (85–248)
	Clone 25	140.5 (79–300)

[a]10 mice/group. Mice were injected IV and killed 18 days later. The number of lung tumor colonies was determined with a dissecting microscope.
[b]5×10^4 viable cells injected IV (see Fidler and Kripke [9]).
[c]1×10^5 viable cells injected IV (see Kripke et al [10]).

TABLE II. In Vitro Growth Rate of B16 Melanoma Parent and Cloned Lines of Varying Metastatic Potential

Tumor lines	Metastatic potential[a]	Doubling time[b] (hours)
B16 Clone 16	Low	12.4
B16 Clone 15	Low	13.5
B16 Clone 12	Low	12.2
B16 Parent	Intermediate	12.4
B16 Clone 9	High	12.4

[a]Based on the number of pulmonary tumor colonies present at 21 days in mice injected IV with 5×10^4 cells [9].
[b]Doubling times calculated form the slope of a 96-h growth curve of cells in logarithmic growth. The differences in doubling time were not significant within a confidence limit of 95%.

Since the growth rate of tumor cells in culture need not reflect the rate of growth of the cells in an animal host, we also measured the growth rate of the tumors at a subcutaneous site in syngeneic mice. Again there was no direct relationship between the average tumor size at various weeks and the metastatic behavior of the tumors (Table III). Clones of low metastatic potential also exhibited a slow growth rate subcutaneously; however, the rapid growth of tumors subcutaneously was not necessarily associated with high metastatic potential. For example, clone 25, which is highly metastatic, grew more slowly than the less metastatic clone 43.

TABLE III. In Vitro and In Vivo Growth Rates of UV-2237 Fibrosarcoma Clones of Different Metastatic Potential

Clone No.	Metastatic potential[a]	Doubling time[b]	Tumor incidence at following weeks after subcutaneous injection[c]		
			1	2	3
38	Low	17.4	0/5 (0)	0/5 (0)	1/5 (1 ± 1)
15	Low	20.3	0/5 (0)	1/5 (2.2 ± 0.9)	3/5 (3.1 ± 1.3)
43	Intermediate	18.7	4/5 (4.5 ± 1.1)	5/5 (8.0 ± 0.6)	5/5 (11.1 ± 0.6)
39	High	21.7	0/5 (0)	5/5 (5.4 ± 0.6)	5/5 (9.4 ± 2.4)
25	High	24.4	1/5 (0.8 ± 0.8)	3/5 (2.8 ± 1.1)	5/5 (4.8 ± 1.1)

[a]See text for details.

[b]Doubling times in hours calculated from the slope of a 120-h growth curve (cells in logarithmic growth). There were no statistically significant differences among the clones within a confidence limit of 95%.

[c]Average tumor diameter in mm ± SE measured at weekly intervals after the subcutaneous injection of 10^6 cells into syngeneic mice (five mice per group).

Chromosome Patterns vs Metastatic Potential

To determine whether clones of different metastatic potential also differed in chromosome number, we processed clones of UV-2237 and B16 for chromosome counts. Typical chromosome spreads are shown in Figure 1. Clone 43 of UV-2237 is shown at the top of Figure 1 and clone 15 of B16 is at the bottom. None of the UV-2237 clones show gross chromosomal abnormalities. All of the B16 clones examined have four abnormal chromosomes which are metacentric. The chromosome number of several B16 melanoma clones and parental tumor was examined. The mode and range of chromosome number was very similar. For example, for the parental tumor the mode was 79 with a range of 65–88. For clone 15 (low metastatic) the mode was 74 and chromosome range was 68–80. For the highly metastatic clone 9, chromosome mode was 75 and the range was 67–80.

Since the UV-2237 clones are very stable (at least up to 2 months of continuous culture) with regard to their metastatic behavior in vivo (Cifone, unpublished data), extensive chromosome studies were carried out with these clones. One hundred or more spreads were counted per clone. All spreads of a given clone were prepared at the same time from cultures grown for no longer than 7 days after recovery from frozen stocks. The mode and range of the chromosome numbers of the lines are shown in Table IV. With one exception (clone 38), neither the modes of the different clones (which were very similar) nor the differences in ranges (as seen in column 4) correlate with metastasis. Clone 38 exhibits a very different chromosome pattern from the others, ie, hyperploidy, with a wide range in chromosome number (Fig. 2c). Nonetheless, clone 38 is virtually nonmetastasizing. The ranges in chromosome number from at least 100 cells of clones 25 and 15 (highest and lowest metastatic potential, respectively) are indistinguishable, as shown in Figure 2. The data for the UV-2237 clones were analyzed statistically, and no individual clone differed significantly from the general population of all clones (except clone 38) by either the Student t test, the Mann-Whitney test, or the Median test.

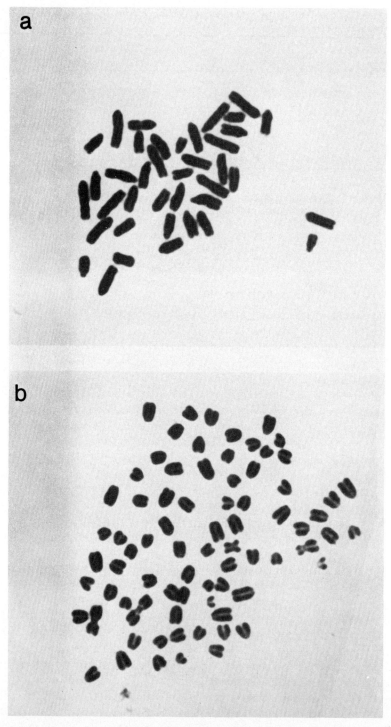

Fig. 1. Metaphase of UV-2237 and B16 lines. a: UV-2237 clone 43 (× 1,000); b: B16 clone 15 (× 1,000).

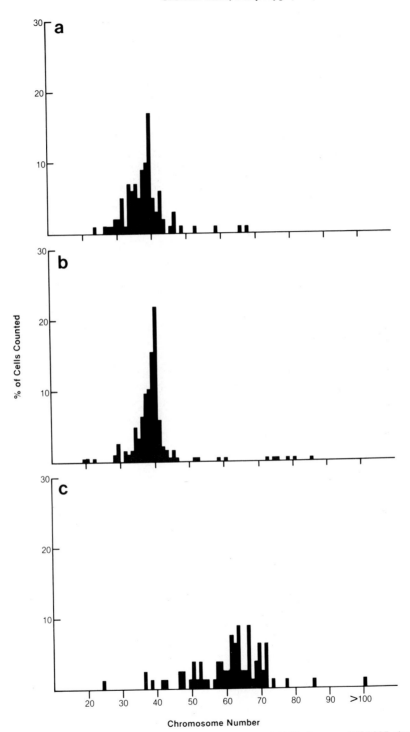

Fig. 2. Distribution of chromosome numbers of three UV-2237 clones. a: UV-2237 clone 15; b: UV-2237 clone 25; c: UV-2237 clone 38.

TABLE IV. Chromosome Mode and Range of UV-2237 Fibrosarcoma Clones With Different Metastatic Potential

		Percentage of cells at the mode	
Clone No.	Metastatic potential	Chromosome mode[a]	Chromosome range[a]
15	Low	39	23–68
38	Low	61–66	24–> 100
42	Low	40	21–71
31	Intermediate	39	27–72
26	Intermediate	41	19–63
25	High	40	19–85

[a]Average of 100 or more chromosome spreads per clone. Where no definite mode is apparent, a range where the highest percentage of chromosomes occurs is given.

DISCUSSION

These studies were designed to evaluate whether the metastatic potential of cloned murine tumor cell lines correlated with a deviation in chromosome number and/or an accelerated growth rate in vivo or in vitro. Many investigators have attempted to determine whether a change in chromosome number from diploidy is associated with the neoplastic malignant transformation of normal cells. Although the DNA content and chromosome number of neoplastic cells often differ from that of normal cells, such changes are by no means characteristic of all tumors. In fact, in some tumor cells no such abnormalities can be demonstrated [5–8]. In some systems chromosome alterations also occur in the later stages of tumor progression [6, 7, 15, 16]. Even with tumors that were found to be aneuploid initially, additional chromosome changes were observed that were associated with an increased growth rate [6, 7, 17]. Thus, a change in chromsome number from diploidy to aneuploidy has been implicated in the progression of tumors to a malignant stage. The progression to malignancy, however, is not always associated with an increase in mean chromosome number. The chromosome number of cells obtained from different patients with either dysplasia, carcinoma in situ, or invasive carcinoma of the cervix was determined, and a decrease in the mean chromosome number was associated with the progression of tumors from carcinoma in situ to invasive carcinoma [16].

Our analysis of the chromosome number of cloned populations of cells with differing metastatic potential reveals no correlation between metastasis and chromosome number and range. The one case of hyperploidy, observed in cells of UV-2237 clone 38, was not associated with a high metastatic potential, since clone 38 does not metastasize. Further, hyperploidy was not required for nonmetastatic behavior, because UV-2237 clones 15 and 42, which are also nonmetastasizing, are near diploid. In the case of the B16 melanoma, cells with either low or high metastatic potential were hyperploid. Thus, systematic alterations in chromosome number were not associated with metastatic behavior in the two tumor systems that we studied. It is important to note that the analysis used here (chromosome counts) is indeed gross. Systematic changes in chromosomes of metastatic cells could perhaps be demonstrated by more sophisticated techniques such as chromosome banding. In some tumor systems, such as murine lymphoma induced by radiation leukemia virus [18] and a murine T-cell leukemia induced by 7, 12-

dimethylbenz-(a)-anthracene [19], constant chromosome changes, ie, trisomies No. 15, No. 17, and trisomy No. 15, respectively, were associated with neoplastic cells. In contrast, consistent chromosomal changes were not reported in earlier studies of nine primary and 14 transplanted rat leukemias and lymphomas [20]. Therefore, if changes more subtle than chromosome number and range are indeed associated with increased malignancy, they were not detected here.

An increased growth rate could be responsible for the eventual dominance of tumor variants with an increasingly malignant character. We tested this possibility by measuring the growth rates in vitro of a variety of cell lines from two different tumor systems and comparing them with the metastatic behavior of these tumor lines. No correlation was detected between these parameters in either tumor system. However, measuring the doubling time of cells in vitro does not take into account the possible involvement of host factors that could alter the rate of tumor growth. For this reason, we also measured the rate of growth of several UV-2237 clones in syngeneic mice. As expected, there was no direct correlation between growth rate of a cell line in vivo and its doubling time in vitro. Furthermore, there was no simple relationship between metastatic behavior of the cell lines and their growth rate in animals. Although the nonmetastatic clones grew slowly in animals after subcutaneous injection, the highly metastatic clones did not necessarily grow more rapdily in vivo.

In summary, we did not find a correlation between increasing malignancy and gross changes in chromosome number or tumor growth rate. Although these parameters may be associated with malignant progression in some instances, it does not appear that such changes are requisite for the progression of murine fibrosarcoma or melanoma tumors from a benign to a malignant phenotype.

ACKNOWLEDGMENTS

This research was sponsored by the National Cancer Institute under contract No. NO1-CO-75380 with Litton Bionetics, Inc.

We thank Mr. C. Riggs and Ms. Lenita Thibault for their help in the statistical analysis of the data and Ms. Joan Connors for her technical assistance.

REFERENCES

1. Foulds I: "Neoplastic Development." New York: Academic, 1969, pp 69–75.
2. Klein G, Klein E: Proc Natl Acad Sci USA 74:2121, 1977.
3. Medina D: In Becker FF (ed): "Cancer: A Comprehensive Treatise." New York: Plenum, 1975, vol 3, pp 149–250.
4. Prehn RT: In LaVia MF, Hill RB (eds): "Principles of Pathobiology." London: Oxford University Press, 1975, pp 203–245.
5. Koller P: "The Role of Chromosomes in Cancer Biology." Recent Results in Cancer Research Series. New York: Springer-Verlag, 1972, p 38.
6. Nowell PC: In Becker FF (ed): "Cancer: A Comprehensive Treatise." New York: Plenum, 1975, vol 1, pp 3–31.
7. Nowell PC: Science 194:23, 1976.
8. Wolman SR, Horland AA: In Becker FF (ed): "Cancer: A Comprehensive Treatise." New York: Plenum 1975, vol 3, pp 155–198.
9. Fidler IJ, Kripke ML: Science 197:893, 1977.
10. Kripke ML, Gruys E, Fidler IJ: Cancer Res 38:2962, 1978.
11. Fidler IJ: Nature New Biol 242:148, 1973.
12. Fidler IJ: Cancer Res 25:218, 1975.

13. Fel Giudice RA, Hopps HE: In McGarrity GJ et al (eds): "Mycoplasma Infection of Cell Cultures." New York: Plenum, 1978, pp 57–69.
14. Fidler IJ: In Busch H (ed): "Methods in Cancer Research." New York: Academic, 1978, vol 15, pp 399–439.
15. Al-Saadi A, Beierwaltes WH: Cancer Res 27:1831, 1967.
16. Cellier KM, Kirkland JA, Stanley MA: J Natl Cancer Inst 44:21, 1970.
17. Nowell PC, Morris HP, Potter VR: Cancer Res 27:1565, 1967.
18. Weiner F, Ohno S, Spira J, Haran-Ghera N, Klein G: J Natl Cancer Inst 60:227, 1978.
19. Weiner F, Spira J, Ohno S, Haran-Ghera N, Klein G: Int J Cancer 22:447, 1978.
20. Mori M, Sasaki M: J Natl Cancer Inst 52:153, 1974.

Journal of Supramolecular Structure 11:477–483
Tumor Cell Surfaces and Malignancy 319–325

Cholesterol Levels and Plasma Membrane Fluidity in 3T3 and SV101-3T3 Cells

Carl J. Scandella, James A. Hayward, and Nancy Lee

Department of Biochemistry, State University of New York, Stony Brook, New York, 11794

Polyene antibiotics such as filipin selectively inhibit wheat germ agglutinin-induced agglutination of transformed and malignant cells compared to normal cells (Hatten ME, Burger MM: Biochemistry 18:739, 1979). Since filipin binds specifically to cholesterol, we measured cholesterol levels in 3T3 cells and SV101-3T3 cells. SV101-3T3 cells contained 50–100% more cholesterol per cell than 3T3 cells. Both cell types were starved for cholesterol by growth in lipid-depleted medium plus 25-hydroxycholesterol. The cholesterol level of SV101-3T3 cells decreased by 30–50%, while the level in 3T3 cells remained constant. Filipin-stained SV101-3T3 cells revealed bright patches of filipin under fluorescence microscopy. These patches were absent in 3T3 cells and in SV101-3T3 and 3T3 cells starved for cholesterol. We selectively labeled plasma membranes of these cells with a spin label analog of phosphatidylcholine. The spin label indicated differences in plasma membrane fluidity that may be related to the different cholesterol levels in 3T3 and SV101-3T3 cells.

Key words: virus transformation, membrane fluidity, plasma membrane, filipin, cholesterol, spin label, lectin agglutination

Hatten and Burger [1] found that polyene antibiotics such as filipin inhibit wheat germ agglutinin-induced agglutination of transformed or tumor cells but not normal cells. In addition, transformed cells are more sensitive to lysis by filipin. The polyene antibiotics bind specifically to membrane cholesterol [2]. The intrinsic fluorescence of filipin allows one to visualize bound filipin by fluorescence microscopy. Transformed or tumor cells stained with filipin reveal fluorescent patches, while normal cells stain diffusely. These observations prompted us to investigate cholesterol levels in mouse fibroblasts (Swiss 3T3) and their SV-40 virus-transformed derivative, SV101-3T3.

Received April 24, 1979; accepted July 25, 1979.

We find that SV101-3T3 cells have 50–100% more cholesterol per cell than 3T3 cells. The regulation of cholesterol levels in the transformed cell appears less stringent, as judged by the response of cells to cholesterol starvation. Cholesterol is mainly localized in the plasma membrane [3] and it alters membrane fluidity [4]. We measured plasma fluidity in intact, viable fibroblasts using a spin label phospholipid:

```
H₂C————C(CH₃)₂                    O
   |        |                      ‖
   O        N–O      H₂  C–O–C–(CH₂)₁₄–CH₃
    \      /      O    |
CH₃–(CH₂)₁₂–   C–(CH₂)₃–C–O–CH    O
                            |      ‖                    +
                           H₂C–O–P–O–CH₂–CH₂–N(CH₃)₃
                                  |
                                  O–
```

This spin label analog of phosphatidylcholine (SLPC) carries a 5-doxylstearate spin label in the β position. After incubating cells with a sonicated dispersion of SLPC and washing away unbound spin label, the SLPC was preferentially incorporated into the plasma membrane fraction. Plasma membrane fluidity measured with SLPC differed in 3T3 and SV101-3T3 cells. This difference in fluidity may be related to the elevated cholesterol levels in the transformed cell.

METHODS

Cells

Swiss 3T3 and SV101-3T3 cells were grown in Dulbecco's modified Eagle's medium (DMEM) plus 10% calf serum or 10% lipid-depleted serum as described earlier [5].

Lipid Analysis

Lipids were extracted from cells by the method of Bligh and Dyer [6]. Phospholipid was measured by the method of Rouser et al [7]. Cholesterol was measured by gas-liquid chromatography with a Hewlett-Packard model 5830 gas chromatograph equipped with 1.8-m glass columns containing 3% OV-17 on 100/120 mesh Gas Chrom Q (Applied Science Laboratories, State College, Pennsylvania). Cholesterylacetate served as an internal standard.

Fluorescence Microscopy

Cells grown on collagen-coated coverslips were fixed with 0.1% osmium tetroxide in phosphate-buffered saline (PBS) (0.15 M NaCl–0.01 M sodium phosphate, pH 7.4), stained with filipin (20 μg/ml) in PBS for 30 min at 22°C, then washed with PBS. Filipin was the generous gift of Dr. G. B. Whitfield, Jr., Upjohn Co., Kalamazoo, Michigan. Stained cells were examined with a Zeiss Photomicroscope III fluorescence microscope equipped with epi-illumination.

Spin Labeling

A sonicated dispersion of SLPC was prepared as previously described [8]. Washed cells (5×10^8) were suspended in 0.01 M Tris-HCl (pH 7.5)–0.02 M NaCl–0.1% NaN_3 (0.2 ml). A sonicated dispersion of SLPC (0.4 ml) was added and the cells were incubated for 1 h at 22°C. Additional spin label (0.4 ml) was added and the cells were incubated for 30 min at 22°C. Cells were washed with PBS to remove unbound spin label, collected by centrifugation (600 rpm, 3 min, 22°C), and used for electron spin resonance (ESR) measurements or membrane fractionation.

Membrane Fractionation

Membrane fractions were isolated from spin-labeled cells by a modification of published procedures [9–11]. The details of our method will be published elsewhere. Marker enzymes used were 5'-nucleotidase (plasma membrane) [12], nicotinamide adenine dinucleotide dehydrogenase (NADH) (endoplasmic reticulum) [13], succinic dehydrogenase (mitochondria) [13]. After fractionation, spin label was extracted into chloroform [6] for quantitation by ESR spectroscopy.

RESULTS

Cholesterol Levels

Cholesterol and phospholipid levels in lipid extracts of whole cells are listed in Table I. The cholesterol content of SV101-3T3 cells was approximately twice that of 3T3 cells (15 fmoles/cell vs 7 fmoles/cell). SV101-3T3 had a correspondingly higher phospholipid content so the cholesterol: phospholipid ratio was the same (0.27) in these two cell types. Other investigators have reported values of 0.26–0.30 for the cholesterol: phospholipid ratio [1, 14].

Cells were starved for cholesterol by growth in lipid-depleted medium containing 25-hydroxycholesterol, a specific inhibitor of cholesterol biosynthesis [15]. Starvation for cholesterol reduced the cholesterol level in SV101-3T3 cells to 9.2 ± 2.3 fmoles/cell, while the level in 3T3 cells remained 9.0 ± 3.3 fmoles/cell (Table II).

Filipin Staining

We also observed the differential staining of SV101-3T3 cells reported by Hatten and Burger [1] (Fig. 1a, b). SV101-3T3 cells regularly displayed fluorescent patches, often near the perimeter of the nucleus. By focusing through the cell it was apparent that these patches reside near the upper or lower surface of the cell. 3T3 cells, in contrast, stained diffusely with filipin and rarely showed fluorescent patches. After cholesterol starvation 3T3 and SV101-3T3 cells rarely displayed fluorescent patches (a typical SV101-3T3 cell is shown in Fig. 1c).

TABLE I. Cholesterol and Phospholipid Levels in 3T3 and SV101-3T3

Cell type	Cholesterol per cell (fmoles)	Phospholipid per cell (fmoles)	Cholesterol:phospholipid molar ratio
SV101-3T3	15.1 ± 2.6	56 ± 10	0.27
3T3	6.9 ± 0.9	26 ± 3	0.27

Mean cholesterol and phospholipid levels (± SD) for cells grown in DMEM + 10% calf serum. The results of 12 trials for each cell type are represented.

TABLE II. Effect of Cholesterol Starvation on Growing Cells

Experiment	25-Hydroxycholesterol (nM)	$\triangle$ Cholesterol level, %	
		3T3	SV101-3T3
1	50	23	-26
2	10	-13	-54
	50	-25	-48
3	10	24	-22
	50	-27	lysis

Cells were starved for cholesterol by growth in DMEM + 10% lipid-depleted serum + 25-dydroxycholesterol as indicated. The cholesterol level was compared to that of a parallel culture grown in DMEM + 10% calf serum. High levels of 25-hydroxycholesterol sometimes lysed SV101-3T3 cells.

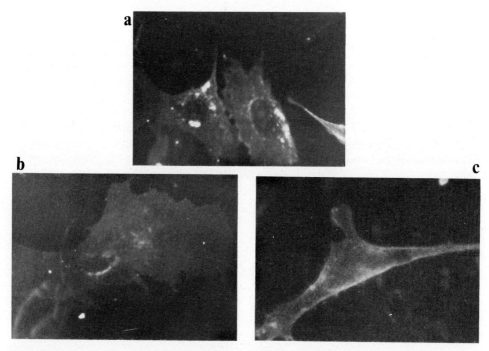

Fig. 1. Fluorescence micrographs of filipin-stained cells. a: SV101-3T3 cells grown in DMEM + 10% calf serum (× 1,600). b: 3T3 cells grown in DMEM + 10% calf serum (× 1,000). c: SV101-3T3 cells starved for cholesterol by growth in DMEM + 10% lipid-depleted serum + 50 nM 25-hydroxycholesterol (× 1,600).

Fluidity Measurements on Plasma Membranes of Intact Cells

We synthesized a spin label analog of phosphatidylcholine (SLPC) and found conditions that allowed us to incorporate this label into 3T3 and SV101-3T3 cells (see Methods). The cells were intact and viable after the labeling procedure, as judged by phase contrast microscopy and trypan blue exclusion. The ESR spectra of labeled cells showed that the label was incorporated into membranes and not adsorbed to cells [8]. The phospholipid label was not degraded, as judged by extraction and thin-layer chromatography. Isolation of plasma membrane, mitochondria, and endoplasmic reticulum fractions from spin-labeled cells showed that the spin label is mainly localized in the plasma membrane fraction (Table III). The temperature dependence of the spectral parameter $2T_\parallel$ differed for 3T3 and SV101-3T3 cells (Fig. 2).

TABLE III. Membrane Fractions From Spin-Labeled SV101-3T3 Cells

Fraction	5'-Nucleotidase		Succinic dehydrogenase		NADH dehydrogenase		ESR signal intensity	
	Units/mg Protein	% of total	Units/mg protein	% of total	Units/mg protein	% of total	Units/mg protein	% of total
Homogenate	15	(100)	0.55	(100)	0.13	(100)	12	(100)
Mitochondria	9	3	3.6	45	0.19	1	13	5
Pellet	26	13	0.13	4	0.43	65	32	26
Plasma membrane	65	37	0.35	3	0.53	22	30	27

SV101-3T3 cells were spin-labeled and fractionated as described in Methods. Four fractions were analyzed: the crude homogenate, mitochondria, pellet (endoplasmic reticulum plus unbroken cells), and plasma membrane.

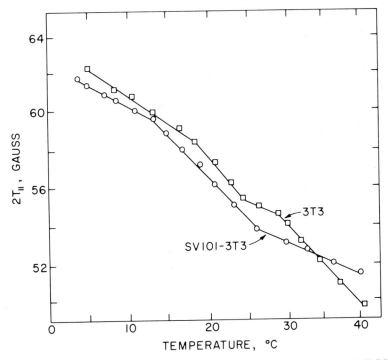

Fig. 2. Temperature dependence of $2T_\parallel$ in 3T3 cells and SV101-3T3 cells labeled with SLPC. Cells were spin-labeled as described in Methods. ESR measurements were carried out as described elsewhere [5].

DISCUSSION

We found consistently higher levels of cholesterol in SV40-transformed 3T3 cells compared to 3T3 cells. This result is particularly interesting in light of the alterations of cholesterol levels and cholesterol metabolism frequently observed in tumor cells [16] and the correlation of filipin staining with the transformed or tumor state [1]. From the response of SV101-3T3 cells to cholesterol starvation it seems clear that filipin staining is related to plasma membrane cholesterol levels.

SV101-3T3 cells are enriched for phospholipid as well as cholesterol. This result is surprising considering the smaller size of SV101-3T3 cells [14]. The excess membrane lipid may be related to the abundance of microvilli on the transformed cell surface [17] or to the elaboration of membrane vesicles [18].

Altering the fatty acyl composition of membrane phosphatides affects the temperature dependence of concanavalin A-induced and wheat germ agglutinin-induced agglutination of 3T3 and SV101-3T3 cells [19]. Spin label measurements revealed lipid structural changes occurring at temperatures corresponding to the agglutination effects [5]. The appearance of the cytoskeleton, as seen with immunofluorescent actin, myosin, and tubulin stains, was not altered (Buttrick, Hayward and Scandella, unpublished results), so we suspect that plasma membrane fluidity may regulate the function of lectin receptors directly. The previous measurements of membrane fluidity utilized fatty acid spin probes which partition into the lipid phase of cell membranes and probably label all cell membranes. These measurements indicated that bulk membrane fluidities in SV 101-3T3 and 3T3 cells are identical [5]. In contrast, plasma membrane fluidity measured here with SLPC differs. The difference in fluidity may be related to elevated cholesterol levels in the plasma membrane of the transformed cell. Recent work on cultured animal cells has shown that the sodium-potassium ATPase and adenyl cyclase activities are strongly influenced by cholesterol levels and membrane fluidity, as measured by lipid spin labels (M. Sinensky, personal communication).

Our studies of membrane fluidity in sea urchin eggs show that membrane fluidity changes after activation by sperm or parthenogenic agents [20]. The egg regulates plasma membrane fluidity and bulk membrane fluidity independently (Campisi, Galson, and Scandella, unpublished results). From the fibroblast agglutination studies it appears that the plasma membrane is heterogeneous with respect to fluidity. Taken together, these results show that membrane fluidity is complex. Changes in plasma membrane fluidity may have a crucial role in cell activation and transformation.

ACKNOWLEDGMENTS

This work was supported by National Institutes of Health grant GM-23218 to C.J.S. and by NIH Training grants GM-07212 and CA-09176.

REFERENCES

1. Hatten ME, Burger MM: Biochemistry 18:739, 1979.
2. de Kruijff B, Demel RA: Biochim Biophys Acta 339:57, 1974.
3. Rothblat GH: In Rothblat GH, Cristafalo VJ (eds): "Growth, Nutrition and Metabolism of Cells in Culture." New York: Academic, 1972, 297.
4. Demel RA, de Kruyff B: Biochim Biophys Acta 457:109, 1976.
5. Hatten ME, Scandella CJ, Horwitz AF, Burger MM: J Biol Chem 253:1972, 1978.
6. Bligh EG, Dyer WJ: Can J Biochem Physiol 37:911, 1959.

7. Rouser G, Fleischer S, Yamamoto A: Lipids 5:494, 1969.
8. Scandella CJ, Devaux P, McConnell HM. Proc Natl Acad Sci USA 69:2056, 1972.
9. Brunette DM, Till JE: J Membr Biol 5:215, 1971.
10. Quinlan DC, Hochstadt J: J Biol Chem 251:344, 1976.
11. Harshman S, Conlin G: Anal Biochem 90:98, 1978.
12. Avruch J, Wallach DFH: Biochim Biophys Acta 233:334, 1971.
13. Hochstadt J, Quinlan DC, Rader RL, Li C, Dowd D: In Korn E (ed): "Methods in Membrane Biology." New York: Plenum, 1975, vol 5, p 117.
14. Adam G, Alpes H, Blaser K, Neubert B: Z Naturforsch 30c:638, 1975.
15. Kandutsch AA, Chen HW, Heiniger HJ: Science 201:498, 1978.
16. Chen HW, Kandutsch AA, Heiniger HJ: Progr Exp Tumor Res 22:275, 1978.
17. Willingham MC, Pastan I: Proc Natl Acad Sci USA 72:1263, 1975.
18. van Blitterswijk WJ, Emmelot P, Hilkmann HAM, Hilgers J, Feltkamp CA: Int J Cancer 23:62, 1979.
19. Horwitz AF, Hatten ME, Burger MM: Proc Natl Acad Sci USA 71:3115, 1974.
20. Campisi J, Scandella CJ: Science 199:1336, 1978.

Journal of Supramolecular Structure 11:485–492 (1979)
Tumor Cell Surfaces and Malignancy 327–334

Ganglioside Patterns of Metastatic and Non-Metastatic Transplantable Hepatocellular Carcinomas of the Rat

Thomas M. Kloppel, D. James Morré, and Linda B. Jacobsen

Department of Biological Sciences (TMK, DJM), Department of Medicinal Chemistry and Pharmacognosy (DJM), and the Purdue Cancer Center (DJM, LBJ), Purdue University, West Lafayette, Indiana 47907

In previous investigations, we correlated levels of sialic acid, gangliosides, and ganglioside glycosyltransferases with tumorigenesis over a 24-week continuum of growth of hepatocellular neoplasms of the rat induced by the carcinogen N-2-fluorenylacetamide. However, metastatic tumors developed only rarely and were not analyzed. To investigate surface changes associated with metastasis, well-differentiated and poorly differentiated hepatocellular carcinomas were transplanted to syngeneic recipient rats. From those, several metastatic and nonmetastatic isolates were obtained and compared. Both total and ganglioside sialic acid amounts in transplantable hepatomas were elevated above control liver values but were significantly lower for metastatic lines than for nonmetastatic lines. The nonmetastatic lines were characterized by ganglioside patterns depleted in the precursor ganglioside G_{M3} (sialic acid-galactose-glucose-ceramide) and elevated in the products of the monosialoganglioside pathway. In contrast, metastatic isolates exhibited a restoration of G_{M3} and nearer normal amounts of other gangliosides. The findings point to differences in sialic acid-containing glycolipids, comparing metastatic and nonmetastatic hepatocellular carcinomas, and further extend the concept that ganglioside alterations do not cause tumorigenesis but are the end result of a cascade of events which apparently continue beyond the onset of metastasis.

Key words: carcinoma, cell surface, ganglioside, hepatoma, metastatis, sialic acid

Both neutral glycosphingolipids and sialoglycosphingolipids (gangliosides) appear altered in amount and composition when a cell undergoes neoplastic transformation [1, 2]. The alterations frequently correlate with changes in activity of one or more glyco-

Received March 18, 1979; accepted August 3, 1979.

syltransferases responsible for the single sugar additions required for the biosynthesis of these glycoconjugates [3]. Not infrequently, the alteration appears as a deletion or reduction of the complex glycolipids concomitant with an increase in the simpler, precursor glycolipids [4, 5]. Particularly with liver cancer, the overall effect is to increase total glycolipid constituents including total ganglioside sialic acid [6] and neutral glycolipids [7].

While ganglioside amount and composition have been analyzed for a variety of hepatic neoplasms and contrasted with values from normal rat liver [4, 7–15], comparisons of metastatic and nonmetastatic hepatoma lines have not been reported. Metastasis of tumors is a phenomenon related to the cell surface [16, 17]. Gangliosides represent informational-type molecules enriched at the cell surface [18, 19], which function as receptors and antigens [20] and exhibit compositional alterations during the course of the tumorigenic progression [1–15]. In the present study, ganglioside profiles of metastatic and nonmetastatic transplantable hepatoma lines were compared in an effort to extend information on the tumorigenic cascade of glycolipid changes in liver cancer to and beyond the initial metastatic events.

MATERIALS AND METHODS

Animals and Tumors

The carcinogen, N-2-fluorenylacetamide (Aldrich) was administered orally at a level of 0.025% in a low-protein diet to male inbred rats (CDF; Charles River Breeding Laboratories, Wilmington, Massachusetts). After 6–12 months, hepatocellular carcinomas were removed from the liver, minced into 1- to 2-mm fragments and injected subcutaneously using a trocar into syngeneic recipients or processed for tissue culture (see Kloppel et al [21]; and Kloppel and Morré, submitted for publication). Tumorigenicity of tissue culture cells was monitored by injecting saline-washed cells into syngeneic animals. Pulmonary metastasis was confirmed by observing hepatocellular foci on the surface of the lungs. Tumor growth rates were estimated from measurements of tumor dimensions [22].

Hepatomas growing subcutaneously were aseptically removed and cleared of necrotic tissue prior to mincing for subsequent passages. Nonnecrotic samples for biochemical analysis were frozen at −20°C. All tissues were fixed with 10% buffered formalin for light microscopy. Regenerating liver was obtained 1 week following partial hepatectomy of sodium pentobarbital-anesthetized rats.

Analysis of Sialic Acid and Gangliosides

Hepatomas, control livers, or regenerating livers were homogenized in 1 volume of 1 mM sodium bicarbonate prior to protein [23] and total sialic acid [24] determinations. Homogenates were extracted over night at 4°C with 10 volumes of chloroform: methanol (CM) (1:1, v/v), filtered over medium porosity sintered glass, and the residue reextracted with CM (2:1) to remove gangliosides. Gangliosides were purified from the combined filtrates using DEAE-Sephadex (Sigma) and Unisil (Clarkson) chromatography [25]. The ganglioside content of purified fractions was determined by sialic acid quantitation [24] prior to composition analysis by thin-layer chromatography (Fig. 1) [26].

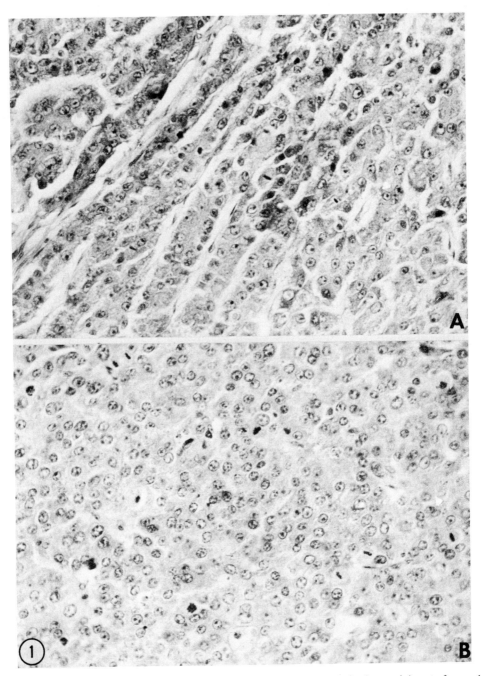

Fig. 1. A: Well-differentiated hepatocellular carcinoma with cellular organization reminiscent of normal liver; cells and nuclear sizes are near normal in appearance. B: Poorly differentiated hepatoma with overall loss of cellular organization, irregular cell and nuclear sizes, and multiple and prominent nucleoli. Hematoxylin and eosin; × 700.

TABLE I. Total and Ganglioside Levels of Sialic Acid in Liver and Transplantable Hepatomas

Tissue[b]	Sialic acid (nmoles/mg protein)[a]	
	Total	Ganglioside
Normal liver	4.5 ± 1.5 (12)	0.22 ± 0.08 (5)
Regenerating liver	3.4 ± 0.4 (3)	0.27 ± 0.12 (3)
Transplanted hepatomas		
Nonmetastatic		
T_2 (PD)	16.0 ± 6.9 (4)	1.12 ± 0.08 (4)
T_7 (PD)	9.2 ± 2.9 (3)	0.76 (1)
T_{10} (WD)	19.2 (1)	0.40 (1)
H_7 (PD)	25.3 ± 9.8 (3)	
Ave	17.9 ± 8.0 (11)[c]	0.94 ± 0.31 (6)[d]
Metastatic		
T_1 (PD)	15.6 ± 3.9 (3)	0.43 (1)
T_3 (HD)	8.3 (2)	0.28 (1)
T_8 (WD)	6.2 (2)	0.55 (1)
Ave	11.8 ± 4.4 (7)[c]	0.42 ± 0.14 (3)[d]

[a]Values are means ± standard deviations. Numbers in parentheses indicate number of samples analyzed in duplicate.

[b]Letters following hepatoma designations indicate histologic classification.
PD = poorly differentiated; WD = well-differentiated; HD = highly differentiated.

[c]Means are significantly different ($P < 0.10$).

[d]Means are significantly different ($P < 0.01$).

RESULTS

Characteristics of Transplantable Hepatomas

A variety of hyperplastic nodules and hepatocellular carcinomas of the liver were obtained following carcinogen treatment. However, only the hepatomas were successfully transplanted to syngeneic recipients. Following the scheme of Reuber [27], those hepatomas scored as well-differentiated displayed some cell order reminiscent of normal liver and cells and nuclei of relatively normal size and appearance (Fig. 1A). Poorly differentiated hepatomas lacked cell order, demonstrated irregular cell and nuclear sizes, and contained multiple and prominent nucleoli (Fig. 1B).

Growth rates of the transplanted hepatomas ranged from 0.1 to 0.8 mm/day. There was no obvious correlation between growth rate and degree of differentiation or between either of these two parameters and the ability to metastasize. Both slow- and fast-growing hepatomas of either well-differentiated or poorly differentiated lines demonstrated the ability to metastasize during the course of this study. Correspondingly, there was no correlation between ability to metastasize and degree of histologic deviation from normal.

Total Sialic Acid and Gangliosides

Sialic acid was increased in total amount in most transplantable hepatocellular carcinomas compared to normal or regenerating livers (Table I). Interestingly, total sialic

TABLE II. Percentage Composition of Gangliosides in Liver and Transplantable Hepatomas

Gangliosides[a]	Liver[b]		Transplantable hepatomas[b]	
	Normal	Regenerating	Nonmetastatic	Metastatic
	(N = 4)	(N = 2)	(N = 4)	(N = 3)
G_{M3} Gal-Glc-Cer	46 ± 8	63	7 ± 4	40 ± 8
NAN				G_{M3}
Monosialoganglioside pathway				
G_{M2} GalNAc-Gal-Glc-Cer	10 ± 2	10	2 ± 2	5 ± 5
NAN				
$G_{M1} + G_{D1a}$ Gal-GalNAc-Gal-Glc-Cer + Gal-GalNAc-Gal-Glc-Cer 30 ± 3		16	77 ± 6	37 ± 6
NAN NAN NAN				
Disialoganglioside pathway				
G_{D3} Gal-Glc-Cer	7 ± 3	3	7 ± 4	16 ± 8
NAN-NAN				
$G_{D1b} + G_{T}$ Gal-GalNAc-Gal-Glc-Cer + higher homologs	8 ± 6	8	8 ± 4	2 ± 1
NAN-NAN				
$\dfrac{G_{M2} + G_{M1} + G_{D1a}}{G_{D3} + G_{D1b} + G_{T}}$ Ratio[c]	2.6	2.4	5.3	2.5

Based on densitometer (Varicord) tracings of resorcinol-positive bands corrected for number of sialic acid residues per molecule. Values represent the mean ± standard deviation.

[a] Identified by comparison with standards. Cer = ceramide; Gal = galactose; Glc = glucose; GalNAc = N-acetylgalactosamine; NAN = N-acetylneuraminic acid (sialic acid); G_T = trisialogangliosides and higher homologs of G_{D1b} and G_{T3}. Use of a different solvent system (n-propanol: ammonium hydroxide; 7:3) resolved the G_{M1} and G_{D1a} bands; spots were approximately 70–80% G_{D1a}.

[b] N = number of samples analyzed in duplicate.

[c] Ratio of monosialoganglioside pathway products and intermediates to those of the disialoganglioside pathway.

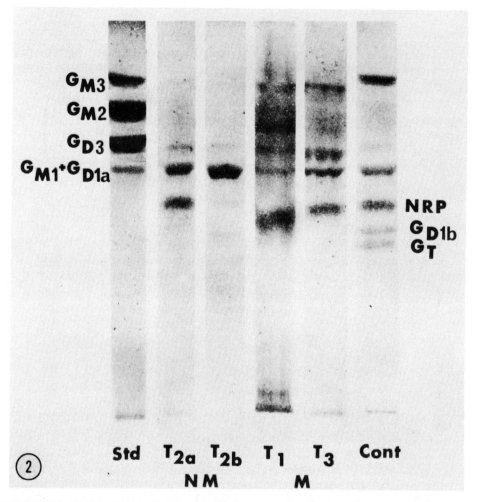

Fig. 2. Gangliosides from normal rat liver and metastatic (M) and nonmetastatic (NM) transplanted hepatomas. Tumors 2a and 2b represent the same transplantable line at two different generations. Silica gel G (Analtech) thin-layer plates were developed in chloroform:methanol:ammonium hydroxide:water (65:30:7:2.5, v/v) and sprayed with resorcinol reagent to detect sialic acid-containing glycolipids. NRP, nonresorcinol-positive band. Std, ganglioside standards. See Table II for an explanation of ganglioside terminology.

acid was lower in two or three metastatic lines and the mean for the metastatic lines was significantly lower than the mean of the nonmetastatic lines.

Ganglioside sialic acid was increased at least two-fold in all transplantable hepatomas when contrasted with the control average of 0.22 nmoles ganglioside sialic acid per milligram protein (Table I). As with total sialic acid, ganglioside sialic acid was significantly reduced in the metastatic lines.

Total and ganglioside sialic acid levels were similar comparing control and regenerating livers (Table I).

Ganglioside Composition

All transplantable hepatoma tissues exhibited different ganglioside patterns when contrasted with control tissues. A major difference, however, was observed between metastatic and nonmetastatic lines. Nonmetastatic lines were depleted in G_{M3} and enriched in G_{D1a}, while metastatic lines, although different from normal, exhibited a more normal pattern (Table II; Fig. 2). An elevation of the ratio of the gangliosides in the monosialoganglioside pathway to those in the disialoganglioside pathway was observed only in the nonmetastatic lines.

Regenerating liver yielded a relatively normal ganglioside pattern. The differences noted were, if anything, an enrichment in G_{M3} and a decrease in $G_{M1} + G_{D1a}$.

DISCUSSION

The development of hepatocellular carcinomas of N-2-fluorenylacetamide-treated livers was slow and progressive as observed by previous investigators [28]. That only certain hepatocellular foci of livers of carcinogen-treated animals were capable of transplantation is indicative of a critical transformation event which separates or distinguishes transplantable hepatomas from other premalignant forms of neoplasms [29]. Within the population of transplantable hepatomas, some eventually formed metastases while others did not.

Ganglioside patterns of rat liver change markedly during both development and tumorigenesis [4, 6]. The patterns of change are relatively complex in an apparent cascade of events in which levels of various ganglioside intermediates vary depending on the stage of development. Deletions or reductions in G_T and accumulations of G_{M3} or G_{D1a} [10–12] have been noted; G_{D1b} has also been observed to be increased in tumor tissue [8] as has G_{M1} [4]. There appears to be no common alteration in ganglioside profiles that characterizes all hepatomas in all stages of development [13–15]. What may happen is a sequence of ganglioside changes as summarized by Merritt et al [4]. In this sequence, a "cross-over" point was predicted at or about the time of metastasis where the levels of monosialogangliosides, at least, should approach control levels. The lower total and ganglioside sialic acid in metastatic lines has also been observed in metastatic and nonmetastatic cell lines derived from murine lung tumors (unpublished results). In this context, the apparent "return to normalcy" of the metastatic lines of transplantable hepatomas is of interest. To what extent the relatively normal ganglioside pattern of metastatic lines observed in the present study relates to the cells' ability to dislodge from the primary tumor mass and survive in metastatic isolation remains to be investigated.

ACKNOWLEDGMENTS

This study was supported in part by grants from the National Cancer Institute CA 18801 and CA 21958. Ganglioside standards were provided by Dr. T.W. Keenan. The assistance of Dorothy A. Werderitsh, Dorien Sarles, Paula Fink, D.M. Morré and J. Michael Cherry is gratefully acknowledged.

REFERENCES

1. Hakomori S: Adv Cancer Res 18:265, 1974.
2. Richardson CL, Baker SR, Morré DJ, Keenan TW: Biochim Biophys Acta 417:175, 1975.

3. Merritt WD, Morré DJ, Keenan TW: J Natl Cancer Inst 60:1329, 1978.
4. Merritt WD, Richardson CL, Keenan TW, Morré DJ: J Natl Cancer Inst 60:1313, 1978.
5. Mora PT, Brady RO, Bradley RM, McFarland VW: Proc Natl Acad Sci USA 63:1290, 1969.
6. Morré DJ, Kloppel TM, Merritt WD, Keenan TW: J Supramol Struct 9:157, 1978.
7. Dnistrian AM, Skipski VP, Barclay M, Stock CC: Cancer Res 27:2182, 1977.
8. Dyatlovitskaya EV, Novikov AM, Gorkova NP, Bergelson LD: Eur J Biochem 63:357, 1976.
9. Dnistrian AM, Skipski VP, Barclay M., Essner ES, Stock CC: Biochem Biophys Res Commun 64:367, 1975.
10. Brady RO, Borek C, Bradley RM: J Biol Chem 244:6552, 1969.
11. Siddiqui B, Hakomori S: Cancer Res 30:2930, 1970.
12. Cheema P, Yogeeswaran G, Morris HP, Murray RK: FEBS Lett 11:181, 1970.
13. van Hoeven R, Emmelot P: In Wood R (ed): "Tumor Lipids: Biochemistry and Metabolism." Champaign, Illinois: American Oil Chemists Society, 1973, p 126.
14. Leblond-Larouche L, Morais R, Nigram VN, Krasaki SA: Arch Biochem Biophys 167:1, 1975.
15. Yogeeswaran F, Sheinin R, Wherrett JR, Murray RK: J Biol Chem 247:5146, 1972.
16. Gasic G, Gasic T: Proc Natl Acad Sci USA 48:1172, 1962.
17. Hagmar B: In Garanttini S, Franchi G (eds): "Chemotherapy of Cancer Dissemination and Metastasis." New York: Raven, 1973, p 261.
18. Dod BJ, Gray GM: Biochim Biophys Acta 249:81, 1971.
19. Klenk HD, Choppin PW: Proc Natl Acad Sci USA 66:57, 1970.
20. Miller HC, Esselman WJ: J Immunol 115:839, 1975.
21. Kloppel TM, Sarles D, Jacobsen LB, Morré DJ: Proc Ind Acad Sci 87:131, 1978.
22. Sedlacek HH, Meesman H, Seiler FR: Int J Cancer 15:409, 1975.
23. Lowry OH, Rosebrough NJ, Farr AL, Randall RJ: J Biol Chem 193:265, 1951.
24. Warren L: J Biol Chem 234:1971, 1959.
25. Ledeen RW, Yu RK, Eng LF: J Neurochem 21:829, 1973.
26. Svennerholm L: Biochim Biophys Acta 24:604, 1957.
27. Reuber MD: Gann Monographs 1:43, 1966.
28. Morris HP: Adv Cancer Res 9:227, 1965.
29. Farber E, Okita K, Kligman LH: In Schultz J, Leif RC (eds): "Critical Factors in Cancer Immunology." New York: Academic, 1975, p 71.

Journal of Supramolecular Structure 11:493–502 (1979)
Tumor Cell Surfaces and Malignancy 335–344

Lectin Affinity Chromatography of Cell Surface Proteins of Novikoff Tumor Cells

John R. Glenney, Jr. and Earl F. Walborg, Jr.

The University of Texas Health Science Center at Houston, Graduate School of Biomedical Sciences, Houston, Texas 77025, and The University of Texas System Cancer Center, Science Park—Research Division, Smithville, Texas 78957

Novikoff hepatocellular carcinoma cells were radioiodinated by a cell surface-specific method using lactoperoxidase/^{125}I. The iodinated proteins were solubilized in 0.5% Nonidet P-40 and subjected to affinity chromatography on Sepharose-conjugated lectins (Ricinus communis agglutinins I or II, soybean agglutinin, concanavalin A, or wheat germ agglutinin) and analyzed by polyacrylamide gel electrophoresis in the presence of sodium dodecyl sulfate. Almost all the iodinated proteins bound to one or more of the Sepharose-conjugated lectins, presumptive evidence that these peptides are glycosylated. Lectin affinity chromatography resolved defined subsets of iodinated glycoproteins and suggested that certain glycoproteins could be fractionated on the basis of heterogeneity of their heterosaccharide moieties. Incubation of the iodinated cells with neuraminidase resulted in increased binding of iodinated proteins to Sepharose-conjugated Ricinus communis agglutinins I and II and soybean agglutinin and decreased binding to Sepharose-conjugated wheat germ agglutinin. Binding of iodinated proteins to concanavalin A was unaffected by neuraminidase treatment of the cells. These studies demonstrate the utility of lectins for the multicomponent analysis of plasma membrane proteins.

Key words: cell surface, plasma membrane, glycoproteins, affinity chromatography, lectins, Novikoff hepatocellular carcinoma, neuraminidase

Transformation of epithelial cells to the malignant phenotype is accompanied by the acquisition of new surface properties that influence cell-cell adhesion and communication [1, 2]. These altered functional properties of the plasma membrane presumably result from alterations in the composition, structure, topography, and/or dynamics of cell surface components, including the plasma membrane glycoproteins [3, 4]. Lectins, sugar-binding

Received April 23, 1979; accepted August 13, 1979.

proteins, have been used to probe the properties of cell surface glycoproteins of normal and malignant epithelial cells [5, 6]; for example, studies in this laboratory, using rat hepatocytes and Novikoff rat ascites hepatocellular carcinoma cells, showed that cell surface receptors for the lectin concanavalin A (Con A) exhibited differential lability to cleavage from the cell surface by papain, the Con A receptors of Novikoff cells being more labile [2, 7]. Although controlled proteolysis yielded valuable information regarding cell surface heterosaccharide moieties, it precluded the characterization of individual plasma membrane glycoproteins. The investigations reported here have been designed to identify and characterize the plasma membrane glycoproteins of Novikoff tumor cells. Cell surface proteins have been radiolabeled using a lactoperoxidase/^{125}I method and the glycoproteins resolved by affinity chromatography on carrier-bound lectins and by polyacrylamide gel electrophoresis.

METHODS

Tumor Cells

Novikoff hepatocellular carcinoma [8] cells were propagated in the ascitic form by transplantation in 6- to 9-week-old female Sprague Dawley rats (A. R. Schmidt, Inc., Madison, Wisconsin). Tumor cells were harvested 5–8 days following inoculation of 1 ml of ascitic fluid. Cells were washed (55g, 5 min) three times in phosphate-buffered saline (PBS), pH 7.4.

Lactoperoxidase-Catalyzed Iodination

Cells were iodinated by a modification of the method of Keski-Oja et al [9]. Briefly, cells were washed (50g, 5 min) with PBS containing 10^{-6} M KI. To the cell suspension (10^7 cells in 0.5 ml PBS, containing 10^{-6} M KI) in a 1-ml plastic tube (Fisher Scientific Co., Houston, Texas, Cat. No. 4-978-145) was added 10 μl of lactoperoxidase in PBS (1 mg/ml), 5 μl of D-glucose (D-Glc) oxidase in PBS (40 units/ml), 0.5 ml PBS containing 10 mM D-Glc and 1.5 mCi Na^{125}I. The tube was capped and placed on a tube rotator (Scientific Equipment Products, Baltimore, Maryland, Cat. No. 60448) at 20 rpm for 10 min at 23°C. The cells were washed (500g, 1 min) three times with PBS containing 5×10^{-3} M KI. Chemicals were obtained from the following sources: lactoperoxidase and D-Glc oxidase from Sigma Chemical Co., St. Louis, and Na^{125}I (17 Ci/mg) from New England Nuclear, Boston.

In some cases iodinated cells were treated with Vibrio cholera neuraminidase, a protease-free preparation obtained from Calbiochem, La Jolla, California. In such cases cells were washed two additional times with PBS containing 1 mM CaCl$_2$ and resuspended in 1 ml of the same buffer. To the iodinated cell suspension was added 0.1 ml of neuraminidase (500 units/ml in 0.05 M Na acetate buffer containing 0.9% NaCl and 0.1% CaCl$_2$, pH 5.5) or buffer alone. The tubes were capped and incubated at 37°C for 1 h on a tube rotator. Following incubation, the cells were washed (500g, 1 min) three times with PBS.

Following iodination cells were analyzed for viability by exclusion of trypan blue [10] and loss of cells by counting in a hemocytometer. At the conclusion of the labeling procedure cell viability was >90% and cell loss was <25%.

Preparation of Carrier-Bound Lectins

Ricinus communis agglutinins I and II (RCA$_I$ and RCA$_{II}$) were prepared essentially by the method of Nicolson and Blaustein [11]. Soybean agglutinin (SBA) was prepared using the methods of Liener [12] and Lis et al [13]. Wheat germ agglutinin (WGA) was prepared by the method of Nagata and Burger [14] as described previously [15]. The lectins were coupled to Sepharose 4B (Pharmacia Fine Chemicals, Piscataway, New Jersey) using the method of Cuatrecasas [16]. Coupling was performed in the presence of 0.2 M saccharide inhibitors: lactose (Eastman Kodak Co., Rochester, New York) for RCA_I and RCA_{II}, 2-acetamido-2-deoxy-D-galactose (D-GalNAc) for SBA and 2-acetamido-2-deoxy-D-glucose (D-GlcNAC) (Sigma) for WGA. Con A coupled to Sepharose was purchased from Pharmacia. The Sepharose-conjugated lectins contained 7–10 mg of covalently bound lectin per milliliter of settled gel. Carrier-bound lectins were washed three times with PBS containing 0.5% Nonidet P-40 (NP-40) and stored at 4°C in PBS containing 0.5% NP-40 and 0.02% NaN_3.

Affinity Chromatography of Solubilized Plasma Membrane Glycoproteins on Sepharose-Bound Lectins

To the radiolabeled cell suspension (10^7 cells per 0.5 ml PBS) was added an equal volume of PBS containing 1% NP-40. The suspension was vortexed for 15 sec and after standing 30 min the suspension was centrifuged at 15,500g for 30 min. Solubilization of the glycoproteins was performed at 4°C.

Affinity chromatography was performed on columns (0.6 cm internal diameter) containing 0.25 ml of carrier-bound lectin equilibrated with PBS containing 0.5% NP-40. The NP-40-solubilized cell components from 2×10^6 cells were applied to the column at a flow rate of 0.5 ml/h. The column was then eluted with 7 ml of PBS containing 0.5% NP-40 at a flow rate of 1.5 ml/h. Material bound to the affinity column was eluted with PBS, containing either 0.2 M lactose for carrier-bound RCA_I and RCA_{II}, 0.1 M D-GalNAc for carrier-bound SBA, 0.2 M D-GlcNAc for carrier-bound WGA, or 0.2 M methyl α-D-mannoside (Sigma) for carrier-bound Con A, at a flow rate of 5 ml/h. Fractions (0.5 ml) were collected and monitored for radioactivity using a Packard Auto Gamma Scintillation Spectrometer. Affinity chromatography was performed at 4°C. The three fractions from each peak containing the highest amounts of radioactivity were pooled for subsequent electrophoretic analysis.

Resolution and Visualization of Radiolabeled Glycoproteins

Polyacrylamide gel electrophoresis in the presence of sodium dodecyl sulfate (SDS) was performed according to the procedure of Laemmli [17], using a Model 221 slab gel electrophoresis apparatus (BioRad Laboratories, Richmond, California). Samples adjusted to 2% SDS, 1% β-mercaptoethanol, 10% glycerol, 62.5 mM Tris, pH 6.8, were heated at 100°C for 3 min prior to application to the gel. Electrophoresis was performed in 1.5-mm slabs at constant current (25 mA per gel). The gels were stained overnight in 0.2% Coomassie Blue R250 in methanol:acetic acid:water [23:4:23 (v/v)]. The gels were destained for 5–7 h in the above solvent.

Molecular weight standards used to calibrate the gels were myosin (a gift from Dr. D. Via), β-galactosidase from Escherichia coli (Worthington Biochemical Corp., Freehold, New Jersey), rabbit muscle phosphorylase A (Worthington), bovine serum albumin (Sigma), hen ovalbumin (Sigma), Con A (a highly purified preparation obtained from Dr. D. C. Hixson) and bovine hemoglobulin (Pentex, Inc., Kankakee, Illinois). These proteins or their monomeric peptides have molecular weights of 200,000, 130,000, 98,000, 68,000, 43,000, 25,000, and 15,500, respectively. Other chemicals used for polyacrylamide gel electrophoresis were electrophoresis grade obtained from BioRad Laboratories.

The gels were swollen in methanol:acetic acid:glycerol:water [5:7.5:2:85.5 (v/v)] and dried under vacuum. Autoradiography was performed using calcium tungstate intensify-

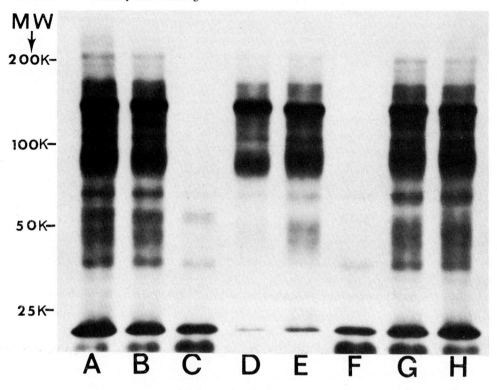

Fig. 1. SDS polyacrylamide gel electrophoresis of ^{125}I-labeled plasma membrane proteins subjected to affinity chromatography on Sepharose-RCA$_I$. Radiolabeled proteins were visualized by autoradiography. Each lane contains radiolabeled components derived from the same number of cells, ie, $(2.5-3) \times 10^4$ cells. Lanes A–D: cells not treated with neuraminidase; lanes E–H: cells treated with neuraminidase; lanes A, H: SDS-solubilized whole cells; lanes B, G: components solubilized by 0.5% NP-40; lanes C, F: components not retained on Sepharose-RCA$_I$; lanes D, E: components retained on Sepharose-RCA$_I$.

ing screens and incubation at −70°C according to the procedure of Swanstrom and Shank [18]. X-ray film (RP-5 Xomat) was purchased from Kodak and X-ray intensifying screens (Cronex, Lightning Plus) were obtained from DuPont, Wilmington, Delaware.

RESULTS

Radioiodination and Solubilization of Cell Surface Proteins

Novikoff cells were effectively labeled by the lactoperoxidase/^{125}I method. At least ten major components having apparent molecular weights of 35,000–250,000 could be distinguished (Fig. 1). In addition, a component which migrated in front of the tracking dye was also resolved. The specificity of the reaction was demonstrated by controls in which lactoperoxidase or D-Glc oxidase were omitted in which no radiolabeled components were observed (data not shown).

As demonstrated by Swanstrom and Shank [18] the use of calcium tungstate intensifying screens and low temperature (−70°C) greatly enhanced the detection of ^{125}I by autoradiography. This was accomplished without loss of resolution of the radiolabeled components.

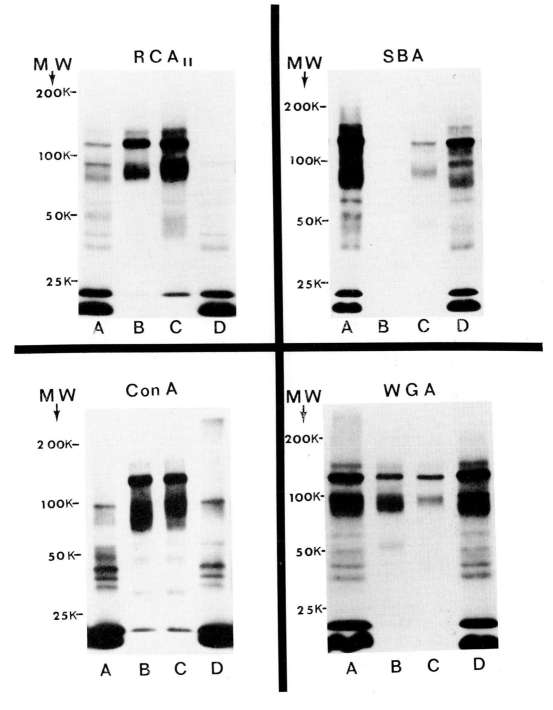

Fig. 2. SDS polyacrylamide gel electrophoresis of ^{125}I-labeled proteins subjected to affinity chromatography on Sepharose-bound RCA$_{II}$, SBA, Con A, and WGA. Each lane contains radiolabeled components derived from the same number of cells, ie, $(2.5-3) \times 10^4$ cells. Radiolabeled proteins were visualized by autoradiography. Lane A: unbound components; lane B: bound components; lane C: bound components; neuraminidase-treated cells; lane D: unbound components; neuraminidase-treated cells.

Over 85% of the ^{125}I-labeled cell surface components were solubilized in 0.5% NP-40. Furthermore, the autoradiographic pattern of SDS polyacrylamide gels of iodinated cells solubilized in sample buffer containing 2% SDS immediately following iodination was identical to the pattern of the 0.5% NP-40 extracts (Fig. 1), indicating that proteolysis during solubilization did not introduce artifacts.

Affinity Chromatography of Radioiodinated Components on Carrier-Bound Lectins

Affinity chromatography of the components solubilized in 0.5% NP-40 resulted in fractionation of the radiolabeled components (Figs. 1 and 2). Furthermore, affinity chromatography on carrier-bound lectins resolved the radiolabeled components from the bulk of the Coomassie Blue-stained peptides. This suggests that the vast majority of Coomassie-stained peptides are not glycoproteins, as demonstrated previously [20]. Recovery of radioactivity from the carrier-bound lectin columns was 80–85% and duplicate columns always agreed to within ±2%.

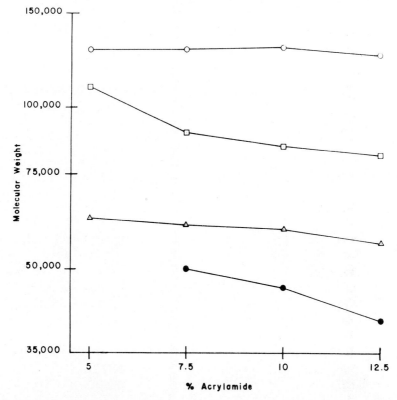

Fig. 3. The effect of acrylamide concentration on apparent molecular weight of peptides that bind to Sepharose-conjugated SBA after neuraminidase treatment. Cells were labeled within ^{125}I, treated with neuraminidase, solubilized in PBS containing 0.5% NP-40, and subjected to affinity chromatography on Sepharose-SBA. The iodinated components eluted with 0.1 M GalNAc were submitted to SDS polyacrylamide gel electrophoresis. Five to seven peptides of known molecular weights were used to estimate the molecular weights of the iodinated peptides. The data represent the average of three separate determinations. The apparent molecular weights agreed within ±4%. Individual lines are peptides having apparent molecular weights of 128,000 (○—○), 90,000 (□—□), 61,000 (△—△), and 50,000 (●—●) in 7.5% gels (see Fig. 3).

Estimation of the Molecular Weight of the Major Peptides That Bind to Sepharose-SBA

Glycoproteins that contain more than 10% carbohydrate behave anomalously on SDS polyacrylamide gel electrophoresis, the degree of anomaly being some direct function of its percent carbohydrate [19]. Segrest and Jackson [19] have demonstrated that a more accurate estimate of the molecular weight may be obtained by using several gels of different acrylamide concentrations. Such an analysis has been performed on four iodinated peptides derived from neuraminidase-treated cells. These glycoproteins were bound to Sepharose-SBA and eluted with D-GalNAc (Fig. 3). Exposure of the X-ray film to the gel for longer periods of time still showed only the four radiolabeled bands seen in Figure 3 (SBA, lane C). Five to seven molecular weight standards were used to calibrate the gels. An accurate estimate of the molecular weight is approached using gels of higher acrylamide concentration; thus the SBA-binding components have molecular weights of 124,000 (±3,000), 80,000 (±2,000), 55,000 (±2,000), and 40,000 (±1,000) in 12.5% gels. Furthermore, whereas the molecular weight of the largest of these glycoproteins did not vary appreciably between 5% and 12.5% acrylamide, the molecular weight of the next largest component varied from 109,000 (±3,000) in 5% gels to 80,000 (±2,000) in 12.5% gels.

Effect of Neuraminidase Treatment of Radioiodinated Cells on Lectin Binding of Cell Surface Proteins

Previous investigations [15] indicated that lectin binding to the cell surface was altered by treatment of Novikoff cells with neuraminidase; therefore the effect of neuraminidase treatment on the lectin binding of the iodinated peptides was investigated (Table I, Figs. 1 and 2). The incubation conditions employed for neuraminidase treatment of Novikoff cells yield maximal release of cell surface sialic acid [15]. Whereas there was no effect of neuraminidase treatment on binding of the iodinated proteins to Sepharose-Con A, significant alterations in binding to Sepharose-conjugated RCA$_I$, RCA$_{II}$, SBA, and WGA were observed. Neuraminidase treatment of the cells was accompanied by increased binding to RCA$_I$, RCA$_{II}$, and SBA, as evidenced by the percentage of total label bound to the Sepharose-con-

TABLE I. Effect of Neuraminidase on the Binding of ^{125}I-Labeled Plasma Membrane Proteins to Sepharose-Conjugated Lectins

Lectin	% [125]I bound to Sepharose-conjugated lectins	
	Without neuraminidase	With neuraminidase
RCA$_I$	58	73
RCA$_{II}$	29	60
SBA	<0.1	13
Con A	26	26
WGA	19	14

Novikoff cells were labeled with ^{125}I and treated with neuraminidase or buffer alone as described in Methods. Cells were then solubilized in PBS containing 0.5% NP-40 and subjected to lectin affinity chromatography on Sepharose-conjugated lectins. Equivalent amounts of trichloroacetic acid-precipitable radioactivity from control or neuraminidase-treated cells were loaded on duplicate lectin affinity columns and eluted under identical conditions. The column fractions (0.5 ml) were assayed for radioactivity. The amount of ^{125}I bound to the column and eluted with saccharide is expressed as a percentage of the total trichloroacetic acid-precipitable radioactivity recovered from the column.

jugated lectins and the disappearance or diminution of iodinated components from fractions not bound to the lectin affinity columns. Particularly striking was the increase in binding of iodinated components to RCA_{II} and SBA. On the other hand, neuraminidase treatment of the cells was accompanied by decreased binding to WGA.

DISCUSSION

Cell surface radiolabeling techniques, coupled with lectin affinity chromatography, represent a powerful tool to study the composition and structure of plasma membrane glycoconjugates. By use of lectins possessing different saccharide specificities information can be gained concerning the structure and heterogeneity of the heterosaccharide moieties of the plasma membrane glycoproteins. Our previous studies [20] using saccharide-specific labeling techniques to radiolabel plasma membrane glycoconjugates, ie, reduction with NaB^3H_4 following oxidation by $NaIO_4$ or D-galactose oxidase, have now been extended to a cell surface labeling method using radioiodination. In addition the number of lectins used for affinity chromatography has been increased to include lectins specific for many of the saccharide structures present in glycoproteins, including D-Gal by RCA_I [11], D-Gal/D-GalNAc by RCA_{II} [11], D-GalNAc by SBA [13], α-D-manno- or α-D-glucopyranosyl residues by Con A [21], and D-GlcNAc or sialic acid by WGA [14, 22].

Binding of almost all major iodinated proteins to one or more of the Sepharose-conjugated lectin columns is strong evidence that these components are glycoproteins. This conclusion is corroborated by previous studies in which most of these components were labeled by saccharide-specific cell surface labeling techniques [20]; however, since noncovalent multimeric associations of plasma membrane proteins and glycoproteins resistant to disruption by nonionic detergents have been reported [23], this conclusion must be considered tentative. Comparative analysis of the iodinated proteins and the plasma membrane glycoproteins labeled using the $NaIO_4/NaB^3H_4$ or D-Gal oxidase/NaB^3H_4 method must await analysis by high-resolution two-dimensional gel electrophoresis [24]. One major iodinated protein did not bind to any of the Sepharose-conjugated lectins and therefore may be a nonglycosylated protein. This protein had a molecular weight of 40,000 in 7.5% gels.

Juliano and Li [25] demonstrated that plasma membrane glycoproteins can be resolved on the basis of their binding to lectins. They used immunoprecipitation by lectins to resolve two of the major plasma membrane glycoproteins of CHO cells. Plasma membrane glycoproteins of Novikoff tumor cells were fractionated using five lectins of differing saccharide specificities: RCA_I, RCA_{II}, SBA, Con A, WGA. For example, a glycoprotein having an apparent molecular weight of 125,000 in 7.5% gels bound completely to Sepharose-conjugated RCA_I and Con A but did not bind to Sepharose-conjugated SBA. This same glycoprotein was fractionated into bound and unbound forms by affinity chromatography on carrier-bound RCA_{II} and WGA, suggesting heterogeneity in its heterosaccharide moiety or moieties. Such heterogeneity could not be detected using the ^{125}I-lectin overlay technique [26] or precipitin formation in Ouchterlony-type double diffusion [27].

Treatment of cells with neuraminidase affects the surface properties of tumor cells, including alteration of cell surface charge [28], exposure of new saccharide moieties [29, 30], and enhancement of immunogenicity [31]. For example, Nicolson [30] reported that neuraminidase treatment of erythrocytes, lymphoma cells, and fibroblasts was accompanied by an increase in RCA_I-induced cytoagglutination and binding of labeled lectin to the cell surface. Previous studies in this laboratory demonstrated that the immunogenicity of Novikoff tumor cells was not affected by neuraminidase [32], even though this treatment resulted in a loss of cell surface charge [33], and the exposure of D-Gal and/or D-GalNAc residues on cell surface heterosaccharide moieties [15]. The significant increase in the binding of iodinated proteins to Sepharose-conjugated RCA_I, RCA_{II}, and SBA confirms these previous findings. Lectin affinity chromatography and SDS polyacrylamide gel electrophoresis of the glycoproteins bound to Sepharose-conjugated RCA_I, RCA_{II}, and SBA allowed assignment of this increased lectin receptor activity to specific glycoprotein species. It should be noted, however, that this experimental approach only allows identification of new lectin-binding species of glycoproteins. For example, neuraminidase may expose new RCA_I binding sites on particular glycoproteins, but if these glycoproteins already contain RCA_I binding sites, the new binding sites will not be detected.

These studies demonstrate the utility of lectins as saccharide-specific probes for the multicomponent analysis of plasma membrane glycoproteins and suggest methodology for the resolution and partial structural characterization of glycoproteins present at the surface of other normal and malignant cells.

ACKNOWLEDGMENTS

This research was supported by grants from The National Cancer Institute (CA 18829), The Paul and Mary Haas Foundation, and The George and Mary Josephine Hamman Foundation. John R. Glenney, Jr. was the recipient of predoctoral fellowships from the Rosalie B. Hite and J. S. Abercrombie Foundations. The authors gratefully acknowledge the able technical assistance of Ms. Phyllis J. Kaulfus.

REFERENCES

1. Loewenstein WR: Biochim Biophys Acta 560:1, 1979.
2. Walborg EF Jr, Starling JJ, Davis EM, Hixson DC, Allison JP: In Griffin AC, Shaw CR (eds): "Carcinogens: Identification and Mechanisms of Action," Raven Press, New York 1979, pp 381–398.
3. Nicolson GL: Biochim Biophys Acta 457:57, 1976.
4. Nicolson GL: Biochim Biophys Acta 458:1, 1976.
5. Sharon N, Lis H: Science 177:949, 1972.
6. Nicolson GL: Int Rev Cytol 39:89, 1974.
7. Starling JJ, Capetillo SC, Neri G, Walborg EF Jr: Exp Cell Res 104:170, 1977.
8. Novikoff AB: Cancer Res 17:1010, 1957.
9. Keski-Oja J, Mosher DF, Vaheri A: Biochem Biophys Res Commun 74:699, 1977.
10. Phillips HJ: In Patterson MK, Kruse PF (eds): "Tissue Culture Methods and Applications." New York: Academic, 1973, pp 406–408.
11. Nicolson GL, Blaustein J: Biochim Biophys Acta 266:543, 1972.
12. Liener IE: J Nutr 49:527, 1953.
13. Lis H, Sela BA, Sachs L, Sharon N: Biochim Biophys Acta 211:583, 1975.
14. Nagata Y, Burger MM: J Biol Chem 247:2248, 1972.
15. Neri G, Giuliano MC, Capetillo S, Gilliam EB, Hixson DC, Walborg EF Jr: Cancer Res 36:263, 1976.
16. Cuatrecasas P: J Biol Chem 245:3059, 1970.
17. Laemmli UK: Nature 227:680, 1970.
18. Swanstrom R, Shank PR: Anal Biochem 86:184, 1978.
19. Segrest JP, Jackson RL: Methods Enzymol 28(part B):54, 1972.
20. Glenney JR Jr, Allison JP, Hixson DC, Walborg EF Jr: J Biol Chem 254:9247, 1979.
21. Goldstein IJ, Hollerman CE, Smith EE: Biochemistry 4:876, 1965.
22. Greenaway PJ, Levine D: Nature New Biol 241:191, 1973.
23. Vitetta ES, Poulik MD, Klein J, Uhr JW: J Exp Med 144:179, 1976.
24. O'Farrell PH: J Biol Chem 25:4007, 1975.

25. Juliano RL, Li G: Biochemistry 17:678, 1978.
26. Burridge K: Proc Natl Acad Sci USA 73:4457, 1976.
27. Carter WG, Hakomori S-I: Biochem Biophys Res Commun 76:299, 1977.
28. Weiss L: J Natl Cancer Inst 50:3, 1973.
29. Rosen SW, Hughes RC: Biochemistry 16:4908, 1977.
30. Nicolson GL: J Natl Cancer Inst 50:1443, 1973.
31. Prager MD, Baechtel FS: Methods Cancer Res 9:339, 1973.
32. Neri G, Mastromarino P, Seminara D, Walborg EF Jr: Cancer Immunol Immunother 5:229, 1979.
33. Neri G, Giuliano MC, Capetillo S, Gilliam EB, Hixson DC, Walborg EF Jr: Acta Med Romana 14: 432, 1976.

Journal of Supramolecular Structure 11:503—515 (1979)
Tumor Cell Surfaces and Malignancy 345—357

Human Placental Cell Surface Antigens: Expression by Cultured Cells of Diverse Phenotypic Origin

Thomas A. Hamilton, H. Garrett Wada, and Howard H. Sussman

Laboratory of Experimental Oncology, Department of Pathology, Stanford University School of Medicine, Stanford, California 94305

The present work examined the expression of cell surface glycoprotein antigens in cultured human cell lines. The set of glycoproteins studied was defined by their immunoreactivity with antiserum developed to Triton-solubilized extracts of placental brush border membranes. Studies were performed using cell lines of trophoblastic (BeWo, JEG-3) and nontrophoblastic (Chang liver cells) origin, as well as diploid fibroblast cell lines (WI-38, GM-38).

Antiplacental brush border antiserum reacts with at least 19 distinct antigens present in placental membrane preparations, each of which can be resolved and identified in two-dimensional electrophoresis. The subunit molecular weight and isoelectric point for all components were defined by their positions in the two-dimensional matrix. Thirteen of these could be detected among the five cell lines examined by lactoperoxidase-catalyzed cell surface iodination.

One of these 13 antigens has been identified as the placental isoenzyme of alkaline phosphatase (PAP). The expression of this component is limited to choriocarcinoma cells and Chang liver cells and it is not present in diploid fibroblasts. Under normal circumstances expression of PAP is unique to the differentiated placenta but has been frequently demonstrated in both trophoblastic and nontrophoblastic neoplasms.

Two other antigens are variably expressed among the different cell types examined in the present study and their presence or absence was independent of the trophoblastic, epithelial nontrophoblastic, or fibroblastic origin of the cells.

Ten surface antigens were expressed in all five cell lines. Six of these had previously been found common to membranes from three adult differentiated tissues, including liver and kidney, as well as placenta (Wada et al, J Supramol Struc 10(3):287—305, 1979). The presence of this set of antigens in cultured cells as well extends the possibility that these are ubiquitously expressed on human cell surfaces. Two other antigens observed in all cultured cells had been found in both placental and either kidney or liver membranes and may represent common functions shared by many tissues which are also necessary for growth in vitro. The two remaining placental antigens seen in all cultured cells have previously been shown to be absent in adult tissues. Their presence in cultured cells but not in the membranes of resting differentiated tissues may signify the expression of glycoproteins characteristic of trophoblasts in all cells adapted to growth in culture.

Received March 18, 1979; accepted August 1, 1979.

Key words: glycoproteins, two-dimensional electrophoresis, differentiation

Cell surface glycoproteins have been the subject of intense study in recent years because of their direct interaction with the cell's immediate external environment. Consequently, they may play a major role in dictating cellular behavior in response to specific environmental stimuli. Trophoblastic and neoplastic cells share some behavioral properties including invasiveness [1], escape from immunosurveillance [2,3], and cell surface charge properties [4,5] which may be determined by their surface glycoproteins. The identification of the placental isoenzyme of alkaline phosphatase on both trophoblastic and neoplastic cell surfaces [6] provides evidence of biochemical similarity as well. Other presumptive placental specific membrane antigens have been demonstrated on the surface of several tumor cell lines grown in tissue culture [7], but precise identification of such components is necessary for their further analysis. Our interest in this area has focused on the brush border membrane of the human placenta with the intent of defining the tissue distribution of glycoprotein components found in this organ.

Previous work from this laboratory described a set of 33 sialoglycoprotein subunits in purified brush border membranes utilizing high-resolution two-dimensional electrophoresis in polyacrylamide gel slabs [8]. Antiserum prepared against detergent-extracted membranes (anti-placental brush border serum [APBB]) in combination with two-dimensional electrophoresis demonstrated 18 of the original 33 presumptive glycoproteins to be antigenic [9]. For comparison with other tissues, the glycoprotein antigen content of human liver and kidney membranes were similarly examined. This analysis identified four glycoprotein subunits which were present only in the placental membranes. In addition, we identified ten of the original 18 subunits in liver or kidney, and seven of these were found in all three tissues examined. Those studies thus defined three groups of placental surface antigens: a) those which appear unique to placenta; b) those which exhibit limited but not unique tissue distribution; and c) those which appear common to all tissues and which may perform essential functions.

The present study considers the frequency with which glycoproteins that fit into these three categories are expressed in selected human cell lines. Using the xenogenic antiserum described above to compare the glycoprotein antigen content of trophoblastic and nontrophoblastic tumor cells or diploid fibroblastic cells, we can evaluate how the expression of such surface components relates to the specific cellular phenotype. In this study, we used two cell lines (BeWo, JEG-3) developed from human gestational choriocarcinomas which have been shown to retain a variety of biochemical properties characteristic of the differentiated trophoblast [10–13], the Chang liver cell line, which is nontrophoblastic in origin and has been in continuous culture for 25 years [14], and two diploid fibroblastic lines (WI-38, GM-38). A remarkably similar set of placental membrane antigens was expressed by these distinct cell lines. In concert with previous work, the present study defines a set of antigenic glycoproteins which may be ubiquitously expressed on human cell surfaces.

METHODS

Cell Culture

BeWo cells were obtained from the American Type Culture Collection ([ATCC], CCL 98). JEG-3 cells were kindly provided by Dr. Saul Rosen of the National Institutes of Health. Both cell lines were grown as previously described [15]. Chang liver cells were provided by Dr. R. S. Chang of the University of California at Davis, and were grown as described earlier [16]. WI-38 cells were obtained from the ATCC (CCL 75) and GM-38 were a gift from Dr. Jon Williams of the Department of Pathology at Stanford University. Both fibroblast cells were subcultured at intervals of 3–4 days by 1:2 splits in minimum essential medium (MEM) and 10% fetal calf serum. Antibiotic-Antimycotic (Gibco) was present at a 1:100 dilution. Both fibroblasts were used at passage levels of 15–25. All cells were grown until confluent (3–4 days following subculture) before use. Cell culture media and fetal calf serum were from Gibco. Cells were grown in polystyrene T-flasks (Corning).

Lactoperoxidase-Catalyzed Cell Surface Labeling

Monolayers of cells were washed twice with Earle's balanced salt solution without Ca^{++} and Mg^{++} followed by two washes with 10mM Na phosphate-buffered saline (PBS), pH 7.5. The monolayers were then thoroughly drained and 1 ml of PBS containing 50 μg lactoperoxidase (Sigma Chemical Co.) and 100–200 μCi of ^{125}I (New England Nuclear, carrier-free) was added. Iodination was started by addition of 10 μl of 250 μM hydrogen peroxide followed by an additional 10 μl after 5 min. Following a total incubation period of 10 min at room temperature, the labeling reaction was terminated by addition of 50 μl of 0.5 M NaI followed by two washes with PBS containing 50 mM NaI. A final wash of the monolayer was done with PBS. Examination of viability by Trypan Blue exclusion showed such cells to be > 90% viable. After the flasks were drained of excess PBS, the cells were scraped from the plastic surface with a rubber policeman into 1 ml of PBS per T-75 flask. The resulting cell suspension was made 1% in Triton X-100 and extracted at 4°C for 10 min. The extracts were centrifuged at 1000g for 10 min to remove nuclei and cell debris and at 110,000g for 60 min. The trichloroacetic acid-precipitable radioactivity in the resulting supernatant was measured in a gamma counter.

Immunoprecipitation and Two-Dimensional Electrophoresis

The preparation and characterization of APBB serum as well as adsorption of this antiserum with liver microsomes has been previously described [9]. Between 200,000 and 400,000 cpm of iodinated cell extracts were reacted with 20 μl of APBB serum or 100 μl of liver-adsorbed APBB serum in the presence of 0.1% sodium dodecyl sulfate (SDS). After 1 hr at 4°C, the APBB-bound labeled antigens were precipitated by the addition of 200 μl of a 10% suspension of heat-killed, glutaraldehyde-fixed S. aureus according to Kessler [17]. After 1 h at 4°C, the mixture was centrifuged at 6000g for 10 min and the resulting pellet was washed twice in NET buffer (150 mM NaCl, 5 mM EDTA, 50 mM Tris-HCL, pH 7.2, 0.5% v/v Triton X-100) containing 1 mg/ml ovalbumin (Sigma Chemical Co.) and 50 mM NaI. A final wash of the pellet was done in NET buffer. The washed pellet containing specific APBB-adsorbed antigens was extracted with 5 mM Na phosphate (pH 8.1), 8 M urea, and 2% Triton X-100 for 10 min at room temperature. The extracted material was subjected to sequential isoelectric focusing and SDS polyacrylamide gel electrophoresis as fully described in Wada et al [8].

Alkaline Phosphatase Assay

Alkaline phosphatase activity was measured in unlabeled crude sonicates of cells according to Bessey et al [18] and the placental isoenzyme was identified in Triton X-100 extracts with a previously described immunochemical assay [19]. Protein was measured by the method of Schaffner and Weissmann [20].

RESULTS

Figure 1 is a schematic representation of a two-dimensional electropherogram of placental brush border glycoproteins selected by immunoprecipitation with anti-placental brush border antiserum. Eighteen distinct components are present. Those components represented by open spots are potentially specific to placental tissue (P) by virtue of their absence in either liver or kidney. Those represented by filled spots are found in liver and kidney as well as placenta (PKL). The crosshatched spots are common to kidney and placenta but were not observed in liver plasma membranes (PK). The numbering system used in this figure and throughout this report corresponds to the originally identified components present in the total placental brush border membrane preparation [8,9]. Table I gives the subunit molecular weight (m_r) and isoelectric point (pI) for each component in Figure 1.

The components described in Figure 1 were initially identified by radiolabeling of sialic acid moieties using [^{3}H] sodium borohydride reduction of periodate oxidized mem-

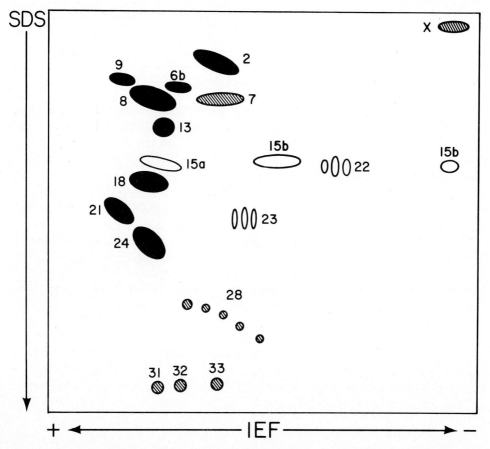

Fig. 1. Schematic diagram of two-dimensional electropherogram of placental brush border glycoprotein antigens. The relative positions and number assignments as well as the indicated tissue distribution are derived from a previous publication. Solid spots: subunits common to placenta, liver, and kidney; crosshatched spots: subunits common to placenta and kidney only; open spots: subunits potentially specific to placenta.

branes. All except 28 and X were also labeled by lactoperoxidase-catalyzed incorporation of ^{125}I. Each component that labeled with both ^{3}H and ^{125}I was considered to be a glycoprotein. Component P23 was shown by coelectrophoresis of ^{32}P$_i$ and ^{3}H-labeled membranes to be placental alkaline phosphatase [8]. Component P22 was identified as membrane-bound human transferrin by coelectrophoresis and radioimmunoassay [9]. Of the 18 components in Figure 1, only 12 will be considered below: PK X and 28 are not labeled with ^{125}I; 31, 32, and 33 are not adequately resolved for evaluation; and P22 is not an integral membrane protein.

Initially, we wished to examine a cell line of trophoblastic origin known to express placenta-specific functions. For this purpose, we selected the BeWo line, originally grown by serial transplantation of a human gestational choriocarcinoma in the hamster cheek pouch [10] and later adapted to growth in tissue culture [11]. As a nontrophoblastic cell, we chose the Chang liver cell line [14] because it is known to make at least one placental membrane glycoprotein (placental alkaline phosphatase) [16]. Lactoperoxidase-catalyzed iodination was used to label cell surface proteins and it was demonstrated that the incorporated iodine label banded at the same buoyant density as the alkaline phospatase-containing plasma membrane vesicles in sucrose density gradients. This indicated the cell surface specificity of the labeling method (data not shown).

TABLE I. Coordinates of Placental Brush Border Sialoglycoprotein Subunits in Two-Dimensional Maps

Spots	Apparent pI	Apparent M_r (k)
X[a]	8.15	308.0
2	5.80	235.0
6b	5.68	170.0
7[b]	5.88	161.0
8	5.68	148.0
9	5.18	175.0
13	5.86	123.0
15a	5.82	100.0
b	6.57	100.0
18	5.65	92.4
21	4.60	72.5
22a	7.10	74.6
b	7.19	74.6
23a	6.22	66.2
b	6.30	66.2
c	6.39	66.2
24	5.60	64.2
28a	5.79	47.0
b	5.89	46.0
c	6.00	44.0
d	6.12	42.0
e	6.22	41.0
31	4.60	< 40.0
32	5.45	< 40.0
33	5.66	< 40.0

[a]X was only detectable after immunoprecipitation with APBB serum.
[b]7 was only detectable after immunoprecipitation with liver-adsorbed APBB serum.

Figure 2A shows a two-dimensional map of iodinated BeWo cell surface components immunoprecipitated with APBB serum. Nine of the 12 components under consideration could be identified in this gel. All three putative placenta-specific subunits are expressed by this cell line. Components P15a and P15b are easily seen. However, component P23 (placental alkaline phosphatase) is not seen in BeWo cells by surface labeling with ^{125}I. Previous studies using two-dimensional electrophoresis of ^{32}P$_i$ active center labeled subunits have demonstrated this enzyme in membranes of BeWo cells [15]. Table II gives the specific activity of the placental isoenzyme of alkaline phosphatase in each of the cell lines examined in this study. In addition to the P-type subunits, six of eight PKL-type subunits were positively identified (PKL 26b, 8, 9, 21, 24), while 13 and 18 were not seen. Component 2, whose tissue distribution was previously undefined, is also present. Two components not previously described are observed in this autoradiogram; one (7a) focusing at a pI of 5.9 and having a M_r of 130,000 daltons, and a second (2a) which runs directly above component 2. Subunit 7a is observed at low levels in placental membranes labeled with ^{125}I.

Figure 2B presents a two-dimensional map of iodinated Chang liver cell surface components precipitated with APBB. This cell line expresses 11 of 12 original placental brush border antigens as well as 7a. The only apparent difference between the trophoblastic BeWo line and the nontrophoblastic Chang cell line is the presence of PKL 18 and the absence of 2a in Chang. All three putative placental subunits (P15a, P15b, and P23) are expressed in Chang cells. P15a is easily identified. A subunit which runs at the same M_r as P15b (100,000) but which does not enter the focusing gel is seen as the basic pole of the map. We have tentatively designated this component as P15b because it appears to be immunochemically related to P15b (see below) and in placental membrane preparations P15b has shown a similar failure to migrate from the basic pole in the isoelectric focusing dimension. The failure of this subunit to enter the focusing gel may be due to higher structure order which is not sufficiently disrupted by the 8 M urea present in the first-dimension buffer. P23 is not easily seen in Figure 2B but could be detected in the original autoradiogram. Previous studies have clearly identified this specific enzyme in Chang liver cells [16]. Table II shows that the placental alkaline phosphatase specific activity is nearly ten times higher in Chang cells than in BeWo cells.

The identity of the glycoprotein subunits present either in BeWo or Chang cells is confirmed by two-dimensional electrophoretic analysis of iodinated material immunoprecipitated with APBB serum that has been adsorbed four times with human liver microsomes. As shown in Figure 2 (C,D), components also found in liver membranes are either eliminated or reduced in intensity (PKL 6b, 8, 9, 21, 24), while those not previously observed in liver are unaffected or relatively enhanced (PK 7, P15a, 15b). Antibodies to PAP (P23) are not removed by absorption [9], but this component is very difficult to visualize when present at the low levels seen in these cultured cells. Component 7a is also eliminated by liver adsorption. The enhanced intensity of the 100,000-dalton polypeptide at the basic pole supports our suggestion that this corresponds to P15b. Because both 2 and 7a are removed by adsorption we conclude that these components are also present in liver tissue. The intensity of PKL 18 is seen to be unreduced in the Chang cell map using adsorbed antiserum (Fig. 2D). PKL 18 is found in liver and kidney membranes but antibodies to this antigen are not removed from APBB serum by adsorption with liver or kidney tissue or with cultured cells which contain this component (data not shown). This suggests that the antigenic determinants of PKL 18 recognized by APBB serum are not exposed when this glycoprotein is in the membrane.

The remarkable similarity demonstrated between BeWo and Chang liver cells in the results described above prompted our examination of other cultured cell lines in order to determine whether the expression of placental antigens is a common phenomenon in cells adapted to growth in vitro. We have examined the surface antigen composition of a second choriocarcinoma cell (JEG-3, a clonal cell line isolated independently of BeWo but from the same transplantable tumor [13]), as well as two fibroblastic cell lines of embryonic (WI-38) and adult (GM-38) origin. Table III provides a summary of the glycoprotein antigen composition for each cell line examined. Figure 3A–C shows three autoradiograms of APBB-precipitated ^{125}I-labeled material from these cells. Figure 3A is a map of JEG-3 which demonstrates that the two choriocarcinoma cell lines (BeWo and JEG-3) contain a qualitatively identical set of placental membrane antigens, an observation which is not unexpected considering their identical origin (see also Table II).

Figure 3 (B and C) shows electropherograms of iodinated cell surface antigens from WI-38 and GM-38 cells, respectively. These cell lines also expressed most of the placenta-related surface antigens. Six of eight PKL-type subunits and two of the three P-type subunits were detected. PKL 13 is seen only in WI-38. PKL 24 is not seen in this photograph of the WI-38 map (Fig. 3B) but was seen in other gels. P23 was not present, either in the map or by enzymatic assay (see Table II), but both 15a and 15b were readily visible for either cell line. The identity of the various antigenic subunits was confirmed in each of these additional cell lines (WI-38, GM-38, JEG-3) by means of two-dimensional gels of liver microsome-adsorbed APBB immunoprecipitates, as had been done for BeWo and Chang cell membrane antigens (see Fig. 2C, D). In addition, all gel patterns were reproducible using cells grown and labeled on separate occasions.

TABLE II. Placental Alkaline Phosphatase Specific Activities

Cell line	Specific activity (Units × 10^{-3}/mg protein)
BeWo	23
Chang	170
JEG-3	7
WI-38	–
GM-38	–

TABLE III. Summary of Plasma Membrane Antigen Compositions

Tissue or cell line						Antigens						
	2	6b	7a	7	8	9	13	15a	15b	18	21	23	24
Placenta	+	+	+	+	+	+	+	+	+	+	+	+	+
Liver	+	+	+	–	+	+	+	–	–	+	+	–	+
Kidney	–	+	ND	+	+	+	+	–	–	+	+	–	+
BeWo	+	+	+	+	+	+	–	+	+	–	+	+	+
JEG-3	+	+	+	+	+	+	–	+	+	–	+	+	+
Chang	+	+	+	+	+	+	–	+	+	+	+	+	+
WI-38	+	+	+	+	+	+	+	+	+	–	+	–	+
GM-38	+	+	+	+	+	+	–	+	+	–	+	–	+

ND – Not determined.

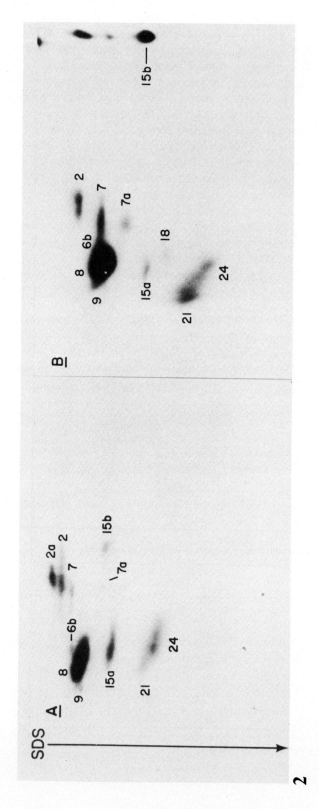

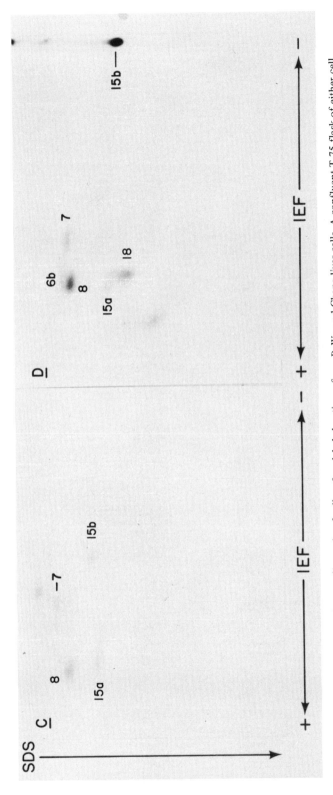

Fig. 2. Two-dimensional autoradiographs of cell surface labeled antigens from BeWo and Chang liver cells. A confluent T-75 flask of either cell type was iodinated as described in Experimantal Procedures; 300,000 acid-precipitable cpm of iodinated detergent-solubilized proteins was then precipitated with either APBB serum or liver-adsorbed APBB serum and finally subjected to two-dimensional electrophoresis. Gels were dried and exposed for four days at −76°C using Dupont "Lightening-Plus" intensifying screens. A) BeWo vs APBB; B) Chang liver vs APBB; C) BeWo vs liver-adsorbed APBB; D) Chang liver vs liver-adsorbed APBB.

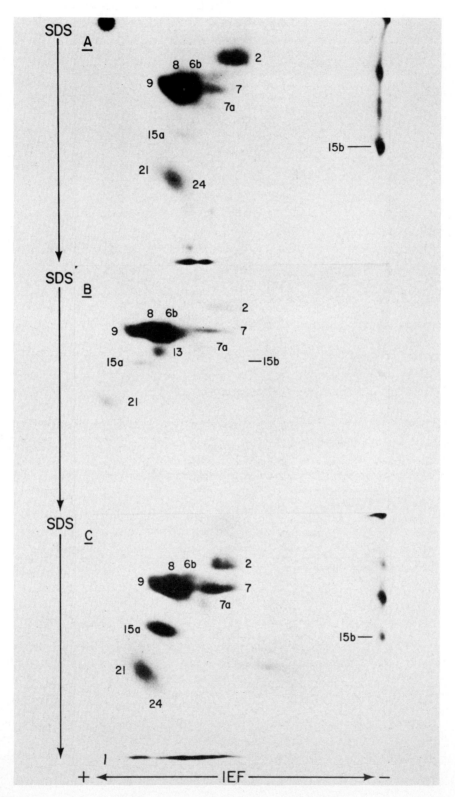

Fig. 3. Two-dimensional autoradiographs of cell surface antigens of JEG-3, WI-38, and GM-38. JEG-3 (300,000 cpm) and WI-38 or GM-38 (200,000 cpm) were immunoprecipitated with APBB serum. Two-dimensional electrophoretic analysis was as described in Figure 2. A) JEG-3; B) WI-38; C) GM-38.

DISCUSSION

The experiments described in the present report focus on the expression of a defined set of surface antigens in cell lines derived from gestational choriocarcinoma as well as in other transformed or diploid cells growing in culture. The application of lactoperoxidase-dependent ^{125}I-labeling in the present study convincingly demonstrates that nearly all of the antigens previously identified in placental brush border membranes are in fact located on the exterior surface of the cell and are in direct contact with the environment. These cell surface components were also shown to be glycoproteins by virtue of their coincident labeling with reagents directed toward both the protein and carbohydrate moiety of the molecules [8,9]. Whether PK 28, X, 31, 32, and 33 are located on the plasma membrane could not be assessed because they were either not labeled by ^{125}I or could not be adequately resolved. Components 2 and 7a, which labeled with ^{125}I, had not been demonstrated previously by specific labeling of sialic acid groups, and consequently they may not be sialoglycoproteins. Both components may also be present in liver membranes because adsorption of APBB serum with liver microsomes removes these components from immunoprecipitates.

The resolving potential of two-dimensional electrophoresis has been thoroughly documented [21]. Because glycoproteins especially exhibit heterogeneity in both focusing and SDS dimensions, the individual spots have unique morphology, facilitating identification in the two-dimensional matrix. The certainty of individual component identification is further improved by the application of immunologic criteria. By using a multivalent antiserum to preselect the antigenic proteins and then adsorbing this antiserum with a membrane-enriched fraction of human liver, each component considered must fit these four objective criterial before identity is confirmed (ie, pI, $M_{\bar{r}}$, antigenicity, loss of immunoreactivity following adsorption of the antiserum).

The two-dimensional autoradiographic technique used to separate and visualize the membrane antigens is a qualitative rather than a quantitative method. However, we are able to provide an estimate of its lower limit of detection by using placental alkaline phosphatase as a specific example. In Chang liver cells this enzyme is barely visible by autoradiography at a level of approximately 150–300 ng/mg total cell protein as estimated both from enzyme activity measurements and radioimmunoassay (Hamilton and Sussman, unpublished data). Hence, any cell surface component which represents 0.015–0.03% or more of the total cell protein should be detectable in the current system. Such sensitivity is of course also dependent upon the relative intensity of radiolabeling for the component under consideration.

Consideration of the antigenic complement of all five cell lines examined here shows them to be remarkably similar. All five express 10 of 14 components in common (2, 7, 7a, 6b, 8, 9, 15a, 15b, 21, 24). The only major distinctions are: 1) the presence of placental alkaline phosphatase in BeWo, JEG-3, and Chang detected by enzymatic immunochemical assay, and its absence in WI-38 and GM-38; 2) the expression of PKL 13 in WI-38, which was not detected in either choriocarcinoma cells or in Chang liver cells; and 3) the expression of PKL 18 in Chang cells but not in choriocarcinoma or fibroblasts.

Our previous work showed that six (7a, 6b, 8, 9, 21, 24) of these common antigens were also found in human kidney and liver membranes (see Wada et al [9]; and unpublished data). With the exception of human lymphocytes and lymphoblastoid cell lines (Hamilton et al [21a]), these components appear to be ubiquitously expressed on human cell surfaces. Two other components among the 10 common antigens (PKL 2 and PK 7) are also present on liver and kidney membranes, respectively. These may represent relatively common entities expressed by most but not all tissues whose functions are also necessary for in vitro growth. It has been observed that xenogenic antisera prepared against human membrane-bound antigens detect many common antigens [22,23]. The predominance of commonly expressed components among these antigens bound by APBB serum may result from this phenomenon. These common antigens may be minor components in some cell types and consequently would be masked in whole-membrane extracts by the major membrane components. However, the use of immunoprecipitation enhances their detectability.

Neville and Glossman [24, 25] have studied the plasma membrane protein and glycoprotein composition of three adult rat tissues in one-dimensional SDS polyacrylamide gel electrophoresis and observed that the pattern for each tissue was largely distinct. In our previous study the two-dimensional maps of total plasma membrane glycoproteins from human placenta and liver also demonstrated distinct patterns [9]. These results suggested that cell surface phenotypes may result principally from a display of a unique combination of components on the plasma membrane. However, quantitative expression of common antigens as indicated by relative spot intensity varies considerably among different cell and tissue types. This variation could be partially responsible for some phenotypic differences between highly differentiated cell types.

Several laboratories have identified common human cell surface antigens in cultured cells and defined the chromosome segments coding for their expression [23, 26, 27]. For the most part, these antigens have been demonstrated and studied by immunologic methods and their molecular characteristics have not been determined. Consequently, the relationship between these antigens and those described in the present report remains to be determined.

Several of the antigens commonly expressed in the cultured cell lines studied here were not detected at any level in kidney or liver membranes (P15a and P15b). The presence of these two components on all five cell lines examined could be accounted for by the stringent selective pressures applied to cells adapting to growth in vitro. The re-expression of functions repressed during differentiation and the loss of luxury functions normally expressed in the original differentiated tissue locale are commonly observed phenomena in cultured cells [28].

The present study clearly defines a set of commonly expressed human cell surface antigens according to the criteria of M_r and pI. Additionally, components which may show a more limited tissue distribution are identified and characterized. This work provides a firm data base for the further study of both the tissue distribution and functional identity of each glycoprotein entity. This approach should prove to be of value in the understanding of molecular events occurring at the cell-environment interface.

ACKNOWLEDGMENTS

This work was supported by contract CB74086 and grant CA13533 from the National Cancer Institute of the National Institutes of Health. T.A.H. was supported by a postdoctoral traineeship from the National Institutes of Health. We wish to express our appreciation to Agnes Tin for her technical assistance in cell culture, and to Philip Hass for his technical assistance in electrophoretic analysis.

REFERENCES

1. Billington WD: In Bishop MWH (ed): "Advances in Reproductive Physiology." New York: Academic, 1971, vol 5, No. 2, pp 27–66.
2. Beer AE, Billingham RE: Sci Am 230:36, 1974.
3. Nicolson GL: Biochim Biophys Acta 458:1, 1976.
4. Gasic G, Baydak T: In Brennan MJ, Simpson WL (eds): "Biological Interactions in Normal and Neoplastic Growth." Boston: Little, Brown, 1961, pp 709–719.
5. Hause LL, Pattillo RA, Sances A Jr, Mattingly RF: Science 169:601, 1970.
6. Sussman HH: In Ruoslahti E, Engvall E (eds): "Chemistry of Tumor-Associated Antigens." Scand J Immunol (Suppl 6), 1978, pp 126–140.
7. Faulk WP, Temple WP, Lovins RE, Smith N Proc Natl Acad Sci USA 75:1947, 1978.
8. Wada HG, Górnicki S, Sussman HH: J Supramol Struct 6:473, 1977.
9. Wada HG, Hass PE, Sussman HH: J Supramol Struct 10(3):287–305, 1979.
10. Hertz R: Proc Soc Exp Biol Med 102:77, 1959.
11. Pattillo RH, Gey GO: Cancer Res 28:1231, 1968.
12. Pattillo RH, Story MT, Hershman JM, Delfs E, Mattingly RF: In Anderson NG, Coggin JH Jr, Cole E, Holleman JW (eds): "Embryonic and Fetal Antigens in Cancer." Proceedings of the Second Conference, Springfield, VA: National Technical Information Service, vol 2, 1972, pp 45–52.
13. Kohler PO, Bridson WE: J Clin Endocrinol Metab 32:683, 1971.
14. Chang RS: Proc Soc Exp Biol Med 87:440, 1954.
15. Hamilton TA, Tin AW, Sussman HH: Proc Natl Acad Sci USA 76:323, 1979.
16. Ludueña MA, Iverson GM, Sussman HH: J Cell Physiol 91:119, 1977.
17. Kessler SW: J Immunol 115:1617, 1975.
18. Bessey OA, Lowry OH, Brock MJ: J Biol Chem 164:321, 1946.
19. Sussman HH, Small PA, Cotlove E: J Biol Chem 243:160, 1968.
20. Schaffner W, Weissmann C: Anal Biochem 56:502, 1973.
21. O'Farrell PH: J Biol Chem 250:4007, 1975.
21a. Hamilton TA, Wada HG, Sussman HH: Scand J Imm (in press).
22. Williams AF: In Ada GL, Porter RR (eds): "Contemporary Topics in Molecular Immunology," 1977, vol 6, pp 93–116.
23. Barnstable CJ, Bodmer WF, Brown G, Galfre G, Milstein C, Williams AF, Ziegler A: Cell 14:9, 1978.
24. Neville DM, Glossman H: J Biol Chem 246:6335, 1971.
25. Glossman H, Neville DM: J Biol Chem 246:6339, 1971.
26. Buck DW, Bodmer WF: Cytogen Cell Gen 14:257, 1974.
27. Kao FT, Jones C, Puck TT: Somatic Cell Gen 3:421, 1977.
28. Schwarz RI, Bissell MJ: Proc Natl Acad Sci USA 74:4453, 1977.

Journal of Supramolecular Structure 11:517–528 (1979)
Tumor Cell Surfaces and Malignancy 359–370

Selection of Malignant Melanoma Variant Cell Lines for Ovary Colonization

Kenneth W. Brunson and Garth L. Nicolson

Department of Developmental and Cell Biology, University of California, Irvine, California 92717

Murine melanoma line B16-F1, which shows some specificity for metastatic organ colonization of lung but rarely metastasizes to ovary, was used to select variant cell lines with increased preference for experimental ovary metastasis. Ovary-colonizing melanoma cell lines were sequentially selected in syngeneic C57BL/6 mice by repeated intravenous administration and surgical recovery of ovarian melanoma tumors for tissue culture. After ten selections for experimental ovary metastasis, line B16-O10 was established which formed experimental metastatic ovary tumors in almost every test animal. In tissue culture B16-O10 cells grew in circular colonies with rounded, smooth cell peripheries compared to B16-F1 cells which were flatter, grew in irregular patterns, and exhibited long cellular projections. Ovary-selected B16 lines contained less melanin pigment (B16-O10 < B16-O5 < B16-O1 ≅ B16-F1) compared to the parental melanoma line. Together with previous cloning and selection data, these results are consistent with the preexistence of highly malignant cells in the parental tumor population that possess the ability to metastasize to specific organs.

Key words: cell variants, electron microscopy, malignant melanoma, melanin, metastasis

Tumor cells are characteristically uncontrolled because of their abilities to proliferate in an unregulated fashion, circumvent normal differentiation processes, and thwart normal cellular interactions that maintain proper cell positioning and movement [1, 2]. In malignant neoplasms these properties lead to invasion of surrounding normal tissues and dissemination to form new tumor colonies (metastases) at near and distant host sites [3–5]. Distant metastatic colonization occurs when invading malignant cells penetrate and are released into the lymphatics, coelmoic cavities, or circulating system. However, many of these transported malignant cells die and only a small fraction are thought to survive to form new tumor colonies [6–8].

K. W. Brunson is now at the Department of Microbiology and Immunology, Indiana University School of Medicine, Gary, IN 46408.

Received May 31, 1979; accepted July 16, 1979.

Metastasis via blood-borne dissemination does not always result in tumor coloniza-tion of tissues and organs based strictly on circulatory tracks. In many experimental animal models of metastatic tumor spread, the locations of gross metastases are non-random and do not parallel malignant cell distribution or the initial capillary beds en-countered [9–18], suggesting that factors other than nonspecific trapping in the micro-circulation are involved in tumor cell arrest. After their initial arrest malignant cells may die, invade and grow, or detach and recirculate to colonize other sites [12, 13, 19, 20]. During circulatory transport a variety of cellular interactions take place such as homotypic adhesion of tumor cells to form multicell emboli [21–23], heterotypic adhesion of tumor cells to platelets [24], lymphocytes [25, 26], and noncirculating host cells [23, 27], and these may affect subsequent malignant cell arrest and survival.

In order to study tumor cell and host properties important in metastatic tumor spread, animal tumor models have been developed that show reproducible metastatic be-havior in syngeneic hosts and where low or nonmetastatic tumor lines are available for direct comparison [5, 28]. Several of these models have been based on Fidler's sequential selection procedures [29] to obtain metastatic variant lines of B16 melanoma with altered preference for lung [25, 29] or brain [14–16] tumor colonization. Here we de-scribe in vivo selection of B16 melanoma variants that show increased preference for ex-perimental ovary metastasis.

MATERIALS AND METHODS

Cells

The murine melanoma line (B16-F1, selected once for lung colonization [29], was obtained from Dr. I. J. Fidler (National Cancer Institute–Frederick Cancer Research Center, Frederick, Maryland). This cell line, which shows some specificity for lung but also forms experimental metastases at a variety of extrapulmonary sites [12–14], was used for subsequent in vivo selection of melanoma cell lines that preferentially colonize brain [14–16] or ovary. Cells from tumor minces were grown in tissue culture dishes or flasks (Corning Plastics) in Dulbecco-modified Eagle's medium (DMEM) supplemented with 10% fetal bovine serum, nonessential amino acids, and antibiotics (either 50 μg/ml) gentamicin or 100 units/ml penicillin plus 100 μg/ml streptomycin). Cell cultures which had just attained confluency were used for biologic assays, usually between the second and tenth passage in vitro.

Biologic Assays

Cells were detached from tissue culture surfaces with 2 mM ethylenediaminetetra-acetic acid (EDTA) in Ca^{2+}-free, Mg^{2+}-free phosphate-buffered saline and suspended in serum-free DMEM. Viable cells (2.5×10^4) were injected in a volume of 0.2 ml into tail veins of ten female C57BL/6 mice, and the animals were sacrificed after 3–4 weeks. Lungs were injected via the trachea with 10% buffered formalin for fixation prior to scoring for lung melanoma colonies; all other organs were removed and examined under a dissecting microscope and the body cavities were examined for presence of gross tumor colonies.

Histology

Organs of animals previously injected with parental or ovary-selected B16 melanoma lines were surgically removed and fixed in 10% buffered formalin for 3–4 weeks. Organs were routinely processed for paraffin embedding and sectioning (5–10 μm), and mounted sections were stained with hematoxylin-eosin and examined.

Phase Contrast and Scanning Electron Microscopy

B16 malanoma cell lines were plated at various densities in T-25 tissue culture flasks (Corning Plastics) and grown for 3 days in DMEM plus 10% fetal calf serum. Sparse and confluent cultures were photographed with phase contrast optics (Nikon) at 100×.

For scanning electron microscopy B16 lines grown on glass cover slips were fixed in 1.5% glutaraldehyde in phosphate buffered saline, pH 7.2, for 10 min at 37°C and then 1–3 h at 22°C. The glutaraldehyde-fixed monolayers were postfixed in 1% osmium tetroxide in 1 mM $CaCl_2$ –0.1 M sodium phosphate buffer, pH 7.2 for 1 h at 22°C. Monolayers were dehydrated through a graded series of ethanol, transferred to Freon 113 and critical-point-dried. After coating with 50–100 Å gold-palladium, the samples were observed in a Hitachi model S500 scanning electron microscope.

RESULTS

Selections, Biologic Assays, and Histology

Ovary-colonizing B16 melanoma variant lines were sequentially selected from B16-F1 by intravenous (tail vein) injection of single-cell suspensions of line F1 (100,000 cells per inoculum). Four weeks later rare ovary tumors were surgically removed and adapted to tissue culture to form line B16-01, which was further selected five and ten times to obtain lines B16-05 and B16-010, respectively. The number of cells per inoculum was gradually decreased with the latter sequential selections; the last injections for ovary selection employed approximately 20,000 cells. Assays for organ colonization were conducted by intravenous (tail vein) injection of 25,000 viable melanoma cells followed by examination after 4 weeks. In this assay B16-F1 yields an average of approximately 40–50 lung tumors per animal, but often fails to form ovary tumors (Table I). Line B16-01 shows similar biologic behavior to B16-F1; however, lines B16-05 and B16-010 form experimental ovary metastases in almost all animals injected and dramatically fewer lung tumor colonies (Table I).

Histologic examination of ovary tumors was performed on animals injected with the various melanoma lines. The rare ovary tumors formed in mice injected with lines

TABLE I. Experimental Metastasis After Intravenous Injection of B16 Melanoma Variant Lines

| Cell line | Experimental metastases[a] | | |
	Ovary tumors	Average no. lung tumors (range)	Other tumors
B16-F1	0/10	47 (22–200)	2/10 thoracic 1/10 liver 1/10 adrenal
B16-01	0/10	53 (1–256)	3/10 thoracic
B16-05	8/10	32 (30–155)	2/10 thoracic 1/10 liver
B16-010	8/9	7 (1–17)	2/10 liver 1/10 adrenal

[a]25,000 viable B16 melanoma cells were inoculated intravenously into groups of ten animals and experimental metastases were determined after 4 weeks.

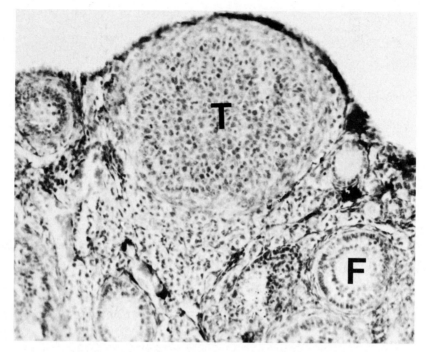

Fig. 1. Histology of ovary from B16-010-injected animal. T, tumor; F, follicle. × 248.

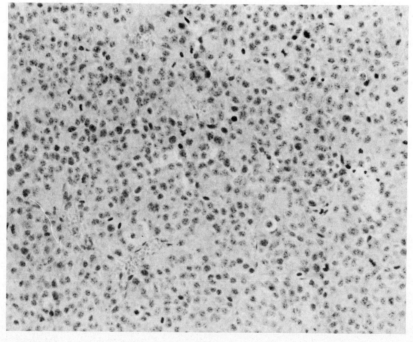

Fig. 2. Histology of ovary from B16-010-injected animal. Amelanotic tumor has obliterated ovary.
× 248.

B16-F1 or B16-01 were pigmented and easily identified in ovary sections (Fig. 1). Ovaries from animals injected with B16—010 cells were greatly enlarged owing to the presence of amelanotic tumors, and examination of these ovaries revealed that the 010 tumors had obliterated the normal ovary structure (Fig. 2).

Cell Morphology and Pigmentation

Colony and cell morphology was assessed in vitro by phase contrast and scanning electron microscopy. Sparse B16-F1 cells were irregularly spaced and shaped with long

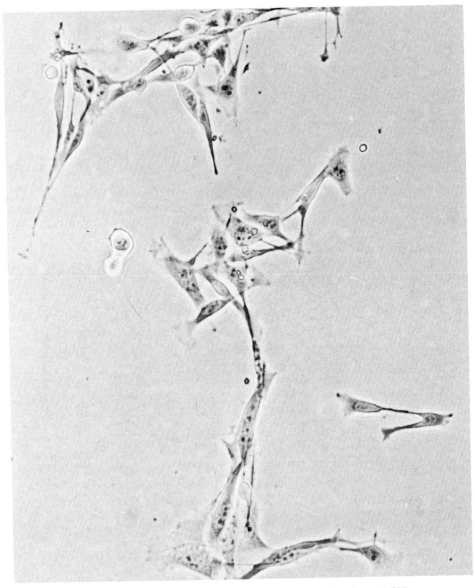

Fig. 3. Phase contrast micrograph of sparse B16-F1 cells in culture. × 300.

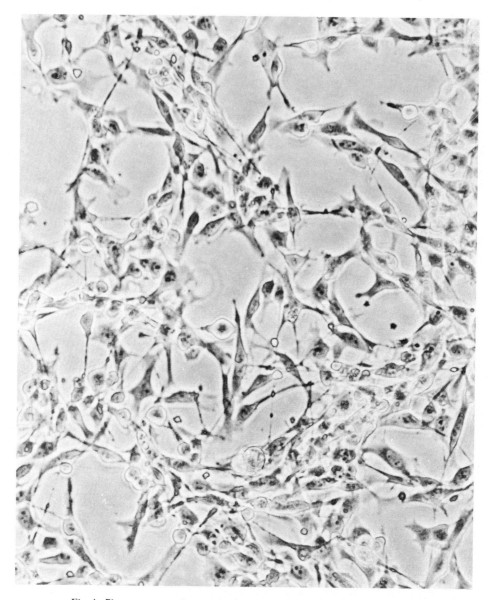

Fig. 4. Phase contrast micrograph of confluent B16-F1 cells in culture. × 300.

cytoplasmic extensions which often under- and overlapped adjacent cells (Fig. 3). At confluency this same pattern of irregular cell placement and multilayering was apparent (Fig. 4). Sparse B16-010 cells were flatter with fewer cytoplasmic extensions and grew in round-shaped colonies (Fig. 5). When B16-010 cells grew to confluency, this same pattern of growth persisted, and the cells seemed to form multilayers less readily than B16-F1 cells (Fig. 6). When examined by scanning electron microscopy, these morphologic differences were even more apparent. B16-F1 cells appeared very irregularly shaped at confluency, with numerous long cell projections and microvilli (Fig. 7), while B16-010 cells were rounder and contained fewer pseudopodia (Fig. 8).

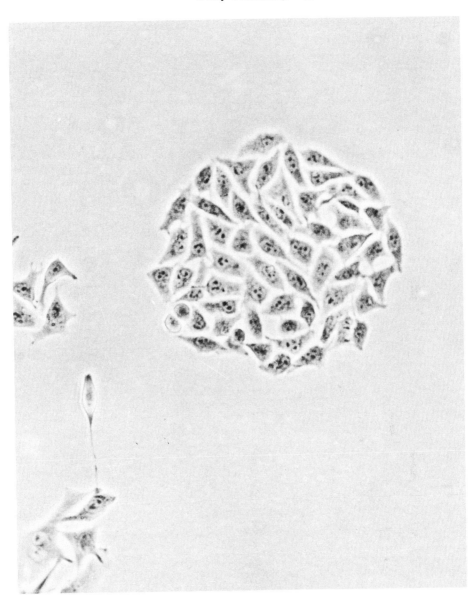

Fig. 5. Phase contrast micrograph of sparse B16-010 cells in culture. × 300.

The relative pigmentation in various B16 melanoma lines was examined by comparing cell pellets for the black pigment melanin. When line B16-F1 was compared to brain- and ovary-selected variant lines, only the latter selections showed dramatic differences (Fig. 9). Lines B16-05 and B16-010 exhibited a progressive loss of pigmentation with selection for ovary preference. That this is related to the number of in vivo selections was unlikely, since brain-selected lines B16-B5 and B16-B10N were similar in pigmentation to B16-F1 (Fig. 9).

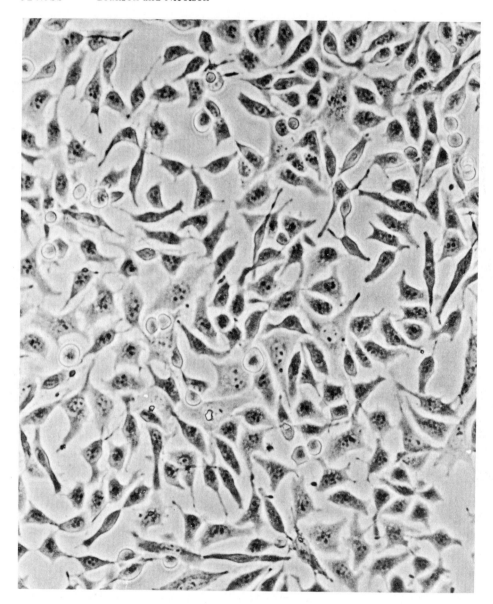

Fig. 6. Phase contrast micrograph of confluent B16-010 cells in culture. × 300.

DISCUSSION

Sequential selection for ovary-preferring B16 melanoma lines yielded increasingly more ovary-specific lines. Although line B16-010 was not totally specific for ovary and gave some experimental metastases at other sites, we have recently obtained a clone of B16-010 that appears to be quite specific in colonizing ovaries (K. W. Brunson and G. L. Nicolson, unpublished). In the biologic assays utilized here tumor cells were intravenously injected via the tail vein so that they had to pass through pulmonary

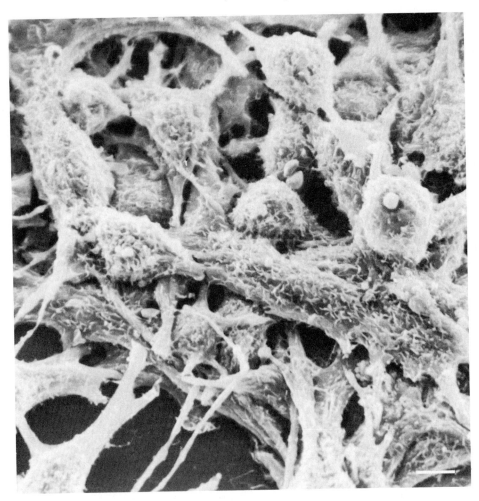

Fig. 7. Scanning electron micrograph of B16-F1 cells at confluency. Bar equals 5 μm.

capillaries and recirculate to reach the ovaries. Similar assays for brain-selected B16 lines have also shown that variant cell lines can be selected that are capable of recirculating from sites of initial arrest and finding their way to target organ sites [15, 16].

The in vivo and in vitro properties of ovary-selected lines suggest that they may represent a subpopulation of the parental B16-F1 melanoma cells. Cell and colony morphology in vitro are distinctly different from B16-F1 in the ovary-selected series, and there is a marked difference in melanin pigmentation. Preliminary cell surface labeling studies using lactoperoxidase-catalyzed ^{125}I-iodination techniques indicate that lines B16-05 and B16-010 have two exposed surface proteins that differ in amounts or exposures compared to parental line B16-F1. When analyzed by sodium dodecyl sulfate-polyacrylamide electrophoresis autoradiography, lines B16-05 and B16-010 show increased ^{125}I-incorporation in surface proteins of approximately 140,000 and 150,000 mol wt, which correlates with the number of in vivo selections and preference for ovary

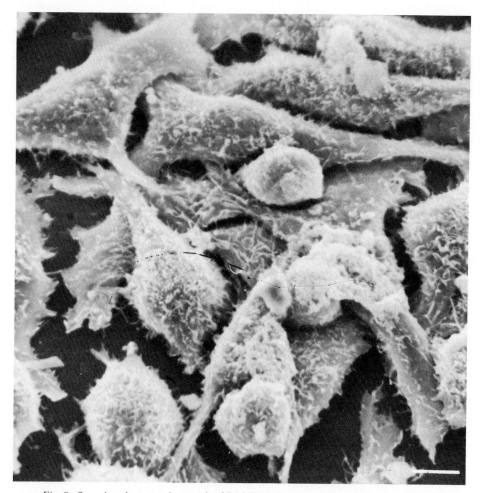

Fig. 8. Scanning electron micrograph of B16-010 cells at confluency. Bar equals 5 μm.

metastasis. In contrast, variants selected for brain colonization show different changes which correlate with their in vivo properties. Lines B16-B5 and B16-B10N show increased exposure to lactoperoxidase-iodination in proteins of approximately 95,000 and 100,000 mol wt which correlates with the number of in vivo selections and preference for brain metastasis [15]. Therefore, certain identifiable surface proteins are different in each of the selected series, and these changes may be important in directing implantation at specific organ sites in vivo [27].

The successful selection of metastatic variants with altered organ preference suggests that the original parental line B16-F1 and perhaps its precursor may be hetero-geneous with respect to its phenotypic properties. Either these highly metastatic variant cells preexisted in the primary tumor population, or the phenotypic variants could have arisen by a process of organ adaptation during the selection process. Two different types of experiments have been performed to answer this question. First, primary tumor cell populations have been cloned and fluctuation tests carried out to determine whether highly metastatic variant cells preexist in the parental population. Experiments with B16

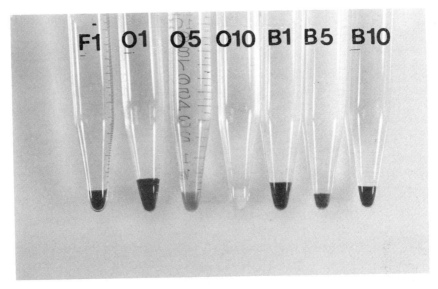

Fig. 9. Relative melanin contents of various B16 melanoma lines shown by pigmentation intensities of cell pellets.

melanoma [30], a UV-induced sarcoma [31], and a vasoformative sarcoma [5, 28] indicate that tumor cell clones differ widely in their metastatic properties, and some rare clones exist that possess highly metastatic phenotypes. Subcloning experiments ruled out the possibility that the in vitro cloning techniques caused the variations in phenotypic properties [30]. The second type of experiment was an attempt to adapt cells to grow at a specific organ location by direct inoculation [16]. This experiment was performed using line B16-F1, which was sequentially adapted to grow in brain for a series of ten cycles of similar durations in vivo and in vitro to the brain-selected line B16-B10N. After ten sequential adaptations for brain survival, adaptation, and growth, the adpated line B16-ICer10 was tested for its ability to metastasize to brain. Line B16-ICer10 was no more effective in colonizing brain after intravenous administration than its original parental line B16-F1, suggesting that adaptation per se is not responsible for generating variants with increased metastatic potential [16]. These data suggest that highly malignant, organ-preferring cells preexist in the unselected parental tumor cell population and that in vivo selection of variant lines yields new populations enriched in cells with highly malignant phenotypes.

ACKNOWLEDGMENTS

We thank A. Brodginski, R. Davis, and D. Welch for assistance. These studies were supported by US Public Health Service National Cancer Institute grant R01-CA-15122 and contract NO1-CB-74153 and a grant (BC-211B) from the American Cancer Society to G.L.N.

REFERENCES

1. Nicolson GL, Poste G: New Engl J Med (Part 1) 295:197, 1976, (Part 2) 295:253, 1976.
2. Nicolson GL: Biochim Biophys Acta 458:1, 1976.

3. Zeidman I: Cancer Res 17:157, 1957.
4. Fidler IJ: In Becker FF (ed): "Cancer: A Comprehensive Treatise," vol 4: "Biology of Tumors: Surfaces, Immunology, and Comparative Pathology." New York: Plenum, 1975, p 101.
5. Nicolson GL: Bio Science 28:441, 1978.
6. Fidler IJ: J Natl Cancer Inst 45:773, 1970.
7. Proctor JW, Auclair BG, Rudenstam CM: Int J Cancer 18:255, 1976.
8. Fidler IJ: In Day SB et al (eds): "Cancer Invasion and Metastasis." New York: Raven, 1977, p 277.
9. Dunn TB: J Natl Cancer Inst 14:1281, 1954.
10. Potter M, Rahey JL, Pilgrim HI: Proc Soc Exp Biol Med 94:327, 1957.
11. Parks RC: J Natl Cancer Inst 52:971, 1974.
12. Fidler IJ, Nicolson GL: J Natl Cancer Inst 57:1199, 1976.
13. Fidler IJ, Nicolson GL: J Natl Cancer Inst 58:1867, 1977.
14. Nicolson GL, Brunson KW: Gann Monogr Cancer Res 20:15, 1977.
15. Brunson KW, Beattie G, Nicolson GL: Nature 272:543, 1978.
16. Brunson KW, Nicolson GL: In Weiss L, Gilbert H, Posner JB (eds): "Brain Metastasis." Boston: GK Hall & Co. (in press).
17. Brunson KW, Nicolson GL: J Natl Cancer Inst 61:1499, 1978.
18. Conley FK: Cancer Res 39:1001, 1979.
19. Zeidman I: Cancer Res 21:38, 1961.
20. Fisher B, Fisher ER: Cancer Res 27:421, 1967.
21. Fidler IJ: Eur J Cancer 9:223, 1973.
22. Liotta LA, Kleinerman J, Saidel GM: Cancer Res 36:889, 1976.
23. Nicolson GL, Winkelhake JL, Nussey AC: In Weiss L (ed): "Fundamental Aspects of Metastasis." Amsterdam: North-Holland, 1976, p 291.
24. Gasic GJ, Gasic TB, Galanti N, Johnson T, Murphy S: Int J Cancer 11:704, 1973.
25. Fidler IJ: Cancer Res 35:218, 1975.
26. Fidler IJ, Bucana C: Cancer Res 37:3945, 1977.
27. Nicolson GL, Winkelhake JL: Nature 255:230, 1975.
28. Nicolson GL, Brunson KW, Fidler IJ: Cancer Res 38:4105, 1978.
29. Fidler IJ: Nature New Biol 242:148, 1973.
30. Fidler IJ, Kripke ML: Science 197:893, 1977.
31. Kripke ML, Gruys E, Fidler IJ: Cancer Res 38:2962, 1978.

Journal of Supramolecular Structure 11:529–538 (1979)
Tumor Cell Surfaces and Malignancy 371–380

Growth Control of Normal and Transformed Cells

Veronica G.H. Riddle, Arthur B. Pardee, and Peter W. Rossow

Laboratory of Tumor Biology, Sidney Farber Cancer Institute, Boston, Massachusetts 02115 and Department of Pharmacology, Harvard Medical School, Boston, Massachusetts 02115

Both serum factors and protein synthesis are required for normal cell growth. Swiss 3T3 cells require the serum growth factors insulin and EGF (epidermal growth factor) during the initial part of the G_1 period, until they pass a restriction point about 2 h before the initiation of DNA synthesis. Concentrations of cycloheximide that inhibit protein synthesis by as much as 70% dramatically lengthen the cell cycle before the restriction point, while the cell cycle after the restriction point remains nearly constant. These results are consistent with a model in which labile proteins are required for transit of cells past the serum-sensitive restriction point. The relation of these findings to the growth control of transformed cells is discussed.

Key words: 3T3 cells, transformed cells, restriction point, labile proteins, growth factors

A central question regarding cancer is how normal cells differ from transformed cells. Tumorigenic cells have been reported to differ from nontumorigenic ones in many ways. The differences can be divided into four groups: 1) growth properties in culture (for example, transformed cells require lower serum concentrations for optimal growth, grow to higher density, grow into mutlilayers, do not arrest in a state with a G_1 DNA content (G_0) at high density or in low serum, and grow without anchorage); 2) metabolic properties (for example, transformed cells produce a protease called the plasminogen activator and have altered surface components and higher transport rates of several nutrients); 3) morphologic changes; and 4) karyotypic changes. Most of these differences have been observed by comparisons of normal and DNA virus-transformed cells, although there have been a few studies with RNA virus-transformed cells, and a very few with chemically transformed cells.

Cell populations in vivo exist in a steady-state condition in which most cells are quiescent and cell replication is balanced by cell death. Two broad models can be considered for the control of normal cell growth and the loss of this control upon transforma-

Received May 11, 1979, accepted July 29, 1979.

tion. The first model proposes that transformed or tumor cells arise in the population as cells that can escape from the quiescent state in some abnormal way. Thus the process of transformation is an initation of growth in an otherwise resting cell. An alternative, equally plausible, model is that cells in the steady-state, resting condition require a starting event as suggested in the first model but the difference is that once in the cycle, the transformed cells are unable to stop growing.

The growth of normal cells is regulated in the G_1 phase of the cell cycle. It has been proposed that the regulatory event occurs at a specific "metabolic place" in G_1 called the restriction point (R point) [1]. Thus each cell carries out certain early G_1 processes and then must undergo a special event at the restriction point in order to carry out further biochemical processes leading to DNA synthesis. If the cell cannot carry out this restriction point event, it passes off into the G_0 state. This event can be considered a sort of "switch" at which a choice is made between proliferation and quiescence. A variety of conditions that control growth appear to involve the same restriction event. That is, only one control point exists and is responsive to many growth-restrictive conditions.

Some sort of crucial G_1 event was also suggested earlier (see Baserga [2] and Prescott [3]). Temin's experiments [4] showed serum to be dispensable to the growth of chick fibroblasts about halfway through G_1; he suggested that all serum-dependent events were accomplished at that time. Hershko et al [5] proposed a pleiotypic control, meaning that when cells are arrested in a variety of ways they always show several characteristic changes, including slower transport of some nutrients, diminished macromolecular synthesis, and enhanced protein breakdown. By analogy with the stringent response of bacteria, Hershko et al proposed that these effects were mediated by a pleiotypic modulator compound of low molecular weight. This compound has yet to be identified. Smith and Martin's concept [6] comes close to the idea of a restriction point; they propose a point (in G_1) at which all cells under all conditions become arrested and from which they escape probabilistically, either rapidly or slowly, depending on growth conditions.

Lower organisms also show a cell-cycle specific control event prior to DNA synthesis initiation. Hartwell [7] showed that yeasts are arrested at a specific point, under conditions of poor nutrition, or when they are exposed to mating factor peptide made by the opposite mating type. A temperature-sensitive mutant arrested at this event has been isolated. In Bacilli there is also a critical event at which the decision is made as to whether the bacteria continue vegetative growth or form a spore [8].

The growth behavior of cells in culture is central to the entire cancer problem, since growth changes characteristic of transformed cells are similar to the altered growth kinetic properties observed with malignant cells in vivo. In this article we describe some of our recent results on the regulation of normal cell growth. We also relate these findings to growth control in transformed cells.

MATERIALS AND METHODS

Materials

Epidermal growth factor (EGF) was the generous gift of Dr. Tom Maciag, Collaborative Research, Inc. Radiochemicals were obtained from New England Nuclear. Colcemid was purchased from Gibco. All other chemicals were obtained from Sigma.

Cell Culture

Swiss 3T3 cells were originally obtained from Dr. Howard Green, Massachusetts Institute of Technology, and Balb/c 3T3 clone A31 were obtained from Dr. Charles D. Sher, Sidney Farber Cancer Institute.

Cells were routinely grown at $37°C$ in a water-saturated $10\% \; CO_2 : 90\%$ air atmosphere in Dulbecco's modified Eagle's medium (DME, Gibco H21, high glucose) supplemented with 10% calf serum (Flow Laboratories), 100 units/ml of penicillin, and 100 μg/ml streptomycin. Both cell lines were determined to be free of mycoplasma by the ratio of ^{3}H-uridine to ^{3}H-uracil incorporation into RNA [9].

Cell Counting

Cells were removed from duplicate plates or flasks using trypsin (0.05%)/EDTA (0.5 mM) (in 138 mM NaCl, 2.67 mM KCl, 1.47 mM KH_2PO_4, 8.10 mM Na_2PO_4) and were resuspended in 20 ml Hanks' balanced salt solution (BSS) containing 0.5% formalin to fix them. Cell numbers were determined with a Coulter Counter model B.

Cell Synchrony

A modification of the technique of Hamlin and Pardee [10] was used. Cultures in 75-cm^2 Falcon flasks were arrested in G_0 by exposure to medium containing 0.5% serum for 40 h. These quiescent cells were then stimulated to grow by the addition of medium containing 10% serum, and 8 h later, before cells had begun to synthesize DNA, 0.1 mM hydroxyurea was added for 8 h to block the cells at the G_1/S boundary. In order to obtain mitotic populations, the cells were released from the G_1/S block by replacing the medium containing hydroxyurea with regular medium. After a further 8 h, cells began to enter mitosis and these cells were shaken off the culture flask every 20 min for 2 h and pooled on ice; $10^4 - 10^5$ mitotic cells were plated into 8-cm^2 culture dishes in medium containing 10% serum.

Cytofluorimetry

Cells were prepared for cytofluorimetry by a modification of the method of Fried et al [11]. Cells were removed from the culture flasks (Falcon, 75 cm^2) with trypsin/ EDTA and resuspended in DME supplemented with 10% calf serum. After pelleting at $4°C$ the cells were resuspended in 3 ml of hypotonic staining solution [12] containing 50 μg/ml propidium iodide in 0.1% sodium citrate. The suspension was maintained on ice for at least 15 min prior to cytofluorimetry.

Cytofluorographic analysis was performed with a model 4800 Cytofluorograf equipped with a model 2102 multichannel analyzer with a distribution integration capability (Biophysics Systems, Ortho Instruments).

Autoradiography

Cells were labeled with 2 μCi/ml methyl ^{3}H-thymidine (45 Ci/mmole). The fraction of labeled cells was determined by fixing the cells onto the culture dish with MeOH:HOAc fixative, 2:1. Dried plates were then coated directly with Kodak NTB2 emulsion, exposed for three days, and then developed. A minimum of 400 total cells were counted for each determination.

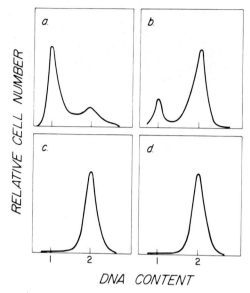

Fig. 1. Effect of cell density on the arrest of Swiss 3T3 cells in G_1. DNA histograms of (a) an exponential cell population at a density of 2.4×10^4 cells/cm^2; (b) a cell population, initially at 2.4×10^4 cells/cm^2, 24 h after shiftdown into medium containing 0.5% serum and 0.05 μg/ml colcemid; (c) a cell population, initially at 2.2×10^3 cells/cm^2, 24 h after shiftdown into medium containing 0.5% serum and 0.05 μg/ml colcemid; (d) a cell population, initially at 2.5×10^4 cells/cm^2, 24 h after addition of 0.05 μg/ml colcemid directly to culture medium.

RESULTS

Time and Growth Factor Requirements of the R Point

Recently Yen and Pardee [13] have described a technique to differentiate between cells that are located either before or after the serum-sensitive R point in G_1. In this technique, exponentially growing cells are placed in medium containing 0.5% serum and 0.05 μg/ml colcemid. Cells that have already passed the serum-requiring point at the time of shiftdown go on to mitosis, where they all stop owing to the presence of colcemid (see Fig. 1a,b). After 20–24 h of this treatment the initial exponential population has separated into two fractions that are easily resolvable by cytofluorography; one has a G_1 DNA content representing those cells initially in G_1 and prior to the serum-sensitive step, and the other has a G_2 DNA content representing cells initially beyond the serum-sensitive step.

Yen and Pardee showed that the R point is about 2 h before S phase in Swiss 3T3 cells. It is important to note, however, that the method requires cells to experience serum starvation immediately following shiftdown. Figure 1b, c shows the results of taking exponentially growing cultures of 3T3 cells at two densities differing nearly tenfold and shifting down as described above. At the higher density, which was in the range used by Yen and Pardee, a comparable arrest was obtained. Thus the small quantities of serum factors provided by the low serum were rapidly utilized by the cells and a large, definite fraction of cells were arrested in G_1. Cells at this high density were not already arrested in G_1 at the time of shiftdown, since addition of colcemid alone with no serum reduction resulted in the accumulation of all cells in the G_2 peak (see Fig. 1d). At tenfold lower density, all of the cells that had been in G_1 phase at the time of shiftdown were able to pass around the cell cycle and were arrested at the colcemid block. In this case, residual serum factors must have permitted those cells prior to the restriction point at shiftdown to traverse the cell cycle. The cell density dependence of growth arrest illustrated by these results suggests that specific serum factors are required for R point transit.

Insulin and epidermal growth factor (EGF) appear to be able to replace the serum-derived growth factors that become limiting when cell growth is arrested. Almost complete relief from the restrictive condition of 0.5% serum was observed after Swiss 3T3 cells were subjected to the above procedure in the presence of insulin (10 μg/ml) and EGF (10 ng/ml) [14]. This suggests that these factors, or factors closely related to them structurally, are required for the transit of G_1 phase.

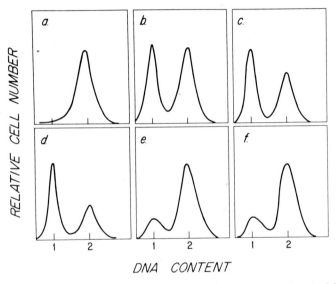

Fig. 2. Effect of serum and purified growth factors on the G_1 transit of synchronized Swiss 3T3 cells. DNA histograms of G_2 cells (1.2×10^4 cells/cm^2) placed in medium containing (a) 10% serum; (b) 0.5% serum; (c) 0.2% serum; (d) 0% serum; (e) 0.5% serum, 10μg/ml insulin, and 10 ng/ml EGF; (f) 0.2% serum, 10 μg/ml insulin, and 10 ng/ml EGF. In all cases 0.05 μg/ml colcemid was added 4 h after the G_2 cells were shifted into the media indicated above and cells were prepared for cyto-fluorography 20 h after addition of colcemid.

TABLE I. Effect of Serum and Purified Growth Factors on G_1 Transit of Synchronized Swiss 3T3 Cells

	Fraction of cells with G_1 DNA content
0% serum	0.58
0.2% serum	0.50
0.5% serum	0.43
0.2% serum + insulin + EGF	0.23
0.5% serum + insulin + EGF	0.23

These values were obtained by integrating the peaks in the DNA histograms shown in Figure 2.

The insulin and EGF requirement for Swiss 3T3 cells to pass the R point can be demonstrated with a larger fraction of the population using synchronized cultures. Cells were synchronized by slight modification of the hydroxyurea (HU) technique developed for CHO cells [10]. At 6 h after release from HU, when the cells were in G_2, they were shifted into serum-deficient medium; and 4 h later, when most of the cells had completed division and were in early G_1, 0.05 μg/ml colcemid was added to arrest at mitosis all cells able to escape the serum deprivation. When G_2 cells were shifted into medium completely lacking serum factors, nearly 60% of the cells were arrested in the G_1 phase after 20 h (Fig. 2 and Table I). However, as little as 0.2% or 0.5% serum in the shiftdown medium provided sufficient amounts of the limiting growth factors to permit a further 8% or 15% of the cells, respectively, to escape arrest and synthesize DNA. Addition of insulin (10 μg/ml) plus EGF (10 ng/ml) to medium containing either 0.2% or 0.5% serum allowed approximately 75% of cells to escape G_1 arrest. It is not known why 25% of the cells were arrested in G_1 even in the presence of insulin and EGF. Possible explanations — for instance, that concentrations of insulin and EGF were not optimal for R point transit of G_2 cells — will require further study.

The observation that both 0.5% and 0.2% serum were equally effective when supplemented with insulin and EGF is of special interest. This implies that only these two factors and no others became limiting when the serum concentration was reduced to 0.2%. If other factors had become limiting, then the fraction of cells able to escape from the 0.2% restriction would have been smaller than the fraction able to escape 0.5%, upon the addition of insulin and EGF. From this result it follows that other essential growth factors in serum besides insulin and EGF do not become limiting until their concentration is at least two times lower than in 0.5% serum

Effect of Protein Synthesis Inhibition

Transit throughout the G_1 phase depends not only on serum factors but also on the synthesis of proteins. Inhibitors of protein synthesis added at high concentration block entry into S phase [2, 3]. Low doses of streptovitacin A specifically arrest the transit from G_0 to S of baby hamster kidney (BHK) cells [15], whereas low concentrations of the related compound cycloheximide slow the transit of Swiss 3T3 cells though the same process [16]. Schneiderman et al [17] presented evidence, from the effects of time exposures to high concentrations of cycloheximide, that progress of CHO cells through G_1 depends on the synthesis of labile protein(s) (half-life 2 h) that must be made in sufficient amount before the cells are able to proceed to make DNA.

If transit through G_1 depends on the synthesis of labile proteins, we might expect this part of the cell cycle to be preferentially inhibited by low doses of cycloheximide. We therefore examined the effect of low doses of cycloheximide on Swiss 3T3 cell cycle transit. Growth remained exponential, but there was a progressive increase in the cell doubling time as the concentration of cycloheximide increased (Fig. 3). This effect was observed with cycloheximide concentrations that inhibited protein synthesis by up to 70%. The diminution of the growth rate was as might be expected from the inhibition of protein synthesis. Surprisingly, however, the elongation was not uniform around the cell cycle.

The elongation of the cell cycle occurred mainly in G_1. When cytofluorographic DNA histograms were obtained from Swiss 3T3 cells growing exponentially in the presence of various concentrations of cycloheximide, the proportion of cells with a G_1 DNA content increased as the cycloheximide concentration increased (Fig. 4). The aver-

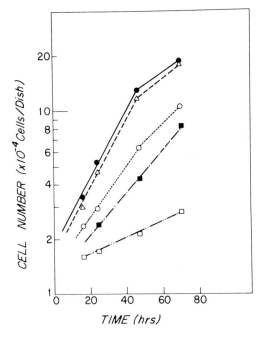

Fig. 3. Effect of cycloheximide on cell doubling time. Swiss 3T3 cells were plated in 8-cm² culture dishes in the presence of cycloheximide and the doubling time was obtained from the increase in cell number, determined using a Coulter Counter, over time. ●, no cycloheximide; △, 0.01 μg/ml cycloheximide; ○, 0.03 μg/ml cycloheximide; ■, 0.05 μg/ml cycloheximide; □, 0.1 μg/ml cycloheximide.

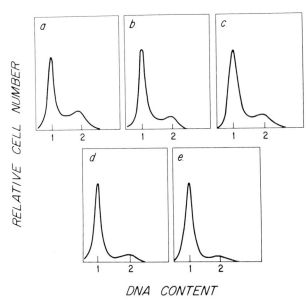

Fig. 4. Effect of cycloheximide on cell-cycle distribution. DNA histograms of exponential populations of Swiss 3T3 cells in (a) no cycloheximide; (b) 0.01 μg/ml cycloheximide; (c) 0.03 μg/ml cycloheximide; (d) 0.05 μg/ml cycloheximide; and (e) 0.1 μg/ml cycloheximide.

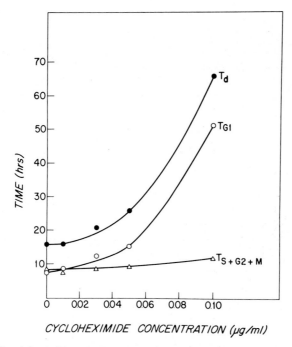

Fig. 5. Effect of cycloheximide on cell-cycle parameters. •, doubling time, T_d; ○, duration of G_1, T_{G1}; △, duration of $S + G_2 + M$, $T_{S + G_2 + M}$.

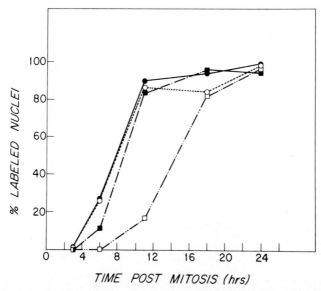

Fig. 6. Effect of cycloheximide on the entry of mitotic Balb/c 3T3 cells into DNA synthesis. Mitotic cells (10^4) were plated into 8-cm^2 culture dishes in the presence of cycloheximide and 2 μ Ci/ml ^{3}H-thymidine. Plates were processed for autoradiography at the indicated times. •, no cycloheximide; ○, 0.03 μg/ml cycloheximide; ■, 0.05 μg/ml cycloheximide; □, 0.1 μg/ml cyclo-heximide.

age durations of G_1 and of the remainder of the cycle were calculated from these histograms using the Von Foerster equation [18], which takes into account the decreasing number of cells with increasing age in the cycle. The values are shown in Figure 5. Almost all of the increase in cycle duration caused by cycloheximide occurs in the G_1 period, while the $S + G_2 + M$ duration is only slightly changed. Using the shiftdown technique of Yen and Pardee, we have shown elsewhere that this elongation of the G_1 phase occurs primarily before the serum-sensitive R point [19]. These experiments support the idea that labile proteins are required for cell passage past the serum-sensitive R point.

Timing of Cycloheximide-Sensitive Events

We were interested in determining whether synthesis of the labile proteins is accomplished only during the G_1 period in which they are utilized or whether some synthesis of the proteins occurs during the preceding cycle. If some of the labile proteins are produced in the preceding cycle, then cells collected at mitosis should be less delayed by low concentrations of cycloheximide present only during the following G_1 transit than are cells inhibited throughout the entire cycle. If, however, the synthesis of these proteins does not start until after mitosis, then mitotically collected cells should be just as delayed as cells grown for several generations in cycloheximide. Balb/c 3T3 cells were used for these experiments because Swiss 3T3 cells adhere to culture dishes more tenaciously and thus give extremely low yields of mitotic cells following a shake procedure. Labile protein synthesis similar to that described in Swiss 3T3 cells has also been demonstrated in Balb/c 3T3 cells [19]. Figure 6 shows the entry into S phase as determined autoradiographically for Balb/c 3T3 cells collected by a mitotic shake procedure. The duration of G_1 after shifting into low doses of cycloheximide was little changed. At the highest concentration of cycloheximide (that inhibits protein synthesis by 70%), the duration of the first G_1 after exposure was almost doubled. This elongation, however, was still not as great as that found in cells grown for several generations with the same concentration of cycloheximide. Thus at least some of the protein synthesis involved in regulation of R point transit may occur in the preceding cycle.

DISCUSSION

Both serum factors and protein synthesis are required for normal cell growth. Lowering the serum concentration to 0.2% stops the growth of Swiss 3T3 cells mainly by limiting their supply of insulin and EGF. Under these conditions cells are unable to pass a growth restriction point located 2 h before the initiation of DNA synthesis. Experiments using the protein synthesis inhibitor cycloheximide indicate that labile proteins are involved in cell transit past this serum-sensitive restriction point in G_1 phase. Indeed, results from experiments with cycloheximide can be used to quantitiatively support a model in which an initiator protein with a half-life of 2.2 h has to be synthesized at a constant rate and built up to a specific level before a cell can pass the restriction point [19].

Transformed cells are generally thought to have a markedly lowered serum requirement. Recent work, however, shows that this is not always so. Dubrow et al [20] found that the ability of Balb/c 3T3 cells and seven transformed derivatives (DNA virus, RNA virus, and chemical) to grow in media containing low serum concentrations was a function of the mode of transformation. DNA virus-transformed lines remained distributed throughout the cell cycle whereas RNA virus-transformed and chemically transformed cells accumulated in G_1. Cherington et al [21] have examined the growth requirements of various hamster cell lines using a chemically defined medium containing the purified growth hormones insulin, EGF, fibroblast growth factor (FGF), and transferrin. They found that a DNA virus-transformed line had lost the requirement for insulin, FGF, and EGF. In contrast, chemically and spontaneously transformed cell lines retained the insulin requirement and had a diminished requirement for EGF. Transformed cells requiring insulin but not EGF were arrested in G_1 on withdrawal of insulin.

The mode of transformation appears to determine the amount of growth control exhibited by transformed cell lines. The behavior of a single transformed line cannot be taken to represent the behavior of all transformed lines. In particular, transformation by DNA tumor viruses such as polyoma and SV40 is an extreme sort, with abolished growth control and few growth factor requirements. In contrast, transformation with RNA viruses and chemicals generally has much less drastic consequences for growth regulation.

ACKNOWLEDGMENTS

This work was supported by US Public Health Service grant GM 24571 to A.B. Pardee and National Cancer Institute Fellowship 5-F32-CA 05595-02 to P.W. Rossow. V.G.H. Riddle is an Aid for Cancer Research Fellow.

We acknowledge the assistance of David S. Schneider in preparing the manuscript for publication, and that of Mary Addonizio for care in handling technical procedures.

REFERENCES

1. Pardee AB: Proc Natl Acad Sci USA 71:1286, 1974.
2. Baserga R: "Multiplication and Division in Mammalian Cells." New York: Marcel Dekker, 1976.
3. Prescott DM: "Reproduction of Eukaryotic Cells." New York: Academic Press, 1976.
4. Temin HM: J Cell Physiol 78:161, 1971.
5. Hershko A, Mamont P, Shields R, Tomkins GM: Nature New Biol 232:206, 1971.
6. Smith JA, Martin L: Proc Natl Acad Sci USA 70:1263, 1973.
7. Hartwell LH: Bacteriol Rev 38:164, 1974.
8. Mandelstam J, Higgs SA: J Bacteriol 120:38, 1974.
9. Schneider EL, Stanbridge EJ, Epstein CJ: Exp Cell Res 84:311, 1974.
10. Hamlin JL, Pardee AB: Exp Cell Res 100:265, 1976.
11. Fried J, Perez AG, Clarkson BD: J Cell Biol 71:172, 1976.
12. Krishan AJ: J Cell Biol 66:188, 1975.
13. Yen A, Pardee AB: Exp Cell Res 116:103, 1978.
14. Rossow PW, Pardee AB: Nature (In press).
15. Pardee AB, James LJ: Proc Natl Acad Sci USA 72:4994, 1975.
16. Brooks, RF: Cell 12:311, 1977.
17. Schneiderman MH, Dewey WC, Highfield DP: Exp Cell Res 67:147, 1971.
18. Von Foerster H: In Stohlman F (ed): "The Kinetics of Cellular Proliferation." New York and London: Grune & Stratton, 1959, p 382.
19. Rossow PW, Riddle VGH, Pardee AB: Proc Natl Acad Sci USA (In press).
20. Dubrow R, Riddle VGH, Pardee AB: Cancer Res 39:2718, 1979.
21. Cherington PV, Smith BL, Pardee AB: Proc Natl Acad Sci USA 76:3937, 1979.

Journal of Supramolecular Structure 11:539—546 (1979)
Tumor Cell Surfaces and Malignancy 381—388

Tumorigenicity of Revertants From an SV40-Transformed Line

Bettie M. Steinberg, Daniel Rifkin, Seung-il Shin, Charles Boone, and
Robert Pollack

*Department of Biological Sciences, Columbia University, New York, New York 10027 (B.M.S.
and R.P.), Department of Cell Biology, New York University Medical School, New York,
New York 10016 (D.R.), Department of Genetics, Albert Einstein College of Medicine,
Bronx, New York, 10461 (S.S.), and Cell Biology Section, Laboratory of Viral Carcinogenesis, National Cancer Institute, Bethesda, Maryland 20014 (C.B.)*

A syndrome of in vitro properties correlates with the tumorigenicity of SV40-
transformed rodent cells. These properties are: plasminogen activator production, loss of large actin cables, and anchorage-independent growth. An
established rat fibroblast line, its SV40 transformant, several T-antigen negative revertants, and a spontaneous retransformant isolated from one of the
revertants were analyzed in vivo for their tumorigenicity and in vitro for the
syndrome. The two transformed lines were highly tumorigenic, and had clearly
abnormal in vitro properties. The parental rat line was weakly tumorigenic
in nude mice and demonstrated a slightly transformed response in the in vitro
assays. The revertants were completely nontumorigenic. Expression of the
in vitro syndrome was not uniform for all revertants; however, most cell lines
maintained the correlation of the syndrome and tumorigenicity.

Key words: SV40 transformation, tumorigenicity, anchorage independence

SV40-transformed murine cells demonstrate a number of cellular properties which
differ from normal cells and can be studied in vitro. Selective characteristics include a reduced need for serum [1], density-independent growth [2], and the ability to grow without anchorage [3]. Among the nonselective changes which occur are decreased organization of the actin-containing cytoskeleton [4], increased production of proteolytic enzymes [5], and a reduction of cell surface fibronectin [6]. Anchorage independence is
the change that best correlates with tumorigenicity [7], although there is also a fairly
good correlation with plasminogen activator production and with disruption of intracellular
actin cables [7—9]. This syndrome of changes would appear to be interrelated, since a
change in any one characteristic usually results in changes in the others (Fig. 1).

Received May 14, 1979; accepted July 25, 1979.

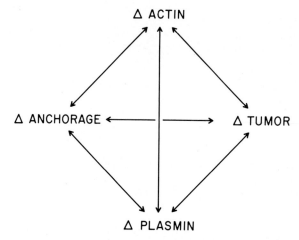

Fig. 1. Tumorigenicity syndrome. The relationship of changes in tumor forming ability to changes in anchorage independence, the structure of actin cables, and the production of plasminogen activator is shown. Double-headed arrows indicate that the changes are coordinate in both directions.

Revertants from transformed cells which have been previously isolated regained some of the normal in vitro growth properties and showed a reduced degree of tumorigenicity [10–12]. We have isolated a group of revertants from an SV40-transformed rat line which contained a single copy of the SV40 genome [13]. These revertants have lost detectable large T and small t antigens and regained the in vitro growth control of the non-transformed grandparental line. In this article we report on the tumorigenicity, and the in vitro characteristics which best correlate with tumor formation, of revertants and of a spontaneously occuring retransformed clone derived from one of the revertants.

MATERIALS AND METHODS

Cells and Culture Procedure.

The cell line 14B, the revertants F1[1] 1-4, 3-3, 3-5, 3-7 and 3-8, and parental line Rat-1 have been previously described [13]. 1-4 MCA was a spontaneous retransformant of F1[1] 1-4. It was isolated by picking a single large colony growing in methocel, and recloned by plating in microtiter wells (Falcon). 14B/nu 1 and T 14B were isolated from tumors excised from a nude mouse and a neonatal Fisher rat respectively. All cells were cultured in Dulbecco's modified Eagle's Medium (Gibco H21), supplemented with 10% fetal calf serum (Reheis) and 100 units/ml of penicillin and streptomycin (Gibco).

Plasminogen Activator Levels.

Assay methods for plasminogen activator have been previously described [14].

Actin Containing Cytoskeleton.

Presence of large actin cables was determined by indirect immunofluorescence. Cells seeded on glass coverslips at $10^3/mm^2$ were grown for 2 days, fixed with 10% formalin for 15 minutes, treated with 1% NP40 in PBS for 20 minutes at room temperature, and stained with rabbit anti-actin serum (gift of K. Burridge, CSH) followed by goat anti-rabbit IgG (Cappel) [15].

Anchorage Independence.

Cells were plated in triplicate at 10^5, 10^4, and 10^3 cells/60mm dish in 3 ml DME plus 10% FCS containing 0.33% Agarose (Difco) over a 2 ml layer of 0.9% agarose in the same medium. Cultures were fed twice weekly with an additional 2 ml of the soft agar-DME-10% FCS and cultured for 3 weeks. Large colonies greater than 0.2mm in diameter were scored using a dissecting microscope. Total colony volume (CVI) increase in agar was determined as described [16].

Tumorigenicity.

Ability of cells to form tumors in nude mice and Fisher rats was previously described [17, 18]. Briefly, cells for injection into nude mice were trypsinized, resuspended in phosphate buffered saline (PBS) at the desired concentration and 0.2 ml injected subcutaneously at a single site.

Tumorigenicity in rats was determined by trpsinizing cells, suspending in DME at the desired concentration and injecting 0.2 ml subcutaneously. Newborn rats were inoculated within 48 hours of birth.

Chromosome Number

Determination of chromosome number was carried out by the method of Vogel et al [19].

RESULTS

In Vitro Properties

Table I shows 3 in vitro properties of the cells: plasminogen activator production, the presence of well defined actin cables, and the ability to grow in soft agar. Rat-1, an established rat fibroblast cell line, produced low levels of plasminogen activator, in any

TABLE I. Syndrome of In Vitro Properties Which Correlate With Tumorigenicity

| Cells | Production of plasminogen activator (% counts released) | | | Cytoskeletal organization | Anchorage independence | |
	Fibrin plates	Cell extract	Harvest fluid	% Cells with actin cables	Relative EOP agarose/plastic	Colony volume increase in agarose[a]
Rat 1	8	4	0	59	7.0×10^{-5}	1.3×10^{1}
14B	43	27	0	17	1.5×10^{-1}	3.8×10^{2}
FI 1-4	74	51	44	64	3.0×10^{-5}	2.1×10^{1}
FI 3-3	29	21	0	78	5.0×10^{-5}	ND
FI 3-5	ND	ND	0	72	4.0×10^{-5}	ND
FI 3-7	13	10	0	81	3.0×10^{-5}	ND
FI 3-8	9	6	0	90	4.0×10^{-5}	1.0
1-4 MCA	72	ND	ND	2	5.4×10^{-2}	4.2×10^{3}

[a] 10^5 cells plated.

ND, not determined.

of the 3 assays. The majority of Rat-1 cells contained large actin cables. This line did not grow well in soft agar when scored for the presence of large (> 0.2mm) colonies ($7 \times 10^{-3}\%$ relative plating efficiency). However, this arbitrary criterion of colony size does not detect a significant increase in cell volume if most or all of the colonies are smaller than the threshold at the time they are measured. Therefore we also determined the line's colony volume increase (CVI), defined as the (average colony volume $\times$ total number of colonies)/(total initial volume of the cells plated in agar [16]. There was a 10-fold increase in colony volume when Rat-1 was grown in soft agar.

14B, an SV40 transformant of Rat-1, grew in low serum, grew to a high density on plastic and contained both large and small T-antigens [13]. It produced approximately 6 times more plasminogen activator than Rat-1, with all of the enzyme cell-associated. There was no detectable plasminogen activator released in the harvest fluid. This cell line showed a reduction in actin cables, compared to Rat-1, but a significant percentage of the cells still contained some cables. 14B formed colonies in soft agar with a 15% relative plating efficiency. The CVI of 14B was 3.8×10^2. For comparison, the CVI of a clone of rat embryo fibroblasts transformed by wild-type SV40 was 1.6×10^3 when 10^5 cells were inoculated into soft agar [16]. 14B has a CVI capability appropriate for a fully transformed line.

The revertants FI^1 1-4, 3-3, 3-5, 3-7 and 3-8 were all isolated from 14B [13]. They were all contact inhibited and did not contain either large or small T antigen. FI^1 1-4 appeared to contain the intact SV40 genome, while 3—3 and 3—5 had undergone deletions within the SV40 early region, and 3—7 and 3—8 lacked detectable viral sequences [13]. Base sequence analysis will be necessary to determine whether FI^1 1-4 contains a point mutation in the early region, or a deletion too small to be detected by the methods used.

The cured cells 3-7 and 3-8 were at least as growth controlled as Rat-1. They produced very little plasminogen activator, contained large numbers of well defined cables, and had a very low plating efficiency in soft agar. In fact, the CVI of 3-8 was 10-fold lower than Rat-1. No cell growth in agar by 3-8 was detectable.

FI^1 3-3, containing a large deletion in the early region of SV40, produced a significant amount of plasminogen activator. The counts released by growing the cells on fibrin coated plates were less than for 14B, but extracts from the cells were comparable. FI^1 3-3, and FI^1 3-5 contained fewer actin cables than the cured revertants, but more than Rat-1. Neither line was able to form large colonies in agar. The CVI of these cells has not been determined.

FI^1 1-4 contains a full sized SV40 genome, as measured by the Southern blotting technique [13]. This revertant produced twice the plasminogen activator of 14B, as assayed by growth on fibrin-coated plates or assay of cell extracts. It was the only cell line of this set to release significant amounts of enzyme into the surrounding media. As with many other PA secreting cell lines, FI^1 1-4 growth in agar was enhanced by the presence of dog serum [16]. FI^1 1-4 had an actin cable composition comparable to Rat-1. Like the other revertants, FI^1 1-4 had a very low plating efficiency when counting large colonies in agar. Its CVI was 2.1×10^1, more like Rat-1 than like 3-8.

The last cell line described in Table 1 is 1-4 MCA. This line was isolated from a rare colony of FI^1 1-4 growing in methocel. It had no fixed saturation density. When plated sparesely, it formed very dense colonies, but if plated at 1/10 confluence, the saturation density of this line in 10% FCS was only 2.3×10^5 cells/cm^2. Its doubling times in 1% and 10% FCS were 58 hours and 33 hours respectively, compared to 22 and 14 for 14B, and 56 and 25 for $FI^1$1-4 [14]. 1-4 MCA was negative for nuclear T-antigen as measured by indirect immunofluorescence.

TABLE II. Tumorigenicity of 14B, Revertants and a Spontaneous Retransformant in Nude Mice

Cells	Inoculum	No. of tumors / No. of animals	Days after inoculation
Rat 1	2×10^6	0/4	$> 150^a$
Rat 1	1×10^7	2/3	84
14B	1×10^7	3/3	15
14B	1×10^6	2/2	60
14B	1×10^5	1/1	90
FI 1-4	1×10^7	0/4	$> 150^a$
FI 3-3	1×10^7	0/4	$> 150^a$
FI 3-5	1×10^7	0/4	$> 150^a$
FI 3-7	1×10^7	0/4	$> 150^a$
FI 3-8	1×10^7	0/4	$> 150^a$
1-4 MCA	5×10^6	3/3	28

[a]Discontinued at 150 days — still free of tumors.

When assayed for those in vitro properties which correlate with tumorigenicity, 1-4 MCA was found to more like 14B than like F^1 1-4 (Table 1). The plasminogen activator activity of live 1-4 MCA cells on fibrin plates was 72%. This cell line contained almost no actin cables. If formed large colonies in soft agar with a relative efficiency of 5.4%, and a total CVI of 4.2×10^3. The CVI of 1-4 MCA was greater than the CVI of 14B. Also, although the total number of 1-4 MCA colonies larger than 0.2 mm was fewer than 14B, the 1-4 MCA colonies grew to a significantly larger size. Based on these results, 1-4 MCA had a highly transformed phenotype.

Tumorigenicity

The ability of the various cell lines to form tumors in the nude mouse was determined (Table II). Rat-1 did not form tumors at an inoculation density of 2×10^6 cells. It did slowly form tumors if 10^7 cells were injected. None of the revertants were able to form tumors, even at the higher inoculation density. 1-4 caused the formation of small nodules which eventually regressed. The SV40 transformed parent, 14B, was able to generate a tumor with an inoculation as small as 10^5 cells. The time of appearance of 14B tumors in nude mice was inversely proportional to cell number at inoculation. 1-4 MCA was highly tumorigenic, forming tumors with an efficiency comparable to 14B. This correlated well with its CVI, anchorage independence, disorganization of actin, and production of plasminogen activator (Table I).

We also measured the ability of 14B and the revertants to form tumors in inbred Fisher rats (Table III). 14B generated tumors in both newborn and weanling rats, but not in adults. Four months after inoculation, there were still no tumors in any of the newborn rats injected either with Rat-1 or the revertants. These experiments are being continued, but at the present time we conclude that the tumorigenic pattern of 14B and the revertants is the same in nude mice and in syngenic rats.

TABLE III. Tumorigencity of 14B and Revertants in Fisher Rats

Cells	Inoculum	No. of Tumors/ No. of animals		
		Newborn	Weanling	Adult
Rat 1	1×10^7	0/3	0/3	0/3
14B	1×10^7	5/5	6/6	0/3
14B	1×10^6	3/3	2/5	0/3
14B	1×10^5	0/3	ND	ND
FI 1-4	1×10^7	0/3	ND	ND
FI 3-3	1×10^7	0/3	ND	ND
FI 3-8	1×10^7	0/3	ND	ND

ND: not determined.

TABLE IV. Properties of Cells Isolated From Tumors

Cells	Tumor source	Doubling time (1%FCS/10%FCS)	Relative plating efficiency[a] (agarose/plastic)	Average No. of chromosomes
14B	–	0.44	0.14	41 (36–50)
TI4B	Fisher rat	0.32	0.27	33 (31–38)
14B/nu	Nude mouse	0.45	0.38	52 (48–60)

[a]agar colonies > 0.2mm

Characteristics of Tumor Cells

Since 14B can spontaneously revert to a non-tumorigenic, stable "normal" cell [13], we considered the possibility that this cell line is markedly heterogenous, and that a small, highly transformed subset of the population actually gave rise to the tumors. We therefore isolated 14B tumor cells from both a Fisher rat and a nude mouse. A comparison of these tumor cells to the original 14B is shown in Table IV. The relative doubling time in 10% FCS and 1% FCS was comparable for the 3 lines, although not identical. Both tumor lines grew somewhat better than 14B in soft agar, using the standard assay of large colony formation. This selection is not suprising, since cells recovered from rare tumors which arose in nude mice after injection with other revertants had an increased capacity to grow in agar [12]. Here however, plating efficiency in soft agar of 14B/nu is increased only 2.7-fold over that of 14B because the plating efficiency in soft agar of 14B is already quite high.

Klinger et al [20] reported that both anchorage-independent growth and tumorigenicity in the nude mouse were accompanied by an increased ploidy in aneuploid Chinese hamster cells. We determined the chromosome numbers for 14B, T-14B, and 14B/nu (Table IV). As previously reported [13] 14B has a near diploid number of chromosomes. 14B/nu showed an increase in chromosomes, but not to a tetraploid number. T-14B had undergone a reduction in total chromosomes. A complete karyotype will have to be done to determine whether the ratios of specific chromosomal sections were consistently altered.

DISCUSSION

We have shown that the series of T-antigen negative revertants isolated from 14B have not only regained normal growth properties in vitro, but have lost the ability to form tumors after injection into nude mice or Fisher rats.

As already reported by us and others [7, 8, 12] the best in vitro correlation of tumorigenicity is anchorage-independent growth (Table I). Determination of CVI provides more information than simply scoring visible agar colonies. The lines studied here show a consistent correlation of CVI with tumorigenicity. We have recently observed with other cell lines that there can be a very large discrepancy between CVI and the formation of colonies greater than 0.2mm [16].

Rat-1 was capable of a 10-fold increase in cell volume while suspended in agarose. Although its ability to form large colonies was very low, this cell line was weakly tumorigenic. F[1] 1-4 had a CVI comparable to Rat-1. While it did not form tumors, it did form long-lasting nodules at the site of the injection. FI 3-8 had a CVI as low as REF [16] and was not tumorigenic. 1-4 MCA and 14B were comparable and high in tumorigenicity.

Many factors can affect the ability of a given line to grow in agar. Folkman and Moscona [21] recently observed that a minimal degree of endothelial or fibroblast cell spreading in vitro was critical for DNA synthesis. O'Neill et al [22] reported that the growth of Nil 8 hamster fibroblasts in agarose was a linear function of serum concentration. Some hamster lines require additional purines for anchorage-independent growth [P. Kahn and S. Shin, personal communication]. Regardless of the underlying cause(s), it is clear that in the group of cells we studied, there is a gradation of anchorage-independent growth, and that this gradation tends to parallel the observed tumorigenicity.

The presence of actin cables also paralleled both the tumorigenicity of these cells and their ability to grow without anchorage. Plasminogen activator levels correlated well with tumorigenicity, with the exception of 1-4. This revertant line had very high levels of this enzyme by all 3 assays but contained a large number of actin cables, did not grow well in agar, and did not form tumors.

The re-transformant 1-4 MCA has regained all of the in vitro properties which correlate with tumorigenicity (Table I), and is highly tumorigenic (Table II). It contains neither of the early SV40 viral proteins [24]. It is clear that, while FI[1] 1-4 is non-tumorigenic, it can give rise to a tumorigenic variant. We have not yet determined if 1-4 MCA contains any SV40 sequences different from those in 1-4.

The revertants we have described have almost completely regained normal phenotype. This is in contrast to earlier SV40 revertants that continue to express SV40 T-antigens [9, 11, 23]. Most significantly, the revertants described here are not only less tumorigenic than their transformed parent, but are less tumorigenic than the original grandparental line.

ACKNOWLEDGMENTS

B.M.S. and R.P. were supported by grants CA 25096 and CA 25066 from the National Cancer Institute, S.S. by grant CA 21054 from the National Institutes of Health and a Faculty Research Award from the American Cancer Society, D.R. by grants from the National Institutes of Health and the American Heart Association. We would like to thank Katy Smith for her excellent assistance and Marisa Bolognese for her help in the preparation of this manuscript.

REFERENCES

1. Dulbecco R: Nature 227:802–806, 1970.
2. Todaro GJ, Green H: Virology 23:117–119, 1964.
3. MacPherson I, Montagnier L: Virology 23:291–294, 1964.
4. Pollack R, Osborn M, Weber K: Proc Natl Acad Sci USA 72:994–998, 1975.
5. Unkeless JC, Tobia A, Ossowski L, Quigley JP, Rifkin D, Reich E: J Exp Med 137:85–111, 1953.
6. Hynes RO, Wyke JA: Virology 64:492–504, 1975.
7. Barrett JC, Crawford BD, Mixter LO, Schectman LM, Ts'o PO, Pollack R: Cancer Res 39:1504–1510, 1979.
8. Kahn P, Shin S: J Cell Biol, 82:1–16, 1979.
9. Pollack R, Risser R, Conlon S, Freedman V, Shin S, Rifkin D: In "Proteases and Biological Control." New York: Cold Spring Harbor Laboratory Press, pp 885–899, 1975.
10. Marin G, MacPherson I: J Virol 3:146–149, 1969.
11. Pollack RE, Green H, Todaro GJ: Proc Natl Acad Sci USA 60:126–133, 1968.
12. Shin S, Freedman V, Risser R, Pollack R: Proc Natl Sci USA 72:4435–4439, 1975.
13. Steinberg B, Pollack R, Topp B, Botchan M: Cell 13:19–32, 1978.
14. Crowe R, Ozer H, Rifkin D: In "Experiments with Transformed Cells." New York: Cold Spring Harbor Laboratory Press, pp 77–82, 1979.
15. Pollack RE, Rifkin D: Cell 6:495–506, 1975.
16. Steinberg B, Pollack R: Virology, in press, 1979.
17. Shin S: In Jacoby W, Pastan I (eds): "Cell Culture Techniques." Methods in Enz LVIII. New York: Academic Press, 1979.
18. Boone CW: Science 188:68–70, 1975.
19. Pollack R, Wolman S, Vogel A: Nature 228:967–970, 1970.
20. Klinger HP, Shin S, Freedman VH: Cytogenet Cell Genet 17:185–199, 1976.
21. Folkman J, Moscona A: Nature 273:345–349, 1978.
22. O'Neill CH, Riddle PN, Jordan PW: Cell, 16:909–18, 1979.
23. Vogel A, Risser R, Pollack R: J Cell Physiol 82:181–188, 1973.
24. Pollack R, Lo A, Steinberg B, Smith K, Shure H, Blanck G, Verderame M: Cold Spring Harbor Symposium, in press, 1980.

Journal of Supramolecular Structure 11:547—561 (1979)
Tumor Cell Surfaces and Malignancy 389—403

Alteration of Insulin Binding and Cytoskeletal Organization in Cultured Fibroblasts by Tertiary Amine Local Anesthetics

Mohan K. Raizada and Robert E. Fellows

Department of Physiology and Biophysics, The University of Iowa College of Medicine, Iowa City, Iowa 52242

Tertiary amine local anesthetics cause a time- and dose-dependent, reversible increase in insulin binding sites in cultured chick embryo fibroblasts. Incubation of fibroblasts with 0.2 mM dibucaine for 3 h at $37°C$ results in a twofold to threefold increase in insulin binding, with an increase in average number of binding sites ($K_a = 3.0 \times 10^7 M^{-1}$) from 9×10^3 to 29×10^3 per cell. Trypsin or ethyleneglycoltetraacetic acid (EGTA) alone increases insulin binding twofold to threefold, but fails to further increase ^{125}I-insulin binding in cells pretreated with dibucaine. Transformation of chick embryo fibroblasts with Rous sarcoma virus causes a threefold to fivefold increase in insulin binding, which is not further increased by incubation with dibucaine. As demonstrated by transmission electron microscopy, dibucaine and trypsin also induce changes in the cytoskeleton of chick embryo fibroblasts, characterized by disorganization and disappearance of microfilament and microtubule bundles. These alterations are accompanied by gross morphologic changes, including rounding of cells and appearance of numerous ruffles and blebs on the cell surface. These observations are consistent with the hypothesis that expression of surface receptors in cultured chick embryo fibroblasts is related to the organization and disorganization of cytoskeletal structures.

Key words: insulin receptors, ^{125}I-insulin binding, microtubules and microfilaments, cultured fibroblasts, local anesthetics

The changes in distribution of cell surface receptors after binding of ligands, a two-step process involving clustering of receptors into patches and accumulation of these patches at one pole of the cell, demonstrate the importance of fluidity of plasma membranes and the movement of membrane components in receptor processing [1, 2]. In turn, the movement of membrane receptors (and cytoplasm) in cells has been shown to be a function of the organizational pattern of microfilaments and microtubules [3].

Received March 18, 1979; accepted July 30, 1979.

In previous studies of the growth-promoting action of insulin, we have demonstrated that cultured chick embryo fibroblasts (CEF) have specific insulin receptors, the occupancy of which is closely correlated with the magnitude of the pleiotypic responses to insulin [4, 5]. Brief incubation with trypsin or transformation of CEF by Rous sarcoma virus (RSV) results in a severalfold increase in the number of these receptors [6]. Similarly, treatment of untransformed CEF with cytochalasin B causes an increase in the number of insulin receptors as well as changes in cell shape and surface morphology. Cytochalasin B fails to increase these receptors in transformed CEF [7], which already have a round cell shape, numerous ruffles, and disorganized cytoskeletal structure.

Recently it has been reported that tertiary amine local anesthetics are able to produce structural and organizational changes in both microtubules and microfilaments, and alter ligand-induced distribution of concanavalin A receptors [8, 9]. In this study, we have examined the effects of local anesthetics in cultured CEF with regard to cytoskeletal integrity and insulin binding. Our observations demonstrate that tertiary amine local anesthetics, like other agents that alter cell shape and cytoskeletal organization, have major effects on the expression of insulin receptors in cultured CEF.

MATERIALS AND METHODS

Fertilized eggs were supplied by Spafes, Inc. (Norwich, Connecticut). Modified Eagle's medium (Temin) and fetal bovine serum were purchased from Grand Island Biological Company (Grand Island, New York). Bovine serum albumin (fraction V) and and cytochrome C were from Sigma Chemical Co. (St. Louis), trypsin (190 units/mg) was from Worthington Biochemical Corp. (Freehold, New Jersey), Rous sarcoma virus (Schmidt Ruppin subgroup A) from American Type Culture Collection (Rockville, Maryland), and ^{125}I-insulin (specific activity $\sim 100~\mu Ci/\mu g$) from New England Nuclear (Boston). Dibucaine-HCl was obtained from Ciba Pharmaceuticals (Worchester, Massachusetts), and mepivacaine-HCl, procaine-HCl, and tetracaine-HCl from Sterling Winthrop Laboratories, Worcester, Massachusetts). Porcine insulin was a gift from Dr. R.E. Chance, Eli Lilly Company (Indianapolis).

Cell Culture

Chick embryo fibroblasts, prepared from 12-day-old embryos according to a previously published procedure [10] were cultured in modified Eagle's medium (Temin) containing 4% fetal bovine serum at 37°C with 5% CO_2. Primary cultures were dissociated with 0.25% trypsin, and 2.5×10^5 cells were subcultured in 35-mm Falcon tissue culture dishes in the same medium. Cells were fed on day 2 and used for experiments 24 h later.

Infection of CEF With Rous Sarcoma Virus

Primary cultures of CEF were dissociated with trypsin, and 1×10^6 cells were incubated in 100-mm Falcon tissue culture dishes with modified Eagle's medium (Temin) without serum for 6 h. CEF were infected with Rous sarcoma virus, Schmidt Ruppin subgroup A, as described previously [11]. After 4 days, confluent cultures of infected CEF were dissociated with trypsin, and 2.5×10^5 cells were plated in 35-mm dishes. Cells were fed on day 2 and used for experiments 24 h later.

Measurement of ^{125}I-Insulin Binding

The specific binding of ^{125}I-insulin to confluent cultures of untransformed and transformed CEF was measured with intact cells attached to culture dishes as described elsewhere [4]. All binding assays were performed in triplicate, with the results expressed as femtomoles of ^{125}I-insulin bound per milligram cell protein. Specific binding was obtained by subtracting the amount of radioactivity bound to cells in the presence of 16.6 μM unlabeled insulin from that bound in the absence of unlabeled insulin. The protein content of cultures was determined by the method of Lowry, with a bovine serum albumin standard.

Transmission Electron Microscopy

For visualization of cytoskeletal organization, cultured fibroblasts were treated with Triton X-100 by the method of Small and Celis [12]. Approximately 2.5×10^5 CEF were seeded and grown in 35-mm culture dishes containing four gold electron microscope grids which had been precoated with carbon, incubated at 110°C overnight, and sterilized with ultraviolet radiation. On day 3, grids were removed, rinsed twice with phosphate-buffered saline, pH 7.4 (PBS), and immersed in 0.1% Triton X-100 in Pipes buffer. Cells were fixed with 2.5% glutaraldehyde for 30 min at room temperature. Samples were negatively stained and prepared for microscopic examination essentially as described by Small and Celis [12]. Cytoskeletal structures were examined and photographed with a Hitachi HV-125E electron microscope at 75 kV.

For visualization of microtubules and microfilaments in thin sections of CEF, cells grown in 35-mm culture dishes were fixed with 2.5% glutaraldehyde, postfixed with osmium tetraoxide and tannic acid, stained with uranyl acetate, dehydrated, and infiltrated in Spurr's low-viscosity resin according to previously described procedure [7]. Sections of 500 Å were cut perpendicularly to the dish, poststained with uranyl acetate and lead citrate, and examined under a Hitachi HV-125E electron microscope at 50 kV.

RESULTS

Effect of Anesthetic Agents on ^{125}I-Insulin Binding

Treatment of confluent cultures of untransformed CEF with tertiary amine local anesthetics of varying hydrophobicity caused a twofold to threefold increase in the specific binding of ^{125}I-insulin (Fig. 1). The concentration required to produce maximum binding differed from each anesthetic (Table I), dibucaine being the most and procaine the least potent. The concentration required to produce the maximum effect on ^{125}I-insulin binding in CEF was similar to that required for redistribution of concanavalin A receptors in 3T3 cells [8, 9], and was related to the hydrophobicity of the anesthetic (reviewed in Seeman [13]).

Specific binding increased with increasing concentration of anesthetic. A 2.7-fold increase was observed with 0.2 mM dibucaine (Fig. 2a), a concentration which did not affect attachment of cells to plates. Although treatment of CEF with 0.4 mM dibucaine produced a threefold increase in binding, it also resulted in a 60–65% decrease in the amount of protein per plate, due to detachment and loss of cells. The increase in binding was time-dependent, reaching a maximum 3 h after incubation of cultures at 37°C with 0.2 mM dibucaine (Fig. 2b).

The increase in ^{125}I-insulin binding induced by dibucaine was due to an increase in the total number of binding sites, determined by Scatchard analysis, from 9×10^3 to 29×10^3 per cell (Table I). The affinity constant for binding ranged from 3.0 to $3.6 \times 10^7 M^{-1}$, and was indistinguishable from the constant for low-affinity binding sites of untreated CEF (Table II). Treatment of untransformed CEF with either trypsin or cytochalasin

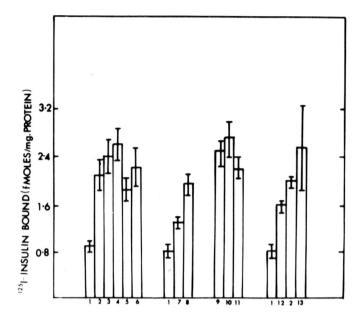

Fig. 1. Effect of tertiary amine local anesthetics, trypsin, and EGTA on ^{125}I-insulin binding in cultured chick embryo fibroblasts. Confluent cultures of untransformed CEF were incubated with modified Eagle's medium (Temin) containing 4% fetal bovine serum (1,12), 0.2 mM dibucaine (2,13), 0.5 mM tetracaine (3), 5 mM lidocaine (4), 5 mM mepivacaine (5), 10 mM procaine (6) for 3 h at 37°C; and containing 4 and 10 mM EGTA (7, 8) for 40 min at 37°C. Similarly, cultures of RSV-transformed CEF were incubated with growth medium (9), 0.2 mM dibucaine (10), and 5 mM procaine (11) for 3 h at 37°C. Cultures were washed twice with PBS and used for ^{125}I-insulin binding, except groups 12 and 13, which were treated with 10 µg/ml trypsin for 7 min at room temperature prior to insulin binding as described previously [4]. Data are given as the mean ± SEM of triplicate determinations.

B [7] also caused an increase in the number of low-affinity binding sites; a similar increase in specific binding was observed when confluent cultures of untransformed CEF were treated with EGTA, 5–10 nM, for 40 min at 37°C (Fig. 1).

The effect of removing dibucaine from the medium on binding of ^{125}I-insulin by CEF was investigated. Fibroblasts were incubated with 0.2 mM dibucaine for 3 h at 37°C, washed twice with modified Eagle's medium (Temin) containing 4% fetal bovine serum, and incubated up to 6 h in the same medium. A decrease in ^{125}I-insulin binding was observed 2 h after removal of dibucaine. Binding fell to control levels within 6 h (Fig. 2c), with a $T_{1/2}$ of approximately 2.5 h.

Virus-transformed CEF have been shown to have a threefold to fivefold increase in the number of low-affinity binding sites. Treatment of transformed cells with either 0.2 mM dibucaine or 10 mM procaine for 3 h at 37°C did not lead to a further increase in binding (Fig. 1).

Effect of Trypsin on ^{125}I-Insulin Binding

Treatment of confluent cultures of untransformed CEF with trypsin, 10 µg/ml, causes a twofold to threefold increase in specific binding of ^{125}I-insulin [4]. This is due to an increase in the number of low-affinity binding sites from 9×10^3 to 29×10^3 per cell [5]. The effect of sequential treatment of CEF with local anesthetics and trypsin was

TABLE I. Effect of Tertiary Amine Local Anesthetics on ^{125}I-Insulin Binding in Cultured Chick Embryo Fibroblasts

Local anesthetics	Concentration (mM)	^{125}I-Insulin bound (fmoles/mg protein $\pm$ SEM)
None	–	0.9 ± 0.08
Dibucaine	0.2	2.0 ± 0.05
Tetracaine	0.25	1.7 ± 0.10
Tetracaine	0.50	2.4 ± 0.20
Lidocaine	2.5	1.5 ± 0.08
Lidocaine	5.0	2.7 ± 0.27
Mepivacaine	5.0	2.3 ± 0.10
Mepivacaine	10.0	2.2 ± 0.30
Procaine	5.0	1.8 ± 0.10
Procaine	10.0	2.0 ± 0.50

Experimental conditions are described in legend to Figure 1.

TABLE II. Affinities and Number of Insulin Binding Sites in Chick Embryo Fibroblasts Treated With Dibucaine and Cytochalasin B

Treatment	Affinity constant K_1 ($\times 10^8 M^{-1}$)	K_2 ($\times 10^7 M^{-1}$)	Binding sites ($\times 10^3$)
Untreated	2–6	0.8–3	8.5–9
Dibucaine, 0.2 mM, 3 h at 37°C	–	3.0–3.6	20–29
Cytochalasin B, 10 μg/ml, 24 h at 37°C	–	0.8–3.6	18–22

The affinity constants and number of ^{125}I-insulin binding sites per cell were determined by Scatchard analysis for confluent cultures of untreated CEF [4], of CEF treated with CB [7], and of CEF treated with dibucaine.

studied. Since local anesthetics and trypsin each disrupt the organization of cytoskeletal structure, the effect of sequential treatment was investigated. Although treatment of CEF with trypsin or dibucaine alone caused a (2–2.5)-fold increase in ^{125}I-insulin binding (Fig. 1), no further increase was observed when cultures were treated with dibucaine followed by trypsin. Similarly, no increase in binding was observed when CEF were sequentially treated with other local anesthetics and trypsin.

Effect of Dibucaine and Trypsin on CEF Morphology and Cytoskeletal Structure

In previous studies we have demonstrated that treatment of confluent cultures of CEF with cytochalasin B caused an increase in the number of low-affinity insulin binding sites. The increase in receptors was accompanied by changes in cell shape from flat and

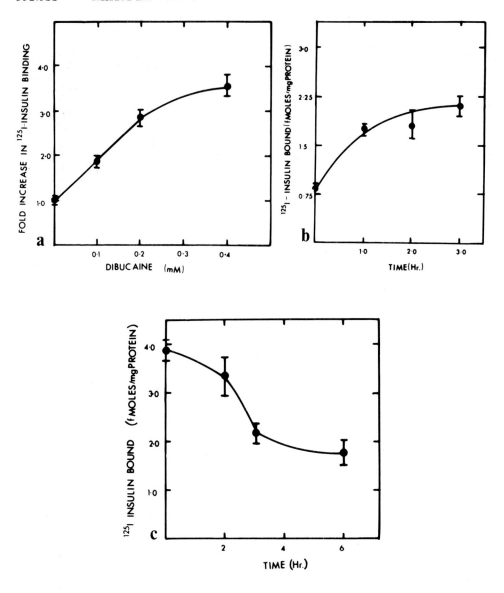

Fig. 2. Effect of dibucaine on ^{125}I-insulin binding to chick embryo fibroblasts. a: Concentration dependence. Confluent cultures of CEF were incubated with several concentrations of dibucaine for 3 h at 37°C. Specific binding is given as mean of triplicates ± SEM. b: Time dependence. Confluent cultures of CEF were incubated with 0.2 mM dibucaine in PBS for indicated time periods and specific binding of ^{125}I-insulin was determined as described in text as a mean of triplicates ± SEM. c: Effect of dibucaine removal on ^{125}I-insulin binding. Confluent cultures of CEF were incubated with 0.2 mM dibucaine for 3 h at 37°C, washed twice, and incubated in modified Eagle's medium (Temin) containing 4% fetal bovine serum. At indicated time periods, specific binding of ^{125}I-insulin was determined; untreated cultures (not shown) bound 1.8 fmoles ^{125}I-insulin/mg protein.

fusiform to round, by development of numerous ruffles and blebs on the cell surface, and by disruption and disorganization of cytoskeletal structures, including microfilament bundles [7]. Since local anesthetics cause an increase in specific binding of ^{125}I-insulin, we have investigated the effects of dibucaine on cell shape and cytoskeletal organization.

Examination of Triton X-100-treated intact CEF by transmission electron microscopy after negative staining shows a well-organized cytoskeleton with filaments running parallel to the plasma membrane (Fig. 3) and particularly prominent near the periphery of the cell. The cytoskeleton, as visualized by this method, consists of actin- and tubulin-containing fibers of various sizes in a three-dimensional array [12, 14]. Although in untreated CEF these appear as a highly organized network of banded and unbanded filaments (Fig. 3a), there is a prominent loss of cytoskeletal organization after treatment with 0.2 mM dibucaine for 3 h at 37°C (Fig. 3c). Observation of the cytoskeleton of untreated cells at high magnification reveals multiple filamentous structures joined together in bundle-like arrays (Fig. 3b). In dibucaine-treated cells, the remaining filament bundles show a significant decrease in thickness (Fig. 3d).

Electron microscope examination of thin sections of untreated CEF demonstrated a fusiform cell shape and relatively smooth cell surface (Fig. 4a). At high magnification, bundles of microfilaments predominently are seen close to the plasma membrane and running parallel with it (Fig. 4b). Microfilaments of different sizes (Fig. 4c), as well as microtubules (Fig. 4d), are also seen throughout the cytoplasm.

Treatment of CEF with trypsin, 10 μg/ml (Fig. 5a), or with 0.2 mM dibucaine (Fig. 4e) results in significant modification in cell shape and surface morphology, including rounding of fibroblasts and development of large and small ruffles and blebs. These changes are accompanied by disappearance of membrane-associated microfilament bundles and a significant reduction of microtubules and microfilaments in the cytoplasm (Fig. 4f and 5b).

DISCUSSION

The present investigation supports our earlier finding [7] that polymerization and depolymerization of cytoplasmic microfilaments and microtubules are associated with changes in the expression of insulin binding sites on the cell surface. Other investigators have shown that in 3T3 and BHK-21 cells, tertiary amine local anesthetics cause an alteration in the organization of microtubules and microfilaments and affect the ligand-induced distribution of concanavalin A receptors [8, 9]. In this study, treatment of confluent cultures of CEF with these agents caused a time- and dose-dependent increase in low-affinity insulin binding sites, the occupancy of which stimulates pleiotypic responses in the target cell [4]. An increase in these sites was accompanied by changes in the cell shape from fusiform to round, with development of numerous ruffles and blebs on the cell surface and disappearance of microfilament bundles closely associated with the plasma membrane. Brief treatment of cells with trypsin also caused a similar change in cell shape, surface morphology, and insulin receptor number, but incubation with both dibucaine and trypsin did not have an effect greater than either agent alone. In addition, RSV-transformed CEF, which have a greater number of insulin binding sites, a rounded cell shape, irregular cell surface morphology, and disorganized cytoskeletal structures, do not increase number of receptors in response to local anesthetics.

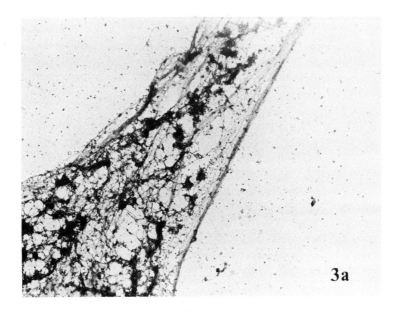

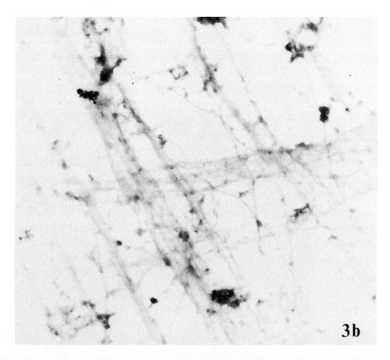

Fig. 3. Distribution of cytoskeletal structures in untreated and dibucaine-treated chick embryo fibroblasts. Confluent cultures were incubated with 0.2 mM dibucaine for 3 h at 37°C, treated with Triton X-100, and processed for electron microscope examination as described in Methods. a: Untreated CEF, region near cell periphery (× 5,500). b: Filaments of untreated CEF (× 47,200). c: Dibucaine-treated CEF, nucleus stains dark (× 5,500). d: Filaments of dibucaine-treated CEF (× 47,200).

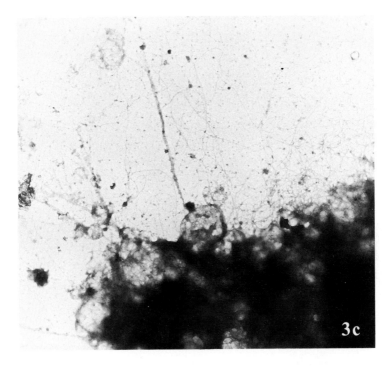

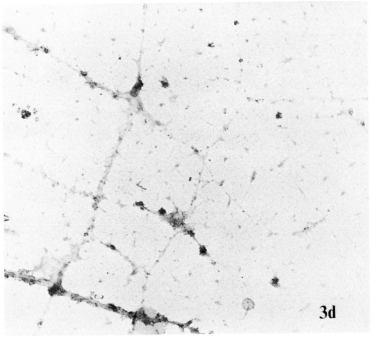

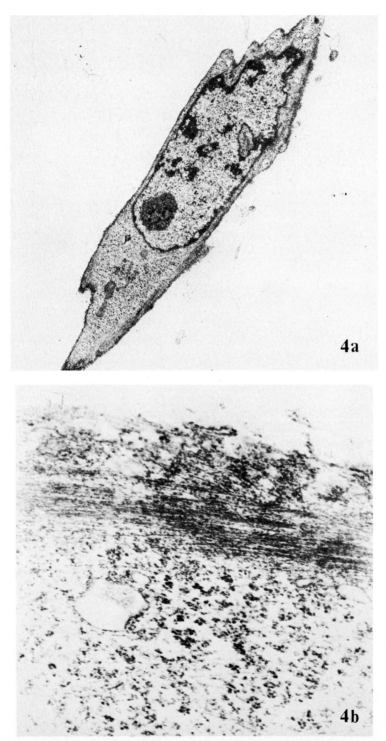

Fig. 4. Electron photomicrographs of thin sections of untreated and dibucaine-treated chick embryo fibroblasts. a: Untreated CEF demonstrating fusiform shape and relatively smooth cell surface (× 5,500). b: Untreated CEF with prominent microfilament bundles in close association with plasma membrane (× 47,200).

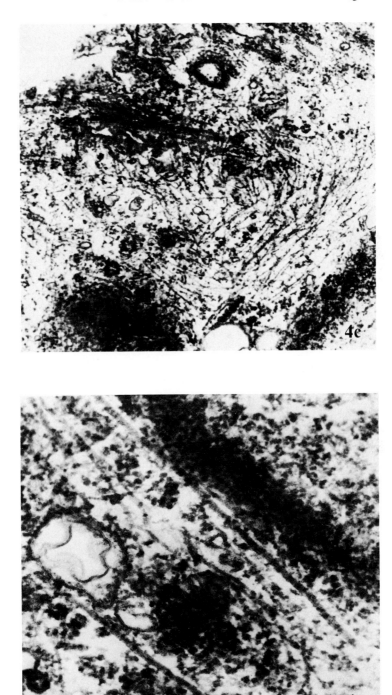

Fig. 4. Electron photomicrographs of thin sections of untreated and dibucaine-treated chick embryo fibroblasts continued. c: Untreated CEF with microfilaments present in the cytoplasm and away from the plasma membrane ($\times$ 47,200). d: Untreated CEF showing prominent microtubules ($\times$ 64,000).

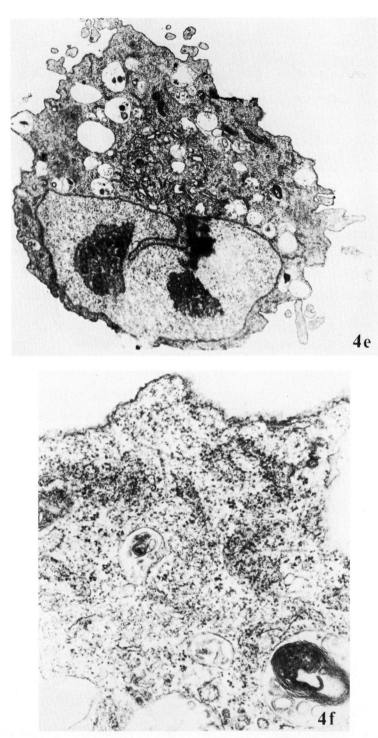

Fig. 4. Electron photomicrographs of thin sections of untreated and dibucaine-treated chick embryo fibroblasts continued. e: Dibucaine-treated CEF demonstrating round cell shape with numerous micro-villi and blebs on the cell surface (× 5,500). f: Dibucaine-treated CEF representing the absence of microfilament and microtubules (× 47,200).

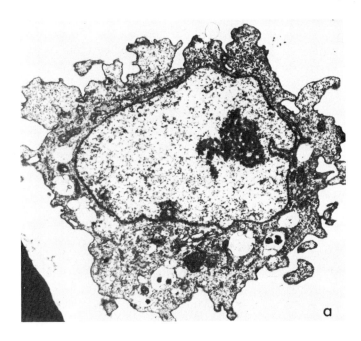

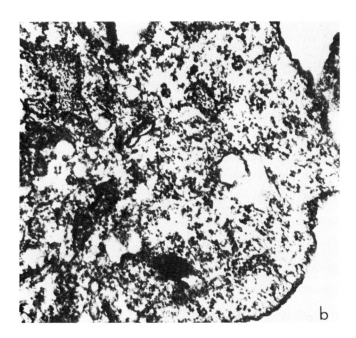

Fig. 5. Electron photomicrographs of thin section of trypsin-treated chick embryo fibroblasts. a: Trypsin-treated CEF demonstrating round cell shape with numerous microvilli and blebs on the cell surface (× 5,500). b: Trypsin-treated CEF showing the absence of microfilament bundles (× 47,200).

The finding that tertiary amine local anesthetics, trypsin, EGTA, and viral transformation produce similar effects on cytoskeletal organization and insulin binding sites suggests that the effect on insulin binding sites is mediated by a common cellular mechanism dependent on cytoskeletal integrity. The mechanism by which changes in the cytoskeleton might bring about changes in insulin binding sites is speculative at this time. It is possible that disorganization of these structures by local anesthetic inhibits the rate of endocytosis of cell surface receptors, resulting in an increase in their number. It is also possible that receptors "hidden" in the membrane are exposed as a result of disorganization.

Insulin receptor macromolecules on the cell surface may be directly linked to the cytoskeleton by a structure or structures which can be modified by chemical agents, transformation, or rapid growth. This type of organized relationship between cell surface macromolecules and cytoskeleton has been proposed by Ash et al [15]. Schlessinger and co-workers have demonstrated that movement of concanavalin A receptors in the plane of plasma membrane involved microtubules and microfilaments [16, 17]. It is reasonable to suggest that this relationship exists where receptor exposure and movement can be related to the organization of cytoskeletal structures, although the molecular evidence for such a linkage and the mechanism by which it may bring about changes in the expression of receptors has not been established.

It is possible that such a mechanism may involve a cellular "messenger." A likely candidate for this is calcium, since it is involved in many aspects of membrane function, as well as in the organization and disorganization of microtubules and microfilaments [8, 18, 19]. The effects of local anesthetics and cytochalasin B [7] on mitogen receptors, cell shape, and surface morphology are indistinguishable from those produced by EGTA. Thus, displacement of membrane-bound calcium by EGTA may, by raising cytoplasmic levels, cause depolymerization of the cytoskeleton. This is supported by the report of Poste et al [9] that elevation of intracellular calcium by calcium ionophore A 23187 has an effect on concanavalin A receptor mobility similar to that of colchicine or vinblastine.

ACKNOWLEDGMENTS

This research was supported in part by a grant from Milheim Foundation for Cancer Research to M.K. Raizada.

We thank Mrs. Wen-shen Wu for expert technical assistance.

REFERENCES

1. Taylor RB, Duffus WPH, Raff M, DePetris S: Nature New Biol 233:225–229, 1971.
2. DePetris S, Raff M: Eur J Immunol 2:523–535, 1972.
3. Schreiner GF, Uanue ER: Adv Immunol 24:38–165, 1976.
4. Raizada MK, Perdue JF: J Biol Chem 251:6445–6455, 1976.
5. Perdue JF, Raizada MK: Progr Clin Biol Res 9:49–64, 1976.
6. Raizada MK, Perdue JF: Proc Am Assoc Cancer Res 17:86, 1976 (Abstract).
7. Raizada MK, Fellows RE: Submitted for publication.
8. Poste G, Papahadjopoulos D, Jacoson K, Vail WJ: Nature 352:552–554, 1975.
9. Poste G, Papahadjopoulos D, Nicholson GL: Proc Natl Acad Sci USA 72:4430–4434, 1975.
10. Temin HM: Virology 10:182–191, 1960.

11. Bradley WEC, Culp LA: Exp Cell Res 84:335–350, 1974.
12. Small JV, Celis JE: Cytobiologie 16:308–325, 1978.
13. Seeman P: Pharmacol Rev 24:583–655, 1972.
14. Webster RE, Henderson D, Osborn M, Weber K: Proc Natl Acad Sci USA 75:5511–5515, 1978.
15. Ash JF, Louvard D, Singer SJ: Proc Natl Acad Sci USA 74:5584–5588, 1977.
16. Schlessinger J, Koppell DE, Axelrod D, Jacobsen K, Webb WW, Elson EL: Proc Natl Acad Sci USA 73:2409–2413, 1978.
17. Schlessinger J, Elson EL, Webb WW, Yahara I, Ruteschauser V, Edelman GM: Proc Natl Acad Sci USA 74:1110–1114, 1977.
18. Poste G, Paphadjopoulos D, Jacobson K, Vail WJ: Biochim Biophys Acta 394:504–519, 1975.
19. Nicolson GL: Biochim Biophys Acta 457:1–57, 1976.

Journal of Supramolecular Structure 11:563–577 (1979)
Tumor Cell Surfaces and Malignancy 405–419

Production of Monoclonal Antibodies Against a Cell Surface Concanavalin A Binding Glycoprotein

James J. Starling, Charles R. Simrell, Paul A. Klein, and Kenneth D. Noonan

Department of Biochemistry and Molecular Biology (J.J.S., K.D.N.) and Department of Pathology (C.R.S., P.A.K.), J. Hillis Miller Health Center, University of Florida, Gainesville, Florida 32610

Concanavalin A-binding (Con A)-binding cell surface glycoproteins were isolated, via Con A-affinity chromatography, from Triton X-100-solubilized Chinese hamster ovary (CHO) cell plasma membranes. The Con A binding glycoproteins isolated in this manner displayed a significantly different profile on sodium dodecyl sulfate–polyacrylamide gels than did the Triton-soluble surface components, which were not retarded by the Con A-Sepharose column. [^{125}I]-Con A overlays of the pooled column fractions displayed on sodium dodecyl sulfate–polyacrylamide gel electro-phoresis (SDS-PAGE) demonstrated that there were virtually no Con A receptors associated with the unretarded peak released by the Con A-Sepharose column, whereas the material which was bound and specifically eluted from the Con A-Sepharose column with the sugar hapten α-methyl-D-mannopyranoside contained at least 15 prominent bands which bound [^{125}I]-Con A.

In order to produce monoclonal antibodies against various cell surface Con A receptors, Balb/c mice were immunized with the pooled Con A receptor fraction. Following immunization spleens were excised from the animals and single spleen cell suspensions were fused with mouse myeloma P3/X63-Ag8 cells. Numerous hybridoma clones were subsequently picked on the basis of their ability to secrete antibody which could bind to both live and glutaral-dehyde-fixed CHO cells as well as to the Triton-soluble fraction isolated from the CHO plasma membrane fraction. Antibody from two of these clones was able to precipitate a single [^{125}I]-labeled CHO surface component of ∿265,000 daltons.

Key words: plasma membrane, lectin receptors, affinity chromatography, membrane proteins, hybridoma, monoclonal antibody

A great deal of work over the last decade has dealt with the structure and function of the plasma membrane. Many investigators have used lectins as probes to study cell surface architecture [1–3]. While much useful information concerning membrane structure

J.J. Starling is now at the Department of Biochemistry, Eastern Virginia Medical School, PO Box 1989, Norfolk, VA 23501.

Received May 18, 1979; accepted July 24, 1979.

and function has been obtained with use of lectins, a problem remains in that although the binding of lectins to cell surface components occurs through specific carbohydrate-lectin interactions, a given lectin may bind to a variety of different molecules at the cell surface, all of which possess the appropriate carbohydrate determinant. This problem in specificity is particularly vexing if one is interested in studying a single molecule on the cell surface as opposed to analyzing the characteristics of a class of cell surface components. This problem can be circumvented by using a more specific probe to investigate cell surface structure.

The probe most frequently used to answer questions regarding individual surface components is an antibody prepared against a specific membrane component. Unfortunately, owing in part to the extreme complexity of membrane structure [4] relatively few membrane proteins have been purified to homogeneity and therefore the production of monoclonal antibodies against surface proteins has been achieved in only a very few instances. Fortunately, the pioneering work of Kohler and Milstein [5,6] has recently provided a technology which offers the potential of preparing monoclonal antibody against a variety of membrane proteins and glycoproteins. In Kohler and Milstein's approach, monoclonal antibody production is achieved by cloning cell hybrids produced between membrane protein activated spleen cells and a myeloma cell line maintained in vitro. This technology has an extreme advantage over more traditional approaches to antibody production in that a single membrane protein does not have to be isolated and purified to homogeneity in order to produce a homogeneous antibody. Furthermore once a hybridoma clone producing a desired antibody has been established, the actively secreting clone can serve as a source of large amounts of the particular antibody. In this manuscript we report the application of the hybridoma technology of Kohler and Milstein [5,6] to the production of monoclonal antibodies against a specific Con A receptor localized to the cell surface of Chinese hamster ovary (CHO) cells.

MATERIALS AND METHODS

Cell Lines

The H-7$_W$ subclone of Chinese hamster ovary cells was maintained in McCoy's 5A medium + 10% (v/v) fetal calf serum as previously described [7].

The myeloma cell line P3/X63-Ag8 [8] was maintained in Dulbecco's modified Eagle's medium containing 7.5% (v/v) heat-inactivated fetal calf serum, 7.5% (v/v) gamma-globulin-free horse serum, and 1% penicillin-streptomycin (DME-P). The cells were routinely passaged 1:20 upon reaching a cell density of 5×10^6 to 1×10^7 per milliliter.

Hybridomas derived from the fusion of spleen cells and myeloma cells were maintained in medium consisting of 7 parts DEM-P and 3 parts DME-P conditioned by the myeloma cells (designated DME-PC). The hybridoma nomenclature used throughout this manuscript follows the nomenclature recently described by Springer et al [9] except that the hybridomas derived from mice immunized with the Con A receptors (peak B, Fig 2) carry the prefix BI.

Whole-Cell Labeling Procedures

H-7$_W$ cells were removed from the substratum using CMF-PBS-EDTA containing 1 gm/liter glucose as previously described [7]. Following removal from the substratum, the cells were washed three times with phosphate-buffered saline (PBS, pH 7.4) and resuspended in PBS to a final density of 2×10^7 cells per milliliter. Cell surface sialoglycoproteins were labeled using the $NaIO_4/NaB^3H_4$ technique described by Gahmberg and Anderson [10], while membrane proteins containing accessible tyrosine residues were labeled with [^{125}I] using the lactoperoxidase technique described by Phillips and Morrison [11]. Immediately after labeling with either reagent the cells were washed extensively with PBS.

Plasma Membrane Isolation and Solubilization

Subcellular fractions enriched in plasma membrane were isolated according to the aqueous two-phase polymer techniques of Brunette and Till [12]. Following isolation the membrane fraction was resuspended in 1 mM Tris-HCl (pH 7.4) containing 10 mM EDTA and incubated for 10 min at room temperature in order to remove excess Zn^{2+}. The membrane fraction was then pelleted at 11,000g for 10 min in a Sorvall HB-4 rotor. The membranes were then resuspended (at a concentration of 1−2 mg protein per milliliter buffer) in 50 mM sodium borate (pH 7.4) containing 0.5% Triton X-100 and were incubated for 30 min at room temperature. Finally the insoluble material was pelleted at 11,000g (10 min) in a Sorvall HB-4 rotor and the Triton-soluble (T_s) fraction was collected.

Electron Microscopy

Membranes were prepared for electron microscopy as previously described [7].

Con A Affinity Chromatography

Sepharose 4B (Pharmacia, Piscataway, New Jersey) was activated with cyanogen bromide according to the procedure of Cuatrecasas [13]. A 30-ml portion of a solution containing 100 mg affinity-purified Con A, 1 mM α-methyl-D-mannopyranoside (α-MM), 1 M NaCl, and 0.13 M $NaHCO_3$ was added to 30 ml activated Sepharose 4B and gently agitated over night at 4°C. Following the overnight incubation, 0.5 ml ethanolamine was added to the reaction mixture and the agitation was continued for 2 h at 4°C. The Con A-Sepharose resin was then washed sequentially with 1 liter of each of the following: 0.1 M $NaHCO_3$; 1 M NaCl; Tris-Triton buffer (0.1 M NaCl, 0.1% Triton X-100, 0.7 mM $CaCl_2$, 0.01% NaN_3, 10 mM Tris-HCl, pH 7.4 [14]); Tris-Triton buffer containing 100 mM α-MM; and finally Tris-Triton buffer. This procedure produced a Con A-to-Sepharose coupling efficiency of at least 90%.

Following coupling the Con A-Sepharose was poured into a column and washed over night with 50 mM sodium acetate containing 4.5 M urea, pH 6.5 [15]. The column was subsequently re-equilibrated in Tris-Triton buffer prior to application of the sample. The radiolabeled T_s fraction derived from the isolated plasma membrane was allowed to percolate onto the column matrix and then the column flow was stopped. The sample was incubated with the Con A-Sepharose for 1−3 h prior to resumption of flow. After the nonretarded fractions were eluted from the affinity matrix, Tris-Triton buffer containing 100 mM α-MM was added and the Con A-receptor glycoproteins were eluted. The hapten-released material was pooled and dialyzed against Tris-Triton buffer at 4°C.

SDS Polyacrylamide Gel Electrophoresis

Membrane proteins and glycoproteins were separated on slab gels according to the discontinuous technique of Laemmli [16]. The stacking gel consisted of 5.6% acrylamide (w/w), while the separating gel was a linear gradient of 7.5−12.5% acrylamide. Following electrophoresis the gels were fixed in trichloroacetic (TCA) acid, stained with Coomassie blue, and destained as previously described [7].

[^{125}I]-Con A Overlays

Con A was iodinated by the lactoperoxidase/[^{125}I] technique of Martinozzi and Moscona [17] and subsequently affinity-purified on a Sephadex G-100 column [18]. [^{125}I]-Con A overlays of the slab gels were performed according to the method of Burridge [19]. After extensive washing of the overlaid gels to remove unbound [^{125}I]-Con A, the gels were dried and an autoradiogram was produced.

Immunization and Cell Fusion

T_s membrane proteins (peak A or peak B, Fig. 2) were concentrated (10–20-fold) using polyethylene glycol (mol wt 6,000) and mixed with an equal volume of complete Freund's adjuvant. Balb/c mice were initially immunized with 20 μg of protein via subcutaneous and intramuscular injections. The mice were boosted at 7 and 14 days with a single injection of 20 μg of the concentrated T_s membrane proteins (minus the Freund's adjuvant) via intraperitoneal and intravenous injections, respectively. Three days after the last injection the spleens were excised aseptically and a spleen cell suspension was prepared as described by Simrell and Klein [20]. The spleen cells were then fused with the mouse myeloma P3/X63-Ag8 cells according to procedures previously described [21,22]. The hybrids were initially seeded (in 0.1-ml aliquots) into 96 well microtiter plates in hypoxanthine/aminopterin/thymidine (HAT) selective medium. The hybridoma cultures were maintained in HAT medium for $\sim$3 weeks and then gradually transferred to DME-P.

Poly-L-lysine Attachment of Cells to Microtiter Plates and Radioimmunoassay

Hybridoma colonies were screened for the production of antibodies specific for the CHO cell surface by assay of the capacity of components from the medium in which the hybridomas were growing to bind to glutaraldehyde-fixed H-7$_w$ cells using the radioimmunoassay (RIA) described by Simrell and Klein [20]. Briefly, 25 μl of poly-L-lysine (PLL) in PBS was added to each well of a U-bottom flex vinyl microtiter plate and incubated for 45 min at room temperature (RT). The PLL was then aspirated from the wells and the plates were washed twice with PBS. A CHO cell suspension (50 μl) containing 3×10^6 cells per milliliter PBS was added to each well and the cells were allowed to attach to the PLL-coated microtiter plates for 60 min (RT). The attached cells were subsequently washed three times with PBS. Then 25 μl of PBS containing 10% gamma-globulin-free horse serum and 0.1% NaN$_3$ was added to each well and the incubation was continued for 10 min. Each well was then washed twice with PBS and the cells were fixed with 25 μl of 0.1% glutaraldehyde in PBS (5 min, RT). Following fixation the cells were washed three more times with PBS, and 25 μl of 100 mM glycine in PBS was added to each well (5 min, RT). Finally the cells were washed twice with PBS and stored (4°C) in 25 μl of PBS containing 10% gamma-globulin-free horse serum and 0.1% NaN$_3$. Live (ie, nonfixed) cells were prepared for the RIA as above except both the glutaraldehyde fixation and the subsequent wash with glycine were omitted. In our "live cell" RIA the cells were maintained at 0°C throughout the binding assay. The ability of hybridoma supernates to detect soluble antigen was determined by using as the target membrane proteins or glycoproteins (peak A or B, Fig. 2) dried (37°C) over night onto individual microtiter wells and then fixed with absolute methanol (5 min at RT) prior to use in the RIA.

In order to quantitate antibody production, 25 μl of the test solution (hybridoma supernatant, whole serum, ascites fluid, etc) was added to the attached cells and allowed to incubate for 90 min at either room temperature (for fixed cells) or 0°C (for "live" cells). Following incubation with the test solution, the cells were washed three times with

PBS containing 1% gamma-globulin-free horse serum and 0.1% NaN_3. Then 25 μl of affinity-purified [23] $[^{125}I]$-labeled [24] rabbit anti-mouse IgG serum was added to each well (40,000 cpm/well) and the incubation was continued for 90 min at either room temperature or 0°C. Subsequently the cells were washed three more times with PBS containing 1% gamma-globulin-free horse serum and 0.1% NaN_3. Finally the individual wells were cut out of the microtiter plate and counted in a gamma counter.

Cloning

Hybridoma colonies were cloned in soft agar [25] using a stock solution of 2% (w/v) agar without a cellular feeder layer. The hard agar underlayer was composed of Dulbecco modified Eagle's medium containing 25% DME-PC, 7% heat-inactivated fetal calf serum, 7% gamma-globulin-free horse serum, and 1% penicillin-streptomycin. The soft agar overlay in which the cells were suspended was composed of 0.33% (w/v) agar containing the same nutrients as the hard agar.

Immunoprecipitation

Immunoprecipitations of $[^{125}I]$-labeled, T_S membrane components were performed with whole antisera and hybridoma-secreted monoclonal antibody.

In our immunoprecipitation protocol four 150-μl aliquots of inactivated Staphylococcus aureus (Pansorbin, Calbiochem, La Jolla, California) were centrifuged for 3 min in 1.5-ml Eppendorf cups in an Eppendorf microfuge. Aliquots (475 μl) of $[^{125}I]$-labeled T_S membrane proteins ($\sim 2.2 \times 10^6$ aliquot) were added to each of the Pansorbin pellets and mixed well. After incubation at 4°C for 30 min the material was pelleted and the supernates were placed into new Eppendorf cups. This step "cleared" $\sim 1\%$ of the T_S counts, suggesting that a minor component(s) of the T_S membrane fraction bound to the Pansorbin. A ten-fold concentrated DME-PC solution (100 μl) was then added to the Pansorbin-cleared, $[^{125}I]$-labeled membrane components and incubated 6 h at 4°C. Then 10 μl rabbit anti-mouse IgG serum (IgG fraction, Miles Yeda, 1.6 mg antibody per milliliter) or another appropriate antiserum was added, and the samples were mixed well and incubated over night at 4°C. The next day the samples were transferred to Eppendorf cups containing the pellet from 150 μl of Pansorbin and were incubated for another 1.5 h (4°C). Following this incubation the material was again pelleted in a microfuge and the supernates were collected. Finally 100 μl of the antibody to be used in the immunoprecipitation was added to the Triton-soluble $[^{125}I]$-labeled membrane proteins and incubated 6 h (4°C). After 6 h, 10 μl of rabbit anti-mouse IgG (or another appropriate second antibody) was added to the solution and the samples were again incubated over night at 4°C. The following day the supernates were added to a pellet from 150 μl Pansorbin and incubated 1.5 h at 4°C, and the immunotitrated material that adsorbed to the Pansorbin was pelleted. The supernates were removed, the pellets were washed twice with 500 μl Tris-Triton buffer containing 5 mg/ml ovalbumin, and then the adsorbed material was removed from the Pansorbin by boiling for 5 min in Laemmli sample buffer [16].

RESULTS

A plasma membrane-enriched fraction was isolated from the $H-7_W$ subclone of CHO cells according to a modification [7] of the two phase aqueous polymer membrane isolation technique of Brunette and Till [12]. This membrane fraction has been extensively characterized in a previous publication [7], where it was shown to be highly enriched in plasma membrane. An electron micrograph of the isolated material is displayed in Figure 1.

In order to solubilize the majority of the membrane fraction, the membranes were incubated in 1 mM Tris-HCl (pH 7.4) containing 10 mM EDTA (to remove excess Zn^{2+}), pelleted, and then resuspended for 30 min at RT in 50 mM sodium borate (pH 7.4) containing 0.5% Triton X-100. Finally the insoluble material was pelleted at 12,000g for 15 min and both the Triton-soluble (T_s) and Triton-insoluble (T_i) fractions were collected. Using this solubilization protocol $\sim$ 80% of the membrane fraction is solubilized. Figure 3A displays a Coomasie blue-stained SDS-PAGE in which it can be seen that the plasma membrane-enriched fraction as well as the T_s and T_i fractions are easily distinguishable from each other.

The T_s fraction was concentrated approximately ten-fold and then applied to a urea-stripped Con A-Sepharose affinity column (see Materials and Methods). Figure 2 presents the elution profile from the affinity column. Three peaks can be collected from the column. Peak A is the nonretarded fraction which is eluted in the Tris-Triton buffer (see Materials and Methods) without α-MM. Peak B is eluted with Tris-Triton buffer containing 100 mM α-MM, while peak C can only be eluted with Tris-Triton buffer containing 4.5 M urea. Peak C contains both non-Con A-binding proteins and Con A receptors as well as a large amount of Con A (data not shown). Peak A accounts for $\sim$65% of the radioactivity applied to the column, peak B accounts for $\sim$25% of the applied material, and peak C accounts for another 5% of the applied material. Approximately 5% of the T_s fraction remains bound to the column even after the 4.5 M urea wash.

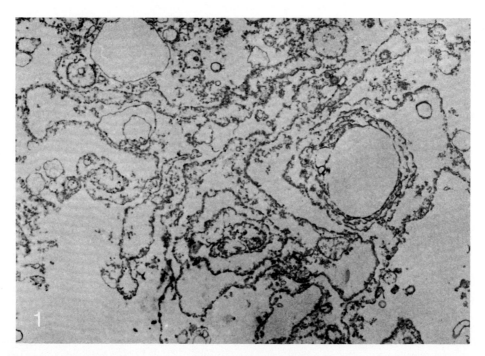

Fig. 1. Electron micrograph of H-7$_w$ membrane fraction ($\times$ 5,000). The "particles" seen attached to the membranes do not have the dimensions of ribosomes. The "particles" probably represent aggregates of actin associated with the inner face of the surface membrane [26].

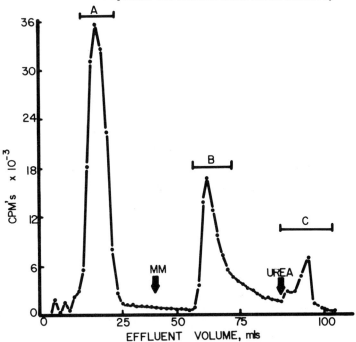

Fig. 2. Elution profile of Con A-Sepharose Column. The column was prepared and run as described in Materials and Methods. In this experiment 2×10^7 H-7$_W$ cells were labeled with [^{125}I]/lactoperoxidase [26] prior to membrane isolation and then the radiolabeled membrane was used as a "tracer" with membrane isolated from 1.6×10^8 H-7$_W$ cells. In the particular experiment shown, 5.4 mg of protein was applied to the column and 1.8-ml fractions were collected. Peak A represents the nonretarded membrane components, peak B the Con A-binding membrane components, and peak C the nonspecifically adsorbed membrane components which could be eluted with 4.5 M urea.

Figure 3A contains the Coomasie blue staining profile on an SDS-PAGE of the material recovered from the affinity column. As can be seen, peaks A and B are clearly distinguishable from each other as well as from the T_S fraction and the isolated membrane. The profile presented in Figure 3Ae resolves approximately 15 major Con A receptors. Two-dimensional analysis of this fraction according to the technique of O'Farrell [27] resolves peak B into at least 50 distinct spots, all capable of binding [^{125}I]-Con A (data not shown). Figure 3B is an [^{125}I]-Con A overlay [19] of the SDS-PAGE displayed in Figure 3A. Figure 3B demonstrates that the majority of the Con A receptors present in the membrane-enriched fraction are soluble in Triton (lane b) and that virtually all of them can be recovered in peak B of the Con A affinity column (lane e, Fig. 3B).

Following isolation, the Con A-binding glycoproteins (peak B, Fig. 2) were concentrated and used as a complex antigen for the production of antiserum and hybridomas against the Con A-binding glycoproteins.

Production of Antiserum

Balb/c mice were injected with concentrated peak B material as described in Materials and Methods. Following the completion of the immunization protocol the animals' sera were collected and the spleens excised for subsequent fusion with the myeloma cells.

The serum derived from clotted whole blood was tested for its ability to bind to glutaral-

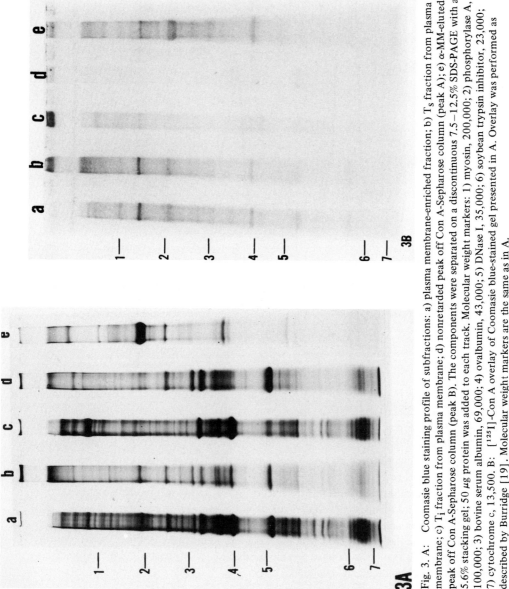

Fig. 3. A: Coomasie blue staining profile of subfractions: a) plasma membrane-enriched fraction; b) T_s fraction from plasma membrane; c) T_i fraction from plasma membrane; d) nonretarded peak off Con A-Sepharose column (peak A); e) α-MM-eluted peak off Con A-Sepharose column (peak B). The components were separated on a discontinuous 7.5–12.5% SDS-PAGE with a 5.6% stacking gel; 50 μg protein was added to each track. Molecular weight markers: 1) myosin, 200,000; 2) phosphorylase A, 100,000; 3) bovine serum albumin, 69,000; 4) ovalbumin, 43,000; 5) DNase I, 35,000; 6) soybean trypsin inhibitor, 23,000; 7) cytochrome c, 13,500. B: [125I]-Con A overlay of Coomasie blue-stained gel presented in A. Overlay was performed as described by Burridge [19]. Molecular weight markers are the same as in A.

Table I. Antiserum Binding to CHO cells

Antiserum	cpm [^{125}I]-anti-IgG bound to glutaraldehyde-fixed cells
Preimmune	1,500
Immune serum (peak B)	12,000
Immune serum (10 × Tris-Triton)	1,700
Immune serum (nuclear envelope)	1,600

Preimmune serum was drawn from a nonimmunized mouse. Antisera against peak B (Fig. 2) and Tris-Triton were prepared as described in Materials and Methods. Immune serum was also prepared against a Triton-solubilized fraction of CHO cell nuclear envelopes [28].

dehyde-fixed CHO cells and the soluble antigens in peaks A and B (Fig. 2) as described in Materials and Methods. Table I demonstrates that antiserum derived from peak B-injected animals binds to glutaraldehyde-fixed CHO cells significantly more efficiently than do pre-immune sera, immune sera produced against ten-fold concentrated Tris-Triton (the carrier of peak B), or antisera produced against a T_S fraction derived from the nuclear envelope of CHO cells [28]. Furthermore, antisera derived from animals injected with peak B material preferentially recognize peak B material relative to peak A in the soluble antigen assay described in Materials and Methods (Fig. 4). Conversely antisera derived from animals injected with concentrated peak A material preferentially recognize soluble peak A antigen (Fig. 4). Immunoprecipitation of iodinated T_S surface components with antisera to peak A or peak B results in the recovery of different radio-labeled components in the precipitate. These components can be matched to specific peak A or peak B components displayed in Figure 3 (data not shown).

Production of Hybridomas

The spleen cell suspension derived from the peak B-immunized Balb/c mice was fused with mouse myeloma cells P3/X63-Ag8 as previously described [21,22] and distributed into microtiter test plate wells. Approximately 2 weeks later the supernates from those wells that showed good growth were tested for the presence of antibody which could cross-react with glutaraldehyde-fixed CHO cells. In the particular fusion being described in this manuscript only 9 of 101 growing hybridoma cultures produced an antibody capable of cross-reacting with glutaraldehyde-fixed CHO cells (Fig. 5). The average fusion we now do in the laboratory routinely results in a fusion in which ∿30% of the growing colonies secrete antibody which cross-reacts with glutaraldehyde-fixed CHO cells (data not shown).

Figure 6 displays a titration of the antibody secreted by one of the hybridoma colonies (BI41) against soluble peak A and peak B antigen. As can be seen, the antibody secreted by this colony shows virtually no binding to peak A even at a 1:1 dilution, while the midpoint in the titration curve against soluble peak B occurs between a 1:64 and a 1:128 dilution. A similar titration curve has been derived for the other eight colonies which were scored as positive in their ability to bind to glutaraldehyde-fixed CHO cells.

Selection and Characterization of Clones

Colonies BI41 and BI69 proved to be most efficient in producing clones in soft agar, and therefore the data to be discussed in this manuscript will be limited to the results obtained with these two clones. As can be seen in Table II, colony BI41 produced

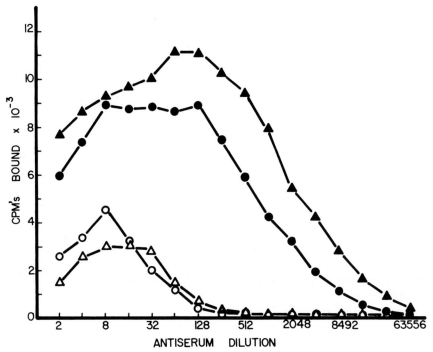

Fig. 4. Antiserum binding to soluble peaks A and B. Peaks A and B were isolated as described in Materials and Methods and Figure 2. The soluble proteins and glycoproteins from each fraction were dried down and fixed to microtiter wells as described in Materials and Methods. Finally an RIA on the soluble antigens was performed as described in Materials and Methods. ▲, peak B antiserum binding to peak B; △, peak B antiserum binding to peak A; ●, peak A antiserum binding to peak A; ○, peak A antiserum binding to peak B.

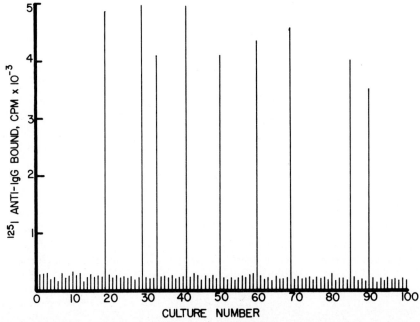

Fig. 5. Hybridoma supernate binding to glutaraldehyde-fixed CHO cells. Culture fluid (25 μl) was aseptically removed from the growing hybridoma cultures approximately 2 weeks after the initial fusion and tested for its ability to bind to glutaraldehyde-fixed CHO cells in the RIA described in detail in Materials and Methods.

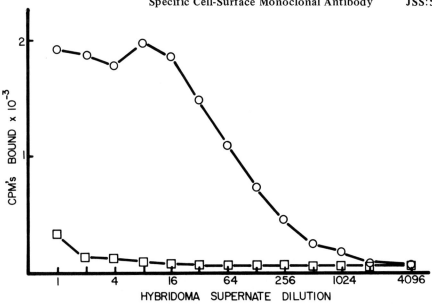

Fig. 6 Hybridoma supernate binding to peaks A and B. Peaks A and B were isolated as described in Materials and Methods and Figure 2. The soluble proteins and glycoproteins were dried down and fixed to microtiter wells as described in Materials and Methods. Finally an RIA on the soluble antigens was performed as described in Materials and Methods. ○, Supernate binding to peak B; □, supernate binding to peak A.

TABLE II. Binding of Clonal Supernates

	Glutaraldehyde-fixed CHO cells	[^{125}I]-anti-IgG bound			
		Live cells (0°C)	Peak A	Peak B	Fetuin
BI41.1	240	160	150	150	100
BI41.2	270	300	100	100	100
BI41.3.	270	250	100	100	100
BI41.4	4,500	2,500	1,700	10,600	100
BI69.1	4,000	3,000	1,800	7,800	100
BI69.2	280	300	100	100	100
BI69.3	250	200	100	100	100
BI69.4	4,600	2,910	1,600	10,120	100

The RIAs were performed as described in Materials and Methods. Among the other 21 clones selected from the BI41 colony, 18 showed positive binding to glutaraldehyde-fixed CHO cells.

23 clones that were subsequently picked and grown to high cell density in vitro. Clone BI69 produced two actively growing clones that were also picked (Table II). Both clones secreted antibodies of the gamma-globulin class 1 variety.

It is worth noting that in those cases where it has been studied the clonal supernates show an apparently higher efficiency of binding to glutaraldehyde-fixed CHO cells than to live cells maintained at 0°C (Table II). This may result from a glutaraldehyde-mediated preservation of the antigenic structures recognized by the particular antibody or to down-modulation of surface antigens on the live cells subsequent to antibody binding. It should also be

TABLE III. Antibody Binding to CHO, 3T3 (Balb/c A-31), and NIL 8 M-2 Cells

Clonal supernate	Cell line	cpm [^{125}I]-anti-IgG bound
BI41.4	CHO (H-7$_{\text{w}}$)	5,000
	NIL 8 M-2	3,790
	Balb/c A-31	147
BI69.1	CHO (H-7$_{\text{w}}$)	4,000
	NIL 8 M-2	2,800
	Balb/c A-31	125

Antibody binding to glutaraldehyde-fixed cells was determined as described in Materials and Methods.

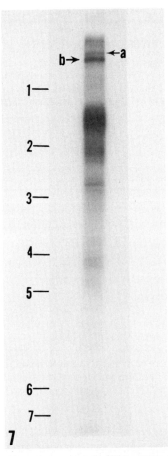

Fig. 7. Iodination of surface proteins and glycoproteins. H-7$_{\text{w}}$ cells were iodinated according to the technique of Phillips and Morrison [11]. A plasma membrane-enriched fraction was then isolated [12], the membranes were solubilized in SDS, and the proteins and glycoproteins were separated on a 7.5–12.5% Laemmli discontinuous SDS-PAGE [16]. Approximately 100,000 cpm was applied to the gel. After separation the gel was dried and an autoradiograph was prepared. Molecular weight markers [1–7] as in Figure 3. Arrow (a) identifies the 265,000-dalton component, arrow (b) the 250,000-dalton component.

noted that where it has been tested the clonal supernates that have proved active in their ability to bind to glutaraldehyde-fixed CHO cells were capable of efficiently distinguishing between peak A and peak B material in the soluble antigen assay (Table II). None of the active supernates tested showed any binding to fetuin (an excellent Con A receptor, [29]), which suggests but by no means proves that the antigenic determinant recognized by the monoclonal antibody is the peptide rather than the oligosaccharide portion of the Con A-binding glycoprotein.

Table III demonstrates that the antibody secreted by BI41.4 and BI69.1 binds efficiently to CHO cells and NIL 8 M-2 cells (another hamster-S derived cell line provided to us by Dr. Richard Hynes). Interestingly the antibody secreted by these two clones does not bind to a mouse-derived permanent cell line, Balb/c A-31 (a 3T3 clone, Table III). These antibodies also show no binding to a wide variety of chicken, mouse, and human cell lines (data not shown). These data clearly suggest that the antibodies secreted by BI41.4 and BI69.1 are "hamster-specific."

Figure 7 is an autoradiograph of iodinated surface components of the H-7$_w$ CHO cell clone. As can be seen, the pattern of surface iodination is complex [7]; however, one band does clearly stand out. This band electrophoreses with a molecular weight of $\sim$250,000 daltons and can be labeled with [^{3}H]-glucosamine or with $NaIO_4/NaB^3H_4$ as previously described [7]. Above this major band is a more minor band which displays an apparent molecular weight of $\sim$265,000. Figure 8 is an autoradiograph of an immunoprecipitate of iodinated T$_s$components (see Fig. 3A) that had been incubated with antibodies derived from clone BI41.4, as described in Materials and Methods. As can be seen, the antibodies secreted by clone BI41.4 precipitate an iodinated species which runs at $\sim$265,000 daltons. This band represents 2–3% of the T$_s$ iodinated surface components and almost certainly corresponds to the more "minor" high-molecular-weight band identified in Figure 7 that has an apparent molecular weight of $\sim$265,000. The same iodinated species is precipitated by the supernate derived from clone BI69.4 (data not shown) as well as the other clones derived from BI41 (Table II).

DISCUSSION

The data presented in this manuscript clearly demonstrate that one can use Con A affinity chromatography to isolate cell surface Con A-binding glycoproteins from a Triton X-100-soluble fraction of a plasma membrane-enriched organelle isolate. Furthermore the data clearly demonstrate that immunization of Balb/c mice with *all* of the T$_s$ Con A receptors followed by fusion of the spleen cells with mouse myeloma cells will produce a series of hybridoma clones which secrete antibodies capable of recognizing Con A receptors associated with the CHO cell surface as well as T$_s$ Con A receptors. Furthermore the antibodies derived from the clonal hybridoma supernates can be used, in conjunction with S aureus protein A, to immunoprecipitate specific Con A receptors from the T$_s$ fraction of the iodinated surface membranes.

The work described in this manuscript demonstrates that we have been able to select a series of hybridoma clones which secrete a monoclonal antibody against a surface component of $\sim$265,000 mol wt. Extensive work in our laboratory has demonstrated that this high-molecular-weight glycoprotein is not fibronectin. Among the evidence we have gathered to support this conclusion are the following points: 1) anti-fibronectin antibody does not precipitate the 265,000-dalton CHO cell surface component; 2) the monoclonal antibodies described in this manuscript precipitate a 265,000-dalton NIL cell surface component but not

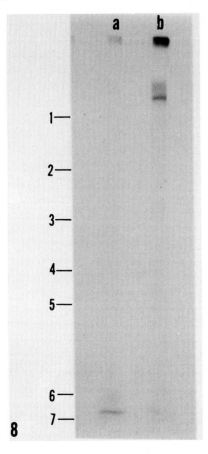

Fig. 8. Immunoprecipitation with clone BI41.4. H-7$_w$ cells were labeled with [^{125}I], the surface membrane was isolated, and the T$_s$ fraction prepared. The immunoprecipitation was performed as described in Materials and Methods. a: T$_s$ fraction was taken through the immunoprecipitation protocol as outlined in Materials and Methods using supernate from myeloma cells that had not been fused with spleen cells as the source of antibody ($\sim$7,000 cpm applied). Supernate from spleen-myeloma fusions which showed no binding to the CHO cells also failed to precipitate any surface component. b: Immunoprecipitation with BI41.4 supernate ($\sim$7,000 cpm applied). None of the "clearings" which occurred prior to the addition of the antibody precipitated any components that could be detected on SDS-PAGE.

NIL cell fibronectin which can be precipitated by an antibody prepared against NIL cell fibronectin; and 3) the monoclonal antibodies do not precipitate purified NIL cell fibronectin. All of these data as well as an extensive characterization of the synthesis, turnover, and topologic localization of this 265,000-dalton CHO cell surface component are the subject of a manuscript about to be submitted for publication (Starling and Noonan, manuscript in preparation).

Finally we would like to point out that we also have derived monoclonal antibodies against other Con A-binding surface glycoproteins as well as some non-Con A-binding surface components. It is our intention to utilize these monoclonal antibodies to study the lateral mobility of individual membrane proteins and glycoproteins. We also intend to use these antibodies in efforts to isolate CHO cell variants lacking specific surface receptors.

It is our hope that such cell variants might provide us with information relating to the physiologic role of some membrane components in such biologically important phenomena as cell-cell and cell-substrate adhesion.

ACKNOWLEDGMENTS

This work was supported by US Public Health Service grants GM-0994 from the National Institutes of Health and PCM 76-15327 from the National Science Foundation.

The authors gratefully acknowledge the expert technical assistance of Mr. William Elmquist. We would also like to thank Dr. Richard Hynes (Massachusetts Institute of Technology) for providing us with both the NIL8 M2 cell line and the anti-fibronectin antiserum.

REFERENCES

1. Nicolson GL: Int Rev Cytol 39:89, 1974.
2. Goldstein IJ, Hayes CE: Adv Carbohydr Chem Biochem 35:127, 1978.
3. Noonan KD: In Nicolau C (ed): "Virus-transformed Cell Membranes." London: Academic, 1978, pp 281–371.
4. Singer SJ: Ann Rev Biochem 43:805, 1974.
5. Kohler G, Milstein C: Nature 256:495, 1974.
6. Kohler G, Milstein C: Eur J Immunol 6:511, 1976.
7. Noonan KD: Biochim Biophys Acta 551:22, 1979.
8. Kohler G, Milstein C: Nature 244:42, 1973.
9. Springer T, Galfne G, Secher DS, Milstein C: Eur J Immunol 8:539, 1978.
10. Gahmberg CG, Anderson LC: J Biol 252:5888, 1977.
11. Phillips, DE, Morrison M: Biochem Biophys Res Commun 40:284, 1970.
12. Brunette DM, Till JE: J Membr Biol 5:215, 1971.
13. Cuatrecasas P: J Biol Chem 245:3059, 1977.
14. Findley JB: J Biol Chem 249:4398, 1974.
15. Jacobs S, Schechter Y, Bissel K, Cuatrecasas P: Biochem Biophys Res Commun 77:981, 1977.
16. Laemmli UK: Nature 227:680, 1970.
17. Martinozzi M, Moscona A: Exp Cell Res 94:253, 1975.
18. Agrawal BBS, Goldstein IJ: Biochem J 96:23c, 1965.
19. Burridge K: Proc Natl Acad Sci USA 73:4457, 1976.
20. Simrell CR, Klein PA: J Immunol. In press.
21. Koprowski H, Gerhard W, Croce CM: Proc Natl Acad Sci USA 74:2985, 1977.
22. Gerhard W, Croce CM, Lopes D, Koprowski H: Proc Natl Acad Sci USA 75:1510, 1978.
23. Guimezanes A, Fridman WH, Gisler RH, Korrilsky FM: Eur J Immunol 6:69, 1976.
24. Hunter R: Proc Soc Exp Biol Med 133:989, 1970.
25. Coffins P, Scharff MD: Proc Natl Acad Sci USA 68:2A, 1971.
26. Moore PB, Ownby CL, Carraway KL: Exp Cell Res 115:331, 1978.
27. O'Farrell PH: J Biol Chem 250:4007, 1975.
28. Noonan NE, Noonan KD: In preparation.
29. Sela BA, Wang JL, Edelman GM: J Biol Chem 250:7535, 1976.

Journal of Supramolecular Structure 11:579—586 (1979)
Tumor Cell Surfaces and Malignancy 421—428

Modulation of Cell Surface Iron Transferrin Receptors by Cellular Density and State of Activation

James W. Larrick and Peter Cresswell

Division of Immunology, Department of Microbiology and Immunology, Duke University Medical Center, Durham, North Carolina 27710

This report describes investigations of plasma membrane transferrin receptors on a variety of lymphoid cell lines and normal peripheral blood lymphocytes during activation and cell growth cycles. Transformed lymphoid cell lines have as many as 1,000 times the number of receptors found on normal resting lymphocytes. The number of iron transferrin receptors on continuous cell lines as well as normal human fibroblasts is down-regulated during the transition from log-phase growth to stationary plateau growth. When normal lymphocytes are transformed by mixed lymphocyte culture or mitogens, they rapidly express a 50-fold increase in the number of transferrin binding sites. This appearance of iron transferrin receptors anticipates nuclear changes during cell activation and subsequent mitosis of normal cells.

Key words: growth factors, transferrin receptors, mitogenesis, mixed lymphocyte culture, cell cycle

A number of investigators have shown that transferrin is among a small group of essential protein growth factors necessary to support serum-free growth of cell lines [1—6]. These studies suggest an important role for transferrin in the metabolism of a number of cell types, a role which is poorly understood at the present time. During the course of biochemical studies of iron transferrin receptors on lymphoblastoid cell lines [7] we noted variation in the number of receptors with growth state of the cell cultures. Although the number of iron transferrin receptors on erythrocyte precursors has been shown to decrease during maturation in the bone marrow [8], variation in numbers of transferrin receptors on other cell types in various metabolic states has not been studied. Furthermore the metabolism of these important cell surface molecules has not been studied in relation to the change from normal to malignant cell growth. Because resting lymphocytes express very few receptor sites and continuous lymphoid cell lines express up to 1,000 times as many receptors the present communication describes investigations of iron transferrin receptors during transformation, during in vitro growth and during the cell cycle.

Received May 7, 1979; accepted August 1, 1979.

MATERIALS AND METHODS

Reagents

Purified transferrin and crystalline bovine serum albumin were purchased from Sigma Chemical Co. (St. Louis). $Na^{125}I$ (carrier-free) was obtained from New England Nuclear (Boston).

Cell Lines

Human lymphoblastoid cell lines which were used had the following origins: HSB, CEM, T cell lymphoma; SB, JOKO, in vitro transformation with Epstein-Barr virus; K562, chronic myelogenous leukemia; U937, histiocytic lymphoma. Cell lines are grown in RPMI-1640 medium containing 10% fetal calf serum. They are maintained in 250-ml polystyrene tissue culture flasks (Corning) at $37°C$ in a humidified incubator with 5% CO_2.

Normal Human Peripheral Lymphocytes

Blood was drawn by venipuncture into heparinized plastic syringes (40 units/ml). It was diluted 10:35 with 0.95% NaCl, layered on Ficoll-Hypaque (LSM, Litton Bionetics, Kensington, Maryland) and spun at 400 g for 30 min. The harvested peripheral mononuclear cells were harvested from the interface above the Ficoll-Hypaque and washed twice in culture medium to remove platelets. All peripheral blood lymphocytes (PBLs) were cultured in the same medium as that used for cell lines.

Mixed Lymphocyte Cultures

For two-way mixed lymphocyte culture (MLC) activation of peripheral blood lymphocytes equal numbers of lymphocytes from two individuals were cultured at a final concentration of 1.5×10^6 cells per milliliter. For one-way MLC activation stimulator cells received 1,500 R prior to being added to an equal volume of responder cells with a final concentration of 1.5×10^6 cells per milliliter.

Mitogen Stimulation

PBLs were mitogen-stimulated by culturing cells at 1.5×10^6/ml in the presence of phytohemagglutinin (PHA) (2 µg/ml) (Kidney Bean Phytohemagglutinin, Burroughs Wellcome Co., Research Triangle Park, North Carolina) or Con A (2 µg/ml) (Concanavalin A Jack Bean lectin, Miles Laboratories, Elkhart, Indiana).

Thymidine Labeling

When cells were prepared for MLC or mitogen activation, 0.2-ml aliquots were plated into round-bottom microtiter plates for subsequent thymidine labeling. Sixteen hours prior to a time point 1 µCi of ^{3}H-thymidine was added to quadruplicate wells. Cells were harvested with a Skatron cell harvester and counted in a Beckman liquid scintillation counter.

Fibroclast Cultures

Passage seven human skin fibroblasts were cultured in 75-cm^2 Falcon tissue culture flasks in Eagle's minimal essential medium (MEM) supplemented with 4 mM glutamine, 10% fetal calf serum, penicillin (100 U/ml), and streptomycin (100 µg/ml). For assay cells were removed with 0.05% sodium bicarbonate (w/v) in phosphate-buffered saline containing 0.02% ethylenediaminetetraacetic acid (EDTA) (w/v). Cells were washed twice in culture medium and assayed for transferrin binding as described above.

Cell Synchronization

A double-thymidine block technique [11, 12] was used to arrest CEM (T cell line) in late G1. Cells were grown in 2 mM thymidine (Sigma Chemical Co., St. Louis) for 16 h, followed by growth for 10 h in thymidine-free medium. Thymidine was added for an additional 14 h and the cells were washed free of thymidine. Transferrin receptors of the synchronized population of cells were measured by the ^{125}I-FeTF binding assay. Cell mitoses were counted in Dif-Quik-stained cytofuge preparations (Harleco, Gibbstown, New Jersey).

Preparation of Transferrin

A 10 mg/ml solution of transferrin in phosphate-buffered saline was saturated with iron by incubation with ferric ammonium citrate (0.1 mg/ml) in 0.01 M Na HCO$_3$ for 4 h at room temperature. Excess ions were removed by dialysis versus phosphate-buffered saline over night at 4°C and the final concentration of iron-saturated transferrin was measured by absorbance at 454 nm.

Iron-saturated transferrin was labeled by a modified chloramine T method [9]. Briefly, 1–2 mCi Na-^{125}I, 100–200 μg saturated transferrin, and 2.5 μg chloramine T were incubated at room temperature in 30 μl 0.05 M phosphate buffer pH 7.4. After 2 min, the reaction was stopped by the addition of 10 μl sodium metabisulfite (0.625 mg/ml) and 100 μg Kl in water (20 mg/ml). Excess iodine was removed by Sephadex G-50 gel filtration chromatography in phosphate-buffered saline. We found that 99% of the labeled transferrin (^{125}I-FeTF) was immunoprecipitable by specific antitransferrin antibody. Labeled transferrin gave a single peak of apparent molecular weight 80,000 on SDS-PAGE run under reducing conditions [10].

Binding Assay

To assess binding of transferrin to cells, various amounts of ^{125}I-FeTF were added to 2.0×10^6 cells in a final volume of 200 μl of RPMI-1640 containing 15 mM Hepes, pH 7.4. Cells were incubated at 37°C for 20 min. Binding was terminated by addition of 12 ml cold phosphate-buffered saline to the conical 15 ml polystyrene tubes used for the incubations. Cells were pelleted and resuspended in additional cold buffer three times and transferred to 12-$\times$ 75-mm glass tubes. After the cells were centrifuged a final time they were counted in a Nuclear-Chicago Model 1185 gamma counter. The washing procedure consistently removed all but about 50 cpm from an initial input as high as 10^6 cpm.

RESULTS

Transferrin Receptors on Normal and Transformed Lymphoid Cells

Table I presents a comparison of the relative amount of binding of iron-saturated transferrin to normal peripheral blood lymphocytes and to cell lines derived from T and B lymphocyte subpopulations. Normal mixed peripheral blood mononuclear cells express very few receptor sites. T lymphoblastoid cell lines derived from patients with acute leukemia bind 3–7 times as much ^{125}I-FeTF as B lymphoblastoid cell lines induced

TABLE I. Binding of ^{125}I-FeTF to Various Human Myeloid and Lymphoid Cells

Name of cell	Origin	^{125}I-FeTF bound (ng/10^6 cells)
CEM	T lymphoblastoid	21.7
HSB	T lymphoblastoid	12.3
SB	B lymphoblastoid	3.5
JOKO	B lymphoblastoid	4.0
K562	Myeloid/erythroid	38.7
U937	Macrophage-like	5.4
Normal PBL[a]		0.1

[a]Mean from eight people.

by Epstein-Barr virus transformation of B cells. U937, a human macrophage-like cell line derived from the pleural effusion of a patient with histiocytic lymphoma [13], binds approximately as much ^{125}I-FeTF as the B cell lines. The cell line binding the most transferrin was K562, derived from a patient with chronic myelocytic leukemia. This is of interest because this human myeloid cell line can be induced to produce hemoglobin and may in fact be of early erythroid origin [14].

Density-Dependent Down-Regulation of Transferrin Receptors

Because of the large difference in transferrin receptor number between transformed and normal cells, it was of interest to determine if the greater receptor number was due to the higher metabolic rate of the neoplastic cells. Using the T cell line CEM, binding of transferrin was measured during log-phase growth at relatively low cell density and during the slowing of growth with the approach of stationary phase (Fig. 1). As the cells slow their metabolic rate and cease dividing, there is a gradual decline in the number of binding sites for iron transferrin. However, even under conditions in which the cells are in stationary phase they express no less than 10% of the number of log-phase binding sites. The amount of ^{125}I-FeTF binding to the stationary lymphoblastoid cell line is approximately 50–100 times that binding to resting lymphocytes.

To determine if a similar phenomenon of down-regulation has relevance to normal cells, transferrin binding was measured on secondary cultures of human skin fibroblasts. Following cell passage these cells grow slowly. At subconfluency their rate of growth is more rapid and they display density-dependent topoinhibition when the culture when the culture becomes confluent. There is a marked decrease in the number of binding sites on cells grown to confluency compared to subconfluent or low-density, recently passaged, cells (Table II).

Normal Lymphocytes Transformed by Mitogens or During MLC Exhibit a Marked Increase in Transferrin Receptors Prior to DNA Synthesis

The plant lectins kidney bean phytohemagglutinin (PHA) and jack bean concanavalin A (Con A) have been used to probe the molecular events associated with lymphoid cell activation. Lymphocytes cultured in the presence of these substances undergo cell division and exhibit many of the cell surface changes characteristic of normally cycling cells. When the kinetics of transferrin binding and cellular DNA synthesis (measured by ^{3}H-

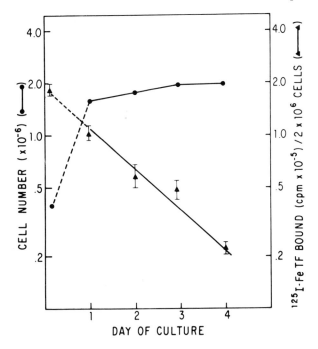

Fig. 1. Modulation of ^{125}I-FeTF binding: CEM cells (T lymphoblastoid) approaching stationary phase (sold lines) are compared to log-phase cells (left of broken lines).

TABLE II. Down-Regulation of Transferrin Receptors on Human Skin Fibroblasts

Cell Density	Cells harvested/cm^2	^{125}I-FeTF bound (ng/10^6 cells)
Confluent	3.0×10^4	3.9
Subconfluent	1.7×10^4	50.0
Sparse	0.9×10^4	29.7

thymidine incorporation) was studied (Fig. 2), there was a marked increase in the number of receptors within 24 h of contact with both lectins, and the peak of receptor expression anticipated the DNA synthesis peak by almost 24 h. Cells cultured in the absence of mitogens demonstrated a small increase in binding consistent with low-level nonspecific activation or bound transferrin released after transfer from in vivo.

Figure 3 presents a comparison of the kinetics of appearance of iron transferrin receptors during one-way and two-way MLCs. The total numbers of cells in each experiment are equal, but in the one-way MLC stimulator cells were irradiated to prevent cell division. In the two-way MLC the transferrin receptor number peaks earlier and is approximately twice the one-way MLC response. In the one-way MLC the transferrin receptor number anticipates DNA synthesis and subsequent cell mitosis in a manner similar to

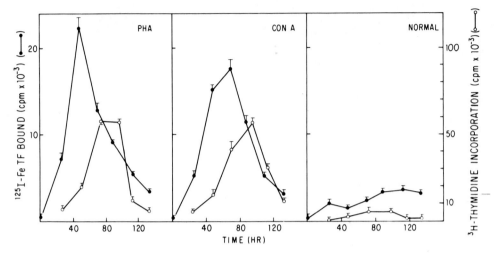

Fig. 2. Mitogen-stimulated peripheral mononuclear cells demonstrate a marked increase in the number of ^{125}I-FeTF binding sites (●—●), which anticipates ^{3}H-thymidine incorporation (○—○).

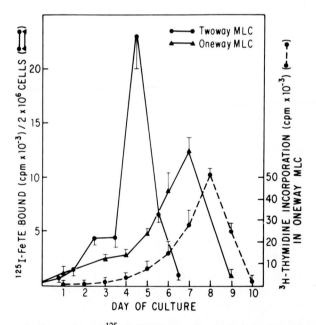

Fig. 3. Increase in the number of ^{125}I-FeTF binding sites during mixed lymphocyte cultures.

that described for mitogen activation. Because cells activated by plant lectins or allogeneic lymphocytes (MLC) express transferrin receptors prior to the ^{3}H-thymidine incorporation peak, it is possible to substitute binding of transferrin as the end point for these assays.

Increase in Transferrin Receptors in the Late GI Phase of the Cell Cycle

The appearance of iron transferrin receptors was studied in synchronized populations of lymphoblastoid cells because the kinetic studies of mitogen-activated cells suggested a possible correlation with the cell cycle. These studies showed that the blocked synchronized cells (0.2% mitoses) had 54% of the binding sites of the unsynchronized randomly growing cells. When the thymidine blockage was removed the number of transferrin receptors remained constant for 24 h. At 31 h, when 8% of the cells were in mitosis, the number of iron transferrin binding sites had increased to 93% of control levels.

DISCUSSION

These studies demonstrate that the number of cellular iron-transferrin binding sites is modulated by the growth rate of cells. Cells which are rapidly proliferating, such as a variety of leukemia and continuous lymphoid cell lines, have many receptors. Normal resting lymphocytes have very few receptors. Density-dependent arrest of normal fibroblasts was accompanied by a significant decline in the number of receptors. Likewise slowly proliferating cells in stationary-plateau cultures demonstrated one-tenth as many receptors as rapidly growing log-phase lymphoblastoid cells. These studies suggest that rapidly dividing cells which require one of the metals which transferrin is capable of delivering will express more cell surface receptors than slowly growing or nonproliferating cells.

Early studies of mitogens showed that cultured human lymphocytes release a substance which is required for an optimal PHA response [15]. Tormey et al [16] demonstrated that a protein factor from human serum could substitute for this substance and identified it as transferrin. These same investigators subsequently reported that a subpopulation of mitogen-stimulated lymphocytes as well as cells activated by other means develop a requirement for transferrin 5–6 h prior to the onset of DNA synthesis in late G1 [17]. Our preliminary cell synchronization studies and mitogen studies showing increased numbers of transferrin receptors prior to DNA synthesis complement these findings. In contrast to these studies the original studies describing appearance of insulin receptors on mitogen-stimulated lymphocytes showed that their appearance was a late event which coincided with uptake of ^{3}H-thymidine [18]. It can be hypothesized that during late G1, prior to commitment to DNA synthesis, the cell has a programmed expression of transferrin receptors because critical metabolic pathways require one of the metals transferrin transports. This could be iron [19] (multiple critical biochemical pathways require heme proteins) or zinc [20], which is required as a cofactor in nucleic acid metabolism. Whether transferrin itself has a mitogenic or growth factor role in cell proliferation independent of its transport role for metals is under current investigation. None of the published studies on the requirement of transferrin for serumless growth of cells in vitro suggest what its precise role in cell growth is [1–6].

Investigations of other receptor molecules demonstrate no single pattern of response to a state of increased cellular growth. For example, studies by Smith et al [21] do demonstrate an increase in glucocorticoid receptors (by a factor of 2–6) in blast transformation and Lippman et al [22] have reported that lymphoblasts from patients with acute lymphoblastic leukemia have higher levels of receptors than normal peripheral lymphocytes. Studies of BALB/3T3 mouse embryo fibroblasts showed that insulin binding was low in growing cells and increased 2–9 times in confluent stationary cultures [23]. The same authors showed that viral transformation caused the number of insulin receptors to decrease. Westermark compared epidermal growth factor binding in sparse and dense cultures of normal human glial cells [24]. Sparse cultures had 20,000 sites per cell and dense, contact-inhibited cells had 35,000 sites per cell.

The expression of an increased number of iron transferrin receptors may be a useful marker of cellular activation for studying subpopulations of cells in vitro. Mitogen stimulation of lymphocytes or the blastogenesis which accompanies an MLC results in the expression of as many as 50 times the number of receptors expressed by resting peripheral mononuclear cells. Not only is this enhanced expression of a cell surface marker many times the increase reported for insulin receptors [25] but the demonstrated high affinity of the receptor for transferrin [7] ($K_{affinity} = 10^{11} M^{-1}$) suggests that it may be possible to separate activated and unactivated subpopulations by affinity techniques.

ACKNOWLEDGMENTS

This work was supported by National Institutes of Health training grant GM-07171 (Medical Scientist Training Program) to JWL and US Public Health Service grant AI-14016.

REFERENCES

1. Hayashi I, Sato GH: Nature 259:132, 1976.
2. Hamilton WG, Ham RG: In Vitro 13:537, 1977.
3. Hutchings SE, Sato GH: Proc Natl Acad Sci USA 75:901, 1978.
4. Allegra JC, Lippman ME: Can Res 38:3823, 1978.
5. Rizzino A, Sato GH: Proc Natl Acad Sci USA 75:1844, 1978.
6. Iscove NN, Melchers F: J Exp Med 147:923, 1978.
7. Larrick JW, Cresswell P: Biochim Biophys Acta 583:483, 1979.
8. Kailis SG, Morgan EH: Br J Haem 28:37, 1974.
9. Hunter WM, Greenwood FC: Nature 194:495, 1962.
10. Laemmli AK: Nature 227:680, 1970.
11. Bootsma D, Budke L, Vos O: Exp Cell Res 33:301, 1964.
12. Griffin MJ, Ber R: J Cell Biol 40:297, 1969.
13. Sundstrom C, Nilsson K: Int J Can 17:565, 1976.
14. Anderson LC, Jokinen M, Galinberg CG: Nature 278:364, 1979.
15. Sasaki MS, Norman A: Nature 210:913, 1966.
16. Tormey DC, Imrie RC, Mueller GC: Exp Cell Res 74:163, 1972.
17. Tormey DC, Mueller GC: Exp Cell Res 74:220, 1972.
18. Krug U, Krug F, Cuatrecasas P: Proc Natl Acad Sci USA 69:2604, 1972.
19. Worwood M: Sem Haematol 14:3, 1977.
20. Phillips JL: Cell Immunol 35:318, 1978.
21. Smith KA, Crabtree GR, Kennedy SJ, Munck AU: Nature 267:523, 1977.
22. Lippman ME, Halterman RH, Leventhal BG, Perry S, Thompson EB: J Clin Invest 52:1715, 1973.
23. Thomopoulos P, Roth J, Lovelace L, Pastan I: Cell 8:417, 1976.
24. Westermark B: Proc Natl Acad Sci USA 74:1619, 1977.
25. Helderman JH, Strom TB: Nature 274:62, 1978.

Journal of Supramolecular Structure 12:63–72 (1979)
Tumor Cell Surfaces and Malignancy 429–438

Effects of the Tumor Promoter TPA on the Induction of DNA Synthesis in Normal and RSV-Transformed Rat Fibroblasts

Bruce E. Magun and G. T. Bowden

Department of Anatomy (B.E.M.) and Division of Radiation Oncology (G.T.B.), Arizona Health Center College of Medicine, University of Arizona, Tucson, Arizona 85724

Induction of DNA synthesis by the tumor promoter tetradecanoyl phorbol acetate (TPA) was studied in a line of cultured rat fibroblasts (Rat-1) and their Rous sarcoma virus-transformed derivative (Rat-1(RSV)). Following serum deprivation for 54 h to achieve quiescence, semiconservative DNA replication was measured by incubation of cells in BrdUrd and FdUrd after serum stimulation in the presence or absence of TPA. Optimal concentrations of TPA (0.1–0.5 µg/ml) in serum-free medium induced a small increase (10–15%) in the amount of DNA made over a 30-h period in both Rat-1 and Rat-1(RSV) cells. When Rat-1 cells were stimulated by a 4-h serum pulse, 30% of the DNA was replicated by 30 h. If the serum pulse was followed by TPA addition, 70% DNA replication was observed. If the serum pulse was preceded by TPA addition, the onset of DNA synthesis was delayed by several hours, but stimulation of DNA synthesis occurred. In contrast, the Rat-1(RSV) cells did not show an increase in DNA synthesis induced by TPA in similar protocols, but the serum-induced onset of DNA synthesis was delayed by several hours in the presence of TPA. Therefore, TPA acts as a co-inducer of DNA synthesis in the Rat-1 but not in the Rat-1(RSV) cells. The parent alcohol, phorbol, was inactive in Rat-1 cells, but delayed the onset of DNA synthesis in the Rat-1(RSV) cells. We conclude that the co-inducing and delaying activities of TPA on DNA synthesis appear to be distinct and to act at different points in the G_1 phase of the cell cycle.

Key words: tumor promoter, DNA synthesis, transformed cells, serum stimulation

The concept of tumor promotion was first developed from studies using mouse skin [1–4] and has since been applied to malignant transformation of other tissues [5–7] as well as cells in culture [8–12]. In the classical two-stage system of skin tumor formation,

Abbreviations used: TPA, 12-O-tetradecanoyl-phorbol-13-acetate; BrdUrd, 5′-bromodeoxyuridine; FdUrd, 5′-fluorodeoxyuridine; DMSO, dimethyl sulfoxide; TdR, thymidine; ODC, ornithine decarboxylase.
Received April 17, 1979; accepted August 13, 1979.

a subcarcinogenic dose of a tumor initiator (mutagen) is followed by frequent applications of a tumor promoter to produce both benign and malignant tumors. Tetradecanoyl phorbol acetate (TPA) is the most active tumor-promoting phorbol diester present in croton oil [13], which was used by Mottram [4] to demonstrate the two-stage mechanism of carcinogenesis in mouse skin. Tumor promotion using TPA also has been demonstrated to occur in vitro in 10 $T_{1/2}$ mouse fibroblasts using different initiators [9–11].

In an attempt to elucidate the mechanism of tumor promotion, the effects of TPA on a variety of molecular events in cells in culture have been studied. These include a TPA-induced increase in ODC [14, 15], plasminogen activator synthesis [7], a decrease in epidermal growth factor binding [16, 17], and fibronectin production [18], and the induction of DNA synthesis [11, 14, 19, 20].

Tumor promoters stimulate cell proliferation in epidermal target tissue [21] as well as in primary cultures of mouse epidermal cells [20] and in rodent fibroblasts [11], in which a transient depression in DNA synthesis was also seen. TPA was found to be mitogenic for chick chondroblasts, but not for fibroblasts [22]. TPA has been shown to act as a comitogen with phytohemagglutinin (PHA) in cultures of bovine lymph node lymphocytes [23]. At dose levels of PHA and TPA which were independently inactive as mitogens, when used in combination they were highly effective in promoting lymphocytes to enter into cell replication. It has been suggested that lymphocytes which have been stimulated minimally with PHA depend on TPA to release or activate certain intracellular factors that promote the cell to engage in nuclear and cellular replication processes [22]. In human lymphocytes, however, TPA was found to be mitogenic [23].

Much of the confusion in the literature concerning the mitogenic versus comitogenic capacity of TPA is due, in part, to the addition of TPA to confluent cultures in serum-containing medium. In these instances an apparent mitogenic response might be the result of a TPA-induced sensitization to serum growth factors. In order to begin to investigate these events we studied the effect of TPA on the extent of DNA synthesis in arrested, serum-deprived normal rat fibroblasts (Rat-1 cells), and in cultures which were suboptimally stimulated by serum. DNA synthesis in rat fibroblasts transformed by Rous sarcoma virus (Rat-1(RSV) cells) was also investigated, in order to compare the effect of TPA on cells whose growth control mechanisms are controlled, at least in part, by the *src* gene product.

MATERIALS AND METHODS

Chemicals

TPA was purchased from Dr. Peter Borchert, Chemical Carcinogenesis, Eden Prairie, Minnesota, and phorbol from Consolidated Midland Corp., Brewster, New York. [2-^{14}C]-Thymidine (43 mCi/mmole) was obtained from Research Products International, Elk Grove, Illinois. Fetal bovine serum was purchased from K. C. Biologicals, Inc., Lenexa, Kansas.

Cell Culture Techniques

The Rat-1 line used in these experiments refers to the F2408 established line derived from Fischer rat embryo fibroblasts [24]. Untransformed Rat-1 cells and Rat-1 cells transformed by the B-77 strain of Rous sarcoma virus (Rat-1(wt/RSV)) were kindly supplied by J. A. Wyke. The cell lines were propagated in Dulbecco's minimal essential medium containing 10% heat-inactivated (56°C, 30 min) fetal bovine serum at 39°C in a humidified 5% CO_2, 95% air atmosphere.

Measurement of Replicated DNA

This technique has been described in detail [25]. Briefly, the technique requires labeling exponentially growing cells for several generations with [^{14}C] thymidine. Upon stimulation from the serum-deficient state, the medium was adjusted to contain 50 μg/ml 5′-bromodeoxyuridine (BrdUrd) and 0.1 μg/ml 5′-fluorodeoxyuridine (FdUrd). Newly replicated DNA was then determined after centrifugation of DNA, isolated from these cultures, on neutral CsCl gradients (unsubstituted DNA density 1.70 g/cc, BrdUrd-substituted density 1.75 g/cc). The percentage DNA replicated was then determined by the percentage of DNA which had attained the hybrid density. Under conditions of DNA replication, a complete density shift was observed from 1.70 to 1.75 g/cc, indicating that possible alterations in cell membrane permeability did not cause DNA precursor pool fluctuations which could affect the results reported here.

Each plotted value for percentage DNA replicated, as displayed in the figures, represents the result of a complete CsCl density gradient profile. In several instances three identical culture dishes were analyzed for variations in amount of DNA replicated. Results in our laboratory show the standard error to be less than 1% DNA replicated. It is important to emphasize that neither numbers of cells per plate nor time of isotope incorporation affect the results. All of the values in each figure were determined from cultures that were part of the same experiment.

Experimental Design

Stock solutions of TPA and phorbol were made up in DMSO and added to cultures to give 0.1% DMSO and final concentrations ranging from 1 ng to 1000 ng/ml of culture medium. Cultures were plated out to give 3×10^5 cells per 6-cm culture dish (Flow Labs, Rockville, Maryland). [2-^{14}C] Thymidine was added at 0.1 μCi/ml and 48 h later the medium was exchanged for one lacking serum and isotope. Experiments were begun 54 h later to investigate effects of serum and TPA addition on the induction of DNA synthesis. At this time (t = 0) the cell number reached stable plateau values, and cell viability as determined by colony-forming ability was undiminished. Flow microfluorimetric analysis of both the Rat-1 and Rat-1(RSV) cells demonstrated identical G_1-like contents of DNA per cell [26]. At t = 0 BrdUrd and FdUrd were added for 4 h, at which time the medium was replaced with serum-free medium containing TPA or phorbol. In all experiments BrdUrd and FdUrd were present from t = 0 to t = 30.

RESULTS

Effect of TPA in Serum-Free Medium

When serum-deprived cultures of Rat-1 and Rat-1(RSV) cells were incubated in serum-free medium containing BrdUrd and FdUrd, 5% and 37% of the DNA, respectively, was replicated over a 30-h period (Fig. 1). Upon addition of various concentrations of TPA in serum-free medium, the total amount of DNA replicated was increased in a dose-dependent manner. The optimal concentration (500 ng/ml) increased the amount of DNA replicated in the Rat-1 cells to a level of 16%. In the Rat-1(RSV) cells, the optimal concentration (100 ng/ml) increased the amount of DNA replicated to 53%. In subsequent experiments the optimal concentrations of TPA derived from Figure 1 were used.

The time course of the onset of DNA synthesis after TPA addition in serum-free medium is shown in Figure 2. In the Rat-1(RSV) cells in serum-free medium alone (with

DMSO), the rate of DNA synthesis is higher (1.6%/h, Fig. 2A) than in the untransformed Rat-1 cells (0.3%/h, Fig. 2B). When TPA is included in the serum-free medium, there is an initial inhibition in the onset of DNA synthesis in the Rat-1(RSV) cells, which is followed by an increased rate beginning at 14 h. The total amount of DNA synthesized at 30 h in the Rat-1(RSV) cells was increased from 40% to 50% by the presence of TPA. When TPA was added to the untransformed Rat-1 cells in serum-free medium, an early increase in DNA synthesis was seen (Fig. 2B), without the initial inhibition which occurred in the Rat-1(RSV) cells.

Effect of TPA in Medium Containing 20% Serum

Both TPA and fetal calf serum were added simultaneously to quiescent cultures of Rat-1 (Fig. 3A) and Rat-1(RSV) (Fig. 3B) cells. The presence of TPA had no effect in the onset, rate, or extent of DNA synthesis in the Rat-1 cells. However, in the Rat-1(RSV) cells, the presence of TPA delayed the onset of DNA synthesis by about 6 h. The rate of DNA synthesis in the latter case was the same.

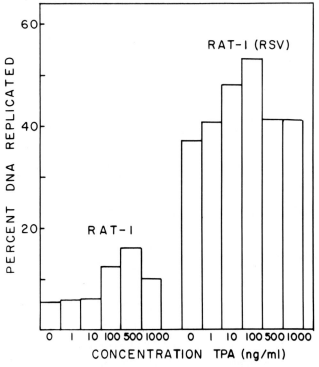

Fig. 1. Stimulation of DNA synthesis in quiescent Rat-1 and Rat-1(RSV) cells by TPA. Cells were seeded at 3×10^5 per 6-cm dish in medium containing 10% serum and 0.10 μCi/ml [^{14}C] thymidine. After 48 h the dishes were rinsed briefly with 5 ml serum-free medium, refilled with fresh serum-free medium, and replaced in the incubator for 54 h. At that time fresh serum-free medium containing BrdUrd, FdUrd, 0.1% DMSO, and varying concentrations of TPA was added to each plate. Control cultures lacked TPA but contained DMSO. Thirty hours later cells were harvested from each dish and prepared for CsCl gradient analysis as described in Materials and Methods. Following density gradient centrifugation of DNA isolated from each sample in CsCl, the ^{14}C activity recovered from the hybrid density peak divided by the ^{14}C activity recovered from the entire gradient was taken as percentage DNA replicated (ordinate). Examples of DNA distribution in CsCl gradients, for conditions similar to those reported here, have been previously published in detail [25, 27].

Effect of TPA Under Suboptimal Serum Conditions

Although addition of TPA and serum simultaneously did not enhance the rate or extent of DNA synthesis in Rat-1 cells, the possibility of synergistic effects of TPA by suboptimal conditions of serum stimulation was investigated. Medium containing 20% serum was added to cultures of Rat-1 and Rat-1(RSV) cells for 4 h, at which time the medium was exchanged for one lacking serum but containing TPA or DMSO (for controls). In cultures of Rat-1 cells a 4-h serum pulse followed by serum-free medium and DMSO resulted in 30% DNA replicated at 30 h compared to 70% when TPA was added in serum-free medium at 4 h (Fig. 4A). If phorbol (1 μg/ml) was added in serum-free medium at 4 h, a delay in the onset of DNA synthesis was seen compared to DMSO controls, although the final amount of DNA replicated at 30 h (30%) was the same as controls. Therefore, in Rat-1 cells TPA but not phorbol acts in a synergistic capacity with serum to induce DNA synthesis.

An identical series of experiments were performed with the Rat-1(RSV) cells. Addition of serum-containing medium for 4 h followed by serum-free medium and DMSO resulted in replication of 60% of the DNA. If TPA was present in the serum-free medium at

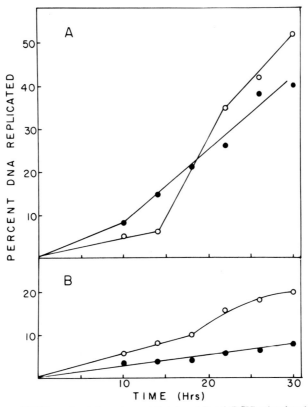

Fig. 2. Time course of DNA synthesis in quiescent Rat-1 and Rat-1(RSV) stimulated by addition of TPA in serum-free medium. Rat-1(RSV) cells (A) and Rat-1 cells (B) were prelabeled in [^{14}C] thymidine for 48 h and serum-deprived for 54 h, as described in Figure 1. At that time (t = 0) the medium was replaced by fresh serum-free medium containing 0.1% dimethyl sulfoxide, BrdUrd, FdUrd with TPA (open circles), and 100 ng/ml for Rat-1(RSV) cells (A) or 500 ng/ml for Rat-1 cells (B). Filled circles represent plates treated identically except that TPA was omitted. Percentage DNA replicated was determined by CsCl density gradient analysis of samples at 10, 14, 18, 22, 26, and 30 h later.

4 h there was no change in the rate or extent of DNA synthesis. Identical results were obtained using 500 ng/ml and 1,000 ng/ml TPA (data not shown). However, in the presence of phorbol (1 μg/ml) in the serum-free medium, the onset of DNA synthesis was delayed by 3 h. Therefore, TPA does not appear to stimulate the onset of DNA synthesis in the Rat-1(RSV) cells.

Effect of Varying Time of TPA Addition

Experiments were performed to determine the time at which TPA was able to exert its comitogenic effect in the Rat-1 cells. When TPA was present in serum-free medium from hour 4 to 5 (Fig. 5A), the amount of DNA replicated was only slightly less (63% versus 70%) than when TPA was present for the entire experiment (Fig. 4A). If the 4-h serum stimulation was preceded by a 1-h treatment with TPA, there was a 4-h delay in the onset of DNA synthesis (Fig. 5A). The amount of DNA synthesized was only slightly less (58% versus 63%). Addition of TPA at 8 h to Rat-1 cells stimulated by serum for 4 h did not alter the rate or extent of subsequent DNA synthesis. From these experiments we conclude that TPA is synergistic with serum when preceded by serum stimulation but is ineffective when added at 8 h. Although TPA is effective as a synergistic inducer of DNA synthesis when addition precedes serum stimulation, a delay in the onset of DNA synthesis occurs.

Experiments similar to the above were conducted using Rat-1(RSV) cells. When the 4-h serum pulse was preceded by a 1-h TPA treatment, the onset of DNA synthesis was de-

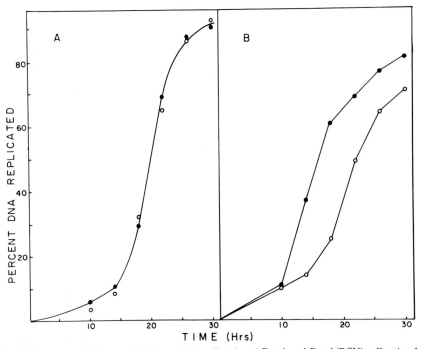

Fig. 3. Time course of DNA synthesis in quiescent Rat-1 and Rat-1 and Rat-1(RSV) cells stimulated by simultaneous addition of TPA and serum. Rat-1 cells (A) and Rat-1(RSV) cells (B) were prelabeled in [14C]-thymidine for 48 h and serum-deprived for 54 h, as described in Figure 1. At that time (t = 0) the medium was replaced by fresh medium containing 20% serum, BrdUrd, FdUrd, 0.1% dimethyl sulfoxide with TPA (open circles, 500 ng/ml in panel A or 100 ng/ml in panel B) or without TPA (filled circles). Percentage DNA replicated was determined by CsCl density gradient analysis of samples at 10, 14, 18, 22, 26, and 30 h later.

layed by 3 h. A delay of 6 h was seen if TPA was added at 8 h. From these results we can conclude that addition of TPA retards the onset of DNA synthesis in Rat-1(RSV) cells. The extent of the retardation is increased when TPA is added closer to the point at which DNA synthesis normally commences (8–12 h).

DISCUSSION

The method which was employed for measuring DNA synthesis using isopycnic density gradient centrifugation of DNA following BrdUrd labeling has been described in several previous publications [25, 27]. The method offers the advantage of measuring the absolute rate of DNA synthesis in cultures over a selected time interval, in contrast to the method of [³H] TdR pulse labeling which provides relative measurements. Such relative measurements do not provide data concerning the amount of DNA replicated. Furthermore, the influence of TPA on the uptake of [³H] TdR into cells must be considered. Comparison of rates of DNA synthesis among different cell lines using [³H] TdR pulse labeling additionally may be complicated by such differential uptake of thymidine.

The same method of analysis of DNA replication employed in the present investigation was used to study the serum requirements for initiation of DNA replication in Rat-1 and Rat-1(RSV) cells [26]. The Rous sarcoma virus transforming function in Rat-1(RSV) cells was able to supplant a serum-dependent process in late G_1 which was necessary for the transformed Rat-1 cells to enter S and complete DNA replication. However, serum was necessary initially for both lines of cells to move toward the G_1/S boundary when a relative state of quiescence had been induced by serum deprivation.

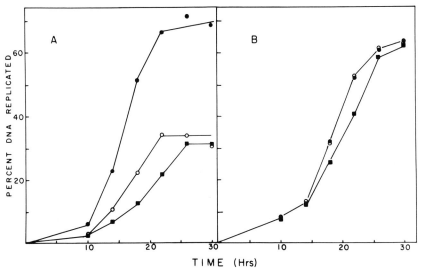

Fig. 4. Time course of DNA synthesis in quiescent Rat-1 and Rat-1(RSV) cells stimulated by a pulse of serum and followed by addition of TPA. Rat-1 cells (A) and Rat-1(RSV) cells (B) were prelabeled in [¹⁴C] thymidine for 48 h and serum-deprived for 54 h, as described in Figure 1. At that time (t = 0), medium containing 20% serum, BrdUrd, and FdUrd was added to all plates. At t = 4, the medium was removed, and plates were filled with fresh serum-free medium containing BrdUrd, FdUrd, and 0.1% dimethyl sulfoxide (○) or with the latter solution containing 1 μg/ml phorbol (■) or TPA (●). The TPA concentration was 500 ng/ml in dishes containing Rat-1 cells (A) and 100 ng/ml in dishes containing Rat-1(RSV) cells (B). Percentage DNA replicated was determined by CsCl density gradient analysis of samples at t = 10, 14, 18, 22, 26, and 30 h.

In serum-free medium, TPA caused a small dose-dependent increase in the rate of DNA synthesis in serum-deprived Rat-1 and Rat-1(RSV) cells.

In contrast, O'Brien and Diamond [14] reported that TPA, when added to confluent quiescent cultures of normal or transformed hamster embryo cells, neither produced an increase in cell number nor in the percentage of [3H] TdR-labeled nuclei, and did not stimulate the incorporation of [3H] TdR. A delay in the onset of DNA synthesis was observed in TPA treated Rat-1(RSV) cells but not in Rat-1 cells. A similar observation was made by Fusenig and Samsel [28], who found that optimal concentrations of TPA in mouse dermal fibroblasts caused an initial short-term inhibition of DNA synthesis followed by stimulation, with a maximum at 24 h after addition, as measured by [3H] TdR incorporation and labeling indices.

In the untransformed Rat-1 cells, the only conditions which led to significant TPA stimulation were those in which addition of TPA was temporally associated with a brief exposure (1 h) to serum. One explanation of the necessary time coincidence of treatment for a co-inducing effect is that TPA could induce sensitization to serum growth factors which might remain associated with the cell after the shift to serum-free medium. In contrast, TPA was unable to stimulate if its addition was delayed until 4 h after the end of the serum pulse. In the above system, DNA replication normally begins at 14 h after serum

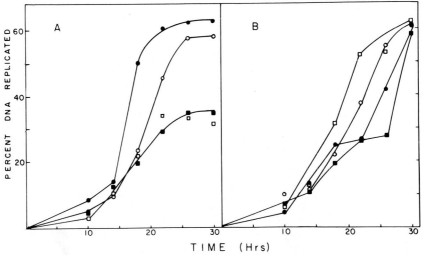

Fig. 5. Time course of DNA synthesis in quiescent Rat-1 and Rat-1(RSV) cells stimulated by a pulse of serum and a 1-h treatment with TPA before or after the serum pulse. Rat-1 cells (A) and Rat-1(RSV) cells (B) were prelabeled in [14C] thymidine for 48 h and serum-deprived for 54 h, as described in Figure 1. For one set of cultures, at 53 h of serum deprivation (t = −1) the medium was changed for fresh serum-free medium containing TPA for 1 h (○). At the end of 1 h, the medium was removed and cultures were stimulated with fresh 20% serum-containing medium containing BrdUrd and FdUrd for 4 h (t = 0 to t = 4). At t = 4, the serum-containing medium was removed and exchanged for an identical medium lacking serum. Experimental groups were stimulated by TPA for 1 h at different times. For each panel, one set of cultures was stimulated with TPA for 1 h prior to addition of serum (t = −1 to t = 0, ○). One set of cultures was stimulated with TPA for 1 h immediately after removal of the serum-containing medium (t = 4 to t = 5, ●). One set of cultures was stimulated with TPA for 1 h from t = 8 to t = 9 (■). One set of cultures was not stimulated at any time by TPA (□). For cultures receiving TPA, the medium contained BrdUrd, FdUrd, and either 500 ng/ml (Rat-1 cells, panel A) or 100 ng/ml (Rat-1(RSV) cells, panel B) TPA in 0.1% dimethyl sulfoxide. Percentage DNA replicated was determined by CsCl density gradient analysis of samples at t = 10, 14, 18, 22, 26, and 30 h.

stimulation [26]. Therefore, the stimulatory effects of TPA on cellular events in the Rat-1 cells do not occur within 6 h prior to the onset of DNA synthesis.

The inhibitory effects of TPA are temporally distinct from the stimulatory effects in the untransformed Rat-1 cells. TPA will inhibit only if present prior to, but not after, serum exposure. Furthermore, the inhibitory actions of TPA affect only the time of onset of DNA synthesis but not the extent. When added before a 4-h serum pulse, therefore, TPA both delays the onset and increases the amount of DNA replicated in the cultures. We therefore suggest that TPA acts on two distinct cellular regulatory mechanisms in the G_1 phase of the cell cycle of untransformed Rat-1 cells.

The RSV-transformed Rat-1 cells were not responsive to the DNA-stimulating effects of TPA with serum, but in serum-free medium a slight stimulation of DNA synthesis was seen when TPA was added to quiescent cultures. Therefore, it appears that RSV-transformed Rat-1 cells are refractory to the DNA-stimulating effects of TPA but do respond to the retardation of DNA synthesis induced by TPA. The mechanisms of DNA synthesis delay in the Rat-1 and Rat-1(RSV) cells may differ, since TPA is most effective in delaying the onset of DNA synthesis when added before serum stimulation in the Rat-1 cells and just before the onset of DNA synthesis in the Rat-1(RSV) cells.

It was of interest to discover that the parent alcohol phorbol, which is inactive as a tumor promotor and comitogen in other systems [21], caused a delay in the onset of serum-induced DNA synthesis in both untransformed and RSV-transformed Rat-1 cells. The possibility exists that in experiments utilizing TPA, the active inhibitor of DNA synthesis is phorbol, which is either present as a contaminant or is produced through metabolism of TPA. Experiments currently are in progress to test these possibilities.

How TPA and other tumor promotors are able to promote the appearance of neoplasms in initiated cells is unknown. It is significant that the two-stage mechanism of carcinogenesis has been demonstrated in cultured cells as well as in animal models. Using cultured 10 $T_{1/2}$ mouse cells, Peterson et al [11] found that TPA treatment of log-phase cells induced a transient inhibition of [^{3}H]TdR incorporation. Since phorbol did not produce these effects, the authors suggested that the inhibition of DNA synthesis was associated with the process of promotion. Although the results of the present investigation do not address the question of tumor promotion per se, the different TPA-induced responses of normal and RSV-transformed cells may help clarify the role of induced DNA synthesis in the conversion of initiated cells to malignantly transformed cells.

ACKNOWLEDGMENTS

This work was supported in part by grants by the US Public Health Service (CA-18273, CA-20913).

The technical assistance of Chris Fennie and Herb Wagner is gratefully acknowledged.

REFERENCES

1. Berenblum I: Cancer Res 1:44, 1942.
2. Boutwell RK: Prog Exp Tumor Res 4:207, 1964.
3. Boutwell RK: CRC Crit Rev Toxicol 2:419, 1974.
4. Mottram JC: J Pathol Bacteriol 56:181, 1944.
5. Hicks RM, Wakefield JStJ, Chowaniec J: J Chem Biol Interact 11:225, 1975.
6. Peraino C, Fry RJM, Staffeldt E, Kisieleski WE: Cancer Res 33:2201, 1973.
7. Wigler M, Weinstein IB: Nature 259:232, 1976.

8. Colburn NH, Vorder Bruegge WF, Bates JR, Gray RH, Rossen JD, Kelsey WH, Shimada T: Cancer Res 38:624, 1978.
9. Mondal S, Brankow DW, Heidelberger C: Cancer Res 36:2254, 1976.
10. Mondal S, Heidelberger C: Nature 260:710, 1976.
11. Peterson AR, Mondal S, Brankow DW, Thon W, Heidelberger C: Cancer Res 37:3223, 1977.
12. Steele VE, Marchok AC, Nettesheim P: In: Slaga TJ, Sivak A, Boutwell RD (eds): "Carcinogenesis," Vol. 2: "Mechanisms of Tumor Promotion and Cocarcinogenesis." New York: Raven Press, 1978.
13. Hecker E: Naturwissenschaften 54:282, 1967.
14. O'Brien TG, Diamond L: Cancer Res 37:3895, 1977.
15. Yuspa SH, Lichti U, Ben T, Patterson E, Hennings H, Slaga T, Colburn N, Kelsey W: Nature 262:402, 1976.
16. Lee LS, Weinstein IB: Science 202:313, 1978.
17. Brown ND, Dicker P, Rozengurt E: Biochem Biophys Res Commun 86:1037, 1979.
18. Blumberg PM, Driedger, Rossow PW: Nature 264:446, 1976.
19. Boynton AC, Whitfield JF, Isaacs RJ: J Cell Physiol 81:25, 1975.
20. Yuspa SH, Ben T, Patterson E, Michael D, Elgjo K, Hennings H: Cancer Res 36:4062, 1976.
21. Baird WM, Sedgewick JA, Boutwell RK: Cancer Res 31:1434, 1971.
22. Lowe M, Pacifici M, Holtzer H: Cancer Res 38:2350, 1978.
23. Mastro AM, Mueller GC: Exp Cell Res 88:40, 1974.
24. Prasad I, Zouzias D, Basilico CJ: Virology 18:436, 1976.
25. Meyn RE, Hewitt RR, Humphrey RM: Exp Cell Res 82:137, 1973.
26. Magun BE, Thompson RL, Gerner EW: J Cellular Physiol (In press).
27. Gerner EW: Radiat Res 71:387, 1977.
28. Fusenig N, Samsel W: In: Slaga TJ, Sivak A, Boutwell RD (eds): "Carcinogenesis," Vol. 2: "Mechanisms of Tumor Promotion and Cocarcinogenesis." New York: Raven Press, 1978, pp 203–220.

Journal of Supramolecular Structure 12:73–114 (1979)
Tumor Cell Surfaces and Malignancy 439–480

Structural and Functional Alterations in the Surface of Vascular Endothelial Cells Associated With the Formation of a Confluent Cell Monolayer and With the Withdrawal of Fibroblast Growth Factor

Israel Vlodavsky and Denis Gospodarowicz

Cancer Research Institute and the Department of Medicine, University of California Medical Center, San Francisco, California 94143

Vascular endothelial cells cultured in the presence of fibroblast growth factor (FGF) divide actively when seeded at low or clonal cell densities and upon reaching confluence adopt a morphologic appearance and differentiated properties similar to those of the vascular endothelium in vivo. In this review, we present some of our recent observations regarding the characteristics (both structural and functional) of these endothelial cells and the role of FGF in controlling their proliferation and normal differentiation. At confluence the endothelial cells form a monolayer of closely apposed and nondividing cells that have a nonthrombogenic apical surface and can no longer internalize bound ligands such as low-density lipoprotein (LDL). The adoption of these properties is correlated and possibly causally related to changes in the cell surface such as the appearance of a 60,000 molecular weight protein (CSP-60); the disappearance of fibronectin from the apical cell surface and its concomitant accumulation in the basal lamina; and a restriction of the lateral mobility of various cell surface receptor sites. In contrast, endothelial cells that are maintained in the absence of FGF undergo within three passages alterations that are incompatible with their in vivo morphologic appearance and physiologic behavior. They grow at confluence on top of each other and hence can no longer adopt both the structural (CSP-60, cell surface polarity) and functional (barrier function, nonthrombogenicity) attributes of differentiated endothelial cells. Since these characteristics can be reacquired in response to readdition of FGF, in addition to being a mitogen FGF may also be involved in controlling the differentiation and phenotypic expression of the vascular endothelium.

Key words: fibronectin, CSP-60, extracellular matrix, thrombogenic properties, low-density lipoprotein, receptor redistribution, asymmetry of cell surfaces, cell morphology, spatial configuration

Endothelial cells constitute the inner lining (intima) of the blood vascular system and play an active role in normal hemostasis. They function as a selective permeability barrier, actively participate in the metabolism of vasoactive substances, and have a nonthrombogenic surface exposed to the bloodstream [1–6]. Abnormalities of the endothelial cell structure

Received April 10, 1979; July 21, 1979.

0091-7419/79/1201-0073$06.80 © 1979 Alan R. Liss, Inc.

and function are therefore prominent in the pathology of a number of blood vessel diseases leading to thrombus formation or to the development of an atherosclerotic plaque. The elucidation of the factors involved in endothelial cell survival, continuity, and differentiation can be best studied using the tissue culture approach. This may shed light on characteristics that enable the endothelial layer to function as an effective permeability barrier, to resist high pressure and sheer forces, and to form a nonthrombogenic surface.

A number of laboratories [4–7] are now routinely maintaining vascular endothelial cells in culture, the only limitation being a short life-span (20–40 generations) and a requirement for a low (up to 1:8) split ratio. In contrast, the use of fibroblast growth factor (FGF) has led us to establish in culture a variety of *cloned* endothelial cell lines derived from vascular territories as diverse as fetal, neonatal, and adult vein, arteries, and heart [8, 9]. These cell lines divide with a high mitotic index when maintained at low or clonal cell densities and when they are confluent, they exhibit the morphologic and metabolic characteristics of vascular endothelial cells in vivo as expressed by the preservation of their shape and spatial organizations, non-thrombogenic apical surface, and ability to produce a basement membrane, as well as by other structural and functional properties which we are presenting here. These cell lines are indistinguishable from their in vivo counterparts in their karyotype, even after being passaged in vitro for 400 generations [1–3].

The endothelial apical surface, being located at the interface between blood and tissue, is expected to fulfill a major role in various differentiated functions of the vascular endothelium (permeability barrier, nonthrombogenicity) and could therefore differ from the basal cell surface, which functions in the production of a basement membrane to which the endothelium is firmly attached [1–3, 5, 10]. Therefore, following the interaction between cells that leads to the adoption of a monolayer configuration one might expect a reorganization of proteins in the cell surface, some of whose synthesis is turned on while that of others is turned off. This will in turn lead to the asymmetric organization of the cell surface characteristic of the vascular endothelium. In the following study, we present our observations a) on changes in the structural organization of cell surface proteins (fibronectin, CSP-60) and in surface receptor (low-density lipoprotein [LDL], concanavalin A) redistribution associated with the formation of a confluent cell monolayer, and b) on cell surface changes (protein organization, surface asymmetry, platelet-binding capacity) associated with maintaining the endothelial cells in the absence of FGF. These observations are discussed in relation to the normal differentiation of the vascular endothelium and to the protective role of the endothelial layer against an uncontrolled uptake of LDL and thrombi formation. We wish to emphasize that we have not attempted to review the pioneering and important studies of other groups working with cultured endothelial cells. Instead, we have chosen to present some of our recent studies, in particular those dealing with changes in the endothelial cell surface, as well as our overall outlook regarding the use and role of FGF in establishing long-term cultures of vascular endothelial cells that adopt the morphologic appearance and differentiated properties of the vascular endothelium in vivo.

MATERIALS AND METHODS

Cells

Bovine endothelial and smooth muscle cells were obtained from the fetal heart and the aortic arches of adult animals [8, 9]. Bovine corneal endothelial cells were obtained from steer eyes [11]. Cells were cloned and cultured in Dulbecco's modified Eagle's medium (DMEM, Gibco, H-16), as previously described except that in some experiments a fibronectin-free serum, rather than regular calf serum, was used. For this purpose, the fibronectin present in serum was first adsorbed by affinity chromatography on gelatin-Sepharose as described [12]. Endothelial cells were passaged weekly at a 1:64 split ratio. Fibroblast growth factor (FGF, 100 ng/ml) was added every other day until the cells were nearly confluent. Similar results were obtained with confluent cultures that were continuously maintained with FGF (added every other day). Presence of factor VIII antigen and the adoption of a highly organized morphology of flattened and closely apposed cells at confluence have been constant features of all subcultures of the vascular endothelial cells [1–3, 8–10]. Cultures were used when sparse (178 cells/mm^2) or subconfluent (458 cells/mm^2), or 8–10 days after reaching confluence (713 cells/mm^2). FGF was purified, as previously described, from bovine pituitary glands [13] and bovine brains [14]. Both pituitary and brain FGF yield single bands in polyacrylamide disk gel electrophoresis at pH 4.5. Endothelial cells that were seeded in the absence of FGF and no longer maintained with FGF, lost within three passages their unique morphologic organization at confluence, became considerably larger, and grew in multiple layers.

Iodination of Cell Surface Proteins

Radioiodination of cell monolayers catalyzed by lactoperoxidase-glucose oxidase was carried out in Dulbecco's phosphate-buffered saline (PBS) in the presence of ^{131}INa (Amersham), lactoperoxidase (Calbiochem), and glucose oxidase (Sigma) as described by Teng and Chen [15]. Iodinated cells were washed five times with Ca^{2+},Mg^{2+}-free PBS and lysed in buffer containing 15% glycerol, 2% sodium dodecyl sulfate (SDS), 75 mM Tris-HCl (pH 6.8), and 2 mM phenylmethylsulfonyl fluoride and 2 mM EDTA to inhibit proteolysis. To block free sulfhydryl groups [16], 1 mM N-ethylmaleimide and 1 mM iodoacetic acid were added. The cell lysates were then boiled for 2 min to denature nucleic acids and proteins. To reduce disulfide bonds, dithiothreitol (DTT) were added to a concentration of 0.1 M before the boiling step [16].

Polyacrylamide Gel Electrophoresis

Samples containing 50,000–100,000 protein-bound cpm were applied to exponential gradient polyacrylamide slab gels with a 3% stacking gel [17]. The standards used for molecular weight determinations were [^{35}S]methionine-labeled T$_4$ phage proteins. For analysis in two dimentions [18], appropriate individual lanes were cut out of the first-dimension slab gel, and each lane was placed on top of a second slab gel and sealed in place with 0.1% (w/v) agarose in electrophoresis buffer. For reduction prior to the second dimension, the agarose contained 5%-mercaptoethanol. After electrophoresis, the slab gels were fixed in 7% (w/v) acetic acid, dried onto filter paper, and subjected to autoradiography on Kodak NS-2T X-ray film for 8–24 h.

Metabolic Labeling and Immunoprecipitation of Fibronectin

Sparse and confluent cultures were labeled with [^{35}S]methionine (20 h, 65 μCi/ml) in DMEM containing 0.5% calf serum and 10^{-5} M L-methionine. The tissue culture medium was then collected, the cell layer was washed, and both were analyzed by SDS polyacrylamide gel electrophoresis (PAGE) before or after immunoprecipitation with antifibronectin antiserum. For this purpose, cells were extracted with Tris-buffered saline (pH 8.0) containing 0.1% SDS, 0.5% Triton X-100, and 1 mM phenylmethylsulfonyl fluoride (PMSF).

Insoluble material was removed by centrifugation of the medium and cell extract at 15,000g for 15 min at 4°C. Rabbit anti-bovine plasma fibronectin antiserum or non-immune rabbit serum (10 μl) was added to 0.25 ml cell extract or to 1 ml of growth medium and after incubation for 2 h at 37°C the antigen-antibody complexes were precipitated by addition of 10 μl of goat anti-rabbit IgG antiserum (1 h at 37°C followed by 16 h at 4°C). The immunoprecipitates were washed and collected by centrifugation as described [19], dissolved in a sample buffer, and analyzed by SDS polyacrylamide slab gel electrophoresis either before or after reduction with dithiothreitol as described above.

Indirect Immunofluorescence Staining

Cells were grown on 12-mm glass coverslips in DMEM supplemented with 10% calf serum first depleted of its fibronectin content. At various times in culture, the coverslips were washed with DMEM containing 0.5% bovine serum albumin, fixed for 5 min with 10% formaldehyde in PBS, and washed extensively with PBS. They were then incubated for 30 min with a 1:40 dilution in the same medium of rabbit anti-bovine fibronectin antiserum, generously provided by Dr. C. R. Birdwell (Scripps Research Clinic, La Jolla, California). This antiserum gave by immunoelectrophoresis one precipitin line against whole bovine plasma or serum and cross-reacted with fibronectin from several species [20]. After three 15-min washes in PBS, the coverslips were incubated for 30 min at room temperature with a 1:20 dilution of fluorescein isothiocyanate-conjugated (FITC-conjugated) goat anti-rabbit IgG (Meloy Co., Virginia) in the same medium. Cultures were rinsed six times in PBS and once in distilled water and mounted for microscopy in buffered glycerol. In all cases where positive fluorescence was observed, the specificity of the staining was determined by control coverslips in which nonimmune rabbit serum was used in place of the anti-bovine plasma fibronectin antiserum. Under these conditions, little or no fluorescence could be observed. Cultures were also extracted with 0.5% Triton X-100 in PBS (5 min at room temperature with gentle shaking) to remove the cell monolayer and expose the extracellular matrix remaining on the coverslip. The coverslips were then subjected to indirect immunofluorescence as described above.

Staining With fl-Anti LDL

All experiments were initiated after cells had been incubated for 48 h in DMEM supplemented with lipoprotein-deficient serum (LPDS). Cell cultures were incubated for 1 h at 37°C with human LDL (50–100 μg/ml), chilled, and washed briefly eight times at 4°C with phosphate-buffered saline (pH 7.4) containing 0.2% bovine serum albumin. Each culture was then incubated (1 h, 4°C) with a 1:30 dilution of fluorescein isothiocyanate-conjugated IgG fraction of rabbit anti-human LDL serum (fl-Anti LDL, Research Plus Co.) and washed eight times at 4°C. Incubations of cells at 4°C and 37°C were in DMEM containing LPDS (2.5 mg/ml), except that at 4°C the bicarbonate was replaced by 10 mM Hepes (pH 7.4). Coverslip cultures were then fixed (30 min, 22°C) with 3.7% formaldehyde in PBS and mounted for microscopy in buffered glycerol. To study the distribution of fl-Anti LDL in a single cell suspension, cells in monolayer were incubated with LDL and fl-Anti LDL as described, dissociated (2–3 min, 37°C) with a 0.03% EDTA solution, and then either fixed or immediately examined by phase contrast and fluorescence microscopy. In some experiments, fl-Anti LDL Fab fragments rather than intact IgG anti-LDL antibodies were used. Exposure of cells at 4°C to fl-Anti LDL, in the absence of an initial exposure to LDL, failed, under the indicated conditions, to stain the cells or gave at most a very slight uniform background of fluorescence. Because intact cells exclude antibody molecules, staining of chilled cells with fluorescein-conjugated anti-LDL rather than with fluorescein coupled directly to LDL permits the selective visualization of the LDL bound to the cell surface.

In order to improve the sensitivity of the immunofluorescence staining, cell monolayers in some experiments were incubated first with LDL, then with a 1:40 dilution of rabbit anti-human LDL antiserum, and finally with fluorescein-conjugated goat anti-rabbit IgG. This procedure also heightened, especially in sparse cultures, the background of fluorescence caused by staining of LDL particles nonspecifically adsorbed to the coverslip.

Cells were incubated, under all conditions, with LDL or with fl-Anti LDL when attached to the tissue culture dish. Washings were performed at 4°C. This allowed rapid washing of the cells and greatly reduced the dissociation and internalization of the bound LDL that occurs in cells that are washed free of unbound molecules.

Staining With fl-Con A

Coverslip cultures or EDTA-dissociated cells in suspension were washed twice in PBS containing 1 mM glucose and incubated (15 min, 37°C) in the same medium with fluorescein isothiocyanate-conjugated Con A (fl-Con A, Yeda Research and Development Co., Rehovoth, Israel) at 50 μg/ml. Coverslips were then washed briefly five times, fixed (3.7% formaldehyde, 30 min, 24°C), and mounted for microscopy in buffered glycerol. Cells in suspension were washed twice (4 min X 300g) and scored for their fluorescence staining pattern either before or after fixation with formaldehyde. Staining was inhibited completely by exposing the cells to fl-Con A in the presence of 0.05 Mα-methyl-D-mannoside.

In order to avoid detection of Con A molecules which are taken into the cells, cells were also incubated with native rather than fluorescein-conjugated Con A, followed by fixation (3.7% formaldehyde, 15 mm, 24°C) and exposure to a 1:15 dilution of fl-anti-Con A (Cappel Laboratories). Fluorescence was observed with a Leitz orthoplan fluorescence microscope under epi-illumination and a planar 63/1.4 oil objective. Photographs were taken on Kodak Tri-X film using a Leitz orthomat camera.

Lipoproteins

Human LDL (1.019 density 1.063 g/cm^3) and human lipoprotein-deficient serum (density 1.21 g/cm^3) were obtained from plasma by differential ultracentrifugation [21]. Chemical modification of LDL with N,N-dimethyl-1,3-propanediamine (DMPA) was performed with ethyl-3,3-dimethylaminopropyl carbodiimide (Sigma) as described [22]. Cationized LDL was optically clear and, when compared to native LDL by electrophoresis in agarose (pH 8.6), remained in the sample well, while the native LDL migrated toward the anode, as previously reported [22]. Cationized LDL gave a precipitin line with anti-human LDL antiserum. Native and cationized LDL were iodinated using a modification of the iodine monochloride method [23] as described [24–26].

Biochemical Assays

Measurements of surface-bound (heparin-releasable) [125] I-LDL as well as internalization and degradation of [125] I-LDL by endothelial and smooth muscle cells were carried out as previously described [24–27]. Incorporation of (1-^{14}C)-acetate and (^{3}H)-oleate into free cholesterol and cholesteryl esters, respectively, was determined after extraction of the cellular lipids by thin-layer chromatography, as described [26].

RESULTS

Surface Changes Associated With the Formation of a Confluent Cell Monolayer

Immunofluorescence and metabolic labeling studies have demonstrated that in vascular endothelial cell cultures, depending on the cell density, large quantities of fibronectin can be found in the tissue culture medium, the plasma membrane of the cells, or the extracellular matrix [1–3]. Since fibronectin has been shown to be involved in cell-cell interaction and cell-substrate adhesion, we have looked for changes in its localization and surface distribution as a function of the cell density and spatial organization.

For these experiments, cells were cultured in the presence of serum that was first depleted in its fibronectin content [12, 20] to avoid detection of fibronectin derived from the calf serum. The importance of cell-cell contacts as a signal for the appearance of fibronectin was reflected by its apparent absence on endothelial cells that are not yet in contact (Fig. 1A) and its presence on cells that contact each other (Fig. 1B). In sparse and subconfluent cultures, thin fibers of fibronectin were seen along the apical cell surface as well as in the areas of cell-cell contacts (Fig. 1B). In subconfluent and not yet organized cultures the fibronectin was localized mainly in areas restricted to cell-cell contact and tended to disappear from the apical cell surfaces. Finally, little or almost no fibronectin was observed late at confluence, after the cells had adopted a closely apposed and tightly packed monolayer configuration (Fig. 1C). Occasionally, with careful focusing, the presence of scattered areas of fluorescence could be observed, and this was in most cases related to areas where the cells retracted and the extracellular matrix became exposed.

Fibronectin is a major component of the extracellular matrix produced by a variety of cell types both in vivo and in vitro [28]. Since fibronectin is resistant to treatment with low concentrations of nonionic detergents, its presence and organziation in the basal lamina can be demonstrated after the cell layer is removed with Triton X-100. Figure ID shows the immunofluorescence staining pattern of fibronectin in the extracellular matrix left on the tissue culture dish after removing a 4-week-old, confluent endothelial cell monolayer. The fibronectin is located in fibrillar structures distributed in correspondance to the organization of the matrix. Radioiodination (lactoperoxidase/glucose oxidase) of the extracellular matrix followed by SDS slab gel electrophoresis revealed (Fig. 2A) that the fibronectin identified by double immunoprecipitation (Fig. 2B) is the major component of the endothelial basal lamina and is extensively disulfide-bonded into dimers and larger aggregates that hardly penetrates the running gels. Reduction with DTT greatly decreased the amounts of these high-molecular-weight complexes and yielded a major band that comigrated with a fibronectin monomer (Fig. 2F). Sparse and subconfluent cultures deposited little or no extracellular material onto the tissue culture dish. These results demonstrate that concomitant with the formation of a confluent vascular endothelial cell monolayer, fibronectin is no longer found on the apical cell surfaces but rather becomes a major component of the extracellular matrix and forms a meshwork of disulfide-bonded fibrils that are closely associated with the basal cell surface. Endothelial cells therefore differ from fibroblasts [28] and smooth muscle cells [29], where the fibronectin not only appears underneath the cells but is also found over the entire cell surface regardless of the degree of confluence. This unique polarity in the production of fibronectin by the confluent vascular endothelium could be indirectly related to the nonthrombogenic properties of the vascular endothelium and reflect a rearrangement of cell surface proteins as cells become confluent and stop dividing.

The production of fibronectin by confluent endothelial cells was further studied by

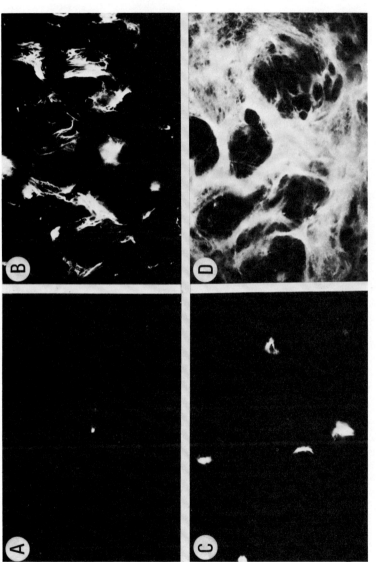

Fig. 1. Indirect immunofluorescence localization of fibronectin in vascular endothelial cell cultures. A) Staining of cells prior to the formation of cell-cell contacts shows the absence of fibronectin. B) Staining of a subconfluent culture showing the distribution of fibronectin on the apical cell surface and preferentially in the areas of contact between cells. C) Staining of a 4-week-old confluent culture with little or no detectable fluorescence. D) Staining of the extracellular matrix left after removal of the confluent cell layer with Triton X-100 (0.5%, 5 min at 37°C). All photomicrographs were at × 400.

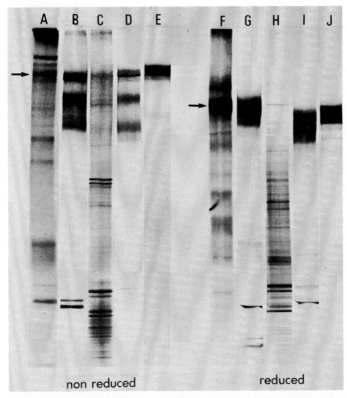

Fig. 2. SDS polyacrylamide gel electrophoresis of the extracellular matrix produced by a confluent vascular endothelial cell monolayer. Vascular endothelial cells maintained in culture for 2 weeks after reaching confluence were treated with 0.5% Triton X-100 to remove the cell layer, and the extracellular matrix thus exposed was then iodinated with iodine 131 and lactoperoxidase. Alternatively, the culture was first incubated with [35S]methionine (65 μCi/ml, 20 h), the medium was collected, and the cell layer was removed with Triton X-100 to expose the underlying basement membrane. The labeled basement membranes were either dissolved in a sample buffer (lanes A, F) or subjected to a double immunoprecipitation with antifibronectin (lanes B, G, and D, I) (rabbit anti-bovine plasma fibronectin followed by goat anti-rabbit IgG, as described under Materials and Methods). Samples were analyzed by a gradient (4.5–16%) polyacrylamide gel electrophoresis either before (lanes A–E) or after (lanes F–J) reduction with 0.1 M DTT. A,F) ^{131}I-labeled vascular endothelial basement membrane. Total extract in 2% SDS (sample buffer). B,G) ^{131}I-labeled basement membrane extracted with 0.5% Triton X-100 and 0.1% SDS and subjected to a double immunoprecipitation with antifibronectin. C,H) [35S]-methionine-labeled vascular endothelial basement membrane. Total extract prior to immunoprecipitation. D,I) [35S]methionine-labeled basement membrane after a double immunoprecipitation with antifibronectin. E,J) [35S]methionine-labeled growth medium precipitated by antifibronectin. Arrows mark the positions of fibronectin dimers (460K, nonreduced samples) and monomers (230K, reduced samples). Iodinated cultures were dissolved in electrophoresis sample buffer (2% SDS) (lanes A, F) to obtain the total protein iodination pattern or in Tris-buffered saline containing 0.1% SDS and 0.5% Triton X-100 (lanes B, G) to allow the immunoprecipitation reaction. In the latter case, insoluble material was first removed by centrifugation, and this may account for the lower amounts or absence of large fibronectin aggregates in the immunoprecipitates. [35S]methionine-labeled cultures were extracted only with the immunoprecipitation medium (0.1% SDS, 0.5% Triton X-100), and the samples were centrifuged before being applied for either gel electrophoresis or immunoprecipitation. Proteolytic degradation of fibronectin seemed to have taken place during the incubation required for immunoprecipitation (lanes B, G and D, I).

exposing cultures to [^{35}S] methionine 2 weeks after they had reached confluence. The newly synthesized fibronectin was then specifically precipitated by a double antibody technique from the growth medium (Fig. 2E, J), cell extract, and the extracellular matrix underlying the confluent cell monolayer (Fig. 2D, I). These experiments have shown that most of the fibronectin produced at a late stage of confluence no longer remains as a cellular component but is instead largely secreted into the tissue culture medium and, to a lesser extent, toward the basement membrane underlying the cell monolayer.

CSP-60 and the Formation of a Confluent Cell Monolayer

Cell surface components are involved in cell-cell interactions and have been shown to undergo structural changes in response to cell contacts [30, 31]. Since cultured vascular endothelial cells mimic their in vivo counterparts in their two-dimensional organization, asymmetry, and barrier function, these cells provide a system with which to study whether changes in the cell surface correlate with the ability of the endothelial cells to adopt at confluence the morphologic appearance of a highly organized monolayer composed of closely apposed and flattened cells. To study whether surface components are involved in the adoption of such a morphology and, if so, what these components are, we have looked for surface proteins that are affected by changes in the cell density or by dissociation and formation of cell-cell contacts. Density-dependent changes in the cell surface were studied by use of the lactoperoxidase catalyzed iodination to label in sparse, subconfluent, and confluent cultures the apical cell surface of vascular endothelial cells. The labeled proteins were analyzed by gel electrophoresis and their pattern was compared with that of such cell types as vascular aortic smooth muscle cells, which in contrast to the vascular endothelium grow at confluence in multilayers (Fig. 3). We also studied whether changes in the appearance of various surface proteins could be induced by disorganization and reorganization of a confluent endothelial cell monolayer (Figs. 4 and 5). Our results indicate a clear correlation between the formation of a highly organized endothelial cell monolayer and the appearance of a 60K molecular weight component which has been named CSP-60 [32]. This correlation is based on the following findings. a) Under various experimental conditions, the formation of a closely apposed and highly organized endothelial cell monolayer was associated with the appearance of CSP-60 as a major cell surface component susceptible to iodination by lactoperoxidase. This occurred under normal conditions, ie, as soon as the culture adopted the configuration of a confluent monolayer composed of tightly packed and cuboidal cells (Fig. 3A, E) or in reconstituted monolayers (Fig. 5B, C, F, G, K, L) derived from cultures that were first dissociated into single cells by urea (Fig. 4D), trypsin, or EDTA. b) In the various cultures studied thus far, CSP-60 was not detected when cells were sparse (Fig. 3B, F and Fig. 5D, H, M) or when no contact between the cells existed (Fig. 5E, J). Likewise, CSP-60 was not present at a subconfluent density (Fig. 6B), when cells contacted each other but were still elongated, overlapped each other, and were not yet organized in a tightly packed cuboidal manner (Fig. 4B). c) Cells which grow in multiple layers at confluence (ie, smooth muscle cells) contained no CSP-60 even after being maintained at confluence for an extended period of time (Fig. 3C, G). d) CSP-60 was not present in a disorganized cell monolayer (Fig. 5E, J) or up to 72 h after reseeding the confluent cells at a low density, nor could it be found in sparse cells that were pooled and reseeded at a high density (Fig. 6D) to yield a confluent but unorganized endothelial culture (Fig. 4H).

After disruption of an already formed cell monolayer, both the appearance of CSP-60 and the adoption of a monolayer configuration required a short time (2—5 h). In comparison,

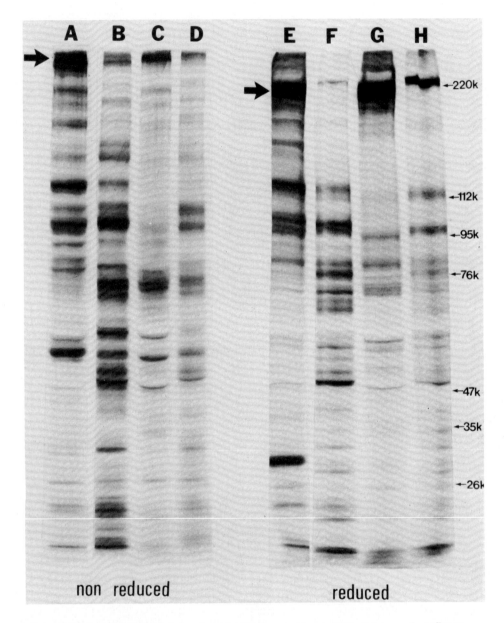

Fig. 3. SDS-polyacrylamide gel electrophoresis of lactoperoxidase-iodinated sparse and confluent cultures of vascular endothelial and smooth muscle cells. Washed cells were radioiodinated, lysed, and analyzed by a gradient (6.5–15%) PAGE either before (lanes A–D) or after (lanes E–H) reduction with 0.1 M DTT. A,E) Confluent monolayers of bovine aortic endothelial cells. B,F) Sparse culture of bovine aortic endothelial cells. C,G) Confluent culture of bovine aortic smooth muscle cells. D,H) Sparse culture of bovine aortic smooth muscle cells. Gels were standardized with T_4 phage [^{35}S] methionine-labeled proteins, and arrows mark the positions of fibronectin and CSP-60.

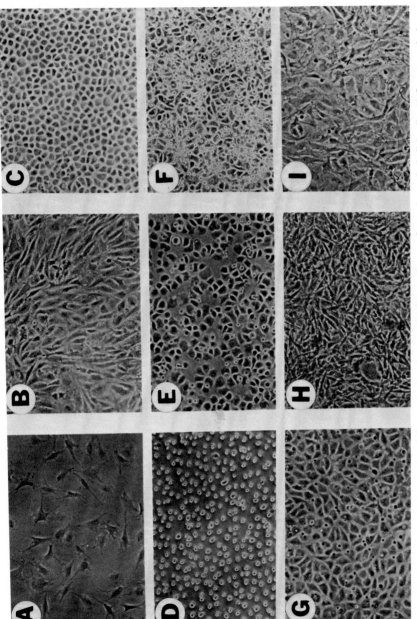

Fig. 4. Phase contrast micrographs of disorganized and reorganized monolayers of vascular endothelial cells. A) Sparse, actively growing culture, two days after seeding. B) Subconfluent culture 5 days after seeding. C) A confluent cell monolayer, 7 days after reaching confluence. D) A confluent cell monolayer treated with urea (1 M in DME, 1 h, 37°C). E) Urea-treated cells at an intermediate stage of reorganization, 1 h after washing the urea out and incubating the culture under growth conditions. F) Urea-treated cells seeded at high density and observed after 5 h. The excess of cells remain round, and do not adhere or grow on top of the attached cells. G) Urea-treated cells seeded at a high cell density and observed 24 h later after washing the excess of cells. H) Cells from a sparse culture that were pooled together, reseeded at a high density, and observed 48 h later. A similar morphology was adopted by the cultures described under E,F,G, and H when calf serum free of fibronectin, rather than normal calf serum, was used. I) Endothelial cells maintained for three passages in the absence of FGF.

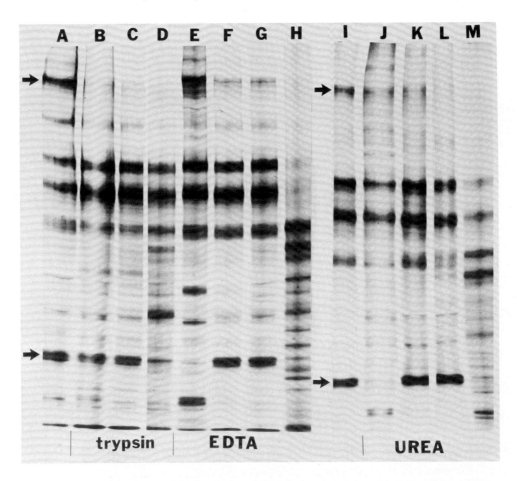

Fig. 5. Appearance of CSP-60 and fibronectin after disorganization and a subsequent reorganization of a confluent cell monolayer. Confluent endothelial monolayers were treated with either trypsin (0.05% Gibco, 3 min, 37°C), EDTA (0.03% in Ca^{2+}, Mg^{2+}-free PBS, 30 min, 37°C), or with urea (1 M in DME, 1 h, 37°C) to dissociate cell-to-cell contacts. The disruptive agent was then washed out and the cells were allowed to reorganize in DME containing a fibronectin-depleted serum on the same plate or reseeded at a high or low density. Disorganized and reorganized cultures were iodinated and analyzed by PAGE (a 6–16% gradient) after the samples were reduced with DTT. A) Confluent endothelial cell monolayer. B) Confluent culture that was first trypsinized into single cells and then washed and incubated in the same plate for 12 h under growth conditions to readopt its original monolayer configuration. C) Cells 12 h after trypsinization and seeding at a high density. The cells fully adopt a monolayer organization and show the presence of CSP-60, but little or no fibronectin. D) Cells 12 h after trypsinization and seeding at a low density. E) Confluent culture treated with EDTA and labeled when the cells detached from each other. CSP-60 is now only slightly or no longer exposed for iodination. F) Confluent culture that was first dissociated by EDTA and then incubated for 5 h under growth conditions to readopt its original morphology. G) Cells 12 h after EDTA dissociation and seeding at a high density. H) Cells 12 h after EDTA dissociation and seeding at a low density. I) Confluent cell monolayer. J) Confluent culture treated with urea and labeled when the cells appeared as single round spheres. K) Confluent culture that was first treated with urea and then allowed to reorganize by a 3-h incubation under growth conditions. L) Cells 24 h after exposure to urea and reseeding at a high density. M) Cells 24 h after treatment with urea and reseeding at a low density. Arrows mark the positions of fibronectin and CSP-60.

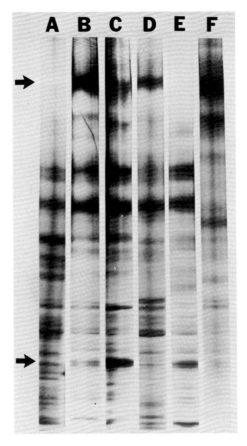

Fig. 6. Appearance of fibronectin and CSP-60 in organized and nonorganized cultures of endothelial cells. Endothelial cultures were labeled with ^{131}I and lactoperoxidase and samples applied onto a gradient (6–16%) polyacrylamide slab gel after reduction with 0.1 M DTT. A) Sparse, actively growing endothelial cells. B) Subconfluent endothelia culture. C) Confluent highly organized cell monolayer. CSP-60 appears as a major band; fibronectin is detected in small quantities compared to subconfluent cultures. D) Cells derived from sparse, actively growing cultures reseeded at a high density and iodinated 48 h later. E) Cells 12 h after trypsinization of a confluent monolayer and reseeding at a high density. F) A confluent but unorganized endothelial culture maintained for three passages in the absence of FGF. Large amounts of fibronectin and little or no CSP-60 can be detected. Arrows mark the positions of fibronectin and CSP-60.

no less than 72 h were required for actively growing cultures to acquire a similar morphology after reaching confluence. This result and the fact that 10^{-4} M cycloheximide did not prevent the reappearance of CSP-60 in a monolayer which was first disrupted and then allowed to reorganize suggest that in cells which have already reached the stage of a confluent monolayer CSP-60 is reexposed rather than resynthesized during the reorganization of the cells into a monolayer.

CSP-60 has been identified in confluent cell monolayers of all the vascular endothelial cell types studied so far, regardless of their origin or age of their donor (Fig. 7). These include endothelial cells from the bovine fetal (lanes C and c), calf (lanes G and g), and adult (lanes D and d) aortic arches; pig aortic arch (lanes B and b); fetal bovine heart (lanes E and e); bovine umbilical vein (lanes F and f); and bovine pulmonary artery (lanes A and a).

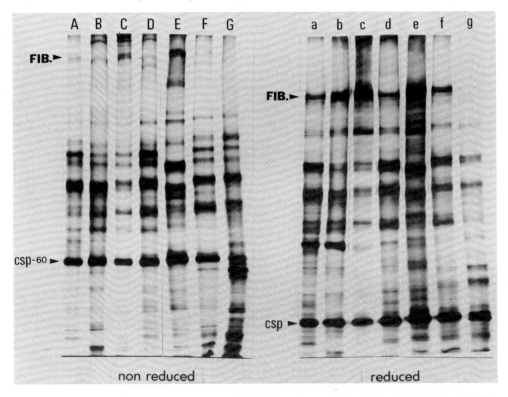

Fig. 7. Appearance of CSP-60 in various types of cultured vascular endothelial cells. Vascular endothelial cells of various origins were obtained, cloned, and maintained in culture as described [8, 9]. Confluent cell monolayers (5–7 days after reaching confluence) were radioiodinated (lactoperoxidase/glucose oxidase) and analyzed by a gradient (5–16%) PAGE before (lanes A–G) or after (lanes a–g) reduction with 0.1 M DTT. Vascular endothelial cells of the following origins were studied: A,a) Bovine pulmonary artery; B,b) adult pig aorta; C,c) fetal bovine aorta; D,d) adult bovine aorta; E,e) fetal bovine heart; F,f) bovine umbilical vein; and G,g) calf bovine aorta. Arrows mark the positions of fibronectin (460K and 230K) and CSP-60 (60K and 30K) before and after reduction of the samples with DTT, respectively.

In order further to characterize CSP-60, we have looked for its electrophoretic mobility before and after reduction with DTT. The results (Figs. 3, 7, and 8) indicate that nonreduced samples contained a 60K component that is characteristic of confluent endothelial cell monolayers and that, after reduction, was missing from its original position and yielded a major band of an apparent molecular weight of about 30K. The dimeric disulfide-bonded nature of CSP-60 was further demonstrated on two-dimensional gels, nonreduced in the first dimension and reduced in the second [18]. Samples derived from confluent vascular endothelial cell monolayers (Fig. 8B) revealed a major, off-diagonal spot that had an apparent molecular weight of about 30K and which, at the first, nonreduced dimension, migrated as a 60K component. Likewise, a similar off-diagonal spot was observed with corneal endothelial cells (Fig. 8E), which at confluence are as organized as vascular endothelial cells (1–3). There were either small amounts of or no such 30K components in samples derived from either sparse, actively growing endothelial cells (Fig. 8C) or from sparse and confluent (Fig. 8F) cultures of smooth muscle cells. Control gels, running either

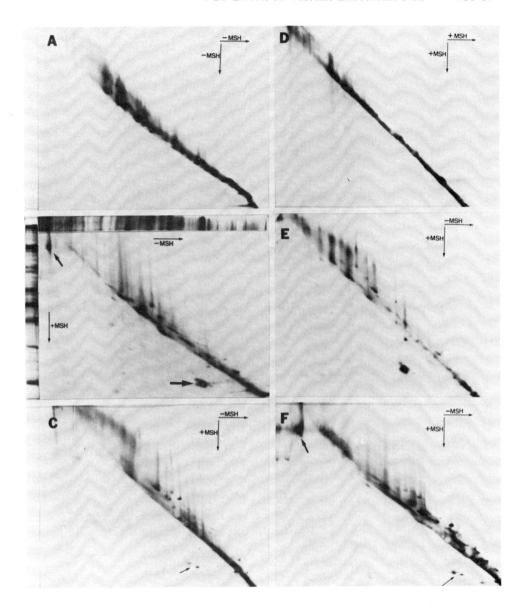

Fig. 8. Two-dimensional gel analysis of lactoperoxidase-iodinated cells. Cultures were iodinated and the cells lysed and harvested under nonreducing conditions. Aliquots were run on a gradient (6.5–16%) polyacrylamide slab gel, and the gel was cut into appropriate narrow strips that were each then placed at the top of another 6.5–16% slab gel. A reducing agent (5% MSH, 2-mercaptoethanol) was present, as shown. A,D) Confluent vascular endothelial cells. A) Both dimensions without reduction. D) Both dimensions with reduction. No off-diagonal spots are present. B) A confluent monolayer of vascular endothelial cells. Arrows mark the position of fibronectin (upper left) and CSP-60 (lower right). C) Sparse, actively growing vascular endothelial cells. Note the absence of fibronectin and CSP-60. E) A confluent corneal endothelial cell monolayer. CSP-60 appears as a major off-diagonal spot. Fibronectin is only slightly or not at all exposed to the lactoperoxidase-catalyzed iodination F) Confluent vascular smooth muscle cells. Note the absence of CSP-60 and the presence of fibronectin.

nonreduced or reduced in both directions, showed no such off-diagonal spots, proving that the appearance of the low-molecular-weight, off-diagonal spot was caused by the reduction step between the two stages of electrophoresis.

The results of these experiments have also demonstrated that fibronectin is not essential for the formation of a highly organized cell monolayer. This conclusion is based on the following observations: a) High amounts of fibronectin were detected in subconfluent but not yet organized endothelial cultures (Fig. 6B) as well as in sparse (Fig. 3D, H) and confluent (Fig. 3C, G) cultures of vascular smooth muscle cells that form multiple layers at confluence; b) Following dissociation of a highly organized vascular endothelial cell monolayer with EDTA, urea, or trypsin and upon removal of the disruptive agent, the cultures resumed their normal configuration within a 2- to 5-h incubation in a fibronectin-free medium despite the partial or nearly total removal of fibronectin from the cell surface (Fig. 5B, F, K). Likewise, when endothelial monolayers were trypsinized and the cells then seeded at a high density in a medium containing no fibronectin, the cultures resumed, within 5–12 h, their original morphology (Fig. 4F, G), despite the removal of fibronectin from the cell surface by trypsin (Fig. 5B, C).

These results indicate that CSP-60, rather than fibronectin, correlates with the formation of a confluent, highly organized cell monolayer, so that its exposure only in cells that adopt such a morphology might play an essential role in the control of contact response phenomena. CSP-60, however, was not required for substrate adhesion and flattening of cells, since it was missing from cells that adhered and spread perfectly well after first disrupting a confluent monolayer and seeding the cells at a low density (Fig. 5D, H, M). These results also suggest that in confluent cultures fibronectin serves mainly as a glue by which the cells are attached to their substratum, since, unlike CSP-60, which is only present as a surface protein, fibronectin is secreted in large quantities and is a major component of the basement membrane produced by endothelial cells.

Restriction of Surface Receptor Lateral Mobility: Relationship to a Protective Fuction of the Endothelium Against an Uncontrolled Uptake of LDL

In previous studies [24–26] we have demonstrated that, as in other cell types examined [33], actively growing vascular endothelial cells bind, internalize, and degrade LDL via a receptor-mediated pathwasy which regulates the synthesis of cholesterol, the formation of cholesterol esters, and the number of surface receptor sites for LDL [24–26]. In contrast, once the growing cells reach confluence and form a cell monolayer, they can no longer internalize the LDL and hence exhibit no lysosomal degradation and its associated regulatory biochemical responses, even though the cells bind the lipoprotein at high-affinity receptor sites [24–26]. This inhibition of internalization, but not of binding, of LDL is due to the formation of highly organized cell monolayer rather than to the inhibition of cell proliferation at confluence, since it was reversed by disrupting the cell monolayer under conditions which did not stimulate cell division [24, 25]. Furthermore, when incubated with cationized LDL rather than with native LDL, the confluent cell monolayers exhibited lysosomal degradation of the lipoprotein as well as the subsequent regulatory effects on cellular cholesterol metabolism, indicating no defect beyond the internalization step [26].

Receptor redistribution is involved in the internalization of various ligand-receptor complexes by various cell types [34–37]. It has also been shown that endocytosis is associated with a directional lateral movement of certain cell surface lectin receptors from their original random distribution into specific membrane regions [38]. These observations led us to postulate that in vascular endothelial cells, as opposed to fibroblasts and vascular smooth muscle cells [39], a certain degree of surface receptor lateral mobility is required for the internalization of LDL. If this were the case, it would be expected that surface receptor lateral mobility in confluent endothelial cell monolayers should be severely restricted in comparison to that of endothelial cells in sparse culture.

Using fluorescein-conjugated anti-LDL (fl-Anti LDL) and fluorescein-Con A (fl-Con A), we have examined the binding and distribution of LDL and Con A molecules in sparse and confluent cultures of aortic endothelial and smooth muscle cells. Our results demonstrate that both LDL receptor and Con A receptor mobility are indeed subject to regulation by changes in the density and organization of endothelial cell cultures. In contrast, vascular smooth muscle cells do not display such density-dependent membrane changes [40].

Cells attached to the tissue culture dish. A nonrandom, splotchy to minicap-like fluorescence pattern was observed in sparse, substratum-attached, endothelial cells that were first incubated with LDL at 37°C and then chilled, washed, and exposed at 4°C to either fl-Anti LDL (Fig. 9A) or to rabbit anti-human LDL followed by fl-anti-rabbit IgG (Fig. 9B). As shown in Table I, these cells also exhibited an active uptake and lysosomal degradation of LDL. In contrast, highly confluent cell monolayers that bind but no longer internalize or degrade LDL (Table I) showed a random, although aggregated, distribution of fluorescence over the entire cell surface under the same conditions (Fig. 9D). A similar randomly distributed staining pattern was obtained with sparse endothelial cells that were preincubated with LDL at 4°C, rather than at 37°C (Fig. 9C), or that were first fixed with formaldehyde to inhibit the internalization of LDL (not shown). These results demonstrate that in actively growing, but not in confluent endothelial cell monolayers the bound LDL molecules are capable of a temperature-dependent lateral movement in the membrane plane which allows them to form large aggregates. Smooth muscle cells, unlike endothelial cells, grow on top of each other at confluence and show a similar degree of LDL internalization and degradation when maintained at either low or high cell densities (Table I) [24–26]. Accordingly, the present experiments revealed no difference between sparse and confluent cultures of smooth muscle cells, which, at both densities, showed a highly aggregated but randomly distributed anti-LDL fluorescence staining after exposure to LDL at 37°C (Fig. 9E). In each of these experiments, cells were incubated with the fluorescent antibodies at 4°C and most of the fluorescence could be removed afterwards by incubation with pronase (3 μg/ml, 30 min, 37°C), thereby demonstrating the surface localization of the LDL molecules thus detected.

Results similar to those observed with LDL were obtained when both endothelial and smooth muscle cultures were exposed to fl-Con A. In sparse cultures of endothelial cells incubated (15–20 min, 37°C) with fl-Con A, the Con A binding sites were drawn into large aggregates to form a "nuclear cap" at the center of the cells (Fig. 9F, G), thereby indicating the occurrence of Con A internalization already within 15–20 min. No such perinuclear caps, but rather a uniform distribution of fluorescence over the entire cell surface, was obtained by fixing the cells before Con A coating (Fig. 9H). In contrast to sparse endo-thelial cultures, confluent cell monolayers showed a random, slightly aggregated but mostly peripheral fluorescence staining pattern over the entire cell surface area (Fig. 9I). Capping by Con A was not induced in smooth muscle cells, and as already observed with fl-Anti LDL, both sparse (Fig. 9J) and confluent cultures showed, under the same conditions, a random distribution of fl-Con A. Similar results (capping under sparse conditions and a uniform distribution at confluence) were obtained when native Con A molecules and fluorescein-conjugated anti-Con A antibodies were used instead of fl-Con A, except that little or no internalization of fluorescence was observed in the latter case.

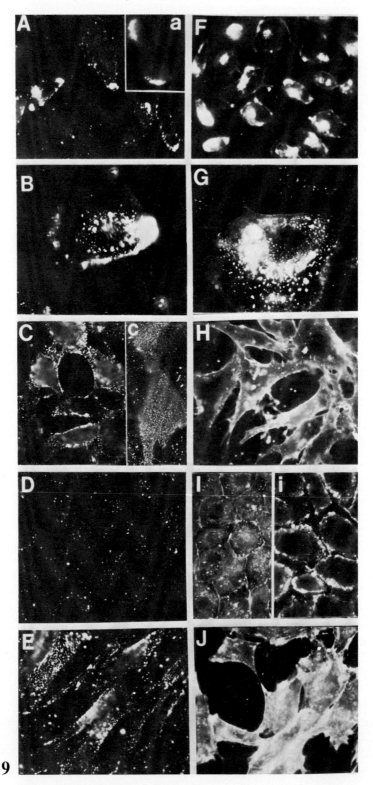

9

TABLE I. Expression of the LDL Pathway in Sparse and Confluent Cultures of Vascular Endothelial and Smooth Muscle Cells

	Endothelial cells		Smooth muscle cells	
	Sparse (84 μg protein per dish)	Confluent (270 μg protein per dish)	Sparse (119 μg protein per dish)	Confluent (407 μg protein per dish)
^{125}I-LDL binding (ng/mg protein)	128	60	91	69
^{125}I-LDL internalization (ng/mg protein)	1,233	113	546	436
^{125}I-LDL degradation (ng/mg protein/6 h)	2,754	68	2,317	1,566
[125]I-cationized LDL degradation (ng/mg protein/6 h)	3,651	1,687	1,849	1,490
Suppression of free cholesterol synthesis (96 inhibition)	73	10	89	90
Activation of cholesteryl ester formation (fold increase)	12.5	1	9	8

Data are mean values obtained from 3–5 experiments carried out under the following conditions. Sparse and confluent cultures of bovine aortic vascular endothelial and smooth muscle cells were preincubated for 48 h in growth medium containing LPDS (4 mg/ml), washed, and incubated for 2.5 h at 37°C with ^{125}I-LDL (50 μg/ml) to measure specific binding (accessible for heparin release) and internalization (heparin-resistant) of LDL [24, 27]. Cultures were also incubated (6 h, 37°C) with either native ^{125}I-LDL (20 μg/ml) or ^{125}I-cationized LDL (7.5 μg/ml) to determine the amounts of acid-soluble lipoprotein degradation products released into the medium [24, 26]. To study the regulation of cholesterol synthesis and esterification, cultures in LPDS medium were incubated (5 h and 12 h, respectively) with or without native LDL (100 μg/ml) and then with either (1-^{14}C)-acetate or (^{3}H)-oleate, respectively. Cells were then washed, harvested, and extracted to determine the content of labeled cholesterol and cholesteryl oleate as described [26].

Fig. 9. Cell surface distribution of LDL and Con A receptor sites in sparse and confluent vascular endothelial and smooth muscle cells attached to coverslips. Coverslip cultures of sparse and confluent bovine aortic endothelial and smooth muscle cells were labeled either with fl-Anti LDL or with anti-LDL and fl-anti-rabbit IgG, after first being incubated with LDL (A–E). Coverslips were also incubated directly with fl-Con A (F–J) and mounted for fluorescence microscopy as described under Materials and Methods.

A–E) Cell surface distribution of receptor sites for LDL. A,B) Sparse endothelial cultures exposed to LDL and then to fl-Anti LDL (A,a) or successively to LDL, rabbit anti-LDL, and fl-goat anti-rabbit IgG (B) as described. The LDL receptor sites are segregated into large aggregates (minicaps) located primarily in one pole of the cell. a) Cells that were rounded up during the incubations but still remained attached to the substrate. c) Sparse endothelial cells that were incubated with LDL at 4°C rather than at 37°C, washed, and stained with fl-Anti LDL at 4°C. A random distribution of fluorescence in small clusters. D) Highly confluent and contact-inhibited endothelial cells after preincubation with LDL at 37°C and with anti-LDL and fl-anti-IgG at 4°C. The LDL receptor sites are distributed in small clusters over the entire cell surface area. E) Sparse culture of smooth muscle cells treated with LDL, anti-LDL, and fl-anti-IgG as in D. A random, uniformly distributed LDL receptor cluster.

F–J) Cultures exposed to fl-Con A. F,G) Sparse culture of endothelial cells. Surface receptor sites for Con A are segregated into large patches and form perinuclear caps (F, G). H) Sparse endothelial culture fixed with formaldehyde (3.7%, 15 min, RT) before exposure to fl-Con A. A diffused fluorescence staining pattern over the entire cell surface area. I) A highly confluent and contact-inhibited monolayer of endothelial cells. A mostly peripheral, slightly aggregated, and random distribution of Con A receptor sites. i) Cells that contract during incubation and washing. J) Sparse culture of smooth muscle cells. Cells display a random, slightly clustered receptor distribution.

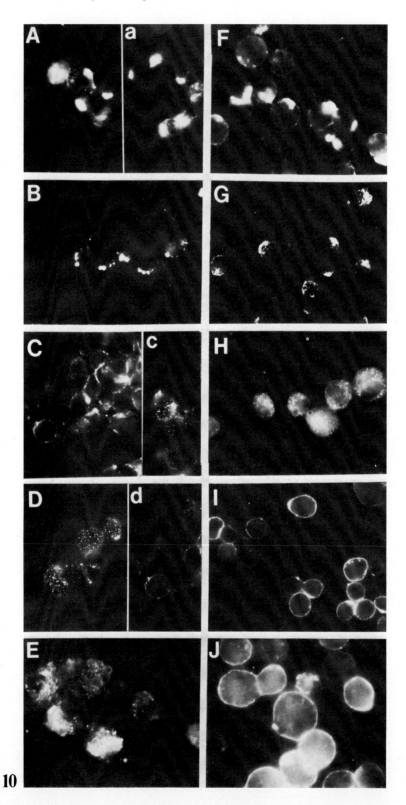

10

Single cells in suspension. The higher degree of receptor lateral mobility in sparse, as opposed to confluent, endothelial cell monolayers or to either sparse or confluent smooth muscle cell cultures was best demonstrated in suspension, after the cells had been released from the restriction imposed by their attachment to the substratum. Sparse endothelial cell cultures that were first incubated with LDL at 37°C and then exposed to fl-anti LDL at 4°C showed a high percentage (up to 70%) of cells with LDL capping when dissociated from their substrate with EDTA (Fig. 10A). Some of the cells showed minicaps or large aggregates similar to those observed with cells attached to a substratum (Fig. 10B). Small clusters randomly distributed over the entire cell surface area and no cap formation were observed in EDTA-dissociated, sparse endothelial cells that were dissociated with EDTA, fixed to prevent the internalization process, and then incubated in suspension with LDL and fl-anti LDL (Fig. 10C). A short (2–3 min) incubation at 37°C is required to dissociate the cell monolayers with EDTA into a single cell suspension. The possibility that the LDL capping observed in sparse endothelial cells could have been induced during the incubation with EDTA by a receptor cross-linking via the polyvalent anti-LDL molecules rather than by the initial incubation with the LDL particles themselves was tested by using fl-Anti LDL Fab fragments. These are monovalent and therefore incapable of receptor cross-linking and cap formation. Sparse endothelial cells that were exposed to LDL followed by incubation with either intact IgG anti-LDL or Fab fragment anti-LDL showed, after EDTA-dissociation, a similar percentage of cells with LDL capping, indicating that the LDL surface receptor sites were, in fact, redistributed in response to the initial incubation of the cells with LDL. In contrast to the results obtained with actively growing cells, cells from confluent endothelial monolayers that were similarly incubated with LDL and fl-Anti LDL showed, even in a single cell suspension, a clustered distribution of fluorescence but no caps (Fig. 10D). Suspensions of smooth muscle cells taken from either sparse or confluent cultures showed,

---

Fig. 10. Cell surface distribution of LDL and Con A receptor sites in EDTA-dissociated sparse and confluent vascular endothelial and smooth muscle cells.

A–E) Labeling with fl-Anti LDL. Cells attached to the tissue culture dish were incubated with LDL and fl-Anti LDL as described, dissociated with 0.03% EDTA solution, and spun; single cells in suspension were observed for their fluorescence staining pattern as described. A,B) represent cells from sparse endothelial cultures showing segregation of the LDL receptor sites into caps (A) or minicaps (B) in one pole of the cells. C) Sparse endothelial cells that were first dissociated with EDTA, fixed (3.7% formaldehyde, 15 min), and then incubated in suspension with LDL and fl-Anti LDL. A clustered but random distribution of fluorescence. D) Cells from a highly confluent and contact-inhibited monolayer of endothelial cells (the LDL receptor cites are randomly distributed in clusters over the entire cell surface area), focused on top (D) and at the cell periphery (d). E) Cells from a sparse culture of smooth muscle cells gave a highly aggregated but randomly distributed staining pattern.

F–J) Labeling with fl-Con A. EDTA-dissociated cells derived from sparse and confluent endothelial monolayers and from sparse cultures of smooth muscle cells were incubated with either fl-Con A or with native Con A followed by fl-anti-Con A, washed, and scored (single cells) for their fluorescence pattern as described. F,G) Sparse endothelial cells. In 70–80% of the cells the Con A receptor sites are segregated into large aggregates (G) or caps (F) at one pole of the cells. A similar percentage of Con A capping was obtained by using fl-anti-Con A rather than fl-Con A. H) Sparse endothelial cells that were fixed before exposure to fl-Con A. Cap formation by Con A is fully inhibited. I) Cells from a confluent endothelial monolayer incubated in suspension with Con A followed by fixation and incubation with fl-anti-Con A. A peripheral, ring-like distribution of Con A surface receptor sites. A slightly clustered distribution but no capping was obtained by a direct incubation with fl-Con A. J) Cells from a sparse culture of smooth muscle cells incubated as in (I). Receptors are slightly segregated and show no cap formation.

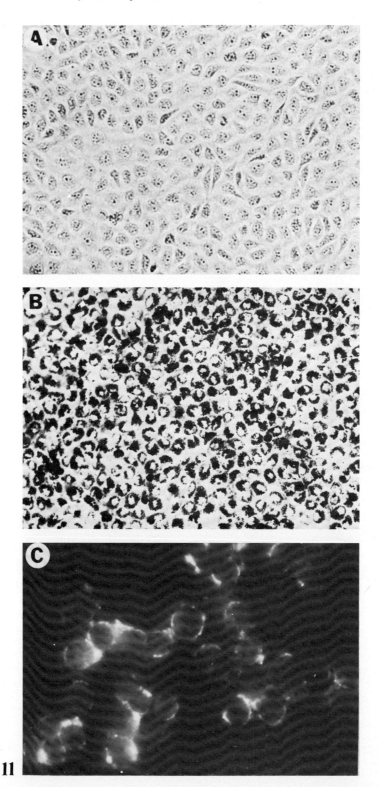

under the same conditions, an aggregated staining pattern distributed over the entire cell surface, and there was no induction of receptor capping (Fig. 10E).

Experiments with Con A- and EDTA-dissociated cells gave results similar to those obtained with fl-Anti LDL. Cap formation by Con A was induced in 60–80% of the cells from sparse, actively growing endothelial cell cultures (Fig. 10F, G), whereas cells from a confluent monolayer showed a uniform ring-like distribution of fl-Con A (Fig. 10I). Cap formation by Con A was prevented by formaldehyde fixation before coating with fl-Con A (Fig. 10H). Patching, but not capping, of Con A receptor sites was observed in EDTA-dissociated smooth muscle cells (Fig. 10J). Similar results (capping with sparse endothelial cells and a ring-like distribution at confluence) were obtained with cells that were incubated directly with fl-Con A or first with Con A and then fixed and incubated with fl-anti-Con A in order that only Con A molecules on the cell surface and not those which might have been taken into the cells would be detected. These results indicate that the formation of a confluent endothelial cell monolayer composed of closely apposed and nonoverlapping cells is associated with a restriction of the lateral mobility of both LDL and Con A cell surface receptor sites [40].

Interaction of endothelial cells with cationized LDL. Experiments with cultured human fibroblasts and smooth muscle cells [22, 33] have indicated that the highly regulated process of LDL uptake can be bypassed by incubating the cells with cationized LDL. These positively charged LDL molecules bind to nonspecific sites on the cell surface from which they are taken up and degraded through a mechanism that does not involve the physiologic LDL receptor sites. Unlike the receptor-mediated binding and internalization of native LDL, the uptake and lysosomal degradation of cationized LDL was not affected by the density and organization of the endothelial cell cultures (Table I). Thus, staining of confluent endothelial cell monolayers with Oil Red 0 revealed substantial intracellular accumulation of lipid droplets after exposure to cationized LDL (Fig. 11B), but not after incubation with native LDL (Fig. 11A). The confluent cells also showed an active lysosomal degradation of ^{125}I-cationized LDL (Table I). As shown in Fig. 11C, a ring-like distribution of fluorescence and little or no receptor capping was observed with confluent endothelial cell monolayers that were incubated with cationized LDL followed by fl-Anti LDL and EDTA-dissociation into a single cell suspension. Therefore, the uptake of cationized LDL by these cells did not correlate with, nor did it induce, capping of the appropriate nonspecific, negatively charged surface receptor sites.

Our results therefore demonstrate that in sparse endothelial cells which internalize LDL the LDL receptor sites can be segregated into large patches or caps. Similar results were obtained when the lectin Con A, rather than LDL, was used as a probe. In contrast, confluent endothelial cell monolayers that can no longer internalize the bound lipoprotein

---

Fig. 11. Oil Red 0 and fl-Anti LDL staining of confluent endothelial cells exposed to cationized LDL. A,B) Confluent monolayers of bovine aortic endothelial cells were exposed (48 h, 37°C) to either native LDL (600 μg/ml) or cationized LDL (15 μg/ml). The cell monolayers were then washed extensively, fixed, and stained with Oil Red 0 and hematoxylin. A) Cell exposed to native LDL. No accumulation of stained lipid droplets. B) Cells exposed to cationized LDL. Large numbers of Oil Red 0-positive inclusions. C) Surface distribution of the cell-bound cationized LDL molecules. Confluent endothelial monolayers were incubated (4 h, 37°C) with cationized LDL (10 μg/ml) and at 4°C with fl-Anti LDL and the fluorescence staining pattern determined after dissociation with EDTA as described under Materials and Methods. The cells display a ring-like distribution of fluorescence.

show no LDL- or Con A-induced receptor redistribution either before or after being released from their attachment to the substrate. These cells revealed at both 4°C and 37°C a clustered distribution of the LDL receptor sites, thereby showing a lack, or a very restricted type, of LDL receptor lateral mobility. A similar aggregated staining pattern was obtained with prefixed, either sparse or confluent, endothelial cells, indicating that surface receptors for LDL are located, even before the addition of LDL, in small clusters which only under sparse conditions and upon the binding of LDL can further move to form larger aggregates (cells attached to a substrate) or caps (cells in suspension) [40]. In contrast, if, instead of native LDL one uses cationized LDL, which binds nonspecifically to the cell surface, this positively charged ligand will be taken into the cells without a redistribution of its binding sites. Internalization of cationized LDL can therefore take place in both sparse and confluent cultures, regardless of the restriction on surface receptor mobility imposed upon vascular endothelial cells when they become highly organized and form a closely apposed cell monolayer.

Changes in the Cell Surface Occurring When Endothelial Cells Are Maintained in the Absence of FGF: FGF and the Normal Differentiation of the Vascular Endothelium

The preceding results demonstrated that the formation of a confluent endothelial cell monolayer is associated with structural (fibronectin, CSP-60) and function-related (receptor lateral mobility, adsorptive endocytosis) alterations in the cell surface. These changes can be looked upon as differentiation events which enable the endothelial cells to adopt in culture the morphologic appearance and metabolic behavior which characterize the endothelium of the large vessels. Of paramount importance to us was to determine the role of FGF in this expression of differentiated properties, ie, whether the presence of FGF during the phase of active cell growth is required for the normal differentiation of the endothelium [41]. For this purpose, cells were cultured in the absence of FGF and tested for growth behavior and surface-associated properties both at a sparse and confluent cell density.

Growth properties and morphologic appearance. Endothelial cells maintained without FGF had a much longer doubling time (60–78 h) than cultures maintained in the presence of FGF (18 h; Fig. 12A) and failed to proliferate when seeded at a high split ratio (Fig. 12B). They also adopt a strikingly different morphology (Fig. 13). The alterations in growth

---

Fig. 12. Growth rate of vascular endothelial cells in the presence and absence of FGF. A) Vascular endothelial cells derived from the adult aortic arch (32 passages; 160 generations) were plated onto 35-mm dishes (2×10^4 cells per dish) in DMEM (H-16) supplemented with 10% calf serum. Duplicate cultures were counted every other day and the medium replaced every four days. ▲, Cells after three passages in the absence of FGF, no FGF was added. △, Cells after three passages in the absence of FGF; FGF was added on the third day after seeding and every other day thereafter. These cells adopted at confluence a perfect monolayer configuration indistinguishable from that of cells that were never subjected to FGF withdrawal. ○, Cells derived from endothelial cultures that were continuously maintained with FGF. FGF was added every other day. B) Confluent endothelial cell cultures maintained with (16 passages) (▲) or without (4 passages). (●) FGF were split at various ratios and cultured in the presence and absence of FGF (added every other day), respectively. The medium (DMEM + 10% calf serum) was replaced after four days and triplicate dishes were counted every other day. The number of cells after 9 days in culture is plotted as a function of the split ratio. The seeding level at a split ratio of 1:2 was 1.65×10^5 and 1.4×10^5 cells per 35-mm dish for cells maintained with and without FGF, respectively.

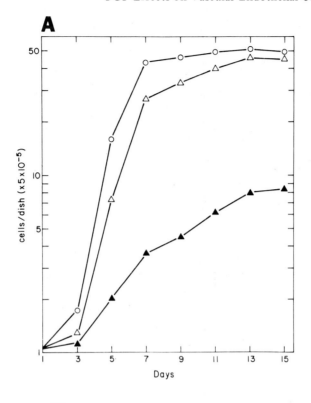

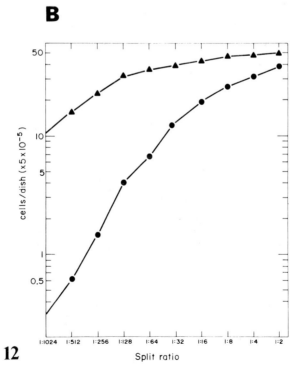

12

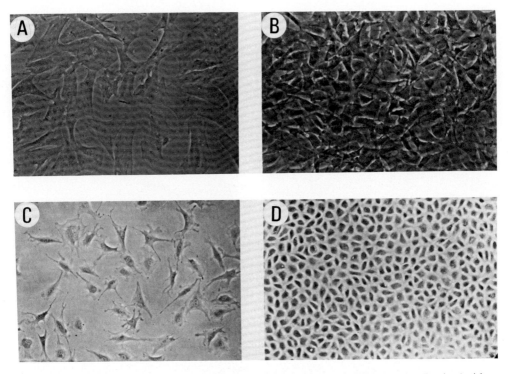

Fig. 13. Morphologic appearance of sparse and confluent vascular endothelial cultures maintained with and without FGF (phase contrast, × 150). A) Sparse endothelial cells maintained in the absence of FGF. The cells are 4–6 times larger and spread farther apart than sparse cells (C) seeded and maintained in the presence of FGF. B) Confluent endothelial cells after four passages (12 generations) in the absence of FGF. The cells grow on top of each other and in various directions. D) A confluent endothelial monolayer formed by cells (100 generations) maintained in the presence of FGF. The cells are highly flattened, closely apposed, and nonoverlapping.

behavior and morphologic appearance were best demonstrated after 3–4 passages (15–20 generations) in the absence of FGF. The cells, by then 4–6 times larger, failed to adopt a nonoverlapping monolayer configuration even after being split at a 1:4 ratio. Instead, at sparse density they were flattened and highly spread (Fig. 13A) and at confluence they grew on top of each other, leaving intercellular spaces (Fig. 13B). These cells exhibited a short lifespan, as reflected by vacuolization and cell degeneration after 30 generations in the absence of FGF. Readdition of FGF at an early passage to sparse or subconfluent cultures, or reseeding the cells at a low density but in the presence of FGF (Fig. 12A), resulted within 2–3 days in a resumption of cell growth and within 5–7 days in a morphologic appearance similar to that observed with endothelial cultures that are continuously maintained with FGF.

Fibronectin. As already described (Fig. 1C), the formation of a closely apposed endothelial cell monolayer is associated with a change in the localization of fibronectin so that it is no longer found on the apical cell surfaces but rather becomes a major component of the extracellular matrix and closely associated with the basal cell surface. In contrast, cells that were cultured in the absence of FGF showed a fibrillar distribution of fibronectin over their apical cell surfaces, both when sparse (Fig. 14B) and even prior to the formation of cell-cell contacts (Fig. 14A) as well as late at confluence (Fig. 14C). Addition of FGF to sparse or subconfluent cultures previously deprived of FGF induced both cell proliferation and reorganization. This was associated with a change in the distribution of fibronectin which was much less or no longer detectable on the apical surface of cells that adopted the flattened, closely apposed, and nonoverlapping configuration typical of cultures maintained in the presence of FGF. In cells that were seeded in the presence of FGF, such a redistribution of fibronectin was revealed by the entire culture 5–7 days after reaching confluence, as previously observed with endothelial cells that were continuously maintained with FGF. When the FGF was added to a culture that had already reached subconfluence in the absence of FGF, the redistribution of fibronectin required a similar time interval (during which only 1–2 cell doublings took place), but was incomplete in those areas (up to 30% of the entire culture) which failed to adopt the appropriate morphology.

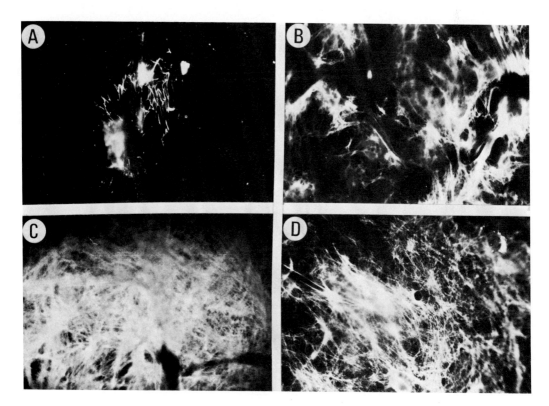

Fig. 14. Indirect immunofluorescence localization of fibronectin in endothelial cultures maintained without FGF. Vascular aortic endothelial cells maintained without FGF (three passages) were stained with rabbit anti-bovine plasma fibronectin and FITC goat anti-rabbit IgG as described in Materials and Methods. A) Sparse cultures prior to the formation of cell-cell contacts. Fibronectin is detected on top of the cells. B) Sparse and subconfluent cultures. Fibronectin is detected on top as well as in the areas of cell-cell contact C) Confluent cultures. Fibronectin is present in large quantities on top of the cells. D) Extracellular matrix left after removing the confluent cell layer with Triton X-100 (0.5%, 5 min, at 37°C).

Sparse and confluent cultures of endothelial cells maintained with or without FGF were subjected to the lactoperoxidase-catalyzed iodination in order to study further the differences in the surface localization of fibronectin and in particular in its quantity relative to other cell surface proteins. As demonstrated in Figure 15, cells that were cultured in the absence of FGF showed, even at a sparse density and even prior to the formation of cell-cell contacts (Fig. 15D, J), more fibronectin than that exposed for iodination in either sparse (Fig. 15A, G) or confluent (Fig. 15B, H) cultures that were maintained with FGF.

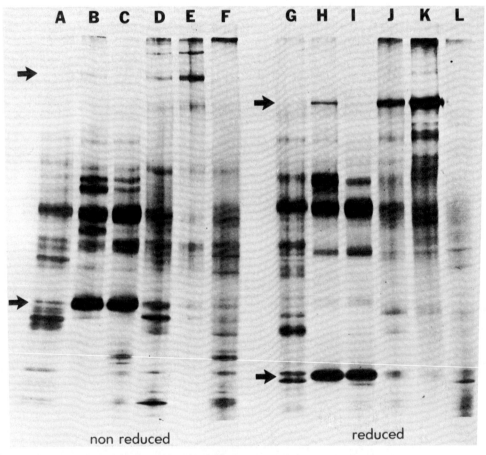

Fig. 15. SDS-polyacrylamide gel electrophoresis of lactoperoxidase-iodinated sparse and confluent endothelial cultures maintained with or without FGF. Washed cultures (maintained with or without FGF in a medium containing a fibronectin-depleted serum) were iodinated with ^{131}I and lactoperoxidase, lysed, and analyzed by a gradient (5–15%) polyacrylamide slab gel electrophoresis either before (lanes A–F) or after (lanes G–L) reduction with 0.1 M DTT. A,G) Sparse cultures maintained in the presence of FGF – almost no contacts among the cells. Fibronectin and CSP-60 are slightly or not detected. B,H) A confluent monolayer of cells cultured in the presence of FGF. Both CSP-60 and fibronectin become susceptible to iodination; CSP-60 appears as a major band. C, I) Confluent cultures exposed to a mild trypsinization (0.2 μg/ml, 45 min, 37°C). Fibronectin is largely removed, whereas CSP-60 is affected little or not at all. D,J) Sparse cultures prior to the formation of cell-cell contacts and maintained in the absence of FGF. Fibronectin is highly susceptible to iodination. E,K) Confluent endothelial cultures maintained in the absence of FGF. Fibronectin appears as the major component, whereas CSP-60 is slightly or not detectable. F,L) Confluent cultures after a mild trypsinization. Fibronectin is largely removed. Arrows mark the positions of fibronectin and CSP-60.

In fact, in cells that were not exposed to FGF, fibronectin was the major component susceptible to iodination either at sparse density and to an even greater extent, late at confluence (Fig. 15E, K). When these cells were reseeded in the presence of FGF, they formed a confluent cell monolayer and showed, like cells that are continuously maintained with FGF, little or no fibronectin accessible to the lactoperoxidase-catalyzed iodination (Fig. 16D, I). In contrast, cultures that were reexposed to FGF after having already reached a high cell density showed only a partial removal of surface-associated fibronectin even after adopting a cell monolayer configuration (Fig. 16C, H). These experiments had also demonstrated that the fibronectin present on the cell surface is bonded by disulfides or otherwise (eg, transglutaminase) to form dimers, trimers, and higher complexes which hardly entered the running gel. Most of these aggregates were precipitated by antifibronectin antiserum and gave rise to a 230K component (fibronectin monomer) after reduction of the samples with DTT (Figs. 15 and 16).

Immunofluorescence staining of the extracellular material left after removal of the confluent cell layer with Triton X-100 had demonstrated a massive accumulation of fibronectin in the extracellular matrix produced by cells maintained with (Fig. 1D) or without (Fig. 14D) FGF. Endothelial cells that were cultured in the absence of FGF therefore resembled fibroblasts [28] or smooth muscle cells [29] in having fibronectin associated with both their upper and lower cell surfaces. The expression at confluence of fibronectin underneath the cell layer but not on the apical cell surface might therefore be a unique differentiated property of endothelial cells that are maintained in the presence of FGF and form a monolayer composed of flattened and nonoverlapping cells [41].

The production of fibronectin by sparse and confluent endothelial cultures maintained with or without FGF was further studied by exposing the cells to [^{35}S] methionine and subjecting both the cell layer (Fig. 17K–N) and tissue culture medium (Fig. 17A–J) to SDS slab gel electrophoresis before and after immunoprecipitation with antifibronectin antiserum. As shown in Table II, antifibronectin precipitated less than 3% of the total [^{35}S]-labeled proteins that were secreted into the medium of cells that were cultured with FGF. In contrast, 20–25% of the total [^{35}S]-labeled proteins were precipitated from the culture medium of cells that were maintained in the absence of FGF. When analyzed on SDS polyacrylamide gels (Fig. 17A, F), more than 90% of the immunoprecipitated radioactivity comigrated with fibronectin. On the basis of the immunoprecipitation values, it can be calculated that sparse and confluent cultures maintained in the absence of FGF secreted into the medium 30 and 50 times more fibronectin per cell than sparse and confluent cells cultured in the presence of FGF, respectively (Table II).

A higher production of fibronectin in the absence of FGF was also observed when cell extracts, rather than the tissue culture medium, were analyzed for the presence of [^{35}S]-labeled fibronectin (Fig. 17M, N). These results, together with the immunofluorescence and surface iodination experiments, indicate that the production and distribution of fibronectin are sensitive to changes in cell organization and growth behavior induced by FGF.

CSP-60. The presence on the cell surface of a specific protein (CSP-60) is a characteristic property of endothelial cells that form a highly confluent cell monolayer (Figs. 3–8). This protein cannot be detected by lactoperoxidase-catalyzed iodination in actively growing and unorganized endothelial cultures. Likewise, CSP-60 was no longer exposed for iodination in disorganized endothelial cell monolayers and was not present in sparse or confluent cultures of vascular smooth muscle cells that grow in multiple layers [32]. As demonstrated in Figure 15, CSP-60 was not detected in sparse cultures maintained with (lanes A and G) or without (lanes D and J) FGF but was largely exposed for iodination in confluent cultures

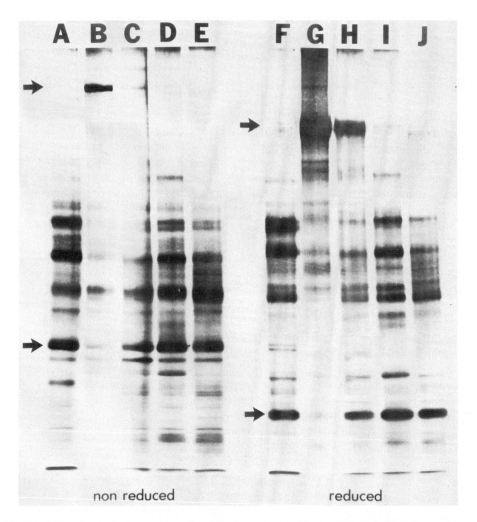

Fig. 16. Cell surface iodination pattern of overlapping and reorganized endothelial cells before and after being reexposed to FGF. Endothelial cells maintained for three passages in the absence of FGF were seeded at a split ratio of 1:8 and FGF was added (every other day) starting on day 2 or day 7 after seeding. Control cultures (not exposed to FGF) and reorganized cultures (reexposed to FGF) were iodinated at confluence (14 days after seeding) and analyzed by gradient (5–15%) polyacrylamide slab gel electrophoresis before (ianes A–E) and after (lanes F–J) reduction with 0.1 M DTT. A,F) A confluent monolayer of endothelial cells that were continuously maintained in the presence of FGF. CSP-60 appears as a major band. B,G) Confluent but unorganized endothelial culture maintained for four passages without FGF. Fibronectin appears as a major band; CSP-60 is missing. C,H) Same cells as in (B) and (G) exposed to FGF at a subconfluent density (7 days after seeding) and labeled 7 days later. Most of the cultures adopt a monolayer configuration, although some unorganized areas (about 20% of the culture) are still present. Both fibronectin and CSP-60 are exposed for iodination. D,I) The same cells as in (B) and (G) exposed to FGF at a sparse density (3 days after being split at a 1:8 ratio) and labeled 12 days afterwards, when the cells were highly organized and closely apposed. CSP-60 appears as a major band, whereas fibronectin is detected in small amounts as in cells that are maintained continuously with FGF. E, J) – FGF culture exposed when subconfluent to a medium conditioned by a confluent monolayer of endothelial cells and iodinated 7 days afterwards. Arrows mark the positions of fibronectin and CSP-60.

TABLE II. Secretion of Fibronectin Into the Growth Medium of Endothelial Cells Maintained With or Without FGF

Cells	Total [^{35}S]-labeled proteins[a] (cpm × 10^{-6} per 10^6 cells)	[^{35}S]-labeled material precipitated with antifibronectin[b] (cpm × 10^{-6} per 10^6 cells)	% Fibronectin in total [^{35}S]-labeled proteins
(+) FGF cultures			
Sparse	11.6	0.195	1.7
Confluent	3.8	0.120	3.2
(−) FGF cultures			
Sparse	26.9	6.45	24.4
Confluent	32.6	5.76	17.7

Sparse and confluent endothelial cultures were maintained with or without FGF and exposed to [^{35}S]methionine (65 µCi/ml, 20 h) in DMEM containing 10 µM methionine and 0.5% bovine serum as described in the legend to Figure 17. Aliquots (10 µl) of the growth medium were taken for precipitation with 10% boiling TCA and the entire 1 ml medium was subjected to double immunoprecipitation with 10 µl of rabbit anti-bovine fibronectin antiserum followed by 10 µl of goat anti-rabbit IgG antiserum as described in Materials and Methods. The same amounts of fibronectin were precipitated by using either 5 µl or 50 µl of each of these antisera preparations.
[a] Sparse and confluent endothelial cells maintained in the presence of FGF contained 320 and 260 µg protein per 10^6 cells, whereas sparse and confluent cells maintained in absence of FGF contained 1,810 and 1,462 µg protein per 10^6 cells, respectively.
[b] Nonspecific precipitation with nonimmune rabbit serum was carried out under each condition and the values were substracted from those obtained with antifibronectin. Nonspecific precipitation did not exceed 1% of the total [^{35}S]-labeled proteins secreted into the medium.

that were maintained in the presence of FGF and had adopted a closely apposed cell monolayer configuration (Fig. 15B, H). In contrast, endothelial cells that were cultured and reached confluence in the absence of FGF showed little or no CSP-60 even at late confluence (Fig. 15E, K). Readdition of FGF to sparse or subconfluent endothelial cultures that were maintained without FGF was associated with a reappearance/exposure of CSP-60 concomitant with the adoption of a closely apposed cell monolayer configuration (Fig. 16C, D and H, I). The presence of CSP-60 on the cell surface was not affected by a mild trypsinization (Fig. 15C, I) which did not disrupt the cell layer. Since under the same conditions fibronectin was largely or completely removed from the cell surface, it is unlikely that CSP-60 is not detected in cells maintained without FGF because of being masked by the meshwork of fibronectin which, under these conditions, is found on top of the cells.

Thrombogenic properties. Like the vascular endothelium in vivo [42], sparse and confluent (Fig. 18A) endothelial cells maintained with FGF have an apical, nonthrombogenic surface to which platelets cannot adhere. Thus, no platelets, or less than one platelet per cell, were found on top of cells that were incubated (30 min, 37°C) with human platelets (2 × 10^8 platelets/m) and washed extensively (Fig. 18B). In contrast, when endothelial cells maintained without FGF (Fig. 18C) were tested for the same property, they exhibited a high platelet-binding capacity (20–50 platelets per cell) both at a sparse and confluent (Fig. 18D) cell density. As shown in Fig. 18D, the platelets were bound singly to the apical surface of these cells and no aggregation of the attached platelets took

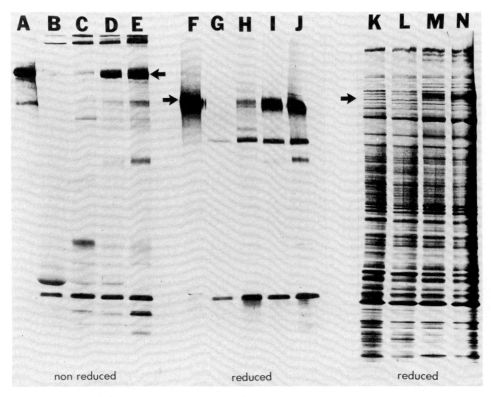

Fig. 17. Electrophoresis of [^{35}S] methionine-labeled proteins present in cell extracts and tissue culture medium of sparse and confluent endothelial cultures maintained with or without FGF. Sparse (actively growing) and confluent (10 days after reaching confluence) endothelial cultures maintained with or without (three passages) FGF were exposed to [^{35}S] methionine (65 μCi/ml, 20 h) in DMEM containing 10 μM methionine and 0.5% bovine serum. Cell extracts (in sample buffer) (lanes K–N) and 5–15 μl aliquots of the medium (lanes A–J) containing 50,000 protein-bound (TCA-precipitable) cpm were then subjected to a gradient (5–16%) polyacrylamide slab gel electrophoresis either before (lanes A–F) or after (lanes F–N) reduction with 0.1 M DTT. A,F) Immunoprecipitation pattern (antifibronectin followed by anti-IgG) of growth medium taken from sparse endothelial cells cultured in the absence of FGF. B, G) Proteins secreted into the medium by sparse cells maintained with FGF. C,H) Proteins secreted by sparse cells cultured in the absence of FGF. D,I) [^{35}S]-labeled proteins secreted into the medium by confluent cells that were maintained with FGF. E,J) Medium of confluent cells cultured in the absence of FGF. K–N) Cell extracts of sparse (K,M) and confluent (L,N) endothelial cultures maintained with (K,L) or without (M,N) FGF. Arrows mark the positions of fibronectin dimers (460K, nonreduced samples) and monomers (230K, reduced samples).

Fig. 18. Adherence of platelets to confluent vascular endothelial cultures maintained with or without FGF. Confluent endothelial cultures maintained in the absence (three passages) or presence (during the phase of logarithmic growth) of FGF were incubated with human platelets (2 × 10^8/ml, 30 min, 37°C), washed, and observed by phase microscopy (× 150) as described under Materials and Methods. A,B) Cells maintained with FGF. Very little or no platelets can be seen (B) attached to the upper surface of cells that adopt a monolayer configuration as in (A). In contrast, most of the upper surface of unorganized cultures (C) maintained in the absence of FGF is covered with platelets which attached singly and do not form aggregates (D).

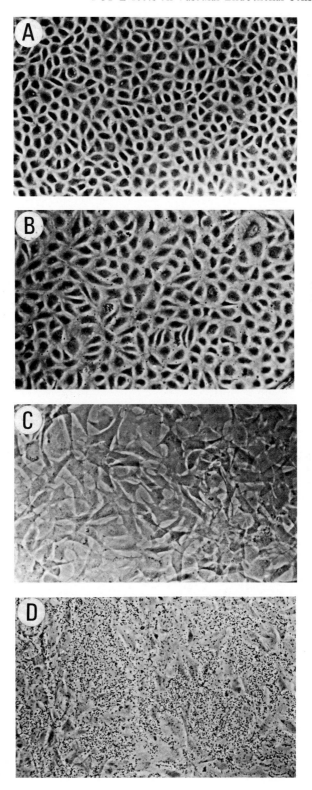

18

place. In order to determine whether this interaction is associated with a release reaction, confluent cultures maintained with or without FGF were incubated with platelets that were prelabeled with ^{14}C-serotonin. The reaction medium containing unattached platelets and any serotonin which might have been released during binding were then removed and the platelets collected by centrifugation. The cell layer was then extensively washed and solubilized in 0.1 N NaOH. The cells, platelets, and platelet-free supernatant were counted separately to determine the distribution of ^{14}C-serotonin. As shown in Table III, the interaction between platelets and endothelial cells maintained with or without FGF was not associated with any serotonin release beyond that spontaneously released during incubation (30 min, 37°C) of platelets in the absence of cells. The lack of serotonin release was not due to defects in the release reaction, since exposure to thrombin (1 IU/ml) induced the platelets to secrete 80–90% of their ^{14}C-serotonin content (Table III). When the radioactivity associated with the cell layer was measured, it was found, as already observed (Fig. 18), that endothelial cells maintained without FGF bind platelets to an extent that is 9 and 25 times higher (when calculated per culture dish and per cell, respectively) than cells that were cultured in the absence of FGF. Trypsinization (0.5 μg/ml, 2 h 37°C), which caused no release or rounding up of cells but removed the fibronectin from the upper surface of cells that were cultured in the absence of FGF (as detected by lactoperoxidase-catalyzed iodination) (Fig. 15F, L), decreased the adherence of platelets by no more than 40%. Cultures maintained in the absence of FGF readopted within 8–10 days after being exposed to FGF the configuration of a highly flattened monolayer composed of closely apposed and nonoverlapping cells. These cells, like cells that were continuously maintained with FGF, exhibited a nonthrombogenic apical surface to which platelets did not adhere.

Barrier function. Vascular endothelial cells, by virtue of their location at the inner surface of blood vessels, are exposed to various substances at concentrations and proportions far different from those found in the extravascular region and are therefore expected to possess unique properties, both as a barrier and as a transport system. Such properties

TABLE III. Binding of Platelets to Vascular Endothelial Cells Maintained With or Without FGF

Cells	Cell-bound platelets (^{14}C-serotonin)		Released ^{14}C-serotonin (cpm/dish)
	cpm/dish	cpm/10^6 cells	
+ FGF cultures	1,192	1,748	5,930
– FGF cultures	9,504	50,553	6,097
– FGF cultures pretreated with trypsin[a]	5,227	27,803	5,944
No cells	–	–	6,311
No cells + thrombin (1 unit/ml)	–	–	87,653

Platelets (2 × 10^8) prelabeled with ^{14}C-serotonin were incubated (30 min at 37°C in DMEM containing 0.25% BSA) with confluent endothelial cultures that were maintained with (during the active phase of growth) or without (three passages) FGF. Platelet binding and serotonin release were determined as described in Materials and Methods. The amount of serotonin release was in all cases equivalent to that spontaneously released by platelets during a 30-min incubation without cells. Treatment of 2 × 10^8 platelets with thrombin (1 unit/ml) induced a 90% release of the ^{14}C-serotonin that was introduced into the platelets.
[a]Worthington twice-crystallized trypsin (0.5 μg/ml, 2 h, 37°C in DMEM).

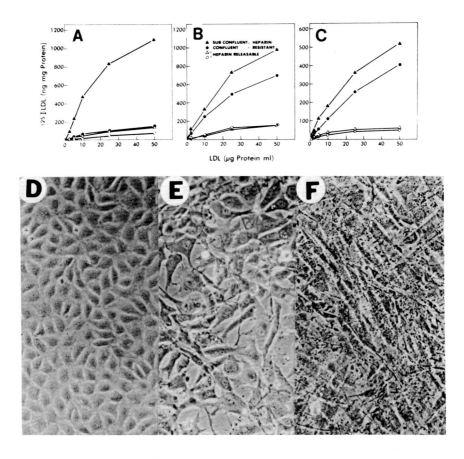

Fig. 19. Binding and uptake of ^{125}I-LDL by sparse and confluent cultures of endothelial and smooth muscle cells. A–C) LDL binding and internalization. A) Adult bovine aortic endothelial cells. B) Adult bovine aortic endothelial cells maintained in the absence of FGF for four passages. C) Adult bovine aortic smooth muscle cells. D–F) Morphologic appearance of the confluent cultures described under (A), (B), and (C) at the time of the experiment, respectively. The endothelial and smooth muscle cells were exposed to LDL before (▲, △) and 8 days after (●, ○) reaching confluence. Cells were seeded, maintained, and tested for specific binding (△ and ○, accessible for heparin release) and internalization (▲ and ●, heparin-resistant) of ^{125}I-LDL, as described under Materials and Methods. The results demonstrate that LDL internalization by different cell types can be correlated with their morphologic appearance at a high density.

are of particular significance in preventing an excess of plasma lipoproteins from accumulating in the subendothelial regions and in the smooth muscle cells of the arterial wall. In previous studies, we have demonstrated that when endothelial cells form a confluent cell monolayer, although the LDL still binds to cell surface receptors, the molecules are no longer internalized and, hence, there is no degradation of the lipoprotein [24–26]. Since morphologic as well as surface changes are induced by maintaining the endothelial cells without FGF, we have studied whether these alterations can in turn be expressed by changes in the permeability barrier function of these endothelial cells. For this purpose, sparse and confluent endothelial cultures maintained with or without FGF were tested for

their ability to bind and internalize ^{125} I-labeled LDL particles. As shown in Figure 19, endothelial cultures maintained without FGF (Fig. 19B) can, like vascular smooth muscle cells
(Fig. 19C), internalize the receptor-bound LDL particles both at a sparse and confluent cell
density. These cells can grow on top of each other and form multiple cell layers at confluence (Fig. 19E, F). In contrast, vascular endothelial cells that are maintained in the
presence of FGF adopt at confluence a monolayer configuration (Fig. 19D) and as a result
can bind but no longer internalize the LDL particles (Fig. 19A). As demonstrated in Figure
19, sparse endothelial cultures exhibited a similar degree of LDL binding and internalization
when maintained either with or without FGF. The difference between the two types of
cultures was expressed only late at confluence and was reflected by the lack of LDL uptake
in cells that were maintained with FGF. Since the cell surface area becomes smaller once
a tightly packed monolayer is formed, cells in a confluent endothelial monolayer showed
up to a twofold to threefold decrease in LDL-binding capacity compared with sparse (+)
FGF cultures or with either sparse or confluent cultures that were maintained without FGF.

DISCUSSION

The present study summarizes various observations on the role of the cell surface in
determining the normal morphologic appearance and physiologic function of the vascular
endothelium. These cells exhibit unique adhesive interactions (both in terms of cell-cell
interactions and adhesion to the basal lamina) as well as a nonthrombogenic apical surface
to which platelets cannot adhere. These apparently contradictory properties imply that a
certain degree of membrane asymmetry has to be achieved as the endothelial cells differentiate to form a monolayer composed of nonoverlapping cells that no longer divide. The
adoption of such a morphology is in turn essential in order that the endothelium function
both as a nonthrombogenic surface and as a regulator of the system's permeability to plasma
constituents. By using FGF and cultured endothelial cells that mimic perfectly their in
vivo counterparts, we have demonstrated that a cell surface asymmetry is in fact acquired
late at confluence and concomitant with the formation of a highly organized cell monolayer. In terms of structural rearrangements, this was reflected by disappearance of fibronectin from the apical cell surface; appearance of a specific cell surface protein (CSP-60)
not detected in actively growing cells; production of a highly thrombogenic basal lamina
composed mostly of a fibronectin-collagen-proteoglycan meshwork; and restriction of the
lateral mobility of various cell surface receptor sites. In terms of physiologic function, the
confluent endothelial cell monolayer fulfills the requirements of having a nonthrombogenic
apical surface and serving as an efficient barrier against the uptake of LDL, which is the
main cholesterol carrier in blood. Both the structural and functional attributes exhibited
by a confluent endothelial cell monolayer can be regarded as differentiated properties and
they have been shown to depend on the presence of FGF during the active phase of cell
growth [41].

Respective Roles of Fibronectin and CSP-60

The presence of large amounts of fibronectin in cells that grow on top of each other,
and the rapid reorganization of trypsinized endothelial cells despite the removal of fibronectin, suggest that fibronectin is not an essential factor in the formation of highly
organized cell monolayer. Fibronectin is a major constituent of the basal lamina produced
at confluence by endothelial cells [1–3]. it is therefore likely that with these cells the
primary function of fibronectin is to enforce cell-to-substrate adhesion rather than to be

involved in determining the final organization of the tissue. If one considers the turbulence, the pressure variation, and the speed of blood flow in the aortic arch, it becomes evident why the endothelial cells must develop a special means of remaining attached as a cell monolayer to their basal lamina. Such a means could be the production of great amounts of extracellular material, such as fibronectin, which primarily functions to enforce cell adhesion [43, 44]. It is therefore suggested that because of their morphology (monolayer), shape (flattened), and situation (inner layer of the arteries and veins), vascular endothelial cells are called upon to make a major contribution to the production of the fibronectin found in the basement membrane of the blood vessels as well as that found in the plasma, where it is present as CIG. In contrast, the appearance on the cell surface of CSP-60 was, under normal and various experimental conditions, always correlated with the formation of a confluent cell monolayer but not with substrate adhesion and flattening of the endothelial cells. This protein can therefore play a role in the interaction between cells which leads to the adoption of a monolayer configuration composed of closely apposed and nonoverlapping cells.

Receptor Restriction, Production of a Fibronectin Meshwork, and Formation of an Endothelial Barrier to Receptor-Mediated Uptake of LDL

Experiments with human fibroblasts have indicated that a lateral receptor mobility is not required for the receptor-mediated uptake of LDL. In these cells the LDL receptor sites are predominantly located in coated regions of the plasma membrane, which can invaginate to form coated vesicles [39]. It has been observed, however, that the internalization of various polypeptides (α_2-macroglobulin, insulin, epidermal growth factor) is preceded by patching, probably into coated pits, of specific receptor sites that are otherwise diffusely distributed over the entire cell surface area [37]. The present results on the inhibition in confluent endothelial cultures of both the uptake of LDL and the lateral mobility of the appropriate cell surface receptor sites suggest that receptor redistribution might also be involved in the internalization of LDL by actively growing vascular endothelial cells. It therefore seems that a requirement for a certain degree of ligand-receptor lateral mobility is the more general mechanism for internalization via adsorptive endocytosis, although various cell types and various receptor sites on a given cell type might require a very limited degree of such receptor distribution or none at all. This has been demonstrated by showing that the internalization of native LDL by vascular smooth muscle cells and of cationized LDL by endothelial cells was not correlated with a detectable receptor redistribution.

Bornstein et al [45] have proposed a model in which an external fibronectin-collagen meshwork interacts, via transmembrane and cytoplasmic peripheral proteins, with microfilaments subjacent to the plasma membrane. This interaction might, among other effects, restrict the lateral mobility of various receptor sites in the membrane plane [45, 46]. Evidence of such an interaction was provided by these [45] and other investigators [47, 48]. There is also evidence of a restricting effect of the extracellular matrix, consisting mostly of fibronectin, on Con A receptor lateral mobility and cell agglutinability [49, 50]. Using indirect immunofluorescence and surface iodination techniques, we have demonstrated that late at confluence fibronectin becomes less exposed on the apical endothelial cell surface and is primarily produced as disulfide-bonded complexes toward the substrate underlying the cell layer. This is associated with a reorganization of the cellular microfibrillar system, which no longer shows any linkage with the apical cell surface but rather lies parallel to both the basal and apical cell surfaces [2]. It therefore seems possible that an "exoskeleton" of the matrix, consisting of fibronectin and perhaps other proteins or glycoproteins, might interact indirectly with cytoskeletal elements or be directly cross-linked to other components of the cell surface [16], thereby leading to a change in membrane dynamics and organization. This might affect not only the freedom of surface receptor lateral mobility but also the rigidity of the membrane in general, thus inhibiting processes such as invagination and formation of endocytotic vesicles. That this could, indeed, be the case is strongly supported by the experiments of Nicolau et al [51], which show a significant stiffening of the cell membrane at a saturation density of growth-controlled cells.

Contact inhibition was shown to inhibit phagocytosis [52] and toxin uptake [53] in cultured epithelial sheets and 3T3 fibroblasts, respectively. We have also observed a two-fold to threefold inhibition of the bulk phase pinocytosis (measured by the uptake of either ^{14}C-inulin or ^{14}C-sucrose) upon the formation of a confluent endothelial cell mono-layer. Experiments with membrane vesicles isolated from rapidly growing and quiescent 3T3 cells have demonstrated that the inhibition of uridine transport at confluence is due to a modification in the structure of the cell membrane rather than in the overall cell metab-olism [54]. In the case of the vascular endothelium, such a structural modification was reflected by the appearance of CSP-60 on the apical cell surface and the redistribution of fibronectin, which was no longer found on top of the cells but rather accumulated in the basal lamina. We have also observed an increased production of a 58,000 MW protein in highly organized and resting endothelial cultures versus sparse and actively growing cells (Fig. 20, protein No. 1). This difference is most significant in view of the greatly reduced synthesis of other cellular proteins (in terms of protein types and total incorporation of [^{35}S] methionine) that occurs late at confluence. Preliminary studies suggest that the 58,000 MW protein migrates in a manner similar to the 58K intermediate (10 nm) filament, which has been shown to be a major cytoplasmic structure of many eukaryotic cells. This protein might play an important role in maintaining the flattened and closely apposed morphology of confluent endothelial cells (Vlodavsky, Savion, and Gospodarowicz, manu-script in preparation).

FGF and the Normal Differentiation of Vascular Endothelial Cells

In previous studies we have emphasized the role of FGF as a potent mitogen for vascular endothelial cells and an essential factor in developing clonal endothelial cell populations. We have now compared endothelial cells maintained with and without FGF in order to study whether changes other than those related to cell proliferation can be induced by the presence of FGF [41]. Of particular interest in this regard is the adoption at confluence of a highly flattened, nonoverlapping and closely apposed cell organization, as well as of a cell surface asymmetry. These properties reflect an advanced stage of dif-ferentiation in which the upper cell surface is nonthrombogenic and no longer covered with fibronectin, whereas the basal cell surface is closely associated with a highly thrombogenic fibrillar matrix composed mostly of fibronectin and collagen. It is important to study how endothelial cells can gain and lose such characteristics in order to elucidate the factors which allow the endothelium of the large vessels to form a nonthrombogenic surface, to resist high pressure and Sheer forces, and to function as a selective barrier against plasma com-ponents and particularly lipoproteins.

The present results have demonstrated that cells maintained in the absence of FGF exhibit, in addition to a much slower growth rate, morphologic as well as structural and functional alterations that are incompatible with their appearance and behavior in vivo. These include: a) a failure to adopt at confluence the configuration of a cell monolayer composed of flattened and nonoverlapping cells; b) a loss of cell surface asymmetry, as

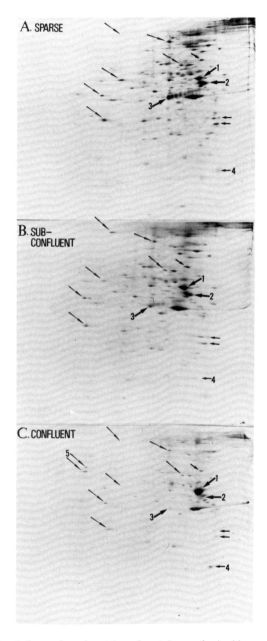

Fig. 20. Two-dimensional electrophoresis pattern of proteins synthesized by sparse, subconfluent, and confluent vascular endothelial cells. Endothelial cultures maintained with FGF were exposed to [^{35}S] methionine (200 μCi/ml, 60 min, 37°C), washed, and lysed with isoelectric focusing sample buffer (9.5 M urea, 2% NP-40, 2% ampholytes, pH 3.5–10,5% β-mercaptoethanol). Then 500,000 protein-bound cpm was subjected to two-dimensional gel electrophoresis (nonequilibrium, pH gradient electrophoresis followed by SDS gel electrophoresis on a 10–16% gradient polyacrylamide slab gel). A) Sparse, actively growing endothelial cells. B) Subconfluent cultures which are not yet organized into a cell monolayer. C) Confluent, highly organized, and resting monolayer of endothelial cells. Arrows mark the main differences between the three autoradiograms (exposure time was 4 days).

demonstrated by the presence late at confluence of fibronectin associated with both the apical and basal cell surfaces, and by thrombogenicity (platelet-binding capacity) of the apical cell surfaces; c) an increased production and secretion of fibronectin by both sparse and confluent cultures; d) a lack of CSP-60 (detected by the lactoperoxidase-catalyzed iodination technique), a cell surface protein susceptible to iodination only in cells that adopt a monolayer configuration; and e) a failure to form an effective barrier against low density lipoprotein. Exposure of the cultures to FGF induces a restoration of the normal endothelial characteristics concomitant with the adoption of a flattened cell monolayer morphology [41]. The physiologic significance of the alterations listed above is in particular demonstrated by the inability of the non-contact-inhibited (minus FGF) endothelial cells to protect the subendothelial layer against an overaccumulation of LDL cholesterol. This might initiate the formation of foam cells and lead later on to the formation of an atherosclerotic plaque. Furthermore, by having a thrombogenic surface exposed to the medium, these cells can serve as a nucleus for platelet adherence, blood clotting, and thrombus formation.

The notion of a factor simultaneously inducing apparently contradictory effects such as cell proliferation and differentiation is quite new. Whether FGF is directly involved, via a mechanism distinct from its mitogenic activity, in the adoption of the monolayer configuration and cell surface polarity characteristic of endothelial cells has yet to be studied. A simple explanation might be that the presence of FGF is required for the formation of a cell monolayer, while the other differentiated attributes are controlled by secondary factors like the unique cell-cell adhesive interactions established at confluence. That this might not be the case is suggested by the finding that some of the FGF-dependent alterations (increased production of fibronectin, platelet-binding capacity) were already observed at a sparse cell density and even prior to the formation of cell-cell contacts, which suggests, in turn, a direct relation to the actual withdrawal of FGF. On the other hand, the appearance of CSP-60 and the removal of fibronectin from the apical cell surface seem to depend more on a prior formation of the appropriate cell-cell contacts. It should also be emphasized in this regard that each of the alterations observed in the absence of FGF represents a phenotypic rather than a permanent genetic modification, because the readdition of FGF was associated with a restoration of a normal growth rate, morphologic appearance, and membrane properties. Endothelial cells maintained in the absence of FGF also showed no chromosomal aberrations insofar as chromosome number and morphology are concerned.

Preliminary results from this laboratory (Fig. 16E, J) indicate that a reversion of highly overlapping endothelial cells can also be induced by a conditioned medium taken from confluent endothelial cells that have adopted a monolayer configuration. This medium is currently being analyzed for the presence of various components of cellular origin which might be responsible for the induced changes in cellular morphology and growth characteristics [55]. Therefore, endothelial cells that are seeded at a high density (1:4 split ratio), unlike cells that are seeded at a low or clonal density, may, by conditioning the medium, adopt a cell monolayer configuration and the associated differentiated properties, even in the absence of an added factor such as FGF.

The present study presents new aspects of the pleiotropic interaction between a mitogen and a given cell type. This is best demonstrated by the observation that FGF can induce both proliferation and differentiation of vascular endothelial cells. A similar observation has already been made for the nerve growth factor (NGF), which has been shown to control the survival as well as the differentiation, of neuronal cells.

However, in the case of NGF, because of the specific nature of its target cells, which lose their proliferative capacity early in their lifespan, the survival and differentiating effects are observed at different times in the cells' lives. Our recent studies with rat pituitary cells have also demonstrated an epidermal growth factor (EGF) effect on gene expression and differentiated functions (synthesis of prolactin and growth hormone) which was not associated with a mitogenic response [56]. In contrast, with vascular endothelial cells FGF can simultaneously be both a proliferative and differentiating agent. Its long-term effects on the differentiation and physiologic function of the vascular endothelium should therefore not be overlooked by studying various immediate and relatively short-term responses such as changes in metabolic behavior and proliferative index.

ACKNOWLEDGMENTS

The authors wish to thank Dr. L. K. Johnson (Endocrine Research Division), Dr. P. E. Fielding (Cardiovascular Research Institute), and G. Greenburg (Cancer Research Institute) of the University of California, San Francisco, for their invaluable contributions. The expert and dedicated help of Mr. G. L. Lui and the assistance of Mr. Harvey Scodel in the preparation of this manuscript are gratefully acknowledged. This work was supported by grants HL 20197 and EY 02186 from the National Institutes of Health.

REFERENCES

1. Gospodarowicz D, Greenburg G, Bialecki H, Zetter B (1978): In Vitro 14:85.
2. Gospodarowicz D, Vlodavsky I, Greenburg G, Alvarado J, Johnson LK, Moran J (1979): Rec Prog Horm Res 35:375–448.
3. Gospodarowicz D, Vlodavsky I, Greenburg G, Johnson LK (1979): In Ross R, Sato G (eds): "Cold Spring Harbor Conferences: Hormones and Cell Culture." Cold Spring Harbor, NY: Cold Spring Harbor Laboratories (In press).
4. Gimbrone MA Jr (1976): In Spaet T (ed): "Progress in Hemostatis and Thrombosis." New York: Grune & Stratton, vol 3, pp 1–28.
5. Macarak EJ, Kirby E, Kirk T, Kefalides NA (1978): Proc Natl Acad Sci USA 75:2621–2625.
6. Weksler BB, Marcus AJ, Jaffe EA (1977): Proc Natl Acad Sci USA 74:3922–3926.
7. Stein O, Stein Y (1976): Biochim Biophys Acta 431:363–368.
8. Gospodarowicz D, Moran J, Braun D, Birdwell C (1976): Proc Natl Acad Sci USA 73:4120–4124.
9. Gospodarowicz D, Moran J, Braun DJ (1977): J Cell Physiol 91:377–386.
10. Birdwell CR, Gospodarowicz D, Nicolson GL (1978): Proc Natl Acad Sci USA 75:3273–3277.
11. Gospodarowicz D, Mescher AR, Birdwell CR (1977): Exp Eye Res. 25:75–89.
12. Engvall E, Ruoslahti E (1977): Int J Cancer 20:1–5.
13. Gospodarowicz D (1975): J Biol Chem 250:2515–2520.
14. Gospodarowicz D, Bialecki H, Greenburg G (1978): J Biol Chem 253:3736–3743.
15. Teng NNH, Chen LB (1976): Nature 259:578–580.
16. Hynes RO, Destree A (1977): Proc Natl Acad Sci USA 74:2855–2859.
17. Laemmli UK: Nature 227:680–685, 1970.
18. Wang K, Richards FM: J Biol Chem 249:8005–8018, 1974.
19. Mosher DR, Saksela O, Vaheri A: J Clin Invest 60:1036–1045, 1977.
20. Gospodarowicz D, Greenburg G, Vlodavsky I, Alvarado J, Jonson LK: Exp Eye Res (In press).
21. Havel RJ, Eder HS, Bragdon JA: J Clin Invest 34:1345–1353, 1955.
22. Basu SK, Anderson RGW, Goldstein JL, Brown MS: J Cell Biol 74:119, 1977.
23. MacFarlane AS: Nature 182:53, 1958.
24. Vlodavsky I, Fielding PE, Fielding CJ, Gospodarowicz D: Proc Natl Acad Sci USA 75:356–360, 1978.
25. Gospodarowicz D, Vlodavsky I, Fielding PE, Birdwell CR: In Littlefield JW, de Grouchy J (eds): "Birth Defects." Amsterdam: Excerpta Medica, 1978, pp 233–271.

26. Fielding PE, Vlodavsky I, Gospodarowicz D, Fielding CJ: J Biol Chem 254:749–755, 1979.
27. Goldstein JL, Basu SK, Brunschede GY, Brown MS: Cell 7:85–95, 1976.
28. Hedman K, Vaheri A, Wartiovaara J: J Cell Biol 76:748–760, 1978.
29. Chen LG, Gallimore PH, McDougall JK: Proc Natl Acad Sci USA 73:3570–3574, 1976.
30. Gahmberg CG: In Poste G, Nicolson GL (eds): "Dynamic Aspects of Cell Surface Organization. Cell Surface Reviews." vol 3. Amsterdam: Elsevier/North-Holland Biochemical Press, 1977, pp 378–412.
31. Roseman S: Chem Phys Lipids 5:270–279, 1970.
32. Vlodavsky I, Johnson LK, Gospodarowicz D: Proc Natl Acad Sci USA 76:2306–2310, 1979.
33. Goldstein JS, Brown MS: Ann Rev Biochem 46:897–930, 1977.
34. Silverstein S, Steinman RM, Cohn ZA: Ann Rev Biochem 46:669, 1977.
35. Ryan GB, Borysenko JZ, Karnovsky MJ: J Cell Biol 62:351–365, 1974.
36. Taylor RB, Duffus WPH, Raff MC, de Petris S: Nature New Biol 233:225–229, 1971.
37. Maxfield FR, Schlessinger J, Schechter Y, Pastan I, Willingham MC: Cell 14:805–810, 1978.
38. Oliver JM, Ukena TE, Berlin RD: Proc Natl Acad Sci USA 71:394–398, 1974.
39. Anderson RGW, Brown MS, Goldstein JL: Cell 10:351–364, 1977.
40. Vlodavsky I, Fielding PE, Johnson LK, Gospodarowicz D: J Cell Physiol 100:481–496, 1979.
41. Vlodavsky I, Johnson LK, Greenburg G, Gospodarowicz D: J Cell Biol 83:468–486, 1979.
42. Weiss HJ, Baumgartner HR, Tschopp TB, Turitto VT: Ann NY Acad Sci 283:293–301, 1977.
43. Yamada KM, Olden K: Nature 275:179–184, 1978.
44. Ali IU, Mautner V, Lanza R, Hynes RO: Cell 11:115–126, 1977.
45. Bornstein P, Duksin D, Balian G, Davidson JM, Crouch E: Ann NY Acad Sci 312:93–105, 1978.
46. Hynes RO, Destree A: Cell 15:875–886, 1978.
47. Heggeness MH, Ash JF, Singer SJ: Ann NY Acad Sci 312:414–419, 1978.
48. Hunt CR, Brown JC: Ann NY Acad Sci 312:418–419, 1978.
49. Furcht LT, Mosher DF, Wendelschafter-Crabb G: Cell 13:263–271, 1978.
50. Skehan P, Friedman SJ: Exp Cell Res 92:350–360, 1975.
51. Nicolau C, Hildenbrand K, Reimann A, Johnson SM, Vaheri A, Friis RR: Exp Cell Res 113:63–73, 1978.
52. Vasiliev JM, Gelfand IM, Domnina LV, Zacharova OS, Ljubimov AV: Proc Natl Acad Sci USA 72:719–722, 1975.
53. Nicolson GL, Lacorbiere MN, Hunter TR: Cancer Res 35:144–155, 1975.
54. Quinlan DC, Hochstadt J: Proc Natl Acad Sci 71:5000–5003, 1974.
55. Greenburg G, Vlodavsky I, and Gospodarowicz D: J Cell Physiol (in press).
56. Johnson LK, Baxter JD, Vlodavsky I, and Gospodarowicz D: Proc Natl Acad Sci USA (in press).

NOTE ADDED IN PROOF

In a recent communication [1], the group of Collaborative Research (CR) has described the identification of a new growth factor, endothelial cell growth factor (ECGF) isolated from brain tissue. They also report, in contrast to our own findings [2], that neither brain nor pituitary FGF had any activity on human umbilical endothelial cells. In this communication, the extraction procedure of pituitary and brain FGF used by CR is described for the first time. Although they claimed in the past that their purification was similar to the one we have described [3, 4], it differs from our own at a single but critical point. Although we insisted that brain and pituitary tissue be extracted at pH 4.5 in the presence of 0.15 M $(NH_4)_2$ SO_4, CR has been extracting the tissues in saline, ie without pH control and probably near neutrality (pH 6.5–7.0). In 1975 we reported the characterization from brain and pituitary tissue of a factor we named by its activity on the first cell type upon which it was tested, viz myoblast growth factor [5]. This factor is in all likelihood the same as the so-called ECGF and is preferentially, if not exclusively extracted at basic (8.5) as well as neutral (7.0) pHs, but not at acidic pHs [5]. In contrast, as already reported [5], FGF can only be extracted at an acidic pH of 4.5. Extraction at neutral or basic pHs results in the solubilization of little or *no* activity [5]. It is therefore not surprising that CR reports that, when a neutral pH of extraction was used, brain or pituitary FGF had no activity on endothelial cells, since this factor was never extracted from these tissues.

1. Maciag T, Cerundolo J, Isley S, Kelley PR, Forand R: Proc Natl Acad Sci USA 76:5674–5678 (1979).
2. Gospodarowicz D, Greenburg G, Bialecki H, Zetter B: In Vitro 14:85–118 (1978).
3. Gospodarowicz D: J Biol Chem 250:2515–2520 (1975).
4. Gospodarowicz D, Bialecki H, Greenburg G: J Biol Chem 253:3736–3743 (1978).
5. Gospodarowicz D, Weseman J, Moran J: Nature 256:216–219.

Journal of Supramolecular Structure 12:115−125 (1979)
Tumor Cell Surfaces and Malignancy 481−491

Ehrlich Ascites Tumor Cell Surface Labeling and Kinetics of Glycocalyx Release

Thomas C. Smith and Charles Levinson

Department of Physiology, The University of Texas Health Science Center, San Antonio, Texas 78284

Ehrlich ascites tumor cells spontaneously release cell surface material (glycocalyx) into isotonic saline medium. Exposure of these cells to tritium-labeled 4,4′-diisothiocyano-1,2-diphenylethane-2,2′-disulfonic acid ($^3H_2$ DIDS) at 4°C leads to preferential labeling of the cell surface coat. We have combined studies of the kinetics of $^3H_2$ DIDS-label release, the effects of enzymatic treatment, and cell electrophoretic mobility to characterize the $^3H_2$ DIDS-labeled components of the cell surface. Approximately 73% of the cell-associated radioactivity is spontaneously released from the cells after 5 h at 23°C. The kinetics of release is consistent with the first-order loss of two fractions; a slow ($\tau_{1/2}$ = 360 min) component representing 33% of the radioactivity, and a fast ($\tau_{1/2}$ = 20 min) component representing 26%. The remaining 14% of the labile binding may reflect mechanically induced surface release. Trypsin (1 μg/ml) also removes approximately 73% of the labeled material within 30 min and converts the kinetics of release to that of a single component ($\tau_{1/2}$ = 5.5 min). The specific activity (SA) of material released by trypsin immediately after labeling is 83% of the SA of the material spontaneously lost in 1 h. However, trypsinization following a 2-h period of spontaneous release yields material of reduced (43%) SA. Neither $^3H_2$ DIDS labeling nor the initial spontaneous loss of labeled material alters cell electrophoretic mobility. However, extended spontaneous release is accompanied by a significant decrease in surface charge density. Trypsinization immediately following labeling or after spontaneous release (2 h) reduces mobility by 32%. We have tentatively identified the slowly released compartment as contributing to cell surface negativity.

Key words: glycocalyx, cell surface, tumor cells, Ehrlich ascites tumor, surface labeling

INTRODUCTION

The external cell surface coat or glycocalyx [1] of animal cells represents a biochemically and functionally separate fraction of the cell membrane. It has been implicated as playing a major role in cell adhesion, cell recognition, and the establishment or modulation of antigenic properties of the cell [2, 3]. Perhaps related to these functions, the oligosaccharide portions of the glycocalyx impart a net surface negative charge to the cell [4].

Comparison of the peripheries from normal and malignant cells have demonstrated differences in the functional activities of glycoproteins [5], glycolipids [6], and surface

Received March 18, 1979; accepted August 17, 1979.

antigens [3, 7]. Alterations in the oligosaccharide composition of cell glycoproteins have also been noted upon transformation of BHK cells [8], leading to the hypothesis that changes in the bound carbohydrates signal malignant behavior. Loss of the glycocalyx may also be involved in tumorigenicity. The glycocalyx is a labile structure which can be removed from a variety of cells, including tumor cells, by mild treatments such as repetitive washing [9]. Malignant cells, in particular, shed glycoproteins into their environment [10]. Consequently, spontaneous shedding of surface antigens may provide a mechanism for avoidance of immunologic destruction [11].

Ehrlich ascites tumor cells have been shown to spontaneously release a variety of surface iodinated glycoproteins and glycosaminoglycans from lactoperoxidase-labeled cells after incubation in physiologic salt solution for 1 h at 4°C [12]. Comparison of enzymatic activity, and protein and sialic acid contents of the glycocalyx, with those of the plasma membrane demonstrated a clear distinction between these cellular fractions.

Recently, we have utilized the transport inhibitor, $H_2 DIDS$ (4',4'-diisothiocyano-1,2-diphenylethane-2,2'-disulfonic acid), to investigate anion transport in Ehrlich ascites tumor cells [13, 14]. Incubation of cells in the presence of $H_2 DIDS$ at 21°C results in an irreversible binding of the agent to components of the cell surface. As a consequence of binding, inhibition of sulfate transport occurs. However, cells incubated with $H_2 DIDS$ at low temperature (1–5°C) irreversibly bind the agent without concomitant transport inhibition.

Furthermore, cells labeled at either low temperature or 21°C spontaneously release $H_2 DIDS$-labeled surface proteins into their environment. In the case of transport-inhibited cells, this spontaneous release does not relieve inhibition. Protein collected from the medium is significantly enriched with respect to $H_2 DIDS$-binding compared to the whole-cell protein under all labeling conditions. These results suggest that $H_2 DIDS$ may be used as a marker for cell surface material under mild conditions which do not compromise cell integrity or viability.

While it is clear that cell surface components of these cells are labile, no studies concerning the rate of loss, or indeed whether all components are equally labile, have been reported. In the present investigation, we have employed tritiated $H_2 DIDS$ ($^3H_2 DIDS$) as a label for cell surface material. We have combined studies of the kinetics of release of $^3H_2 DIDS$-labeled surface components, and the effects of trypsin, on this process to characterize cell surface dynamics. In addition, the effect of glycocalyx removal on cell electrophoretic mobility was determined.

MATERIALS AND METHODS

Cell Suspension

Experiments were performed with Ehrlich-Lettré ascites tumor cells (hyperdiploid strain) which were maintained in Ha/ICR male mice by weekly transplantations. Tumor-bearing animals with growths of 8–11 days were used. Cells were removed from unanesthetized animals by peritoneal aspiration and washed free of ascitic fluid by gentle centrifugation and resuspension. The wash and resuspension solution had the following composition: 135 mM NaCl, 10 mM $Na_2 SO_4$, 7 mM KCl, and 10 mM Hepes-NaOH (pH 7.2–7.3; 296–301 mOsm). All experiments were also carried out in this medium. Cell suspensions (20–40 ml; 100 mg wet mass per milliliter) were placed in Ehrlenmeyer flasks under air atmosphere and incubated in an ice-bath for 5 min prior to use.

Reagents

Tritium-labeled 4,4'-diisothiocyano-1,2-diphenylethane-2,2'-disulfonic acid (^{3}H$_2$DIDS) was synthesized as previously described [14]. Trypsin (twice crystallized), trypsin inhibitor (from soybean), and neuraminidase (from Cl. perfringens) were products of Sigma Chemical Co.

^{3}H$_2$DIDS Labeling of the Cells

Cells, maintained in the resuspension medium, were incubated in the presence of ^{3}H$_2$DIDS (25 μM) for 30 min at 1–4°C. The interaction between ^{3}H$_2$DIDS and the cells was stopped by the addition of ice-cold medium containing 0.5% bovine serum albumin (Sigma Chemical Co.). Usually 40 ml of cold albumin wash solution was added per 10 ml cell suspension. The cells were separated from the medium by centrifugation (1,500g for 1 min) and the packed cells were then washed once in ice-cold albumin solution and twice in ice-cold, albumin-free medium. The labeled, packed cells were resuspended at 23°C. This procedure results in an interaction of ^{3}H$_2$DIDS with the tumor cell which is restricted to the cell surface and membrane, but which does not lead to inhibition of anion transport [14]. Aliquots of the labeled cell suspension were removed for the determination of wet and dry weight [15] and total ^{3}H$_2$DIDS binding [14] as previously described.

Kinetics of ^{3}H$_2$DIDS-Labeled Glycocalyx Release

To assess the spontaneous release of labeled glycocalyx, aliquots (0.2 ml) of the labeled cell suspension were removed periodically (1–120 min) and centrifuged (15,000g; 1 min) and the supernatant was assayed for radioactivity.

The effect of trypsin (1 μg/ml) on glycocalyx release was investigated in two ways. First, cells were permitted to spontaneously release glycocalyx for 2 h; then they were centrifuged (ca. 1,600g; 1 min) and resuspended in fresh medium containing trypsin. Aliquots (0.2 ml) were removed periodically (1–30 min) and the supernatant was assayed for radioactivity. In other studies, freshly labeled, washed cells were resuspended directly into medium containing trypsin (1 μg/ml). Loss of glycocalyx was followed for 30 min as described above.

Aliquots of cell suspensions were taken for analyses of wet and dry weights, protein, and radioactivity.

Collection of the Glycocalyx

Glycocalyx fractions from cell suspensions were prepared by a modification of the method of Rittenhouse et al [12]. Briefly, 10 ml cell suspension was added to 7 ml cold medium. (In the case of trypsin experiments, trypsin inhibitor (5 μg/ml) was included to prevent further proteolysis.) The suspension was then centrifuged (3,000g; 5 min) and the pellet discarded. The supernatant was then centrifuged (twice at 70,000g; 60 min) and the high-speed supernatant was analyzed for protein and radioactivity. Finally, the supernatant was dialyzed (6,000–8,000 MW cutoff) against deionized water (40–44 h; 1–4°C) and subsequently lyophilized. The glycocalyx material was assayed for protein and radioactivity.

Gel Electrophesis

Glycocalyx samples were heated in a boiling water bath for 5 min with 1% sodium dodecyl sulfate (SDS), 1% β-mercaptoethanol, and 0.5 mM EDTA before electrophoresis. SDS-polyacrylamide slab gels (8%) with stacking gel (5%) were prepared and run according to Laemmli [16] . Gels were stained with Coomassie blue [17] and passively destained 24 h in 7.5% acetic acid.

Cell Electrophoretic Mobility

Cell suspension for each test condition was diluted 40-fold with appropriate medium for determination of surface charge density. Mobilities were measured in a microelectro-phoresis apparatus using a cylindrical cell (Rank Bros., Bottisham, England) maintained at 23°C. A voltage gradient of 4.79 V/cm was applied between palladium electrodes, and by reversing the current each cell was timed to traverse 48 μ in both directions.

Surface charge density (σ) was estimated from the mobility by application of the Helmoholtz-Smoluchowski equation [18] . This estimation yields $\sigma = 12.1 \times 10^{-12}$ Eq/cm^2 for a mobility of 1 $\mu \cdot \sec^{-1} \cdot V^{-1} \cdot$ cm.

Analytical Procedures

Radioactivity (^{3}H) of the cell suspension and glycocalyx was assayed by liquid scin-tillation counting as previously described [14] . Protein analysis was carried out according to Hartree [19] . Sialic acid was determined by the method of Warren [20] .

RESULTS

Exposure of Ehrlich ascites tumor cells to 25 μM ^{3}H$_2$ DIDS for 30 min at 1−4°C re-sults in an association of 0.062 ± 0.006 nmoles/mg dry wt (± SEM) which is not removed by the standard washing procedure. Upon resuspension in medium, cells spontaneously lose ^{3}H$_2$ DIDS-labeled cell surface materials. Electrophoretograms of glycocalyxes collected from control (unlabeled) and ^{3}H$_2$ DIDS-labeled cells are shown in Figure 1. There is neither a quantitative nor a qualitative difference in the protein collected in the presence or absence of ^{3}H$_2$ DIDS labeling. This is indicative that the loss of surface material from these cells is not induced by ^{3}H$_2$ DIDS, but rather represents a natural pheno-menon.

The time course of release is shown in Figure 2. There is an initial rapid loss of radio-activity followed by a slower release up to 120 min, at which time 45.9 ± 1.2% of the cell-associated radioactivity has been released into the medium. Experiments extended to 5 h show a total loss of 72.5% of the initial bound ^{3}H$_2$ DIDS.

Addition of trypsin (1 μg/ml) to cell suspension 120 min after resuspension leads to accelerated appearance of additional labeled material in the medium (Fig. 2). Thirty minutes after trypsin addition 71.0 ± 2.1% of total bound ^{3}H$_2$ DIDS has been released from the cells.

Freshly ^{3}H$_2$ DIDS-labeled cells resuspended directly into medium containing trypsin (1 μg/ml) rapidly shed cell surface material (Fig. 3), but not 100% of that bound to the cells. If it is assumed that the release of labeled cell surface material is a first-order process from a single trypsin-sensitive compartment, then the appearance of radioactivity in the medium can be described by:

$$\ln [x(t) - x (\infty)] / [x(0) - x(\infty)] = -kt \qquad (1)$$

where x(0), x(t), and x(∞) are the percentages of total ^{3}H$_2$ DIDS-labeled material released to the medium at times zero, t, and infinity, respectively, and k is the rate constant (min^{-1}) describing the release. Analysis of the data (Fig. 3) provides a best fit (r = 0.99) with k =

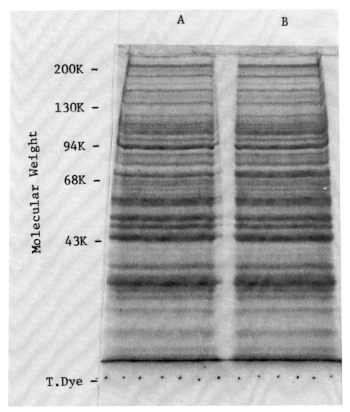

Fig. 1. Electrophoretograms of glycocalyx isolated from unlabeled control (A) and $^3H_2$DIDS-labeled (B) tumor cells. Control and $^3H_2$DIDS-labeled cells were washed and incubated (60 min at 23°C) in fresh medium to permit release of glycocalyx protein. The glycocalyx was collected and analyzed for protein distribution by SDS-polyacrylamide slab gel (8%) electrophoresis. Proteins were stained with Coomassie blue. Control cells released 0.014 mg protein per milligram cell protein in 60 min while $^3H_2$DIDS labeled cells released 0.013 mg protein per milligram cell protein.

0.125 ± 0.012 min^{-1} ($\pm$ SE) and $x(\infty) = 74.3 \pm 1.2\%$ ($\pm$ SE). This is indicative that trypsin will release $74.3 \pm 1.2\%$ of the total $^3H_2$DIDS-labeled cell surface material.

Under all of the conditions studied the maximum release of labeled material approximates 71–74% total bound $^3H_2$DIDS. Consequently, to better define the kinetics of release of the labeled surface components we have analyzed the data according to Equation 1 with $x(\infty) = 0.73 \times$ bound $^3H_2$DIDS. The spontaneous release (Fig. 2) is consistent with loss from at least two surface compartments. Extrapolation of the final four points defines a slow compartment with a half-time ($\tau_{1/2}$) of 360 min, which represents 45% of the labile material (33% of total bound $^3H_2$DIDS). Subtraction of this compartment from the total loss reveals a second compartment ($\tau_{1/2} = 20$ min) which represents 36% of the labile pool (26% of total bound $^3H_2$DIDS). The remaining (14% total bound) labile material may represent a very rapid initial loss of labeled material which occurs upon resuspension of the cells.

Trypsin, added after 120 min of spontaneous release, converts the kinetics to that of a single labile pool with $\tau_{1/2} = 7.2$ min. A similar result is obtained for loss from cells resus-

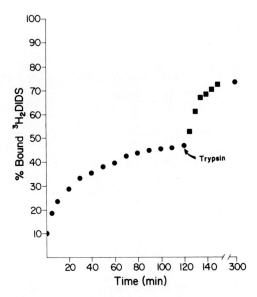

Fig. 2. Release of $^3H_2DIDS$-labeled cell surface components. Cells were exposed to $^3H_2DIDS$ (25 μm) for 30 min at 1–4°C, then washed free of $^3H_2DIDS$ and resuspended in fresh medium at 23°C. Aliquots of the cell suspension were removed at specified times (1–120 min and 5 h) and assayed for radioactivity in the medium. Release to the medium is reported as percentage of the initial total binding. Values shown (●) are the averages for nine experiments. In four of these experiments, trypsin (1 μg/ml) was added to cell suspension after 2 h of spontaneous release and the release of bound $^3H_2DIDS$ was followed for 30 min (■). Standard errors of the mean were smaller than the symbols and are not shown.

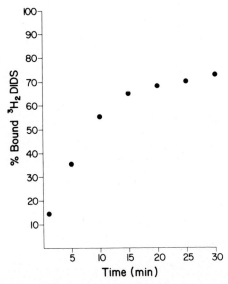

Fig. 3. Effect of trypsin on release of $^3H_2$ DIDS-labeled cell surface components. Cells were exposed to $^3H_2$ DIDS as before (Fig. 1) and resuspended in fresh medium containing trypsin (1 μg/ml) at 23°C. Aliquots of the cell suspension were removed at specified times (1–30 min) and assayed for radioactivity in the medium. Release to the medium is reported as percentage of the total initial $^3H_2$ DIDS bound. Values are averages for four experiments. Standard errors of the mean were smaller than the symbols and are not shown.

pended initially into trypsin. In this case the trypsinization results in a slightly accelerated release of surface label ($\tau_{\frac{1}{2}}$ = 5.5 min).

Glycocalyx Fraction

The glycocalyx fractions collected from cell suspensions used for the kinetic studies were assayed for protein and radioactivity. The results are given in Table I.

Glycocalyx collected from cell suspension (10 ml) incubated for 2 h in medium contains 2.18 ± 0.15 mg protein (1.88 ± 0.23% total cell protein) with a specific activity of 3.85 ± 0.53 × 10^6 cpm/mg protein. This represents a 19.7-fold enrichment of $^3H_2$ DIDS label compared to total cell protein. Resuspension of these cells in trypsin-containing medium (1 μg/ml; 30 min) results in an additional release of protein of 2.47 ± 0.23 mg (2.32 ± 0.29% total cell protein) having specific activity (1.50 ± 0.16 × 10^6 cpm/mg protein).

Glycocalyx derived from cells exposed to trypsin for 1 h immediately after $^3H_2$ DIDS labeling contains 250% more protein than comparable control cells. While the specific activity of glycocalyx from trypsin-treated cells in 83% of control, the difference is not significant for three experiments. However, in each of the experiments the specific activity of control glycocalyx exceeded that after trypsinization.

In a single experiment we compared the sialic acid contents of glycocalyx collected from spontaneous and trypsin-induced release to that released by neuraminidase (100 units/ ml). Glycocalyx collected from control cells contained no detectable sialic acid, while trypsinization resulted in glycocalyx containing 12.5% of the sialic acid available to neuraminidase treatment (0.20 nmoles/mg dry wt versus 1.60 nmoles/mg dry wt).

Cell Electrophoretic Mobility and Surface Charge Density

The electrophoretic mobilities of Ehrlich ascites tumor cells in these studies are shown in Figure 4. The mobiliy of cells washed free of ascitic fluid with medium is 0.86 ± 0.01 μ· $sec^{-1} \cdot V^{-1} \cdot cm$ (±SE) (σ = 1.06 × 10^{-11} Eq/cm^2). An additional wash with medium contain-

TABLE I. Collection of Glycocalyx

Experimental procedure	Protein recovered in supernatant, mg (% cell protein)	SA: Protein recovered in supernatant (cpm/mg protein × 10^{-6})	SA: Total cell protein (cpm/mg protein × 10^{-6})
A. Consecutive Collection (2)[a]			
Control	2.18 ± 0.15 (1.88 ± 0.23)	3.85 ± 0.53	0.20 ± 0.02
Experimental	2.47 ± 0.23 (2.32 ± 0.29)	1.50 ± 0.16	0.09 ± 0.01
B. Simultaneous Collection (3)[a]			
Control	1.08 ± 0.22 (0.88 ± 0.01)	4.21 ± 0.39	0.15 ± 0.03
Experimental	2.65 ± 0.60 (2.16 ± 0.23)	3.50 ± 0.46	0.15 ± 0.03

Collection of glycocalyx. Cells were exposed to $^3H_2$ DIDS (25 μM) for 30 min at 1–4°C, then washed with 0.5% albumin-containing medium. A: Consecutive collection (10 ml cell suspension): Cells were resuspended in fresh medium for 2 h and the supernatant collected (control). The cells were then resuspended in fresh medium plus trypsin (1 μg/ml) for 30 min and the resulting supernatant was again collected (experimental). B: Simultaneous collection: Cell suspension was divided and the cells (10 ml cell suspension) incubated in the absence (control) or presence (experimental) of trypsin (1 μg/ml) for 1 h prior to glycocalyx collection. The supernatants were analyzed for total protein and radioactivity.

[a]Number of experiments. Standard errors of the mean are given.

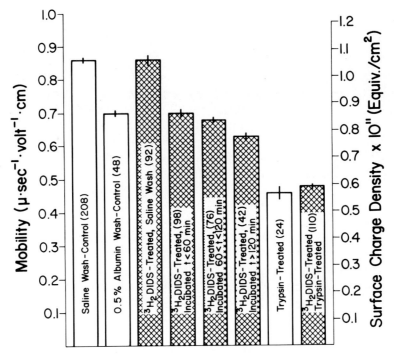

Fig. 4. Effect of $^3H_2$DIDS binding and release on cell electrophoretic mobility and surface charge density. Conditions describing the cell treatment are given in each bar. Cell suspensions were diluted 40-fold with the appropriate media and the electrophoretic mobility was determined at 23°C. Number of determinations for each condition is given in parentheses. Standard errors of the mean are shown.

ing 0.5% albumin reduces the mobility to 0.70 ± 0.01 $\mu \cdot sec^{-1} \cdot V^{-1} \cdot cm$. To determine whether the reduction in mobility after albumin wash reflected an actual loss of surface charge or simply "masking" by absorbed albumin, we determined the mobility of cells washed with medium and resuspended in medium containing 0.5% albumin. The mobility (not shown) was not different from saline-washed cells.

Labeling of cells with $^3H_2$DIDS followed by either medium or albumin-containing wash does not alter the cell mobility compared to the appropriate control. During the first or second hour of spontaneous glycocalyx loss there is no significant change in mobility. However, cells which have been incubated for 2 h (plus 30 min for measurements) have a significantly ($P < 0.05$) reduced mobility (0.63 ± 0.02 $\mu \cdot sec^{-1} \cdot V^{-1} \cdot cm$).

Trypsin treatment of unlabeled cells washed with either medium or 0.5% albumin-containing medium reduces the mobility by 35%. The presence of bound $^3H_2$DIDS does not alter the effect of trypsin on cell mobility.

DISCUSSION

These studies demonstrate that incubation of Ehrlich ascites tumor cells with $^3H_2$DIDS (25 μM; 30 min) at 1–4°C results in an irreversible binding of this agent (0.062 ± 0.006 nmoles/mg dry wt) to the cell surface. Previous studies from our laboratory established that the $^3H_2$DIDS associated with the cell using identical conditions was confined to the surface and did not enter the cells. Furthermore, the cells maintain viability as judged by Trypan blue exclusion ($> 96\%$) and capacity to accumulate amino acid [14].

Resuspension of labeled cells in fresh medium at $23°C$ resulted in the spontaneous release of surface proteins into the medium (Fig. 2). Kinetic analysis of this process indicates the existence of at least three major binding populations. Approximately 27% of the bound $^3H_2 DIDS$ is associated with components of the cell which are not released spontaneously or by mild trypsination. The remaining 73% of bound $^3H_2 DIDS$ is spontaneously released from two major labeled compartments representing 33% ($\tau_{1/2}$ = 360 min) and 26% ($\tau_{1/2}$ = 20 min) of the total binding, respectively.

The existence of two kinetically dissimilar surface compartments does not imply that only two chemical components are spontaneously lost by the cell. The sensitivity of the kinetic analysis does not permit the separation of components which have similar rates of loss. Chemical analysis [12] and polyacrylamide gel electrophoresis [Fig. 1] of glycocalyx derived from Ehrlich ascites tumor cells have shown the presence of a complex mixture of proteins and glycosaminoglycans. Thus it is likely that each of the kinetically identifiable compartments represents a mixture of surface macromolecules which are shed with similar rates.

One possible explanation for the different rates of release is a combination of surface shedding and internalization of cell membrane with subsequent secretion [21]. However, the effect of mild trypsination on the release of labeled material argues against this mechanism. All of the labile $^3H_2 DIDS$-labeled components are readily accessible to trypsin. Since trypsin at the concentration used does not alter cell viability, it is unlikely that it could accelerate the release of internalized membrane components destined for secretion.

The most likely explanation for these findings is that the two labile compartments are spontaneously shed into the environment at different rates. Trypsin has access to both and hydrolyzes them at similar rates. This is reflected by conversion of the kinetics of release to that of a single population.

It is not possible in the present study to identify the source of the shed material. However, Rittenhouse and co-workers [22] have recently shown that approximately 30% of the total protein which is spontaneously shed by these cells is in the form of high-molecular weight aggregates which contain host-derived, tumor-associated immunoglobulin G (TAIg) and a complement component (C3). Numerous tumor-derived glycoproteins are present in shed material, but only one of these (45K) is associated with the host-derived components [23]. Thus, our finding of two kinetic compartments would be consistent with a combined process of release of immune complexes and natural cell surface turnover.

The bound $^3H_2 DIDS$ (27%) which is not subject to either spontaneous release or trypsin hydrolysis may represent an association with surface components inaccessible to trypsin or binding interaction at a site distal to trypsin hydrolysis. In the erythrocyte, $H_2 DIDS$ interaction with the anion transport protein occurs at a site interior to cleavage by trypsin [24]. Similarly, anion transport inhibition by $H_2 DIDS$ in Ehrlich ascites cells is not relieved by spontaneous loss of the glycocalyx [25], suggesting that $H_2 DIDS$ binds to protein components of the cell membrane which are not labile.

Comparison of the glycocalyxes prepared by trypsinization of freshly labeled cells and cells which have been incubated for 2 h prior to trypsin treatment is revealing. Both treatments release equivalent amounts of protein (Table I) and result in the same total loss of bound $^3H_2 DIDS$ (Figs. 2 and 3). However, the specific activity of glycocalyx from cells which had spontaneously shed material prior to trypsin treatment is only 43% of that from freshly labeled cells. This reduction in specific activity might result from an exposure of trypsin-sensitive protein previously masked by the glycocalyx. Since trypsin itself effectively removes the $^3H_2$DIDS-labeled labile components of the glycocalyx within 30 min, the same exposure should occur. If spontaneous release unmasks cryptic protein, we would expect an extended exposure to trypsin to hydrolyze at least an equivalent amount of protein. However, the total protein collected after 2 h of spontaneous release plus 30 min in trypsin exceeds that removed by 1 h in trypsin. This makes an unmasking effect unlikely, in agreement with previous conclusions based on access of the cell surface to iodination [12].

Consequently, the reduction in specific activity after spontaneous release and the increase in total protein subject to spontaneous release plus trypsin suggest that new cell surface material has been incorporated into the glycocalyx during the incubation period (2 h). This suggestion is in concert with the view that surface membrane components are constantly renewed by insertion of newly synthesized molecules to replace those shed into the environment [26]. If this is the case, the kinetic experiments reported here provide an estimate of the rates of turnover of the glycocalyx components.

In an effort to further characterize the interaction of $^3H_2$DIDS with the cell surface, we have examined the effects of labeling and subsequent removal on the cell electrophoretic mobility. Ehrlich ascites tumor cells carry a net negative surface charge. Much of the surface negativity can be abolished by neuraminidase treatment [27], indicating an important contribution from bound sialic acid. In addition, it has been suggested that a large portion of the cellular, negatively charged glycosaminoglycans are located at the cell periphery [12].

In the present studies, the binding of $^3H_2$DIDS to the cell surface is without effect on surface charge density. Subsequent spontaneous loss of the glycocalyx does not alter mobility during the initial phase (Fig. 4). However, after 2 h of incubation there is a significant decline in surface charge density. This temporal pattern of surface charge change can be compared to the kinetics of spontaneous $^3H_2$DIDS label release, suggesting that only the more slowly released population ($\tau_{1/2}$ = 360 min) contributes to the alteration in cell surface charge.

The glycocalyx collected by spontaneous release from these cells contains no sialic acid [12]. Others have demonstrated the presence of glycosaminoglycans in glycocalyx collected by gentle elution [12]. It seems likely, then, that the charge-bearing, slowly released surface material contains significant amounts of glycosaminoglycans.

Trypsin treatment of the cells further reduces the surface charge density and hydrolyzes the labile compartments of the cell surface (Figs. 2 and 3). Glycocalyx collected from these cells contains 12.5% of the sialic acid which can be released by neuraminidase. Whether the sialic acid-containing glycoproteins which are susceptible to trypsin (1 $\mu g/ml$) contributed the cell mobility is not clear. Trypsin, at the concentration used, readily removes glycosaminoglycans from the cell surface [28]. This is consistent with both glycoproteins and glycosaminoglycans contributing to the altered mobility, but does not necessarily indicate that sialic acid-associated glycoproteins constitute part of the slowly desorbed surface components.

Taken together, the results of this investigation demonstrate the applicability of $^3H_2$DIDS as a label for cell surface constituents. $^3H_2$DIDS irreversibly interacts with three major populations of cell surface components. One of these does not dissociate from the surface during the time course of the experiments. The other two are spontaneously released by the cell with measurably different rates. It is likely that this represents different rates of surface protein turnover. Alterations in the cell surface charge density suggest that the more slowly desorbing of these labile compartments is rich in the glycosaminoglycans of the cell surface.

ACKNOWLEDGMENTS

This study was supported by grant CA 10917, US Public Health Service, National Cancer Institute.

We gratefully acknowledge the excellent technical assistance of Mrs. Rebecca Corcoran, Ms. Ellen Edwards, and Mrs. Carmen DuBose.

REFERENCES

1. Bennet HS: J Histochem Cytochem 11:14, 1963.
2. Stuhlmiller GM, Siegler HF: J Natl Cancer Inst 58:215, 1977.
3. Coddington JF, Sanford BH, Jeanloz RW: J Natl Cancer Inst 51:585, 1973.
4. Weiss L: In: "The Cell Periphery, Metastasis and Other Contact Phenomena." New York: Wiley, 1967.
5. Hynes RO, Humphreys KC: J Cell Biol 62:438, 1975.
6. Hakomori S: Adv Cancer Res 18:265, 1973.
7. Baldwin RW: Adv Cancer Res 18:1, 1973.
8. Warren L, Clayton AB, Tuszynski GP: Biochim Biophys Acta 516:97, 1978.
9. Kilarski W: Canc Res 35:2797, 1975.
10. Kim W, Baumler A, Carruthers C, Bielat K: Proc Natl Acad Sci USA 72:1012, 1975.
11. Sjogren HO, Hellstrom I, Bansal SC, Warner GA, Hellstrom KE: Int J Cancer 9:274, 1972.
12. Rittenhouse HG, Rittenhouse JW, Takemoto L: Biochemistry 17:829, 1978.
13. Levinson C, Corcoran RJ, Edwards EH: J Membrane Biol 45:61, 1979.
15. Levinson C, Villereal MV: J Cell Physiol 85:1, 1975.
16. Laemmli UK: Nature 227:680, 1970.
17. Fairbanks G, Steck TL, Wallach DFH: Biochemistry 10:2606, 1971.
18. Abramson HA, Moyer LS, Gorin M: In "Electrophoresis of Proteins and Chemistry of Cell Surfaces." New York: Reinhold, 1942, p. 108.
19. Hartree EA: Anal Biochem 48:422, 1972.
20. Warren L: J Biol Cehm 234:1971, 1959.
21. Scanlin TF, Glick MC: In Jamieson GA, Robinson DM (eds): "Mammalian Cell Membranes." London: Butterworths, 1977, vol 5, pp 1–46.
22. Rittenhouse HG, Ar D, Lynn MD, Denholm DK: J Supramol Struct 9:407, 1978.
23. Rader RL, Rittenhouse HG, Lynn MD, Ar D, Moon MM: J Supramol Struct (Suppl 3) 9:538, 1979.
24. Rothstein A, Grinstein S, Ship S, Knauf PA: Trends Biochem Sci 3:126, 1978.
25. Levinson, C: Ann NY Acad Sci (In press).
26. Hughes RC, Sanford B, Jeanloz RW: Proc Natl Acad Sci USA 69:942, 1972.
27. Wallach DFH, Eylar EH: Biochim Biophys Acta 52:594, 1961.
28. Chiarugi VP, Vannucchi S, Urbano P: Biochim Biophys Acta 345:283, 1974.

Journal of Supramolecular Structure 12:127–137 (1979)
Tumor Cell Surfaces and Malignancy 493–503

Polyoma T (Tumor) Antigen Species in Abortively and Stably Transformed Cells

Thomas L. Benjamin, Brian S. Schaffhausen, and Jonathan E. Silver

Department of Pathology, Harvard Medical School, Boston, Massachusetts 02115

Stable neoplastic transformation of cells by polyoma virus requires the participation of two viral genes, designated *ts-a* and *hr-t*. The effects of mutations in these two genes on the patterns of T-antigen synthesis during productive infection have been previously described: ts-a mutants are affected in the "large" (100K) nuclear T antigen, and hr-t mutants are affected in the "middle" (36K, 56K, 63K) and "small" (22K) T antigens. The latter are associated predominantly with the plasma membrane (56K) and cytosol fractions, respectively.

Here we examine the expression of the various forms of polyoma T antigen in nonproductive infection (abortive transformation) as well as in stably transformed cell lines of different species. The results on abortive transformation are essentially the same as those described above for productive infection. In stably transformed cells, the middle and small T antigens are seen to various extents. The large T antigen, however, is often absent or present below the level of detection. Clones lacking the large T antigen are found most often among mouse transformants, but are also seen among rat transformants. Retention of the 100K species in transformed cells therefore appears to be, at least in part, an inverse function of the level of permissivity of the host toward productive viral infection. These findings indicate that the induction of the transformed phenotype in both abortively and stably transformed cells generally does not require the large T antigen, but rather the products of the hr-t gene.

Key words: polyoma virus; large, middle, and small tumor antigens; ts-a; hr-t; abortive transformation; transformed cells.

Mouse cells undergo predominantly a productive infection by polyoma virus, although occasionally they may become transformed. The reverse is true for rat and hamster cells, which undergo predominantly a nonproductive infection. The latter kind of infection leads first to an abortive transformation in which up to 50% of the cells become transformed within 24–48 h after infection. The majority of these altered cells revert to a normal phenotype after a few cell divisions [1]. A few percent, however, will remain stably transformed. Stable transformants contain integrated viral DNA and express virus-

Received June 26, 1979; accepted June 26, 1979.

specific proteins called T, or tumor, antigens [2]. Although direct evidence is lacking, it is plausible that a failure of stable integration of viral DNA in abortive transformants leads to a loss of the transformed phenotype.

The hr-t and ts-a mutants define two viral gene functions essential for stable transformation [3,4]. While neither type of mutant can stably transform cells, ts-a mutants are capable of abortively transforming cells at the nonpermissive temperature [5,6]. Various cellular parameters of transformation have been used to monitor abortive transformation, such as growth in soft agar, morphologic changes, lectin agglutinability, and loss of stress fibers [3]; hr-t mutants fail to induce these changes [6,7–9], while ts-a mutants induce them in a manner essentially identical to the abortive transformation phase of a wild-type viral infection [5,6,8,10]. These results show a requirement for the hr-t gene function in the induction of abortive transformation. They also suggest a persisting role for these proteins in maintaining the stably transformed state.

The present study describes the T-antigen species induced by wild-type and mutant strains of polyoma virus during abortive transformation, and shows them to be the same as previously described for productive infection. A survey of stably transformed cell lines shows that the hr-t products continue to be expressed, while the 100K product of the ts-a gene may or may not persist, depending in part on the permissiveness of the host for viral DNA replication.

MATERIALS AND METHODS

Cell Lines and Viruses

A derivative of the Pasadena small-plaque strain of polyoma virus was used to transform cells from various established lines of mouse or rat origin. Py-3T3-6 was derived from Swiss mouse 3T3 cells [11]; five polyoma transformants and four SV-40 transformants were obtained from Balb-3T3 clone A-31 cells. Rat cells of the NRK, BN, and F-111 cell lines were transformed by polyoma virus. All transformants were either directly isolated or eventually cloned in soft agar.

De novo infections of rat F-111 cells were carried out with different virus strains at multiplicities of 5–50 plaque-forming units (PFU) per cell to study T-antigen species made during the period of abortive transformation. Wild-type polyoma, hr-t mutants NG-18 and NG-59 [11], and ts-a mutants ts-616 and ts-25D [12,13] were used.

Labeling and Immunoprecipitation

Polyoma anti-T serum was obtained as ascites fluid of brown Norwegian rats inoculated with a syngeneic polyoma virus-transformed cell adapted to grow as a transplantable ascites tumor. Procedures for labeling of cells, extraction, T-antigen immunoprecipitation, and analysis by gel electrophoresis have all been described [14,15]. Briefly, exponential cells were grown in Dulbecco's modified Eagle's medium plus 5% calf serum, and labeled in methionine-free medium with [^{35}S] methionine (20–100 μCi/ml, 400 Ci/mmole) for 2–4 h at 37°C, or as indicated in the figure legends. Labeled cells were washed and extracted with a pH 9 buffer containing NP-40. The clarified extracts were incubated with 5–10 μl of anti-T serum and the immune precipitates collected on Staphylococcus protein A-Sepharose beads. Washed immunoprecipitates were dissociated and electrophoresed on 12.5% acrylamide gels in the presence of sodium dodecyl sulfate (SDS).

TABLE I. Test for the Induction of Abortive and Stable Transformation by Transformation-Defective Mutants of Polyoma Virus*

Virus 5–10 PFU/cell	Abortive transformation[a]		Stable transformation[b]		T antigen[c]	
	33°C	39.5°C	33°C	39.5°C	33°C	39.5°C
Polyoma, wild-type	20	23	120	152	80	80
Polyoma TS-616	17	29	25	0	80	3
Polyoma NG-18	0.3	0.3	0	0	80	80
Control F-111 cells	0.3	0.2	0	0	- -	- -

*Data from Fluck M, Benjamin T [6].
[a]Percentage of population undergoing more than one division, scored after 10 days at 33°C or 5 days at 39.5°C.
[b]Macroscopic clones per 10^4 infected cells, scored after 30 days at 33°C or 18 days at 39.5°C.
[c]Percentage of population with nuclear immunofluorescence.

RESULTS

Abortive Transformation

Table I shows results of tests for abortive and stable transformation of F-111 rat cells by wild-type polyoma virus, hr-t mutant NG-18, or a ts-a class mutant, ts-616 [6]. The mutant ts-616 induces abortive transformation in a temperature-independent way, as shown by the early proliferation of cells in soft agar at the high as well as at the low temperature. Similar results for ts-a were reported earlier by Stoker and Dulbecco using BHK (hamster) fibroblasts [5]. When the same F-111 cultures are scored later for macroscopic clones corresponding to stable transformants, the temperature-sensitivity of the ts-616 infected cells is evident. Thus, the ts-a function is not required to *induce* anchorage-independent growth, but rather to *secure* that property in a stably inherited fashion. A failure of stable integration of the viral DNA in cells abortively transformed by ts-a mutants has been suggested as the basis for these findings [6]. In the same experiment, hr-t mutant NG-18 is unable to induce even transient growth in soft agar, showing that the hr-t function is required for anchorage-independent growth [6,7].

T-Antigen Expression During Abortive Transformation Compared With Productive Infection Infection

Sera from rats or hamsters carrying tumors derived from syngeneic polyoma-transformed cells have been used to immunoprecipitate T antigens from cells productively infected by wild-type polyoma virus and various mutants. Labeling of infected cells with ^{35}S methionine, followed by immune precipitation and SDS-polyacrylamide gel electrophoresis, has led to the identification of a large T antigen (100K), a small T antigen (22K), and one or more middle-sized antigens (36K–63K) [14–17]. Work from several laboratories has shown that the 100K T antigen, localized predominantly in the nucleus, is thermolabile in pulse-chase experiments in ts-a mutant-infected cells [15,16]. The hr-t mutants of the deletion type, such as NG-18, make normal amounts of the 100K species, but fail to make any of the middle or small T antigens [14]. The hr-t mutants of the nondeletion type, such as NG-59, again induce normal 100K, but also induce a 56K

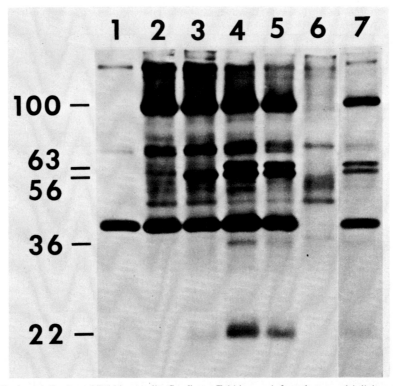

Fig. 1. De novo infection of F-111 rat cells. Confluent F-111 were infected at a multiplicity of infection of 5–20 PFU per cell. Cells at 32°C were pulse-labeled at 44 h after infection for 45 min in Hanks's salts containing 100 μCi/ml[^{35}S]methionine. Cells at 39°C were pulse-labeled at 30 h after infection for 20 min in the same medium. Cells were extracted and T antigens collected as described in Materials and Methods, using either preimmune serum or anti-T ascites. 1, Control cell extracts, 32°C, precipitated with anti-T ascites; 2, NG18-infected cells, 32°C, anti-T ascites; 3, NG-59-infected cells, 32°C, anti-T ascites; 4, ts-25D-infected cells 32°C, anti-T ascites; 5, wild-type-infected cells, 32°C, anti-T ascites; 6, wild-type-infected cells, 32°C, preimmune serum; 7, ts-25D-infected cells, immune serum, 39°C.

middle T species and a 22K small T species, the latter in very reduced amounts [15]. Both NG-18 and NG-59 fail to show two other middle-sized T-antigen species (63K and 36K) made by wild-type virus and ts-a mutants [14,15]. From peptide mapping data, it appears that the hr-t region of the polyoma DNA codes for the C-terminal portion of the small T antigen, and that the same sequences also code for part of the 56K middle T species [18,19]. Cell fractionation experiments have shown the 56K species to be associated with the plasma membrane, and the 22K to be largely in the cytosol fraction [15,17].

To examine the T-antigen patterns in a nonproductive infection, F-111 rat cells were infected by NG-18, NG-59, ts-25D, or wild-type virus. The results of immunoprecipitation followed by gel electrophoresis and autoradiography are shown in Figure 1. Lanes 1–6 are from cells incubated and labeled at 33°C. The results are strictly parallel to those reported earlier for lytic infection: NG-18 (lane 2) induces only 100K; NG-59 (lane 3) induces 100K, a 56K species, and reduced amounts of a 22K species (seen here by overexposing the film); ts-25D (lane 4) and wild-type virus (lane 5) induce all five species – 100K, 63K, 56K, 36K, and 22K. Since ts-25D, like ts-616, abortively transforms F-111 cells at 39.5°C, its T-antigen pattern was also examined at the high temperature; as seen in lane 7, all five T-antigen species are seen. In pulse-chase experiments, the 100K band of ts-25D proved to be thermolabile, as previously shown for lytic infection [15]. The patterns with wild-type virus and hr-t mutants are independent of the temperature. These results show that under conditions of abortive transformation, hr-t and ts-a mutants induce the same T-antigen species as in lytic infection. Thus, anchorage-independent growth occurs only in cell populations expressing hr-t gene products, ie, middle and small T antigens; a normal large T antigen is neither sufficient nor necessary for abortive transformation.

Patterns of T Antigen in Stably Transformed Rat Cells

A series of wild-type polyoma virus-transformed rat cells, isolated as macroscopic clones in soft agar, were examined for their T antigens. Figure 2A shows results with five

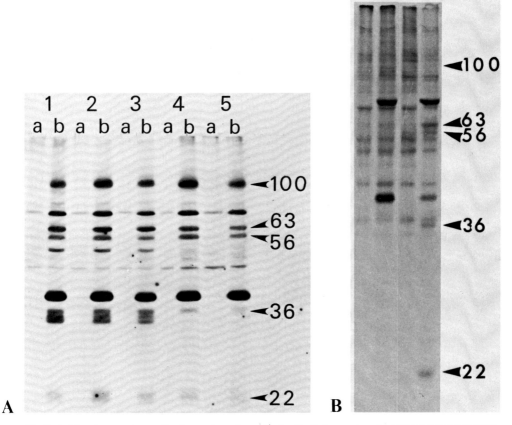

Fig. 2. A: T-antigen patterns of polyoma-transformed rat cells. Polyoma-transformed rat cells were pulse labeled during exponential growth for 1h in phosphate-buffered saline (PBS) containing 20 μCi/ml [^{35}S] methionine. The T antigens were extracted, precipitated, and electrophoresed as described in Materials and Methods. 1, PyB4; 2, PyB4TA; 3, PyB4T; 4, PyF; 5, PyNRK-Cl 1. a, Preimmune serum; b, anti-T ascites. B: Patterns of T antigens in polyoma-transformed normal rat kidney (PyNRK) cells. Cells were labeled for 10 h in Dulbecco's modified Eagle's medium lacking methionine and containing 20 μCi/ml [^{35}S] methionine. T antigens were extracted, precipitated, and separated as described in Materials and Methods. a, NRK, preimmune serum; b, NRK, anti-T ascites. c, PyNRK-Cl 3, preimmune serum; d, PyNRK-Cl 3, anti-T ascites.

such clones isolated from three different established rat embryo fibroblast lines. All show large, middle, and small T antigen species, some with multiple bands around 36K. Retention of the complete set of T-antigen species in transformed rat cells is not an invariable rule, as shown by the polyoma-transformed NRK cell in Figure 2B. This clone shows no detectable 100K species but does show middle and small T antigens. Relatively intense bands with an apparent molecular weight around 75K are seen in de novo infections as well as some transformed cell lines (Fig. 1 and Fig. 2A,B). However, such bands are seen in preimmune and normal cell controls so they cannot represent viral products.

It is our experience that transformed rat cells are positive for nuclear T-antigen immunofluorescence immediately after isolation, but may become negative after continued cultivation or subcloning. This loss of nuclear T antigen upon serial passage is not accompanied by any loss or diminution in any parameter of the transformed phenotype as far as we have been able to determine. That the predominant nuclear T antigen is the 100K species [15,16] provides additional support for the idea that the large T antigen is not required after transformation has been established.

Patterns of T Antigen in Stably Transformed Mouse Cells

A similar investigation of polyoma-transformed mouse cells was carried out. Such transformants are most readily obtained by partially inactivating the virus by X-rays or UV irradiation to produce a preferential loss of replicating over transforming ability [20]. Receptor-destroying enzyme and antiviral antiserum are added after infection to protect the rare transformants from being reinfected and killed [11]. Figure 3A shows the results with five independently derived clones of Balb-3T3 clone A-31 transformed by irradiated virus [21]. All are free of infectious virus, and are capable of growth in soft agar. The 100K T antigen is not detected in any of the five clones, while the middle and small T antigens are present in varying amounts in all of them. The same pattern is seen in Py-3T3-6 cells (Fig. 3B), a derivative of Swiss-3T3 cells used in the original isolation of hr-t mutants [11]. This line, and a second one from Swiss 3T3, are negative for T-antigen nuclear fluorescence. These two clones were obtained with unirradiated virus; thus, the absence of 100K T antigen in the Balb-3T3 transformants is not necessarily due to the use of partially inactivated virus.

It is interesting that virus-specific RNA in Py-3T3-6 cells is homologous only to the proximal part of the early region which includes the hr-t gene, and not to the distal or "ts-a" part [22]. Tests for early viral gene functions in some of these polyoma mouse transformants have shown that they are permissive for hr-t mutant growth [21], and fail to complement ts-a mutant growth at the high temperature [3]. These observations taken together point clearly to the persistence and functioning of the hr-t gene in transformed mouse cells, and to the absence of a functioning ts-a gene.

In a survey of 13 independently isolated clones of mouse cells transformed by polyoma virus, 11 showed no evidence of a 100K T antigen species. The higher frequency of

---

Fig. 3. A: T-antigen patterns of polyoma-transformed Balb/3T3 cells (A31). Cells were labeled for 90 min in Hanks's salt solution containing 5% dialyzed calf serum and 40 μCi/ml [^{35}S] methionine. The T antigens were extracted, precipitated, and electrophoresed as described in Materials and Methods. 1, A31; 2, PyA31-Cl 1; 3, PyA31-Cl 4,PyA31-Cl 6; 5, PyA31-Cl 12; 6, PyA31-Cl 38, a, Preimmune serum; b, anti-T ascites. B: T-antigen patterns of Py-3T3-6 cells. Cells were pulse-labeled for 1 h in Hanks's salt solution containing 10% dialyzed calf serum and 100 μCi/ml [^{35}S] methionine. T antigens were extracted, immuneprecipitated, and electrophoresed as indicated in Materials and Methods. a, Preimmune serum; b, Anti-T ascites.

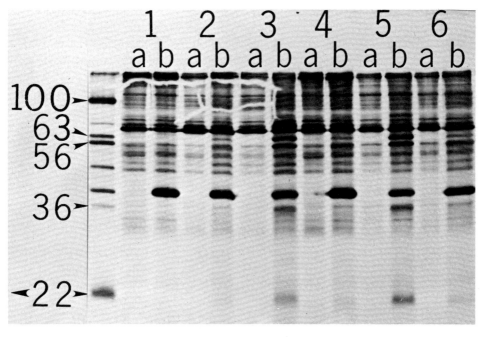

A

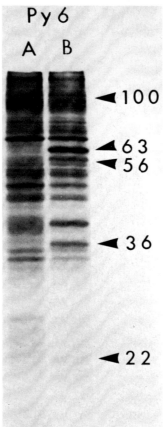

3B

large T antigen-negative clones among mouse compared to rat transformants may be explained by the fact that mouse cells are far more permissive than rat cells to viral DNA replication, a process in which the ts-a gene plays a direct role [23]. Thus, if viral DNA replication were lethal for the cell, one would expect a stronger selection against retention of the 100K T antigen in mouse versus rat transformants.

Retention of the Large T Antigen in SV-40-Transformed Mouse Cells

The argument relating permissivity of the host to selection against expression of large T antigen was tested by examining Balb-3T3 clone A-31 cells transformed by SV-40. These cells are nonpermissive for SV-40 DNA replication. Four out of four clones examined show persistence of the large T antigen (Fig. 4). The 94K protein is the product of the SV-40 "A" gene, and as in the case of the polyoma virus 100K protein, it is required for the initiation of viral DNA synthesis during productive infection [24]. These results lend further support to the idea that the permissivity of the host to viral DNA replication is a major factor in the failure of stably transformed cells to express the large T antigen.

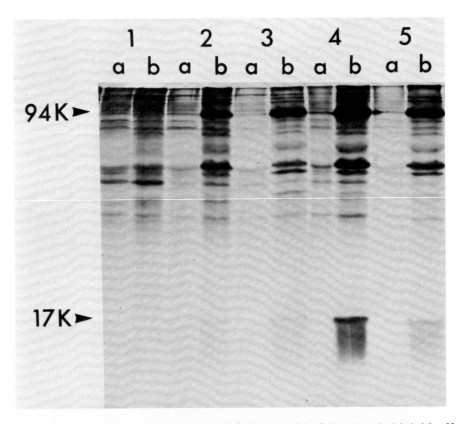

Fig. 4. T-antigen patterns of SV-40-transformed Balb/3T3 cells (A31). Cells were pulse-labeled for 60 min in Hanks's salt solution containing 100 μCi/ml [^{35}S] methionine. T-antigens were collected, immune precipitated, and electrophoresed as described in Materials and Methods. 1, A31; 2, SVA31-Cl 1; 3, SVA31-Cl 5; 4, SVA31-Cl6; 5, SVA31-Cl 8. a, Preimmune serum; b, anti-T hamster serum.

DISCUSSION

Ts-a mutants, which are defective in the large T antigen but make normal middle and small T antigens, induce *abortive* transformation of rat cells at the nonpermissive temperature just as in a wild-type viral infection. The important difference between ts-a mutants and wild-type virus is that ts-a mutants are defective in their ability to induce *stable* transformation. Once transformation is established, the ts-a gene product appears to be no longer required; thus, stable transformants often fail to express large T antigen. The possibility that the 100K protein present in amounts below the level of detection may play a persistent role in transformation cannot be excluded by these data. Although in most 100K antigen-negative clones, there is no indication of fragments of the 100K protein, the existence of such truncated species cannot categorically be ruled out. Among mouse transformants, 100K T antigen-negative clones are the general rule, while in rat transformants such clones occur but less frequently. The difference is most likely related to the greater permissivity of mouse cells to polyoma replication, which brings with it the need for the cells to inactivate the "a" function in order to survive. Hamster (BHK) cells, which are slightly permissive for polyoma replication, also generally fail to show the large T antigen when transformed by polyoma virus [18]. Consistent with this interpretation is the persistence of SV-40 large T antigen in mouse cells, the latter being nonpermissive for SV-40 DNA replication.

The role of the large T antigen of polyoma virus in transformation thus appears to be one of initiating stable transformation, most likely by carrying out steps which lead to the integration of viral DNA into the host genome [6]. Thereafter, there may be selection against cells expressing large T antigen in order that excision and replication not occur. Two recent findings from other laboratories support this view. First, excision and replication of viral DNA in polyoma rat transformants have been shown to depend on the "a" gene function [25]. Second, inactivation of the "a" gene by endonuclease EcoRI cleavage does not impair the ability of viral DNA to induce tumors in hamsters [26], presumably because the host is competent to take up and incorporate the viral DNA, thus bypassing the need for the "a" function. Although it is clear from the existence of large T antigen-negative stable transformants that the 100K protein is not obligatory for the maintenance of the transformed state, the existence of some ts-a transformants with a temperature-sensitive transformed phenotype [27,28] suggests that the large T may in some cases act to control the transformed state.

A functional hr-t gene is both necessary and sufficient for inducing transformed cell properties following de novo infection of rat cells. The hr-t gene codes for the small and middle T antigens in nonproductive as well as productive infection. A role for these viral products in inducing and maintaining the transformed state is supported by the inability of hr-t mutants to abortively or stably transform cells, and by their persistent expression in transformed cells regardless of the species of origin.

Gene expression from the hr-t region is complicated by multiple RNA splicing events leading to the generation of multiple proteins. Current evidence based on peptide mapping (see Hutchison et al [18] and Smart and Ito [19]; B. Schaffhausen and T. Benjamin, unpublished results), DNA sequencing [29–33], and RNA splicing patterns (R. Kamen, personal communication) gives the following picture of the coding sequences corresponding to the hr-t and ts-a genes: 1) Hr-t mutants map in a region which comprises an "intron" for the 100K T antigen, but which forms part of the mRNAs for both the 56K and 22K T antigens; 2) the 56K protein includes essentially all of the 22K protein in its tryptic peptides, but has additional sequences at the C-terminal end which come from

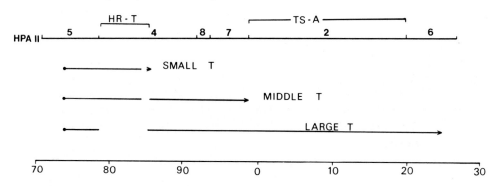

Fig. 5. Schematic diagram of the polyoma virus early region. The coordinates at the bottom refer to the map units defined by the EcoRI cleavage site (0). The map at the top shows the cleavage pattern obtained with HPA II and the positions of the hr-t and ts-a mutations. The sequences coding for small, middle, and large T antigens are shown schematically by the arrows. See Discussion for a more complete description.

reading a portion of the large T coding sequences in a second frame; 3) ts-a mutants map in the distal part of the early region, affecting only the large T antigen in the C-terminal portion downstream from the overlap region with 56K; 4) large, middle, and small T antigens share a common N-terminal sequence which is not directly affected by either hr-t or ts-a mutants. Figure 5 presents these findings schematically.

Besides the normal 56K and 22K products, hr-t mutants fail to induce 63K and 36K species found in wild-type infected cells [14,15]. The relationships of these proteins to the other T-antigen species and to the viral DNA have not yet been determined. An understanding of these relationships may allow the construction of new mutants defective in one but not the other middle or small T antigens, and eventually lead to elucidation of the role of each species in transformation.

ACKNOWLEDGMENTS

The authors gratefully acknowledge the expert technical assistance of Ingrid Lane in the work described here. The work has been supported by grants 19567 and 14723 from the National Cancer Institute.

REFERENCES

1. Stoker M: Nature 218:234, 1968.
2. Habel K: Virology 25:55, 1965.
3. Fluck M, Staneloni R, Benjamin T: Virology 77:610, 1977.
4. Eckhart W: Virology 77:589, 1977.
5. Stoker M, Dulbecco R: Nature 223:397, 1969.
6. Fluck M, Benjamin T: Virology 96:205, 1979.
7. Benjamin T, Norkin L: In "Molecular Studies in Viral Neoplasia." (25th Annual Symposium on Fundamental Cancer Research, M.D. Anderson Hospital and Tumor Institute), Baltimore, Williams and Wilkins, 1972, p 158.
8. Schlegel R, Benjamin T: Cell 14:587, 1978.
9. Benjamin T, Burger M: Proc Natl Acad Sci USA 67:929, 1970.
10. Eckhart W, Dulbecco R, Burger M: Proc Natl Acad Sci USA 68:283, 1971.
11. Benjamin T: Proc Natl Acad Sci USA 67:394, 1970.
12. Eckhart W: Virology 38:120, 1969.

13. DiMayorca G, Callender J, Marin G, Giordano R: Virology 38:126, 1969.
14. Schaffhausen B, Silver J, Benjamin T: Proc Natl Acad Sci USA 75:79, 1978.
15. Silver J, Schaffhausen B, Benjamin T: Cell 15:485, 1978.
16. Ito Y, Spurr N, Dulbecco R: Proc Natl Acad Sci USA 74:1259, 1977.
17. Ito Y, Brocklehurst J, Dulbecco R: Proc Natl Acad Sci USA 74:4666, 1977.
18. Hutchinson M, Hunter T, Eckhart W: Cell 15:65, 1978.
19. Smart J, Ito Y: Cell 15:1427, 1978.
20. Benjamin T: Proc Natl Acad Sci USA 54:121, 1965.
21. Goldman E, Benjamin T: Virology 66:372, 1975.
22. Kamen R, Lindstrom D, Shure H, Old R: Cold Spring Harbor Symp Quant Biol Biol 39:187, 1974.
23. Francke B, Eckhart W: Virology 55:127, 1973.
24. Tegtmeyer P: J Virol 10:591, 1972.
25. Basilico C, Gattori S, Zouzias D, DellaValle G: Cell (In press).
26. Israel M, Chen G, Hourihan S, Rowe W, Martin M: J Virol 29:990, 1979.
27. Seif R, Cuzin F: J Virol 24:721, 1977.
28. Rassoulzadegan M, Seif R, Cuzin F: J Virol 28:421, 1978.
29. Hattori J, Carmichael G, Benjamin T: Cell 16:505, 1978.
30. Friedmann T, Doolittle R, Walter G: Nature 274:291, 1978.
31. Friedmann T, La Porte P, Esty A: J Biol Chem 253:6561, 1978.
32. Soeda E, Griffin B: Nature 276:294, 1978.
33. Carmichael G, Benjamin T: J Biol Chem (in press).

Journal of Supramolecular Structure 12:139–150 (1979)
Tumor Cell Surfaces and Malignancy 505–516

Possible Role of Fibronectin in Malignancy

Lan Bo Chen, Ian Summerhayes, Philip Hsieh, and Phillip H. Gallimore

Sidney Farber Cancer Institute, and Department of Pathology, Harvard Medical School, Boston, Massachusetts 02115 (L.B.C., I.S., P.H.); and Department of Cancer Studies, The Medical School, University of Birmingham, Birmingham, England (P.H.G.)

Frozen sections of tumors induced by injecting virally transformed cells into animals were stained for fibronectin by immunofluorescence. Many tumor cell lines do not express fibronectin in tumors in situ even though some of them express fibronectin in culture. Cell shape and hormones appear to influence the expression of fibronectin in culture; however, it is unclear how fibronectin expression is regulated in vivo.

Key words: fibronectin, tumor, malignancy, cell shape, hormone, embryogenesis

In 1973, Hynes first reported that cell surface fibronectin is greatly reduced in many virally transformed cells [1]. This observation was rapidly confirmed [2]. At Cold Spring Harbor, we followed up Hynes's discovery and investigated in detail the status of cell surface fibronectin on a series of human adenovirus type 2-transformed rat cells. The remarkable feature of these cell lines (developed by one of [PG]) is that even though they are all T-antigen-positive and exhibit a spectrum of transformation phenotypes, there is a gradation of tumorigenicity among these lines. While the key to the difference in tumorigenicity among these lines may reside in the realm of immunology, we were intrigued by the observation that nontumorigenic cells express significant amounts of fibronectin, whereas tumorigenic cells express less than half of the normal level. Some highly tumorigenic cells have no detectable cell surface fibronectin. In the first phase of screening numbers of transformed cell lines, the correlation between the loss of fibronectin and tumorigenicity appeared to be good, even though we already noticed that tumorigenicity in nude mice gave a poorer correlation. For example, F19 (adenovirus-transformed rat cells) express nearly normal levels of fibronectin, are nontumorigenic in normal or immunosuppressed syngeneic rat, and yet are tumorigenic in 2 of 10 nude mice tested [3].

In order to assess whether fibronectin is really involved in the oncogenic potential of transformed cells, we have continued to investigate various aspects of the possible role of fibronectin in malignancy. Here we summarize some of our findings of the last two years.

Received May 17, 1969; accepted September 10, 1979.

DOES LOSS OF FIBRONECTIN STILL CORRELATE WELL WITH ONCOGENIC POTENTIAL?

As noted in the previous summary of our work, there are transformed cells that still express significant amounts of fibronectin [4]. Some of them are highly tumorigenic — for example, mouse 3T12 cells and hamster 333-8-9 cells.

Thus, at the outset, we should say it is impossible to use the expression of fibronectin by transformed cells in culture to predict its tumorigenicity. Even in adenovirus-transformed rat cells, investigation on clonal lines isolated from methylcellulose has shown that the correlation between tumorigenicity and loss of fibronectin in culture is not absolute (Table I).

However, it should be noted that when we used epidemiologic methods to make a statistical assessment of the correlation among the 250 cell lines tested, we found the relationship between the loss of fibronectin in culture and the tumorigenicity to be extremely close (correlation of 0.92). So statistically, the loss of fibronectin in culture may still be a reasonable correlate for predicting tumor induction. But the biologic significance of such a correlation is uncertain at the moment.

FIBRONECTIN IN TUMORS IN SITU

In order to study the relationship between fibronectin and tumors properly we have to be able to study the expression of this protein in tumors in situ. Localization of fibronectin in tissue sections has been reported previously [5—7]. We satisfactorily ran through all the necessary controls and convinced ourselves that fibronectin in tissues can be unambiguously localized. The controls resulting in negative staining include: 1) FITC-conjugated IgG of rabbit anti-goat IgG alone; 2) preabsorption of goat antifibronectin antibody with purified human plasma fibronectin, prior to staining; 3) normal goat serum as a substitute for fibronectin antiserum; 4) incubation, prior to staining with FITC-conjugated second antibody, or the specimen with an excess of unlabeled IgG of rabbit anti-goat IgG, which will saturate all the antigenic sites of the first antibody (goat antifibronectin) available for RITC-conjugated second antibody (rabbit anti-goat IgG).

The key to successful immunofluorescence staining of fibronectin in tissue sections is to avoid using a second antibody that recognizes the IgG of the species of the specimen. An example of successful staining, similar to previous reports [5, 6], is shown in Figure 1, where fibronectin is localized in mouse muscle (A,B), in the stromal region but not the epithelium of the rat lung (C,D), and in blood vessels (distorted by sectioning procedures) of hamster liver (E,F). However, we are still unable to do immunofluorescence localization of fibronectin in frozen sections of skin and cornea, apparently because of nonspecific trapping.

We then procedded to stain frozen sections of tumors. All tumors tested are experimentally induced by injecting tumorigenic cells. We have not tested spontaneous or carcinogen-induced tumors. Figure 2 shows an example of immunofluorescence stain with fibronectin antibody on a frozen section of tumor induced in Swiss mice by injecting 3T12 cells. This cell line expresses a significant level of matrices in culture (C,D). However, no fibronectin can be detected in the tumor section (A,B). When the tumor was dissociated and placed in culture, the expression of fibronectin resumed and was similar to cells prior to the injection of cells into syngeneic rats. This observation indicates that fibronectin-negative cells in tumors do not result from the preferential overgrowth of fibronectin-negative cells in animals.

TABLE I. Fibronectin Expression and Tumorigenicity

Parent cell lines and methylcellulose subclones	% Fibronectin-positive cells at time of inoculation	Syngeneic as rats[a]		2- 3-week old nude mice; Route of inoculation:	
		Newborn	ATS-immuno-suppressed[b]	IP	SC
F4 Parent	63	0/20	5/6	6/6	5/5
F4 M1	5	0/5	5/5	3/3	3/3
F4 M2	70	0/5	0/5	2/3	0/6
F4 M6	3	0/5	4/5	3/3	3/3
F4 M7	8	0/5	5/5	3/3	3/3
F4 M9	0	0/5	5/5	3/3	3/3
F4 M10	27	0/5	5/5	3/3	3/3
F4 M12	4	0/5	4/5	3/3	3/3
F4 M13	0	0/5	5/5	3/3	3/3
F17 Parent	100	0/20	0/10	0/6	0/10
F17`M1	32	0/5	0/5	3/3	2/3
F17 M2	78	0/5	0/5	3/3	4/5
F17 M3	85	0/5	0/5	2/3	1/3
F17 M6	17	0/5	0/5	3/3	2/3
F17 M7	7	0/5	0/5	2/3	1/3
F17 M8	0	0/5	0/5	3/3	4/4
F17 M9	0	0/5	0/5	4/4	3/4
F19 Parent	100	0/20	0/10	3/3	5/5
F19 M1	0	0/5	0/5	2/3	2/5
F19 M2	5	0/5	0/5	2/6	1/6
F19 M3	0	0/5	4/5	6/6	3/3
F19 M4	0	0/5	0/5	0/6	0/6
F19 M5	90	0/5	0/5	2/3	0/3

[a] All animals received 2×10^6 cells in 0.1 ml Ham's F10 medium.
[b] ATS given IP when rats were 8, 9, 10, 11, and 12 days old.
Adapted from Gallimore et al [17, 18].

Table II summarizes the results of immunofluorescence stain of frozen sections of various tumor. Most tumor cells do not express fibronectin in situ, even if they express fibronectin in culture. It is important to note that all these tumors are small (less than 5 mm in diameter) and poorly vascularized. In some sections blood vessels are found and, of course, are fibronectin-positive, but adjacent tumor cells are still negative. In a large tumor (2 cm in diameter) normal stromal fibroblasts frequently participate in tumor formation. For example, tumors induced in nude mice by HeLa cells often consist of as much as 70% host normal cells (Stiles, C., personal communication). Often in these tumors the fibronectin-negative tumor cells and fibronectin-positive stromal fibroblasts are intermingled. All tumor sections studied here used tumors of small size, thus minimizing the incidence of normal cell participation.

It is most noteworthy that 3T6 and 3T12 cells express significant levels of cell surface fibronectin in confluent culture yet produce no detectable fibronectin in frozen sections of their tumors. It is also important to note that some of the tumor cells in tumors induced by 333-8-9, Herpes simplex virus (type II)-transformed hamster cells, do express some detectable fibronectin (Fig. 3). So far this is the only definitive exception in which fibronectin can be localized unambiguously in tumor cells in situ. Work in progress indicates

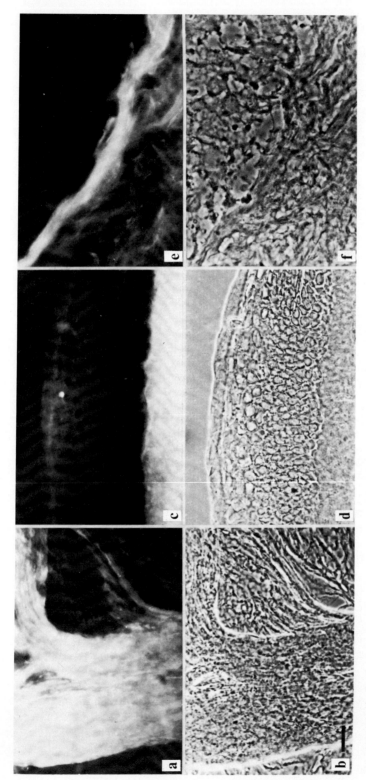

Fig. 1. Immunofluorescence stain of fibronectin in frozen section of normal tissue. (a,b): Mouse muscle; (c,d): rat lung; (e,f): hamster liver. Bar represents 15 μm.

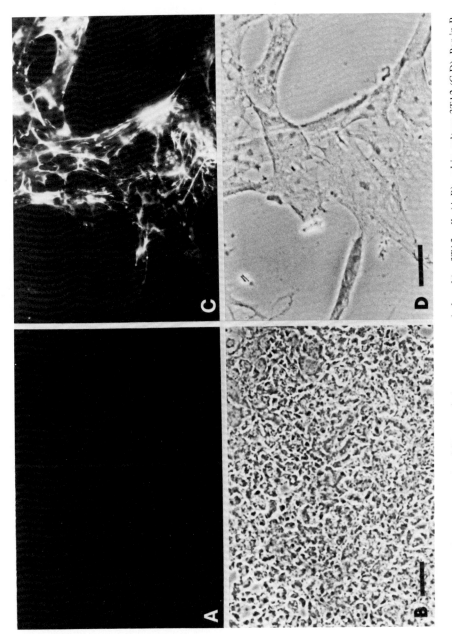

Fig. 2. Immunofluorescence stain of fibronectin in mouse tumor induced by 3T12 cells (A,B) and in culture 3T12 (C,D). Bar in B represents 15 μm and in D represents 10 μm.

TABLE II. Fibronectin in Tumor Frozen Section

Cell lines	Solid tumor induction	Metastasis to:	Fibronectin matrices in culture	Fibronectin in tumor
333-8-9, hamster	+	None	+	+
SV-3T3, mouse	+	None	+	−
Py-3T3, mouse	+	None	+	−
3T6, mouse	+	None	+	−
3T12, mouse	+	None	+	−
SVRE, rat	+	None	+	−
THE, hamster	+	Intestine, liver, kidney	−	−
2Tul, hamster	+	Lung, intestine	−	−
CCL49, hamster	+	Lung	−	−
MSV-3T3, mouse	+	Intestine, lung, liver	−	−
CCL47, rat	+	liver, stomach, intestine	−	−
T2C4, rat	+	Liver, lung, intestine	−	−
T8, rat	+	Liver	−	−
F4M1, rat	+	Liver	−	−
F4M9, rat	+	Liver	−	−
F4M12, rat	+	Lung, liver, lymphatics	−	−
F17M2, rat	+	Liver	−	−
F17M3, rat	+	Lung	−	−
F17M9, rat	+	Lung	−	−

that some mouse bladder epithelial cells transformed by chemical carcinogens do express small amounts of fibronectin in their tumors.

WHY IS THERE A DIFFERENCE BETWEEN FIBRONECTIN EXPRESSION BY TUMOR CELLS IN SITU AND IN CULTURE?

At this writing we offer no explanation as to why some cells will express fibrillar fibronectin in culture and, on the other hand, no fibronectin at all in tumors. For those who are trying to use cells in culture as a model for the behavior of cells in vivo, it is alarming that these two environments exert quite different effects on the cells. To extrapolate observations made on cells in culture to cells in vivo may be more difficult than anticipated. Fibronectin may be a significant example.

Although at the moment it is impossible to answer why there is such a difference in fibronectin expression in vivo and in culture, we offer two possible explanations to account for it. One is the influence of cell shape to fibronectin assembly; the other is the effect of hormones on fibronectin expression. It is possible that tumor cells in vivo may assume quite different shapes as opposed to fully spread cells on a plastic substratum. It is also possible that the set of hormal factors interacting with cells differs in vivo from in culture. Cells in vivo normally do not interact with serum unless there is a wound and blood clotting. Cells in culture, on the other hand, are exposed to many hormones at the same time, some of which may never be encountered in vivo with the type of cells we grow in culture. Conceivably, a different differentiation program may be induced when cells suddenly see nonphysiologic combinations of hormones in culture. It may not be surprising that in physiologic conditions tumor cells do not express fibronectin but upon the stimulation by unusual hormones in an alien environment they start to do so.

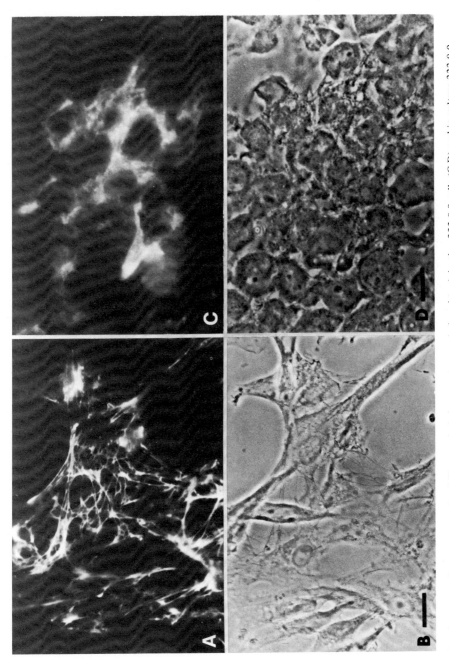

Fig. 3. Immunofluorescence stain of fibronectin in hamster tumors induced by injecting 333-8-9 cells (C,D) and in culture 333-8-9 cells (A,B). Bar represents 10 μm in B and 15 μm in D.

EFFECT OF CELL SHAPE ON FIBRONECTIN ASSEMBLY

Inspired by Folkman's studies on the effect of cell shape on DNA synthesis of normal fibroblastic cells and the possibility that tumor cells may assume quite a different shape in vivo than in culture, we undertook an investigation on the relationship between cell shape and fibronectin expression. Figure 4 shows that when 3T6 cells were kept round-shaped by placement on a bacterial dish, essentially no fibrillar fibronectin was to be detected by immunofluorescence with fibronectin antibody. However, when 3T6 cells were maintained in a well-spread shape by placement on a charged surface such as glass, massive networks of fibrillar fibronectin were detected by immunofluorescence. Cells (3T6) placed on a culture dish coated with a high concentration of hydron (1–10) dilution of stock poly(2-hydroxyethyl methacrylate, which is 12 g/100 ml in ethanol), which prevents cell spreading [8], also do not assemble fibronectin on the cell surface. But it returns to normal expression when 3T6 cells are grown on a culture dish coated with a low concentration of hydron, $1-10^{-4}$ dilution of stock solution, which supports fully spread cells.

INFLUENCE OF HORMONAL GROWTH FACTORS ON CELL SURFACE FIBRONECTIN

In 1977, we reported that Cohen's epidermal growth factor (EGF) stimulates the expression of fibronectin matrices in 3T3 cells [9]. Conceivably, if cells in culture interact with EGF-like hormones (EGF indeed is present in the serum) but not in vivo, then the difference in fibronectin expression in vivo and in culture can be conveniently explained. Unfortunately, little progress has been made as to what kind of hormones cells actually interact in vivo, in particular, the fibroblasts or epithelial cells that we study most frequently in culture. Thus, investigations on the effect of hormones on fibronectin expression provide only a few clues as to what extent the expression of this differentiated product of fibroblasts can be influenced by hormones.

Continuing this aspect of the work, we have now found, in collaboration with Drs. C. Scher and C. Stiles (Sidney Farber Cancer Institute), that platelet-derived growth factor (PDGF) has an effect opposite to that of EGF in that cell surface fibronectin completely disappears from Balb 3T3 (A31) cells treated with PDGF (5 ng/ml) for 24 h. It appears that both anabolic and catabolic hormones exist for the expression of cell surface fibronectin in 3T3 cells.

WHY DO IN CULTURE FIBRONECTIN-ABUNDANT TUMOR CELLS STILL HAVE ABNORMAL MORPHOLOGY IN CULTURE?

There are fibronectin-abundant tumor cells (1 week old in culture) that still have abnormal morphology and intercellular organization. These cells often overlap and criss-cross one another on the culture dish. Based on published information about fibronectin, one would predict that if fibronectin matrices were abundantly produced by the cells, the overall morphology of confluent monolayers would behave like primary cultured fibro-blasts, aligned in parallel array. Why, then, do the in culture fibronectin-abundant tumor cells still have abnormal morphology and intercellular organization?

One possibility is that fibronectin matrices are not the overriding factor in cellular morphology and intercellular organization. Although they are producing fibronectin matrices, cells still have an option to assume abnormal morphology in culture. If this is the

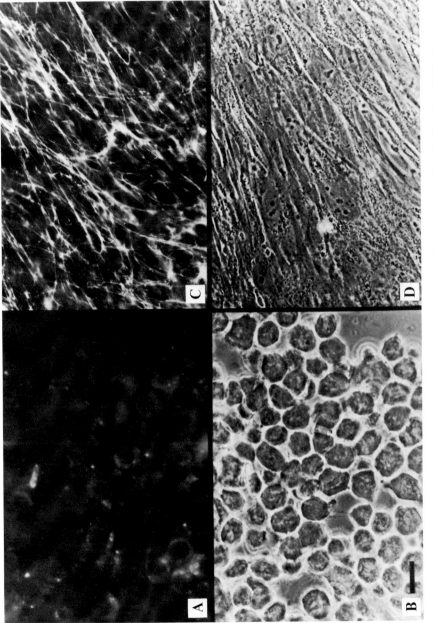

Fig. 4. Immunofluorescence stain of fibronectin in 3T6 cells one day after seeding on bacterial dish (A,B) or glass (C,D). Bar represents 15 μm.

case, one has to search for factors essential for determining cellular morphology and social behavior of cells other than fibronectin. In this regard, it is of interest to note that some mitogenic hormones such as fibroblast growth factor do alter the morphology and social behavior of 3T3 cells in a direction similar to SV-3T3 or Py-3T3 [10]. More intriguingly, conditioned medium of some of the transformed cells, which contains proteins such as sarcoma growth factor (SGF), can convert cellular morphology and intercellular organization of normal cells into transformed-like cells [11]. We have recently used conditioned medium of feline sarcoma virus-transformed mink cells (64F3clone7) to alter the morphology of chick embryo fibroblasts. When these cells were assayed for fibronectin matrices, only some alterations in distribution and organization of fibronectin matrices, but not drastic reduction in matrices, were detected (Fig. 5). Is it possible that in conditioned medium there are SGF-like molecules that influence the key "morphology regulator" which is not the fibronectin matrices? Since the effect exerted by conditioned medium takes 16 h to detect and is dependent upon protein synthesis, it is unlikely that SGF-like molecules directly interact with "morphology regulator." Rather, through hormone-like action, a new morphologic program is induced, for example, by changing gene expression. At the moment, of course, we know nothing about the molecular basis of cellular morphology. Perhaps fibronectin research represents the beginning of a long-term endeavor to understand the molecular equation of cell morphology.

While it takes 16 h for conditioned medium to induce transformed-like morphology in chick embryo fibroblasts, protease can mimic such effects within a few minutes. In most cases the loss or reduction of the fibronectin matrix is accompanied by morphologic changes [12]. However, an important exception was noted. When resting chick embryo fibroblasts were treated with highly purified thrombin they underwent a morphologic change similar to certain types of oncogenic transformation without losing or altering fibronectin matrices [13]. This is another example indicating that cells can undergo transformation-like morphologic change without affecting fibronectin matrices. Perhaps, one can conclude that the correlation between fibronectin matrices and the normal intercellular organization of cultured cells is not absolute. Therefore, one is not surprised to find fibronectin-abundant tumor cells still having abnormal morphology.

Although the above discussion tends to argue against a dominant role for fibeonectin matrices in cellular morphology, the involvement of fibronectin in morphology, intercellular organization, and "social behavior" of cultured cells is beyond any doubt [14, 15]. The question is what role it plays. Is it the cell-substratum adhesion, as suggested by numerous reports, see review by Yamada and Olden [16]?

IS THERE A ROLE FOR FIBRONECTIN IN MALIGNANCY?

In regard to human cancer, the role of fibronectin is not too encouraging. Since the normal epithelium of adult tissues rarely has fibronectin associated with it, it is difficult to argue about the significance of the "loss" of fibronectin. However, during metastasis, transformed cells have to penetrate the various basement membranes, which often contain fibronectin; this interaction of tumor cells with fibronectin may be significant in the development of a malignancy. In order to study this we have to first understand the structure and chemistry of basement membranes; unfortunately, we know very little.

For experimental tumors, where fibroblasts are often the host for oncogenic transformation, fibronectin is clearly a good cell surface marker to follow. But does it have a

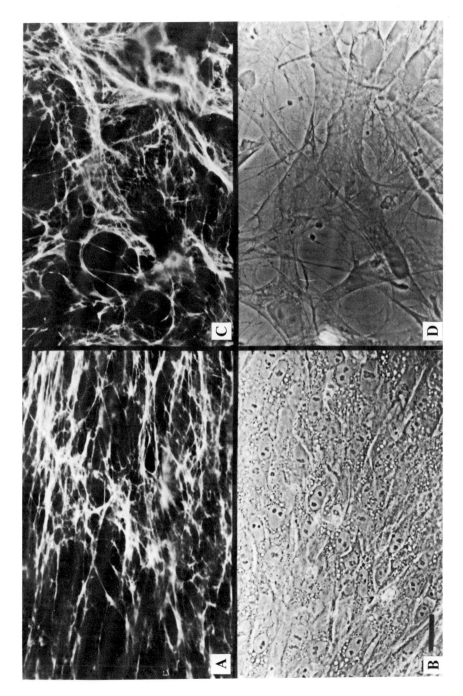

Fig. 5. Immunofluorescence stain of fibronectin in chick embryo fibroblasts (A,B) or treated with conditioned medium of FeSV-transformed mink cells (C,D). Bar represents 15 µm.

role in malignant development? The answer seems to depend on how the untransformed normal parent cells behave in vivo. At present, we don't know how cells such as 3T3, CEF, Nil or BHK, that produce fibronectin in culture behave with respect to fibronectin expression in a physiologic environment. Perhaps one can place 3T3 cells on glass beads, inject or implant them subcutaneously into animals, and then examine whether fibronectin is expressed. If that is true, then the fact that SV-3T3, Py-3T3, 3T6, and 3T12 do not express fibronectin in their tumors is of the utmost significance from an oncogenic transformation standpoint. We really need such data before we can assess whether there is any role for fibronectin in clinical tumors.

In in vitro studies of oncogenic transformation in the cell system, fibronectin is undoubtedly involved. However, as mentioned earlier, we still don't know how. But the rapid progress in this area may soon lead us to an understanding of the pathway of oncogenic transformation induced by either src gene product of T antigen. We are most hopeful that the role of fibronectin in that process will then become clear.

ACKNOWLEDGMENTS

This research was supported by grants from the National Cancer Institute and the American Cancer Society to L.B.C., and by the Cancer Research Campaign (England) to P.H.G. Frozen sections of rabbit cornea were provided by Dr. Charles Cintron, Eye Research Institute, Boston. Goat antifibronectin antibody was a gift of Dr. Ken Yamada, National Institutes of Health, Bethesda Maryland.

REFERENCES

1. Hynes RO: Proc Natl Acad Sci USA 70:3170, 1973.
2. Hynes RO: BBA Rev Cancer 458:73, 1976.
3. Chen LB, Gallimore PH, McDougall JK: Proc Natl Acad Sci USA 73:3570, 1976.
4. Chen LB, Burridge K, Marray A, Walsh ML, Copple CD, Bushnell A, McDougall JK, Gallimore PH: Ann NY Acad Sci 312:366, 1978.
5. Linder E, Vaheri A, Ruoslahti E, Wartiovaara J: J Exp Med 142:41, 1975.
6. Schachner M, Schoonmaker G, Hynes RO: Brain Res 158:149, 1978.
7. Zetter BR, Daniels TE, Guillen C, Greenspan JS: J Dent Res (In press).
8. Folkman J, Moscona A: Nature 273:345, 1978.
9. Chen LB, Gudor RC, Sun TT, Chen AB, Mosesson MW: Science 197:776, 1977.
10. Gospodarowicz D, Moran JS: Proc Natl Acad Sci USA 71:4548, 1974.
11. DeLarco JE, Todaro GJ: Proc Natl Acad Sci USA 75:4001, 1978.
12. Zetter BR, Chen LB, Buchanan JM: Cell 7:407, 1976.
13. Chen LB, Murray A, Segal RA, Bushnell A, Walsh ML: Cell 14:377, 1978.
14. Yamada KM, Yamada SS, Pastan I: Proc Natl Acad Sci USA 73:1217, 1976.
15. Ali IU, Mautner V, Lanza R, Hynes RO: Cell 11:115, 1977.
16. Yamada KM, Olden K: Nature 275:179, 1978.
17. Gallimore PH, McDougall JK, Chen LB: Cell 10:669, 1977.
18. Gallimore PH, McDougall JK, Chen LB: Int J Cancer 24:477, 1979.

Journal of Supramolecular Structure 12:185–194 (1979)
Tumor Cell Surfaces and Malignancy 517–526

7-Acetylcytochalasin B: Differential Effects on Sugar Transport and Cell Motility

Andrew Lees and Shin Lin

Department of Biophysics, Johns Hopkins University, Baltimore, Maryland 21218

Cytochalasin B (CB) is a potent inhibitor of sugar transport and cell motility in animal cells. We have synthesized and characterized the CB derivative 7-acetylcytochalasin B (CBAc) and have found that it has differential effects on transport and motile processes in fibroblasts. The derivative inhibited sugar transport in human red cells, 3T3 cells, and chicken embryo fibroblasts at micromolar concentrations, although it was less potent than its parent compound. Unlike CB, which causes fibroblasts to round up and arborize at less than 10 μM, CBAc had no effect on fibroblast morphology and membrane ruffling at concentrations as high as 90 μM. Competitive binding experiments using [^{3}H]CB showed that the affinity of CBAc for sites related to sugar transport in the red cell membrane is about one-fourth of that of CB. In contrast, similar experiments using [^{3}H] dihydrocytochalasin B (a derivative which inhibits cell motility but not sugar transport) showed that the affinity of CBAc for sites associated with red cell spectrin and actin is only about 1/20 of that of dihydrocytochalasin B. This study demonstrates that acetylation of the C-7 hydroxyl group of CB reduces its effect on cell morphology and motility much more than its ability to inhibit sugar transport. This observation, together with our earlier work with dihydrocytochalasin B, establishes that the pharmacologic effects of CB on fibroblasts result from the binding of the drug to two distinct classes of receptors and that these receptors interact with different parts of the cytochalasin molecule.

Key words: cytochalasin B derivative, cell motility, sugar transport

Cytochalasin B (CB) (the numbering of the carbon atoms is according to Tanenbaum [1]) exerts two major classes of effects on animal cells. At 0.1–1 μM, the drug inhibits facilitated diffusion of sugars into mammalian and avian cells [1]. At 1–100 μM, the drug affects cell morphology and inhibits many types of motile processes, such as cell locomotion, membrane ruffling, and cytokinesis [1].

Abbreviations used: CB, cytochalasin B; H$_2$CB, dihydrocytochalasin B; CBAc, 7-acetylcytochalasin B; CBAc$_2$, 7, 20-diacetylcytochalasin B; DME, Dulbecco's modified Eagle's medium; DMSO, dimethyl sulfoxide; DOG, 2-deoxy-D-glucose.

Received May 17, 1979; accepted August 16, 1979.

0091-7419/79/1202-0185$02.00 © 1979 Alan R. Liss, Inc.

While the inhibitory effect of CB on sugar transport in the human red cell can be explained by the direct competition of the drug with sugars for binding to the transport protein [2–6], the molecular basis of cytochalasin action on cell motility is not well understood. Recently, we have shown that dihydrocytochalasin B (H_2CB), a derivative of CB which lacks the double bond between C-21 and C-22, is similar to its parent compound in its effects on cell morphology and motility, but is ineffective at blocking sugar transport [7, 8]. Utilizing the binding of [^3H]H_2CB as an assay, we were able to isolate from human red cells a class of high-affinity binding sites located in supramolecular complexes containing actin and spectrin [9, 10].

Cytochalasin binding to cultured fibroblasts is more complicated than to human red cells. Sugar transport in fibroblasts is a challenging system to cell biologists because it is regulated according to the physiologic state of the cell (eg, contact inhibition, starvation, viral transformation [11]). However, the use of CB as a probe in the fibroblast is complicated by the finding that there are at least three classes of CB-binding sites in this type of cell and that the majority of the sites are apparently unrelated to sugar transport [8]. Moreover, D-glucose displacement cannot be used as a reliable criterion to define transport-related sites because the sugar displaces bound CB from some cell types [12] but not from others [13, 14]. It appears, therefore, that the availability of cytochalasin derivatives which are specific only for sugar transport would greatly facilitate research in this area.

In this paper we report that the CB derivative, 7-acetylcytochalasin B (CBAc), has properties complementary to that of H_2CB. CBAc blocks sugar transport but has little effect on cell motility and morphology. These results corroborate previous results obtained with H_2CB, that the effects of CB on sugar transport and cell motility are mediated by different receptors [7, 8].

EXPERIMENTAL PROCEDURES

Materials

Unlabeled CB was purchased from Aldrich Chemical Co.; [^3H]CB (7.6 Ci/mmole) and [^{14}C] inulin (2.55 mCi/g) were bought from New England Nuclear. [^3H]-Labeled and unlabeled H_2CB were prepared from the corresponding forms of CB by reduction with $NaBH_4$, as previously described [3, 9]. Stock solutions of cytochalasins were made up in dimethyl sulfoxide (DMSO) and stored at 4°C. Unlabeled 2-deoxy-D-glucose (DOG) was obtained from Sigma Chemical Co. [1-^3H] DOG (19 Ci/mmole) was purchased from Amersham/Searle Corporation. Unless otherwise specified, human red cells were from blood generously donated by the Baltimore Red Cross Blood Center and used within two weeks after the blood was drawn. All reagents were of analytical grade and used without further purification.

Preparation and Characterization of CBAc

The synthesis of CBAc, presented schematically in Figure 1, follows the procedure of Masamune et al [15]. CB is first acetylated to 7,20-diacetylcytochalasin B ($CBAc_2$), which is then selectively hydrolyzed to CBAc. A typical preparation was done in the following manner. $CBAc_2$ was prepared by the slow addition of 100 μl of acetic anhydride to a stirred solution of 19.4 mg of CB in 200 μl of pyridine. The reaction was allowed to proceed overnight at room temperature, quenched by the addition of xylenes and the reagents were removed in vacuo. The product was purified by thin-layer chromatography (see below) to give 15.9 mg of $CBAc_2$. Selective hydrolysis was performed by adding 120

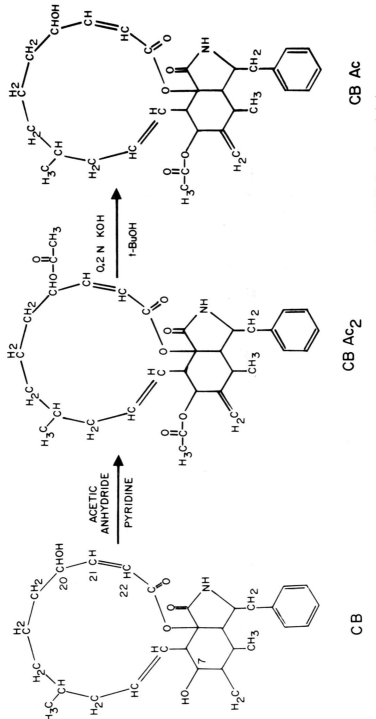

Fig. 1. Synthesis of 7-acetylcytochalasin B from cytochalasin B by the selective hydrolysis of 7,20-diacetylcytochalasin B. Numbering of carbon atoms is according to Tanenbaum [1].

μl of 0.2 N KOH to a solution of 12.7 mg of CBAc$_2$ in 750 μl of t-butanol and 250 μl of water at room temperature for 12 h. The progress of the hydrolysis reaction was followed by thin-layer chromatography. The crude reaction mixture was extracted into ether and washed with saturated NaCl, and the organic phase was dried in a stream of nitrogen. Purification by repeated thin-layer chromatography yielded 7 mg of CBAc.

Purity of the CBAc preparation was confirmed by reversed-phase high-pressure liquid chromatography, which gave a single peak of material. Low-resolution mass spectrometry of the purified product gave a molecular weight (Mr = 521.5) and a spectrum consistent with the structure of CBAc. That this procedure gave a CBAc preparation that contained less than 1% CB and CBAc$_2$ was also shown by using [^{3}H]CB as a tracer through the above synthesis and isolation procedure. Reduction of 7-acetylcytochalasin A with NaBH$_4$ to CBAc, using the procedure described for reduction of cytochalasin A to CB [16], gave a compound indistinguishable by thin-layer chromatography from the CBAc prepared by the hydrolysis method.

Thin-layer chromatography was performed on Analtech silica gel GF plates of 250 μm thickness. The plates were developed with chloroform/ethyl acetate (1:1). In this system the R$_f$ values for CB, CBAc, and CBAc$_2$ are 0.4, 0.5, and 0.6, respectively. The compounds were revealed by charring with chromic acid/sulfuric acid/water (1:1:2). Material to be isolated was revealed by UV quenching of the fluorescent plates and eluted from scraped spots with the same solvent mixture as was used to develop the chromatogram.

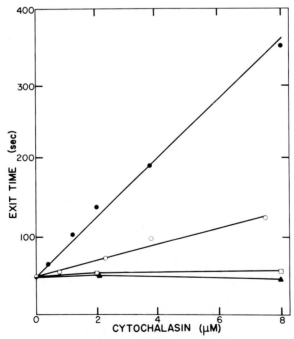

Fig. 2. Effect of cytochalasins on exit of D-glucose from preloaded human red cells. Washed red cells from freshly drawn blood were preloaded with sugar by incubation with 0.1 M D-glucose in 5 mM sodium phosphate buffer, pH 8, with 150 mM NaCl, for 30 min at 37°. Cells were then equilibrated to 25°. At zero time, 50 μl of the cell suspension (10% hematocrit) were added to a cuvette containing 2.5 ml of glucose-free buffer with the specified concentrations of CB (●), CBAc (○), H$_2$CB (□), CBAc$_2$ (▲), or 5 μl DMSO (◓). The exit time, measured as described by Sen and Widdas [17], was monitored by following the change in optical density at 700 nm using a Cary 16 recording spectrophotometer.

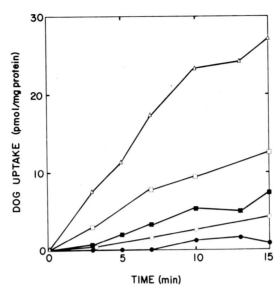

Fig. 3. Effect of cytochalasins on DOG uptake in 3T3 cells. Uptake was measured at 37° on approximately 10^5 cells, grown as monolayers on 35-mm dishes as described previously [8]. The assay medium contained Hanks' balanced salt solution without glucose, buffered with 10 mM N-2-hydroxyethyl-piperazine-N'-2-ethane sulfonic acid to pH 7.3, 0.4 mM DOG, and 1.1 μCi of [^{3}H]DOG. Uptake was measured in the presence of 4 μM CBAc ($\square$), 10 μM CBAc ($\blacksquare$), 4 μM CB ($\circ$), 10 μM CB ($\bullet$), and in the absence of any drug ($\triangle$).

RESULTS

Effect of Cytochalasins on Sugar Transport

CB inhibits sugar transport at micromolar concentrations in mammalian and avian cells [1]. In the three cell types examined in this study, CBAc was also found to be an effective inhibitor of sugar transport, although not as potent as its parent compound.

The Sen and Widdas exit time method [17] was used to estimate the relative potency of several cytochalasins on sugar transport in human red cells. As shown in Figure 2, increasing the amount of CBAc in the assay medium caused the exit time of D-glucose to increase, although the effect was less than that of CB. In contrast, H_2CB and $CBAc_2$ had no effect on transport.

The effects of CB and CBAc on sugar uptake in 3T3 cells are shown in Figure 3. Based on the amount of sugar taken up by the cells at 10 min, CBAc at 4 and 10 μM inhibited the uptake process by 59 and 77%, respectively. In agreement with the results for the red cells, equivalent amounts of CB produced higher levels of inhibition (88 and 94%, respectively). Similar results were obtained with chicken embryo fibroblasts, cultured according to Vogt [18]: CBAc at 4 and 9 μM produced inhibition of 48 and 62%, respectively, as compared to to 88% produced by 4 μM CB.

Effect of Cytochalasins on Cell Morphology and Motility

3T3 cells show a distinct series of morphologic changes when treated with CB or H_2CB. With increasing concentrations of the drugs, the cells elongate, exhibit zeiosis, and finally round up and arborize [8]. As shown in Figure 4a–c, cells treated with 10 μM CB were fully

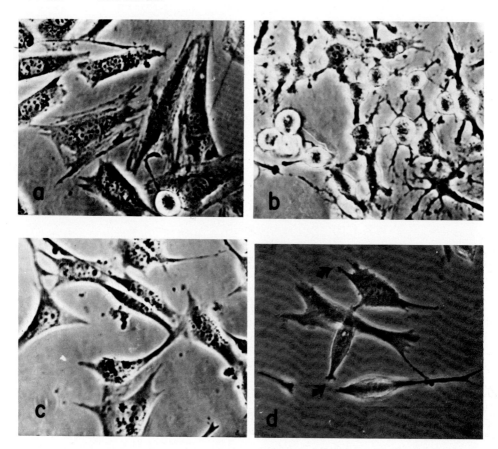

Fig. 4. Effects of cytochalasins on 3T3 cell morphology and motility. The cells were incubated at 37°
for 1 h in the presence of DMSO or cytochalasin and then photographed [8]. a: DMSO-treated cells
showing normal morphology. b: Cells rounded up and arborized in the presence of 10 μM CB. c: Cells
showing normal morphology in the presence of 90 μM CBAc. d: Cells, in the presence of 90 μM CBAc,
showing membrane ruffling (arrows) as judged by time-lapse video recording, performed with a Pana-
sonic video recorder (model No. Nv-8030) and camera (model No. WV 1350) attached to a Nikon MS
inverted scope. M X 300.

arborized, whereas cells treated with 90 μM CBAc had normal morphology. $CBAc_2$ at 90 μM
also had no effect on cell morphology (not shown). However, when $CBAc_2$ was converted
to CB by alkaline hydrolysis, it caused the cells to arborize, indicating that acetylation of the
hydroxyl groups blocked the action of the cytochalasin. Results similar to that seen with
3T3 cells were obtained with chicken embryo fibroblasts. These cells were more sensitive
to CB than 3T3 cells: 1–3 μM CB induced arborization whereas 50 μM CBAc did not significantly affect cell morphology even after 5 h.

Time-lapse video recording of membrane ruffling was used to study the effects of
cytochalasins on motility of 3T3 cells. In control experiments (ie, cells were treated with
DMSO), many areas of the membrane edges of the cells were seen to ruffle with an undulating movement when the video recording was played back at 108 X actual time; membrane
ruffling was especially vigorous when cells were spreading. When cells were treated with
10 μM CB, membrane ruffling was inhibited within a few minutes. This inhibition was ac-

companied by the retraction of the cell margins towards the center of the cells, causing the cells to take on the arborized morphology as shown in Figure 4b. CBAc and CBAc$_2$, on the other hand, had no effect on membrane ruffling or on cell morphology at concentrations as high as 90 μM. This was true for both spreading cells and cells that had been plated the previous day. Figure 4d shows a photomicrograph of CBAc-treated cells which had been shown to exhibit membrane ruffling by time-lapse video recording.

Competitive Binding of Cytochalasins to Red Cell Membrane and Extract

The studies described in the preceding sections showed that CBAc inhibits sugar transport without affecting cell morphology and motility. The following experiments were designed to determine whether this kind of specificity reflects the affinity of CBAc for different types of high-affinity CB binding sites. The human red cell was used as a test system because the binding sites related to sugar transport can be separated from those related to motility and both types of sites have been previously characterized.

Membranes containing only transport-related CB binding sites were prepared by removal of motility-related sites by extraction of ghosts with EDTA at low ionic strength [9]. The relative affinity of CBAc compared with CB for the transport-related sites was estimated by measuring the displacement of [^{3}H] CB bound to the extracted membranes at various concentrations of the unlabeled forms of the two compounds. At 10^{-7} M [^{3}H] CB (a concentration approximately the same as the K$_{dissociation}$(Kd) of CB for transport-related sites [2]), 50% displacement of the labeled compound occurred at 0.24 μM CB compared with 1 μM CBAc (Fig. 5). This indicates that the affinity of the derivative for the transport-related sites is approximately 1/4 that of the parent compound. In a similar experiment,

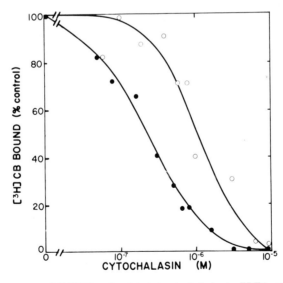

Fig. 5. Competitive binding of [^{3}H] CB and unlabeled cytochalasins to EDTA-extracted red cell membranes. EDTA-extracted membranes [9] derived from 5×10^8 cells were incubated in 600 μl of 5 mM sodium phosphate buffer, pH 8, containing the specified amounts of the unlabeled form of CB ($\bullet$) or CBAc ($\circ$). After 10 min, [^{3}H] CB was added to the assay medium to a concentration of 10^{-7} M and the amount of labeled drug bound to the membrane was determined with the centrifugation assay [2] after another 10 min of incubation. High-affinity binding was defined as the portion of the total binding that was displaceable by 10^{-4} M unlabeled cytochalasin, after correcting for trapped counts measured in [^{14}C] inulin controls.

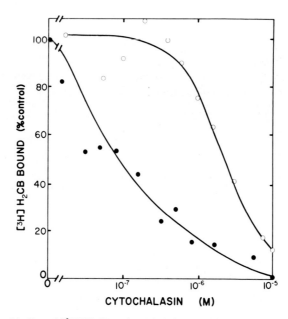

Fig. 6. Competitive binding of [^{3}H]H$_2$CB and unlabeled cytochalasins to sealed red cell ghosts. Sealed ghosts [9] prepared from 5×10^8 cells were incubated in 600 μl of 5 mM sodium phosphate buffer, pH 8, with 150 mM NaCl, containing the specified amounts of unlabeled H$_2$CB ($\bullet$) or CBAc ($\circ$). After 10 min, [^{3}H]H$_2$CB was added to the assay medium to a concentration of 10^{-8} M and the amount of labeled drug bound to the membrane was determined with the centrifugation assay [2] after another 10 min of incubation.

the relative affinities of CBAc and H$_2$CB for motility-related sites were estimated by measuring displacement of [^{3}H]H$_2$CB from red cell ghosts by the two compounds. At 10^{-8}M [^{3}H]H$_2$CB (a concentration close to the K$_d$ of H$_2$CB for motility-related sites [9]), 50% displacement of the labeled compound was observed at 0.1 μM H$_2$CB and at 2.2 μM CBAc (Fig. 6). This indicates that CBAc is only 1/20 as effective as H$_2$CB in competing for motility-related sites.

In order to test whether the higher levels of CBAc required to displace [^{3}H]H$_2$CB resulted from the lower affinity of the drug for motility-related sites or were due to a reduction in its free concentration caused by its binding to transport-related sites and nonspecific partitioning into the membrane, we performed a competitive binding assay on solublized motility-related sites in a low-salt extract of red cell membranes [9]. This experiment was performed with the isoelectric precipitation assay [10] at 5×10^{-9} M [^{3}H]H$_2$CB, a concentration approximately equal to the K$_d$ of this drug for motility-related sites measured under the conditions used for this assay (D.C. Lin and S. Lin, unpublished results). We found that 50% displacement of the [^{3}H]H$_2$CB was observed at 0.02 μM H$_2$CB and 0.45 μM CBAc, indicating that removing the membrane and transport sites did not cause CBAc to be a more effective competitor in this assay; the derivative is still only about 1/20 as effective as H$_2$CB.

DISCUSSION

Since CB affects both membrane transport and motile functions of the cell, it has been proposed that the drug acts in a rather nonspecific way by partitioning into membrane lipids

[19] or binding to hydrophobic regions of membrane-associated proteins in general [14]. The data presented here show that modification of the C-7 hydroxyl group of CB has a much greater effect on its action on cell motility than on its ability to inhibit sugar transport. In an earlier study, we have shown that saturation of the C-21-22 double bond of CB abolishes its ability to block sugar transport without significantly affecting its ability to inhibit cell motility [7, 8]. These two groups of experiments demonstrate that the inhibition of sugar transport and cell motility in fibroblasts by CB are independent events, mediated by separate receptors. The CBAc experiments, in particular, argue against the suggestion that inhibition of sugar transport may be mediated by the interaction of CB with cytoskeletal structures[20].

The competitive binding experiments provide an explanation for the effect of acetylation of the C-7 hydroxyl group on the pharmacologic activity of CB. The human red cell was used as the test system in this study because it is possible to measure cytochalasin binding to sugar transport proteins and to cytoskeletal proteins independently. Consistent with its effectiveness in inhibiting sugar transport in red cells and fibroblasts, CBAc was found to displace $[^3H]$CB from transport-related sites with an efficiency about 1/4 of that of CB. In contrast, the derivative was estimated to be only 1/20 as effective as H_2CB in displacing $[^3H]H_2CB$ from sites located in cytoskeletal proteins. This finding is in keeping with the observation that CBAc, at a concentration about 10 times higher than the effective level for CB, does not affect fibroblast morphology and motility. Therefore, one can conclude from the data of the competitive binding experiments that the lower potency of CBAc in inhibiting sugar transport and cell motility is a direct result of its lower affinity for CB binding sites which have a high degree of structural specificity for their substrates.

Our present knowledge of the pharmacologic properties of several cytochalasin analogs suggests that the two types of CB effects on fibroblasts can be chemically dissected: the C-7 hydroxyl group is essential for activity against cell motility and the C-20 hydroxyl group is important for activity against sugar transport. As demonstrated in this study, acetylation of the first hydroxyl group produced a derivative (CBAc) which is active only against sugar transport, whereas acetylation of both hydroxyl groups yielded a compound ($CBAc_2$) which is inert against both transport and motile processes. These results complement our earlier observation that H_2CB is effective in inhibiting cell motility but does not inhibit sugar transport [7, 8]. Although this derivative has the C-7 and C-20 hydroxyl groups, the saturation of its double bond at C-21-22 may cause sufficient movement of the oxygen atom at C-20 from its original position that the drug can no longer bind to the sugar transport protein in the manner proposed by Taylor and Gagneja [21].

Our finding that blocking the C-7 hydroxyl group of CB has a relatively minor effect on its activity against sugar transport opens up several possibilities for the preparation of derivatives which could be useful for studying sugar transport in fibroblasts. For instance, the product obtained by linking CB to a solid support (eg, sepharose beads) using a synthetic route similar to that used for preparing CBAc would be useful in affinity chromatography for isolating detergent-solubilized membrane proteins involved in sugar transport. Similarly, the coupling of radioactive, fluorescent, and photoaffinity reagents to the C-7 hydroxyl group could yield compounds helpful for the identification of cytochalasin binding components in experiments in vivo and in vitro.

ACKNOWLEDGMENTS

We thank Dr. Satoru Masamune for his suggestions on the synthesis of CBAc, James Evans for performing the mass spectrometry analysis, and Dr. Gary H. Posner for the use of his high-pressure liquid chromatography equipment. A. L. is a Predoctoral Trainee and S. L. is a Research Career Development Awardee of the National Institute of General Medical Sciences. This work was supported by a grant from the American Cancer Society (VC-288) and a grant from the National Institutes of Health (GM-22289).

REFERENCES

1. Tanenbaum SW: "Cytochalasins. Biochemical and Cell Biological Aspects." Amsterdam: Elsevier/North-Holland Biomedical Press, 1978.
2. Lin S, Spudich JA: J Biol Chem 249:5778, 1974.
3. Lin S, Snyder CE: J Biol Chem 252:5464, 1977.
4. Jung CY, Rampal AL: J Biol Chem 252:5456, 1977.
5. Baldwin SA, Baldwin JM, Gorga FR, Lienhard GE: Biochim Biophys Acta 552:183, 1979.
6. Sogin DC, Hinkle PC: J Supramol Struct 8:447, 1978.
7. Lin S, Lin DC, Flanagan MD: Proc Natl Acad Sci USA 75:329, 1978.
8. Atlas SJ, Lin S: J Cell Biol 76:360, 1978.
9. Lin DC, Lin S: J Biol Chem 253:1415, 1978.
10. Lin DC, Lin S: Proc Natl Acad Sci USA 76:2345, 1979.
11. Weber MJ, Hale AH, Yau TM, Buckman T, Johnson M, Brady TM, LaRossa DD: J Cell Physiol 89:711, 1976.
12. Salter DW, Weber MJ: J Biol Chem 254:3554, 1979.
13. Atlas SJ, Lin S: J Cell Physiol 89:751, 1976.
14. Plagemann PGW, Graff JC, Wohlhueter RM: J Biol Chem 252:4191, 1977.
15. Masamune S, Hayase Y, Schilling W, Chan WK, Gordon SB: J Am Chem Soc 99:6756, 1977.
16. Lin S, Santi DV, Spudich JA: J Biol Chem 249:2268, 1974.
17. Sen AK, Widdas WF: J Physiol 160:392, 1962.
18. Vogt PK: In "Fundamental Techniques of Virology." Habel K, Salzman NP (eds): New York: Academic Press, 1969, p 198.
19. Spooner BS: Dev Biol 35:f13, 1973.
20. Lever JE: J Biol Chem 254:2961, 1979.
21. Taylor NF, Gagneja GL: Can J Biochem 53:1078, 1975.

Journal of Supramolecular Structure 12:195–208 (1979)
Tumor Cell Surfaces and Malignancy 527–540

Action of Phorbol Esters in Cell Culture: Mimicry of Transformation, Altered Differentiation, and Effects on Cell Membranes

I. Bernard Weinstein, Lih-Syng Lee, Paul B. Fisher, Alan Mufson, and Hiroshi Yamasaki

Division of Environmental Sciences and Cancer Center/Institute of Cancer Research, Columbia University, New York, New York 10032

The carcinogenic process is usually multifactor in its causation and multistep in its evolution. It is likely that entirely different molecular mechanisms underlie the many steps in this process. In contrast to initiating carcinogens, the action of the tumor-promoting phorbol esters does not appear to involve covalent binding to cellular DNA and they are not mutagenic. Recent studies in cell culture have revealed two interesting biologic effects of the phorbol esters and related macrocyclic plant diterpenes. The first is that at nanomolar concentrations they induce several changes that resemble those seen in cells transformed by chemical carcinogens or tumor viruses. These include altered morphology and increased saturation density, altered cell surface fucose-glycopeptides, decrease in the LETS protein, increased transport of deoxyglucose, and increased levels of plasminogen activator and ornithine decarboxylase. In transformed cells exposed to phorbol esters the expression of these features is further accentuated. Phorbol esters do not induce normal cells to grow in agar but they do enhance the growth in agar of certain transformed cells. The second effect of the phorbol esters is inhibition of terminal differentiation. This effect extends to a variety of programs of differentiation and is reversible when the agent is removed. With certain cell culture systems induction of differentiation, rather than inhibition, is observed. Both the transformation mimetic and the differentiation effects are exerted by plant diterpenes that have tumor-promoting activity but not by congeners that lack such activity. The primary target of phorbol esters appears to be the cell membrane. Early membrane-related effects include enhanced uptake of 2-deoxyglucose and other nutrients, altered cell adhesion, induction of arachidonic acid release and prostaglandin synthesis, inhibition of the binding of epidermal growth factor to cell surface receptors, altered lipid metabolism, and modifications in the activities of other cell surface receptors. A model of "two stage" carcinogenesis encompassing the known molecular

Received June 6, 1979; accepted August 15, 1979.

and cellular effects of initiating carcinogens and tumor promoters is presented. According to this model, initiating carcinogens induce stable alterations in the cellular genome but these are not manifested until tumor promoters modulate programs of gene expression and induce the clonal outgrowth of the initiated cell.

Key words: tumor promoters, phorbol esters, plasminogen activator, epidermal growth factor, carcinogenesis

It is likely that most human cancers do not result from simple exposure to a single exogenous agent but rather a complex interaction between multiple environmental (exogenous) and host (endogenous) factors. The carcinogenic process is often a multistep one occurring over an appreciable fraction of the lifespan of the host. It is probable that each of these steps reflects qualitatively different biologic and biochemical events and that they may be mediated by different types of agents. In other words, the simple exposure of an individual to a DNA-damaging agent may not be sufficient to induce cancer if the subsequent steps in a multistep process are rate-limiting. This has obvious implications for cancer prevention. It may, for example be possible to reduce the incidence of certain human cancers by preventing (or reversing), not the initial step, but the later steps in a multistep carcinogenic process.

The existence of at least two distinct phases in chemical carcinogenesis, termed "initiation" and "promotion," is well illustrated in studies on mouse skin. There is also increasing evidence that a process similar to promotion occurs during tumor induction in certain other tissues and in other species (for review, see refs. 1–6). It is of interest that the most potent promoters on mouse skin, the phorbol esters and related diterpenes, are naturally occurring substances. Although there has been the impression that the action of the phorbol esters as tumor promoters is confined to mouse skin, recent studies indicate that this is not the case (Table I).

One wonders to what extent other promoters and carcinogenic cofactors occur in our diet, in other aspects of the natural environment, or in industrial products, and to what extent they are limiting determinants in the causation of specific human cancers.

The identification of such factors requires better knowledge of their mechanisms of action as well as simple in vitro assays that can be used for their detection. Table II contrasts the biologic properties of carcinogens and tumor promoters on mouse skin.

It should be stressed that although many carcinogens undergo metabolic activation and bind covalently to DNA (and are therefore mutagenic) this is not true for the tumor promoters. A few years ago we became interested in developing cell culture systems which could be used to study the mechanism of action of tumor promoters and which might

TABLE I. Examples in Which Phorbol Esters Enhance Carcinogenesis in Tissues Other Than Mouse Skin

Type of tumor	Species	Agents	Reference
Ovary, intestine	Mouse	DMBA or urethane (diaplacental) + TPA (postnatal)	2
Forestomach	Mouse	DMBA + TPA	3
Stomach	Rat	MNNG + croton oil	4
Esophagous[a]	Human	? + diterpene from croton flavens	6

[a] Suggestive evidence.

TABLE II. Comparison of Biologic Properties of Initiating Agents and Promoting Agents

Initiating agents	Promoting agents
1. Carcinogenic by themselves — "solitary carcinogens"	1. Not carcinogenic alone
2. Must be given *before* promoting agent	2. Must be given *after* the initiating agent
3. Single exposure is sufficient	3. Require prolonged exposure
4. Action is irreversible and additive	4. Action is reversible (at early stage) and not additive
5. No apparent threshold	5. Probable threshold
6. Yield electrophiles that bind covalently to cell macromolecules	6. No evidence of covalent binding
7. Mutagenic	7. Not mutagenic

Reproduced from Weinstein et al [10], with permission.

serve as rapid assays for screening environmental substances for promoting activity. This article will summarize studies from our own laboratory and from other laboratories on the biologic and biochemical effects of the phorbol esters in various cell culture systems. Aspects of this subject have recently been reviewed elsewhere [7].

MIMICRY OF TRANSFORMATION

One of the first effects we observed was that 12-O-tetradecanoyl-phorbol-13-acetate (TPA), and several related macrocylic plant diterpenes, are extremely potent inducers of plasminogen activator (PA) synthesis in both chick embryo fibroblasts (CEF) and HeLa cultures [8–11]. We have previously presented evidence that this effect is highly specific, that it involves de novo macromolecular synthesis, and that it correlates with the tumor-promoting potency of a series of phorbol ester analogs [7–11].

In view of the results obtained with PA, it was natural to ask whether TPA and related compounds also enhance the expression of other biologic markers frequently associated with transformation and tumorigenicity. Elsewhere we have summarized data from several laboratories indicating that TPA does induce several properties in normal cells that mimic those often seen in transformed cells [7–10]. This mimicry includes changes in cell morphology, growth properties, cell surfaces properties, and specific enzymes. We must stress, however, three aspects of the effects obtained when normal cells not previously exposed to an initiating carcinogen are incubated with TPA. 1) Not all cells display the full set of phenotypic changes of mimicry. 2) TPA-treated normal cells do not mimic all of the properties of fully transformed tumorigenic cells. It is of particular importance that they do not acquire the capacity for growth in agar. The stimulatory effects of TPA on the growth in agar of adenovirus-transformed cells are described below. 3) In contrast to fully malignant cells, the maintenance of transformation properties in normal cells is dependent upon the continuous presence of the promoting agent, and the cells revert to normal when the agent is removed from the medium. In mouse skin previously exposed to a carcinogen the repeated application of TPA, however, can lead to "autonomous" malignant tumors. TPA can enhance the stable transformation of fibroblast cultures previously exposed to a chemical carcinogen, UV, or x-irradiation [12–14] or an adenovirus [15, 16]. The latter results indicate that "initiated" cells have a qualitatively different response to TPA than completely normal cells.

PHENOTYPIC ENHANCEMENT AND EFFECTS ON ADENOVIRUS TRANSFORMATION

An intriguing aspect was our finding that TPA causes a further increase in PA synthesis in transformed cells that are already synthesizing high levels of PA [8–10]. We refer to this phenomenon as "enhancement." Studies with chick embryo fibroblasts transformed by a temperature-sensitive mutant of Rous sarcoma virus (RSV) showed that enhancement of TPA-induced PA synthesis required continuous expression of the sarc gene of RSV [8–10]. This finding has been confirmed and extended by other investigators [17, 35]. The results suggest that there is an interaction between products of the sarc gene and cellular events triggered by TPA. We are currently studying the nature of this interaction. Other examples of an enhanced response to TPA by transformed cells have now been seen in terms of morphologic changes [8–10, 17], ornithine decarboxylase (ODC) induction [18], and prostaglandin synthesis [19]. The phenomenon of enhancement may be a useful model for understanding tumor promotion and progression, since it provides examples in which previous changes in phenotype alter a cell's subsequent response (both quantitatively and qualitatively) to a tumor-promoting agent.

The results obtained with RSV-transformed cells suggested that tumor promoters could interact with oncogenic viruses in the transformation process. There are several examples in which chemical and physical agents interact synergistically with viruses in the carcinogenic process both in vitro and in vivo (for review see refs. 15, 20, and 21). Indeed, it seems likely that certain human cancers may be due to interactions between chemical agents and types of viruses which alone would have little or no oncogenic potential. This is important to keep in mind in the search for viruses that might play a role in human cancer causation. These agents may not have all of the properties of oncogenic viruses seen in experimental animal systems and, when assayed alone, they may not be capable of cancer induction in the absence of chemical cofactors.

To explore these aspects of chemical-viral interactions we have recently developed an in vitro system in which the transformation of rat embryo (RE) cells is markedly enhanced when, after infection with a mutant (ts125) of adenovirus type 5, the cells are grown in the presence of TPA [15, 16]. The presence of TPA caused an increased number of foci of transformation. Foci also appeared earlier and were larger than those obtained with adenovirus in the absence of TPA. Phorbol, 4αPDD, and 4-0-MeTPA were inactive in this system. The addition of TPA could be delayed until after viral uptake and integration of adenovirus sequences into the host genome had occurred, thus indicating that the enhancement by TPA was not exerted on these steps. This is in contrast to the ability of certain initiating carcinogens to enhance DNA virus transformation [15,16,21,22].

One of the best in vitro markers for the tumorigenicity of transformed fibroblast or epithelial rodent cells is anchorage independence, ie, ability to grow in agar or agarose suspension, although there are a few exceptions (for review see Fisher et al [16]). It was of interest, therefore, to examine the effects of TPA on this property in adenovirus-transformed cells. In recent studies, we have found that although TPA does not enhance the growth in agar of normal RE cells, it does induce the growth in agar of morphologically transformed adenovirus-infected RE cells [16] (Table III).

This effect appears to be inductive and not due to simple cell selection [81]. Yet it is irreversible, since when the TPA is removed the cells now grow in agar with a higher efficiency than prior to exposure to TPA. Colburn et al [23] have found that certain

TABLE III. Effect of TPA on Growth in Agar of Normal and Adenovirus-Transformed Rat Embryo Cells

Cell type	Agar-cloning efficiency (%)		Ratio (+TPA/−TPA)
	− TPA	+ TPA	
Normal			
Secondary rat embryo	< 0.001	< 0.001	−
Adenovirus-transformed			
Ad-A18-E	< 0.001	0.1	> 100
Ad-A18-L	0.1	0.5	5.0
Ad-E7-E	< 0.001	0.2	>200
Ad-E7-L	1.2	2.7	2.3

Morphologically transformed clones were isolated from cultures of secondary rat embryo cultures previously infected with a mutant of human adenovirus type 5 (H5ts125) and tested for growth in agar in the presence and absence of 100 ng/ml TPA. E, early passages (<10) of these clones; L, later passages (> 25). For additional details see Fisher et al [16].

serially passaged mouse epidermal cell cultures also undergo an irreversible increase in anchorage-independent growth when exposed to TPA. This phenomenon may represent a useful in vitro model system for studying the process of tumor progression.

EFFECTS ON DIFFERENTIATION

Since it is likely that carcinogenesis involves major disturbances in differentiation, it was of interest to determine whether TPA would affect the differentiation of certain well-defined tissue culture systems. Table IV summarizes examples from our own laboratory and from the literature indicating that TPA is a highly potent inhibitor of terminal differentiation in a variety of cell systems.

This effect on differentiation is not simply a consequence of toxicity or growth inhibition, and, in certain cases, is reversed when TPA is removed from the culture. Nor is the effect limited to a specific program of differentiation or species (Table IV). Evidence has also been obtained that, as with the phenomenon of mimicry of transformation, the relative potencies of a series of phorbol ester analogs as inhibitors of differentiation correlates with their potencies as promoters on mouse skin [24].

Recently, cell systems have been found in which TPA induces rather than inhibits differentiation. This has now been seen with a certain clone of murine erythroleukemia cells [34], murine and human myeloid leukemia cells [36, 37, 79, 80], and a human melanoma cell culture [38]. Reciprocal effects of the same agent on differentiation, depending on the type of cell culture, have been seen with other agents, including glucocorticoid hormones, cyclic AMP, and BUdR. It is possible that the ability of TPA either to induce or inhibit differentiation depends on the nature of the membrane, and/or membrane constituents of the target cell. The late Dr. Morris Kupchan and his colleagues found that certain macrocyclic plant diterpenes inhibited the growth of a transplantable mouse lymphoma [39]. We wonder whether this was due to an inductive effect on differentiation and whether this approach can be further exploited in the therapy of certain neoplasms which retain the capacity for differentiation [40].

TABLE IV. Examples of TPA Inhibition of Differentiation

Cell system	Type of differentiation	References
Murine erythroleukemia	Erythroid	24, 25, 72
Chicken embryo myoblasts	Myogenesis	26
Chicken embryo chondroblasts	Chondrogenesis	27, 49
Murine 3T3	Lipocytes	28
Murine neuroblastoma	Neurite	29, 71
Murine melanoma	Melanogenesis	30
Sea urchin	Embryogenesis	31, 32, 33

EFFECTS ON MEMBRANES AND THE CELL SURFACE

Early studies on the effects of TPA in cell culture suggested that the cell surface membrane may be the major target of TPA action [75]. More recent studies have reinforced this hypothesis. Table V is a list of effects of TPA on cell surfaces and membranes.

We have studied the uptake of ^{3}H-TPA by cells in culture and found that it is linear across a wide range of TPA concentration and does not appear to be saturable [55]. Thus far, we have been unable to demonstrate a specific high-affinity saturable receptor, although we are still pursuing this aspect. Cell fractionation studies indicated that the uptake was almost entirely into the membranous fractions of the cell and appeared to be a simple partitioning of the highly hydrophobic compound into the lipid phase of the membrane. Uptake by the nucleus was extremely low. Cellular uptake was not inhibited by a large excess of nonradioactive TPA, inhibitors of energy metabolism, inhibitors of macromolecular synthesis, or cytochalasin. There was no evidence of covalent binding to cellular macromolecules and almost all of the cell-associated ^{3}H-TPA was released when the cells were placed in serum containing medium lacking TPA or when cells were extracted with lipid solvents [55]. Thus the detection of a specific TPA receptor is complicated by the extensive non-specific binding.

In view of the evidence that TPA is concentrated largely in the lipid phase of cell membranes, in collaboration with D. Schachter's laboratory at Columbia University, we have looked for evidence of a change in the physical properties of cell membranes by studying the fluorescence polarization of an asymmetric chromophore, 1,6-diphenyl-1,3,5-hexatriene (DPH) [45]. Concentrations of TPA as low as 0.1 ng/ml (10^{-10}M) produced a reproducible decrease in fluorescence polarization of DPH. The change was detected within less than 1 h and was not blocked by cycloheximide or actinomycin D, suggesting that it occurs directly at the membrane level. Other phorbol esters having tumor-promoting activity (PDD and PDB) also exerted this effect, whereas the compounds phorbol and 4αPDD, which lack tumor-promoting activity, were inactive. These results suggest that TPA produces a generalized change in the physical properties of the lipid phase of cellular membranes and that this effect appears to be a direct one. A similar effect of TPA on fluorescence polarization of DPH has been found in human lymphoblastoid cells [46]. One interpretation is that TPA results in an increase in membrane fluidity, but other interpretations have not been excluded [45].

Additional evidence that an early site of action of TPA is the cell membrane comes from studies with murine erythroleukemia cells. We have found that, whereas these cells usually grew in suspension, within 30–120 min after exposure to TPA they become adherent to tissue culture plates and take on an epithelioid or fibroblastic appearance [48].

TABLE V. Effects of TPA on Cell Surfaces and Membranes in Cell Culture

	References
Altered Na/K ATPase	41
Increased uptake 2-DG, ^{32}P, ^{86}RB	42, 43, 57
Increased phospholipid synthesis	44, 74
Increased membrane lipid "fluidity"	45, 46
Increased release arachidonic acid, prostaglandins	19, 47
Altered morphology and cell-cell orientation	8, 17, 41, 42
Altered cell adhesion	48, 49, 73
Altered fucose-glycopeptides	9, 10
Decreased LETS protein	50
"Uncoupling" of β-adrenergic receptors	51, 52, 53
Inhibition of binding of EGF to receptors	54, 60

The induction of adhesion is not blocked by inhibitors of RNA or protein synthesis, although it is temperature-dependent. Studies in progress indicate that when a series of diterpenes are assayed for induction of adhesion, in a sensitive clone of murine erythroleukemia cells, their relative potency generally correlates with their activity as promoters on mouse skin. Thus, this assay may provide a simple rapid screening test for this class of tumor promoters. The fact that this process also does not appear to require macromolecular synthesis suggests that it is due to a primary effect of TPA on cell membranes. Effects on cell adhesion have also been seen with chondroblasts and lymphoblastoid cultures [49, 73].

Another early response to TPA is the release from membrane phospholipids of arachidonic acid, which is associated with a stimulation of prostaglandin synthesis. This effect was recently described by Levine and Hassid [19] and we have extended this finding to CEF and 10T½ cell cultures [47]. The response in CEF cultures is shown in Figure 1. It occurs rapidly, is not seen with nonpromoting diterpenes, and is inhibited by transretinoic acid. The latter compound is an inhibitor of tumor promotion on mouse skin [56]. A curious aspect is that although the TPA-induced release of arachidonic acid and prostaglandins is not inhibited by actinomycin D it is inhibited by cycloheximide or puromycin [47]. The significance of TPA-induced membrane phospholipid deacylation in terms of the other effects of TPA on cell function are not clear at the present time. The fact that it is inhibited by inhibitors of protein synthesis, whereas certain other early responses to TPA such as increased 2-deoxyglucose uptake [57] and altered membrane "fluidity" [45] are not, suggests that it is not the initial or primary effect of TPA on cells.

We have previously postulated that the phorbol ester tumor promoters may act by usurping the function of a cell surface receptor whose normal function is to mediate the action of a growth regulator or homone yet to be identified [9, 54]. Consistent with this hypothesis are (i) the low concentrations at which TPA acts in cell culture (approximately 10^{-8} to 10^{-10}M); ii) the remarkable similarity in structural requirements seen when a variety of phorbol esters and related macrocyclic diterpenes are tested in diverse systems; and iii) the highly pleiotropic and reversible effects of these compounds. Since the earliest effects of TPA appear to occur at the cell membrane, we further postulated that the putative receptors are on the cell surface and the endogenous growth regulator may be a polypeptide hormone.

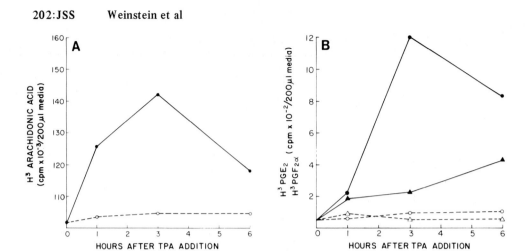

Fig. 1. The accumulation of arachidonic acid and prostaglandins E_2 and $F_{2\alpha}$ in culture medium from CEF. TPA (8×10^{-8}M) or 0.1% DMSO was added in 2 ml of serum-containing medium to cultures prelabeled with [^{3}H]-arachidonic acid and aliquots of the media were collected at the specified times. Control cultures received 0.1% DMSO as vehicle control. Radioactivity was extracted and analyzed by thin-layer chromatography for arachidonic acid and prostaglandins E_2 and F_2. Results are the means from two different cultures. A) Arachidonic acid released, plus TPA (●——●) or 0.1% DMSO (○— — —○). B) Prostaglandin E_2 released, plus TPA (●——●) or 0.1% DMSO (○— — —○); prostaglandin F_2 released, plus TPA (▲————▲) or 0.1% DMSO (△— — —△). For additional details see Mufson et al [47].

A possible candidate for the polypeptide hormone is epidermal (EGF), since it shares a number of biologic effects with TPA [54]. We have shown that EGF, like TPA, is a potent inducer of plasminogen activator in HeLa cell cultures [58]. In addition, we found that TPA and related tumor promoters are extremely potent inhibitors of the binding of ^{125}I-EGF to its cell surface receptors [54]. This effect is seen with a variety of human, rat, and murine cell cultures and is preferential for the EGF receptor [59]. For example, TPA does not inhibit the binding of insulin to its receptors [59]. These findings have been confirmed and extended by other investigators [60, 77].

There is evidence that the concentration of EGF required for maximum biological effect is considerably lower than that required to saturate receptor binding [70, 78]. Therefore, in most of our studies we have used a low concentration of ^{125}I-EGF (approximately 0.04 nM) to provide assurance that we were dealing with physiologic concentrations and to maximize sensitivity to the TPA effect. Under these conditions with HeLa cells the inhibitory effect of TPA is noncompetitive with EGF [54]. This is also true with the macrocyclic diterpene mezerein (Lee and Weinstein, unpublished studies). On the other hand, recent studies by other investigators [60, 77] using 3T3 cells suggest that the TPA inhibition of EGF-receptor binding is competitive with EGF. This apparent discrepancy may relate to differences between HeLa and 3T3 cells or to the much higher concentrations of EGF used in the latter studies. The finding that cells transformed by murine sarcoma viruses have a decrease in EGF receptors and actually synthesize a polypeptide growth factor [61] suggests that changes in the EGF effector system may play an important role not only in the carcinogenic process but also in maintenance of the transformed state.

Figure 2 shows that when ^{125}I-EGF was added to HeLa cultures there was rapid binding which was linear for about 30 min. The amount of bound material declined after 90 min [59]. When TPA (30 ng/ml) was added simultaneously with the EGF, there was rapid inhibition of ^{125}I-EGF binding which was apparent within 15 min and persisted for at least 150 min. The preincubation of cells with TPA 10 min prior to the addition of EGF gave results similar to those obtained when the two were added simultaneously.

The effects of delayed addition of TPA are also shown in Figure 2. The addition of TPA either during the phase of linear binding of ^{125}I-EGF, or the plateau phase, resulted in a rapid decline of ^{125}I-EGF binding. This effect was apparent within 5–10 min of addition of the TPA. In a separate experiment cells were incubated with ^{125}I-EGF for 50 min to achieve plateau binding. The medium was removed and either TPA (33 ng/ml) or DMSO was added and the rate of loss of radioactivity was measured during a subsequent 90-min period. In the control culture there was a gradual decline, whereas in the TPA-treated culture there was a rapid decline, in cell associated radioactivity [59]. Thus TPA is capable of reversing the initial binding of ^{125}I-EGF to cells and also enhances the loss of cell-associated EGF that normally occurs at later time points.

Additional studies indicated that the radioactivity released from the cells by TPA was largely intact ^{125}I-EGF rather than degraded material, as judged by chromatography on Biogel P-6 columns [59]. These results provided evidence that TPA does not exert its effect on cellular binding of EGF by enhancing the degradation of EGF either via direct proteolysis or enhanced cellular internalization and proteolysis.

The influence of temperature on the ability of TPA to affect EGF binding is summarized in Table VI. Although at 37°C TPA caused approximately a 77% inhibition of ^{125}I-EGF binding, at 22°C the inhibition by TPA was 60% and at 4° it was only 26%, compared to the control values at the same temperatures. Additional studies indicated that when ^{125}I-EGF binding was studied over a period of several hours at either 22° or 4°C in the absence or presence of TPA, the percentage inhibition by TPA was greater at all times at 22° than at 4°C. Although TPA had only a small effect on EGF binding when added to cells at 4°C, if cells were preincubated with TPA at 37° (in the absence of EGF) there was a marked inhibition in their capacity to subsequently bind ^{125}I-EGF at 4°C compared to the binding obtained at 4°C with cells not previously exposed to TPA at 37°.

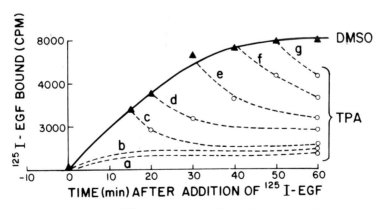

Fig. 2. Time course of binding of ^{125}I-EGF to HeLa cells at 37°C and the effects of addition of TPA at various times. ^{125}I-EGF was added at time zero and cell-associated material was determined at various time intervals in the absence (▲———▲) or presence (○– – –○) of 33 ng/ml TPA. The TPA was added at different times as indicated: a) −10 min; b) time 0; c) time 15 min; d) time 20 min; e) time 30 min; f) time 40 min; g) time 50 min. All plates received 11,488 cpm ^{125}I-EGF (specific activity 77 μCi/μg). For additional details see Lee and Weinstein [59].

TABLE VI. Effect of Temperature on TPA Inhibition of EGF Binding

Temperature	^{125}I-EGF bound (cpm)		% of Control
	Control	+TPA	
4°	3,110	2,295	73.8
22°	6,634	2,612	39.4
37°	7,499	1,687	22.5

HeLa cells were incubated with ^{125}I-EGF (22,727 cpm, specific activity 57 μCi/μg) plus or minus TPA (22 ng/ml) for 60 min at the indicated temperature and the amoung of cell-bound material was measured as described in Lee and Weinstein [54].

To determine the effect of temperature on the ability of TPA to enhance the loss of previously bound EGF from cells, we first allowed cells to bine ^{125}I-EGF at 37° for 50 min, shifted them to either 4° or 22°, added either DMSO or TPA, and then measured the rate of loss of cell-associated ^{125}I-EGF. We found that at 22°C TPA induced a rapid loss of cell-associated ^{125}I-EGF, whereas at 4°C it did not [59].

Taken together, the above results suggest that TPA inhibits EGF binding not by binding directly to the "active site" of the EGF receptor but by indirectly altering the conformation or inducing the clustering of EGF receptors. This could reflect the binding of TPA to sites on the EGF receptor which have an allosteric effect, or TPA-induced changes in the lipid microenvironment in which the EGF receptors are embedded. Conformational changes and temperature-dependent receptor clustering are known to markedly affect the function of various hormones receptors [62, 69, 70, 76].

MODELS OF TPA ACTION AND THEIR RELEVANCE TO TUMOR PROMOTION

Figure 3 integrates the various cellular effects of TPA into a comprehensive model. The primary action of TPA appears to be at the cell surface membrane. Changes in cell surface morphology and cellular adhesion and an apparent increase in membrane lipid fluidity provide evidence that TPA produces a generalized change in cell membrane structure. These early effects do not appear to require de novo RNA and protein synthesis, but their physical and biochemical basis remains to be elucidated. These structural changes presumably account for several effects of TPA on membrane function including an alteration in membrane-associated Na/K ATPase, increased transport of ^{86}Rb, ^{32}P, and 2-deoxyglucose, enhanced phospholipid synthesis, and phospholipid deacylation (Table V). The functions of β-adrenergic receptors [51–53], the receptor for epithelial growth factor [54, 60], and perhaps other receptors involved in growth control are also altered. There are also alterations in cell surface glycoproteins [9, 10, 50], although these appear to occur later than the changes in membrane phospholipids. The ability of retinoids to antagonize certain actions of TPA [47, 74], to inhibit tumor promotion on mouse skin [56], and to inhibit certain other forms of carcinogenesis [63], may be due to reciprocal effects of the retinoids at the membrane level. Since a number of the effects of TPA resemble those of hormonal agents, it is possible that TPA acts by usurping, or disturbing, the function of a cellular receptor-response pathway normally used by an endogenous growth regulatory substance. Studies with TPA may therefore provide clues to the general phenomenon of hormonal carcinogenesis. In addition, the compound provides a useful probe for studies on membrane structure and function.

MOLECULAR MODEL OF TPA ACTION

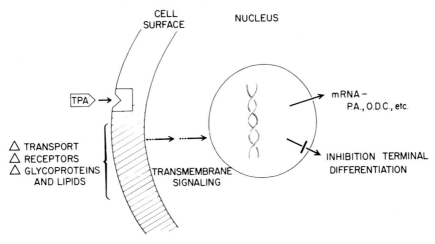

Fig. 3. Schematic model of the primary action of TPA on the cell surface with secondary effects on nuclear function. Reproduced from Weinstein et al [7].

Following the above early effects of TPA on cell membranes, there are a series of later or secondary cellular responses which require RNA and protein synthesis and therefore may reflect the action of "transmembrane signals" on nuclear and cytoplasmic functions. As in the case of certain polypeptide hormones and mitogens that exert their primary effects at the cell surface, the nature of these transmembrane signals is not well understood at the present time. These later responses to TPA include induction of plasminogen activator and ornithine decarboxylase synthesis, inhibition or stimulation of DNA synthesis, altered cell surface glycoproteins and effects on the expression of pre-existent programs of terminal differentiation (Table IV).

We must emphasize that cell types differ considerably in terms of their responses to TPA. Differences in response to the same hormone by different target cells are well known in endocrinology. Clonal variants of murine erythroleukemia cells that are resistant to TPA inhibition of terminal differentiation have recently been isolated [64] and these may prove useful in dissecting out the diverse actions of TPA. Since the transformation process itself leads to changes in cell surface structure and function, one might anticipate that cells previously altered by exposure to a chemical or viral carcinogen would have quantitatively and/or qualitatively different responses to TPA compared to completely normal cells. This aspect could in part explain the phenomenon of "enhancement" observed when transformed cells are exposed to TPA. Mechanisms involving sequential alterations in the response of the same cell type to tumor promoters and growth-controlling substances may underlie the stepwise process of tumor promotion and progression.

A number of years ago, Berenblum [65] postulated that tumor promoters act by inducing disturbances in differentiation and several observations in mouse skin provided indirect support for this hypothesis [66, 67, 68]. The results in cell culture systems provide direct evidence that the phorbol esters can be potent modifiers of terminal differentiation (Table IV). This effect may be an important clue to their ability to act as tumor promoters on mouse skin. A possible model is illustrated schematically in Figure 4. The stem cells in the epidermis are continually dividing; yet the tissue as a whole is in a stage of balanced

EFFECTS OF TPA ON STEM CELL DIVISION

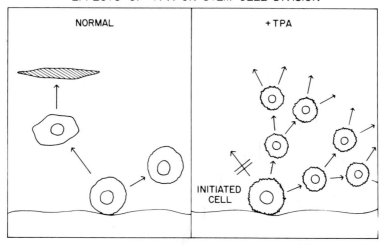

Fig. 4. Schematic representation of the normal mode of asymmetric stem cell division in epidermis and of the hypothesis that TPA induces exponential growth of an initiated stem cell, thus yielding a clone of such cells from which tumors can arise. Reproduced from Weinstein et al [7].

growth and a stable stem cell pool size is maintained. This is probably achieved by a regular asymmetric division of the stem cell. One daughter cell becomes a stem cell and the other daughter cell is committed to keratinize and terminally differentiate, thus irreversibly losing its growth potential. If an "initiated" stem cell were restrained to the stem cell mode of division, it could not increase its proportion in the stem cell pool. If, however, the stem cell division mode were interrupted by the action of a promoting agent, the initiated cell could undergo exponential division, thus yielding a clone of similar cells. Since TPA can also induce phenotypic changes in cells that mimic those of transformed cells, the micro-environment of a clone of such cells might itself enhance their further outgrowth and development into a tumor.

The fact that TPA can induce rather than inhibit differentiation in certain cell systems may, in part, explain its tissue specificity as a tumor promoter. In addition, this action might be exploited as a novel approach to cancer therapy in those tumors in which this type of compound induces terminal differentiation.

Although the above the speculations provide plausible models for thinking about mechanisms by which the phorbol esters enhance the induction of papillomas on mouse skin previously exposed to an initiating agent, they do not readily explain why repeated applications of these agents to mouse skin eventually result in the formation of malignant tumors that do not regress even after application of TPA has been stopped. Stated in other terms, the question is: How is a cellular response mechanism that is normally inductive converted to one which is constitutive or autonomous? This remains one of the major dilemmas in carcinogenesis. It seems likely that the answer to this question relates to the nature of the irreversible change in cells produced by the initiating carcinogens. Elsewhere, we have raised the question of whether the latter lesion is a simple random point mutation or a more complex change in genome structure related to normal mechanisms of cellular differentiation [7]. One hypothesis of two-stage carcinogenesis is that the initiating agent results in the acquisition of an aberrant program of differentiation, but this program remains dormant until expression of the related genes is induced by the promoting agent. With repeated induction the expression of this program becomes "locked in" by a mechanism (yet to be discovered) similar to those that provide stability to normal states of differentiation [7].

ACKNOWLEDGMENTS

The authors wish to acknowledge the valuable contributions made to these studies by Drs. D. Schachter, Eitan Fibach, Paul Marks, and Richard Rifkind.

This investigation was supported by contract No. NO-1-CP-23234 awarded by the National Cancer Institute, Department of Health, Education and Welfare, and grant No. RD-50 awarded by the American Cancer Society.

REFERENCES

1. Slaga TJ, Sivak A, Boutwell RK (eds): "Carcinogenesis," vol 2, "Mechanisms of Tumor Promotion and Cocarcinogenesis." New York: Raven, 1978.
2. Goerttler K, Laerhke H: Virchows Arch A Pathol Anat Hist 376:117–122, 1977.
3. Goerttler K, Laerhke H, Schweizer J, Hesse B: Cancer Res. 39:1293–1297, 1979.
4. Sugimura T, Kawachi T, Nakayasu N: In "Abstracts of Papers, Cold Spring Harbor Meeting." Cold Spring Harbor, New York: Cold Spring Harbor Laboratory, 1978, p 30.
5. Sivak A: Biochem Biophys Acta 560:67–89, 1978.
6. Weber J, Hecker E: Experentia 34:679, 1978.
7. Weinstein IB, Yamasaki H, Wigler M, Lee LS, Fisher PB, Jeffrey AM, Grunberger D: In Griffin AC, Shaw CR (eds): "Carcinogens: Identification and Mechanisms of Action." New York: Raven, 1979, pp 399–418.
8. Wigler M, Weinstein IB: Nature 259:232–233, 1976.
9. Weinstein IB, Wigler M, Pietropaolo C: In Watson JB, Winston JA (eds): "Origins of Human Cancer." Cold Spring Harbor Conferences on Cell Proliferation, vol 4. Cold Spring Harbor, New York: Cold Spring Harbor Laboratories, 1977, pp 751–752.
10. Weinstein IB, Wigler M, Fisher P, Sisskin E, Pietropaolo C: In Slaga TJ, Sivak A, Boutwell RK (eds): "Carcinogenesis," Vol. 2, "Mechanisms of Tumor Promotion and Cocarcinogenesis." New York: Raven, 1978, pp 313–333.
11. Wigler M, DeFeo D, Weinstein IB: Cancer Res 38:1434–1437, 1978.
12. Mondal S, Brankow DW, Heidelberger C: Cancer Res 36:2254–2260, 1976.
13. Mondal S, Heidelberger C: Nature 260:710–711, 1976.
14. Kennedy A, Mondal S, Heidelberger C, Little JB: Cancer Res 38:439–443, 1978.
15. Fisher PB, Weinstein IB, Eisenberg D, Ginsberg HS: Proc Natl Acad Sci USA 75:2311–2314, 1978.
16. Fisher PB, Goldstein NI, Weinstein IB: Cancer Res 39:3051–3057, 1979.
17. Goldfarb RH, Quigley JP: Cancer Res 38:4601–4609, 1978.
18. O'Brien TG, Diamond L: In Slaga TJ, Sivak A, Boutwell RK (eds): "Carcinogenesis," vol 2, "Mechanisms of Tumor Promotion and Cocarcinogenesis." New York: Raven, 1978, pp 273–287.
19. Levine K, Hassid A: Biochem Biophys Res Commun 79:477–483, 1977.
20. Weinstein IB: In Nieburgs HE (ed): "Proceedings of the Third International Symposium on Detection and Prevention of Cancer." New York: Marcell Dekker, 1978.
21. Casto BC, Pieczynski WJ, DiPaolo JA: Cancer Res 33:819–824, 1973.
22. Hirai K, Defendi V, Diamond L: Cancer Res 34:3497–3500, 1974.
23. Colburn NH, Former BF, Nelson KA, Yuspa SH: Nature 281:589–591.
24. Yamasaki H, Fibach E, Nudel U, Weinstein IB, Rifkind RA, Marks PA: Proc Natl Acad Sci USA 74:3451–3455, 1977.
25. Rovera G, O'Brien TA, Diamond L: Proc Natl Acad Sci USA 74:2894–2898, 1977.
26. Cohen R, Pacifici M, Rubenstein N, Biehl J, Holtzer H: Nature 266:538–540, 1977.
27. Pacifici M, Holtzer H: Am J Anat 150:207–212, 1977.
28. Diamond L, O'Brien TG, Rovera G: Nature 269:247–248, 1977.
29. Ishii DN, Fibach E, Yamasaki H, Weinstein IB: Science 200:556–559, 1978.

30. Mufson RA, Fisher PB, Weinstein IB: Cancer Res 39:3915–3919, 1979.
31. Laskin J, Weinstein IB: (Unpublished studies).
32. Bresch H, Arendt U: Naturwissenschaften 65:660–662, 1978.
33. Esumi H, Troll W: (Personal communication).
34. Miao RM, Fieldsteel HA, Fodge DW: Nature 274:271–272, 1978.
35. Bissell MJ, Hatie C, Calvin M: Proc Natl Acad Sci USA 76:348–352, 1979.
36. Sachs L: Nature 274:535–539, 1978.
37. Huberman E, Callahan MF: Proc Natl Acad Sci USA 76:1293–1297, 1979.
38. Huberman E, Heckman C, Langenbach R: Cancer Res 39:2618–2624, 1979.
39. Kupchan SM, Uchida I, Branfman AR, Dailey RG, Fei BY: Science 191:571–572, 1976.
40. Weinstein IB: In Fenoglio CM, King DW (eds): "Advances in Pathobiology," vol 4, "Cancer Biology. II: Etiology and Therapy." New York: Stratton Intercontinental, 1976, pp 106–117.
41. Sivak A, Van Duuren BL: Science 157:1443–1444, 1967.
42. Driedger PE, Blumberg PM: Cancer Res 37:3257–3265, 1977.
43. Moroney J, Smith A, Tomel LD, Wenner CE: J Cell Physiol 95:287–294, 1978.
44. Suss R, Kreibich G, Kinzel V: Eur J Cancer 8:299–304, 1972.
45. Fisher PB, Flamm M, Schachter D, Weinstein IB: Biochem. Biophys Res Commun 86:1063–1068, 1979.
46. Castagna M, Rochette-Egly C, Rosenfeld C, Mishal Z: FEBS Lett 100:62–66, 1979.
47. Mufson RA, DeFeo D, Weinstein IB: "Molecular Pharmacology" 16:569–578, 1979.
48. Yamasaki H, Weinstein IB, Fibach E, Rifkind RA, Marks PA: Cancer Res 39:1989–1994, 1979.
49. Lowe ME, Pacifici M, Holtzer H: Cancer Res 38:2350–2356, 1978.
50. Blumberg PM, Driedger PE, Rossow PW: Nature 264:446–447, 1976.
51. Grimm W, Marks F: Cancer Res 34:3128–3134, 1974.
52. Mufson RA, Simsiman RC, Boutwell RK: Cancer Res 37:665–699, 1977.
53. Garte SJ, Belman S: Proc Am Assoc Cancer Res 20:52, 1979. (Abstract).
54. Lee LS, Weinstein IB: Science 202:313–315, 1978.
55. Lee LS, Weinstein IB: J Environ Pathol Toxicol 1:627–639, 1978.
56. Verma AK, Boutwell RK: Cancer Res 37:2196–2201, 1977.
57. Lee LS, Weinstein IB: J Cell Physiol 99:451–460, 1979.
58. Lee LS, Weinstein IB: Nature 274:696–697, 1978.
59. Lee LS, Weinstein IB: Proc Natl Acad Sci USA 76:5168–5172; and unpublished studies.
60. Brown KD, Dicker P, Rozengurt E: Biochem Biophys Res Commun 86:1037–1043, 1979.
61. Todaro G, DeLarco JG: Cancer Res 38:4147–4154, 1978.
62. DeMeyts P, Bianco AR, Roth J: J Biol Chem 251:1877–1888, 1976.
63. Sporn MB, Newton DL, Smith JM, Acton N, Jacobson AE, Brossi A: In Griffin AC, Shaw CR (eds): "Carcinogens: Identification and Mechanisms of Action." The University of Texas System Cancer Center, 31st Annual Symposium on Fundamental Cancer Research. New York: Raven, 1978, pp 441–453.
64. Fibach E, Yamasaki H, Weinstein IB, Marks PA. Rifkind RA: Cancer Res 38:3685–3688, 1978.
65. Berenblum I: Adv Cancer Res 2:129–175, 1954.
66. Raick AN: Cancer Res 34:2915–2925, 1974.
67. Yuspa SH, Ben T, Patterson E, Michael D, Elgio K, Hennings H: Cancer Res 36:4062–4068, 1976.
68. Colburn NH, Lau S, Head R: Cancer Res 35:3154–3159, 1975.
69. Schlessinger J, Schechter Y, Cuatrecasas P, Willingham MC, Pastan I: Proc Natl Acad Sci USA 75:5353–5357, 1978.
70. Das M, Fox CF: Proc Natl Acad Sci USA 75:2644–2648, 1978.
71. Ishii DN: Cancer Res 38:3886–3893, 1978.
72. Fibach E, Gambari R, Shaw PA, Maniatis G, Reuben RC, Sassa S, Rifkind RA, Marks PA: Proc Natl Acad Sci USA 76:1906–1910, 1979.
73. Castagna M, Rochette-Egly C, Rosenfeld C: Cancer Lett 6:227–234, 1979.
74. Wertz PW, Mueller GC: Cancer Res 28:2900–2904, 1978.
75. Van Duuren BL: Prog Exp Tumor Res 11:31–68, 1969.
76. Singer SJ: In Bradshaw RA, Frazier WA, Merrell RC, Gottlieb DI, Hogue-Angelitti RA (eds): "Surface Membrane Receptors." New York: Plenum, 1976, pp 1–24.
77. Shoyab M, DeLarco JE, Todaro GJ: Nature 279:387–391, 1979.
78. Shechter Y, Hernaez L, Cuatrecasas P: Proc Natl Acad Sci USA 75:5788–5791, 1978.
79. Nakayasu M, Shoji M, Aoki N, Sato S, Miwa M, Sugimura T: Cancer Res: 39:4668–4672, 1979.
80. Rovera G, O'Brien TG, Diamond L: Science 204:868–870.
81. Fisher PB, Bozzone JH, Weinstein IB: Cell 18:695–705, 1979.

Journal of Supramolecular Structure 12:209—226 (1979)
Tumor Cell Surfaces and Malignancy 541—558

Biosynthesis and Maturation of Cellular Membrane Glycoproteins

Lawrence A. Hunt

Department of Microbiology, University of Kansas Medical Center, Kansas City, Kansas 66103

The biosynthesis and the processing of asparagine-linked oligosaccharides of cellular membrane glycoproteins were examined in monolayer cultures of BHK21 cells and human diploid fibroblasts after pulse- and pulse-chase labeling with $[2\text{-}^3H]$ mannose. After pronase digestion, radiolabeled glycopeptides were characterized by high-resolution gel filtration, with or without additional digestion with various exoglycosidases and endoglycosidases. Pulse-labeled glycoproteins contained a relatively homogenous population of neutral oligosaccharides (major species: $Man_9GlcNAc_2ASN$). The vast majority of these asparagine-linked oligosaccharides was smaller than the major fraction of lipid-linked oligosaccharides from the cell and was apparently devoid of terminal glucose. After pulse-chase or long labeling periods, a significant fraction of the large oligomannosyl cores was processed by removal of mannose units and addition of branch sugars (NeuNAc-Gal-GlcNAc), resulting in complex acidic structures containing three and possibly five mannoses. In addition, some of the large oligomannosyl cores were processed by the removal of only several mannoses, resulting in a mixture of neutral structures with 5—9 mannoses. This oligomannosyl core heterogeneity in both neutral and acidic oligosaccharides linked to asparagine in cellular membrane glycoproteins was analogous to the heterogeneity reported for the oligosaccharides of avian RNA tumor virus glycoproteins (Hunt LA, Wright SE, Etchison JR, Summers DF: J Virol 29:336, 1979).

Key words: membrane glycoproteins, human diploid fibroblasts, BHK21 cells, exoglycosidases and endoglycosidases, asparaginyl-oligosaccharides, gel filtration, processing of oligomannosyl core

Biochemical studies of cellular membrane glycoproteins of animal cells in tissue culture [1, 2] have suggested that these polypeptides have asparagine-linked oligosaccharides that are similar to the carbohydrate chains of a number of well-characterized serum glycoproteins [3] with respect to both heterogeneity in oligomannosyl core size and the presence of both acidic and neutral structures. The common structural feature of

Abbreviations: ASN — asparagine; Fuc — fucose; Gal — galactose; Glc — glucose; GlcNAc — N-acetyl-glucosamine; Man — mannose; NeuNAc — sialic acid, N-acetylneuraminic acid.

Received April 23, 1979; accepted August 16, 1979.

these carbohydrate chains is a cluster of mannose units linked to the asparaginase residue in the polypeptide by a N,N-diacetylchitobiose structure $[(Man)_n GlcNAc-GlcNAc-ASN]$, with complex, acidic chains differing from high-mannose neutral chains by the size of the oligomannosyl core and the presence of branch structures terminating in sialic acid (NeuNAc±Gal-GlcNAc−) [3]. The specific function of these oligosaccharides in cellular membrane glycoproteins is not clear, but growth-dependent changes in both the size distribution of oligomannosyl cores and the ratio of acidic to neutral chains have been detected in studies of [³H] mannose-labeled human diploid fibroblasts [2]. These differences may have represented either changes in the carbohydrate composition of individual glycoproteins or changes which were secondary to a new population of polypeptides.

Recent studies with vesicular stomatitits and Sindbis virus-infected cells strongly suggested that viral membrane glycoproteins acquired large oligomannosyl core structures by the en bloc transfer of a preformed oligosaccharide from lipid-linked intermediates (dolichol-phosphate-oligosaccharide), and these asparagine-linked oligosaccharides were subsequently processed to complex acidic structures by the trimming of mannose and sequential addition of branch sugars [4–6]. Because these viral glycoproteins were being synthesized and processed by cellular enzymatic machinery and because the lipid-linked oligosaccharides from a number of virus-infected and uninfected tissue culture cell lines have been shown to have a fairly common structure [4, 7, 8], the heterogeneous array of asparagine-linked oligosaccharides of cellular membrane glycoproteins must be synthesized and matured by similar, if not identical, intracellular processes.

The aim of these studies was to confirm this prediction using [2-³H] mannose pulse- and pulse-chase labeling of the asparagine-linked oligosaccharides of membrane glycoproteins of BHK21 cells and human diploid fibroblasts. The specific objectives were threefold: 1) to determine the size and structure of the asparagine-linked oligosaccharides of pulse-labeled glycoprotein and compare these "precursor" structures with the lipid-linked oligosaccharides; 2) to demonstrate the processing of "precursor" glycoproteins into glycoproteins with "mature" carbohydrate structures containing smaller oligomannosyl cores; and 3) to determine the size of the oligomannosyl cores of these mature asparagine-linked oligosaccharides and their distribution between the complex acidic structures and high-mannose neutral structures.

METHODS

HeLa S3 cells were grown in suspension culture, and the BHK21 cells and human embryonic lung fibroblasts were grown in monolayer culture [5]. The human diploid fibroblasts were provided by Noël Jarnevic of the Department of Pathology and Oncology. Suspension cultures of HeLa cells or monolayer cultures of the human diploid fibroblasts and BHK21 cells were pulse-labeled with 100 μCi/ml [2-³H] mannose (2 Ci/ml, Amersham) in glucose-deficient medium [5, 9]. Pulse-chase labeling was similar except that the radioactive medium was removed at the end of the pulse-labeling and replaced with medium containing 2 mM unlabeled mannose for the duration of the "chase" period. Previous studies with virus-infected cells in culture [5] and uninfected cells in culture (unpublished observations) indicated that the incorporation of [³H] mannose into trichloroacetic acid-precipitable material reached a plateau within approximately 5 min of the initiation of the "chase" after "pulse" labeling for 30–60 min, and then decreased with increasing chase periods. The medium for the overnight labeling of BHK21 cells contained 60 μCi/ml [2-³H] mannose and one-third the normal amount of glucose.

The preparation of membrane glycoproteins and the digestion with pronase (grade B, Calbiochem) were identical to procedures previously employed for vesicular stomatitis virus-infected tissue culture cells [5, 9]. Lipid-linked oligosaccharides (dolichol-phosphate-oligosaccharides) were isolated by selective organic extraction of whole cells with chloroform/methanol (2:1) and chloroform/methanol/water (10:10:3), and the oligosaccharides were released from the lipid by mild acid hydrolysis [7, 10].

Glycopeptides and oligosaccharides were digested with exoglycosidases and endo-β-N-acetylglucosaminidases as previously described [5, 9, 11]. Endo-β-N-acetylglucosaminidase H from Streptomyces plicatus, endo-β-N-acetylglucosaminidase D and exoglycosidases from Streptococcus pnemoniae, and jack bean α-mannosidase were provided by Dr. James Etchison, University of Utah. Clostridium perfringens neuraminidase (type IX) and yeast α-glucosidase (type III) were purchased from Sigma Chemical Company.

Glycopeptides and oligosaccharides were analyzed before and after glycosidase digestions by gel filtration through a BioGel P-4 column [5, 9]. The elution positions of various neutral oligomannosyl cores (Man$_n$GlcNAc$_1$) of known composition were used to calibrate the BioGel P-4 column in the gel filtration of endo-β-N-acetylglucosaminidase digestion products from [2-^{3}H]mannose-labeled cellular membrane glycopeptides [5, 11, 12].

RESULTS

Lipid-Linked and Protein-Linked "Precursor" Oligosaccharides

The newly synthesized asparagine-linked oligosaccharides of cellular glycoproteins were analyzed and compared with the corresponding lipid-linked oligosaccharides after pulse-labeling of BHK21 cells with [2-^{3}H]mannose and isolation of lipid-linked and peptide-linked oligosaccharide fractions from whole cells. [2-^{3}H]mannose was used in the labeling experiments because this sugar was incorporated into the lipid-linked oligosaccharides along with glucosamine and glucose, and was added to glycoprotein only at the initial stage of en bloc glycosylation in the rough endoplasmic reticulum [9]. Additional glucosamine and other radiolabeled sugars (galactose, fucose) would have been immediately added to pre-existing oligosaccharides at the second stage of glycosylation in Golgi-like intracellular membranes [9], and could therefore not have been used to examine the initial glycosylation and processing.

Pronase-digested glycopeptides and oligosaccharides released from the lipid fraction by mild acid hydrolysis were analyzed by gel filtration on BioGel P-4, with or without prior digestion with endo-β-N-acetylglucosaminidase H (Fig. 1B,D). The gel filtration profile of the radiolabeled BHK21 glycopeptides (Fig. 1B) contained a single major peak eluting after the [^{14}C]acetylated asparaginyl-oligosaccharide and a second minor peak eluting before the [^{14}C] marker, and was almost identical to the gel filtration profile for pulse-labeled glycopeptides from HeLa cells (Fig. 1A). After digestion with endo-β-N-acetyl-glucosaminidase H, radiolabel in both major and minor peaks of HeLa and BHK21 glyco-peptides was shifted to a single peak with lower apparent molecular weight, consistent with the release of the radiolabeled oligomannosyl core from the N-acetylglucosaminyl-peptide. As illustrated in Figure 2, the site of hydrolysis of this enzyme was between the two N-acetylglucosamine residues proximal to the peptide moiety of particular oligo-mannosyl di-N-acetylchitobiose structures [13–15] and between the two N-acetylglucos-amine residues of lipid-derived oligosaccharides [4]. The radiolabeled products from the

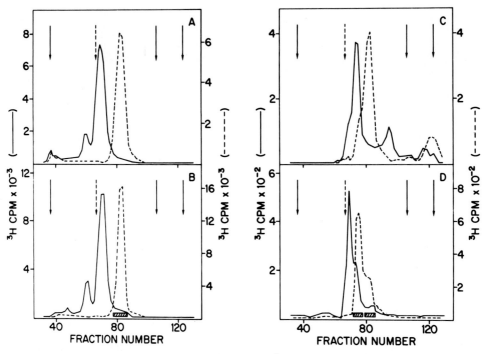

Fig. 1. BioGel P-4 gel filtration of oligosaccharides from [^{3}H] mannose-labeled lipid and protein fractions of BHK21 and HeLa cells. The pulse-labeling times were 60 min for the HeLa cells and 40 min for the BHK21 cells. Pronase-digested glycopeptides from HeLa (A) and BHK21 cells (B) were analyzed before (————) and after (- - - - - -) endo-β-N-acetylglucosaminidase H treatment, and the profiles of radioactivity were superimposed by alignment of the peak elution positions of four column markers (from left to right: blue dextran (void volume), [^{14}C]-acetylated-asparaginyl oligosaccharide from ovalbumin, stachyose, and mannose). Radiolabeled products from the mild acid hydrolysis of lipid-linked oligosac-charides of HeLa (C) and BHK21 cells (D) were analyzed before (————) and after (- - - - - - -) endo-β-N-acetylglucosaminidase H treatment, and the profiles were also superimposed. The boxes with diagonal lines at the bottom of panels B and D indicate the representative fractions pooled from similar preparative BioGel P-4 chromatography of equivalent endoglycosidase-treated samples for further structural analysis (Fig. 3).

endoglycosidase-digested BHK21 and HeLa cell glycopeptides were demonstrated by Dowex ion-exchange chromatography [12] to be neutral oligosaccharides, and the elution positions were indicative of an oligomannosyl core with 8–9 mannoses and one N-acetyl-glucosamine [5, 16]. These results suggested that essentially all of the radiolabel in these glycopeptides was in the form of mannose, since [^{3}H] label incorporated into glyco-proteins in the form of fucose, galactose, sialic acid, or N-acetylglucosamine would have been incorporated directly into higher-molecular-weight, endo-β-N-acetylglucosamine-H-resistant glycopeptides [9]. In addition, if significant radiolabel had been incorporated into N-acetylglucosamine, radiolabel would have been detected in later eluting fractions cor-responding to the GlcNAc-peptide product of endoglycosidase digestion in Figure 1 A,B.

More recent analysis of the peptide-derived neutral oligosaccharides on a different BioGel P-4 column that was capable of resolving a mixture of high-mannose structures differing by one or more hexoses confirmed that the vast majority of radiolabel eluted with Man$_9$GlcNAc$_1$. Very small amounts of radiolabel eluted in the positions expected

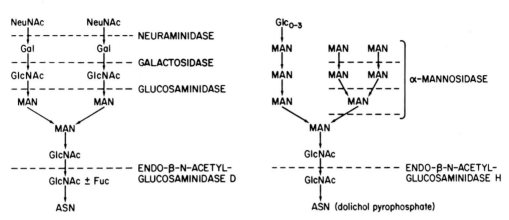

Fig. 2. Typical neutral and acidic asparaginyl oligosaccharide structures and their susceptibility to glycosidases. The acidic structure is identical to that reported for the complex asparaginyl oligosaccharides of Sindbis virus glycoproteins [19], and the neutral structure is identical to that reported for the lipid-linked "precursor" oligosaccharide from vesicular stomatitis virus-infected cells [8], with specific sugar linkages omitted. Horizontal dashed lines show the positions of hydrolysis by enzymes. Neuraminidase, galactosidase, and glucosaminidase from Streptococcus pneumoniae [17] and jack bean α-mannosidase are exolglycosidases that remove the appropriate sugars only when they are at the non-reducing termini of the oligosaccharides. The two forms of endo-β-N-acetylglucosaminidase, D and H, differ in their substrate requirements [13–15]. Both peptide-linked and lipid-derived oligosaccharides (dolichol-phosphate-oligosaccharides) are susceptible to the appropriate glycosidases. With mild acid hydrolysis, the oligosaccharide is released from the dolichol-phosphate.

for oligosaccharides with one less hexose ($Man_8GlcNAc_1$) and one additional hexose (data not shown).

The lipid-derived, [2-^{3}H] mannose-labeled oligosaccharides from BHK21 cells eluted in a single major peak and in an apparent unresolved minor peak on the lower-molecular-weight "shoulder" of the major peak (Fig. 1D). After endo-β-N-acetylglucosaminidase H digestion the oligosaccharides eluted in higher-numbered fractions, as expected from the removal of one of the two N-acetylglucosamines from the radiolabeled oligomannosyl structure (Fig. 2). The major species of lipid-linked oligosaccharide from BHK21 cells was apparently several monosaccharide residues larger than the major species of [2-^{3}H] mannose-labeled oligosaccharide linked to protein, based upon the relative elution positions of the endo-β-N-acetylglucosamine H-released neutral oligosaccharides (Fig. 1B,D). In addition, the lipid-derived oligosaccharides from HeLa cells were smaller before and after endoglycosidase treatment than the corresponding BHK21 oligosaccharides (Fig. 1C,D), the major radiolabeled products of endoglycosidase digestion of both protein and lipid-derived material from the HeLa cells eluting in the same relative position from the BioGel P-4 column (Fig. 1A,C).

Several investigators have presented evidence of terminal glucose residues in radio-labeled asparaginyl-oligosaccahrides and corresponding lipid-linked oligosaccharides extracted from various tissue culture cells [4, 6, 8]. In order to test whether the presence or absence of terminal glucose residues might have accounted for the differences in gel filtration of the major lipid- and protein-derived oligosaccharides, the sensitivity of radiolabel in these structures to jack bean α-mannosidase was examined. If glucose or some monosaccharide other than mannose was present at one or more of the nonreducing termini of the oligomannosyl cores, less of the [3H] label would be released as free mannose, and the decrease in size between the original undigested oligosaccharides and the residual oligosaccharides after exoglycosidase digestion would not be as great (Fig. 2). A more direct method for determining the presence or absence of terminal glucose in both the peptide- and lipid-derived oligosaccharides from the same labeled BHK21 cell culture was not readily available because 1) there was no specific way to radiolabel the glucose (in contrast to the cell-free glycosylation studies using GDP-[3H/14C]glucose [4] or the studies utilizing virus-infected, lectin-resistant cell lines that incorporate [3H]- or [14C] galactose into glycoproteins as [3H]- or [14C]glucose rather than directly as galactose into acidic asparagine-linked oligosaccharides and serine/threonine-linked oligosaccharides [8]); and 2) no well-characterized glucosidases were available to remove terminal glucose residues. In contrast to a previous report of yeast α-glucosidase-mediated removal of terminal glucose from lipid-derived oligosaccharides [18], yeast α-glucosidase had no effect on the gel filtration profiles of the lipid- and peptide-derived oligosaccharides from BHK21 cells (data not shown) or lipid-derived oligosaccharides from Chinese hamster ovary cells in studies by other workers [6].

Neutral oligomannosyl cores corresponding to the major peak of peptide-derived material and the major and minor peaks of lipid-derived material from BHK21 cells were isolated by preparative gel filtration and reanalyzed before and after α-mannosidase digestion (Fig. 3). Prior to α-mannosidase treatment the peptide-derived oligosaccharides and the lipid "shoulder"-derived oligosaccharides eluted in similar positions, distinct from the earlier elution position of the major lipid-derived oligosaccharides. After α-mannosidase digestion a large fraction of the [3H] label of the peptide-derived material and the minor lipid-derived material ("shoulder") eluted in the position of free mannose (Fig. 3, middle and bottom panels). The residual peptide-derived oligosaccharides eluted in a broad peak centered at the psition expected for $Man_3GlcNAc_1$ and in a minor peak just after the position of undigested oligosaccharide (Fig. 3, bottom panel). The α-mannosidase digestion apparently did not go to completion, since the expected products for complete digestion would have been free mannose and the dissacharide, mannose-N-acetylglucosamine ($Man^{\beta}GlcNAc$, reference [8]). This apparent incomplete α-mannosidase digestion of the oligomannosyl core (with $Man_3GlcNAc$ as a major residual product instead of $Man_1GlcNAc_1$) has been previously observed for similar peptide-derived oligosaccharides from vesicular stomatitis virus-infected cells [5, 6]. Similarly, the residual lipid "shoulder"-derived material eluted in the position of $Man_{3-5}GlcNAc_1$ and in a major peak just after the position of undigested material (Fig. 3, middle panel).

In contrast, only a small fraction of radiolabel was released as free mannose by α-mannosidase from the peak of lipid-derived oligosaccharide, and the remaining oligosaccharides eluted in a sharp peak with a slightly decreased apparent molecular weight (Fig. 3, top panel). The significant differences in both the relative amount of free mannose released and size of residual oligosaccharides between the major lipid- and peptide-derived samples after α-mannosidase digestion were most likely due to substrate differences rather than incomplete digestion because of limiting enzymes. The small amounts of apparent high-molecular-weight residual oligosaccharide observed in the digestion products of the lipid-derived "shoulder" material and the peptide-derived material (fractions 80–90 in Figure 3, middle and bottom panels) suggested that a fraction of these samples was also partially protected from α-mannosidase digestion.

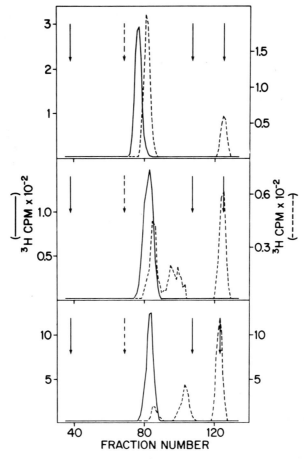

Fig. 3. BioGel P-4 gel filtration of endo-β-N-acetylglucosaminidase H-digested products of [^{3}H] mannose-labeled oligosaccharides from lipid and protein fractions of BHK21 cells. Neutral oligosaccharides were isolated by preparative BioGel P-4 gel filtration, with the representative pooled fractions indicated in Figure 1B and 1D. Aliquots of the radiolabeled oligosaccharides were rechromatographed on the column either before (————) or after (- - - - - -) further treatment with jack bean α-mannosidase, and the profiles were superimposed. Upper panel, peak of lipid-derived oligosaccharides; middle panel, lower-molecular-weight "shoulder" of lipid-derived oligosaccharides; lower panel, peak of peptide-derived oligosaccharides.

The combined results of α-mannosidase digestion and gel filtration were similar to those of other investigators [4, 6], and indicated that the major radiolabeled species of the lipid-derived oligosaccharides 1) contained several more monosaccharide residues than the major radiolabeled species of peptide-derived oligosaccharide (Man$_9$GlcNAc), and 2) was significantly more resistant to α-mannosidase digestion. A logical explanation was that these lipid-derived oligosaccharides contained several residues of glucose at a nonreducing terminus as reported by other investigators [4, 6, 8], whereas most of the peptide-derived "precursor" oligosaccharides from the same radiolabeled BHK21 cell cultures were deficient in terminal glucose. Much of the lower-molecular weight "shoulder" fraction of the lipid-derived oligosaccharides was also apparently deficient in terminal glucose, whereas a small fraction of the peptide-derived oligosaccharides may have contained a single terminal glucose residue (Fig. 3, middle and bottom panels). The proposed "precursor" oligosaccharide structures shown in Figure 4 were consistent with the experimental results presented here and previously published studies on the detailed structure of lipid-linked oligosaccharides from virus-infected chinese hamster ovary cells [8].

Processing of "Precursor" Asparagine-Linked Oligosaccharides

The question of whether a relatively homogenous population of asparagine-linked "precursor" oligosaccharides ($Glc_{0-1}Man_{8-9}GlcNAc_2ASN$) could be processed into a number of distinct oligosaccharide structures was addressed experimentally by pulse-chase labeling of BHK21 cells (45-min pulse, 0,2,4,24-h chase) with [2-^{3}H] mannose. Total cell membrane glycoprotein was isolated from the cell cultures, digested with pronase, and analyzed by gel filtration on a BioGel P-4 column before and after digestion with endo-β-N-acetylglucosaminidase H (Fig. 5). The gel filtration profile of the 0-h "chase" material before and after endoglycosidase digestion (Fig. 5A,E) was similar to that previously observed for oligosaccharides from the protein fraction of pulse-labeled BHK21 and HeLa cells in Figure 1A and 1B, with essentially all of the radiolabeled glycopeptide converted to neutral oligosaccharides eluting from the column in higher-numbered fractions.

With increasing "chase" periods, a significant fraction of the radiolabeled oligosac-

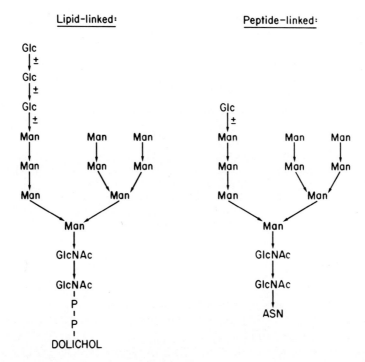

Fig. 4. Structures proposed for the lipid-linked and peptide-linked "precursor" oligosaccharides. The number and arrangement of mannose and glucose units were derived from previously proposed structures for the oligomannosyl core of unit A asparagine-linked carbohydrates of calf thyroglobulin [14] and the lipid-linked oligosaccharides from vesicular stomatitis virus-infected chinese hamster ovary cells in tissue culture [8], and were consistent with the combined gel filtration and glycosidase studies with the BHK21 cellular membrane glycopeptides.

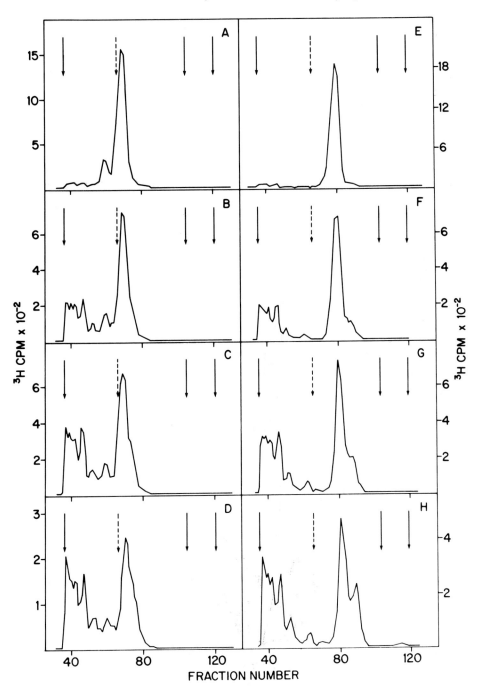

Fig. 5. BioGel P-4 gel filtration of membrane glycopeptides from pulse-chase labeling of BHK21 cells. Monolayer cultures were pulse-labeled with [2-^{3}H] mannose for 45 min and then "chased" in unlabeled medium for 0, 2, 4, and 24 h. Radiolabeled glycopeptides were analyzed either before (A–D) or after (E–H) treatment with endo-β-N-acetylglucosaminidase H. A, E, O-h chase; B, F, 2-h chase; C, G, 4-h chase; D, H, 24-h chase.

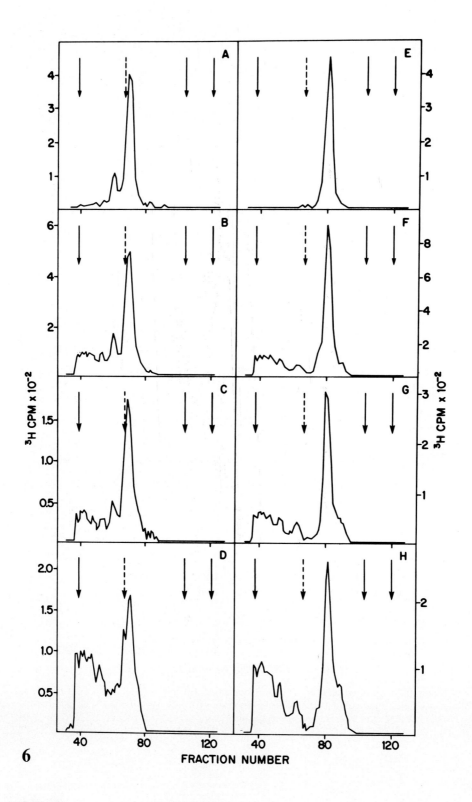

charides was apparently converted to endo-β-N-acetylglucosaminidase H-resistant structures and appeared in a more heterogenous distribution of glycopeptides with apparently higher molecular weights. In addition, some of the asparagine-linked "precursor" oligosaccharides were apparently converted during the incubation in unlabeled medium to smaller oligomannosyl structures ($Man_{5-7}GlcNAc_2ASN$) that were also sensitive to digestion by endo-β-N-acetylglucosaminidase H (fractions 85–95 in Fig. 5H).

An analogous experiment with human diploid fibroblasts gave very similar results (Fig. 6): With increasing "chase" periods radiolabel appeared in a heterogenous population of apparently larger-molecular-weight, endo-β-N-acetylglucosaminidase H-resistant glycopeptides and smaller, endo-β-N-acetylglucosaminidase H-sensitive oligomannosyl core structures.

Structure of "Mature" Asparagine-Linked Oligosaccharides

The resistance to endo-β-N-acetylglucosaminidase H of the apparent high-molecular-weight glycopeptides that appeared after increasing "chase" periods in the labeling of both BHK21 and human diploid fibroblast cells suggested, but did not prove, that these glycopeptides contained complex, acidic oligosaccharides with smaller oligomannosyl core structures. Because more detailed analysis of these oligosaccharide structures required significantly greater amounts of radioactivity than were present in the 24-h chase samples, [2-^{3}H] mannose-labeled glycopeptides were isolated from the membranes of BHK21 cells after a continuous labeling period of 24-h. BioGel P-4 analysis of these radiolabeled glycopeptides before (Fig. 7A) and after (Fig. 7C) digestion with endo-β-N-acetylglucosaminidase H resulted in gel filtration profiles that were virtually indistinguishable from the corresponding profiles of the 45-min pulse–24-h chase sample (Fig. 5D,H). The results of oligosaccharide structural analysis of the 24-h labeled cellular membrane glycoproteins were therefore presumed to be applicable to the "mature" asparagine-linked oligosaccharides derived from the high-mannose "precursor" structure during the 45-min pulse–24-h chase labeling (Fig. 5).

The major peak of radiolabeled glycopeptides eluting after the [^{14}C] column marker in Figure 7A was demonstrated to be a mixture of high-mannose, neutral glycopeptides on the basis of sensitivity to both endo-β-N-acetylglucosamindase H (Fig. 7C) and jack bean α-mannosidase (Fig. 7B). The partial digestion with α-mannosidase released a large amount of radiolabel that coeluted with free mannose, and the residual neutral glycopeptide peak was in the position expected for glycopeptides with smaller oligomannosyl core structures, consistent with the original neutral glycopeptides containing terminal mannose residues (Fig. 2). In contrast, the glycopeptides of higher apparent molecular weight were unaffected by these exoglycosidase and endoglycosidase digestions, but were affected by digestion with Clostridium perfringens neuraminidase (Fig. 7D). This indicated that these glycopeptides contained terminal sialic acid (Fig. 2), but still exhibited considerable heterogenity upon gel filtration in the asialo form.

Fig. 6. BioGel P-4 gel filtration of membrane glycoproteins from pulse-chase labeling of human diploid fibroblasts. Monolayer cultures were pulse-labeled for 30 min with [2-^{3}H] mannose and then "chased" for 0, 2, 4, and 24 h. A–D, not treated with glycosidase; E–H, treated with endo-β-N-acetylglucosaminidase H; A, E, 0-h chase; B, F, 2-h chase; C, G, 4-h chase; D, H, 24-h chase.

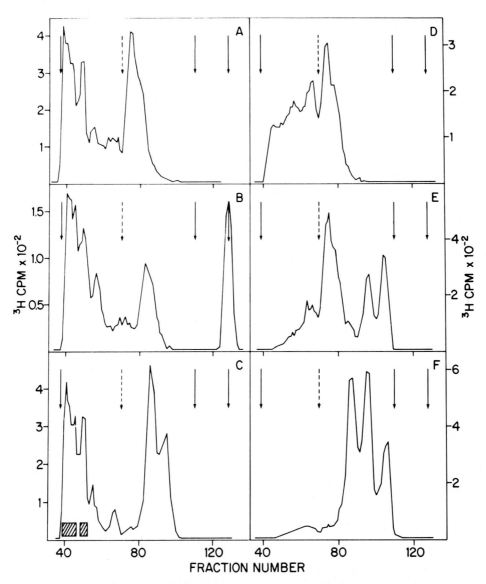

Fig. 7. BioGel P-4 gel filtration of glycosidase-treated membrane glycopeptides from a BHK21 mono-layer culture labeled for 24 h with [2-³H] mannose. Aliquots of a sample of pronase-digested glyco-peptides were analyzed by gel filtration, either without further treatment (A) or after treatment with various glycosidases (B–F). B, α-mannosidase-treated glycopeptides; C, endo-β-N-acetylglucosaminidase H-treated glycopeptides; D, neuraminidase-treated glycopeptides; E, exoglycosidase and endo-β-N-acetylglucosaminidase D-treated glycopeptides; F, glycopeptides after treatment first with endo-β-N-acetylglucosaminidase H and then with the mixture of exoglycosidases and endo-β-N-acetylglucosa-minidase D. The two small boxes with diagonal lines at the bottom of panel C indicate the regions of a similar preparative gel filtration profile of endoglycosidase-treated glycopeptides from which radio-labeled acidic glycopeptides were isolated and analyzed in more detail (Fig. 8).

Digestion with the mixture of exoglycosidases and endo-β-N-acetylglucosaminidase D from Streptococcus pneumoniae should have converted the [2-^{3}H] mannose label in the complex, acidic glycopeptides to neutral oligomannosyl cores (Man$_n$GlcNAc$_1$) while not affecting the neutral glycopeptides with large oligomannosyl cores (Fig. 2) [13, 17]. Digestion with these glycosidases did indeed convert the radiolabel in the large, sialic acid-enriched glycopeptides (but not the major and minor peaks of "precursor"-like neutral glycopeptides) to two new peaks that eluted in the positions expected [5, 12, 16] for Man$_5$GlcNAc$_1$ and Man$_3$GlcNAc$_1$ neutral oligosaccharides (Fig. 7E). Digestion first with endo-β-N-acetylglucosaminidase H and then with the mixture of glycosidases containing endo-β-N-acetylglucosaminidase D (Fig. 7F) converted almost all of the radioactivity in glycopeptides to neutral oligosaccharides with a gel filtration profile identical to the sum of the neutral oligomannosyl core products from the individual endoglycosidase digestions (Fig. 7C and 7E), as expected if essentially all of the radiolabel was in mannose. This indicated that the majority of radiolabeled product eluting in the position of Man$_5$GlcNAc$_1$ after the combined exoglycosidase and endo-β-N-acetylglucosaminidase D digestion (Fig. 7E) was derived from the large, sialic acid-enriched glycopeptides rather than from the smaller neutral glycopeptides with intermediate-size oligomannosyl core structures. In addition, the absence of radiolabel eluting in the positions of free N-acetylglucosamine (between stachyose and mannose gel filtration markers) and galactose (same position as free mannose) or small-molecular-weight glycopeptides (GlcNAc($\pm$fucose)-asparaginyl peptide) expected after the combined endo- and exoglycosidase digestions (Fig. 7E,F) indicated that essentially all of the radiolabel incorporated into membrane glycoproteins during the 24-h labeling period was in the oligomannosyl core of asparagine-linked oligosaccharides.

The apparent heterogeniety in oligomannosyl core size for complex acidic oligosaccharides linked to asparagine in cellular membrane glycoproteins was a rather unusual result when compared to the commonly reported 3-mannose core for asparagine-linked acidic oligosaccharides [3], and was therefore examined in more detail by isolation and analysis of subclasses of these apparent high-molecular-weight acidic glycopeptides. Two individual regions of the preparative gel filtration profile of endo-β-N-acetylglucosaminidase H-resistant glycopeptides were isolated, as indicated by the diagonally lined boxes at the bottom of the analogous analytical profile in Figure 7C, and rechromatographed on the BioGel P-4 column either before or after additional glycosidase treatments (Fig. 8). Neuraminidase digestion shifted the elution positions of both the largest (Fig. 8, top) and next-to-largest (Fig. 8, bottom) acidic glycopeptides to higher-numbered fractions, indicating that both individual subclasses were enriched for terminal sialic acid. The gel filtration profiles after the combined exoglycosidase and endo-β-N-acetylglucosaminidase D digestion of each subclass indicated that the largest glycopeptides were enriched for the larger core structure(s) (Fig. 8, top), whereas the next-to-largest glycopeptides were enriched for the Man$_3$GlcNAc$_1$-size core (Fig. 8, bottom).

In summary, the "mature" glycopeptides from the 24-h labeling of BHK21 membrane glycoproteins contained two major classes of asparagine-linked oligosaccharides (with proposed structures shown in diagrammatic form in Fig. 9): 1) a mixture of neutral oligosaccharides, the major fraction containing 8–9 mannoses and a lesser fraction containing 5–7 mannoses, represented by the broad peak of glycopeptides eluting after the [^{14}C] column marker in Figure 7A,E; and 2) a mixture of acidic oligosaccharides with three and possibly five mannoses, represented by the large apparent molecular weight peaks eluting after the void volume in Figure 7A,C.

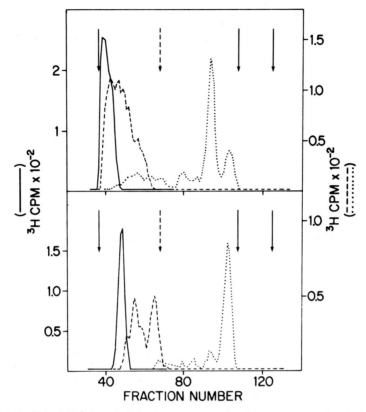

Fig. 8. BioGel P-4 gel filtration of acidic glycopeptides from a BHK21 monolayer culture labeled for 24 h with [2-^{3}H] mannose. Glycopeptides were pooled from two regions of apparent high-molecular-weight, endo-β-N-acetylglucosaminidase H-resistant glycopeptides in a preparative gel filtration profile, as indicated at the bottom of Figure 7C. Aliquots of the first, largest glycopeptide peak (upper panel) and the second glycopeptide peak (lower panel) were analyzed by gel filtration before or after glycosidase treatments, and the profiles of radioactivity superimposed: untreated (————); neuraminidase-treated (- - - - - - -); exoglycosidase- and endo-β-N-acetylglucosaminidase D-treated (. . . . . . .).

DISCUSSION

These studies with [2-^{3}H] mannose-labeled BHK21 cells and human diploid fibroblasts have demonstrated that the processes involved in the biosynthesis and maturation of the asparagine-linked oligosaccharides of cellular membrane glycoproteins are analogous to those processes previously described for vesicular stomatitis and Sindbis virus membrane glycoproteins in virus-infected cells [4—6] and the heavy chain of IgG in murine plasmacytoma cells [6]. Although the pulse-labeled glycoproteins from the membranes of the BHK21 and human cells were a mixture of multiple polypeptide species, the newly synthesized asparagine-linked oligosaccharides were as homogenous in structure (Man$_9$GlcNAc$_2$-ASN, with lesser amounts of a possible glucose-containing oligosaccharide, Glc$_1$Man$_9$GlcNAc$_2$-ASN, and a slightly smaller oligosaccharide, Man$_8$GlcNAc$_2$ASN) as those observed in virus-infected cells with only a single major species of pulse-labeled membrane glycoprotein [5, 21]. The "precursor" forms of the cellular membrane glycoproteins subsequently underwent maturation of their asparagine-linked oligosaccharides as they were processed through intracellular

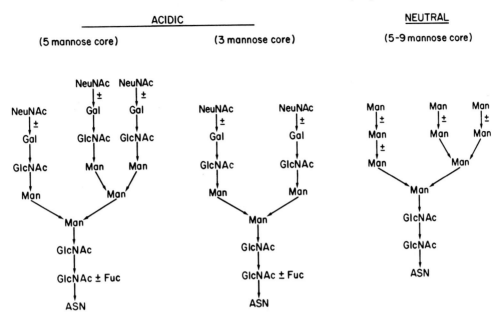

Fig. 9. Structures proposed for the "mature" asparagine-linked oligosaccharides of cellular membrane glycoproteins. The mannose-chitobiose-asparaginyl structure and the number of mannose units for the neutral oligosaccharides were based upon the gel filtration results and the sensitivity to endo-β-N-acetylglucosaminidases H or D. The proposed three-mannose acidic structure was derived from the glycosidase and gel filtration studies and previously proposed three-mannose core structures for immunoglobulin [3] and Sindbis virus glycoproteins [19]. The actual number of branch structures (NeuNAc-Gal-GlcNAc-) may have been either two or three, based upon analysis of the asparagine-linked oligosaccharides of the vesicular stomatitis virus glycoprotein [11, 20], the Sindbis virus glycoproteins [19] and several serum glycoproteins [3, 26]. The proposed five-mannose acidic oligosaccharide structure was consistent with the gel filtration and glycosidase studies of the high-molecular-weight BHK21 glycopeptides and the five-mannose core structure previously reported to be an intermediate in the biosynthesis of the three-mannose acidic oligosaccharides [27].

membranes, with two alternative pathways: 1) removal of mannoses and sequential addition of branch sugars (NeuNAc-Gal-GlcNAc-), to give acidic structures with three, and possibly five, mannoses; or 2) limited removal of mannoses, resulting in a mixture of neutral structures with 5–9 mannoses. This observed heterogenity in oligomannosyl core size and the presence of both acidic and neutral structures in the "mature" membrane glycoproteins from BHK21 and human cells confirmed the results of previous long-term (24- to 48-h) labeling studies with rat and human fibroblasts [1,2]. This heterogenity was also surprisingly similar to that reported recently for the oligosaccharides of avian RNA tumor virus glycoproteins [16].

These present studies further demonstrated that the relatively common high-mannose structure observed for the lipid-linked oligosaccharides in virus-infected and uninfected cells [4, 6–8] could indeed serve as the "precursor" for essentially all asparagine-linked oligosaccharides of cellular and viral membrane glycoproteins. Since the neutral oligomannosyl cores of most of the pulse-labeled "precursor" glycopeptides from BHK21 cells were apparently deficient in terminal glucose on the basis of size and α-mannosidase sensitivity relative to the major species of lipid-linked oligosaccharides from the same cells, the initial glycosylation products on membrane glycoproteins may have contained additional glucose that was rapidly removed following the en bloc transfer from lipid to protein [4–6]. Although lipid-linked oligosaccharides containing glucose have been shown to be transferred more rapidly and to a greater extent than their corresponding nonglucosylated oligosaccharides to endogenous protein acceptors in a cell-free system [22], it was difficult to rule out the possibilities that 1) some of the glycoprotein may have acquired glucose-deficient oligosaccharides in the en bloc transfer; or 2) some of the glucose may have been removed immediately prior to or during the en bloc transfer in intact cells, so that not all of the asparagine-linked oligosaccharides initially contained two to three terminal glucoses.

The pulse-chase labeling studies (Figs. 5 and 6) indicated that whatever amount of terminal glucose that may have been present in the initial protein linked structure was removed from most of the membrane glycoproteins before significant trimming of mannose and conversion of "precursor" neutral structures to "mature" acidic and neutral structures. This processing of "precursor" to "mature" oligosaccharides proceeded over a period of several hours or more, as demonstrated by the increasing relative amounts of radiolabel in acidic glycopeptides and smaller neutral glycopeptides in the BHK21 and human cells after the 2-, 4-, and 24-h "chase" periods. The necessity of transporting newly synthesized glycoportein through the intracellular membrane system (from the site of en bloc addition in the rough endoplasmic reticulum [9] to the Golgi-membranes prior to trimming of mannose and addition of branch sugars [5, 9]) could have accounted for both the minimal lag of approximately 30 min between the initial glycosylation and final processing of oligosaccharides, and the asynchronous processing of these asparagine-linked oligosaccharides after pulse labeling. These conclusions were consistent with the relative enrichment of several specific α-glucosidases in rough endoplasmic reticulum-like membrane fractions [23] and a specific α-mannosidase (capable of removing four of nine mannoses shown in the neutral structure in Fig. 9 as ±) in Golgi-like membrane fractions [24].

More quantitative analysis of the time course of processing or the ratio of acidic to neutral asparagine-linked oligosaccharides in the "mature" glycopeptides from the pulse-chase labeling experiments was not possible for several reasons 1) the spccific activity of labeling of the different mannoses may not have been identical; 2) some of the residual large neutral cores ($Man_{8-9}GlcNac_1$) in the 4- and 24-h chase samples (Figs. 5 and 6) may have represented unprocessed glycoproteins instead of glycoproteins that were supposed to contain large mannose core structures as their "mature" oligosaccharides; 3) radio-labeled mannose was lost as part of the maturation process; and 4) radiolabel may also have been lost because of protein turnover during the longer "chase" periods. Studies of the turnover of plasma membrane proteins in hepatoma cells [25] suggested that the turnover rate was similar for essentially all membrane proteins (half-life of approximately 100 h), so that one might not expect that neutral or acidic oligosaccharides would be lost preferentially by membrane glycoprotein turnover.

Although a number of acidic oligosaccharides with three mannose cores (Fig. 9, middle structure) have been well characterized for serum and membrane glycoproteins [3, 12, 19, 20], acidic oligosaccharides with five mannose cores have not been previously reported for cellular membrane glycoproteins. The asparaginyl-oligosaccharide with five mannoses shown in Figure 9 (left panel) was the most logical structure for the high-molecular-weight glycopeptides from the [2-^{3}H]mannose-labeled BHK21 cells if one assumed that the mixture of exoglycosidases had trimmed all of the complex acidic oligosaccharides to side chain-free structures ($Man_nGlcNAc_2$(± fucose)-peptide) prior to endo-β-N-acetylglucosaminidase D digestion. An alternative structure for the Man_5-$GlcNAc_1$-

size neutral oligosaccharide was a three-mannose core with a residual galactose and N-acetylglucosamine, or just N-acetylglucosamine, attached to one of the mannoses, as has been recently reported in studies of the complex acidic oligosaccharides of fetuin [26]. The envelope glycoprotein of vesicular stomatitis virus has oligosaccharides almost identical to those of fetuin [11, 20, 26], but $Man_3GlcNAc_1$ was the only major neutral oligosaccharide obtained from the combined exoglycosidase and endo-β-N-acetylglucosaminidase D digestion of radiolabeled glycopeptides from purified virus or virus-infected BHK21 cells [5, 11]. Because the identity of these larger core structures from cellular membrane glycoproteins and previously reported five-mannose acidic structures for avian RNA tumor virus glycoproteins [16] was based primarily on high-resolution gel filtration and specific glycosidase studies, the actual structure(s) must be considered tentative until more detailed studies are completed using more extensive exoglycosidase digestions (galactosidase, glucosaminidase, α-mannosidase [12]), periodate oxidation, and/or acetolysis [8].

Recent cell-free glycosylation studies have suggested that the three mannose acidic oligosaccharides are derived from five mannose neutral structures by the following ordered steps: 1) addition of the first branch N-acetylglucosamine to a specific α1,3-linked mannose in the five-mannose core; 2) removal of the final two mannoses; and 3) further addition of 1—2 branch N-acetylglucosamines to the three-mannose core [27]. If acidic oligosaccharides with five mannoses did exist, they would presumably occur by the same initial N-acetylglucosamine addition to the specific mannose, followed by further addition of N-acetylglucosamines without mannose removal.

Another uncertainty in the possible acidic structures proposed in Figure 9 was the actual number of branch structures (NeuNAc-Gal-GlcNAc-) linked to the different-size mannose cores. The apparent molecular weight of glycopeptides derived from gel filtration on BioGel P resins may not be especially meaningful in detailed structural determinations because of peptide heterogeneity and the negative charge exclusion property [5, 9, 11]. However, the good correlation between the larger apparent size of acidic glycopeptides and the larger neutral core after combined exoglycosidase and endo-glycosidase treatment (Fig. 8) suggested that the acidic oligosaccharides with larger apparent core size may have contained a larger average number of branch sugars than the three mannose acidic oligosaccharides. Alternatively, the largest glycopeptides may have contained more than one oligosaccharide, such as an additional unlabeled serine- or threonine-linked oligosaccharide, rather than larger individual oligosaccharide structures.

The significance of this extensive heterogeneity for asparagine-linked oligosaccharides in cellular membrane glycoproteins is not clear. Changes in the size distribution of the oligo-mannosyl cores of membrane glycopeptides have been observed between growing and nongrowing human diploid fibroblasts [2]. In addition, differences in gel filtration profiles of fucose- and glucosamine-labeled glycopeptides from whole-cell membrane protein or individual cellular membrane glycoprotein species have been reported between normal and virus-transformed cells [28—30]. These studies, however, did not analyze the actual oligosaccharide structures nor did they rule out possible contributions of serine/threonine-linked oligosaccharides to the differences in gel filtration profiles. More detailed studies of a number of individual membrane glycoproteins and the oligosaccharide structures at specific glycosylation sites (both asparagine- and serine/threonine-linked) within these proteins will be necessary in order to make a significant correlation of growth- and transformation-dependent changes with possible changes in membrane glycoprotein biosynthesis, structure, and function.

ACKNOWLEDGMENTS

These studies were supported in part by Public Health Service grant AI 14757-01 from the National Institute of Allergy and Infectious Diseases and by a Biomedical Research Support grant from the National Institutes of Health to the University of Kansas Medical Center.

The author thanks Dr. James Etchison for various glycosidases and helpful discussions and comments, Alex Yem for technical assistance in part of these studies, and Brenda Smith for typing of the manuscript.

REFERENCES

1. Muramatsu T, Koide N, Ogata-Arakawa M: Biochem Biophys Res Commun 66:881, 1975.
2. Muramatsu T, Koide N, Ceccarini C, Atkinson PH: J Biol Chem 251:4673, 1976.
3. Kornfeld R, Kornfeld S: Ann Rev Biochem 45:217, 1976.
4. Robbins PW, Hubbard SC, Turco SJ, Wirth DF: Cell 12:893, 1977.
5. Hunt LA, Etchison JR, Summers DF: Proc Natl Acad Sci USA 75:754, 1978.
6. Tabas I, Schlesinger S, Kornfeld S: J Biol Chem 253:716, 1978.
7. Sefton B: Cell 10:659, 1977.
8. Li E, Tabas I, Kornfeld S: J Biol Chem 253:7762, 1978.
9. Hunt LA, Summers DF: J Virol 20:646, 1976.
10. Robbins PW, Krag SS, Liu T: J Biol Chem 252:1780, 1977.
11. Etchison JR, Robertson JS, Summers DF: Virology 78:375, 1977.
12. Robertson MA, Etchison JR, Robertson JS, Summers DF, Stanley P: Cell 13:515, 1978.
13. Tai T, Yamashita K, Ogata-Arakawa M, Koide N, Muramatsu T, Iwashita S, Inoue Y, Kobata A: J Biol Chem 250:8569, 1975.
14. Tai T, Yamashita K, Kobata A: Biochem Biophys Res Commun 78:434, 1977.
15. Trimble RB, Tarentino AL, Plummer TH, Maley F: J Biol Chem 253:4508, 1978.
16. Hunt LA, Wright SE, Etchison JR, Summers DF: J Virol 29:336, 1979.
17. Glasgow LR, Paulson JC, Hill RL: J Biol Chem 252:8615, 1977.
18. Herscovics A, Bugge B, Jeanloz RW: J Biol Chem 252:2271, 1977.
19. Burke D, Keegstra K: J Virol 29:546, 1979.
20. Reading CL, Penhoet EE, Ballou CE: J Biol Chem 253:5600, 1978.
21. Kornfeld S, Li E, Tabas I: J Biol Chem 253:7771, 1978.
22. Turco SJ, Stetson B, Robbins PW: Proc Natl Acad Sci USA 74:4411, 1977.
23. Grinna LS, Robbins PW: J Supramol Struct (Suppl 3):205, 1979.
24. Opheim DJ, Touster O: J Biol Chem 253:1017, 1978.
25. Tweto J, Doyle D: J Biol Chem 251:872, 1976.
26. Baenziger JU, Fiete D: J Biol Chem 254:789, 1979.
27. Tabas I, Kornfeld S: J Biol Chem 253:7779, 1978.
28. Fishman PH, Brady RO, Aaronson SA: Biochemistry 15:201, 1976.
29. Van Nest GA, Grimes WJ: Biochemistry 16:2902, 1977.
30. Tuszynski GP, Baker SR, Fuhrer JP, Buck CA, Warren L: J Biol Chem 253:6092, 1978.

Journal of Supramolecular Structure 12:227–243 (1979)
Tumor Cell Surfaces and Malignancy 559–575

Introduction of Metastatic Heterogeneity by Short-Term In Vivo Passage of a Cloned Transformed Cell Line

James E. Talmadge, Jean R. Starkey, William C. Davis, and Arthur L. Cohen

Department of Veterinary Microbiology and Pathology, Washington State University, Pullman, Washington 99164 (J.E.T., J.R.S., W.C.D.), and Electron Microscope Center, Washington State University, Pullman, Washington 99164 (A.L.C.)

An experimental system for the study of metastasis has been developed using an epithelioid cell line of hepatic origin which had previously been chemically transformed in vitro. These metastatic cells were studied in the syngeneic rat strain. The cloned parent cell line metastasizes only to the lungs following intravenous, subcutaneous, or intraperitoneal injection. The metastatic phenotype is stable during in vitro passage, and subclones from the parent clone have a metastatic capacity statistically similar to that of the parent clone. Following ascites passage of the parent cell line, the cell population obtained exhibits the same metastatic ability as the parent clone. However, subclones obtained from the ascites-passaged population exhibit metastatic heterogeneity. This heterogeneity is introduced by the host passage and not by in vitro culture or subcloning. In the case of the two metastatic variants examined, the difference in the metastatic phenotype is found not to be due to differences in arrest or trapping of the cells but appears to be related to long-term survival and proliferation of the tumor cells following their arrest in the lungs. Morphologically the variants are very similar, and growth of the metastatic foci provokes a vigorous inflammatory response by the host.

Key words: cloned hepatic cell line, isolation of metastatic variants, metastatic heterogeneity introduced by ascites passage, metastatic homogeneity and stability, quantitative lung colony assay, scanning electron microscopy, tumor cell arrest and survival

One of the most important events in the pathogenesis of cancer is metastasis. During the development of a tumor it is the process of metastasis (growth of secondary foci at sites distant from the primary tumor) that most commonly defeats therapeutic efforts.

Within the population of cells in the primary tumor, there are subpopulations of cells with differing growth capabilities, degrees of tumorigenicity, and karyotypes [1]. This heterogeneous nature of a tumor cell population may also include differences in drug sensi-

Received April 25, 1979; accepted August 28, 1979.

tivity [2], antigenicity [1, 3, 4], immunogenicity [5], and cytotoxic lymphocyte specificity [6]. The existence of metastatic heterogeneity within parent tumor cell populations was first demonstrated with the B-16 melanoma [7, 8] and, subsequently, in a UV-induced fibrosarcoma (UV-2237) [9] and a methylcholanthrene-induced fibrosarcoma [10].

Methods other than the cloning of variants from the parent cell population have been devised to obtain metastatic variants. These methods have included the selection of successive tumor lines varying in metastatic capabilities by altering cycles of in vivo—in vitro growth [11, 12], and the adaptation of a tumor to ascites growth in a syngeneic [13] or allogeneic host [14]. Variants which metastasize selectively to various organs [15] have been selected from the parent tumor cell population. Another technique which has been used to develop metastatic variants has been to direct in vitro selective pressures against a cell population. The selective pressures used have included selection of lectin-resistant variants [16], selection of variants with decreased adherence to immobilized lectins [17], and variants which are resistant to specific lymphocyte cytotoxicity [18].

In this report, we examine the metastatic diversity introduced by ascites passage of a cloned subline derived from a chemically transformed epithelioid cell line of hepatic origin.

MATERIALS AND METHODS

Cell Lines

IAR6-7, IAR6-1, and IAR6-1-RT7 cell lines were generously donated by Dr. R. Montesano (International Agency for Research on Cancer, Lyons, France). The cell line IAR6-7 is an epithelioid cell line which originated from a primary liver cell culture initiated from a BD-IV rat. IAR6-1 was derived from IAR6-7 following carcinogenic transformation with dimethylnitrosamine. The cell line IAR6-1-RT7 is an intraperitoneal passaged population of IAR6-1 cells. IAR6-1-RT7 has a shorter (3 weeks) average latent period than IAR6-1 (9 weeks). Both lines give rise to pulmonary metastases [19–21].

Animals

BD-IV ($H-1^d$) and BD-IX ($H-1^d$) [22] rats were bred in our animal facility by brother-sister mating. Pedigree stock of BD-IX rats were obtained from Dr. Mayo, Frederick Cancer Research Center. Pedigree BD-IV rats were kindly donated by Professor Rajewsky, Institute for Cell Biology, University of Essen, Germany, and by Dr. Montesano. Animals 6–12 weeks of age were used for these studies. The BD-IV and BD-IX strains are not syngeneic but do have the same major histocompatability loci, and each permanently accepts skin grafts from the other strain [22].

Culture Conditions

The cell lines were grown in Ham's nutrient mixture F-12 (Gibco) supplemented with 10% prescreened fetal bovine serum FBS (Gibco), penicillin (100 units/ml), and streptomycin (100 μg/ml). This was designated complete medium. Other media and buffers used were Dulbecco's modification of Eagle's minimum essential medium (Gibco) supplemented with 5% heat-inactivated (56°C for 30 min) FBS; Tyrode's balanced salt solution (TBSS); and Ca^{2+}, Mg^{2+}-free Tyrode's balanced salt solution (CMF). The cells were subcultured by gentle trypsinization (0.1% trypsin in CMF) for 6 min at 37°C followed by the addition of complete medium to inhibit further trypsin activity. The cells were grown in 100- X 20-mm tissue culture dishes or 75-cm^2 tissue culture flasks (T-75), both from Falcon. The cell lines were subcultered every 7 days with a split ratio of 1:4. The cultures were incubated at $37°C$ in a humidified atmosphere of air and $7\% \ CO_2$.

Cloning Procedures

Cells were harvested by trypsinization, complete medium was added, and the cells were gently pelleted. The cells were resuspended in CMF, counted, and further diluted in CMF to 500 cells per milliliter. Aliquots of 1 ml were added to each of several 100- X 20-mm dishes, and 10 ml of complete medium was added to the cell suspension with agitation. After incubation for 7 days, the positions of several well-isolated colonies were marked on the underside of each dish, the medium was aspirated, cloning cylinders were placed over the colonies, and the cells were removed with trypsin. Each clone was recloned and reisolated a second time to insure the generation of clones of single cell origin.

Primary Cultures

Cultures of transformed cells were initiated from pulmonary nodules as follows: Lungs were aseptically removed from rats 3 weeks after IV injection of IAR6-1-RT7 cells. The metastatic nodules were located with a dissecting microscope and removed aseptically. The nodules from one rat were pooled, minced, and washed twice in complete medium, and small clumps of cells were allowed to attach to 100- X 20-mm tissue culture dishes. Previous experience with IAR6-1-RT7 had demonstrated a marked sensitivity of these cells to dislodgement from the substratum by trypsin treatment. A pure culture of putative tumor cells was obtained by selective detachment from the culture vessels with trypsin treatment for 6 min at room temperature. The resultant detached cells were washed in complete medium and then allowed to attach to tissue culture dishes for 30 min at $37°C$, at which time the cultures were washed twice with complete medium and refed. This technique resulted in the growth of a monolayer of cells morphologically similar to cultures of IAR6-1-RT7 cells.

Cultures of intraperitoneally passaged tumor cells were initiated from tumor ascites fluid which was collected aseptically with a 5-ml syringe and an 18-guage needle. The cells obtained from the ascites fluid were washed three times in complete medium and then plated in 100- X 20-mm tissue cultures dishes. The medium and putative tumor cells were removed after 10 min incubation at $37°C$ and replated, leaving the majority of the peritoneal macrophages attached to the first culture vessel. The cultures of tumor cells were washed and fed every 24 h for the first 4 days of incubation.

Isolation of Metastatic Variants

Monodispersed IAR6-1-RT7 cells (10^5) obtained from cell cultures in the early log phase of growth were injected into the lateral tail vein of a syngeneic rat, and 3 weeks later metastatic pulmonary nodules were removed and established in primary culture. Several clones were isolated from this metastatic tumor cell population and these were recloned twice to ensure genetic homogeneity. Clone RT7-4b was chosen for use on the basis of its intermediate metastatic capabilities and was passaged three times by intraperitoneal injection in adult BDIX rats. The RT7-4b cells ($2 \times 10^7 – 5 \times 10^7$) were injected intraperitoneally and harvested after 5 days. The ascites-passaged cells were propagated in vitro for 2 weeks until sufficient numbers were obtained for a second ascites passage. After the third such passage the cells were somewhat adapted to ascites growth and presumed to have undergone some inductive/selective pressure(s). Clones were isolated from this partially ascites-adapted cell population in order to obtain metastatic variants.

Quantitative Lung Colony Assay

The transformed cells were harvested from subconfluent (60–80% confluence) cultures growing in T-75 flasks by rinsing the cultures once with CMF and then trypsinizing them for 6 min at 37°C. The flasks were then tapped sharply to dislodge the monolayer and complete medium was added. The cells were pelleted, washed with CMF, resuspended in CMF, and counted. This technique of cell harvest resulted in a suspension of single cells with greater than 95% viability (trypan blue exclusion). The suspension was diluted to 10^5 cells per 0.2 ml CMF, which was the inoculum injected into each rat. This cell number resulted in an easily countable number of pulmonary metastases for most cell lines examined in this study.

Rats between 6 and 12 weeks of age were used for the lung colony assay. Prior to injection, the rats were warmed at 37°C for 30 min. The tumor cell suspension was then injected in the lateral tail vein using a 27-guage needle and a 0.25-ml syringe. After 5 weeks the rats were killed and necropsied. Tissues with suspect metastases were rinsed in TBSS and fixed overnight in Bouin's fixative for gross and histologic examination. Superficial nodules were counted using a dissecting microscope. This experimental metastasis assay was repeated a minimum of two times with a minimum of five animals in each assay. A few animals died following the tumor cell injection, or at times more than two groups of animals were injected; therefore the total number of animals necropsied for each assay did not always total 10.

Quantitative Analysis of Tumor Cell Arrest and Survival

Tumor cells were prelabeled by the addition of 0.5 μCi ^{125}IUDR per milliliter of complete medium to subconfluent cultures of cells in T-75 flasks, and incubating for 24 h. This resulted in the incorporation of 1 cpm of ^{125}I per 5–7 cells. These labeled cells were harvested and prepared for inoculation as described above. Representative samples from each labeled cell line were counted in a Beckman 300 gamma counter. Rats were injected with 10^5 viable labeled cells into the lateral tail vein as described earlier. Five rats from each group were killed at intervals from 10 min to 24 h post injection. Lungs, liver, spleen, kidneys, and 0.5 ml of blood were collected from each rat and the organs placed in vials containing 70% ethanol. The ethanol was replaced daily for 5 days to remove ethanol-soluble ^{125}I. The remaining ethanol-insoluble radioactivity is known to be incorporated into the DNA of tumor cells which are viable at the time of organ removal [23]. Cultures of the cell lines RT7-4bA and RT7-4bE labeled in this manner with ^{125}IUDR were found to have greater than 95% viability by trypan blue exclusion, but in comparison to unlabeled control cells they had a somewhat lengthened doubling time in cell cultures.

Scanning Electron Microscopy

Cells to be examined were seeded in 35-mm tissue culture dishes (Falcon) containing two acid-washed 12-mm-diameter round coverglass slips. The cultures were then incubated with complete medium for 48 h. Following incubation the coverglass slips were quickly rinsed in physiologic saline, and the attached cells were fixed for 30 sec in 4% OsO_4 fumes, rinsed in physiologic saline, and further fixed for 1 h in 1.75% glutaraldehyde (in 0.1 M cacodylate buffer, pH 7.3). The cells attached to the coverslips were then rinsed three times in cacodylate buffer and postfixed for 1 h in 1% OsO_4. Following postfixation, the coverslips were rinsed in water and stacked in critical-point dryer containers. The coverslips were gradually dehydrated in ethanol to 100% and flushed with Freon T.F [24]. The dehydrated coverslips were dried in an Omar SPC 1500 critical-point dryer with liquid CO_2. After drying, the coverslips were attached to aluminum stubs, and a drop of conductive paint was placed on the edge of each coverslip and in contact with the stub, thereby greatly increasing conductivity between the coverslip and the stub after coating (Cohen, unpublished observation). The cells attached to the coverslips were coated with gold-palladium using a Technics hummer sputtering device and examined in an ETEC Autoscan SEM at 20 kV.

RESULTS

Development of the Parent Clone

This experimental tumor metastasis system was developed from the transformed hepatic cell line IAR6-1-RT7. We choose to use a cell population that would preferentially seed to the lungs to facilitate enumeration of the metastatic foci. Following intravenous injection and cell growth for 3 weeks, pulmonary metastatic nodules were excised and established in culture. Among the cell types found in these cultures were fibroblasts and macrophages, islands of ciliated bronchial epithelium, normal epithelioid cells of undetermined origin, and putative epithelioid tumor cells with a high nuclear-to-cytoplasmic ratio. The putative tumor cells (selected as described in Methods) were then seeded into tissue culture dishes at very low density, and well-isolated clones were later ring-isolated. The experimental metastatic capabilities of the isolated clones were tested in the lung colony assay, and one clone which had an intermediate metastatic ability, RT7-4, was chosen for further study. After recloning to ensure single-cell origin this clone was designated RT7-4b.

Experimental Metastatic Homogeneity and Stability of the Parent Clone

The parent clone RT7-4b was seeded at low density and well-isolated clones were removed and propagated. The 10 subclones chosen for further study, RT7-4b (1–10), were examined for their experimental metastatic ability by the intravenous injection of 10^5 cells of each clone into a minimum of two different sets of five rats on different days. The metastatic capabilities of these clones were compared with the metastatic capability of the parent clone (RT7-4b) (Table I). The Mann-Whittney U test was used to evaluate statistical significance. No differences in experimental metastatic abilities were demonstrated between the subclones and the parent clone. It was concluded that the cloned parental cell population was homogeneous with respect to its experimental metastatic capability in the lung colony assay, and this in vivo tumor phenotype was not perturbed by the cloning procedures used. The stability of the metastatic phenotype was evaluated by examining the behavior of the parent clone, RT7-4b, in the lung colony assay at various in vitro passages (Table II). The parent clone exhibited a stable metastatic phenotype over 23 tissue culture passages made at a 1:4 split ratio. This in vitro propagation directly followed its initiation as a clone and took place over a period of 9 months.

Development of Metastatic Heterogeneity During Ascites Growth

The parent clone RT7-4b was subjected to three ascites passages of five days each, separated by several days of in vitro propagation. The resulting cell population (thrice ascites-adapted cell line, 3XAA-RT7-4b) was seeded at clonal density, and clones were isolated and propagated. The experimental metastatic abilities of these variant clones were compared to that of the parent clone, RT7-4b, and the uncloned ascites-adapted population, 3XAA-RT7-4b (Table III). Statistically (Mann-Whitney U test) the uncloned ascites-adapted cell line and the original parent clonal cell line, RT7-4b, had the same metastatic capabilities as determined by the lung colony assay. However, a wide range of experimental metastatic capabilities was found among the subclones from the ascites-adapted cell line, 3XAA-RT7-4b. The data presented in Table III are from lung colony counts made on the left lobe only. This was done because the very high number of pulmonary nodules which developed from several of the variant clones made counting the metastatic nodules present in the whole lung tedious. We had previously demonstrated that comparisons obtained from counts on the left lobe are proportional to those for the whole lung (Talmadge, unpublished results).

The parent clone, RT7-4b, produced 110 ± 53 metastatic nodules in the main pulmonary lobe per 10^5 cells injected. The metastatic capabilities of subclones ranged from an average lung colony count of 396 ± 176 metastatic nodules in the left lobe per 10^5 cells injected for RT7-4bE to an average lung colony count of 12 ± 11 metastatic nodules in the left lobe per 10^5 cells injected for RT7-4bA. RT7-4bL, which produced 205 ± 60 metastatic nodules in the left lobe per 10^5 cells injected, was an example of a clone with intermediate metastatic ability compared to RT7-4bA and RT7-4bE.

Of the 10 subclones examined, 3 were statistically indistinguishable from the parent clone, RT7-4b, in the lung colony assay. For example, RT7-4bM produced 89 ± 62 metastatic nodules in the left lobe per 10^5 cells injected. Thus 70% of the subclones were significantly different from the parent clone, RT7-4b, in the lung colony assay. We found that following multiple brief intraperitoneal passages of the cloned, metastatically homogeneous, parental cell population, the character of the tumor cell population was changed such that metastatic heterogeneity was present and metastatic variant subclones could be isolated.

Quantitative Analysis of Tumor Cell Arrest and Fate

To determine whether the differences in metastatic capabilities of the subclones isolated from the ascites-passaged population were due to differences in tumor cell arrest, trapping, and subsequent short-term survival, ^{125}IUDR-labeled tumor cells were traced in vivo following lateral tail vein injection. This was studied using the two clones which had the greatest difference in their metastatic capabilities: RT7-4bA and RT7-4bE (Table III). Tumor cell arrest, trapping, and short-term survival for these two variants is shown in Table IV. At 10 min post injection, no differences were found in the initial trapping rates of the tumor cells in the capillary beds of the various organs examined.

The highly metastatic variant subclone, RT7-4bE, had 74% of the originally injected cells viable and trapped in the lungs at 10 min post injection, while the poorly metastatic variant subclone, RT7-4bA, had 80% of the originally injected cells viable and trapped in the lungs. At 24 h following the injection of the cells, there was still no significant difference in trapping and survival between the two metastatic variant subclones in the lungs. From the originally injected highly metastatic RT7-4bE cells only 2.3% were still viable and trapped in the lungs compared to 2.0% of the poorly metastatic variant subclone RT7-4bA at 24 h. Therefore, there appeared to be no difference in the initial arrest, trapping, and short-term survival characteristics of the metastatic variant subclones examined. The difference in metastatic capabilities could therefore be attributed to a combination of the long-term survival of a small number of cells and their subsequent proliferation to form gross metastases.

Morphology of the Clonal Lines In Vitro

The morphology of the cells in vitro was studied using unfixed cultures by phase contrast microscopy; and methanol-fixed cells stained with hematoxylin. At the midlog phase of growth no difference in morphology could be discerned between the variant

TABLE I. Pulmonary Metastases Resulting From Intravenous Injection of Cells From the Hepatic Origin Tumor Cell Line RT7-4b and Subclones of RT7-4b

Hepatocyte cell line	No. of rats injected	Median No. of metastases	Mean No. of metastases ± SD[a]	Range	Significance[b]
Parent clone RT7-4b	24	318	370 ± 159	152–743	
Subclone 1	8	321	316 ± 52	253–381	NS
2	16	340	362 ± 166	100–437	NS
3	10	415	429 ± 91	315–609	NS
4	8	321	277 ± 202	79–467	NS
5	11	289	349 ± 165	124–635	NS
6	9	251	284 ± 109	120–573	NS
7	18	322	360 ± 116	185–472	NS
8	10	365	347 ± 139	62–507	NS
9	11	357	364 ± 123	257–460	NS
10	13	406	409 ± 123	266–616	NS

[a]Mean number of metastases per rat ± standard deviation obtained by averaging the results for a minimum of two different sets of five animals each.
[b]Probability of difference from pooled data for parent clone RT7-4b (Mann-Whitney U test). NS, no significant difference between parent clone RT7-4b and subclones. Probability more than 0.05.

TABLE II. Stability of the Metastatic Phenotype of the Hepatic Origin Tumor Cell Line RT7-4b, Following In Vitro Propagation

Cell line	No. of rats injected	No. of culture passages[a]	Median No. of metastases[b]	Range
RT7-4b	5	2	318	178–391
RT7-4b	5	9	329	172–362
RT7-4b	5	10	452	143–743
RT7-4b	5	11	288	182–407
RT7-4b	4	18	487	200–620
RT7-4b	5	23	351	211–407

[a]Number of cell culture passages following initiation of RT7-4b as a clone. The cell cultures were subcultured every 7 days at 1:4 ratio.
[b]Median number of pulmonary metastases per rat.

clones (Fig. 1). In general the cells exhibited a high nuclear-to-cytoplasmic ratio and an occasional multinucleated cell was noted. The nuclei usually contained 2–3 nucleoli and often a slight indentation was found on one side of the nucleus. The cytoplasm was slightly granular. Overall the metastatic variant cells presented an appearance of well-attached "pavement block" epithelioid cells, appearing much the same as the parent line, IAR6-1-RT7. Abnormal mitotic figures were not common.

Morphology of the Metastatic Lesion

The morphology of the pulmonary metastases was examined using periodic acid-Schiff (PAS) and hematoxylin-eosin-stained sections. The metastatic nodules (Figs. 2 and 3) were usually present at the periphery of the lung, although in the case of animals with large numbers of metastases, occasional nodules were present in deeper areas. There was a marked inflammatory response to the tumor which was manifested as mononuclear cell perivascular cuffing and mononuclear cell infiltration of the metastatic nodules. Foamy macrophages were often numerous within, and adjacent to, the metastatic nodules. Invari-

TABLE III. Pulmonary Metastases Resulting From Intravenous Injection of Subclones Isolated From the Hepatic Origin Tumor Cell Population 3XAA RT7-4b (obtained following triple adaptation of the parent clone to ascites culture)

Cell line	No. of rats injected	Median No. of metastases	Mean No. of metastases ± SD[a]	Range	Significance[b]
Parent clone RT7-4b	24	98	110 ± 53	46–227	
3XAA RT7-4b	12	104	105 ± 31	57–163	NS
3XAA RT7-4b-A	10	8	12 ± 11	0–29	>0.0001
B	9	176	217 ± 111	151–361	0.0143
E	9	406	396 ± 176	195–694	>0.0001
F	9	195	205 ± 121	49–454	NS
G	12	212	192 ± 72	64–290	0.0015
K	10	192	221 ± 93	118–337	0.0003
L	10	204	205 ± 60	115–286	0.0002
M	9	61	89 ± 62	23–203	NS
N	8	139	129 ± 39	73–176	NS
O	8	210	209 ± 55	130–297	0.0008

[a]Mean number of pulmonary metastases per rat ± standard deviation (left lobe only) obtained by averaging the results from at least two different sets of five animals each.
[b]Probability of difference from pooled data for parent clone RT7-4b (Mann-Whitney U test) P values. NS, no significant difference between parent clone RT7-4b and subclones. Probability more than 0.05.

ably, the metastatic nodules were associated with the microvasculature of the lung, either capillaries or venules. The anaplastic tumor cells were often present within remnants of the pulmonary stroma giving a histologic impression of glandular structure. This stromal outline was observed best with PAS staining, which we have found to be optimal for scanning slides. The majority of the metastatic clones gave rise to morphologically identical lesions to those described above, differing only in the frequency of metastatic nodules observed. The least metastatic clone, RT7-4bA (Fig. 3), differed slightly; histologic lesions were very rare and small, and were not associated with mononuclear cell perivascular cuffing, although there was a mononuclear and foamy macrophage infiltrate present within the metastatic nodules. The tumor cells, in all the histologic sections examined, had indented nuclei, exhibited multiple nucleoli, and were occasionally multinucleated. They had the same general morphology in vivo (Fig. 4) as they did in tissue culture (Fig. 1). Mitotic figures were not frequently seen and abnormal figures were rare in vivo. Margination of the chromatin was common in these cells, although it was not marked. A few PAS-positive granules were present in the cytoplasm. Cells from the different variant subclones could not be distinguished from one another histologically. Morphologically, the metastatic lesions produced by the different variant clones were remarkably similar.

Scanning Electron Microscopy

Scanning electron microscopy was used to examine the surface morphology of the cloned cell lines in culture. Comparisons were made of cells in areas of comparable densities. Cultures of RT7-4b, RT7-4bA, RT7-4bE, RT7-4bL, and RT7-4bM cells were examined. Mycoplasma were not seen by scanning electron microscopy in any of these cultures.

The poorly metastatic subclone, RT7-4bA (Figs. 5 and 6), had the most distinctive surface morphology. Occasionally a large bleb was seen on the surface of a cell while mitotic cells had numerous blebs (Fig. 5). At higher magnification numerous microvilli and filamentous strands were present (Fig. 6). The majority of the cellular margins were free of

TABLE IV. Arrest, Distribution, and Survival of 100,000 Viable Tumor Cells Injected IV Into Normal BD-IX Rats

Time after tumor cell injection	Lung	Spleen	Liver	Kidney	Blood[a]
RT7-4bA					
10 minutes	80,200 ± 10,500	000 ± 00	2,000 ± 706	173 ± 52	434 ± 116
1 hour	38,400 ± 4,100	153 ± 43	827 ± 717	48 ± 44	266 ± 79
2 hours	16,900 ± 4,800	89 ± 29	726 ± 348	36 ± 8	288 ± 63
4 hours	14,800 ± 3,800	32 ± 7	674 ± 217	48 ± 14	209 ± 60
6 hours	11,400 ± 3,000	24 ± 2	621 ± 106	69 ± 10	198 ± 24
24 hours	2,000 ± 400	20 ± 3	117 ± 97	65 ± 10	82 ± 85
RT7-4bE					
10 minutes	73,900 ± 9,800	161 ± 18	389 ± 361	212 ± 60	240 ± 66
1 hour	37,100 ± 2,500	576 ± 88	1,550 ± 915	110 ± 32	624 ± 152
2 hours	14,300 ± 5,500	153 ± 15	1,212 ± 680	000 ± 00	488 ± 153
4 hours	12,600 ± 6,000	147 ± 10	1,280 ± 227	000 ± 00	488 ± 116
6 hours	8,500 ± 2,600	160 ± 27	971 ± 134	000 ± 00	324 ± 87
24 hours	2,300 ± 800	153 ± 20	176 ± 67	000 ± 00	121 ± 217

Data are average number of originally viable injected tumor cells still present ± SD. Five rats per time interval.
[a]0.5 ml of blood per rat.

contact with other cells. The marginal contacts with other cells were overlapping. Ruffling occurred only at marginal cell-cell contact and was slight. Clefts were found between the individual cells. The majority of these clefts had cellular pseudopodia or filamentous strands extending across or into the clefts, suggesting that they were not artifacts. However, in some cases, rifts, an artifact of preparation, were seen as a "jigsaw puzzle" appearance of the separated cells.

The highly metastatic subclone, RT7-4bE (Figs. 7 and 8), exhibited several morphologic differences from the poorly metastatic subclone, RT7-4bA. The RT7-4bE cells had only a few stubby microvilli. Slender strands were found extending across adjacent cells. Blebs were not seen on these flat, well-spread cells. The mitotic cells exhibited only filopodia and ruffled membranes (Fig. 7). Extensive over-underlapping was found at the cellular margins and marginal ruffles were common at regions of cellular contact (Fig. 8).

The other subclones, as exemplified by RT7-4b (Fig. 9), had surface structures intermediate between the two types previously described for RT7-4bA and RT7-4bE. Blebs were occasionally seen in addition to marginal and internal ruffles. Microvilli were numerous and filamentous strands were found. The subclones RT7-4bL and RT7-4bM appeared by scanning electron microscopy to be very similar to RT7-4b. In addition, RT7-4bM had numerous small pits on the surface of each cell.

DISCUSSION

We have developed a cloned cell line of hepatic origin which exhibited a stable metastatic phenotype during in vitro culture. Ten subclones obtained from the parent clone all exhibited the same metastatic phenotype as the parent clone. However, when the cloned parent cell line was grown as an ascites tumor, heterogeneity appeared such that subclones could be isolated with marked differences in their individual ability to metastasize. The lack of metastatic variation found between subclones from the parent tumor line showed that the

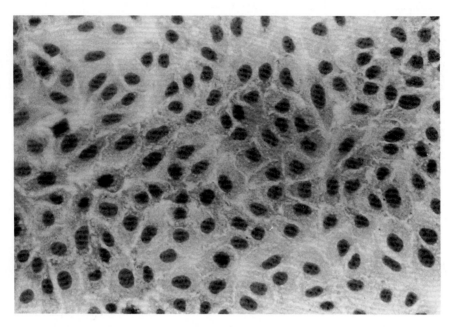

Fig. 1. Micrograph of the RT7-4b cell line. The cells are in log phase of growth. Multiple nucleoli are seen in the slightly indented nuclei. The cells present a "pavement block" pattern of epithelial cells. Hematoxylin; × 1,300.

parent line was homogeneous in this respect and that the high degree of heterogeneity demonstrable by clonal analysis of the ascites-passaged cell population must have resulted from in vivo factors associated with ascites growth, and was not due to subcloning. It is possible that other forms of in vivo passage may also act to introduce similar heterogeneity.

The metastatic capabilities of clones obtained from tumor cell populations has been studied by other workers using several different tumor cell lines. When B-16 melanoma cultures were cloned, the starting population was found to exhibit a heterogeneous metastatic phenotype in either the lung colony assay or following subcutaneous growth [7, 8]. However, subclones obtained from two of these clones exhibited the same metastatic phenotype as the parent clone [7]. Similar results were obtained with a UV-induced fibrosarcoma [8,9] which had been passaged once in a nude mouse and which had limited in vitro passage [25]. As was demonstrated in the B-16 cell system, subclones isolated from one of the fibrosarcoma clones had the same metastatic capability as the parent clone. In both of these tumors the starting tumor populations had previously undergone sufficient cellular proliferation to allow for the induction of genetic and epigenetic variation even without any additional selective pressures.

We introduced metastatic variance into the previously homogeneous tumor cell population, RT7-4b, by partially adapting it to ascites growth. The adaption to ascites growth was achieved by 15 days of intraperitoneal growth, during which time mutational or epigenetic events could have occurred. However, owing to the limited period of ascites growth and the initial poor survival of the tumor cells in this environment, it is likely that restricted numbers of cell divisions occurred in vivo and only a few mutational events would have resulted. Thus, the considerable introduced variance observed is more likely to be of epigenetic origin.

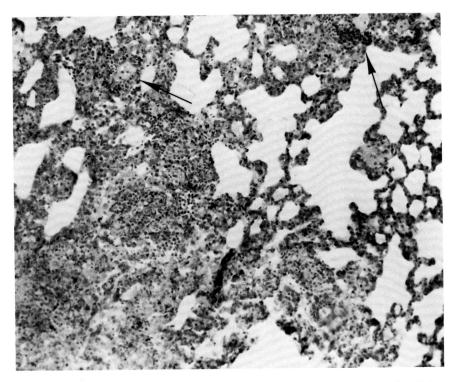

Fig. 2. Histologic appearance of a rat lung 5 weeks after the injection of 100,000 RT7-4b cells into the lateral tail vein. Mononuclear perivascular cuffing (arrow) foci are seen in several areas. The main metastatic nodule, seen here as a dense cellular area, contains tumor cells and a mononuclear infiltrate. Periodic acid-Schiff × 200.

Ascites growth adaptation of cells in syngeneic [13] or allogeneic [14] hosts has been reported to increase the metastatic capabilities of tumor cell populations. However, we found that the ascites-passaged 3XAA-RT7-4b cell population gave, statistically, the same number of lung nodules, as the original non-ascites-passaged parent clone. This may be explained in this system by ascites growth being continued for only 15 days. This was probably insufficient time to have achieved a fully ascites-adapted subpopulation.

Subclones isolated from the ascites-passaged population could be expected to be either homogeneous in their metastatic capabilities, or heterogeneous in their metastatic capabilities as was, in fact, observed. The ascites-passaged cell population was heterogeneous in its metastatic capability, and it might, a priori, be expected that randomly isolated subclones would contain approximately equal numbers of subclones with metastitic capabilities above and below that noted for the ascites-adapted cell population in general. This, however, was not the case. Only one clone tested had a decreased metastatic capability compared to the general population. This would suggest that some selection might have been imposed on the ascites-passaged cells during the cloning process. Perhaps the poorly metastatic cells were less able to survive and grow from single cells in culture than the more metastatic cell lines, thus skewing the resultant isolated clonotypes. Other possibilities are cell interactions that may occur when the heterogeneous ascites-passaged cell population is used in a lung colony

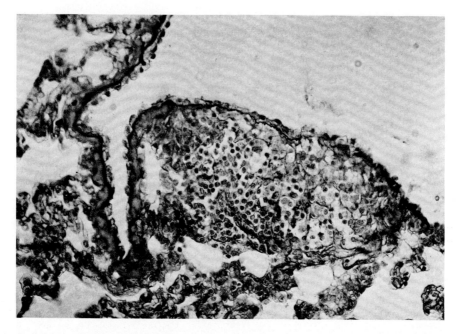

Fig. 3. Pulmonary metastasis from a rat 5 weeks after the intravenous injection of 100,000 RT7-4bA (poorly metastatic subclone) cells. The nodule is found on the periphery of the lung and there is associated with the nodule an infiltrate of inflammatory cells and foamy macrophages. Periodic acid-Schiff × 330.

assay. Such interactions could be postulated to decrease the metastatic expression of the highly metastatic subpopulations.

Adaptation to ascites growth of a tumor cell population appears to be due to the selection of a small (2.5×10^{-6}) subpopulation of phenotypically stable variants which possess a selective growth advantage as an ascites tumor but not as a solid tumor [26]. Adaptation of a tumor population to ascites form occurs at a rate dependent on the number of cells injected and any other enrichment for the ascites phenotype. The role of the ascites environment is selective, not inductive or adaptive, and it enriches for those cells with increased survival capacities in the peritoneal fluid [26].

One of the secondary attributes of tumor cells which can survive in the ascites fluid is an increased ability to metastastize [26]. Because of the short time in the peritoneal cavity and the limited number of serial transfers, the adaptation to ascites growth in our system was not complete nor was the entire cell population converted to being highly metastatic. Thus it appears that the ascites adaptation probably selected those rare cells from the original clonal cell population which had developed some diversity, either genetic or epigenetic, during proliferation.

Morphologically, cells from the subclones and the parent clone appeared quite similar in vitro and in vivo in histologic sections of pulmonary metastases. The vigorous mononuclear inflammatory response observed in the histologic sections is indicative of an immunologic reaction to the cells. This immunologic response was found regardless of the route of injection of the tumor cells (intravenous or intraperitoneal), sex of the animal, or strain of rat injected — BDIV or BDIX (both H-1^d histocompatability type).

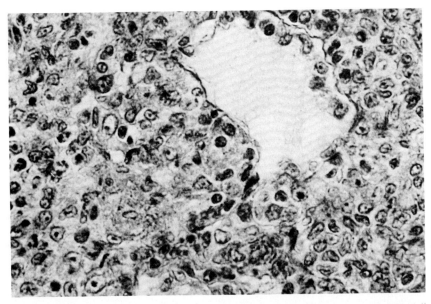

Fig. 4. Photomicrograph of tumor cells from a metastatic nodule in the lung of a rat 5 weeks following the injection of 100,000 RT7-4b cells intravenously. The anaplastic epithelioid cells exhibit slightly indented nuclei and multiple nucleoli and show some chromatin margination. Periodic acid-Schiff × 2,000.

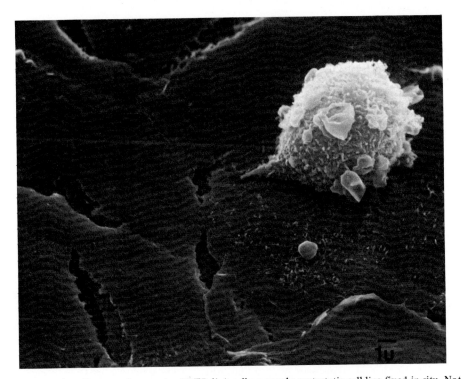

Fig. 5. Scanning electron micrograph of RT7-4bA cells; a poorly metastatic cell line fixed in situ. Note the numerous microvilli and blebs on the mitotic cell. Tilted 45°.

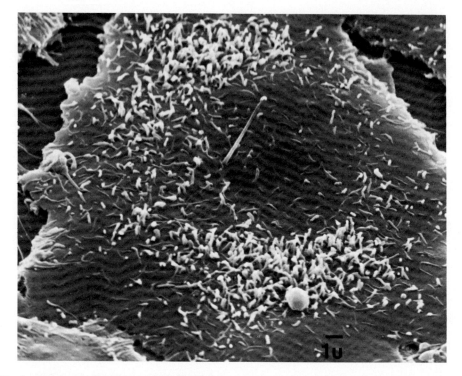

Fig. 6. Scanning electron micrograph of RT7-4bA, a poorly metastatic cell line, fixed in situ. Note the bleb, numerous microvilli, and the short filamentous strands. The cellular margins form spaces between the cells which are characteristic of this subclone. Tilted 45°.

There was one exception to the general histologic picture. Subclone RT7-4bA did not provoke the mononuclear perivascular cuffing found with the other subclones, possibly owing to limited antigenic stimulation following the restricted cell survival and growth. Since, in general, the variants appeared to provoke an active immunologic response as exemplified by the mononuclear and foamy macrophage infiltrate and the mononuclear perivascular cuffing, it is likely that the more metastatic cells are better able to "escape" immune effector cells and so survive to produce gross metastatic lesions. Since cells were well washed in Ca^{2+}-Mg^{2+}-free BSS, an immune reaction to medium components (FBS) is highly unlikely.

Scanning electron micrographs revealed a continuum of membrane morphologic variance which correlated with the subclones' metastatic abilities. The least metastatic subclones exhibited numerous membrane-associated structures including blebbing and extensive microvillus formation, which were indicative of an "active" cell membrane. The most metastatic subclone (RT7-4bE) exhibited less extensive membrane activity, which appeared as only a few stubby microvilli and marginal ruffling. Similar morphologic structures were seen in studies by other workers in which two different solid tumors and their respective ascites-adapted counterparts were examined using scanning electron microscopy [27]. The ascites-adapted cell lines had decreased membrane activity (blebbing, ruffling, and microvilli) compared to the solid tumor cells. Previously it had been reported that the ascites-adapted cells examined by these workers were more metastatic than the solid tumors [13].

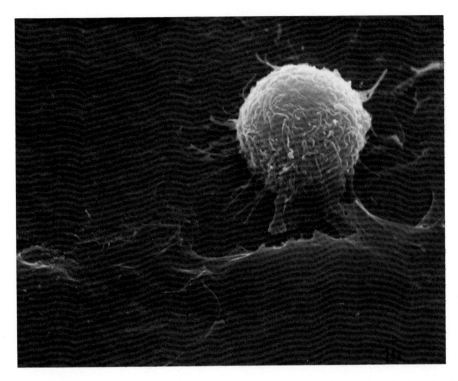

Fig. 7. Scanning electron micrograph of RT7-4bE, a highly metastatic subclone, fixed in situ. Mitotic figures lack blebs and do not exhibit extensive ruffles. The cells appear flat and very adhesive to the substratum. Few microvilli are seen and extensive over-underlapping is found with marginal ruffling. Tilted 45°.

Scanning electron micrographs of the metastatic variant subclones had an appearance suggestive of a tighter adherance to the substratum by the more metastatic subclone (RT7-4bE) as well as increased intercellular contact. The postulated increase in homotypic and substratum attachment suggests that these cells may have greater adhesiveness, which could serve to increase the metastatic capabilities of the tumor by increasing embolus arrest and trapping [28]. However, our studies of the arrest and trapping of ^{125}IUDR-labeled cells show no significant increases in those parameters for RT7-4bE cells over RT7-4bA cells.

Cells labeled with ^{125}IUDR allowed not only the study of tumor cell arrest and trapping, but also short-term tumor cell survival to be evaluated. Using such labeled cells, we studied the mechanism of metastasis of the two subclones (RT7-4bA and RT7-4bE) which exhibited the greatest difference in metastatic abilities. Despite the great difference between these variants in the ultimate yield of lung metastases, there was no discernable difference found in the rate of arrest, the number of cells arrested, or cell survival for 24 h following intravenous injection of the ^{125}IUDR-labeled tumor cells. This suggests that the final metastatic expression was not due to differences in the arrest or trapping of the tumor cells, but to long-term tumor cell survival subsequent to arrest and trapping. Such enhanced survival is postulated to be of particular importance in allowing cell growth to occur and gross metastases to be produced.

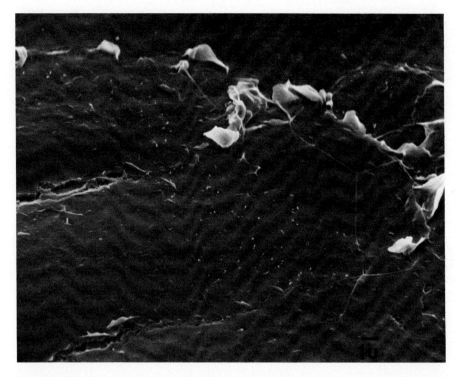

Fig. 8. Scanning electron micrograph of RT7-4bE, a highly metastatic subclone, fixed in situ. Only a few stubby microvilli are found. Extensive over-underlapping is seen with marginal ruffling. Tilted 45°.

Following ascites passage, metastatic diversity could be demonstrated to exist in a cell population which prior to ascites growth had a stable homogeneous metastatic phenotype. The expression of the variant metastatic capabilities does not appear to be due to differences in the arrest and trapping of the tumor cells, but rather to a difference in the subclone's ability to survive to form a gross metastatic nodule. This could to a large extent be due to an ability of the highly metastatic subclone to "escape" the hosts immunologic response [29].

ACKNOWLEDGMENTS

This study was supported in part by the American Cancer Society Institutional Support grant IN-119 and Research Initiation and Support grant NSF SER 77-06943.

REFERENCES

1. Dexter DL, Kowalski HM, Blazar BA, Fligiel Z, Vogel R, Heppner GH: Cancer Res 38:3174, 1978.
2. Heppner GH, Dexter DL, DeNucci T, Millier FR, Calabresi P: Cancer Res 38:3758, 1978.
3. Pimm MV, Baldwin RW: Int J Cancer 20:37, 1977.
4. Byers VS, Johnston JO: Cancer Res 37:3173, 1977.
5. Killion JJ, Kollmorgen GM: Nature 259:674, 1976.
6. Fogel M, Gorelik E, Segal S, Feldman M: J Natl Cancer Inst 62:585, 1979.
7. Fidler IJ, Kripke ML: Science 197:893, 1977.

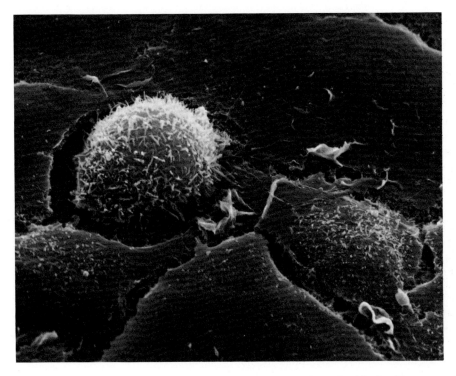

Fig. 9. Scanning electron micrograph of RT7-4b, metastatic parent clone, fixed in situ. Numerous micro-villi are found with occasional blebs and internal and marginal ruffles. The prominent surface characteristic of the mitotic cells are microvilli. Spaces are found between the cellular margins. Tilted 45°.

 8. Fidler IJ: Cancer Res 38:91, 1978.
 9. Kripke ML, Gruys E, Fidler IJ: Cancer Res 38:2962, 1978.
10. Suzuki N, Withers HB, Koehler MW: Cancer Res 38:3349, 1978.
11. Fidler IJ: Nature (New Biol) 242:148, 1973.
12. Brunson KW, Nicolson GL: J Natl Cancer Inst 61:1499, 1978.
13. Hagmar B, Ryd W: Acta Pathol Microbiol Scand Sec A 86:231, 1978.
14. Kerbel RS, Twiddy RR, Robertson DM: Int J Cancer 22:583, 1978.
15. Nicolson GL, Brunson KW, Gann: Monogr Cancer Res 20:15, 1977.
16. Tao TW, Burger MM: Nature 270:437, 1977.
17. Reading CL, Belloni PN, Nicolson GL: J Supramol Struct (Suppl) 3:183, 1979.
18. Fidler IJ, Bucana C: Cancer Res 36:887, 1976.
19. Montesano R, St Vincent L, Tomatis C: Br J Cancer 28:215, 1973.
20. Montesano R, St Vincent L, Drevon C, Tomatis L: Int J Cancer 16:550, 1975.
21. Montesano R, Drevon C, Kuroki T, St Vincent L, Handleman S, Sanford KK, DeFeo D, Weinstein IB: J Natl Cancer Inst 59:1651, 1977.
22. Druckrey H: Arzneim Forsch (Drug Res) 28:1274, 1971.
23. Fidler IJ: J Natl Cancer Inst 45:775, 1970.
24. Cohen AL: In Hayat MA (ed): "Principles and Techniques of Scanning Electron Microscopy." New York: Van Nostrand, vol 1, 1974.
25. Kripke ML: Cancer Res 37:1395, 1977.
26. Klein G, Klein E: Ann NY Acad Sci 63:640, 1956.
27. Ryd W, Hagmar B: Acta Pathol Microbiol Scand Sec A 87:98, 1979.
28. Fidler IJ: Eur J Cancer 9:223, 1973.
29. Fidler IJ, Gersten DM, Riggs CW: Cancer 40:46, 1977.

Journal of Supramolecular Structure 12:245–257 (1979)
Tumor Cell Surfaces and Malignancy 577–589

Direct Linkage of Thrombin to Its Cell Surface Receptors in Different Cell Types

Robert L. Simmer, Joffre B. Baker, and Dennis D. Cunningham

Department of Microbiology, College of Medicine, University of California at Irvine, Irvine, California 92717

When ^{125}I-thrombin was incubated with foreskin fibroblasts, cervical carcinoma cells or fibrosarcoma cells of human origin, or with secondary chick
embryo cells or Chinese hamster lung cells, it became directly linked to its cell
surface receptors. The thrombin-receptor complex (TH-R) was derived exclusively from a pool of ^{125}I-thrombin that had become specifically bound to the
cell surface. The linkage was probably covalent, since the complex was resistant to boiling in sodium dodecyl sulfate and 2-mercaptoethanol. Raising
the pH to 12 disrupted TH-R, but did not affect a similar complex between
epidermal growth factor and its receptor, suggesting that the linkage of these
mitogens to their receptors was different. Mild trypsin treatment removed the
ability of cells to form TH-R; however, after a 24-h incubation in serum-free
medium, trypsin-treated cells recovered the capacity to form TH-R, suggesting
that TH-R resulted from interaction of ^{125}I-thrombin with a cellular rather than
a serum component. The mitogenic response of cells to thrombin was inversely
related to the fraction of specifically bound ^{125}I-thrombin represented by
TH-R. The role of TH-R in mitogenesis may be clarified in future studies by
obtaining clones of Chinese hamster lung cells that vary in their capacities to
form TH-R and to respond to the mitogenic action of thrombin.

Key words: thrombin receptors, epidermal growth factor receptors, cell proliferation, normal and
transformed cells

Recently it has been shown that when ^{125}I-labeled epidermal growth factor (^{125}I-EGF)
was incubated with human [1] or mouse [2] fibroblasts, about 1–10% of the EGF molecules that were specifically bound to cell surface receptors became linked to them. The
EGF-receptor complex (EGF-R) was resistant to boiling in 3% sodium dodecyl sulfate
(SDS) and 1% 2-mercaptoethanol, suggesting that the linkage was probably covalent.

Received June 5, 1979; accepted September 24, 1979.

EGF-R was formed at the cell surface and with time was internalized and cleaved to discrete-molecular-weight forms. The complex and subsequent forms were very similar to ones seen by Das and Fox [3] and Das et al [4], who used a photoactivable derivative of ^{125}I-EGF to crosslink EGF to its receptor and follow the fate of this complex during continued incubation of cells.

It was also reported that incubation of another polypeptide mitogen, ^{125}I-thrombin (^{125}I-TH), with human fibroblasts led to formation of a complex between TH and its cell surface receptor [1]. Like EGF-R, the TH-receptor complex (TH-R) was resistant to boiling in 3% SDS and 1% 2-mercaptoethanol. However, an intriguing difference between EGF-R and TH-R formation in the human cells was that up to 60% of specifically bound TH became linked to its receptor, whereas the corresponding amount for EGF was only 6–9%.

These results prompted the present investigations on TH-R in several kinds of cells. We examined the amounts of TH-R formed and compared this with the ability of the cells to respond to the mitogenic action of TH. We also determined the molecular weights of TH-R in the different cells and showed that TH-R was not derived from a serum component. In addition, we examined the nature of the linkages between the mitogen-receptor complexes, and we report that the linkage for TH-R is different from the EGF-R linkage.

MATERIALS AND METHODS

Purified human thrombin was provided by Dr. John W. Fenton II [5]. EGF was purified from male mouse submaxillary glands by the procedure of Savage and Cohen [6]. MCDB medium 202 was prepared according to Ham and McKeehan [7]. Dulbecco-Vogt modified Eagle's medium (DV) and tryptose phosphate broth were obtained from Flow Laboratories, Inc. Calf serum was purchased from Irvine Scientific. Other medium products, chicken serum, and trypsin solution were purchased from Gibco. Tissue culture dishes were obtained from Falcon Plastics. Na^{125}I was obtained from Amersham, lactoperoxidase from Calbiochem, and bisbenzimide #33258 (Hoechst dye) from American Hoechst.

Normal human fibroblasts (HF cells) prepared from neonatal foreskin explants were maintained as previously described [1]. Cells at passages 7–13 were used for experiments. D98/AH-2 cells (a variant of the Hela human cervical carcinoma line) and HT1080 cells (a human fibrosarcoma cell line) were provided by Dr. Eric J. Stanbridge. Chinese hamster lung (CHL) fibroblasts from the V79 strain [8] were provided by Dr. John J. Wasmuth. Cultures of chick embryo (CE) cells were prepared by the method of Rein and Rubin [9]. Primary cultures were grown in DV medium containing 2% chicken serum and 2% tryptose phosphate broth. Confluent primary cultures were subcultured at 5.7×10^4 cells/cm^2 in fresh medium. After 4 h, these secondary cultures were rinsed with serum-free DV medium (DV-0) and then incubated for 48 h in DV-0 before use in ^{125}I-TH binding experiments. All other cells were grown in DV medium containing 5% calf serum (DV-5). All cultures were incubated at 37°C in an atmosphere of 5% CO$_2$ in air. Stock cultures were seeded at 5.8×10^3 cells/cm^2 (HF cells), 1.5×10^4 cells/cm^2 (CHL and HT1080 cells) and 3.3×10^4 cells/cm^2 (D98 cells). To determine their mitogenic response to TH, CHL and HT1080 cells were plated at 2.3×10^4 cells/cm^2 in DV-5. After 2 days, the medium was replaced with DV-0 or DV medium containing 0.1% calf serum (DV-0.1) for CHL and HT1080 cultures, respectively. Two days later TH was added to final concentrations of 0.3 μg/ml or 3.0 μg/ml, and cell number was determined 48 h later. The effect of TH on cell division was determined by comparing cell number in TH-treated cultures with parallel untreated cultures.

D98, HF, HT1080, and CHL cells were judged to be free of mycoplasma contamination by a modification of the method of Chen [10]. Briefly, subconfluent cultures growing on glass coverslips were fixed in phosphate-buffered saline containing 3% (w/v) formaldehyde, stained in 2 μg/ml Hoechst dye and then analyzed by fluorescence microscopy for mycoplasma.

TH was iodinated by the lactoperoxidase method of Martin et al [11]. EGF was iodinated by the procedure of Carpenter and Cohen [12]. ^{125}I-EGF and ^{125}I-TH total and nonspecific binding to cells was measured as previously described [1] unless noted otherwise. After unbound ^{125}I-EGF or ^{125}I-TH was rinsed from cells with ice-cold phosphate-buffered saline, the cells were solubilized in 0.2 ml solubilization buffer [3% (w/v) SDS, 0.6% (w/v) N-ethylmaleimide, 100 mM Tris-Cl (pH 6.8), 1% (v/v) 2-mercaptoethanol, 5% (v/v) glycerol, 2 mM phenylmethylsulfonyl fluoride, and 0.005% (w/v) bromophenol blue] and placed in a boiling water bath for 5 min. Where protein concentration was determined, the bromophenol blue was omitted. Samples were electrophoresed in 0.1% SDS, 7.5–15% linear gradient polyacrylamide slab or tube gels based on the method of Laemmli [13]. Tube gels were cut into 2-mm slices and the ^{125}I radioactivity in each slice was measured in a gamma counter. The slab gels were fixed, stained, and then dried on Whatman No. 1 chromatography paper. The dried gels were exposed to Kodak X-Omat R film in the presence of Dupont Cronex Lightning Plus intensifying screens. Protein concentrations of nonreduced samples were determined by the method of Lowry et al [14] and those of reduced samples by a modification of the Lowry assay [15].

RESULTS

Formation of TH-R in Different Cell Types

A first step in evaluating the ability of different cells to form TH-R was to determine if they had specific receptors for TH. When HF, HT1080, D98, 2°CE, and CHL cells were incubated with ^{125}I-TH, the fraction of binding that was specific ranged from 25 to 70% and varied with cell type and ^{125}I-TH concentration (Table I). To measure the ability of cells to form TH-R, we incubated them with ^{125}I-TH and solubilized and boiled the extracts in 3% SDS and 1% 2-mercaptoethanol before electrophoresis on SDS polyacrylamide gels. Autoradiographs of slab gels demonstrated that CHL (Fig. 1, lane 1), D98 (Fig. 1, lane 3), HT1080 (Fig. 1, lane 5), and 2°CE (Fig. 2, lane 7) cells formed complexes that were roughly similar in molecular weight to TH-R previously observed [1] in HF cells (Fig. 2, lane 9). We quantitated the contribution of TH-R to specific binding of ^{125}I-TH by electrophoresis of samples on SDS polyacrylamide tube gels and analysis of the distribution of ^{125}I radioactivity in 2-mm slices of the gels (Fig. 3 and Table I). As previously reported for HF cells, most of the nonspecifically bound radioactivity migrated with ^{125}I-TH or smaller-molecular-weight species (presumably due to degradation of ^{125}I-TH), while none of it migrated with TH-R. This suggested that TH-R was formed only from ^{125}I-TH that was specifically bound to cellular receptors. Although all cell types specifically bound ^{125}I-TH and formed TH-R, the percentage of specific binding due to TH-R varied among cell types. With HF and HT1080 cells TH-R formation was generally 4–10 times higher than with 2°CE, CHL, and D98 cells. These differences prompted us to examine the ability of TH to stimulate cell division in these cells.

TH-R and Stimulation of Cell Division

To determine if there was a relationship between TH-R formation and the mito-genic response of cells to TH, we added TH to nondividing cultures of CHL cells in DV-0 and HT1080 cells in DV-0.1, as described in Materials and Methods. Unfortunately, the mito-genic effect of TH could not be determined for D98 cells, since they continued to divide in DV-0.1 and, like HT1080 cells, they began to detach from the plates when placed in DV-0 for 24 h. Exposure of CHL cultures to TH at 0.3 μg/ml or 3.0 μg/ml increased cell number by 39% and 70%, respectively, after two days (Table II). This response was simi-lar in magnitude to that reported by Carney et al [16] for 2°CE and 2° mouse embryo cells. In contrast, HT1080 cells, when treated with 3.0 μg/ml TH, increased in cell num-ber by only 20% after 2 days. This response, albeit faster than that seen with HF cells, was no greater after 4 days of incubation with TH. Thus, HF and HT1080 cells, in which a large fraction of specifically bound ^{125}I-TH became linked to receptors, were mito-genically less responsive to TH than 2°CE and CHL cells, in which less linkage occurred.

Molecular Weights of TH-R in Different Cells

Analysis of autoradiographs such as those in Figures 1 and 2 revealed that the mo-lecular weight of TH-R was not the same in all cell types. TH-R in both normal and trans-formed human cells had a molecular weight of about 68K as determined by comparison of their migration on SDS polyacrylamide gels with that of molecular weight standards. The complex was smallest in 2°CE cells, with an estimated molecular weight of 65K. In CHL fibroblasts the molecular weight of 76K for TH-R was closest to that previously reported [17] for another rodent, mouse, where TH-R was 80K. The cause of these dif-ferences in molecular weights of TH-R is unknown.

TABLE I. Specific Binding of ^{125}I-TH and Formation of TH-R

Cell type	^{125}I-TH concentration (ng/ml)	% Specific binding	% TH-R
A CHL	25	33	19
D98	100	29	11
HT1080	100	64	30
HF	25	67	36
HF	100	63	43
B CHL	200	50	13
D98	200	43	4.3
HT1080	200	25	35
2°CE	200	35	10
HF	200	66	43

Cells were incubated for 60 min at 37°C with the indicated concentrations of ^{125}I-TH. Specific binding was determined by subtracting the cpm bound in the presence of 8 μg/ml nonlabeled TH from the cpm bound in the absence of excess nonlabeled TH and then dividing this value by the cpm bound in the ab-sence of excess nonlabeled TH and multiplying by 100%. Percentage TH-R was quantitated by electro-phoresis of samples on SDS polyacrylamide tube gels, cutting the gels into 2-mm slices, and determining the ratio of specifically bound cpm in slices containing TH-R to the total number of specifically bound cpm in the entire gel (see Fig. 3). A, Cells prepared as in Figure 1; B, cells prepared as in Figure 2.

Complexes Between TH and Serum Components

In the course of our experiments we noted that often two bands, of molecular weights 77K and 90K, were also formed. Since these bands were present when cells growing in 5% serum were used (eg, Fig. 2, lane 3), yet absent when the cells had been in DV-0 or DV-0.1 for one day prior to incubation with ^{125}I-TH (Fig. 1, lane 3), we determined if

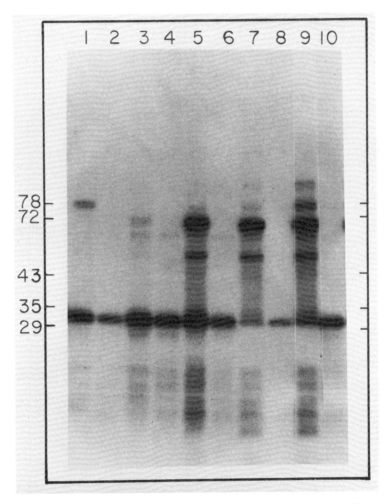

Fig. 1. Cells were seeded at 2×10^5 cells per 35-mm dish in DV-5. After reaching confluence, all cells except HF cells were placed in DV-0 for at least 2 days. Cells were incubated with ^{125}I-TH for 60 min at 37°C at the concentrations noted below. Equal volumes of each sample were used for electrophoresis. Lane 1, CHL cells incubated with 25 ng/ml ^{125}I-TH; lane 2, CHL cells incubated with 25 ng/ml ^{125}I-TH plus 8 μg/ml nonlabeled TH; lane 3, D98 cells incubated with 100 ng/ml ^{125}I-TH; lane 4, D98 cells incubated with 100 ng/ml ^{125}I-TH plus 8 μg/ml nonlabeled TH; lane 5, HT1080 cells incubated with 100 ng/ml ^{125}I-TH; lane 6, HT1080 cells incubated with 100 ng/ml ^{125}I-TH plus 8 μg/ml nonlabeled TH; lane 7, HF cells incubated with 25 ng/ml ^{125}I-TH; lane 8, HF cells incubated with 25 ng/ml ^{125}I-TH plus 8 μg/ml nonlabeled TH; lane 9, HF cells incubated with 100 ng/ml ^{125}I-TH; and lane 10, HF cells incubated with 100 ng/ml ^{125}I-TH plus 8 μg/ml nonlabeled TH.

^{125}I-TH might form complexes with serum components that were resistant to boiling in 3% SDS and 1% 2-mercaptoethanol. Figure 4 shows that 77K and 90K dalton complexes were indeed formed after incubation of 100 ng/ml ^{125}I-TH with 1% calf serum. Moreover, addition of 8 μg/ml nonlabeled TH diminished the amounts of the complexes, indicating that specific binding was involved. Actual identification of the factor(s) in serum that formed these complexes with ^{125}I-TH was not pursued; however, the molecular weights of the complexes and the fact that they were resistant to boiling in SDS and 2-mercapto-ethanol indicated that they might result from linkage of TH with antithrombin III, a well-characterized serum component [18, 19].

Although TH-R formation was observed after maintenance of cells for 2 days in DV-0, the above results indicated that it was important to determine whether ^{125}I-TH was

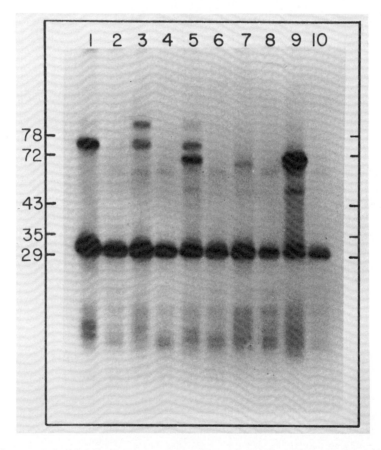

Fig. 2. 2°CE cells were prepared as described in Materials and Methods. All other cells prepared as in Figure 1 except that there was no medium change. Cells were incubated with 200 ng/ml ^{125}I-TH for 60 min at 37°C. Equal volumes of each sample were used for electrophoresis. Lane 1, CHL cells; lane 3, D98 cells; lane 5, HT1080 cells; lane 7, 2°CE cells; and lane 9, HF cells. Lanes 2, 4, 6, 8, and 10 represent binding of ^{125}I-TH under nonspecific binding conditions for CHL, D98, HT1080, 2°CE, and HF cells, respectively.

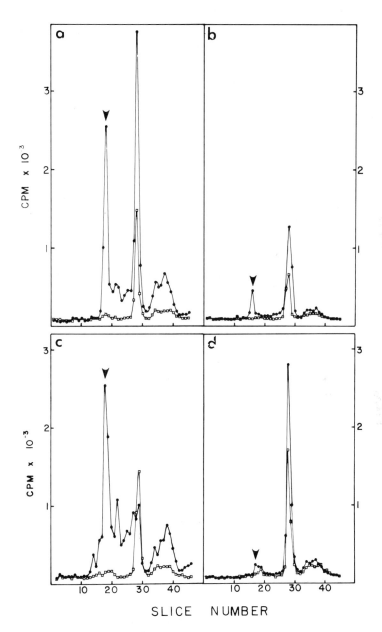

Fig. 3. Distribution of ^{125}I radioactivity in SDS polyacrylamide gels of samples from cells incubated for 60 min at 37°C with ^{125}I-TH at the concentrations noted below. Cells were prepared as in Figure 1. Arrowheads indicate the position of TH-R. Unlinked ^{125}I-TH migrated in gel slices 27–29. Panel a, HT1080 cells incubated with 100 ng/ml ^{125}I-TH; panel b, CHL cells incubated with 25 ng/ml ^{125}I-TH; panel c, HF cells incubated with 25 ng/ml ^{125}I-TH; panel d, D98 cells incubated with 100 ng/ml ^{125}I-TH. ●, total binding of ^{125}I-TH; □, nonspecific binding of ^{125}I-TH.

TABLE II. Stimulation of Cell Division in CHL and HT1080 Cells by Thrombin

Cell type	TH concentration (µg/ml)	Cell number (× 10⁻⁶)	% Increase
CHL	—	1.33	—
CHL	0.3	1.85	39
CHL	3.0	2.26	70
HT1080	—	1.01	—
HT1080	0.3	1.04	3
HT1080	3.0	1.21	20

Cell numbers are averages of duplicate plates.

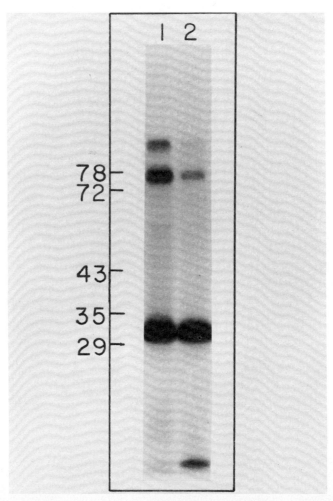

Fig. 4. Binding of ¹²⁵I-TH to calf serum. Lane 1: Binding buffer containing 1% calf serum and 100 ng/ml ¹²⁵I-TH was incubated for 60 min at 37°C. Five volumes of solubilization buffer were added and the sample was heated, electrophoresed, and exposed to film as described in Materials and Methods. Lane 2: Incubation in the presence of 8 µg/ml nonlabeled TH.

forming a complex with a cellular receptor or with a serum component that adsorbed to cells. Since TH-R could be removed by trypsin treatment of cells shortly after binding of ^{125}I-TH [1], it seemed reasonable that pretreatment with trypsin would remove (or change) the receptor for TH and in so doing prevent the formation of TH-R. If cells could then regenerate their capacity to form TH-R in serum-free medium, this would indicate that a cellular component was necessary for TH-R formation. As shown in Figure 5, lane

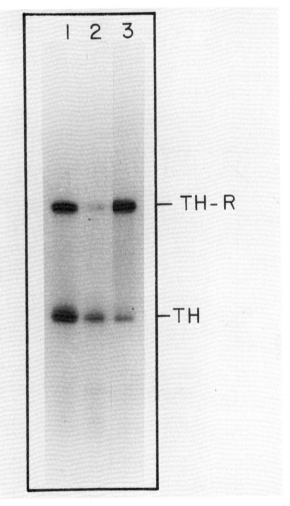

Fig. 5. TH-R formation within 1 h (lane 2) or 25 h (lane 1) after trypsin treatment or in untreated control cells (lane 3). HF cells were seeded at 2×10^5 cells per 35-mm dish in DV-5. Confluent cultures were rinsed once with 2.0 ml DV-0 and then incubated in DV-0 for at least one day. Cells in the recovery group were incubated at 37°C in DV-0 containing 500 μg/ml trypsin. After 5 min, cells were rinsed twice with 1.0 ml DV-0 containing 10 μg/ml soybean trypsin inhibitor (SBTI) and then incubated in a serum-free mixture of DV medium: MCDB 202 medium (2:1). The following day a second group of cells (lane 2) was trypsinized as noted above for 5 min. All trypsin-treated cells were then washed three times in DV-0 containing 10 μg/ml SBTI and incubated for 10 min at 23°C. Next, all three experimental groups of cells were washed three times in DV-0 prior to incubation for 30 min at 37°C with DV-0 containing 0.5% bovine serum albumin and 100 ng/ml ^{125}I-TH. Solubilization and electrophoresis of samples was performed as described in Materials and Methods. An equal amount of protein was loaded in each lane.

2, a 5-min treatment of HF cells with 500 μg/ml trypsin at 37°C drastically reduced the formation of TH-R compared to untreated cells (lane 3) when assayed within 1 h of trypsin treatment. Moreover, when trypsin-treated cells were placed in serum-free medium for 24 h, their ability to form TH-R returned (Fig. 5, lane 1). The simplest interpretation of these results is that TH-R was formed by the interaction of ^{125}I-TH with a cellular rather than a serum component.

Nature of the Mitogen-Receptor Linkage

Since incubation of mouse [2] and human [1] cells with ^{125}I-EGF also resulted in the formation of a mitogen-receptor complex that was resistant to boiling in SDS and 2-mercaptoethanol, it was important to determine whether EGF-R and TH-R were formed by the same or different mechanisms. Although we have not studied the types of chemical bonds involved in the linkage of these mitogens to their receptors, we have found that the linkages are not the same. When ^{125}I-TH or ^{125}I-EGF were incubated with HF cells fol-

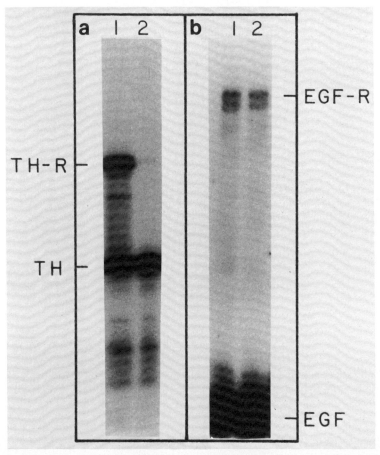

Fig. 6. Stability of TH-R and EGF-R in pH 12 buffer. Confluent HF cultures were incubated in 200 ng/ml ^{125}I-TH (panel a) or 40 ng/ml ^{125}I-EGF (panel b) for 60 min at 37°C. After heating, solubilized samples were dialyzed against 0.1% (w/v) SDS and 50 mM NaCl, then the pH was raised to 12 for 30 min. Samples were then dialyzed against 0.1% SDS, 50 mM Tris-Cl (pH 7.0), 50 mM NaCl before electrophoresis. Lane 1, control, no pH 12 treatment. Lane 2, pH 12 treatment.

lowed by solubilization, electrophoresis, and autoradiography, bands corresponding to TH-R and TH (Fig. 6a, lane 1) and EGF-R and EGF (Fig. 6b, lane 1) were observed. If, however, the pH of the solubilized samples were raised to 12 and then returned to 7.0 before electrophoresis, TH-R disappeared (Fig. 6a, lane 2), whereas EGF-R appeared unaffected (Fig. 6b, lane 2). This strongly suggests that a different type of linkage is involved between these mitogens and their receptors.

Further, it appeared that all of the ^{125}I radioactivity in TH-R was associated with TH, for after disruption by pH 12 virtually all of the radioactivity associated with TH-R migrated with ^{125}I-TH. Figure 6a shows that pH 12 treatment also released ^{125}I-TH from a minor component that was smaller than TH-R. It is not clear whether this component resulted from degradation of TH-R or from linkage of ^{125}I-TH to a different cellular component. The disruption of TH-R by pH 12 suggested that the linkage between TH and its receptor involved an ester bond, based on previous studies of the linkage between TH and antithrombin III [20].

DISCUSSION

We have previously reported that ^{125}I-TH upon incubation with HF cells [1] or 2° mouse embryo cells [17] formed a complex with its receptor. TH-R was resistant to boiling in 3% SDS and 1% 2-mercaptoethanol and was derived exclusively from a pool of ^{125}I-TH that had become specifically bound to the cell surface. Up to 60% of the specifically bound ^{125}I-TH became linked to cellular receptors in HF cells. TH-R formation took place at the cell surface and was an extremely rapid process that preceded by several minutes the accumulation of ^{125}I-TH that was bound but unlinked. These observations suggested that TH-R formation was an important event following ^{125}I-TH binding to cell receptors.

Murine [2] and human [1] cells have also been shown to form a complex between ^{125}I-EGF and its cell surface receptor. Like TH-R, EGF-R was resistant to boiling in SDS and 2-mercaptoethanol, was formed at the cell surface, and was a result of specific binding of ^{125}I-EGF. The amount of EGF-R formed depended upon the concentration of ^{125}I-EGF in the medium and represented a fairly constant portion (6–9%) of the specifically bound ^{125}I-EGF in HF cells.

It appears that the linkages between these mitogens and their receptors are probably covalent, since they survive boiling in SDS and 2-mercaptoethanol. However, the linkages are different, since TH-R but not EGF-R is disrupted by raising the pH to 12. It is noteworthy that the linkage formed between TH and antithrombin III involves an ester bond and is also disrupted at pH 12. Thus, it appears that the linkage between TH and its receptor involved an ester bond. The chemical nature of the linkage between EGF and its receptor is unknown.

EGF-R formation has been reported in HF cells [1], 3T3 cells, SV40-transformed 3T3 cells, A-431 cells (a human tumor cell line), and human placental membranes [2]. Where reported, the molecular weight of EGF-R in the different cell types appeared to be very similar. In the present paper we have shown that TH-R was formed in a variety of cell types that range from avian to rodent and human origin and include normal and malignant cells. The molecular weights of TH-R in these different cells, although very similar, exhibited species-specific differences. Whether these differences are due to amino acid structure, carbohydrate content (if the receptor is a glycoprotein), or modification of TH-R remains to be determined.

Another difference among cell types was the contribution to specifically bound ^{125}I-TH that was due to TH-R. We consistently found that for HF and HT1080 cells TH-R represented a greater proportion of the specifically bound ^{125}I-TH than was seen for $2°$CE, D98, or CHL cells. Since HF, HT1080, and D98 cells were all of human origin, this difference, unlike the molecular-weight differences, did not correlate with the species of origin. To determine if there was a relationship between TH-R formation and the ability to respond to TH, we also examined the mitogenic effect of TH on these cells. We previously reported that addition of TH to nondividing cultures of $2°$CE [16] and HF cells [21] resulted in cell number increases of 60–70% and 20%, respectively. When CHL and HT1080 cells were treated with TH under similar conditions, CHL cultures increased in cell number by as much as 70%, while HT1080 cultures only increased by 20%. Thus, HF and HT1080 cells which formed greater amounts of TH-R did not respond as well mitogenically to TH as did $2°$CE and CHL cells, which formed less TH-R. This suggested an inverse relationship between TH-R and mitogenesis. However, our experiments only measured the amount of TH-R present after 1 h of incubation with ^{125}I-TH. If the rate of degradation relative to rate of formation of TH-R were higher in $2°$CE and CHL cells than in HF and HT1080 cells, this might account for the build-up of TH-R in HF and HT1080 cells compared to $2°$CE and CHL cells. We are presently investigating this possibility.

Previously only human fibroblasts [16, 22] and $2°$CE and $2°$ mouse embryo cells [16] were known to respond mitogenically to thrombin in the absence of serum or other growth factors. Since these were cell strains and thus had a finite life-span, it was not possible to select stable clones that differed in their mitogenic response to TH. In this paper we have reported a mitogenic response to TH by CHL cells in serum-free medium. It should now be possible to produce 1) clones of mitogenically responsive and nonresponsive cells, 2) clones that differ in the number of TH receptors, and 3) clones that have different rates of formation, internalization, or degradation of TH-R. By studying these kinds of variants, it should be possible to obtain a clearer understanding of the role of TH receptors and TH-R in thrombin-stimulated cell division.

ACKNOWLEDGMENTS

This work was supported by a research grant (CA-12306) from the National Cancer Institute. D.D.C. is a recipient of a Research Career Development Award (CA-00171) from the National Cancer Institute.

We thank Cindy Rofer for technical assistance and John W. Fenton II for gifts of human thrombin [5].

REFERENCES

1. Baker JB, Simmer RL, Glenn KC, Cunningham DD: Nature 278:743, 1979.
2. Linsley PS, Blifeld C, Wrann M, Fox CF: Nature 278:745, 1979.
3. Das M, Fox CF: Proc Natl Acad Sci USA 75:2644, 1978.
4. Das M, Miyakawa T, Fox CF, Pruss RM, Aharonov A, Hershman HR: Proc Natl Acad Sci USA 74:2790, 1977.
5. Fenton JW II, Fasco MJ, Stackrow AB, Aronson DL, Young AM, Finlayson JS: J Biol Chem 252:3587, 1977.
6. Savage CR Jr, Cohen S: J Biol Chem 247:7609, 1972.
7. Ham RG, McKeehan WL: In Vitro 14:11, 1978.
8. Ford DK, Yerganian G: J Natl Cancer Inst 21:393, 1958.

9. Rein A, Rubin H: Exp Cell Res 49:666, 1968.
10. Chen TR: Exp Cell Res 104:255, 1977.
11. Martin BM, Wasiewski WW, Fenton JW II, Detwiler TC: Biochem 15:4886, 1976.
12. Carpenter G, Cohen S: J Cell Biol 71:159, 1976.
13. Laemmli UK: Nature 227:680, 1970.
14. Lowry OH, Rosebrough NJ, Farr AL, Randall RJ: J Biol Chem 193:265, 1951.
15. Ross E, Schatz G: Anal Biochem 54:304, 1973.
16. Carney DH, Glenn KC, Cunningham DD: J Cell Physiol 95:13, 1978.
17. Carney DH, Glenn KC, Cunningham DD, Das M, Fox CF, Fenton JW II: J Biol Chem 254:6244, 1979.
18. Rosenberg RD, Damus PS: J Biol Chem 248:6490, 1973.
19. Chandra S, Bang NU: In Lundblad R, Fenton J II, Mann K (eds): "Chemistry and Biology of Thrombin." Ann Arbor, Michigan: Ann Arbor Science, 1977, p 421.
20. Owen GO: Biochim Biophys Acta 405:380, 1975.
21. Baker JB, Barsh GS, Carney DH, Cunningham DD: Proc Natl Acad Sci USA 75:1882, 1978.
22. Pohjanpelto P: J Cell Physiol 91:387, 1977.

Journal of Supramolecular Structure 12:259–272 (1979)
Tumor Cell Surfaces and Malignancy 591–604

Regulation of Dome Formation in Differentiated Epithelial Cell Cultures

Julia E. Lever

Department of Biochemistry and Molecular Biology, The University of Texas Medical School, Houston, Texas 77025

Rat mammary (Rama 25) and dog kidney (MDCK) epithelial cell cultures formed 'domes' of cells due to fluid accumulation in focal regions between the culture dish and the cell monolayer. Addition of ouabain caused collapse of domes, suggesting that transport functions were required for maintenance of domes.

Dome formation in both epithelial cell lines was stimulated by a broad spectrum of known inducers of erythroid differentiation in Friend erythroleukemia cells. Among these inducers were: 1) polar solvents such as dimethylsulfoxide, dimethylformamide, and hexamethylene bisacetamide; 2) purines such as hypoxanthine, inosine, and adenosine; 3) low-molecular-weight fatty acids such as n-butyrate; and 4) conditions expected to elevate levels of cyclic AMP. In the latter group were activators of adenylate cyclase such as cholera toxin and prostaglandin E_1; cyclic AMP phosphodiesterase inhibitors such as theophylline and 1-methyl-3-isobutylxanthine; and analogs of cyclic AMP.

Induction of domes occurred 15–30 h after addition of inducer to the culture medium. Induction by chemicals was serum-dependent and required protein synthesis but not DNA synthesis. Induced dome formation was reversible after removal of inducer, requiring the continuous presence of inducer. Reversal was also observed after either removal of serum or addition of inhibitors of protein synthesis.

These results suggest the hypothesis that domes arise in these epithelial cultures by a process that is similar to cell differentiation and is influenced by cyclic AMP.

Key words: epithelial transport, differentiation, cyclic AMP, cryoprotective solvents

Recently, several tissue culture model systems have been made available for the study of morphogenesis and physiology of transporting epithelia [1–6]. Unique properties of transporting epithelia are expressed in culture by these cell cultures, notably the ability to form cell layers which act as permeability barriers between aqueous compart-

Received March 5, 1979; accepted September 28, 1979.

ments. This property derives from the maintenance of specialized junctional complexes and functional polarization of the plasma membrane after transition to culture and neoplastic transformation [7, 8].

Hemispheres (0.1–1 mm in diameter) of cells, known as domes, blisters, or hemicysts, form spontaneously in densely confluent cuboidal epithelial cell cultures derived from a variety of transporting epithelia [1–9]. Domes rise and fall apparently at random over the culture dish. Domes appear to result from fluid accumulation between the cell monolayer and the plastic dish owing to the manifestation in cell culture of specialized, undirectional epithelial transport and secretory properties. Figure 1 is a schematic representation of a dome.

The focal occurrence of fluid accumulation in domes rather than uniformly under the entire monolayer suggests that dome cells may differ functionally and biochemically from cells in the surrounding monolayer. However, no morphologic features have been found which distinguish dome cells from those in the surrounding monolayer. Pickett et al [10] have demonstrated that the surface of primary mammary epithelial cell cultures in contact with the medium (equivalent to the apical or luminal surface) contained microvilli and well-developed occluding junctions. Gap junctions and desmosomes were also found in the cultures, but the luminal surface membrane of both dome cells and monolayer cells exhibited similar cell and junctional structure.

Active fluid transport is required for the maintenance of domes as shown by observations that domes are collapsed after fluid transport is inhibited by ouabain or when fluid leakage is permitted after a dome is pierced by mechanical means. However, it is important to emphasize that dome formation may represent functional changes unrelated to changes in transport systems in the plasma membrane. Changes in selective adhesion to the culture substratum or in specialized junctional contacts may play a causative role in dome formation.

A remarkable analogy between the development of domes in epithelial cell cultures and processes of cell differentiation was suggested by the following observations. A broad spectrum of compounds known as inducers of differentiation in cell culture systems, such

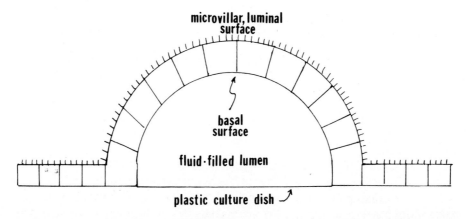

Fig. 1. Schematic representation of a dome. Microvilli are observed on the upper, apical plasma membrane surface of the dome cells and surrounding monolayer, in contact with the culture medium. Domes arise owing to transepithelial fluid transport from the culture medium through the apical membrane to the space between the cell monolayer and the culture dish via the basolateral membrane.

as Friend erythroleukemia cells [11, 12] and neuroblastoma [13], also produced a dramatic increase in both the size and frequency of dome formation in epithelial cultures within 15–30 h after addition [14, 15]. This observation suggested that induced dome formation may result from differentiation of cell types in the culture. Such a possible analogy between dome formation and cell differentiation in vitro in other cell culture model systems is pursued in this report in terms of a parallel study of agonists and antagonists of dome formation in two different dome-forming epithelial cell cultures – the Rama 25 line of rat mammary epithelial cells [6] and the MDCK kidney epithelial cell line [14].

MATERIALS AND METHODS

Cell Culture

Rama 25 (cuboidal), Rama 29 (elongated), and Rama 30 (elongated) clonal epithelial cell lines derived from a dimethylbenzanthracene-induced rat mammary tumor [6] were obtained from Dr. D. Bennett, Imperial Cancer Research Fund Laboratories, London. These cell lines were propagated in Dulbecco's modified Eagle's medium supplemented with 10% calf serum, 50 ng/ml bovine insulin and 50 ng/ml hydrocortisone. It was necessary to replace cultures of Rama 25 from frozen low-passage stocks when they had reached passage numbers above 30 owing to appreciable infiltration by elongated epithelial cell types which arise spontaneously in these cultures [6].

The MDCK epithelial cell line derived from dog kidney [16] was obtained from Dr. R. Holley, Salk Institute. The MDCK cell line, and MDCK clone 4, a subline with a high frequency of spontaneous dome formation, were grown in Dulbecco's modified Eagle's medium supplemented with 10% calf serum, nonessential amino acids, hypoxanthine, putrescine, biotin, lipoic acid, vitamin B-12, ascorbic acid, glutathione, p-aminobenzoic acid, trace metals, and linoleic acid [17].

All cell growth was at $37°C$ in an atmosphere of 10% CO_2 in air.

Quantitation of Domes in Epithelial Cell Cultures

Cultures were fixed with 5% glutaraldehyde in phosphate-buffered saline for 15 min at room temperature. This solution was aspirated, and cells were stained with Giemsa, washed three times with water, and dried in air. This procedure permitted the identification of dome foci on dried monolayers. The number of domes was counted on duplicate 35-mm dishes using 8 to 20 fields of either 0.13 cm^2 (Bausch & Lomb stereozoom microscope) or 0.07 cm^2 (Zeiss stereo microscope). Larger numbers of fields were examined for cultures with an average of fewer than 10 domes per field.

Determination of Intracellular Levels of Cyclic AMP

Medium was removed from epithelial cell monolayers on 5-cm dishes and 1 ml of 50 mM Na acetate, pH 4.75, was added. Harvesting was carried out rapidly at $4°C$. Cells were removed from the dish by scraping with a rubber spatula, the dish was rinsed with an additional 1 ml of buffer, and a tube containing the combined 2 ml of extract was immediately placed in a boiling-water bath for 5 min. Then the extract was cooled and acetylated as described previously [18]. Samples were stored frozen at $-15°C$. Acetylated samples were analyzed for cyclic AMP content by a radioimmunoassay method (New England Nuclear kit NEX-132).

Two-Dimensional Electrophoresis of Labeled Proteins

Epithelial cell cultures on 5-cm dishes were labeled either 2 h or 15 h in the presence of 1 ml of medium containing 0.5 mCi ^{35}S-methionine (Amersham) at 37°. Cultures were washed three times with ice-cold phosphate-buffered saline and then rapidly solubilized by scraping at 4° in the presence of staphylococcal nuclease, 0.3% sodium dodecylsulfate (SDS), 1% mercaptoethanol, deoxyribonuclease I, and ribonuclease A according to the procedure described by Garrels [19]. Samples were lyophilized, dissolved in a sample buffer composed of urea, NP-40, ampholytes (pH 6–8), and dithiothreitol, and then analyzed by the improved high-resolution two-dimensional polyacrylamide gel electrophoresis (PAGE) technique recently described by Garrels [19]. Gels were fixed and stained [20], then processed for fluorography as described by Bonner and Laskey [21]. Dried gels were exposed to flash-presensitized X-ray film (Kodak, XR-5).

Materials

Hexamethylene bisacetamide (HMBA) was generously donated by Dr. R. Reuben, Columbia University, and prostaglandin E_1 was obtained through the courtesy of Dr. J. Pike, Upjohn. Cholera toxin was purchased from Schwartz-Mann. Dimethylsulfoxide (DMSO) was from Mallinckrodt, 1-methyl-2-pyrrolidinone (MPR) was from Eastman, and N-methylacetamide was from Aldrich. Cytochalasin B was obtained from Aldrich. Sodium butyrate was prepared by neutralizing butyric acid (Fisher). Other chemicals were purchased from Sigma.

RESULTS

Cryoprotective Agents as Inducers of Dome Formation

Confluent dense cell cultures of either Rama 25 mammary cells or MDCK kidney cells exhibited a low spontaneous frequency of dome formation – less than 10 domes per 1 cm^2 [14, 15]. Spontaneously occurring domes were dependent on the presence of serum and occurred in patches on the cell monolayer, rather than at random all over the dish.

Addition of certain categories of compounds to dense cultures increased dome formation above the spontaneous level, beginning at 15–30 h (Fig. 2). Table I compares the relative dome-forming response of each cell line at the optimal concentration of each inducer. Polar solvents known as cryoprotective agents [22] and inducers of erythroid differentiation in Friend erythroleukemia cells [11, 12] were among the most effective inducers of dome formation in both the kidney and mammary cell lines. Polar solvent inducers listed in Table I differed in relative potency, both in terms of optimal concentration required for maximal induction, and the magnitude of commitment to dome formation. Thus, dimethylformamide (DMF), hexamethylene bisacetamide, and 1-methyl-2-pyrrolidinone were among the most effective, both on a concentration basis and in terms of response. Dimethylsulfoxide was moderately inductive, and acetamide and diethylene glycol (DEG) were least effective.

The number of dome foci increased quantitatively as a function of polar solvent inducer concentration in both kidney and epithelial cells, as shown in Figure 3 [14, 15]. A maximal number of domes per area was reached, characteristic of the particular inducer

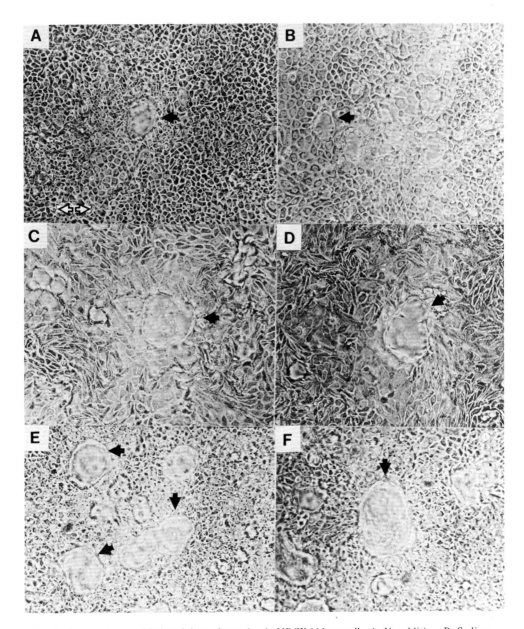

Fig. 2. Spontaneous and induced dome formation in MDCK kidney cells. A: No addition. B: Sodium n-butyrate, 2.5 mM. C: DMF, 190 mM. D: DMF, 190 mM plus cytosine arabinoside, 25 μM. E: Adenosine, 1 mM. F: Cyclic AMP, 1 mM plus theophylline, 1 mM. The indicated compounds were added with medium change to confluent cell cultures. Bar represents 100 μm. From Lever [14], with permission.

TABLE I. Categories of Inducers of Dome Formation in Mammary and Kidney Epithelial Cell Mass Cultures

Compound	Concentration (mM)	Response: Number of domes	
		Mammary cell line (RAMA 25)	Kidney cell line (MDCK)
A. Polar compounds			
Dimethylsulfoxide	200	++	+
N,N'-dimethylformamide	140	++++	++++
N,N-dimethylacetamide	20	++++	0
1,3-Dimethylurea	500	++++	++
Acetamide	1,000	+	0
1-Methyl-2-pyrrolidinone	25	++++	++
N-methylacetamide	100	++	++
Pyridine-1-oxide	50	+++	0
Diethylene glycol	90	+	0
1,1,3,3-Tetramethylurea	10	++++	0
Hexamethylene bisacetamide	5	++++	++++
B. Purines			
Hypoxanthine	1	++	++
Inosine	1	+++	++
Adenosine	1	+++	+++
C. Butyric acid	3	++	++++
D. Cyclic nucleotides			
Cholera toxin, 5 μg/ml		+	+
Prostaglandin E$_1$, 5 μg/ml		+	+
Dibutyryl cyclic AMP, 1 mM, plus theophylline, 1 mM		++++	++++
Dibutyryl cyclic GMP	1	0	0
8-Bromo-cyclic AMP	1	+++	+++
Theophylline	1	+++	+++
1-Isobutyl-3-methylxanthine	1	+++	+++

Symbols: ++++, highest response in terms of numbers and size of domes; +++, good response; ++, moderate response; +, weak but significant response; 0, no detectable induction of domes above spontaneous level.
From Lever [14], with permission.

Induction of domes was reversible, requiring continuous presence of inducer. After removal of inducer, the majority of domes contracted then disappeared over a period of 15–30 h, reaching an incidence corresponding to that observed without addition of in- and the cell line. Above these optimal inducer concentrations decreased dome formation and cell death was observed. The average size of domes showed much less variation with inducer concentration than the number of domes per unit area.
ducer. By contrast, these inducers triggered an irreversible differentiation of Friend erythroleukemia cells [11, 12].

Dome Formation Represents a Specific Cellular Response

Several observations indicated that domes are the result of specific cellular functions, rather than artifacts of toxicity resulting from exposure to these nonphysiologic compounds. First, induction of domes by these chemicals is a property unique to certain epithelial cell lines with the morphologic polarization, electrical resistance, and permea-

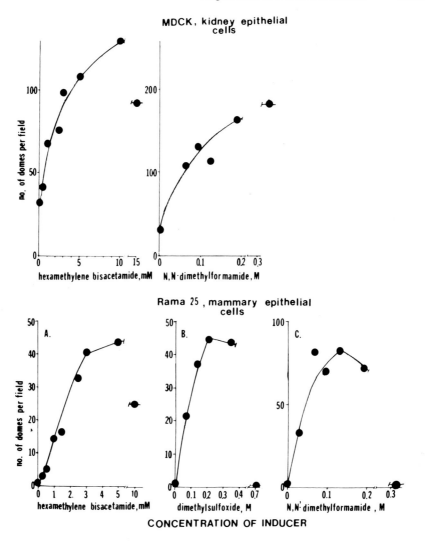

Fig. 3. Induction of domes as a function of inducer concentration. Domes were counted 3 days after addition of the indicated concentrations of inducer to confluent cultures of either Rama 25 mammary epithelial cells or MDCK kidney epithelial cells.

bility properties of transporting epithelia. None of the compounds listed in Table I caused dome formation in either 3T3 fibroblasts, BSC-1 epithelial cells, or certain non-dome-forming cell sublines (Rama 29, Rama 30) which could be isolated from Rama 25 cultures [14, 15].

Second, addition with inducer of inhibitors of protein synthesis (such as cyclohexi-mide or puromycin), or the Na$^+$ pump inhibitor ouabain, or any one of the cytoskeletal disruptive agents cytochalasin B, colcemid, and vinblastine, blocked the chemical induction of domes [14, 15]. If any of these inhibitors were added to cultures after the appearance of domes induced by DMF, domes largely disappeared from the culture. Thus, protein synthesis, cytoskeletal organization, and Na$^+$,K$^+$ ATPase activities were required for induction and maintenance of domes. Finally, domes resulting after chemical induction resembled morphologically those which occurred spontaneously (Fig. 2).

By contrast, DNA synthesis was not a requirement for chemical induction of domes. Thus, DMF converted over 50% of the cells in the culture to participation in dome formation. Addition with DMF of concentrations of hydroxyurea or cytosine arabinoside that inhibited ^{3}H-thymidine incorporation by 99% did not affect the final number of domes in the culture [14, 15].

Dome Formation by Cell Subpopulations

Induction by these chemicals did not occur as the result of selective proliferation of cells which could make domes spontaneously. Rather, additional cell subpopulations were induced to make domes. This conclusion was based on the experiment shown in Table II. Individual colonies were first isolated, then grown without inducer for 11 days. Then colonies were tested for inducibility by these chemicals. Table II shows that 13.5% of colonies tested formed domes in the total absence of inducer in the case of the mammary cell line and 16.6% in the case of the kidney cell line. This indication that only a certain subpopulation of cells can form domes spontaneously may account for the patch-like occurrence of spontaneous dome formation in the parental culture. Addition of either 140 mM DMSO or 190 mM DMF to colonies grown nonselectively greatly increased the incidence of dome-forming colonies in both the mammary epithelial cells and the kidney epithelial cells. Since in this protocol all colonies tested were isolated before exposure to inducer, the inducer is not acting by selecting the survival of colonies. Therefore, the finding that increased numbers of colonies form domes in the presence of inducer compared with spontaneous incidence suggests that these inducers recruit an increased number of preexisting cells in the population to form domes compared with the number capable of forming domes spontaneously. The conclusion that inducers are not acting

TABLE II. Frequency of Colonies Which Form Domes Spontaneously or in Response to Various Inducers

Addition	Number of colonies tested	Average % colonies with domes
A. RAMA 25 (mammary)		
No addition	2,143	13.5
Dibutyryl cyclic AMP, 0.2 mM, plus theophylline, 1 mM	1,091	44.0
Butyrate, 2.5 mM	640	76.5
DMSO, 140 mM	1,097	58.0
DMF, 190 mM	1,099	88.0
B. MDCK (kidney)		
No addition	380	16.6
DMSO, 140 mM	297	44.8
DMF, 190 mM	400	58.3

Isolated colonies were obtained by plating 200 cells per 90-mm dish in the absence of inducer. The cloning efficiency of MDCK cells varied from 60 to 100% and that of RAMA 25 cells varied from 32 to 37%. At 11 days after plating, when colonies were 0.5–1 cm in diameter, the medium was changed and the indicated additions were made. Cultures were fixed and stained after 3 days. Data from Lever [14].

by allowing selective proliferation of cell populations that form domes spontaneously is reinforced also by the observation that inhibition of DNA synthesis does not block the chemical induction of domes.

As a corollary, these data show that certain subpopulations of cells do not make domes in the presence of inducers. For example, Table II shows that 50–60% of MDCK colonies do not form any domes in the presence of either DMSO or DMF.

Another point concerning these data should be noted. Different inducers, including categories discussed below, stimulated different numbers of Rama 25 colonies to form domes. Since the Rama 25 cell line, a putative stem cell line of the mammary gland which undergoes a reproducible differentiation in culture to other cell types [6] was derived from a single cell by two rigorous cloning procedures [6], this observation suggests the possibility that subpopulations of the culture responding to different inducers may arise in vitro with high frequency.

Induction of Domes by Purines

Certain purines and their derivatives caused increased dome formation (Table I). Adenosine was one of the most effective inducers in this category.

Cyclic AMP as a Positive Regulator of Dome Formation

A possible clue to physiologic mechanisms involved in dome formation was provided by the observation that various conditions expected to elevate intracellular levels of cyclic AMP also caused increased incidence of domes in both the mammary and kidney cell culture systems. Thus, compounds known to activate adenylate cyclase activity, such as cholera toxin [23] and prostaglandin E_1 [24] also produced a small but reproducible increase in dome formation. Inhibitors of cyclic AMP phosphodiesterase activity [25], such as theophylline and 1-methyl-3-isobutylxanthine, caused a much more dramatic increase in dome formation. Furthermore, analogs of cyclic AMP, such as $N^6 O^{2'}$-dibutyryl cyclic AMP or 8-bromo-cyclic AMP, caused an increased dome formation which was potentiated after the further addition of phosphodiesterase inhibitors. It seems unlikely that the inductive effects of dibutyryl cyclic AMP are due to breakdown to butyric acid, itself an inducer, since the same concentration of dibutyryl cyclic GMP was ineffective (Table I). Furthermore, this concentration of dibutyryl derivative would yield 1 mM butyric acid upon complete hydrolysis, a concentration of butyrate below the level required for induction.

Interestingly, several, but not all, of the polar solvent category of inducers, as well as n-butyrate, caused an elevation of cyclic AMP levels (Table III). While this unexpected observation may partially explain their inductive effects according to the hypothesis that cyclic AMP levels regulate dome formation, it does not explain the much greater dome-forming response observed with these chemicals compared with that observed to accompany similar levels of cyclic AMP triggered by other agents.

Changes in Synthesis of Specific Proteins Accompanying Dome Formation

Total cellular proteins labeled biosynthetically with ^{35}S-methionine were analyzed by high-resolution two-dimensional polyacrylamide gel electrophoresis. Two narrow pH ranges, pH 5–7 (shown in Fig. 4) and 6–8, were used, each range resolving an average of 395 and 495 spots, respectively, after detection by fluorography – with a region of overlap between the two ranges. Figure 4 compares the pattern obtained after Rama 25 cells were induced to form domes with DMF (50% of the cells in the culture participating in domes) compared with uninduced controls. The arrow indicates a region where major changes in levels of specific proteins were observed in preliminary experiments.

TABLE III. Intracellular Levels of Cyclic AMP in the Presence of Inducers of Dome Formation: RAMA 25 Mammary Cells

Addition	Cyclic AMP[a] (pmoles/mg protein)
Medium change only	1.67 ± 0.15
Theophylline, 1 mM	2.07 ± 0.20
1-Methyl-3-isobutylxanthine, 1 mM	3.06 ± 0.39
Cholera toxin, 5 μg/ml	2.22 ± 0.19
n-Butyrate, 3 mM	3.03 ± 1.1
Dimethylformamide, 190 mM	3.15 ± 0.70
Dimethylsulfoxide, 140 mM	1.77 ± 0.44
Hexamethylene bisacetamide, 5 mM	3.43 ± 1.0

[a]Determinations were made using extracts from confluent RAMA 25 cells 24 h after addition of inducer, as described under Materials and Methods. Values are mean ± SD.

This approach may reveal groups of proteins that are necessary for induction, or that are necessary for maintenance and functional expression of domes, as a preliminary to their biochemical or immunologic identification.

DISCUSSION

Several eukaryotic cell culture systems have been proposed as models to study stages of cell differentiation in terms of molecular events [26]. Whereas in many studies it has not been possible to control either the direction or degree of differentiation, in certain cases several compounds have been identified which trigger a greater magnitude of differentiation of the cell population at a defined time, greatly simplifying experimental approaches.

The pattern of differentiation in these model systems depends on the nature of the cell type rather than the nature of the inducer. Various categories of inducers which promote a program of differentiation in Friend erythroleukemia cells include polar cryoprotective solvents, butyric acid, purines, ouabain, and actinomycin D [11]. Erythroid cultures induced by these compounds undergo a partially normal program of terminal erythroid differentiation leading to heme production, changes in surface glycoproteins, spectrin production, synthesis of globin mRNA and globins, increase in activities of heme synthetic enzymes, and synthesis of hemoglobins. Many of these same inducers also promote neurite extension in neuroblastoma cells [13]. The optimal concentration and relative magnitude of cellular response for each inducer of dome formation in polarized epithelial cell cultures is strikingly similar to their optimal concentration and relative effectiveness in triggering different programs of differentiation characteristic of other cell lines such as neuroblastoma or Friend cells.

Another demonstrated similarity between induction of Friend cell differentiation and induction of domes is that in both cases it has been demonstrated that each inducer triggers only a portion of the cell population to undergo differentiation [11]. These systems differ in that induced dome formation is reversible, whereas erythroid differentiation is terminal [11]. Also, ouabain, a Friend cell inducer [11], blocks dome formation, possibly by direct inhibition of transport systems necessary to maintain domes.

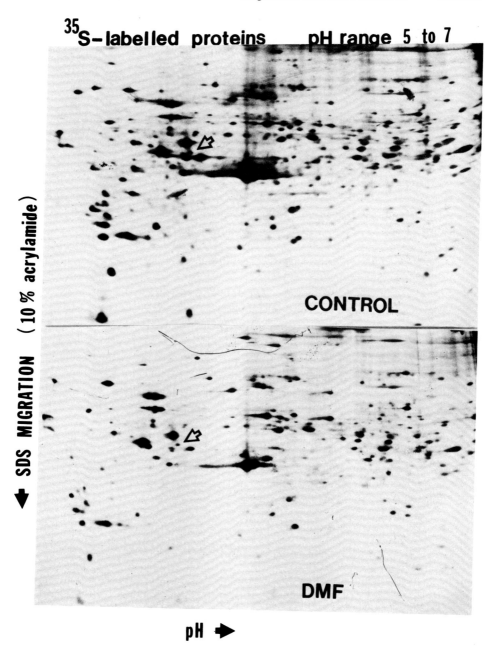

Fig. 4. Two-dimensional polyacrylamide gel electrophoresis of total proteins from Rama 25 mammary epithelial cells after induction of domes by DMF compared with uninduced controls. Cultures were labeled 15 h with ^{35}S-methionine added at 3 days after addition of 1.5% DMF with medium change. Isoelectric focusing was carried out using pH 5–7 ampholytes. Total labeled protein applied to each gel, estimated after precipitation of an aliquot with 5% trichloroacetic acid, was 1.15×10^5 cpm for the control and 8.8×10^4 cpm for the DMF-induced culture.

The degree of experimental manipulation provided by the identification of inducers of dome formation, as well as the use of clonal epithelial cell cultures, should provide a new approach to investigation of differentiation of epithelial cells into polarized fluid-transporting cells. The Rama mammary cell line has been reported to further differentiate in vitro into several morphologically discrete, nonpolarized mammary epithelial cell types [6].

It is not known whether the program of events leading to dome formation in cell culture resembles the normal pattern of secretory epithelial development. Also, it is not known whether changes in any biochemical or functional markers accompany dome formation.

A major question is whether these inducers affect the various patterns of differentiation characteristic of different cell types by similar mechanisms. Furthermore, within a single cell system it is pertinent to ask whether each category of inducer acts by a different mechanism or whether the effects of these compounds intersect within a common pathway.

The polar solvent inducers have nonspecific and generalized effects, making it difficult to identify their obligatory targets. Several mechanisms — including conformational changes in DNA or chromatin proteins [27] or plasma membrane structures [28] induced by solvent effects on water structure — have been proposed. DNA breakage has been proposed to explain their action on Friend cell differentiation [29].

Reuben et al [30] have examined the relationship between structure and activity of the polar solvent inducers of erythroid differentiation. Conclusions from this study were that effective inducers contained both planar and polar components, with optimal activity observed when polar groups were separated by a polymethylene chain of 5—6 methylene residues as in HMBA. Since HMBA can be taken up and metabolized by cells [31], a metabolic product of this molecule may be the active inducer.

Herskovits et al [32] have measured unfolding of globular proteins by monoalkyl- and dialkyl-substituted formamides and ureas. There does not appear to be a direct correlation between the effectiveness of these compounds as inducers of differentiation and their ability to unfold proteins as estimated by solvent denaturation midpoints.

In addition to its effects on erythroid induction in Friend cells [11], sodium butyrate also affects granulopoiesis of mastocytoma cells [33], and causes induction of alkaline phosphatase [34], morphologic transformations, and altered ganglioside sialyltransferase activity [35] in HeLa cells. Sodium butyrate inhibited cytochalasin B-induced multinucleation in NRK (normal rat kidney) cells [36]. Altenberg et al [37] reported that butyrate reversed the morphology of virally transformed cells to normal, accompanied by a striking elaboration of cytoplasmic microfilaments and microtubules. n-Butyrate has been reported to inhibit histone deacetylation [38, 39]. Butyrate and purines such as adenosine may act by elevating cyclic AMP levels, as reported for other cell systems [40, 41].

Observations that some, but not all, inducers caused elevated levels of cyclic AMP, taken together with the finding of sublines of cells which respond to DMF but not to DMSO, suggest that multiple mechanisms may operate. Furthermore, examples could be found where different types of inducers triggered a similar elevation of intracellular cyclic AMP levels but caused a markedly different final response in terms of numbers of domes. However, the possibility remains that different cell types in these cultures may differ in their individual cyclic AMP levels. Therefore, estimations of intracellular cyclic AMP carried out using the total cell population may not reveal a specific response of a target cell.

Although these phenomena are complex, these families of cell lines and categories of inducers will provide a useful experimental system for correlation of biochemical changes which accompany induction of domes. Specific parameters which may be investigated in this model system are 1) the synthesis and regulation of specialized junctions; 2) the synthesis of functionally and structurally polarized plasma membranes; and 3) the coupling of transport and hormone receptor-effector systems that are possibly present on opposite sides of the cell.

ACKNOWLEDGMENTS

I thank Dr. R. Reuben for a generous gift of hexamethylene bisacetamide, Dr. John Pike for providing prostaglandin E_1, Drs. D. Bennett and R. Holley for providing the source of cell cultures, and Marianne Bowman and Ching W. Kalieta for excellent technical assistance. Support was from the US Public Health Service, grants No. GM 25006 and GM 27055.

REFERENCES

1. Leighton J, Brada Z, Estes LW, Justh G: Science 163:472, 1969.
2. Leighton J, Estes LW, Mansukhani S, Brada Z: Cancer 26:1022, 1970.
3. Enami J, Nandi S, Haslam S: In Vitro 8:405, 1973.
4. Visser AS, Prop FJA: J Natl Cancer Inst 52:293, 1974.
5. Owens RB, Smith HS, Hackett AJ: J Natl Cancer Inst 53:261, 1974.
6. Bennett DC, Peachey LA, Durbin H, Rudland PS: Cell 15:283, 1978.
7. Misfeldt DS, Hamamoto ST, Pitelka DR: Proc Natl Acad Sci USA 73:1212, 1976.
8. Cerijido M, Robbins ES, Dolan WJ, Rotunno CA, Sabatini DD: J Cell Biol 77:853, 1978.
9. McGrath CM: Am Zool 15:231, 1975.
10. Pickett PB, Pitelka DR, Hamamoto ST, Misfeldt DS: J Cell Biol 66:316.
11. Marks PA, Rifkind RA: Annu Rev Biochem 47:419, 1978.
12. Marks PA, Rifkind RA, Terada M, Reuben RC, Gazitt Y, Fibach E: In Golde DW, Cline MJ, Metcalf D, Fox CF (eds): "Hematopoietic Cell Differentiation." New York: Academic, 1978, p 25.
13. Palfrey C, Kimhi Y, Littauer UZ, Reuben RC, Marks PA: Biochem Biophys Res Commun 76:937, 1977.
14. Lever JE: In Ross R, Sato G (eds): "Cold Spring Harbor Conference on Cell Proliferation," vol 6. Cold Spring Harbor, New York: Cold Spring Harbor Press, 1979, p 727.
15. Lever JE: Proc Natl Acad Sci USA 76:1323, 1979.
16. Gaush CR, Hard WL, Smith TF: Proc Soc Exp Biol Med 122:931, 1966.
17. Holley RW, Kiernan JA: Proc Natl Acad Sci USA 71:2908, 1974.
18. Harper JF, Brooker GJ: J Cyclic Nucleotide Res 1:207, 1975.
19. Garrels J: J Biol Chem 254:7961, 1979.
20. Fairbanks G, Steck TL, Wallach DFH: Biochemistry 10:2606, 1971.
21. Bonner WM, Laskey RA: Eur J Biochem 46:83, 1974.
22. Nash T: J Gen Physiol 46:167, 1962.
23. Finkelstein RA: Crit Rev Microbiol 2:553, 1973.
24. Kantor HS, Tao P, Kiefer HC: Proc Natl Acad Sci USA 71:1317, 1974.
25. Chasin M, Harris DN: In Greengard P, Robison GA (eds): "Advances in Cyclic Nucleotide Research." New York: Raven, 1976, p 225.
26. Newmark P: Nature 272:756, 1978.
27. Terada M, Nudel U, Fibach E, Rifkind RA, Marks PA: Cancer Res 38:835, 1978.
28. Lyman GH, Preisler HD, Paphadjopoulos D: Nature 262:360, 1976.
29. Scher W, Friend C: Cancer Res 38:841, 1978.
30. Reuben RC, Khanna PL, Gazitt Y, Breslow R, Rifkind R, Marks PA: J Biol Chem 253:4214, 1978.

31. Reuben RC, Marks PA, Rifkind RA, Terada M, Fibach E, Nudel U, Gazitt Y, Breslow R: In Ikawa Y (ed): "Oji International Seminar on Genetic Aspects of Friend Virus and Friend Cells." New York: Academic, 1978.
32. Herskovits TT, Behrens CF, Siuta PB, Pandolfelli ER: Biochim Biophys Acta 490:192, 1977.
33. Mori Y, Akedo H, Tanaka K, Tanigaki Y, Okada M: Exp Cell Res 118:15, 1979.
34. Griffin MJ, Price GH, Bazzell KL, Cox RP, Ghosh NK: Arch Biochem Biophys 164:619, 1974.
35. Simmons JL, Fishman PH, Freese E, Brady RO: J Cell Biol 66:414, 1975.
36. Altenberg BC, Steiner S: Exp Cell Res 118:31, 1979.
37. Altenberg BC, Via DP, Steiner SH: Exp Cell Res 102:223, 1976.
38. Boffa LC, Vidali G, Mann RS, Allfrey VG: J Biol Chem 253:3364, 1978.
39. Candido EPM, Reeves R, Davie JR: Cell 14:105, 1978.
40. Clark RB, Seney MN: J Biol Chem 251:4239, 1976.
41. Storrie B, Puck T, Wenger L: J Cell Physiol 94:69, 1978.

Journal of Supramolecular Structure 12:273–291 (1979)
Tumor Cell Surfaces and Malignancy 605–623

Isolation of Cholera Toxin Receptors From a Mouse Fibroblast and Lymphoid Cell Line by Immune Precipitation

D. R. Critchley, S. Ansell, R. Perkins, S. Dilks, and J. Ingram

Department of Biochemistry, University of Leicester, Leicester LE1 7RH, England

Cholera toxin receptors have been isolated from both a mouse fibroblast (Balbc/3T3) and mouse lymphoid cell line labeled by the galactose oxidase borotritiide technique. Tritiated receptor-toxin complexes solubilized in NP40 were isolated by addition of toxin antibody followed by a protein A-containing strain of Staphylococcus aureus. In both cell types by far the major species of toxin receptor isolated was ganglioside in nature, although galactoproteins were also present in the immune complexes. Whether the galactoproteins form part of a toxin-receptor complex or are artifacts of the isolation procedure is presently unclear.

The relative specificity of cholera toxin for a carbohydrate sequence in a glycolipid suggests that the toxin might prove a useful tool in establishing the function and organization of glycolipids in membranes. For example, interaction of cholera toxin with the mouse lymphoid cell line was shown to result in patching and capping of bound toxin, raising the possibility that the glycolipid receptor interacts indirectly with cytoskeletal elements. Cholera toxin might also be used to select for mutant fibroblasts lacking the toxin receptor and therefore having an altered glycolipid profile. Such mutants might prove useful in establishing the relationship (if any) between modified glycolipid pattern and other aspects of the transformed phenotype. Attempts to isolate mutants, based on the expectation that growth of cells containing the toxin receptor would be inhibited by the increase in cAMP levels normally induced by cholera toxin, proved unsuccessful. Cholera toxin failed to inhibit significantly the growth of either Balbc or Swiss 3T3 mouse fibroblasts although it markedly elevated cAMP levels.

Key words: cholera toxin – receptors, cell growth, glycolipids – transformation, organization in membranes, glycolipids as cell surface receptors

Abbreviations. Ganglioside structure and nomenclature: GM_3, Cer-Glc-Gal-AcNeu; GM_2, Cer-Glc-Gal(AcNeu)-GalNac; GM_1, Cer-Glc-Gal(AcNeu)-GalNac-Gal; GD_{1a}, Cer-Glc-Gal(AcNeu)-GalNac-Gal(AcNeu); GD_{1b}, Cer-Glc-Gal(AcNeu)$_2$-GalNac-Gal; GT, Cer-Glc-Gal(AcNeu)$_2$-GalNac-Gal(AcNeu). Cer, ceramide; Glc, glucose; Gal, galactose; GalNac, N-acetylgalactosamine; AcNeu, N-acetylneuraminic acid. Glycolipids referred to in this paper are glycosphingolipids. PBS, phosphate buffered saline; PMSF, phenylmethylsulphonylfluoride; SDS, sodium dodecylsulphate; SDS-PAGE, SDS-polyacrylamide gel electrophoresis; $PGF_{2\alpha}$, Prostaglandin $F_{2\alpha}$.

Received April 23, 1979; accepted August 29, 1979.

One of the many changes associated with the transformed phenotype is loss of the ability to synthesize the more complex cell surface glycolipids. While the observation is well documented and there are few if any exceptions, the significance of the change has remained obscure (for a review, see Critchley and Vicker [1]). Recent interest has centered around the idea that glycolipids act as cell surface receptors. For example, glycolipids have been implicated as important determinants of cellular interaction [1–5] and as receptors for the glycoprotein hormones and certain bacterial toxins (for reviews see Refs. 1 and 6–8). That glycolipids act as receptors for the glycoprotein hormones appears somewhat surprising in that glycoprotein receptors for thyrotropin and human chorionic gonadotropin have previously been isolated [9, 10]. However, the primary determinant of receptor activity is probably a specific carbohydrate sequence, which may therefore appear on both glycolipids and glycoproteins. Perhaps the best evidence relating to a possible receptor role for glycolipids stems from studies on the interaction of cholera toxin with target cells: a) Ganglioside GM_1 is the best inhibitor of toxin binding to cells [11]; b) cells lacking GM_1 are unresponsive to toxin, and such cells become toxin-responsive following insertion of exogenous GM_1 into their membranes [12, 13]; c) GM_1 but not other glycolipids causes a change in the fluorescence spectrum of the toxin [14, 15]; d) saturating levels of toxin protect the terminal galactose residue of GM_1 from galactose oxidase [14, 16]. However, while the evidence is substantial it is largely indirect, and in light of the apparent dual nature of the glycoprotein hormone receptors, it remains important to establish by a more direct approach the nature of the cholera toxin receptor.

If it were shown that cholera toxin is specific for a carbohydrate sequence in glycolipid, the toxin might prove a useful tool to probe the function and organization of glycolipids in membranes. For example, interaction of cholera toxin with lymphocytes is known to result in capping of the bound toxin (and presumably the toxin receptor) in a manner which is inhibited by azide, colchicine, and cytochalasin [17–19]. If one assumes the glycolipid nature of the toxin receptor, then one of a number of possible explanations for the phenomenon is that the glycolipid receptor is associated with a transmembrane protein which in turn interacts with the cytoskeletal system. In addition the toxin could be used to derive mutant cell lines lacking the toxin receptor and therefore defective in their ability to synthesize complex glycolipids. Such cells would then be monitored for the expression of any parameters of the transformed phenotype which might arise as a consequence of loss of complex glycolipids. This approach would offer a useful alternative to the so-called "add-back" experiments where one attempts to look for reversion of transformed cell characteristics following incorporation of glycolipids into the transformed cell membrane [20, 21]. While such an approach has been extremely important in establishing the significance of loss of a high-molecular-weight cell surface protein (fibronectin) on transformation [22, 23], it has not been particularly helpful in the case of glycolipids.

In this paper we report experiments in which we have isolated the cholera toxin receptor from mouse lymphoid and fibroblast cell lines by immune precipitation. In both cases the *major* species of toxin receptor would appear to be glycolipid in nature.

MATERIALS AND METHODS

Cell Culture

The mouse lymphoid cell line (AT5) was obtained from Dr. M. Boss of the Imperial Cancer Research Fund Laboratories (ICRF), London. It was derived from a tumor formed in an inguinal lymph node following injection of Abelson virus into a Balbc mouse. The cell line was grown in suspension in Dulbecco's modified Eagle's medium containing 10% heat-inactivated calf serum and maintained at densities below 1×10^6/ml. Balbc/3T3 cells (clone A31) were also obtained from ICRF.

Scheme for Isolation of the Cholera Toxin Receptor

Terminal galactose residues are an important determinant of cholera toxin receptor activity [11]. We therefore initially chose to label surface components by the galactose oxidase borotritiide technique (see Fig. 1). Labeled cells were then exposed to an excess of cholera toxin; the mouse lymphoid and fibroblast cell lines used in the study bound approximately 1×10^6 molecules of toxin per cell, which is equivalent to 0.16 μg of toxin bound per 10^6 cells. The amount of toxin added to labeled cells was therefore based on this figure. The apparent dissociation constant for cholera toxin is of the order of 10^{-10} M [24] and although some toxin can be removed by washing, about 50% remains apparently irreversibly bound. Toxin-receptor complexes were then solubilized in 1% NP40 and incubated with toxin antibody, and the immune complexes were adsorbed to a protein A-containing strain of Staphylococcus aureus [25] (Fig. 2). Pilot experiments with a [^{3}H] GM$_1$

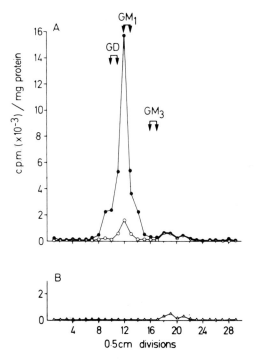

Fig. 1. Surface labeling of the gangliosides of a mouse lymphoid cell line by the galactose oxidase borotritiide technique. Cells (5×10^7) were incubated with galactose oxidase (2 units/ml) with and without neuraminidase (25 units/ml) in 5 ml of Hanks' balanced salt solution (HBSS) at 37°C for 3 h in a 5% CO_2 atmosphere. Cell viability was not significantly impaired under these conditions as monitored by dye exclusion. Following two cycles of washing in HBSS, cells were incubated with 1 mCi of NaB^{3}H$_4$ in 1 ml of PBS, pH 7.8 (stock 10 mCi/ml in 0.01 M NaOH stored at −70°C) for 15 min at 20°C. Cells were washed three times with PBS/1 mM PMSF, pH 7.4, and gangliosides were extracted and separated by thin-layer chromatography on silica gel G precoated plates using the solvent chloroform:methanol: water (60:35:8). Following visualization of glycolipid standards with iodine vapor, the plate was marked in 0.5-cm divisions and the silica gel was transferred to vials for scintillation counting. A: Galactose oxidase alone (o——o); with neuraminidase (●——●). B: No enzyme.

standard, cholera toxin, and toxin antibody showed that 1% NP40 did not reduce the recovery of GM_1 in the bacterial pellets. This suggests that NP40 does not inhibit binding of
GM_1 to toxin or toxin antibody to toxin. In similar experiments, 1% deoxycholate reduced
the recovery of GM_1 by about 50%. Bacterial pellets were then extracted for analysis of
adsorbed lipid or protein. Lipids were extracted and partitioned against water [26] to give
organic-phase lipids (primarily cholesterol, phospholipids, and neutral glycolipids) and
aqueous-phase lipids (primarily gangliosides). The aqueous-phase material was saponified
with 200 μl of 0.1 M NaOH in methanol for 4 h at 20°C prior to desalting and separation of
the gangliosides by thin-layer chromatography. Organic-phase lipids were separated by two-
dimensional thin-layer chromatography [27]. Glycoproteins were extracted by boiling with
2% SDS in electrophoresis sample buffer and the sample was reduced with dithiothreitol
prior to SDS-PAGE [28].

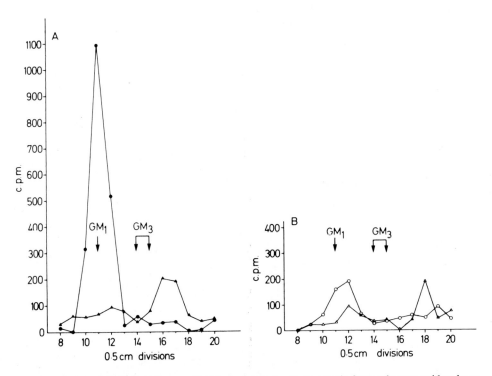

Fig. 2. Isolation of the cell surface ganglioside receptors for cholera toxin from galactose oxidase borotritiide-labeled cells. Galactose oxidase borotritiide-labeled cells (2 × 10⁸) of the mouse lymphoid cell
line were incubated with and without 50 μg of cholera toxin in 1 ml of PBS/0.05% bovine serum albu-
min/1 mM PMSF for 30 min at 20°C. The cells were washed twice with PBS/PMSF, extracted with 8
ml of 1% NP40 in 0.15 M NaCl, 5mM EDTA, 50 mM Tris (NET) buffer, pH 8/PMSF (0°C, 1 h), and centrifuged at 100,000g for 1 h. Aliquots (1 ml) of the supernatant were incubated with 40 μl of toxin
antibody or preimmune serum for 1 h at 4°C, 400 μl of a 10% suspension of a protein A-containing
strain of Staphylococcus aureus (in 0.5% NP40 NET, pH 8, 0.25% gelatin, or bovine serum albumin)
was added [25], and incubation continued for a further 30 min. The bacterial pellet (1,000g, 10 min,
4°C) was washed three times with the same buffer, and gangliosides were extracted and separated as
described in Figure 1. A: Plus toxin; •——•, plus toxin antibody; ▲——▲, plus preimmune serum.
B: Minus toxin; ○——○, plus toxin antibody; △——△, plus preimmune serum.

Antibodies to Cholera Toxin

Rabbit antibodies were prepared by injection of 30 μg of cholera toxin in 1 ml of complete Freund's adjuvant into two subcutaneous and four intramuscular sites. The procedure was repeated 3 weeks later and after a further 10 days the rabbit was bled. Preimmune serum was obtained from the same animal.

Materials

NaB^{3}H$_4$ (7 Ci/mmole), [1-^{14}C] palmitate (50 mCi/mmole), and carrier-free ^{125}I$^-$ were obtained from the Radiochemical Centre. Cholera toxin was purchased from Schwarz Mann, galactose oxidase from Worthington Biochemicals, neuraminidase from Behringwerke, lactoperoxidase from Calbiochem, and ganglioside standards from Supelco.

RESULTS

Isolation of the Cholera Toxin Receptor From a Mouse Lymphoid Cell Line

Galactose oxidase borotritiide labeling profiles of cell surface gangliosides of a mouse lymphoid cell line are shown in Figure 1a. The main peak of radioactivity had a similar mobility on thin-layer chromatograms to a GM$_1$ standard. Other gangliosides known to be synthesized by these cells from metabolic labeling studies (Fig. 3a) were poorly labeled, probably because they lacked terminal galactose or N-acetylgalactosamine residues. The extent of the labeling could be increased approximately tenfold by preincubation of the cells with neuraminidase, which presumably converted some di- and trisialogangliosides to GM$_1$. There was no labeling of gangliosides in the absence of galactose oxidase (Fig. 1b). Cells labeled by this procedure were exposed to cholera toxin and lysed in 1% NP40, and a soluble fraction was obtained by centrifugation at 100,000g for 1 h. Aliquots of the supernatant were incubated with toxin-antibody and the toxin-receptor-antibody (immune) complexes adsorbed to a protein A-containing strain of Staphylococcus aureus. Separation of labeled gangliosides which bound to the bacterial pellets by thin-layer chromatography showed a peak of radioactivity with similar mobility to GM$_1$ (Fig. 2a). Elution of the peak followed by rechromatography in a different solvent (chloroform—methanol—2.5 M ammonium hydroxide containing 20 mg/100ml CaCl$_2$ · 2H$_2$O, 60:35:8) again showed a single major peak of radioactivity coincident with a GM$_1$ standard. The ganglioside was not found adsorbed to the bacterial pellet if cholera toxin or toxin antibody was omitted during the isolation procedure (compare Fig. 2a and b).

Because galactose oxidase borotritiide labeling of cellular lipid is restricted mainly to a component(s) with similar chromatographic properties to GM$_1$, these experiments do not resolve the issue of whether cholera toxin is specific for GM$_1$. We have attempted to answer the question by applying the method of immunoprecipitation described to cells metabolically labeled with [^{14}C] palmitate. Separation of the gangliosides from cells labeled in this manner shows a complex profile including molecules with mobilities similar to gangliosides GM$_3$, GM$_2$, GM$_1$, and GD (Fig. 3a). No one ganglioside species predominates. Analysis of [^{14}C] palmitate-labeled gangliosides in the immune complexes adsorbed to protein A showed a considerably less complex pattern, suggesting that the toxin was interacting specifically with certain cell surface gangliosides (Fig. 3d, e). However, although gangliosides with mobilities similar to GM$_1$ predominated, the profile suggested considerable heterogeneity. Again virtually no ganglioside was found adsorbed to the protein A if cholera toxin or toxin antibody was omitted during the isolation procedure (Fig. 3b, c, f).

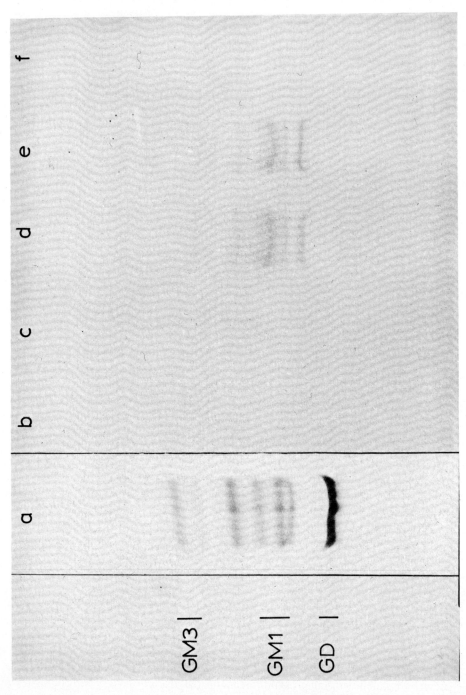

Such experiments strongly suggest that gangliosides, predominantly those with the mobility of GM_1, are at least part of the cholera toxin receptor at the surface of this lymphoid cell line.

During the course of experiments with [^{14}C] palmitate-labeled cells it became clear that other lipids apart from gangliosides were adsorbed to the protein A. Two-dimensional thin-layer chromatography showed that neutral lipids, phosphatidyl choline, and sphingomyelin were the major components (Fig. 4). These lipids were bound to protein A in the absence of cholera toxin or toxin antibody, although levels generally increased when toxin and antibody were included in the isolation procedure. The extent of the increase was variable, however (by a factor of 1.0–4).

A similar experimental approach was used to examine whether any cell surface glycoproteins bind cholera toxin. Galactose oxidase borotritiide labeling profiles of the cell surface glycoproteins separated by SDS-PAGE are shown in Figure 5. As for labeling of gangliosides, labeling of glycoproteins was markedly enhanced by neuraminidase (Fig. 5a, b). Labeling in the absence of enzyme was largely restricted to molecules traveling with the marker dye, much of which probably represents lipid (Fig. 5c). The increased labeling in this region in neuraminidase-treated cells is in accord with increased labeling of gangliosides similar to GM_1 (Fig. 1a). Similar analysis of the toxin-receptor-antibody complexes adsorbed to protein A showed that the major species of toxin receptor traveled with the marker dye and is therefore most likely lipid (Fig. 6). The only lipids found in the immune complexes which are specifically labeled by the galactose oxidase borotritiide technique are gangliosides similar to GM_1. This result therefore suggests that such glycolipids are quantitatively the most important species of toxin receptor. Interestingly, a peak of radioactivity corresponding to a glycoprotein in the molecular weight range 80,000–90,000 has also consistently been found in the immune complexes. The glycoprotein was not adsorbed to protein A if cholera toxin or antibody was omitted during the isolation procedure. Figure 7 shows a more complete analysis of a similar experiment using slab gels and fluorography. Analysis of the immune complexes again shows that quantitatively the major species of toxin receptor travels with the marker dye, and is therefore presumably lipid. Comparison of immune complexes isolated from cells exposed to galactose oxidase with or without neuraminidase shows that recovery of this species is dramatically increased in cells exposed to neuraminidase (Fig. 7f, g). The observation is in agreement with the marked increase in labeling of molecules with similar chromatographic properties to GM_1 following exposure of cells to neuraminidase, and again points to gangliosides as the main species of toxin receptor. As before, a glycoprotein of approximately 80,000–90,000 MW was also found as a minor component of the labeled material present in the immune complexes. This is most clearly seen in cells exposed to neuraminidase (Fig. 7f), although a glycoprotein with a slightly greater apparent molecular weight is also present in the immune complexes isolated from cells treated with galactose oxidase alone (not visible in Fig. 7). This glycoprotein corresponds to one of the major galactose oxidase borotritiide-labeled glycoproteins on this lymphoid cell line. It is indeed the major galactoprotein present in the

---

Fig. 3. Isolation of cell surface ganglioside receptors for cholera toxin from [^{14}C] palmitate-labeled cells. The lipids of the mouse lymphoid cell line were labeled by growing the cells in medium containing 1 μCi/ml [^{14}C] palmitate [27]. The cells were then exposed to cholera toxin and the toxin receptor complexes isolated as described in Figure 2. a, labeling profile of total cell gangliosides; b,c, cells not incubated with cholera toxin; b, plus toxin antibody; c, plus preimmune serum; d–f, cells incubated with toxin; d,e, plus toxin antibody; f, plus preimmune serum.

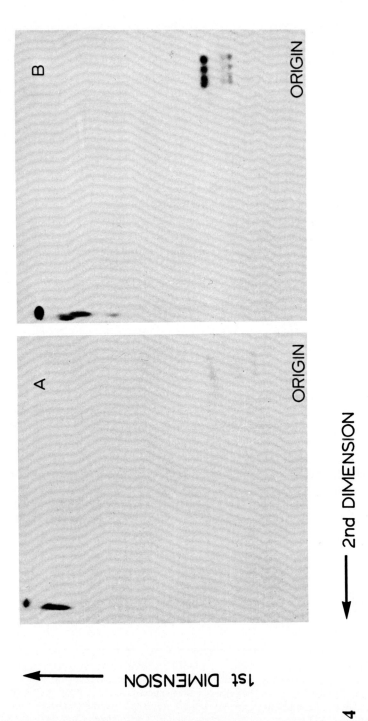

NP40 supernatant, although it is very much less well labeled by lactoperoxidase catalyzed iodination (Fig. 7i), suggesting that it is not quantitatively a major cell surface protein. Analysis of immune complexes isolated from iodinated cells has not as yet revealed the presence of any other cell surface glycoproteins.

Interaction of low concentrations of cholera toxin with the lymphoid cell line leads to patching and some capping of the toxin (Fig. 8a). Such redistribution was not observed if high concentrations of toxin were used (Fig. 8b), a finding that agrees with previous work [17].

Isolation of Cholera Toxin Receptor From Balbc/3T3 Cells

Using methods similar to those described in this paper, we have previously shown that a ganglioside with mobility similar to GM_1 is also at least part of the cholera toxin receptor on mouse fibroblasts [8]. We have recently separated the components present in immune complexes prepared from neuraminidase galactose oxidase-labeled fibroblasts by SDS-PAGE. The major labeled component traveled with the marker dye coincident with a [^{3}H] GM_1 standard, as expected (Fig. 9). Labeling of this component was dependent on galactose oxidase, and the major glycolipid in mouse fibroblasts with terminal galactose has a similar mobility to GM_1 [8]. There is thus little doubt that quantitatively the most important species of toxin receptor on mouse fibroblasts is also a ganglioside. However, as was the case with the lymphoid cell line, a glycoprotein was also present in the immune complexes obtained from mouse fibroblasts. The glycoprotein was not adsorbed to protein A in the absence of antibody.

Examination of One Possible Method of Selection of Mutant Balbc/3T3 Cells Lacking Cholera Toxin Receptors

Our attempts at using cholera toxin to select for mutants of Balbc or Swiss 3T3 cells defective in complex glycolipid biosynthesis have progressed more slowly than expected, owing to unforeseen difficulties with the mutant selection procedure. Cholera toxin has been shown to inhibit mitogen-stimulated DNA synthesis in lymphocytes [17, 32], and serum-stimulated DNA synthesis in a mouse kidney epithelial cell line AL/N [33] and human fibroblasts [34], in accordance with the idea that cAMP is involved in regulation of cell division [35, 36]. One mutant selection procedure tested was therefore based on the assumption that only Balbc/3T3 cells defective in toxin receptor, and therefore complex glycolipid biosynthesis, would be able to grow in the presence of cholera toxin. We were surprised to find that cholera toxin (1 pg–10 μg/ml) failed to markedly inhibit serum-stimulated uridine uptake (data not shown) or DNA synthesis and cell growth in Balbc or Swiss 3T3 cells, two processes previously reported to be inhibited by cAMP [35–37] (Fig. 10). This result may be explained by the observation that cAMP levels elevated (8-fold to

Fig. 4. Characterization of neutral lipids and phospholipids bound to protein A from NP40 extracts of [^{14}C] palmitate-labeled mouse lymphoid cells. A: Cells not exposed to cholera toxin; NP40 extract incubated with toxin antibody. B: Cells exposed to toxin; NP40 extract incubated with toxin antibody. Lipids were separated by two-dimensional chromatography on silica gel G plates and detected by autoradiography as previously described [27]. Neutral lipids travel at the solvent front in both systems; phosphatidyl choline and sphingomyelin stay at the origin in the second dimension. In this experiment toxin antibody led to a fourfold increase in the amount of neutral lipid and phospholipid adsorbed to the bacterial pellet.

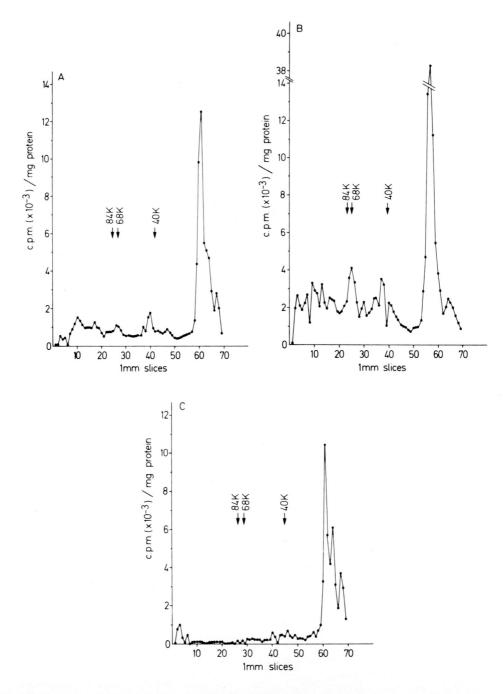

Fig. 5. Surface labeling of the glycoproteins of a mouse lymphoid cell line by the galactose oxidase borotritiide technique. Cells were dissolved by boiling in 2% SDS in electrophoresis sample buffer, aliquots were taken for protein, and the sample was reduced with 0.1 M dithiothreitol. Labeled proteins were separated by SDS-PAGE (7.5% disks) and radioactivity was detected as previously described [29]. A: Cells incubated with galactose oxidase alone; B: neuraminidase and galactose oxidase; C: No enzyme.

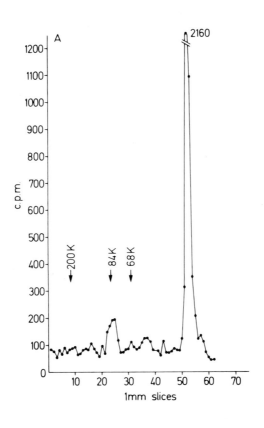

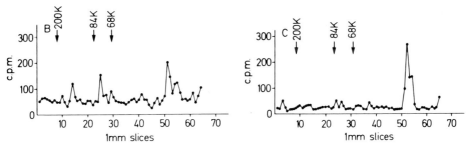

Fig. 6. Analysis of the galactose oxidase borotritiide-labeled glycoproteins which bind to protein A during the isolation of the cholera toxin receptor from a mouse lymphoid cell line. Methodology as described in Figure 2 except that components bound to protein A were solubolized by boiling of the bacterial pellet with 200 μl of 2% SDS in electrophoresis sample buffer plus 0.1 M dithiothreitol. Separation of the extracted material was carried out by SDS-PAGE (7.5% disks) [28, 29]. A: Cells exposed to cholera toxin; NP40 extracts were incubated with toxin antibody; B: as in (A) except preimmune serum was used; C: cells not exposed to cholera toxin; NP40 extracts were incubated with toxin antibody. Identical volumes of the NP40 extracts from equivalent numbers of cells were used during immune adsorption of samples A, B, and C.

30-fold increase) by exposure of cells to cholera toxin in serum-free medium were markedly reduced on addition of serum, although cAMP levels remained substantially elevated over those in quiescent cells (Fig. 11). Inclusion of a phosphodiesterase inhibitor partially prevented the reduction in cAMP levels produced by serum, and markedly elevated levels were maintained for at least 32 h after the addition of complete growth medium. However, although cholera toxin potentiated the inhibition of DNA synthesis produced by low concentrations of a phosphodiesterase inhibitor, the effect was sufficiently incomplete to make this simple approach to mutant selection inapplicable.

DISCUSSION

Our present data strongly suggest that gangliosides with similar chromatographic properties to GM_1 are quantitatively the major species of cholera toxin receptor in both mouse lymphoid and fibroblast cell lines. While GM_1 is the best inhibitor of cholera toxin binding yet reported [11], there is no guarantee that the cell surface receptor will be identical to GM_1. For example, while GD1b is the best commercially available inhibitor of thyrotropin binding to thyroid plasma membranes [14], a more complex ganglioside has recently been isolated from thyroid tissue, which is a far more potent inhibitor of hormone binding [38]. Indeed the apparent heterogeneous nature of the gangliosides in immune complexes isolated from [^{14}C] palmitate-labeled cells might suggest that a number of species of cell surface ganglioside act as the toxin receptor. Such an interpretation is complicated by the fact that gangliosides such as GM_1 tend to resolve into several bands on thin-layer chromatography, probably because of heterogeneity in the sphingosine and fatty acid moieties.

The significance of galactoproteins in the immune complexes obtained from both mouse lymphoid and fibroblast cell lines is somewhat uncertain. Based on an analogy with the ABO blood group system [39], there is no reason to suppose that similar carbohydrate sequences which specify toxin receptor activity might not exist in both glycolipid and glycoproteins. The structure of cholera toxin also has certain similarities to that of the glycoprotein hormones [14, 40], which themselves apparently utilize both glycolipid and glycoprotein receptors [7, 14]. In addition, low levels of a number of cell surface galactoproteins from mouse fibroblasts which cross-react with anti-GM_1 antibodies have recently been tentatively identified [41]. It is therefore perhaps not surprising that a cell surface glycoprotein was present in the immune precipitates. However, there remains some doubt about the validity of this interpretation. First, phospholipid and neutral lipids were adsorbed to the bacterial pellet. A low level of contamination of the bacterial pellet with NP40-extracted [^{14}C]-palmitate-labeled lipid may not be surprising in that they might in some way be retained by the bacterial membrane. However, there was some increase in the level of neutral lipid and phospholipid adsorbed to the bacterial pellets under conditions where specific adsorption of the toxin receptor was expected, although the extent of the increase was variable. One possible conclusion from this result is that mixed micelles of ganglioside, phospholipid, and some protein remain in the supernatant even after centrifugation of the NP40 extract at 100,000g for 1 h. Such micelles containing other components apart from the true toxin receptor may also be adsorbed to the bacterial protein A under these conditions, although the major cell surface proteins labeled by lactoperoxidase-catalyzed iodination were not found in the immune complexes. Alternatively it may be of genuine interest that other lipids apart from gangliosides and a galactoprotein are specifically adsorbed to the bacterial pellet. It is conceivable that a ganglioside-phospholipid-galactoprotein complex exists in the membrane [7], and mild detergents such as NP40 fail to disrupt such complexes. We are presently attempting to use other detergents with different characteristics to resolve this question. A further concern is that the glycoprotein is an artifact of the galactose oxidase procedure. The enzyme creates an aldehyde group on the six carbon of terminal galactose and N-acetylgalactosamine residues. It is therefore possible that the aldehyde created on the terminal galactose of GM_1 formed a Schiff's base with an amino group on a protein in close proximity to GM_1, and the linkage was stabilized and labeled by borotritiide reduction. Under such circumstances one could generate an artifact, ie, a GM_1-containing glycoprotein. However, as the terminal galactose of GM_1 would appear to be an important determinant of its toxin-binding activity, it would seem unlikely that such a protein artifact would bind toxin.

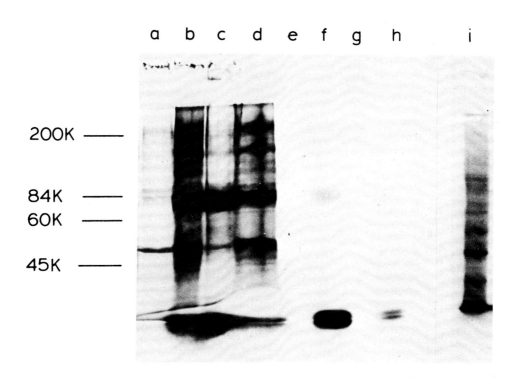

Fig. 7. Fluorographic detection of mouse lymphoid cell surface proteins labeled by the galactose oxidase technique. Methodology as previously described in Figures 2 and 6, except that proteins were separated by SDS-PAGE (7.5% slabs) and labeled proteins detected by fluorography [29, 30]. a, Cells incubated with galactose alone. b, As in (a) plus neuraminidase. c, NP40 extract of cells labeled as in (b). d, NP40 pellet of cells labeled as in (b). e,f, Analysis of glycoproteins from NP40 extracts of cells labeled as in (b) and exposed to cholera toxin, which bound to protein A; e, NP40 extract incubated with preimmune serum; f, Toxin antibody; g,h, As in e,f, except that cells were labeled with galactose oxidase alone; g, NP40 extract incubated with preimmune serum; h, toxin antibody. i, Cells labeled by lactoperoxidase-catalyzed iodination [31]. Tracks (a/b) contained equivalent amounts of protein (140 μg). Track (c) contained half the protein equivalent of track (d), ie, 100 μg and 200 μg, respectively. The amount of NP40 extract used in the immune precipitation procedure was equivalent on a cell basis (e–h).

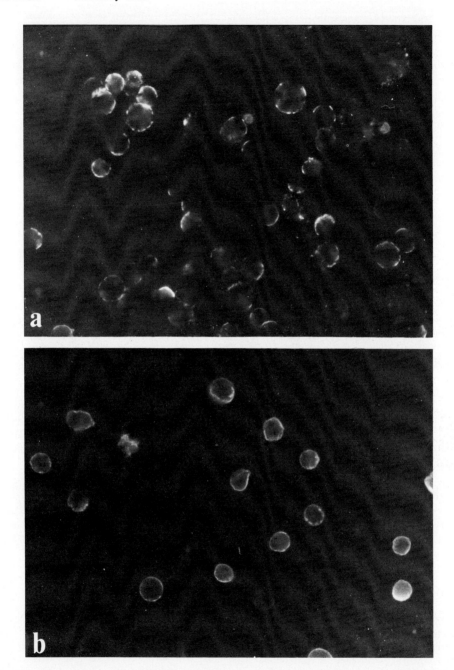

Fig. 8. Detection of cholera toxin bound to the surface of a mouse lymphoid cell line by indirect immunofluorescence. Cells (2×10^6) were incubated with 1 µg/ml (a) or 10 µg/ml cholera toxin (b) in PBS at 0°C for 15 min. Unbound toxin was removed by washing, and the cells were incubated with rabbit anti-cholera toxin (1:10) for 30 min at 20°C. The cells were washed twice and incubated with FITC-labeled goat anti-rabbit antibodies (1:10) for 30 min at 37°C. Excess FITC-labeled antibody was removed by washing, and the cells were suspended in 50% glycerol and viewed in a Zeiss microscope equipped with epifluorescence optics. Photographs were taken on Kodak plus X with exposure times of up to 2 min (× 187).

While it therefore remains somewhat unclear whether we have isolated a genuine glycoprotein toxin receptor, there is little doubt that quantitatively the major species of toxin receptor is ganglioside in nature in both cell lines tested. One is therefore faced with attempting to explain how interaction of cholera toxin with a mouse lymphoid cell line leads to capping. Previous data from other laboratories on capping of toxin in peripheral lymphocytes suggests that the microfilament and microtubule systems are involved [17–19]. As glycolipids are unlikely to interact directly with the cytoskeleton, it is possible that the interaction is mediated by association between the ganglioside receptor and a transmembrane protein which itself is not a toxin receptor. Using the myosin affinity technique, we are presently attempting to see whether gangliosides can be cross-linked to specific proteins in membranes, and whether they indirectly interact with the cytoskeleton [42]. Alternative explanations for capping of toxin ganglioside complexes based on membrane flow [43] should not be ignored, although we have noted that toxin does not cap in

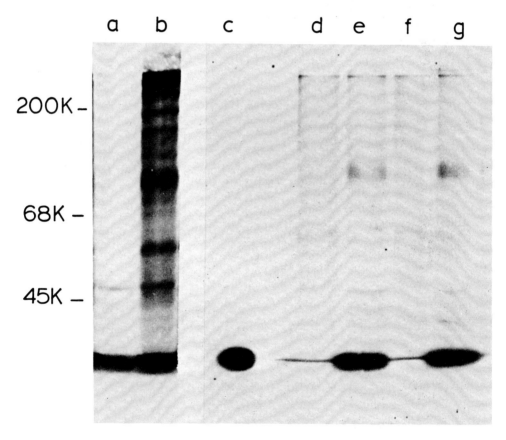

Fig. 9. Fluorographic detection of Balbc/3T3 cell surface proteins labeled by the neuraminidase galactose oxidase borotritiide technique. Cells were labeled in monolayer [29] and labeled proteins were separated and detected as outlined in Figure 7. a, Borotritiide-labeling profile without galactose oxidase; b, labeling profile following incubation with neuraminidase and galactose oxidase; c, [^{3}H]GM$_1$ standard; d–g, Cells labeled as in (b) were exposed to cholera toxin (25 μg in 1 ml PBS, 0.1% BSA), unbound toxin was removed by washing, and the cells were extracted with 4 ml of 1% NP40 in PBS/PMSF for 1 h, 0°C. Toxin-receptor complexes were isolated as described in Figure 2; d,f, NP40 extracts incubated with preimmune serum; e,g, NP40 extracts incubated with toxin antibody.

all cell types tested. For example, a myeloma cell line (MOPC 21) that lacks toxin receptor binds the toxin after incubation of the cells with GM_1. The interaction leads to patching but not capping, as detected by indirect immunofluorescence. Similarly, toxin bound to Balbc/3T3 fibroblasts does not patch or cap under the conditions we have tested so far.

Our results with mouse fibroblasts also suggest that gangliosides represent the predominant species of cholera toxin receptor. It should therefore be feasible to use the toxin to select for mutants defective specifically in glycolipid biosynthesis as outlined in the introduction. The specificity of the toxin offers a major advantage over those approaches previously used to isolate mutants with altered cell surface carbohydrate profiles such as lectin resistance [44, 45] or reduced cell adhesion [46]. The failure of cholera toxin to inhibit serum-stimulated DNA synthesis in Balbc and Swiss 3T3 cells may be related to the rapid reduction in cAMP levels produced when toxin-treated cells are exposed to serum. Assuming that adenyl cyclase is irreversibly activated by cholera toxin [47], then either cAMP was rapidly lost into the medium or it was degraded by an intracellular phosphodiesterase. Although elevated levels of cAMP can lead to a slow increase in phosphodiesterase activity

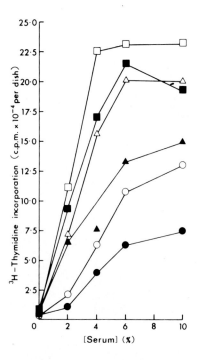

Fig. 10. Effect of cholera toxin and/or a phosphodiesterase inhibitor on serum-stimulated DNA synthesis in Balbc/3T3 cells. Quiescent cells (35-mm dishes) were preincubated for 3 h with serum-free medium alone (□ —— □) or medium containing 100 ng/ml cholera toxin (■ —— ■), 100 μM isobutylmethylxanthine (△——△), 100 μM cholera toxin and 100 μM isobutylmethylxanthine (▲——▲), 500 μM isobutylmethylxanthine (○——○), or 100 ng/ml cholera toxin and 500 μM isobutylmethylxanthine (●——●). Varying concentrations of serum were then added and the cells were pulsed 20 h later for 1 h with 0.4 μCi/ml [methyl-^{3}H] thymidine (28 Ci/mmole). Cells were extracted with 10% trichloracetic acid and ethanol, then solubilized in 0.2 M NaOH. Aliquots were taken for scintillation counting. Each point represents the average incorporation into two separate dishes. Similar results were obtained by autoradiography.

[48, 49], Pledger et al [50–52] have shown that serum rapidly activates a cellular phosphodiesterase in BHK21 cells by an unknown mechanism. However, while a phosphodiesterase inhibitor potentiated the action of cholera toxin in raising cAMP levels in Balbc/-3T3 cells, it did not prevent a significant drop in cAMP levels in response to serum. That this reduction in cAMP levels produced by serum was probably not the key element in the lack of growth inhibition by cholera toxin is suggested by our recent experiments with $PGF_{2\alpha}$, fibroblast growth factor, and insulin. Combinations of these three agents are mitogenic for quiescent Swiss 3T3 cells (eg, percentage nuclei labeled by [^{3}H] thymidine 28 h after addition of $PGF_{2\alpha}$ (200 ng/ml) plus insulin (50 ng/ml) to quiescent cells was 33%) even in the presence of cholera toxin (1 ng–1 μg/ml), yet they failed to produce a rapid reduction in cAMP levels elevated by cholera toxin. Whatever the basis of the serum effect,

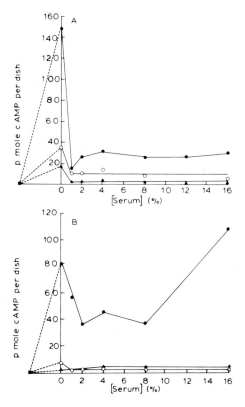

Fig. 11. Effect of serum on the cholera toxin-induced increase in cAMP levels in Balbc/3T3 cells. Quiescent Balbc/3T3 cells (35-mm dishes) were incubated with either cholera toxin or isobutylmethylxanthine, or both, for 3 h in serum-free medium. Twenty minutes after the addition of a variety of concentrations of serum the cells were processed for cAMP determination. A: 1 ng/ml cholera toxin (▲——▲); 10 ng/ml cholera toxin (o——o); 100 ng/ml cholera toxin (●——●). B: 10 ng/ml cholera toxin (o——o); 1 mM isobutylmethylxanthine (▲——▲); 10 ng/ml toxin plus 1 mM isobutylmethylxanthine (●——●). The concentration of cAMP in quiescent untreated cells was approximately 1–2 pmoles/30-mm dish (10–20 pmoles/mg protein). Cyclic AMP was assayed using the system supplied by the Radiochemical Centre. Growth medium was rapidly removed from cell monolayers, 50% acetic acid was added, and the extract was centrifuged prior to freeze-drying. The extract was reconstituted in the Tris/EDTA buffer provided prior to assay. Treatment of samples prepared in this way with cyclic nucleotide phosphodiesterase (Sigma) showed that the material assayed was cAMP.

levels of cAMP in toxin-treated cells (with or without a phosphodiesterase inhibitor) remained substantially elevated for several days after addition of complete growth medium, compared with those in quiescent cells. However, cholera toxin failed to inhibit significantly the growth of either Balbc or Swiss 3T3 cells, a process previously reported to be inhibited by cAMP [35, 36]. Interestingly, cholera toxin and cAMP have recently been reported to be mitogenic for rat Schwann cells [53]. Alternative ways of using cholera toxin as a method of selection for cells deficient in complex glycolipid biosynthesis are presently under study.

ACKNOWLEDGMENTS

The authors would like to thank Drs. M. Boss, M. F. Greaves, and D. Cicco of the Imperial Cancer Research Fund, London, for supplying the mouse lymphoid cell line and cholera toxin antibodies; and Dr. R. O. Thompson of the Wellcome Laboratories, Beckenham, London, for the cholera toxin used in the early stages of this work. The work was supported by a Medical Research Council project grant.

REFERENCES

1. Critchley DR, Vicker M: In Poste G, Nicolson GL (eds): "Cell Surface Reviews." Amsterdam: Elsevier/North-Holland, 1977, vol 3, p 307.
2. Marchase RB: J Cell Biol 75:237, 1977.
3. Obata K, Oide M, Handa S: Nature 266:369, 1977.
4. Lingwood CA, Ng A, Hakomori S: Proc Natl Acad Sci USA 75:6049, 1978.
5. Hakomori S: Biochim Biophys Acta 417:53, 1975.
6. Fishman PH, Brady RO: Science 194:906, 1976.
7. Kohn L: In Cuatrecasas P, Greaves MF (eds): "Receptors and Recognition." London: Chapman Hall, 1978, Series A, vol 5, p 135.
8. Critchley DR, Ansell S, Dilks S: Biochem Soc Trans 7:314, 1979.
9. Tate RL, Holmes JM, Kohn LD, Winand RJ: J Biol Chem 250:6527, 1975.
10. Dufau MI, Ryan DW, Baukal AJ, Catt KJ: J Biol Chem 250:4822, 1975.
11. Cuatrecasas P: Biochemistry 12:3547, 1973.
12. Moss J, Fishman PH, Manganiello VC, Vaughan M, Brady RO: Proc Natl Acad Sci USA 73:1034, 1976.
13. Fishman PH, Moss J, Vaughan M: J Biol Chem 251:4490, 1976.
14. Mullin BR, Fishman PH, Lee G, Aloj SM, Ledley FO, Winand RJ, Kohn LD, Brady RO: Proc Natl Acad Sci USA 73:842, 1976.
15. Fishman PH, Moss J, Osborne JC: Biochemistry 17:711, 1978.
16. Moss J, Manganiello VC, Fishman PH: Biochemistry 16:1876, 1977.
17. Revesz T, Greaves MF: Nature 257:103, 1975.
18. Craig S, Cuatrecasas P: Proc Natl Acad Sci USA 72:3844, 1975.
19. Sedlacek HH, Stark J, Seiler FR, Zeigler W, Weigandt H: FEBS Lett 61:272, 1976.
20. Keenan TW, Schmidt E, Franke WW, Weigandt H: Exp Cell Res 92:259, 1975.
21. Laine RA, Hakomori S: Biochem Biophys Res Commun 54:1039, 1973.
22. Hynes RO, Ali IU, Destree AT, Mautner VE, Perkins ME, Senger DR, Wagner DD, Smith KK: Ann NY Acad Sci 312:317, 1978.
23. Yamada KM, Olden K, Pastan I: Ann NY Acad Sci 312:256, 1978.
24. Cuatrecasas P: Biochemistry 12:3567, 1973.
25. Kessler SW: J Immunol 115:1617, 1975.
26. Fishman PH, Moss J, Manganiello VC: Biochemistry 16:1871, 1977.
27. Critchley DR, Macpherson I: Biochim Biophys Acta 296:145, 1973.
28. Laemmli UK: Nature 222:680, 1970.
29. Critchley DR: Cell 3:121, 1974.
30. Laskey RA, Mills AD: Eur J Biochem 56:335, 1975.

31. Hynes RO: Proc Natl Acad Sci USA 70:3170, 1973.
32. Holmgren J, Lindholm L, Lonnroth I: J Exp Med 139:801, 1974.
33. Hollenberg MD, Fishman PH, Bennett V, Cuatrecasas P: Proc Natl Acad Sci USA 71:4224, 1974.
34. Hollenberg MD, Cuatrecasas P: Proc Natl Acad Sci USA 70:2964, 1973.
35. Pastan I, Johnson GS, Anderson WB: Ann Rev Biochem 44:411, 1975.
36. Willingham MC: Int Rev Cytol 44:329, 1976.
37. Rozengurt E, Jimenez de Asua L: Proc Natl Acad Sci USA 70:3609, 1973.
38. Mullin BR, Pacuska T, Lee G, Kohn LD, Brady RO, Fishman PH: Science 199:77, 1977.
39. Watkins WM: Science 152:172, 1966.
40. Kurosky A, Markel DE, Fitch WM: Science 195:299, 1977.
41. Tonegawa Y, Hakomori S: Biochem Biophys Res Commun 76:9, 1977.
42. Koch GLE, Smith MJ: Nature 273:274, 1978.
43. Bretscher MS: Nature 260:21, 1976.
44. Meager A, Ungkitchanukit A, Nairn R, Hughes RC: Nature 257:137, 1975.
45. Stanley P, Narasimhan S, Siminovitch L, Schacter H: Proc Natl Acad Sci USA 72:3323, 1975.
46. Pouyssegur J, Willingham M, Pastan I: Proc Natl Acad Sci USA 74:243, 1977.
47. Gill DM: Adv Cyclic Nucleotide Res 8:85, 1977.
48. Manganiello V, Vaughan M: Proc Natl Acad Sci USA 69:269, 1971.
49. D'Armiento M, Johnson GS, Pastan I: Proc Natl Acad Sci USA 69:459, 1972.
50. Pledger WJ, Thompson WJ, Strada ST: J Cyclic Nucleotide Res 1:251, 1975.
51. Pledger WJ, Thompson WJ, Strada ST: Nature 256:729, 1975.
52. Pledger WJ, Thompson WJ, Strada ST: Biochem Biophys Res Commun 70:58, 1976.
53. Raff MC, Hornby-Smith A, Brookes JP: Nature 273:672, 1978.

Journal of Supramolecular Structure 12:335—354 (1979)
Tumor Cell Surfaces and Malignancy 625—644

Role of the Microfibrillar System in Knob Action of Transformed Cells

William D. Meek and Theodore T. Puck

Eleanor Roosevelt Institute for Cancer Research and the Florence R. Sabin Laboratories for Genetic and Developmental Medicine, University of Colorado Health Sciences Center, Denver, Colorado 80262

Transformed cells often display knobs (or blebs) distributed over their surface throughout most of interphase. Scanning electron microscopy (SEM) and time-lapse cinematography on CHO-K1 cells reveal roughly spherical knobs of 0.5—4 μm in diameter distributed densely around the cell periphery but sparsely over the central, nuclear hillock and oscillating in and out of the membrane with a period of 15—60 sec. Cyclic AMP derivatives cause the phenomenon of reverse transformation, in which the cell is converted to a fibroblastic morphology with disappearance of the knobs. A model was proposed attributing knob formation to the disorganization of the jointly operating microtubular and microfilamentous structure of the normal fibroblast. Evidence for this model includes the following: 1) Either colcemid or cytochalasin B (CB) prevents the knob disappearance normally produced by cAMP, and can elicit similar knobs from smooth-surfaced cells; 2) knob removal by cAMP is specific, with little effect on microvilli and lamellipodia; 3) immunofluorescence with antiactin sera reveals condensed, amorphous masses directly beneath the membrane of CB-treated cells instead of smooth, parallel fibrous patterns of reverse-transformed cells or normal fibroblasts; 4) transmission electron microscopy (TEM) of sections show dense, elongated microfilament bundles and microtubules parallel to the long axis of the reverse-transformed CHO cell, but sparse, random microtubules throughout the transformed cell and an apparent disordered network of 6-nm microfilaments beneath the knobs; 5) cell membranes at the end of telophase, when the spindle disappears and cleavage is complete, display typical knob activity as expected by this picture.

Key words: knobs or blebs, transformed cells, reverse transformation, time-lapse cinematography, scanning EM, transmission EM, microtubules and microfilaments or microfibrillar system, colcemid, cytochalasin B, dibutyryl cyclic AMP, indirect immunofluorescence, antiactin, antitubulin

Knobs or blebs are a characteristic topographic feature of many transformed cells in culture [1—3], although time-lapse cinematography of other cells growing in vivo also occasionally display similar features [4]. Rounded membrane protuberances or the pro-

Received May 8, 1979; accepted September 10, 1979.

cesses which form them have been described by a variety of names including potocytosis [5], balloon-like structures [6], hyaline bulges or protrusions [7], blisters [8], zeiosis (boiling over) [9], bubbling [10], anaphase bubbling or blebbing [11], bosses [12], and membranous whorls [13]. It is not known to what extent these represent similar or different phenomena. Because of this large variety of observed cell excrescences we adopted the term "knob" for the rounded, oscillating protrusions which characterize the transformed cells studied by us and which display the specific morphologic property of disappearing in response to the addition of agents which increase the level of cyclic AMP in the cell [1,2,14].

Knobs are sparse on normal cells [1–3, 15, 16], but are commonly seen on mammalian cells transformed by viruses [17, 18], chemicals [19], and radiation [15, 20, 21]. This paper describes comparative studies carried out on the transformed Chinese hamster ovary cell (CHO-K1) and two other permanent Chinese hamster cell lines from the ovary (CHO-III) and from the lung (CHL) that display reasonably normal fibroblastic morphology in culture. These studies amplify our previous demonstration that cyclic AMP plays an important role in organizing the microfibrillar structure of particular transformed cells into the pattern resembling that of a normal fibroblast and that knob activity is intimately associated with the microfibrillar structure.

In its native state in normal growth medium CHO-K1 exhibits the following transformation characteristics: 1) The cell is compact, pleomorphic and studded with knobs; 2) single cells grow with virtually 100% plating efficiency, either in agar suspension or on solid surfaces; 3) cells deposited on surfaces produce colonies displaying heavy, three-dimensional growth in the central region and a roughly circular outline, indicating that growth proceeds randomly in all directions. Addition of cyclic AMP derivatives to such a culture causes the following changes: 1) Knobs disappear and the cell becomes elongated, assuming a typical fibroblastic morphology; 2) the capacity to grow in suspension in ordinary serum concentrations disappears; 3) colonial growth on surfaces becomes strongly monolayered, and growth in such colonies displays the typical fibroblastic pattern associated with density-dependent growth inhibition, in which the cells pack closely together in parallel to their long dimension and exhibit loops and whorls resembling stacked sheaves of wheat; 4) cell adhesion to plastic surfaces and to each other is markedly increased so that the satellite colonies which characterize plates grown in normal growth medium virtually disappear [1, 2, 14]. We have named the processes caused by cyclic AMP reverse transformation. Reverse-transformed CHO cells also differ from their native counterparts in resisting the cell-rounding action of antisera against cell surface antigens and the killing action of such antisera in the presence of complement [22]. The reverse-transformed cells are also more resistant to the capping phenomenon which is readily exhibited by the native cells when challenged with lectins [23]. In this paper we present experimental data and interpretations dealing with the knobbing phenomenon that support a picture of this cell surface activity of knobbing as a manifestation of alterations in the microfibrillar structure.

MATERIALS AND METHODS

CHO-K1, CHO-III, and CHL were grown in the standard F12 medium [24] supplemented with 5–20% fetal calf serum (FCS) and an equivalent amount of the macromolecular portion (FCM) of fetal calf serum. All cultures were provided with 100 units/ml of streptomycin and penicillin, and were incubated at 37°C in an atmosphere of high humidity and 5% CO_2 in air. The chemicals used were as follows: N^6,O^2-dibutyryl adenosine 3'-5'-cyclic monophosphoric acid, monosodium salt (Sigma Chemical Co., St. Louis) testololactone

(E. R. Squibb and Sons, Inc., Princeton), colcemid (Sigma Chemical Co.), and cytochalasin B (Sigma Chemical Co.). Several different concentrations of the above reagents were used which included: 0.5–7;5 mM dbcAMP + 10^{-5} M testololactone, 1.4–14 μM colcemid, 1.0–10 μM cytochalasin B. After several experiments with concentrations within these ranges it was found that 1 mM dbcAMP + 10^{-5} M testololactone, 1.4 μM colcemid, and 1.0 μM cytochalasin B yielded optimal results for our particular analysis, as discussed below.

Time-Lapse Microcinematography

For time-lapse cinematography, 3×10^3 cells are inoculated into a growth chamber made by placing a Teflon ring on the bottom of a 35 × 10-mm plastic Petri dish (Lux Scientific Corp., Newbury Park, California) with sterile, Dowex silicone grease as an adhesive. The ring is completely filled with medium. A plastic coverslip (Lux Plastics, No. 5407) is attached to the top of the ring with silicone grease, care being taken to exclude air bubbles. The growth chamber fits snugly into a depression drilled into a brass block, fitted with heater and thermostat so that the temperature is maintained at $37.5 \pm 0.5°$. After the growth chamber is filled, the top of the Petri dish is fitted over the bottom, and 5% CO_2 warmed to 37° is injected continuously into the Petri dish through a fine plastic tube passing through a port in the brass block and through a small hole in the side of the Petri dish. Test solutions are added to the chamber by lifting the coverslip and quickly aspirating the old medium and pipetting the fresh medium containing added agents. It is possible, by this means, to observe the effect of the agent immediately after administration. Agents to be tested are added in growth medium containing the macromolecular fetal calf serum component. It is found that the chamber supports clonal growth of single cells with high efficiency. The entire assembly is placed on the stage of a Wild M40 inverted microscope, with quartz halogen light source, fitted with phase optics and Bolex-Wild variotimer. Exposures are made for 0.5 sec at 30-sec intervals. A Bolex Hl6SBM 16-mm camera and Kodak Plus-X reversal film are used. Films are studied at low speed (1–4 frames per second). Negatives for prints are made from the 16-mm movie film using Kodak Plus-X film. Magnification in all pictures is 260.

Scanning Electron Microscopy

Into 35 × 10-mm plastic tissue culture dishes containing uncoated coverslips (11 × 22 mm) 3×10^4 cells are inoculated and then incubated for 48–72 h in growth medium supplemented with FCM. Agents like 1 mM dbcAMP plus 10^{-5} M testololactone are added and incubation is continued for 3 h. The cultures are washed briefly with saline G (pH = 7.4; 37°C) [25]. Cells are then fixed with 2.5% glutaraldehyde in 0.1 M cacodylate buffer (pH = 7.4; 37°C) for 10 min. The preparations are dehydrated in a graded acetone series (one 5-min change in 1%, 15%, 30%, 50%, 70%, 90%; two 5-min changes in 100%). The cell-attached coverslips are dried in a Sorvall critical-point CO_2 drying apparatus (Ivan Sorvall, Inc., Newton, Connecticut) [26]. Fragments of the coverslips are placed on a stud or specimen holder. These cell-containing coverslip fragments are coated with a thin layer of gold and studied with a Kent Cambridge Stereoscan scanning electron microscope [S4] mounted with a LaB_6 gun. Photographs are taken on a Polaroid P/N Type 55 film at tilt angles of 30–40°.

Transmission Electron Microscopy

CHO-K1 [27, 28] is inoculated at a density of 3×10^3 cells per chamber into four-chamber tissue culture slides (Lab-Tek Products, Westmont, Illinois). Following a 48- to 72-h growth period, the cells are treated for 6 h with 1 mM dbcAMP + 10^{-5} M testololactone in medium either with the macromolecular portion of fetal calf serum, in a concentration equivalent to 5% of that in whole serum, or without any serum supplementation. Cells are next washed and fixed by the same method as used in SEM. Dehydration is performed by a graded ethanol series (one 10-min change in 30%, 50%, 70%, 95%; and two 10-min changes in 100%) followed by two 15-min changes in propylene oxide; followed by a 10-min change in 1:1 propylene oxide : Epon 812 mixture;followed by a 10-min change in Epon 812. The slides are then flat-embedded in Epon 812. Slides are later removed from the plastic by immersion in boiling water for 10—20 sec. Areas of cells, visible with the light microscope, are cut from the plastic and mounted upon Epon bullets for thin-sectioning. Sections are cut with a Porter-Blum MT-2 ultramicrotome and stained with uranyl acetate and lead citrate. The resulting specimens are examined and photographed with a Jeol 100C transmission electron microscope operated at 60 kV.

Immunofluorescence

On the day prior to the experiment, 2.5×10^5 cells (CHO-K1, CHO-III, or CHL) are plated onto 11×22-mm sterile glass coverslips in 35×10-mm Petri dishes and allowed to attach and grow overnight. After overnight incubation the cells are treated with 0.5— 7.5 mM dbcAMP + 10^{-5} M testololactone, 8 μM colcemid, or 2 μM cytochalasin B in growth medium for periods of 1—4 h. Initial gifts of antisera against tubulin and actin, respectively, were kindly furnished to us by B. R. Brinkley and E. Lazarides. The immunofluorescence procedures follow those described by these investigators [29—31].

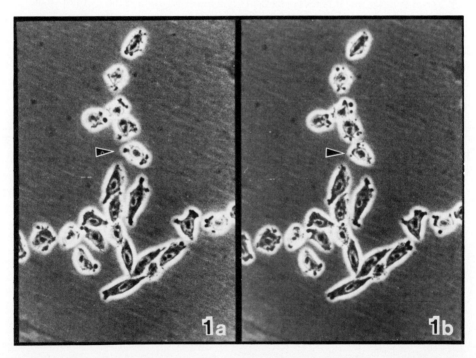

Fig. 1. Time-lapse pictures taken at 30-sec intervals during the growth of CHO-K1 in standard growth medium (F12FCM10). A single cell (arrowhead) is shown in two frames to demonstrate the frequency at which the round protuberances or knobs extrude from and then return to the cell body. Each knob can be seen to form and disappear during a 30-sec period. $\times$ 260.

RESULTS

Time-Lapse Microcinematography

The knobs on the CHO-K1 cell extend from the main body of the cell membrane to a distance of approximately 2 μ and move in and out with a period of approximately 30 sec (Fig. 1). This rapid oscillatory activity is confined to distinct positions and so is clearly different from ruffling that appears in time-lapse movies as an extended waving or undulating motion of a large portion of the membrane. Knobs are exhibited by CHO-K1 cells throughout the entire life cycle except during the first part of mitosis, when the cells are almost completely spherical. At the end of telophase or early G1, knob activity is resumed and is more intense than that which occurs throughout the rest of interphase. The knobs characteristic of the cells just completing cytokinesis are frequently seen in the polar region, but are not necessarily restricted to these areas (Fig. 2).

The addition of cyclic AMP derivatives to CHO-K1 cultures produces virtually complete disappearance of the knobs in all parts of the cell life cycle (Fig. 3 and Table I). Concomitantly the membrane loses its oscillating foci and becomes much more tranquilized. Knob formation is also virtually completely suppressed in the telophase/ early G1 cells under conditions of high cyclic AMP concentration ($>$ 1 mM), although transient knob action may occasionally be visible at this particular period. By the use of 0.5–1 mM dibutyryl cyclic AMP plus 10^{-5} M testololactone knobbing can be suppressed without interference with normal cell division of the CHO-K1 cell (Table I).

Even smooth-surfaced cells can exhibit knob action at the telophase/G1 boundary of the life cycle in normal growth medium (Table II). Addition of cyclic AMP to CHO-III

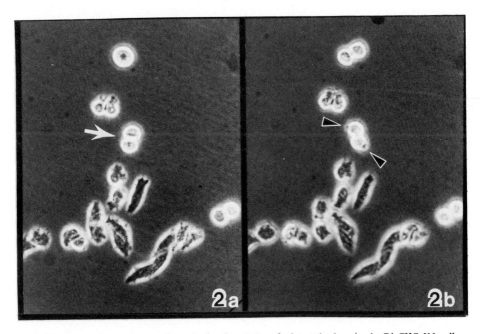

Fig. 2. These time-lapse pictures show the knob activity of a late telophase/early G1 CHO-K1 cell (arrow in a) in standard medium (F12FCM10). The first frame (2a) is 6.5 min after anaphase and 2b is 6.5 min later. Knobs (arrowheads) begin to form in the polar regions 13.0 min after anaphase (2b). Compare with the same colony at a later time in Figure 3. × 260.

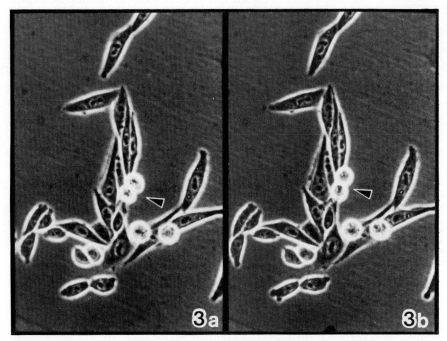

Fig. 3. These time-lapse pictures show the same field as in Figure 2 after the cells have been treated with 1 mM dibutyryl cyclic AMP + 10^{-5}M testololactone in F12FCM10. The first frame (a) is 4.3 h after the addition of the agent and 6.5 min after anaphase; frame b is 6.5 min later. The cells are elongated and possess no knobs. The knob formation as seen in Figure 2 also fails to occur in the late telophase/early G1 cell (arrow). × 260.

TABLE I. Demonstration of Knob Activity in CHO-K1 After Various Concentrations of dbcAMP, Colcemid, and Cytochalasin B Treatment

	Knobbed cells (%)	Smooth-surfaced elongated cells (%)
Normal medium (F12FCMS)	81	19
1 mM dbcAMP + 10^{-5}M testololactone	15	85
3 mM dbcAMP + 10^{-5}M testololactone	8	92
10^{-2}M dbcAMP + 10^{-5}M testololactone	3	97
2.7 μM Colcemid	96	4
2.7 μM Cytochalasin B	99	1

Elongated = one dimension at least three times greater than the other.

or CHL fibroblasts produces little, if any, change in their overall morphology as determined by viewing with time-lapse cinematography (Table II).

Addition of colcemid at a concentration 1.4–14 μM to smooth-surfaced CHO-III or CHL fibroblasts or to CHO-K1 cells that have been reverse-transformed by the presence of cyclic AMP derivatives causes an outbreak of typical knob activity in most points of the

TABLE II. Knob Activity by Culture Condition as Viewed by Time-Lapse Microcinematography

Cell type	Normal medium		1 mM dbcAMP +10^{-5} M testololactone		Colcemid (1.4−14 μM)		Cytochalasin B (1.0−10 μM)	
	Inter-phase	Telo-phase-G1	Inter-phase	Telo-phase-G1	Inter-phase	Telo-phase-G1	Inter-phase	Telo-phase-G1
CHO-K1	+	+	−	±	+	X	+	+
CHO-III	−	±	−	±	±	X	+	+
CML	−	±	−	±	+	X	+	+

Symbols: + = knob presence or formation; − = no knob presence or formation; X = no cell observed in that portion of the cell cycle because of the mitotic arrest produced by colcemid.

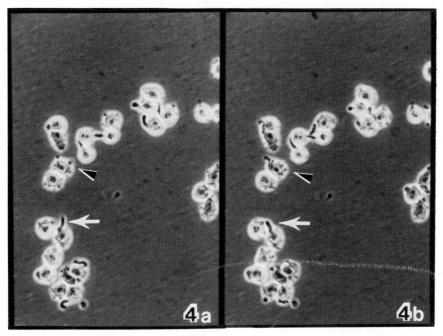

Fig. 4. In the time-lapse pictures a and b, changes are depicted that occur when 1.4 μM colcemid is added to the growth medium (F12FCM10) of CHO-K1. The first frame is 2.2 h after addition of colcemid; frame b is 1 min later. Elongated knobs (arrows), as well as the more spherical type (arrowheads), are seen emanating from the cells. The former wave around in the medium over the period pictured. × 260.

life cycle. CHO-III and CHL cells become almost indistinguishable from the appearance of CHO-K1 in the presence of ordinary growth medium (Table II), and an increase in knob formation is seen in colcemid-treated K1 cells (Table I). Colcemid can also cause extrusion of elongated sausage-shaped knobs from the cell surface (Fig. 4a,b), which undergo waving movements in the medium. When cultures of CHO-K1 are treated with a combination of colcemid and dbcAMP + testololactone, the two sets of reagents antagonize each other's action [1, 2, 14]. In appropriate concentrations the dbcAMP + testololactone can prevent both the knob activity that occurs normally and that which is stimulated by colcemid. Under these circumstances, ruffling is commonly seen along the cell borders (Fig. 5a,b). The addition of cAMP derivatives to cells in colcemid also produces some cell elongation, although

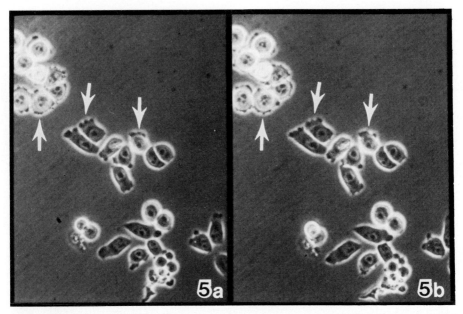

Fig. 5. In these two pictures (a and b) taken at 1-min intervals, another CHO-K1 culture is seen 1.5 h after treatment with both 1.4 μM colcemid and 1 mM dbcAMP + 10^{-5}M testololactone in growth medium (F12FCM10). Knob formation does not occur but lamellipodia or ruffles (arrows) are present along cell borders, and these structures persist over the 1-min period. Some cells have assumed a more flattened appearance. × 260.

not as much as that produced by dbcAMP + testololactone alone. Lamellipodia or ruffles are distinguished from knobs by their restriction to the cell periphery, by their undulating or wavy appearance, and by their continuous existence in contrast to the knobs, whose pulsations cause them to appear and disapper.

Cytochalasin B administered to cell cultures also increases the number of knobs on CHO-K1 (Table 1), causes knobs to form on CHO-III and CHL (Table II and Fig. 6a,b), and appears to increase the frequency of the oscillatory knob action on K1 as viewed by time-lapse cinematography. The knobs are somewhat smaller than those normally present in CHO-K1 (compare with Fig. 1) and form so quickly that the cell topography changes appreciably in periods smaller than 30 sec. Cytochalasin B treatment at low concentrations may leave the general shape of the cell unchanged, so that one may obtain a typical spindle-shaped or epithelioid cell studded with knobs. At higher concentrations of CB, cells with a stellate appearance can result. DbcAMP plus testololactone added with the CB erases the knobs and some ruffling is observed (Fig. 7a,b).

These experiments demonstrate that knob activity exists throughout most of the life cycle for the transformed CHO-K1 cell, but only at the telophase/G1 boundary in smooth-surfaced fibroblastic cells like CHO-III or CHL; it can be diminished or removed from cells in which it is present by reagents which increase the concentration of cyclic AMP; it can be induced in some smooth-surfaced cells in which it is absent by either colcemid or cyto-chalasin B. Knob activity is associated with production of a hyperactive membrane. The substrate attachment of CHO-K1 cells exhibiting such activity is diminished considerably [32, 33]. The oscillatory knob activity may explain at least in part why cells possessing knobs grow in random fashion rather than in specifically oriented patterns in colonies developing on solid surfaces.

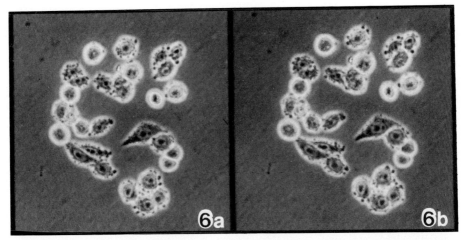

Fig. 6. In these time-lapse pictures (a and b), a culture of CHO-K1 is seen after addition of 1.0 μM cytochalasin B to the growth medium (F12FCM10). Knobs are prevalent over most cells including the elongated ones, and these cells still remain in the shape characteristic of CHO-K1. Frame a is 2.2 h after addition of CB; frame b is 1 min later. Most knobs form and disappear over the 1-min interval. × 260.

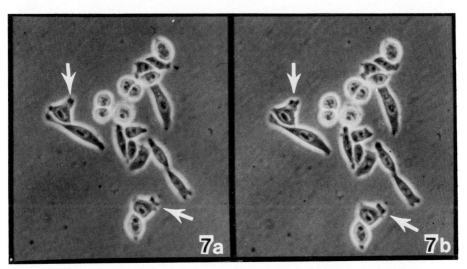

Fig. 7. In these time-lapse pictures (a and b) taken at 1-min intervals, a culture of CHO-K1 is seen 1.5 h after treatment with both 1 μM cytochalasin B and 1 mM dbcAMP + 10^{-5}M testololactone in growth medium (F12FCM10). Knobs are not seen and some cells have elongated. Ruffles (arrows) replace the knobs as surface features. × 260.

Scanning Electron Microscopy

The production of knobs in the CHO-K1 cell by the action of microtubule dis-organizing agents like colcemid and vinblastine — or by cytochalasin B, which disorganizes or disrupts the 6-nm microfilaments — indicates that the integrity of both sets of fibrils is required in order to maintain the smooth, knob-free surface of the fibroblastic cell. SEM studies of native CHO-K1 cells reveal that the shape of the knob is roughly spherical, with occasional indentations (Fig. 8). Continuity between knobs and the cell body is

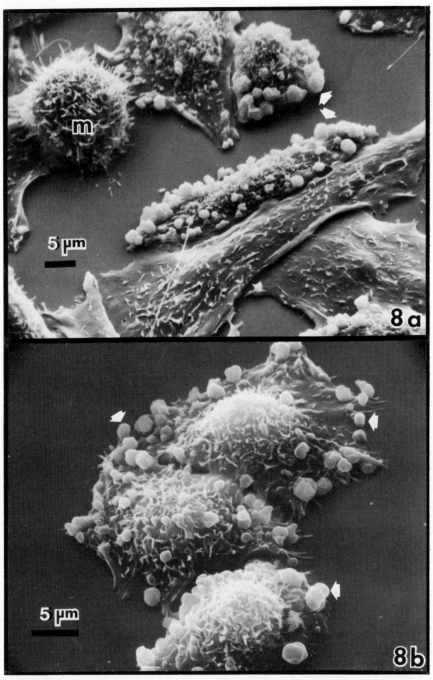

Fig. 8. a: Knobs (arrows) are present over most of the surface of the CHO-K1 cell in the center of the micrograph and along the base of one rounded cell. Other surface features include microvilli, characteristic of the rounded, mitotic cells (m). Some cells are either elongated or flat and noticeably devoid of knobs. F12FCM5 medium; 40° tilt. × 2,000. b: Knobs (arrows) are arranged around the periphery of these cells, while the central, nuclear hillock is covered mainly with microvilli. The two upper cells appear to be in early G1, still connected by the cytoplasmic bridge. F12FCM5 medium; 30° tilt. × 2,625.

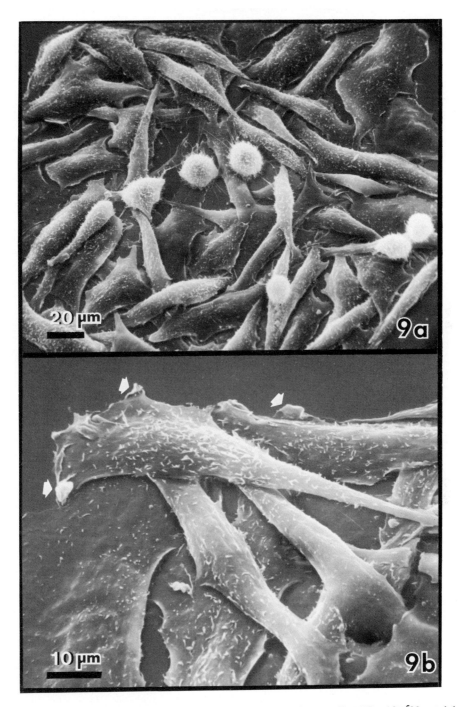

Fig. 9. a: In this low-magnification view of CHO-K1 treated with 0.5 mM dbcAMP + 10^{-5}M testololactone for 3 h, the absence of knobs is noted. Several mitotic cells are present in this colony and most of the other cells are spindle-shaped. F12FCM5 medium; 40° tilt. × 600. b: Lamellipodia or ruffles (arrows) are present in CHO-K1 cells following treatment as in (a). Such higher-magnification micrographs show the detail of the surface as smooth, with scattered microvilli. F12FCM5 medium; 40° tilt. × 1,729.

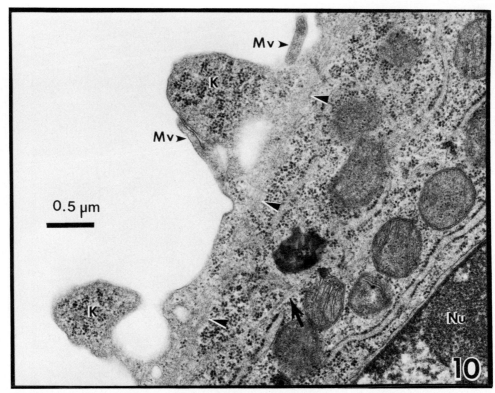

Fig. 10. A high-magnification transmission electron micrograph of CHO-K1 shows knobs (K) and microvilli (Mv) along the surface. Beneath the ribosome-filled knobs and in the cortical cytoplasm, a microfilament bundle (arrowheads) is seen. The filaments are closely related to the cell membrane, and ribosomes are present on both sides of the bundle. A microtubule is seen at the arrow. Nu, Nucleus. F12 medium. × 26,000.

evident. There are always a few CHO-K1 cells visible which lack knobs, particularly in densely packed cultures. These include elongated cells, and some broad, flattened cells, as well as mitotic cells (Fig. 8a). The knobs in the transformed CHO-K1 cells are commonly distributed around the cell periphery while the central, nuclear hillock region contains a dense distribution of microvilli, with a somewhat lower knob density than that found in peripheral areas (Fig. 8b).

The effect of the addition of dbcAMP plus testololactone is shown in Figure 9. The knobs are removed with the appearance of ruffles. Microvilli seem to be little affected (Fig. 9). At the reagent concentrations pictured, most of the cells are elongated within 3h. More rapid and complete response can be achieved with higher drug concentrations, resulting in elongated, spindle-shaped cells (Table I). The change in surface activity observed in

Fig. 11. In this transmission electron micrograph of a CHO-K1 cell, a bundle of microfilaments (arrowheads) is seen near the base of a knob (k) and courses at an oblique angle to the cell membrane. F12 medium. × 39,000.

Fig. 12. This section of CHO-K1 passes through one knob (K*) at its attachment site. Subplasmalemmal filaments (arrowheads) have a felt-like pattern seemingly in a disarranged state. Vesicles (V) are also present in this area. Ribosomes are separated by the filamentous mass, and it can be seen that other organelles such as mitochondria (Mi) and rough endoplasmic reticulum (rER) are not present in the knobs. F12 medium. × 39,866.

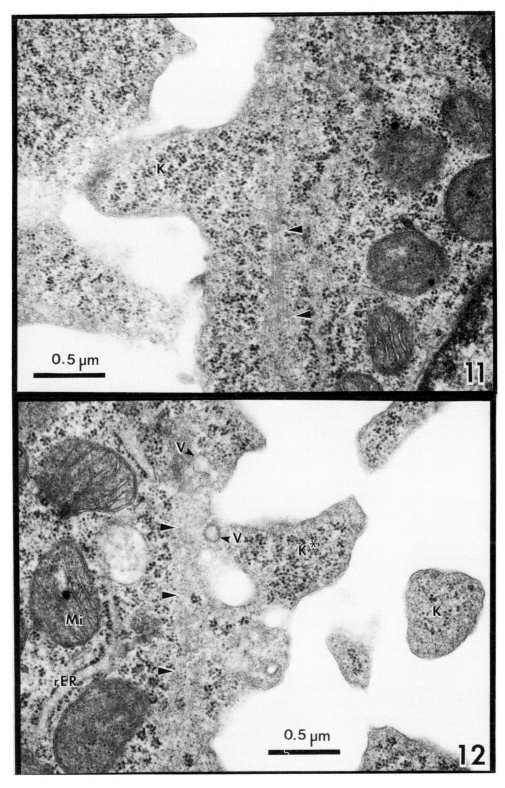

the time-lapse microcinematography appears to be a direct result of the elimination of the knobs which form the foci of oscillatory movement in the cell membrane.

Transmission Electron Microscopy

The knobs of the CHO-K1 cell contain large numbers of free ribosomes (Figs. 10, 11, 12). A zone of material containing either intact filaments or a fuzzy, poorly organized meshwork of filaments often separates the knobs from the body of the cytoplasm (Figs. 10, 11, 12). This meshwork resembles the amorphous material commonly seen in the sub-plasmalemmal region after cytochalasin B treatment [34, 35]. Dense accumulations of ribosomes appear on both sides of the filamentous region and pinocytotic vesicles are some-times present in the cortical regions near the base of knobs (Fig. 12).

After a 6-h exposure of cells to 1 mM dbcAMP plus 10^{-5} M testololactone, the knobs have disappeared (Fig. 13a), and there appears a new, highly ordered arrangement of micro-filament bundles, arranged in parallel to the cell membrane together with a parallel array of microtubules adjacent to the filament bundles (Fig. 13b). Some microtubules run at oblique angles to the others but the overall effect is of a much more dense and orderly pattern of microfibrils than that of the transformed cell. The pattern of the reverse-transformed cell resembles that of the fibroblastic cell. The microfibrils tend to be more closely packed and more nearly paralleled to each other and to the long axis of the cell; the more this is so, the longer, more narrow, and more spindle-shaped is the resulting fibroblast.

Indirect Immunofluorescence

Use of indirect immunofluorescence with antibodies against tubulin and actin pro-vides a means of studying microtubules and 6-nm-diameter microfilaments; this serves as an independent check of the electron micrograph data and also furnishes a different level of magnification for examination of these structures.

Treatment of native CHO-K1 cells with antibodies against tubulin reveals a cytoplasmic microtubular network. Cells that are compact or rounded usually display diffuse fluores-cence, although most cells exhibit at least some recognizable microtubule patterns, which in the transformed cell frequently involve tubules randomly oriented with respect to each other (Fig. 14a; also see Porter et al [36]). Treatment of these cells with dbcAMP plus testololactone greatly increases the number of stretched cells which display dense strands of tubules parallel to each other and to the long axis of the cell (Fig. 14b).

Treatment of such cells with colcemid destroys the tubular patterns and produces only a diffuse fluorescence throughout the cell cytoplasm (Fig. 14c). The knobs that be-come more prominent under these circumstances may contain tubulin because of their faint fluorescence (Fig. 14c). Wherever parallel studies were carried out, our data agree with the results described by Brinkley and his co-workers [29].

Immunofluorescence examination of CHO-III and CHL cells that display a reasonably normal fibroblastic shape demonstrates their microtubular patterns to resemble that ob-tained in CHO-K1 cells treated with dbcAMP plus testololactone. Using antibodies to actin, parallel stress fibers are seen throughout the cytoplasm of the normal CHO-III cell (Fig. 14e). Treatment of the CHO-III cell with CB prior to staining with antiactin reveals localized patches of fluorescence often concentrated through the cell in a fashion similar to that of the knobs that these cells display under such circumstances (Fig. 14f and Table II). Control experiments were performed in identical fashion except for use of normal rabbit

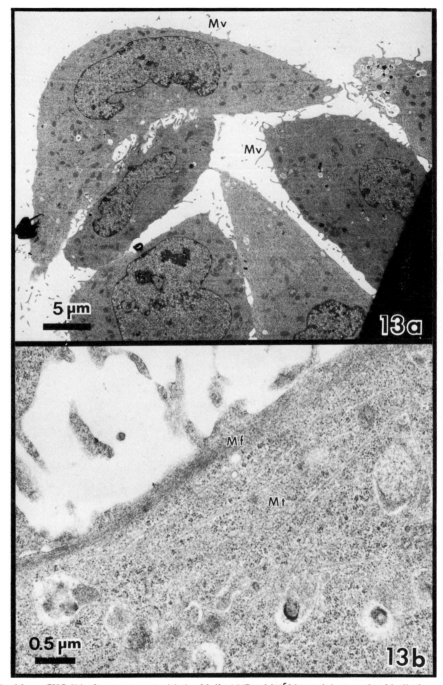

Fig. 13. a: CHO-K1 after treatment with 1 mM dbcAMP + 10^{-5} M testololactone for 6 h displays microvilli (Mv) as the only surface feature. F12 medium. × 3,000. b: A higher magnification of a CHO-K1 cell as treated in panel a shows a compact bundle of microfilaments (Mf) directly beneath the cell membrane. Microtubules (Mt) run generally parallel to the filament layer in the nearby cytoplasm. F12 medium. × 24,000.

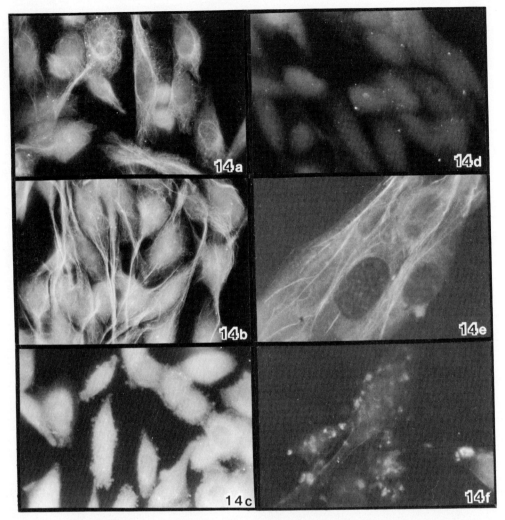

Fig. 14. a: The network of microtubules in CHO-K1 is apparent when cells are labeled with antitubulin sera. × 1,800. b: Parallel bundles of microtubules are seen in many CHO-K1 cells treated with 7.5 mM dbcAMP + 10^{-5}M testololactone for 1 h. × 1,800. C; CHO-K1 cells show a diffuse fluorescence when exposed to 8 μM colcemid for 1 h prior to treatment with antitubulin sera. Knobs are visible along the periphery of the cells. × 1,800. e: CHO-III cells, which display morphology of normal fibroblasts, reveal bundles of stress fibers when treated with serum prepared against the contractile protein actin. Branching bundles are seen in the cytoplasm of these cells. × 2,400. f: Foci of fluorescence appear when CHO-III cells are treated with 2 μM cytochalasin B for 1 h prior to exposure to the antiactin sera. The actin cables are not present as in panel e × 2,400. d: No specific staining was observed in cells treated with normal sera × 1,800.

serum instead of antiserum to actin, and they are presented in Figure 14d. Similar results are obtained in such control experiments carried out with CHO-III and CHL.

Use of Other Fibroblastic Cells

While each cell type has its unique features, the general pattern of findings that we have reported for the fibroblastic CHO-III cell is exhibited by other long-term, cultured fibroblastic cells such as the CHL cell and the V79 cell described earlier [2]. In normal medium these exhibit smooth, knob-free cell membranes except for a brief interval at the telophase/G1 boundary. Addition of dbcAMP plus testololactone produces no effect except for occasional slight cell elongation. Either colcemid or cytochalasin B causes knob extrusion although the concentrations and the times required may vary somewhat with the different cells employed.

DISCUSSION

This paper constitutes part of a continuing study designed to illuminate the relationship between cyclic AMP metabolism and microfibrillar structure in mammalian cells and the relevance of these to cell transformation.

It has been demonstrated by us that in CHO-K1, cyclic AMP is necessary for organization of microtubules into a parallel network, with concomitant effects on the overall shape of the cell. The pattern assumed under these circumstances appears to be genetically or epigenetically predetermined [1, 37].

The fact that the addition of cytochalasin B, colcemid, or other microfibril-disrupting compounds to a stretched, fibroblastic cell [2] can cause it to assume the condensed, pleomorphic structure characteristic of transformed cells implies that the fibroblastic structure is dependent on the integrity of cellular microfilaments and microtubules. This conclusion is strengthened by the fact that in the fibroblastic morphology, which is achieved by cells like CHO-K1 on the addition of cyclic AMP derivatives, microtubules are arranged in parallel to each other and to the long dimension of the stretched cell [36]. A similar dependence of cellular morphology on microtubular integrity in brain cell hybrids that send out nerve-like processes on treatment with dbcAMP supports this general thesis. Ultrastructural studies described elsewhere demonstrate these processes to contain bundles of microtubules parallel to the long dimension of the process [38].

The role of knob formation, which occurs when either microtubules or microfilaments are disrupted, requires more intimate elucidation. We have proposed the working hypothesis that the relatively smooth membranes of normal fibroblasts are not a reflection of the absence of forces operating at the membrane but rather of the fact that such forces are in balance so as to produce a smooth, stretched membranous configuration. The contractile tendency of the actin-containing filaments is balanced by the opposition of the rigid microtubules, the possible opposition of 10-nm filaments, and elastic constraints of the membrane. Disruption of the microtubules or of cytochalasin B-sensitive microfilaments upsets this balance of forces and permits random shortening and relaxation of the remaining contractile elements. Contraction initiated by elements parallel to the membrane would cause the membrane to bulge out to form the typical knob-like structure, which would return into its unstretched position when the contraction is succeeded by relaxation. The tentative model shown in Figure 15 demonstrates how this motion could occur.

The role of the cellular filaments appears to be more complex than that of the microtubules. Apparently treatment with cytochalasin B does not eliminate all activity of contractile elements associated with the cell membrane, since cytochalasin B treatment can cause the appearance of oscillating knob activity. It is possible that cytochalasin B in the concentrations used here, affects only part of the organized contractile activity associated with the cell membrane and permits the remainder to act in unbalanced fashion, which results in the knobbed oscillations. The cytochalasins may also cause a hypercontraction of the actin filaments, an action which might underlie the amorphous deposits of filamentous material in the cortical regions [39]. Other, more complex actions cannot yet be ruled out.

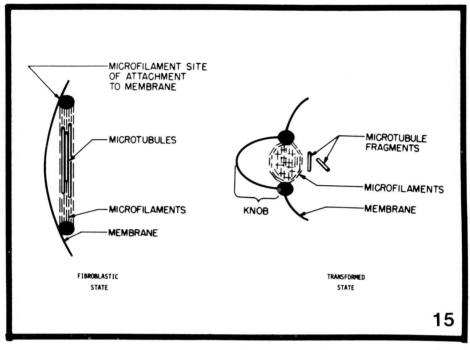

Fig. 15. A highly simplified model of how the knob activity of the cell membrane might occur. In the left diagram microfilaments are pictured as attached to specific membranous sites. The tendency of longitudinal microfilaments to contract is opposed by other forces, such as the rigidity of the associated microtubules, and possible antagonistic action of other contractile elements. In the right diagram, the balance of forces is upset by disorganization of the microtubule or of counteracting contractile 6-nm microfilaments. Random contraction and relaxation of longitudinal filaments may occur, causing the membrane to bulge at a particular point

We have pointed out how these considerations afford a natural explanation of the knob activity that is observed even in normal cells during the brief period between the end of telophase and the initiation of G1 [40]. In mitosis all or most of the cellular tubulin is mobilized into the spindle, and the cell becomes spherical. At the end of telophase, the spindle dissociates and its component tubulin moieties begin to reform the microtubules of the interphase cytoskeleton. The cellular microfilaments also play important roles in the complex events associated with mitosis [41, 42]. Until the interphase cytoskeleton structure is completed the microtubular and microfilamentous elements are partially disorganized in a state similar to that of the interphase CHO-K1 cell. Consequently knob activity is to be expected during this brief interval.

That both microtubules and microfilaments are involved in knob activity is strengthened by the newly discovered microtrabeculae [43]. This network resembles the lattice-like architecture of spongy bone and connects or joins various elements of the cyto-plasm, including microfilaments and microtubules with the cell membrane. Hence, it becomes apparent that when one of the cytoskeletal elements is influenced by destabiliz-ing agents, the remainder may also experience organizational change that will be transferred to the cell membrane. The involvement of the microtrabeculae in cell topography has not been described, but its presence in a large number of cultured cells investigated by Wolosewick and Porter [43], and its intimate relationship with the microfibrillar system, seem to make this network a candidate for a role by which knob activity is expressed.

Of the various transformation characteristics that are reversed by the action of cAMP derivatives, the removal of the knob action appears to be the one that is most rapid and that promises to lend itself readily to precise kinetic experiments.

These considerations imply that every transformed cell that displays knob activity throughout its interphase period suffers from a defective cytoskeletal structure. We have elsewhere suggested as a working hypothesis that this structure plays a role in cellular regulation of growth [1, 14] and in the evolutionary development of a malignant cell from a premalignant form [44].

ACKNOWLEDGMENTS

This project was supported in part by grant No. RR-00592 from the Division of Research Resources, National Institutes of Health; grant No. CA-20810 from the National Institutes of Health, Cancer Institute; and by grant No. HD-02080 from the National Institutes of Health, Child Health and Human Development Institute. This is contribution No. 290 from the Eleanor Roosevelt Institute for Cancer Research and the Florence R. Sabin Laboratories for Genetic and Developmental Medicine.

The authors wish to acknowledge the excellent technical assistance of Bob Johnson in time-lapse microcinematography, to Stan Nielson, Donna Kelley, and Susan Keesee in immunofluorescence experiments, to Bob McGrew in scanning and transmission EM, and to Cynthia Trombly in quantitation data. We are grateful to Dr. Bill Brinkley for gifts of antitubulin IgG used in the early stages of this work.

REFERENCES

1. Hsie AW, Jones C, Puck TT: Proc Natl Acad Sci USA 68:1648, 1971.
2. Puck TT, Waldren CA, Hsie AW: Proc Natl Acad Sci USA 69:1943, 1972.
3. Porter K, Prescott D, Frye J: J Cell Biol 57:815, 1973.
4. Trinkaus JP: J Supramol Struct Suppl 3:166, 1979.
5. Meltzer KJ: Am Med 8:191, 1904.
6. Hogue MJ: J Exp Med 30:617, 1919.
7. Chambers R: J Cell Comp Phys 12:149, 1938.
8. Zollinger HU: Am J Pathol 24:545, 1948.
9. Costero I, Pomerat CM: Am J Pathol 89:405, 1951.
10. Boss J: Exp Cell Res 8:181, 1955.
11. Dornfield EJ, Owczarzak A: J Biophys Biochem Cytol 4:243, 1958.
12. Miranda AF, Godman GC: Tissue Cell 5:1, 1973.
13. Luchtel D, Bluemink JG, DeLatt SW: J Ultrastruct Res 54:406, 1976.
14. Hsie AW, Puck TT: Proc Natl Acad Sci USA 68:358, 1971.
15. Borek C, Fenoglio CM: Cancer Res 36:1325, 1976.
16. Gonda AM, Aaronson SA, Ellmor N, Zeve VH, Nagashima K: J Natl Cancer Inst 56:245, 1976.
17. Porter KR, Fonte VG: In Johari O, Corvin I (eds): "Scanning Electron Microscopy." Chicago: IIT Research Institute, p 683, 1973.
18. McNutt NS, Culp LA, Black PH: J Cell Biol 56:412, 1973.
19. Malick LE, Langenbach R: J Cell Biol 68:654, 1976.
20. Fogh J, Biedler JL, Denues ART: NY Acad Sci 95:758, 1961.
21. Hendee WR, Zebrun W, Bonte FJ: Tex Rep Biol Med 21:546, 1963.
22. Oda M, Puck TT: J Exp Med 113:599, 1961.
23. Storrie B: J Cell Biol 66:392, 1975.
24. Ham RG: Proc Natl Acad Sci USA 53:288, 1965.
25. Puck TT, Cieciura JJ, Robinson A: J Exp Med 108:945, 1958.
26. Anderson TF: Trans NY Acad Sci 13:130, 1951.
27. Kao FT, Puck TT: Proc Natl Acad Sci USA 60:1275, 1968.
28. Kao FT, Puck TT: J Cell Physiol 80:41, 1972.

29. Brinkley BR, Fuller GM, Highfield DP: Proc Natl Acad Sci USA 72:4981, 1975.
30. Lazarides E, Weber K: Proc Natl Acad Sci USA 71:2268, 1974.
31. Goldman RD, Lazarides E, Pollack R, Weber K: Exp Cell Res 90:333, 1975.
32. Puck TT, Jones C: In Braun W, Lichtenstein LM, Parker CW (eds): "Cyclic AMP, Cell Growth, and the Immune Response." New York: Springer-Verlag, 1974, pp 338–348.
33. Cox DM, Puck TT: Cytogenetics 8:158, 1969.
34. Meek BD: Anat Rec 181:423, 1975.
35. Wessells NK, Spooner BS, Ash JF, Bradley MD, Luduena MA, Taylor EL, Wrenn JT, Yamada KM: Science 171:135, 1971.
36. Porter KR, Puck TT, Hsie AW, Kelley D: Cell 2:145, 1974.
37. Kao FT, Faik P, Puck TT: Exp Cell Res 122:83, 1979.
38. Meek WD, Porter KR, Puck TT: J Cell Biol 79:295a, 1978.
39. Miranda A, Godman GC, Deitch AD, Tanenbaum SW: J Cell Biol 61:481, 1974.
40. Puck TT: Proc Natl Acad Sci USA 74:4491, 1977.
41. Fujiwara K, Pollard TD: J Cell Biol 77:182, 1978.
42. Schroeder TE, Mikrosk Z: Anat Forsch 109:431, 1970.
43. Wolosewick JJ, Porter KR: J Cell Biol 82:114, 1979.
44. Puck TT: Somatic Cell Genet 5:973, 1979.

Journal of Supramolecular Structure 12:355–367 (1979)
Tumor Cell Surfaces and Malignancy 645–657

Alteration of Human Breast Tumor Cell Membrane Functions by Chromosome-Mediated Gene Transfer

Razia S. Muneer and Peter N. Gray

Department of Biochemistry and Molecular Biology, University of Oklahoma Health Sciences Center, Oklahoma City, Oklahoma 73190

BOT-2 cells (human breast tumor origin) have an impaired ability to utilize exogenous thymidine. Previous studies revealed this deficiency to be the permeation event rather than phosphorylation, since the cells have active thymidine kinase. Chromosome-mediated gene transfer was used to transfer genetic information in the form of metaphase chromosomes, from HeLa-65 cells to the BOT-2 cells, correcting the permease deficiency. Poly-L-ornithine or lipochromes were used for facilitation of chromosome uptake. After selection on HAT medium, transferant clones were isolated at a frequency of 4×10^{-5} and 1×10^{-5}, respectively. Transferants MGP-1 and MGL-1 are stable after 18 months and have been characterized on the bases of purine and pyrimidine nucleoside uptake, relative thymidine kinase activities, alkaline phosphatase activities, and hydrocortisone-induced alkaline phosphatase activity. MGP-1 demonstrates positive thymidine uptake and incorporates radiolabeled thymidine into DNA. MGL-1 remains thymidine transport-deficient and survives on HAT by increasing endogenous dihydrofolate reductase activity. Alkaline phosphatase activity in MGL-1 is similar to HeLa-65, 2% of that in BOT-2, and in addition, is inducible 25–30-fold by 3 μM hydrocortisone. We have separated, genetically, a thymidine permease function from phosphorylation in cells of human origin and have transferred genetic information for the regulation of alkaline phosphatase.

Key words: Alkaline phosphatase, chromosome-mediated gene transfer, human breast tumor cells, hydrocortisone, lipochromes, membrane bound enzymes, nucleoside uptake, thymidine kinase, thymidine transport

BOT-2 cells are a clonal continuous cell line derived from a human mammary ductal cell carcinoma [1]. They have specific breast tumor antigens [2, 3], are not hormone dependent [4], and have high levels of endogenous alkaline phosphatase (AP) [1]. Previous studies in our laboratory have demonstrated these cells to have low uptake of pyrimidine nucleosides. There is a specific deficiency for thymidine uptake [4, 5], which is not correctable by treatment with estradiols and testosterone. These hormones have proved to be stimulatory effectors of thymidine uptake in other breast tumor cultures [6]. BOT-2 cells are unable to radiolabel DNA with exogenous ^{3}H-thymidine and do not show nuclear (or cytoplasmic) labeling by autoradiography for labeling periods shorter than 15 h. Thymidine kinase (TK) is active in cell-free extracts, yet the cells fail to grow on HAT medium [7].

Received April 23, 1979; accepted August 24, 1979.

The lack of thymidine uptake (presumably transport) (TT^-) in the presence of TK supports the concept of separation of the permeation and phosphorylation events in human cells [8–10] and provides a mechanism to separate genetically the two functions, as was done with haploid frog cells [11, 12]. Following desired treatments of the cultures, selection of TT^+ cells can be achieved on HAT medium.

To alter the TT^- phenotype we used the established method of chromosome-mediated gene transfer (CMGT) for stable genetic transfer of genes from a donor cell type, which is TT^+. The donor in these studies also had very low AP activity levels. CMGT has been reported to transfer genetic information from one type of cultured mammalian cell to another with transfer frequencies from 10^{-5} to 10^{-8} [13–17]. Transfer frequencies have been increased by entrapping purified metaphase chromosomes into phospholipid vesicles (lipochromes) [16] rather than by using other facilitators such as poly-L-ornithine [13]. Treatment of recipient cells, BOT-2, with metaphase chromosomes from a donor cell line (HeLa-65, see below) followed by selection on HAT medium yielded stable and nonstable transferant cell populations expressing genetic information that corrected the original defect, TT^-.

HeLa-65 was selected as the donor cell system [19, 52] due to its growth on HAT medium in monolayer, its human origin, and several additional morphological and biochemical differences that distinguish it from BOT-2 [1]. In addition, HeLa-65 has extremely low alkaline phosphatase activity, which is inducible by hydrocortisone [19–24]. The increased AP activity in HeLa-65 appears to occur by a stimulation of catalytic activity [25] rather than de novo synthesis of new AP, which may occur in other AP inducible systems [24, 25–29]. HeLa cells grow in suspension culture, are subject to metaphase block by usual procedures, and have been used extensively as a donor for CMGT experiments [13, 30–32].

In this report we present evidence of successful transfer of genetic information from HeLa-65 correcting the BOT-2 thymidine transport deficiency. Both lipochromes and poly-L-ornithine were facilitators for the CMGT. The frequencies of transfer were 1×10^{-5} and 4×10^{-5}, respectively. Several transferant clones were isolated, and two, MGP-1 and MGL-1, were used for further study. MGP-1 and MGL-1 are stable transferants. MGP-1 transports thymidine sufficiently to survive on HAT medium, and MGL-1, whose selection was due to methotrexate resistance rather than thymidine transport, has AP activities 2% of BOT-2, and the AP can be induced approximately 25-fold by hydrocortisone. Dihydrofolate reductase activity in MGL-1 was three times greater than the activities in the other cell lines.

Both transferants demonstrate alteration of membrane-associated activities by genetic supplementation. The TT^-, TK^+, BOT-2 modification to MGP-1 genetically separates thymidine transport from thymidine kinase, providing a mechanism for analyzing a specific nucleoside carrier. The MGL-1 transferant representing a change from AP constitutive to AP repressed, but inducible, enables further study of the mechanism for steroid hormone regulation in cells of human origin.

MATERIALS AND METHODS

Cell Cultures

BOT-2 cells were kindly provided by Dr. Robert Nordquist. HeLa-65, the chromosome donor cell line, was a gift from Dr. Martin J. Griffin and has a modal chromosome number of 65. HeLa-65 grows in suspension culture as well as monolayer. The recipient cells, BOT-2, and the donor cells, HeLa-65, differ with respect to the following characteristics: modal chromosome number (BOT-2 has 63), glucose-6-phosphate dehydrogenase isoenzyme patterns [1], alkaline phosphatase activity, tumor antigen specificity, morphology, and growth characteristics (see Table I). Both cell lines were found to be mycoplasma-free as determined by the double-labeling technique of Schneider [33] with ^{14}C-uracil and ^{3}H-uridine.

Other cell cultures described are transferants derived by chromosome transfer. MGP-1 was selected, with poly-L-ornithine as the uptake facilitator. MGL-1 was obtained with lipid coated chromosomes, lipochromes.

Conditions for Cell Growth

Monolayer cultures were grown in plastic tissue culture flasks (Corning, NY) using a Dulbecco's modified Eagle's medium, DPM (72214, GIBCO, Grand Island, NY). This was supplemented with 10% heat-inactivated fetal calf serum (FCS) (GIBCO, Grand Island, NY) and 50 μg/ml gentamicin (Schering, Kenilworth, NJ). Cultures were incubated at 36.5°C in an humidified atmosphere of 6% CO_2, 94% filtered air. For the preparation of metaphase chromosomes cells were grown as spinner cultures in Eagle's phosphate medium (69191 GIBCO, Grand Island, NY) supplemented with 10% FCS and gentamicin.

Growth studies, doubling times, and plating efficiencies were done in 35 mm plastic tissue culture dishes in DPM and DPM-HAT media. Doubling times were determined over a 9-day period, with feeding every third day. Cell counts were made every 24 h with a Coulter particle counter (Hialeah, FL). Plating efficiency was determined 24 h after plating of cells. Multicellular tumor spheroid (MTS) [34] formation was determined for all cell lines in 25 cm^2 tissue culture flasks. When necessary, 3μM hydrocortisone (Sigma Chem Co., St. Louis, MO) was added directly to the culture medium for required times.

Donor Cell Synchronization and Chromosome Isolation

Metaphase chromosomes were prepared from HeLa-65 cells growing in suspension culture. As cells in the exponential growth phase reached a density of 2×10^5 cells/ml, they were synchronized by a double thymidine block [35]. Synchronized cultures were arrested at metaphase, with an efficiency of 95–98%, by addition of colcemid, 0.03 μg/ml, for 15 h.

Metaphase-arrested cells were harvested, under sterile conditions, for chromosome preparation. Chromosomes were isolated by using the pH 10.5 method of Wray [36, 37] and fractionated into small- and large-sized populations by sucrose density gradient centrifugation [37].

Chromosome-Mediated Gene Transfer and Transferant Selection

Two transfer systems were used for fusion of chromosomes with the recipient BOT-2 cells.

First, recipient cell suspensions in DPM without serum, 2×10^6 cells/ml, were mixed with cellular equivalents of metaphase chromosomes and poly-L-ornithine, 12 μg/ml, in siliconized 12 ml glass centrifuge tubes. The tubes rotated slowly, 20 rpm, for 2.5 h on a roller apparatus at 37°C. This suspension was supplemented with fetal calf serum to 10% and placed in plastic tissue culture flasks for plating and subsequent selection. Medium was changed at 24 h with DPM plus 10% FCS to remove nonattached cells, debris, and nonfused chromosomes. After 48 h, cells were switched to HAT selection medium for at least 5 weeks, with biweekly medium changes.

Second, sized metaphase chromosomes were mixed with lipids to form lipochromes [18, 38]. A sterile mixture of lecithin, stearylamine, and cholesterol (4:1:3) dissolved in chloroform and methanol was evaporated to dryness on the walls of a 12 ml sterile siliconized glass tube with nitrogen; 4.4 mg of lipid were used for 2×10^6 cell equivalents of chromosomes. Chromosomes in DPM were added to the lipid-coated tube, and the tube was mixed on a Vortex mixer for 3 min at room temperature. Cellular equivalents of lipochromes were added to monolayer cultures at 1.33×10^4 cells/cm^2 in DPM + 10% FCS. The medium was replaced with DPM + 10% FCS after 8 h to remove excess lipids and nonbound lipochromes. After 24 h the medium was changed to DPM-HAT, and for the next 5 weeks cells were fed biweekly with HAT medium.

In both CMGT systems control flasks of cells were carried through similar manipulations, except for chromosomes, and with chromosomes but no facilitators. After 5 weeks no colonies were detected in control flasks. After a few days there were a few giant bizarre nondividing cells that did not detach as did the majority of the cells. Chromosome-treated cells were observed microscopically at weekly intervals. After 5 weeks the number of colonies surviving selection pressure were determined. Selected colonies were recovered and transferred to individual culture flasks and grown in HAT medium until confluence. Cultures then were split and maintained in DPM as well as HAT medium. A pilot study to measure thymidine uptake in the transferent cultures was done to aid in selection of cultures to be used for further study.

Nucleoside Uptake Measurements

Uptake of purine and pyrimidine nucleosides was determined for donor and recipient cells, as well as for the stable transferants MGP-1 and MGL-1. MGX-100, a nonstable transferant, was also included. The following radioisotopically labeled nucleosides (Amersham, Arlington Heights, IL) were used: [methyl-^{3}H] thymidine, 50 Ci/mmole; 5-[^{3}H] uridine, 2 Ci/mmole; 5-[^{3}H] cytidine, 27 Ci/mmole; 5-[^{3}H]-deoxycytidine, 20 Ci/mmole; 2-[^{3}H]-adenosine; 20 Ci/mmole, G-[^{3}H]-deoxyadenosine, 12 Ci/mmole; 8-[^{3}H]-guanosine, 8 Ci/mmole; and 8-[^{3}H]-deoxyguanosine, 3 Ci/mmole. Each cell type was plated at 1×10^4 cells/cm^2 in 35 mm plastic tissue culture dishes in DPM plus 10% FCS. Following 36 h of incubation, labeled nucleosides were added to a concentration of 2×10^{-5} M, 1 μCi/ml, and incubated for an additional 18 h. Cultures were washed 3 times with cold Tris-Cl saline, pH 7.3 (ST), drained, and lysed with 0.5 ml 0.2M NaOH. The lysate was neutralized, mixed with Redisolv-HP (Beckman, LaJolla, CA), and counted in a liquid scintillation spectrometer (Intertechnique, Englewood, NJ). Parallel cultures were used for cell counts in a Coulter particle counter. All experiments were done in triplicate and repeated a minimum of three times.

DNA Synthesis

To determine to what extent the intracellular labeled thymidine could be phosphorylated and incorporated into DNA, cells were plated and labeled as described above. After rinsing cells three times with ST and lysing with 0.5 ml of 0.2M NaOH, the lysate was mixed with 5 ml of cold 15% trichloracetic acid and set in an ice bath for 60 min. The precipitate was collected on nitrocellulose filter discs, washed with 5% TCA, rinsed with 95% ethanol, dried, and the radioactivity counted in a liquid scintillation spectrometer.

Enzyme Assays

Thymidine kinase (TK) activity was measured with DEAE-52 paper disks [39, 40]. Results are expressed as pmoles phosphorylated thymidine per mg cell protein.

Alkaline phosphatase (AP) activity was measured with para-nitrophenyl phosphate as the substrate [41]. AP activity was determined on whole lysates prepared in 0.5% sodium deoxycholate.

Protein concentrations were determined by the method of Zak and Cohen [42].

Specific breast tumor antigens were monitored by fixed-cell immunofluorescence with antitumor antibodies from human breast cancer sera [2].

RESULTS

Recipient and Donor Cell Characteristics

BOT-2 recipient cells were originally described to be distinct from HeLa-65, the chromosome donor, with respect to morphology, glucose-6-phosphate dehydrogenase isoenzymes, alkaline phosphatase activity, alkaline phosphatase isoenzymes, karyotype, and cell surface antigens [1, 2]. We have repeated these studies on both cell lines and on the transferant clones described, except for the glucose-6-phosphodehydrogenase analysis. These results, along with others presented here, are summarized in Table I. We reported preliminary results indicating a difference in the utilization of pyrimidine nucleosides between the BOT-2 and HeLa-65 cells [4, 5]. The differences between the two cell lines of particular interest in this study are the low levels of thymidine uptake by BOT-2, the inability of BOT-2 to survive in HAT medium, the high activity of AP in BOT-2 cells, and the breast tumor-specific antigens. These parameters, as well as characteristic morphology, modal chromosome number, and multicellular tumor spheroid formation, were used initially to differentiate BOT-2 from HeLa-65 and later to verify the ancestry of transferants selected on the basis of their altered thymidine utilization and alkaline phosphatase regulation.

CMGT and Selection of Transferants

Treatment of BOT-2 cells with metaphase chromosomes was followed by selection on HAT medium. More than 99% of the recipient cells were killed after 5–8 days. HAT-resistant colonies, after 5 weeks of exposure, were counted, and the frequency of transference was found to be 4×10^{-5} for the poly-L-ornithine facilitated transfer method and

TABLE I. Characterization of Parental and Transferant Cells

Cell lines	Chromosome number	Growth on hat	Thymidine uptake[a]	AP[b]	AP in HC[c]	Thymidine kinase[d]	MTS[e]	BOT-2[f] Antigen
BOT-2[g]	63	–	0.20	++++	++++	244 ± 17	+	+
Hela-65[h]	65	+	0.45	+	++	273 ± 25	–	–
MGP-1	63	+	1.00	++++	++++	299 ± 29	+	+
MGX-100	63	+,–	0.20	+++	ND	242 ± 19	+	+
MGL-1	63	+	0.11	+	+++	169 ± 17	+	+

[a]Results expressed as nanomoles thymidine/10^6 cells.
[b]AP = relative alkaline phosphatase activity; see text for values.
[c]Relative alkaline phosphatase activity after treatment of cells with 3 μM hydrocortisone.
[d]Values expressed as picomoles TMP formed/mg protein ± SEM.
[e]MTS = multicellular tumor spheroid formation.
[f]Human breast tumor-specific antigen determined by immunofluorescence.
[g]Parental recipient.
[h]Parental chromosome donor.
ND = value not determined.

1×10^{-5} for the lipochrome technique. No surviving colonies were detected for untreated BOT-2 cells in HAT or for cells mixed with poly-L-ornithine or liposomes without chromosomes.

Transferant colonies were selected for further study after screening for thymidine uptake and alkaline phosphatase activity. MGP-1, MGL-1, and MGX-100 were grown in DPM and HAT media with periodic changes to the alternative medium. MGP-1 and MGL-1 were stable transferants maintaining resistance to HAT and other characteristics described later. MGX-100 was unstable, as determined by exponential increases in sensitivity to growth on HAT medium after removal of selection pressures. The instability of MGX-100 was typical of the majority of original transferants.

The population doubling times and plating efficiencies were measured in nonselective and selective media. Doubling times for MGP-1 and MGL-1 were 28 and 50 h, respectively, whereas the doubling time, using the same conditions, for BOT-2 was 32 h and that for HeLa-65 was 22 h.

Doubling time in HAT medium were extended to 43 h for MGP-1, 72 h for MGL-1, and approximately 30 h for HeLa-65. BOT-2 does not grow in HAT. The plating efficiency after 24 h for each cell type was nearly 98% in nonselective medium. This high efficiency was maintained for MGP-1 and MGL-1.

Nucleoside Uptake Studies

Purine and pyrimidine nucleoside uptake by transferants was compared to the donor and recipient cell lines. MGP-1 demonstrated a 5-fold increase in thymidine incorporation over that of the BOT-2 cells (Fig. 1) and more than twice the level for HeLa-65 cells. MGL-1 did not show a similar increase, and its HAT resistance has been shown to be due

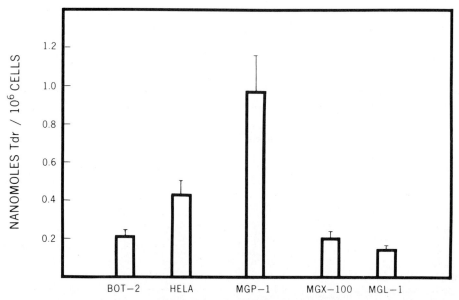

Fig. 1. Thymidine uptake by parental and transferant cells. Cells were grown in monolayer for 18 h in the presence of 1×10^{-5} M [methyl-^{3}H]-thymidine. Whole cell lysates in 0.2 M NaOH were used to determine total uptake. Levels in BOT-2 cells are much lower than for other nucleosides (see Fig. 2). MGP-1 transports sufficient thymidine for survival on HAT medium BOT-2 cells are the parental recipient; HeLa-65 the parental chromosome donor; MGP-1 and MGL-1 are stable transferants; MGX-100 is an unstable transferant.

to other mechanisms (results not shown). The very low levels of thymidine uptake (0.2 nmoles/10^6 cells) in BOT-2 may actually represent plasma membrane-bound (but not incorporated) thymidine. Autoradiography did not demonstrate ^{14}C-labeled thymidine in the cytoplasm or nucleus, whereas similar experiments with cytidine and uridine did (unpublished observation).

MGP-1 has the ability to incorporate uridine and cytidine, whereas no increase in deoxycytidine was noted. The results for nucleoside uptake, except thymidine, are summarized in Figure 2. All transferants were able to transport adenosine and deoxyadenosine equally well, except for MGL-1, with a 50% decrease in adenosine uptake. MGX-100, the unstable transferant, showed an increased ability, compared to BOT-2, to incorporate guanosine and deoxyguanosine. However, this change was unstable with increasing reversion of MGX-100. Likewise, the increases in uridine and cytidine uptake of MGX-100 are difficult to interpret, since no increase in thymidine was noted.

MGP-1, alone, showed a specific alteration in pyrimidine uptake. The 5-fold increase in thymidine uptake is critical for MGP-1 survival in HAT medium. Even though uridine and cytidine incorporation were improved, the parental BOT-2 cells incorporated both of these nucleosides into macromolecules at levels 5 to 10 times greater than thymidine, indicating a membrane specificity for thymidine.

Incorporation of Exogenous ^{3}H-Thymidine Into DNA and Thymidine Phosphorylation

Differences in thymidine incorporation were paralleled in the labeling of DNA as determined by acid precipitation of cells after long-term incubation with ^{3}H-thymidine (Fig. 3). The transferant, MGP-1, had nearly a 5-fold increase over the recipient cells.

To determine whether the low levels of thymidine incorporation into DNA by BOT-2 and the higher levels by MGP-1 were due to an altered transport deficiency or to a modified ability to phosphorylate exogenous thymidine initially, the activity of thymidine kinase was determined for each cell line (Table I). Both parental cell types demonstrated equivalent TK activity. Likewise, the transferants possessed TK activity sufficient to permit cell growth in HAT medium, provided exogenous thymidine entered the cell. We previously demonstrated that BOT-2 cells made permeable to thymidine by gentle hypotonic treatment were able to phosphorylate ^{3}H-thymidine and subsequently utilize this in DNA synthesis [53].

Alkaline Phosphatase

A primary biochemical difference between the recipient and donor cells was that of alkaline phosphatase. This parameter was one of several used to distinguish BOT-2 cells from HeLa-65. It was also used to ascertain the relatedness of the transferants to the parental recipient. Normal levels of alkaline phosphatase activity in HeLa-65 are quite low (approximately 7–10 nmoles Pi/min/mg protein), and can be increased to 50–60 nmoles Pi/min/mg protein by induction with 3 μM hydrocortisone. Alternatively, BOT-2 has relatively high activity levels of alkaline phosphatase (approximately 750 nmoles Pi/min/mg protein), which are not significantly increased by hydrocortisone. Screening of the transferants revealed that MGL-1 shows alkaline phosphatase activity nearly identical to HeLa-65 (12 nmoles Pi/min/mg protein). This AP activity in MGL-1 can be increased nearly 30 times to 356 nmoles Pi/min/mg protein by growing the cells in 3 μM hydrocortisone (Fig. 4). The time course of the induction is similar to that for HeLa-65, including the lag period. Similar changes in AP activity were not seen in MGP-1.

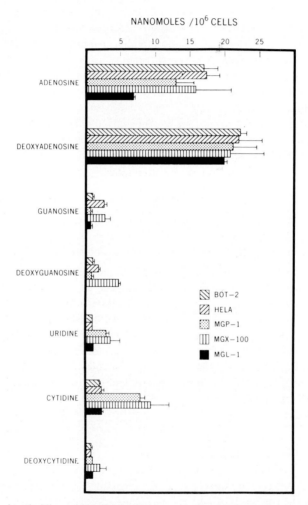

Fig. 2. Purine and pyrimidine nucleoside uptake by parental and transferant cells. All values are significantly higher than for BOT-2 (TT⁻) (see Fig. 1). Uptake was determined after 18 h of growth in radioactive medium (see Methods), followed by whole cell lysis.

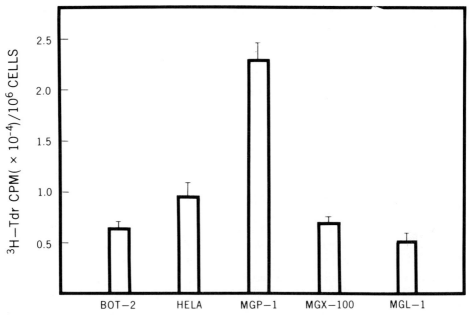

Fig. 3. Incorporation of ³H-thymidine into DNA. Cells were grown as in Figure 1, lysed, and DNA-precipitated with 15% trichloracetic acid (see Methods). Incorporation parallels thymidine uptake. BOT-2 nuclei do not show labeling by autoradiography after 15 h, whereas HeLa-65 nuclei do.

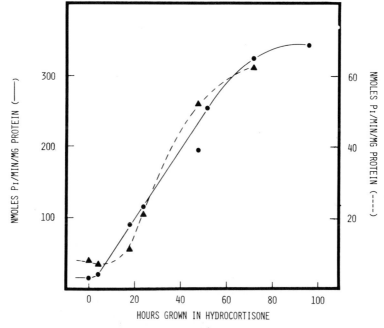

Fig. 4. Alkaline phosphatase induction by hydrocortisone in HeLa-65 and MGL-1. Cells in monolayer culture were grown in the presence of 3μM hydrocortisone for the times indicated. Alkaline phosphatase activity was determined as described in Methods. (————) MGL-1 cells. (- - - - - -) HeLa-65 cells. Both cell types show similar patterns of induction; however, MGL-1 alkaline phosphatase activity is induced nearly 30-fold, whereas HeLa-65 activity is induced only 5–6-fold.

Chromosome Analysis and MTS Formation

Karyotype analyses of the parental cell-lines confirmed a modal chromosome number of 65 for HeLa-65 and 63 for BOT-2, with BOT-2 having 2 minichromosomes [1]. All transferants had the same modal chromosome number as the recipient BOT-2 cells, 63. No major chromosome alterations were detected.

Multicellular tumor spheroid formation was monitored for all cell types. HeLa-65 did not form three-dimensional cellular aggregates; whereas, BOT-2 and all transferant cells presented the cellular aggregates characteristic of mammary tumor cells (Table I). In addition, the transferant cells retained the cell surface antigen specific to breast tumor cells as described for BOT-2 cells [2, 3].

DISCUSSION

The transfer of genetic information, via metaphase chromosomes, between two human cell lines has led to the alteration in the recipient cells of two membrane-associated cellular activities. Activation of thymidine transport and regulation of alkaline phosphatase catalytic efficiency have been stabilized genetically in a human breast tumor cell line originally thymidine transport-deficient and alkaline phosphatase-constitutive. Both modifications reflect the normal phenotype of the parental donor, HeLa-65.

Recipient BOT-2 cells grow well under normal culture conditions; however, exposure to methotrexate, 4×10^{-7} M, completely inhibits cell survival [7]. Addition of thymidine and hypoxanthine to make HAT medium does not increase survival. The reversion frequency for BOT-2 cells in HAT medium is less than 2×10^{-9}, and we have not yet been able to isolate a spontaneous revertant. Following treatment of BOT-2 cells with metaphase chromosomes in the presence of poly-L-ornithine or a mixture of lipids (see Methods), surviving cells appeared after 5 weeks of selection pressure with a frequency in the order of 1×10^{-5}. The majority of the transferants were unstable, as would be expected using these techniques [13, 14, 16]. Several clones were stable after alternate subculturing in selective and nonselective growth medium. Two of the stable transferants, MGP-1 and MGL-1, resembled the parental recipient, except for increased thymidine uptake by MGP-1 and very low levels of alkaline phosphatase activity in MGL-1. No differences in morphology, specific cell-surface tumor antigens, or multicellular tumor spheroid formation were detected. BOT-2 sensitivity to HAT medium could be accounted for by defective thymidine transport, and the resistance of MGP-1 to HAT could be accounted for by thymidine uptake and incorporation into DNA. The resistance of the MGL-1 to HAT apparently was due to another mechanism. MGL-1 cell extracts had a 3.5-fold increase in dihydrofolate reductase activity [5, 43] when measured in the presence of endogenous methotrexate. MGX-100 was unable to incorporate methotrexate (results not published).

The uptake of thymidine by eukaryotic cells in culture includes a permeation event. This event may be mediated by a specific carrier component in the cell membrane and/or by simple diffusion. Transport is followed by a phosphorylation event to a nucleoside monophosphate, with subsequent metabolism and incorporation into macromolecules [8, 44, 45]. Separation of these events in mammalian systems has been reported through the use of thymidine kinase deficient (TK⁻) mutants [9, 11, 46, 47], rapid transport studies [8, 48–50], and ATP depletion to prevent phosphorylation [51]. Actual genetic separation of these events with thymidine transport-deficient (TT⁻) cells having normal TK activity has been limited to a few studies, including those in Chinese hamster ovary cells [10] and haploid frog cells [11]. Whereas correction of TK⁻ with

DNA [47], viral genome [47], and chromosome transfer [12] has become nearly routine, the reversion of TT⁻ to TT⁺ using genetic material, without affecting TK, has been demonstrated satisfactorily only in the haploid frog cell system [11, 12]. Our data now provide similar evidence for genetic regulation of nucleoside transport and its separation from phosphorylation in human-derived cells in culture. This is supported by results showing equivalent TK in vitro activities in all cells studied and by the in vivo TK activity and nucleotide incorporation into DNA in cells "force fed" thymidine by mild hypotonic treatment [53]. Our results support the current concept that permeation and phosphorylation are separate events in mammalian cells and that transport is not necessarily kinase mediated. Recent studies with nitrobenzylthioinosine probes also suggest transport to be the rate-limiting factor in nucleoside uptake [51, 54].

The specific carrier system for transport of purine and pyrimidine nucleosides across the plasma membrane may be either permanent or transient components of the membrane [44]. Transport capacity has been linked to both the cell cycle [44, 55] and malignant transformation [44, 56]. The nucleoside specificity of these carriers appears to be more complex and to a certain degree genus specific. There are systems that generally differentiate between purine and pyrimidine nucleosides and those that show specificities for individual nucleosides [48, 57, 59, 60]. HeLa cells are of the latter classification, having different carriers for thymidine than for uridine [58]. This has been corroborated for our donor HeLa-65 and recipient BOT-2 cells.

The lack of thymidine transport in BOT-2 may be due to a primary structural alteration of the thymidine carrier itself. It may be absent or inactivated through one or more defective functional modifications. It also could be due to a modification in a secondary membrane component that plays a role in localization and activation of the carrier. At this time we have no conclusive evidence for either hypothesis, although the specificity of the BOT-2 defect and its correction suggest a primary alteration to be more probable.

Alkaline phosphatase is found in most tissues and cells in cultures at various endogenous levels of activity and several isoenzyme forms [27, 61]. This can be readily demonstrated in the BOT-2 and HeLa-65 cells used for this study. BOT-2 cells in culture normally demonstrate relatively high activity, and HeLa-65 cells generally have quite low activity, with the activity ratio of BOT-2:HeLa-65 approaching 50. HeLa-65 alkaline phosphatase activity can be induced nearly 10-fold by addition of hydrocortisone [41, 63], 5-bromo-deoxyuridine [62], choline chloride [26], 5-iodouridine [64, 65], sodium butyrate [23], phospholipase A₂ [24], and Rosenthal's inhibitor [66]. Similar results have been obtained with other cells in culture such as skin fibroblasts [67], H.Ep-2 [62], mouse L-cells [28], human placental cells [29], aortic endothelial cells [68], and embryonic chick intestine [69]. In vivo, alkaline phosphatase activity has been used extensively in clinical procedures [27] and induced in rat liver by colchicine [70]. It appears initially that induction can occur with nearly any membrane perturbation. However, induction has been repeatedly linked to a requirement for protein synthesis [22, 25, 28, 70] and, possibly, DNA synthesis [63]. Induction of AP activity may occur by catalytic activation of preexisting AP polypeptides [25] or by de novo synthesis of more AP. A constitutive AP and a different inducible AP have also been suggested [71]. It is likely that both mechanisms exist.

Our experiments showing the stable transfer of AP repression in MGL-1, a decrease to nearly 2% of BOT-2 AP, and its subsequent 25-fold increase by hydrocortisone treatment suggest a specific genetic locus having positive expression that modulates AP activity. While nonspecific stimuli indirectly affect AP activity, it is now possible to examine induced cells for specific regulatory components and mechanisms for induction. In systems with large increases in stimulated AP activity such as MGL-1 and mouse L-cells [28] one may not have induction, but rather specific gene amplification [72].

Altered alkaline phosphatase expression was found in the stable transferants selected from HAT medium. MGP-1 had AP activity greater than either parental cell line and, like the parental donor, was TT$^+$. MGL-1 had AP activity similar to the parental donor but remained TT$^-$, a characteristic of the parental recipient. Since there is a HeLa variant, HeLa-75, with high AP activity, which is also TT$^+$[22], it is difficult to postulate a linkage between the two genes. Based on the characteristics of only two transferants, it is also premature to link HAT resistance with some aspect of AP expression.

The different AP isoenzyme patterns for HeLa-65 and BOT-2 [1] enable us to determine whether MGL-1 and MGP-1 now contain, via gene transfer, either an additional HeLa-65 isoenzyme or a new or altered regulatory protein. Indeed, there may be a transition among the isoenzymes similar to that seen in human placenta during the first and third trimesters [29].

In summary, we have shown stable genetic transfer of information necessary to alter correctively a specific pyrimidine nucleoside carrier function in human cell plasma membranes. This function is genetically distinct from phosphorylation by thymidine kinase. We have also been able to transfer genetic information for regulation of alkaline phosphatase activity. The complex nature of the interaction these two functions have with cell membranes does not enable us, at this time, to specify the chemical nature of the modified behavior. At present, we do not believe there to be a necessary link between thymidine transport and alkaline phosphatase.

ACKNOWLEDGMENTS

We wish to express our sincere gratitude to Dr. Robert Nordquist for providing the BOT-2 cells, performing the tumor antigen studies, and independently corroborating the nucleoside uptake studies. We also wish to thank Dr. Robert Wohlhueter for his helpful discussion of the thymidine experiments, Dr. Martin J. Griffin for his help with the alkaline phosphatase studies, and Dr. O. Wesley McBride for discussions concerning CMGT. This research was supported by the Elsa U. Pardee Foundation.

REFERENCES

1. Nordquist RE, Ishmael DR, Lovig CA, Hyder DM, Hoge AF: Cancer Res 35:3100, 1975.
2. Nordquist RE, Schafer FB, Manning NE, Ishmael DR, Hoge AF: J Lab Clin Med 89:257, 1977.
3. Lerner MP, Anglin JH, Nordquist RE: J Natl Cancer Inst 60:339, 1978.
4. Gray PN: Biophys J 17:189a, 1977.
5. Muneer RS, Gray PN: J Cell Biol 79:321a, 1978.
6. Lippman ME, Bolan G, Huff K: Nature 258:339, 1975.
7. Littlefield JW: Science 145:709, 1964.
8. Wohlhueter RM, Marz R, Graff JC, Plagemann PGW: J Cell Physiol 89:605, 1976.
9. Ungemach FR, Hegner D: Hoppe-Seylers Z Physiol Chem 359:846, 1978.
10. Breslow RE, Goldsby RA: Exp Cell Res 55:339, 1969.
11. Freed JJ, Mezger-Freed L: J Cell Physiol 82:199, 1973.
12. Rosenstein BS, Ohlsson-Wilhelm BM: Somatic Cell Genet 4:341, 1978.
13. McBride OW, Ozer HL: Proc Natl Acad Sci USA 70:1258, 1973.
14. Willecke K, Ruddle FH: Proc Natl Acad Sci USA 72:1792, 1975.
15. Spandidos DA, Siminovitch L: Proc Natl Acad Sci USA 74:3480, 1977.
16. Spandidos DA, Siminovitch L: Cell 12:235, 1977.
17. Spandidos DA, Siminovitch L: Cell 12:675, 1977.

18. Mukherjee AB, Orloff S, Butler J, Triche T, Lalley P, Schulman JD: Am J Hum Genet 29:80a, 1972.
19. Eagle H: Science 130:432, 1965.
20. Cox RP, MacLeod CM: J Gen Physiol 45:439, 1962.
21. Griffin MJ, Ber R: J Cell Biol 40:297, 1969.
22. Cox RP, Elson NA, Tu SH, Griffin MJ: J Mol Biol 58:197, 1971.
23. Griffin MJ, Price GH, Bazzell KL, Cox RP, Ghosh NKA: Arch Biochem Biophys 164:619, 1974.
24. Hung SC, Melnykovych G: Biochem Biophys Acta 428:409, 1976.
25. Bazzell KL, Price G, Tu SH, Griffin MJ: Eur J Biochem 61:493, 1975.
26. Wharton W, Goz B: Cancer Res 38:3764, 1978.
27. Fishman WH: Am J Med 56:617, 1974.
28. Firestone GL: Fed Proc 38:791a, 1979.
29. Sakiyama T, Chow JY: Fed Proc 38:813a, 1979.
30. Burch JW, McBride OW: Proc Natl Acad Sci USA 72:1797, 1975.
31. McBride OW, Athwal RS: In Vitro 12:777, 1976.
32. Athwal RS, McBride OW: Proc Natl Acad Sci USA 74:2943, 1977.
33. Schneider EL, Stanbridg EJ, Epstein CJ: Exp Cell Res 84:311, 1974.
34. Yuhas JM, Li AP, Martinez AO, Ladman AJ: Cancer Res 37:3639, 1977.
35. Firket H, Mahieu P: Exp Cell Res 45:11, 1967.
36. Wray WE, Stubblefield E, Hymphrey R: Nature (New Biol) 238:237, 1972.
37. Wray WE: In Prescott DM (ed): "Methods in Cell Biology," vol. VI New York: Academic Press, 1973 pp 283–315.
38. Papahadjopoulos D, Vail WJ, Jacobson K, Poste G: Nature 252:163, 1974.
39. Kit S, Dubbs DR, Piekarski LJ, Hsu TC: Exp Cell Res 31:297, 1963.
40. Kit S, Leung WC, Jorgenson GN, Trukula D, Dubbs DR: Cold Spring Harbor Symp Quant Biol 39:703, 1975.
41. Cox RP, Ghosh NK, Bazzell K, Griffin MJ: Isozymes I: "Molecular Structure" New York: Academic Press, 1975, pp 343–365.
42. Zak B, Cohen J: Clin Chem Acta 6:665, 1961.
43. Gray PN, Muneer RS: J Supramol Struct Suppl 3:220, 1979.
44. Berlin RD, Oliver JM: Int Rev Cytol 1973, pp 283–315.
45. Paterson ARP, Kim SC, Bernard O, Cass CE: Ann NY Acad Sci 255:402, 1975.
46. Willecke K, Mierau R, Kruger A, Lange R: Mol Gen Genet 161:49, 1978.
47. Wigler M, Pellicer A, Silverstein S, Axel R: Cell 14:725, 1978.
48. Plagemann PGW, Erbe J: J Cell Physiol 81:101, 1972.
49. Plagemann PGW, Erbe J: J Cell Physiol 83:337, 1974.
50. Wohlhueter RM, Marz R, Graff JC, Plagemann PGW: In Prescott DM (ed): "Methods in Cell Biology," Vol. XX, New York: Academic Press, 1978.
51. Wohlhueter RM, Marz R, Plagemann PGW: J Memb Biol 42:247, 1978.
52. Kuebbing D, Werner R: Proc Natl Acad Sci USA 72:3333, 1975.
53. Kidd V, Muneer RS, Gray PN: Proc Okla Acad Sci, 1978.
54. Cass CE, Paterson ARP: Exp Cell Res 105:427, 1977.
55. Hopwood LE, Dewey WC, Hejny W: Exp Cell Res 96:425, 1975.
56. Berlin RD, Oliver JM, Ukena TE, Yin HH: Nature 247:45, 1974.
57. Schuster GS, Hare JD: In Vitro 6:427, 1971.
58. Mizel SB, Wilson L: Biochemistry 11:2573, 1972.
59. Scholtissek C: Biochim Biophys Acta 158:435, 1968.
60. Stambrook PJ, Sisken JE, Ebert JD: J Cell Physiol 82, 267, 1972.
61. Briere RO: CRC Crit Rev Clin Lab Sci 10:1, 1979.
62. Bulmer D, Stocco DM, Morrow J: J Cell Physiol 87:357, 1976.
63. Morrow J, Stocco DM, Fralick JA: J Cell Physiol 98:427, 1979.
64. Goz B: Cancer Res 34:2393, 1974.
65. Goz B, Walker KP: Cancer Res 36:4480, 1976.
66. Melnykovych G, Lopez IC: J Cell Physiol 92:91, 1977.
67. Walters MD, Summer GK: Proc Soc Exp Biol Med 133:926, 1970.
68. Arbogast BW: Fed Proc 38:1452a, 1979.
69. Black BL, Moog F: Dev Biol 66:232, 1978.
70. Ikehara Y, Mansho K, Kato K: J Biochem 84:1335, 1978.
71. Vanneuviue FJ, Vanelsen AF, Leroy JG: Biochem Soc Trans 5:1117, 1977.
72. Alt FW, Kellems RE, Bertino JR, Schimke RT: J Biol Chem 253:1357, 1978.

Journal of Supramolecular Structure 12:369–384 (1979)
Tumor Cell Surfaces and Malignancy 659–674

The Regional Association of Actin and Myosin With Sites of Particle Phagocytosis

Richard G. Painter and Ann T. McIntosh

Research Institute of Scripps Clinic, La Jolla, California 92037

Contractile proteins are thought to play a causative role in motile processes such as phagocytosis. In order to investigate their role in phagocytosis further, simultaneous immunofluorescence localization of F-actin and myosin was carried out in resident mouse peritoneal macrophages after phagocytosis of opsonized zymosan particles. Both actin and myosin appeared to concentrate rapidly at sites of particle phagocytosis. The observed concentration of both proteins at such sites preceded ultimate particle engulfment. Cytochalasin B, a drug which was shown to block pseudopod extensions around the particle, did not prevent the concentration of the two contractile proteins at cell-particle binding sites. This result ruled out path-length effects as an explanation for the observed concentration of actin and myosin at phagocytic sites. Kinetic analysis showed that actin rapidly concentrates at particle-cell binding sites within minutes (or less) of contact with cell surface. The two proteins are present throughout the engulfment phase until and after ingestion is complete. Finally, at later times the particles become clustered over the cell nucleus and the particle-associated actin-myosin seen earlier is no longer evident.

Key words: phagocytosis, actin, myosin, macrophages, immunofluorescence

Contractile proteins are known to play a role in cell movement along substrate surfaces (see Korn [1] for a review). Several lines of evidence exist that implicate both actin and myosin and perhaps other contractile proteins in cell movement along surfaces. However, gross cell movement along infinite surfaces necessarily involves intimate contact of a large portion of the cell surface with the substratum, making interpretation of morphologic data obtained by immunofluorescence or electron microscope techniques difficult at best.

Phagocytosis of particles by contrast is a motile process possessing several unique features which simplify the analysis of immunofluorescence data particularly with respect to the localization of the contractile apparatus (for a review see Stossel [2] and Silverstein

Abbreviations used: B-HMM, biotinyl-heavy meromyosin; F1-Av, fluorescein-labeled egg white avidin; IgG, immunoglobulin G; F(ab′)$_2$, pepsin fragment of IgG; Rh-Con A, rhodamine-labeled concanavalin A; CB, cytochalasin B; MEM, minimal essential medium; PBS, phosphate-buffered saline.

Address reprint requests to Richard G. Painter, PhD, Research Institute of Scripps Clinic, La Jolla, CA 92037.

Received May 21, 1979; accepted October 2, 1979.

et al [3]). For example, Silverstein and his colleagues have shown that pseudopod extension around a particle is receptor-dependent and involves only those regions of the membrane in close opposition to the particle being ingested [4, 5]. This strict regional responsiveness allows sites of particle-membrane interaction to be compared with uninvolved regions of the cell.

Actin has been detected in pseudopod extensions by both electron microscope and immunocytochemical methods [6, 7]. Myosin, which would be expected to participate in any postulated work-producing contraction, has not thus far been reported at sites of phagocytosis.

For the above reasons, we have determined the intracellular distributions of both actin and myosin by simultaneous immunofluorescence techniques. Our data show that myosin and actin are present at particle-membrane binding sites *prior* to pseudopod extension and ultimate particle ingestion.

MATERIALS AND METHODS

Preparation of F-Actin-Specific Fluorescent Reagents

Biotinyl-heavy meromyosin (B-HMM) and fluorescein-labeled egg white avidin (F1-Av) were prepared and characterized as described by Heggeness and Ash [8]. The preparations used in these studies had 10–12 moles biotin/mole HMM and 2–3 moles fluorescein/mole avidin.

Preparation of Uterine Myosin and Rabbit Antimyosin Antibodies

Human uterine myosin was prepared from surgical specimens, within 3–4 h of removal, essentially as described by Pollard et al [9]. The protein was further purified by DEAE-Sephadex A-50 chromatography as described by Wang [10].

Rabbit antibodies were prepared with this material by subcutaneous injection of 100 μg of the protein homogenized in an equal volume of Freund's complete adjuvant into the footpads. Animals were boosted again at monthly intervals with 100 μg of immunogen emulsified in Freund's incomplete adjuvant. Bleedings were taken 10–14 days after the last boost and the IgG fraction was prepared by DEAE-cellulose chromatography.

F(ab')$_2$ fragments of the IgG fraction of immune or preimmune IgG were prepared by limited pepsin digestion as described by Nisonoff et al [11].

Preparation of Affinity-Purified Antiuterine Myosin

Affinity-purified antibodies were prepared by affinity chromatography of 20 mg of immune IgG on a human uterine myosin-Sepharose 4B column that contained a total of 2.5 mg myosin per 2.5 ml of packed gel bed which was prepared with CNBr-activated Sepharose 4B (Pharmacia, Piscataway, New Jersey) in accordance with the instructions of manufacturer. The column was exhaustively washed with 0.5 M NaCl and the bound antibodies were eluted with 0.1 M acetic acid. The eluted antibodies were neutralized immediately with 1/10 volume of 1 M Na acetate, dialyzed versus 0.14 M NaCl/0.02 M Na phosphate (pH 7.3) and ultracentrifuged for 30 min (100,000g) to remove denatured protein aggregates.

For some experiments the affinity-purified antibody was radioiodinated with ^{125}I by the chloramine-T method of McConahey and Dixon [12].

Preparation of Mouse Peritoneal Macrophage Monolayers and Phagocytosis of Zymosan Particles

Peritoneal exudate cells were isolated from Balb/cSt mice as described by Russell et al [13] and allowed to adhere to 16-mm-diameter glass coverslips by culturing of the washed cells for 3–4 h at 37°C in HEPES-buffered Eagles' minimum essential medium (MEM) containing 10% fetal calf serum (Gibco, Inc., Santa Clara, California) followed by vigorous rinsing with Tyrode's balanced salt solution containing 0.1% bovine serum albumin (Tyrode's-BSA) prior to use as described below.

When stimulation of particle phagocytosis was desired, cells were covered with 200 μl of zymosan particles (2×10^7 per milliliter) which had been previously opsonized with fresh human serum. Uptake was allowed to proceed at ambient temperature for up to 90 min. The reaction was terminated at specified time intervals by immersion of the coverslips in Tyrode's-BSA for a few seconds followed by fixation with 2% formaldehyde solution buffered with 0.1 M Na phosphate buffer (pH 7.4) for 20 min. Duplicate coverslips were either immunofluorescently stained for actin and myosin or assayed for degree of particle engulfment as described below.

Drug Inhibition Experiments

When drugs were used as inhibitors of phagocytosis, the cells were pretreated with the indicated concentration of drug for 15 min prior to zymosan challenge. During the 30-min particle incubation period, drug was included in the medium. In order to determine if inhibitory drug effects were reversible, parallel coverslips were washed free of excess zymosan and drug and were incubated in drug-free medium for an additional 30 min.

Immunofluorescence Staining Procedures

Simultaneous immunofluorescence staining for actin and myosin was carried out on coverslips essentially as described by Heggeness and Ash [8] and Heggeness et al [14], except that F(ab')$_2$ fragments (200 μg/ml) of the IgG fraction of antimyosin or preimmune sera were substituted for intact IgG. Briefly, formaldehyde fixed cells were made permeable with 0.1% Triton X-100 (no detectable staining was seen if this step was omitted), rinsed with buffer and incubated with B-HMM (100 μg/ml) and anti-myosin F(ab')$_2$ fragments (200 μg/ml) for 20 min. After extensive washing with buffer the cells were stained with Fl-Av (50 μg/ml) and rhodamine-labeled sheep anti-rabbit IgG (100 μg/ml). After washing, the coverslips were mounted on slides and viewed with a Zeiss microscope equipped with FL-IV epi-illumination optics with filter combinations that allowed for selective viewing of fluorescein and rhodamine fluorescence. Micrographs were recorded on Kodak Tri-X film.

Assay of Particle Engulfment

Zymosan particles that had been completely engulfed by cells were distinguished from surface-bound particles by incubation of formaldehyde-fixed but intact cells with rhodamine-labeled Con A (Rh-Con A) at a concentration of 100 μg/ml for 5 min. After washing, zymosan particles assessible to the extracellular millieu were brightly labeled while those which were completely engulfed were unstained. The percentage engulfment was obtained by calculating the ratio of unstained to total particles times 100. Partially stained particles were not considered to be engulfed. At least 200 particles were scored in each case. All data are the average of three separate experiments.

In experiments designed to relate actin distribution to the degree of particle engulfment, cells which had been first stained with Rh-Con A in an intact state as described above were made permeable with 0.1% Triton X-100 and then stained for F-actin as described above.

Electron Microscopy

Cells were prepared for electron microscopy by immersion of coverslips in Ca^{2+}-free Karnovsky's formaldehyde-glutaraldehyde fixative for 30 min at room temperature. The fixed cells were embedded in Epon in situ by the procedures of Maupin-Szamier and Pollard [15]. After curing, the coverslips were removed and the Epon blocks were remounted for ultrathin sectioning. Silver-colored thin sections were cut on an LKB Ultramicrotome 3 Model 8800 in a plane that was perpendicular to the original plane of cell growth. The sections were mounted on grids and stained with uranyl acetate and Pb citrate. Specimens were examined in a Hitachi 12A electron microscope.

Analytical Procedures

Polyacrylamide electrophoresis in sodium dodecyl sulfate (SDS PAGE) was performed as described by Laemmli [16] in 1.5-mm-thick slabs of 7% acrylamide with a Bio Rad Model #220 slab gel electrophoresis apparatus (Bio Rad, Richmond, California). Samples for SDS PAGE were prepared as described by Wang [10].

Direct staining of Coomassie Blue-stained SDS polyacrylamide gels strips with ^{125}I-labeled anti-human myosin was performed exactly as described by Burridge [17] as modified by Wallach et al [18]. The specific activity of the labeled antibody was 1.22×10^6 cpm/μg protein.

Ouchterlony analysis was carried out in 0.5% agarose gels containing 20 mM Na PP_i/0.5 M KCl (pH 7.0).

Reagents and Chemicals

Paraformaldehyde was obtained from Polysciences (Warrington, Pennsylvania) and fresh formaldehyde solutions were prepared immediately prior to use. Cytochalasin B was obtained from Sigma (St. Louis). Biotinyl-N-hydroxysuccinimide ester was prepared as described by Heitzmann and Richards [19]. All other reagents were reagent grade or better.

RESULTS

Characterization of Antimyosin Antibodies

The myosin antigen used to elicit the antibodies used in these studies was prepared from human uterine muscle as described by Pollard et al [9] and further purified by DEAE Sephadex A-50 chromatography. SDS-PAGE analysis (Fig. 1C) of the final purified protein (DM) shows the characteristic heavy-chain band with the light chains running in the dye front in this system. Actin, which was present at earlier stages of the purification, was not detected in this preparation. Traces of proteolytic degradation products are apparent just below the major heavy-chain band. These trace components are clearly proteolytic products, since they slowly increased during prolonged storage of the purified protein.

Anti-human uterine myosin was prepared by immunizing rabbits with the DEAE-Sephadex-purified protein. This antibody preparation was analyzed by Ouchterlony gel diffusion in 0.5% agarose gels containing 20 mM sodium pyrophosphate/0.5 M KCl (pH 7.0). In Figure 1A, a crude 0.6 M KCl/20 mM $NaPP_i$-1 mM dithiothreitol (DTT) extract (EX) of human uterine tissue is compared with the DEAE-Sephadex A-50-purified myosin (DM) preparation. A single fused precipitin line is seen between the crude extract and the purified protein. When the antibody preparation was preabsorbed with myosin-Sepharose 4B, no detectable reaction was seen in either case (Fig. 1B).

To further verify the specificity of the antimyosin preparation, the Coomassie Blue-stained gels shown in Figure 1C were cut out as strips, neutralized with PBS, and directly stained with affinity-purified ^{125}I-anti-human myosin by the direct labeling technique of Burridge [17] as modified by Wallach et al [18]. Figure 2 shows an autoradiograph of the dried gels obtained after this procedure. Only one major band of radioactivity was seen in the crude uterine extract (EX); it has a mobility that is identical to that of the heavy chain of Sepharose 4B-purified myosin (SM). The lower-molecular-weight bands seen with the purified protein presumably represent antibody reaction with proteolytic fragments of the heavy chain, since they are not detected in the original extract. Thus, by a number of sensitive immunochemical criteria the anti-human uterine myosin used in these studies is monospecific for myosin.

Immunofluorescent Distribution of Actin and Myosin in Resting Macrophages

Figure 3 shows the immunofluorescence staining patterns observed in the same normal resting macrophage for F-actin (3A) and myosin (3B). The spread cell shows a fine network-like distribution of actin (3A) throughout the cell cytoplasm in addition to some areas of punctate staining. The so-called "stress" fibers seen in other adherent cells such as 3T3 fibroblasts were rarely seen in such macrophage preparations even after 24 h of culture.

The myosin distribution (Fig. 3B) is more or less uniformly punctate and shows some areas with an apparent periodicity.

Specificity of the Immunofluorescence Staining Reactions

As seen in Figure 4B, the reaction of B-HMM with the cell is completely inhibited by its specific inhibitor, sodium pyrophosphate. Although not shown, the staining of cells with B-HMM and F1-Av was also blocked by free biotin, a potent competitive inhibitor of avidin binding to B-HMM. Neither inhibitor had any apparent effect on the antimyosin-myosin staining reaction.

The cytoplasm-associated rhodamine staining reaction was not seen if preimmune F(ab')$_2$ fragments were substituted for specific antimyosin F(ab')$_2$ fragments (Fig. 4C). In addition, no reaction was observed if the antibodies were preabsorbed with myosin-Sepharose 4B (not shown).

Actin and Myosin Distributions in Macrophages Phagocytosing Zymosan

Figure 5B,C show the actin and myosin distributions, respectively, in a cell that had been exposed to serum-treated zymosan (Z) for 30 min. A thin ring of bright actin-associated staining is observed which is uniformly and intimately associated with the engulfed zymosan particle (Fig. 5B). The myosin (Fig. 5C) staining pattern in the same cell is also closely associated with the engulfed particle but, unlike the actin pattern, shows a discontinuous or "patchy" distribution. It should be noted that the apparent lack of staining of other cell cytoplasmic regions is due to the fact that the cell body is below the focal plane of the particles. When the cell body was brought into focus, the staining patterns in regions removed from particle engulfment sites were similar to those seen in resting cells.

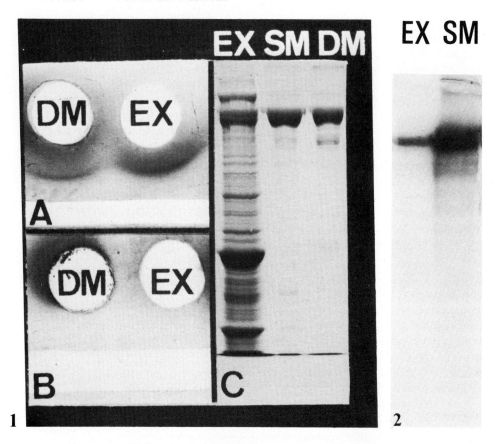

Fig. 1. Characterization of antimyosin antibodies and antigens. A: DEAE-Sephadex A-50-purified human myosin (DM; 6 μg) and 0.6 M KCI/20 mM NaPP$_i$/1 mM DTT extract of human uterine muscle (EX; 126 μg) were placed in Ouchterlony wells as indicated and tested against 1.3 mg rabbit antimyosin immunoglobulin G (trough). Single Coomassie Blue staining lines of immunoprecipitation between the purified myosin and the crude extract which show apparent immunochemical identity are seen. B: As in A except that the antimyosin immune globulin was preabsorbed with myosin-Sepharose 4B (50 μg myosin). No detectable reaction is revealed with Coomassie Blue. C: SDS PAGE electrophoresis of the antigens used in A and B; 50 μg of human uterine extract (EX), 4 μg of human uterine myosin after Sepharose 4 B chromatography (SM), and 4 μg of final DEAE-Sephadex A-50-purified protein (DM) were electrophoresed on 7% SDS PAGE gels in the presence of 1% β-mercaptoethanol and 0.1% SDS. Stained with Coomassie Brilliant Blue.

Fig. 2. Direct staining of SDS gels with ^{125}I-anti-human myosin antibodies. The gels labeled EX and SM are the same as those shown in Figure 1C and were cut out as strips and neutralized by incubation in PBS (pH 8.0). After treatment of the gels with preimmune IgG (1 mg/ml) and BSA (1 mg/ml) for 2 h, affinity-purified ^{125}I-antihuman myosin (2.2 × 10^6 cpm/μg) was added at 1 μg/ml and incubated for 18 h at room temperature. Unbound antibody was removed by exhaustive washing as described by Wallach et al [18] prior to autoradiography of the dried gel strips.

Effect of Cytochalasin B on the Actin-Myosin Distributions in Particle-Treated Macrophages

It is conceivable that the bright actin and myosin staining results from a path-length effect due to viewing long pseudopod extensions which extend out around the particle along their vertical axis. To evaluate this possibility, cells were pretreated with cytochalasin B, a drug known to block particle ingestion and pseudopod extension, and then were

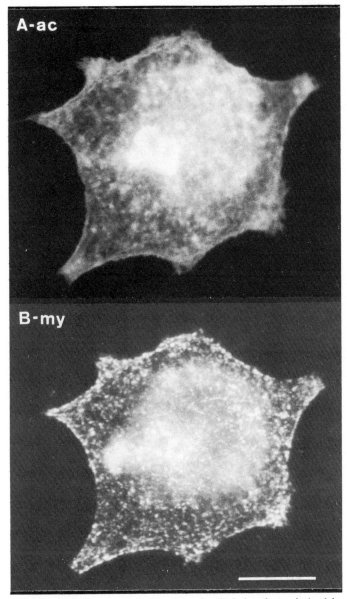

Fig. 3. Simultaneous immunofluorescence localization of actin (ac) and myosin (my) in resting mouse peritoneal macrophages. A: Actin distribution; B: myosin distribution. × 2,400; bar equals 10 μm.

challenged with particles in the presence of the drug. As shown in Figure 5D–F, after staining for actin (Fig. 5E) and myosin (Fig. 5F) both proteins are found in a focal plane which appears to underly the peripheral region of the zymosan particle (Z). As in the case of non-drug-treated cells the myosin distribution is "patchy" or punctate. Occasionally, particles are lost from such sites*, one of which is also shown in Figure 5D–F (arrowhead). A corresponding "oval-shaped" area of phase density (Fig. 5D) is also seen at such sites, which is consistent with the accumulation of protein at these regions of the cell.

*This was rigorously proved by examination of identical fields of cell before and after immunofluorescence staining procedures.

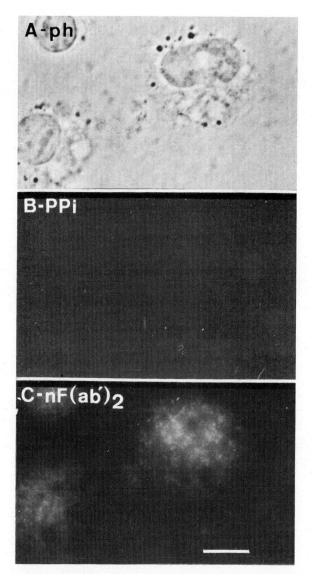

Fig. 4. Immunofluorescence specificity controls. A: Phase contrast (ph); fluorescein staining obtained with B-HMM and F1-Av with B-HMM in the presence of 10 mM NaPP$_i$/2 mM MgCl$_2$ in the same cells; C: staining of the same cells with F(ab')$_2$ fragment of preimmune IgG (200 μg/ml) in the place of F(ab')$_2$ fragments of antimyosin IgG followed by Rh-sheep anti-rabbit IgG. No detectable cytoplasmic staining is seen in either case. × 1,250; bar = 10 μm.

An electron micrograph of CB-treated cells which had been subsequently challenged with particles is shown in Figure 6. Such cells show no evidence of pseudopod extension around the particle surface (inset), a result which rules out path-length considerations as a viable explanation of the immunofluorescent results. Furthermore, in the region of the cell underlying the particle periphery, a dense zone of microfilaments (MF) is clearly evident (arrow).

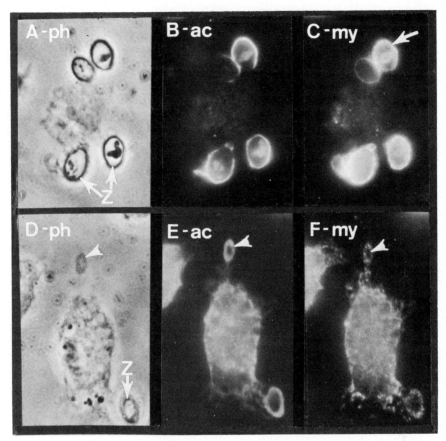

Fig. 5. Simultaneous immunofluorescence localization of actin (ac) and myosin (my) in mouse peritoneal macrophages 30 min after exposure to zymosan (Z) particles in the absence (A–C) and presence (D–F) of CB. A: Phase contrast (ph) micrograph showing macrophages and zymosan (Z); B: actin distribution in same cell as A; C: myosin distribution in same cell as A. Note the patchy distribution of the myosin-associated staining in comparison with the more uniform actin pattern. D: Phase contrast micrograph of a CB-treated cell which has been subsequently exposed to zymosan for 30 min. The cell was pretreated with drug (10 μg/ml) for 15 min, followed by addition of zymosan for an additional 30 min. The cells were then fixed and stained for actin and myosin as before. E: Actin distribution in same cell as D; F: Myosin distribution in same cell as D. The fluorescence associated with the particle core is a nonspecific autofluorescence. A–F × 1,250.

Thus, immunofluorescence and electron microscope examination of phagocytosing cells indicate that both F-actin and myosin concentrate at particle-binding sites even in CB-treated cells which have not extended pseudopods or engulfed the particle.

The Relationship of the Actin Response to the Degree of Particle Engulfment

As seen in Figure 5B, the actin staining regions do not always completely surround the zymosan particle. At early times after particle challenge especially, crescent-shaped profiles of actin staining are commonly seen, indicating that the contractile response occurs before complete ingestion of the particle.

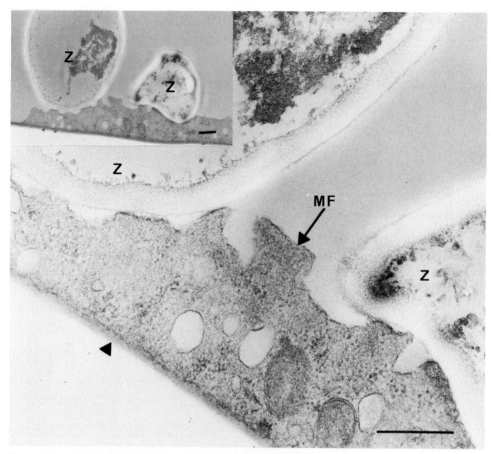

Fig. 6. Transmission electron micrograph of a thin section of Epon-embedded CB-treated macrophage exposed to zymosan (Z) for 30 min. Note the lack of long pseudopod extensions (inset) around the particles. At higher magnification, dense zones of microfilaments (MF) are apparent which lie in areas that are in close proximity to the particle-binding sites and that clearly underly the plasma membrane. The arrowhead indicates the substratum surface. × 55,000; inset × 12,000; bar = 0.2 μm.

In order to investigate the relationship between the degree of ingestion and the actin staining pattern, we took advantage of the fact that those areas of the particle in direct contact with the macrophage membrane did not appear to stain with Rh-Con A in *intact* cells. Thus, particles that are 50% ingested by the cell show a crescent-like staining profile when treated with Rh-Con A (Fig. 7B, dashed arrow).

The cells with Rh-Con A-labeled particles shown in Figure 7 were subsequently stained for actin after being made permeable to the B-HMM/F1-Av reagents with detergent. This staining protocol allows a direct comparison of the extent of engulfment as judged by the Rh-Con A pattern with the intracellular actin distribution. Particles in every phase of engulfment are seen even within the same cell, ranging from those which are completely inaccessible to Rh-Con A (Fig. 7B, solid arrow), intermediate forms (Fig. 7B, broken arrow) and particles which are totally accessible to reagent (Fig. 7E, solid arrows).

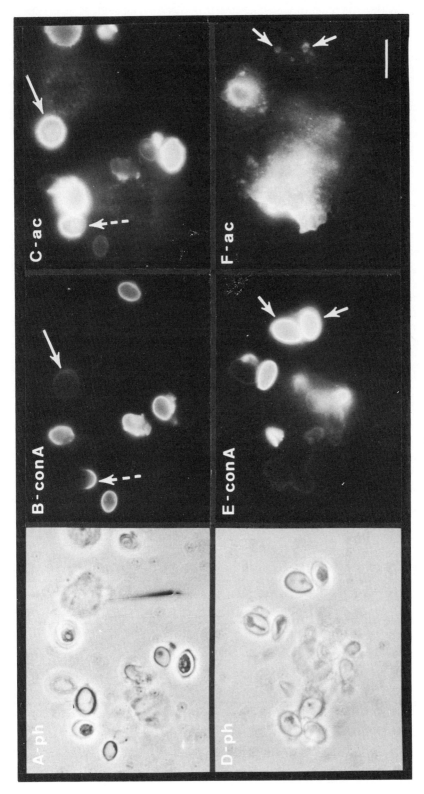

Fig. 7. Relationship of degree of particle phagocytosis to the cytoplasmic actin distribution. Macrophages which had been exposed to zymosan for 15 (D–F) or 30 (A–C) min were fixed with formaldehyde and stained with Rh-Con A immediately after rinsing. After rinsing, the cells were then rendered permeable with 0.1% Triton X-100 and stained for F-actin as described in Materials and Methods. Particles in various stages of engulfment are seen, ranging from initial surface contact (E, F, solid arrows) to 50% ingested (B, C, broken arrows), and finally to completely ingested (B, C, broken arrows).

The actin patterns in order of increasing degree of ingestion range from small rings of fluorescence that lie in a focal plane underlying the particle, and are the first recognizable response of the contractile system to the particle's presence at the cell surface, to the rings seen at later stages of ingestion (Fig. 7C, broken arrow), which lie within the focal plane of the particle and are in all probability pseudopod extensions that have advanced around the particle periphery. Finally, there are particles that are totally inaccessible to Rh-Con A and show actin "rings" that completely envelope the particle, indicating that the particle-associated actin staining persists for some time after the ingestion phase is completed (Fig. 7C, solid arrow).

Kinetics of Engulfment of Zymosan Particles by Macrophages

Through the accessibility of zymosan particles to Rh-Con A labeling in formaldehyde-fixed but intact macrophages, the kinetics of engulfment were followed over a 90-min incubation period at ambient temperature. As seen in Table I, the percentage of cell-associated particles that were *totally inaccessible* to Rh-Con A (an example of which is shown in Figure 7B, solid arrow), and were therefore completely engulfed by the cell, increased with time, plateauing approximately 60–90 min after particle challenge at levels of about 40% engulfment of total cell-bound zymosan. When these cells were rendered permeable with Triton X-100 *prior* to staining with Rh-Con A, >99% of cell-associated particles were stained, confirming that totally engulfed particles were capable of being stained by Rh-Con A.

As expected, CB was found to completely and reversibly block engulfment as measured by this assay (Table I). In addition, no partial engulfment profiles like those noted in Figure 7 were found.

Kinetics of the Actin-Myosin Response

Figure 8 shows a kinetic analysis of the particle-associated actin and myosin response to the presence of particles in phagocytosing macrophages. These data were obtained by immunofluorescently staining cells for actin and myosin at the indicated time points after particle challenge. In each case 200 or more cell-associated particles were microscopically scored for either 1) actin staining alone (o——o), 2) myosin alone (△——△), 3) both actin and myosin (●——●), or 4) no detectable associated staining (▲——▲).

TABLE I. Engulfment of Zymosan (Z) by Macrophages as Assayed by Accessibility of Zymosan to Rh-con A in Intact Cells*

Treatment	Time after Z addition (min)	Total Z/cell[a] (SEM)	% Engulfment[a] (SEM)
No drug	30	5.7 (0.9)	26 (6)
	60	5.4 (0.8)	38 (3)
	90	7.8 (0.6)	40 (5)
CB (10 μg/ml)	30	6.0 (0.4)	0.4 (0.07)
30 min after CB removal	60	ND	23 (4)

*Peritoneal macrophage monolayers on glass coverslips were pretreated with the indicated concentration of drug in Tyrode's-BSA medium 15 min prior to zymosan addition. Drug was included during the zymosan exposure period. To test for drug reversibility cells were rinsed in drug-free medium and incubated an additional 30 min. At the indicated time, cells were rinsed and fixed, and surface-accessible zymosan was stained with Rh-Con A as described in Materials and Methods. ND — not determined.
[a]Mean of three separate experiments.

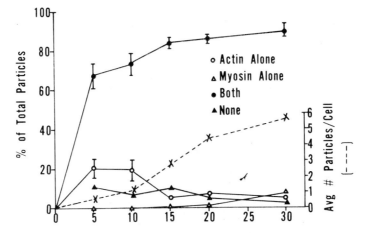

Fig. 8. Kinetic analysis of the actin-myosin response to zymosan challenge in mouse macrophage monolayers. Adherent cells on glass coverslips were challenged with serum-treated zymosan at time zero. At indicated times, cells were fixed with 2% formaldehyde for 20 min and immunofluorescently stained for actin and myosin. At least 200 particles were microscopically scored for a dectable response for actin alone (o——o); myosin alone (△——△); both actin and myosin (●——●); or no detectable staining (▲——▲). The average number of cell-associated particles was likewise determined (– – –). Average of three separate experiments ± SEM.

    The data indicate that the two contractile proteins accumulated rapidly at regions associated with adherent particles at a time prior to any significant engulfment by the cell (see Table I). In addition, the data suggest that actin may associate slightly faster than myosin, since there is a significant and reproducible percentage (20%) of particles at 10–15 min which have only actin associated with them.* At later times this value diminished nearly to zero with a corresponding increase in the percentage of particles with both proteins associated. Particles with associated myosin but no detectable actin (△——△) were only rarely seen.

    At later times after particle addition (> 30 min) cells contained too many particles for accurate quantitation. However, at these later time points, clusters of particles were seen (generally over the cell nucleus) which no longer stained for actin or myosin (Fig. 9).

DISCUSSION

    The data presented here indicate that two major macrophage contractile proteins, F-actin and myosin, accumulate rapidly at phagocytic sites. Detailed kinetic analysis and morphologic evidence further suggest that the observed regional contractile protein response clearly precedes the ultimate engulfment of membrane-associated particles (Figs. 7 and 8).

    The specificity of the reagents used in these studies is worthy of comment. First, the BHMM/F1-Av technique has been shown to be highly specific for actin [8]. In addition, unlike antiactin antibodies which have been used by others [7, 20] to localize actin, the B-HMM reagent is specific for F-actin but not G-actin [21].

---

*Such a result could also be explained by a difference in the sensitivities of the two fluorescent reagents for their respective target proteins.

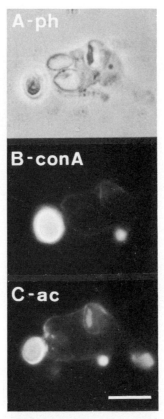

Fig. 9. Con A (B) and actin (C) distributions in a macrophage containing a cluster of zymosan. (A, phase contrast.) This cell was fixed and stained 1 h after particle challenge. Note that the adjacent particle at the cell periphery is stained for actin while those within the cluster are completely unstained. The fluorescence associated with the particle core is a nonspecific autofluorescence. × 1,250; bar = 10 μm.

The use of antibodies for the localization of myosin by immunofluorescence has led to conflicting results in some cases. For example, myosin has been detected on the surface of platelets [22] and fibroblasts [23] by some investigators but not by others using different antibody preparations [24, 25]. The latter result was also found to be the case in these studies. Since these differences could be explained by the presence of antibodies to trace impurities, such as glycolipids, we have extensively characterized the antibody preparation used in these studies. The evidence for monospecificity includes the demonstration of a single line of identity between the highly purified antigen and the crude extract used for preparation of the antigen (Fig. 1A). This reacting antibody species is removed by pre-absorbsion of the antibody with myosin-Sepharose 4B (Fig. 1B). Furthermore, direct staining of SDS gels of the crude extract with ^{125}I-antimyosin labeled only one major protein species which comigrated with myosin heavy chain (Fig. 2). Since this technique is probably an order of magnitude more sensitive than immunofluorescence we conclude that myosin is the major fluorescent species detected in our studies.

The actin and myosin distributions seen in mouse peritoneal macrophages is similar to those noted by others in cultured fibroblasts [8, 20]. The only striking difference that we have noted is the absence of actin-containing "stress fibers" seen in many other cultured cell types. The reason for this is unclear but could conceivably be related to the higher motility rate of this cell type compared with fibroblasts.

In macrophages that are phagocytosing particles the data show that both myosin and actin are associated with and concentrate at phagocytic sites. Unlike the more uniform actin distribution around the phagosome vacuole, the myosin distribution seen is discontinuous or "patchy" (Fig. 5C). This pattern is somewhat reminiscent of myosin staining patterns seen directly underlying capped Ig receptors [26] in B lymphocytes, and it is consistent with the suggestion that phagocytosis and capping are related processes [7].

Our data indicate that actin concentrates at sites in close opposition to particle-cell interactions shortly after the particle has made receptor-mediated contact with the cell surface (Fig. 7F). This initial response of the contractile apparatus continues to propagate outward from the point of initial contact as more of the particle surface comes in contact with the cell surface. Pseudopods, rich in actin and myosin, begin to extend around the particle, becoming so firmly attached to membrane receptors that Rh-Con A is unable to penetrate such regions (Fig. 7B, broken arrow). The close association of the contractile apparatus at phagocytic sites from the point of first contact throughout all phases of the engulfment process is consistent with a major role for this cytoplasmic system in the engulfment phase of the process. Our data also suggest that, in addition to an involvement in the engulfment phase per se, the contractile apparatus may also function to move completely ingested particles within the cell cytoplasm since their association with the phagosome persists after ingestion is completed.

It could be argued that the apparent concentration of actin and myosin with phagosomal vacuoles is due to a path-length effect. Thus, a large particle surrounded by long vertical pseudopodal extensions which contain normal cytoplasmic concentrations of actin and myosin would be expected to show an increased fluorescence when compared to other thinner cell regions. This possibility is ruled out by several lines of evidence. First, cytochalasin B (a drug which prevents pseudopod extension but not particle adhesion to the cell surface [27]) does *not* block the concentration of actin or myosin at cell regions directly underlying the peripheral regions of particle-binding sites (Fig. 5D–F). Second, electron microscope studies of CB-treated cells with attached zymosan show little evidence of pseudopod extension around the particle surface and in fact contain dense regions of microfilaments which underly the vicinity of the particle-membrane binding site (Fig. 6). Finally, increased concentrations of actin are seen which underly particles well before significant pseudopod extension has occurred (Fig. 7F, arrow).

Thus, the observed concentration of these two contractile proteins at particle-binding sites which lack pseudopod extensions rules out gross path-length effects and indicates that particle binding is associated with a localized increase in actin and myosin which *precedes* pseudopod extension and ultimate ingestion.

At present, it is unclear whether the observed actin concentration at such sites represents assembly of F-actin filaments or simply a redistribution of filaments from other cell regions. Nevertheless, the observed highly regional response of the contractile system to a local membrane perturbation places severe restraints upon the nature of any transmembrane signal(s) which may exist to communicate the particle's presence to the contractile apparatus of the cell. Our current data are consistent with a recent suggestion advanced by Bourguignon and Singer [28] that aggregation of surface receptors by a multivalent ligand (a large particle in this case) induces the association of an as yet unidentified actin-binding membrane component (X) with such receptor "patches" leading in turn to actin binding at that site. If their suggestions are correct, on the basis of our data, one would expect to find X in high concentration in isolated phagosomal membranes.

ACKNOWLEDGMENTS

This study was supported in part by grant AI-07007; this article is publication No. 1805 of Scripps Clinic and Research Foundation. RGP is the recipient of National Institutes of Health Research Career Development Award No. AM-00437.

The authors would like to thank Drs. Mark Ginsberg and Charles Cochrane for their critical comments and suggestions. We also thank Mr. Jim Smith and Ms Linda Kitabayashi for their expert help with the electron microscope studies.

REFERENCES

1. Korn ED: Proc Natl Acad Sci USA 75:588, 1978.
2. Stossel TP: J Reticuloendothel Soc 19:237, 1976.
3. Silverstein SC, Steinman RM, Cohn ZA: Annu Rev Biochem 46:669, 1977.
4. Griffin FM Jr, Silverstein SC: J Exp Med 139:323, 1974.
5. Griffin FM Jr, Bianco C, Silverstein SC: J Exp Med 141:1269, 1975.
6. Keyserlingk DG: Exp Cell Res 51:79, 1968.
7. Berlin RJ, Oliver JM: J Cell Biol 77:789, 1978.
8. Heggeness MH, Ash JF: J Cell Biol 73:783, 1977.
9. Pollard TD, Thomas SM, Niederman, R: Anal Biochem 60:258, 1974.
10. Wang K: Biochemistry 16:1857, 1977.
11. Nisonoff A, Wissler FC, Woernley DL: Biochem Biophys Res Commun 1:318, 1959.
12. McConahey P, Dixon FJ: Int Arch Allergy Appl Immunol 29:185, 1966.
13. Russell SW, Doe WF, Hoskins RG, Cochrane CG: Int J Cancer 18:322, 1976.
14. Heggeness MH, Wang K, Singer SJ: Proc Natl Acad Sci USA 74:3883, 1977.
15. Maupin-Szamier P, Pollard TD: J Cell Biol 77:837, 1978.
16. Laemmli UK: Nature 227:680, 1970.
17. Burridge K: Proc Natl Acad Sci USA 73:4157, 1976.
18. Wallach D, Davies PJA, Pastan I: J Biol Chem 253:3328, 1978.
19. Heitzmann H, Richards FM: Proc Natl Acad Sci USA 71:3537, 1974.
20. Pollack R, Osborn M, Weber K: Proc Natl Acad Sci USA 72:994, 1975.
21. Offer G, Baker H, Baker L: J Mol Biol 66:435, 1972.
22. Puszkin EG, Maldonado R, Spaet TH, Zucker MB: J Biol Chem 252:4371, 1977.
23. Willingham MC, Ostland RE, Pastan I: Proc Natl Acad Sci USA 71:4144, 1974.
24. Pollard TD, Fujiwara K, Handin R, Weiss G: Ann NY Acad Sci 283:218, 1977.
25. Painter RG, Sheetz M, Singer SJ: Proc Natl Acad Sci USA 72:1359, 1975.
26. Schreiner GF, Fujiwara K, Pollard TD, Unanue ER: J Exp Med 145:1393, 1977.
27. Axline SG, Reaven EP: J Cell Biol 62:647, 1974.
28. Bourguignon LY, Singer SJ: Proc Natl Acad Sci USA 74:5031, 1977.

Journal of Supramolecular Structure 12:385—402 (1979)
Tumor Cell Surfaces and Malignancy 675—692

Tumor-Associated Antigenic Differences Between the Primary and the Descendant Metastatic Tumor Cell Populations

Eliezer Gorelik, Mina Fogel, Shraga Segal, and Michael Feldman

Department of Cell Biology, The Weizmann Institute of Science, Rehovot, Israel

The existence of antigenic differences between cell populations in the local growth of the 3LL tumor (L-3LL) and its lung metastases (M-3LL) was studied. Normal C57BL/6 spleen cells sensitized in vitro for 5 days against L-3LL monolayers lysed preferentially L-3LL targets but not M-3LL tumor cell targets. Conversely, anti-M-3LL-sensitized lymphocytes killed M-3LL targets more efficiently than they killed L-3LL targets. Furthermore, spleen cells from mice bearing subcutaneous L-3LL tumors were significantly more cytotoxic to L-3LL targets than to M-3LL targets and vice versa. M-3LL cells were found also to be more resistant in vitro and in vivo to natural killer cells than were L-3LL tumor cells. M-3LL cells were more resistant than L-3LL cells to hybrid resistant mechanisms when they were inoculated into F_1 (C3Heb $\times$ C57BL/6) or F_1 (BALB/c $\times$ C57BL/6) mice. Anti-M-3LL lymphocytes generated both in vitro and in vivo, but not anti-L-3LL lymphocytes, admixed with L-3LL or M-3LL tumor cells and inoculated into footpads of syngeneic recipients suppressed the development of lung metastases. These results suggest that metastatic cells are indeed phenotypic variants of the local growing tumor cell populations. Presumably, these variants are selected for their capacity to home to and grow in the lungs, and for their resistance to specific immune effects initially evoked against the local tumor and to nonspecific natural killer cells. These data may prove to be of importance with respect to any rational approach to the problem of immunotherapy.

Key words: hybrid resistance, NK cells, cytotoxic lymphocytes, tumor-associated antigens, primary and metastatic tumor cells, immunoselection

The hope that immunologic methods may become extremely effective in the treatment of cancer patients is based on the notion that specific tumor-associated antigens are expressed on the tumor cell surface and that the host responds specifically against the progressing tumor.

Abbreviations used in this text: CL, cytotoxic lymphocytes; FCS, fetal calf serum; FUdR, fluorodeoxyuridine; ^{125}IUdR, ^{125}I-deoxyuridine; L-3LL, local growing 3LL tumor; M-3LL metastasis-derived tumor cells; NK, natural killer cells; SMS, syngeneic mouse serum; TBM, tumor-bearing mice.

Received May 30, 1979, accepted October 22, 1979.

One may expect that these methods will be specially effective in the prevention of metastatic progression following surgical removal of the primary tumor mass. The search for appropriate immunotherapeutic methods has been intensified [1]. Modern immuno-therapeutic approaches are based either on nonspecific stimulation of the immune system of the host or on the specific immunization of the organism against tumor cells originating in the surgically removed tumor. These immunization procedures are expected to stimulate the development of cytotoxic lymphocytes or antibodies which are capable of inhibiting tumor growth and destroying metastatic tumor cells. Another experimental approach to immunotherapy is based on the adoptive transfer to the diseased host of lymphocytes sensitized in vitro against tumor cells [1, 18].

All of the above-mentioned specific immunotherapeutic methods are based on the assumption that tumor cells originating in metastases are copies phenotypically identical to those tumor cells found in the primary tumor tissues and therefore that tumor cells originating in primary and metastatic tumors are expected to share identical tumor-associated cell surface antigens. Despite that attractive assumption, given the fact that most of the malignant tumors are heteroploid, one is forced to reexamine the validity of the above concept. Obviously the question is raised whether indeed metastatic cells are random representatives of the primary tumor cell population or whether they are selected out of a diverse population. The fact that tumor cells are characterized by impaired chromosome replication and segregation furnishes the basis for the generation of diversity among the primary tumor cell population. Such diversity may determine heterogeneity in genetic and phenotypic properties which in turn may furnish the basis for selective processes. In view of the above-mentioned immunotherapy goals, this question is of obvious importance. Variant cells with a higher probability of metastasis formation could be selected out [2]. Such an increased capacity for metastatic growth could be based a) on an increased probability of cell migration, b) on increased affinity for certain tissues, c) on preferential growth in the new tissue environment [2–5], and d) on resistance of the metastatic cells to the host's immune response directed against the primary tumor [6].

Indeed, recent studies have indicated that metastases may differ from the primary tumor cell population in a number of properties. Thus, differences in drug susceptibility [7], affinity to various organs [4, 5], chromosome number [8, 9], and some biochemical properties [10] have been observed.

The progression of metastasis may be a function of properties both of the host and of the neoplastic cells. Thus, it has been demonstrated that activation or suppression of the host's immune reactivity may result in decrease or increase of metastatic progression [11–13].

Metastatic spread may conceivably take place in organisms which respond immunologically against the primary tumor. The initial small populations of metastatic cells could escape immune destruction if their cell surface tumor antigens were different from those of the primary cell population. Immunoselection, as the basis for metastatic spread, would then predict that cells of tumor metastases differed antigenically from cells of the primary tumor. Furthermore, it has become clear in recent years that in addition to specific antigen-reactive lymphocytes, other lymphocytes manifesting cytotoxic effects against various types of tumors exist in the circulation and in various lymphoid organs [14–17]. These natural killer (NK) cells could then be effective against circulating tumor cells which could otherwise develop metastatic nodules. It seemed, therefore, of interest to test whether cells derived from established metastatic nodules are different from tumor cells of the local primary growth in their susceptibility to the harmful effects of specific cytotoxic lymphoid cells as well as to NK cells. Such differences may be relevant to the control mechanisms involved in metastatic spread and growth.

We approached the problem of the possible diversity existing among primary and metastatic tumor cells by investigating the highly metastasizing Lewis lung carcinoma (3LL). Our investigation was aimed at testing a) antigenic and immunogenic differences existing between cells obtained from the local site of transplantation (L-3LL) and those cells obtained from metastases (M-3LL) which generally appear in the lungs of tumor-bearing mice; and b) the existence of differences in susceptibility of L-3LL and M-3LL tumor cells to the harmful activity of NK cells.

MATERIALS AND METHODS

Mice

Inbred male C57BL/6, C3H/eB, BALB/c mice (2–3 months old) and their F_1 hybrids F_1 (C3HeB × C57BL/6) or F_1 (BALB/c × C57BL/6) and C3H/eB/nu$^+$/nu$^+$ mice, were supplied by the Animal Breeding Center of the Weizmann Institute of Science. In some experiments C57BL/6 "B" mice were used. These were prepared as follows: Two-month-old C57BL mice were thymectomized; 1 month later they were irradiated (850 R) and reconstituted with $2 × 10^6$ normal bone marrow cells. Two months following reconstitution, the presence of NK cells in the spleen was tested.

Tumors

Lewis lung carcinoma (3LL) was maintained by subcutaneous (SC) transfers of $1 × 10^6$ tumor cells into syngeneic mice. The 3LL tumor produces metastases in the lungs following SC, intramuscular or intra-footpad (IFP) transplantation. Cell suspensions from solid tumors were prepared by treatment of minced tumor tissue with a solution of 0.3% trypsin (hog pancrease; Nutritional Biochemicals Corp., Cleveland, Ohio) [18]. The trypsin-treated cells were washed three times with phosphate buffered saline (PBS), pH 7.4, and resuspended in PBS for inoculation.

To obtain metastasis-derived tumor cells (M-3LL), $1 × 10^5$ 3LL tumor cells were inoculated in the hind footpads of C57BL/6 mice. Twenty-one days later mice were sacrificed and the developed pulmonary metastases were excised. In some experiments metastases were obtained from the lungs of mice 10–12 days following surgical removal of the local IFP growing tumor (8–10 mm in diameter). Tumor cell suspensions were prepared by trypsin treatment as above, and after PBS washing $1 × 10^6$ tumor cells were inoculated SC into normal C57BL/6 mice. The cells derived from these tumors after a single SC transfer only were used as M-3LL. In parallel, $1 × 10^6$ tumor cells obtained from the local 3LL SC transplanted tumor were inoculated SC to another group of mice and provided a source for the isolation of the local tumor growth (L-3LL).

Preparation of Sensitizing Monolayers

Subcutaneously growing M-3LL and L-3LL tumors were excised and suspensions of tumor cells were obtained by trypsin digestion The cells were washed three times with PBS and suspended in Waymouth's medium; then $5 × 10^6$ tumor cells were seeded in 50-mm tissue culture plates (Falcon, 3002).

Preparation of Spleen Cells

Spleens from normal mice were removed aseptically, placed in cold PBS, and pressed through a fine stainless steel mesh. The cell suspensions obtained were washed twice with PBS, counted, and resuspended in RPMI-1640. The medium was supplemented with 1% fresh syngeneic mouse serum (SMS) [19].

Sensitization of Spleen Cells

The tumor cell monolayers were treated with 40 μg/ml of mitomycin C for 2 h, then washed twice with PBS and incubated for another 2 h with RPMI plus 1% syngeneic mouse serum. Then 30–40 $\times$ 10^6 splenic lymphocytes were suspended in 4 ml of RPMI-1640 and supplemented with 1% fresh SMS and 5 $\times$ 10^{-5} M 2-mercaptoethanol and seeded on top of the sensitizing monolayers. The lymphocytes were sensitized for 5 days at 37°C in a 10% CO_2 humidified air incubator.

On the 5th day, the sensitized lymphocytes were collected by gentle pipetting and separated from contaminating tumor cells by centrifugation in fetal calf serum. The collected cells were centrifuged and resuspended in undiluted fetal calf serum at a concentration of 10^7 cells/ml. This suspension was sedimented by centrifugation for 4 min at 6.5g and the cells in the supernatant were collected. These lymphocytes were washed three times with PBS and counted by trypan blue exclusion. By this process 15–30% of the initial number of lymphocytes cultured were usually recovered. Control normal lymphocytes were cultured for 5 days in the absence of a sensitizing monolayer.

Cytotoxic Activity of Cytotoxic Lymphocytes Generated In Vivo

The cytotoxic activity of splenic lymphocytes originating in tumor-bearing mice was tested following their precultivation for 2 days in vitro in the absence of sensitizing monolayers to "unmask" their cytotoxic activity [20].

In Vitro Assay of Natural Killer (NK) Cell Activity

The cytotoxicity exerted by normal spleen cells was tested against L-3LL and M-3LL target tumor cells by the same methods used in the assay of immune cytotoxic lymphocytes.

In Vitro Assay of Lymphocyte Cytotoxicity

We used the method described by Takasugi and Klein [21], as modified by More et al [22]. Briefly, 100,000 trypsinized tumor cells were pipetted into wells of microtiter plates (Nunclon-Delta flat-bottom Micro-Test tissue culture plates No. 1480). The cells were incubated for 24 h to permit adherence. The medium was then discarded and the target cells were washed three times with PBS. Following the last PBS wash, 10 control wells were trypsinized and the number of adherent cells was determined. Under these conditions, approximately 10% of the initial cell inoculum adhered to the bottom of the culture wells. Then the sensitized and control unsensitized lymphocytes were seeded (at various ratios relative to the final number of monolayer cells) into the wells. Cultures were incubated for 18 h at 37°C, the supernatants were removed, and each well received 50 μl Na$_2$ ^{51}CrO$_4$ solution (Radiochemical Centre, Amersham, Bucks., UK), diluted in 0.4 M sucrose (5 μCi ^{51}Cr). The cultures were then incubated for 45 min at 37°C. The plates were stored on ice, washed, and then treated with 100 μl of 0.1 N NaOH for 10 min. The percentage of cytotoxicity was calculated according to the following formula:

$$\% \text{ lysis} = 1 - \frac{\text{cpm with test lymphocytes}}{\text{cpm with medium}} \times 100.$$

The percentage of cytotoxicity was expressed in negative values. Positive values represent increased uptake of isotope in test wells compared to control wells. Each percentage lysis value is based on six replicate samples.

In Vivo Assay for Tumor Growth

The immune or normal spleen cells were mixed with 2×10^4 M-3LL or L-3LL tumor cells at various ratios and the mixtures were grafted into hind footpads of syngeneic mice. Control mice were grafted with tumor cells alone. The grafted mice were examined daily and the number of animals with visible palpable tumors were measured. Mice were sacrificed on day 21 following tumor inoculation; their lungs were removed and fixed in Bouin's solution. Visible metastases detected on the surface of the lungs were counted.

In some experiments the development of pulmonary metastases was assessed by determination of the degree of incorporation of ^{125}IUdR into the tested lungs; in these experiments we used mice in which the local IFP growing tumors, 8–10 mm in diameter, were surgically removed. Eleven days following tumor excision mice were inoculated with 25 μg/mouse of FUdR and 30 min later with 1 μCi of ^{125}IUdR [23]. Twenty-four hours following ^{125}IUdR injection the weight of lungs with metastases was determined and in parallel the degree of ^{125}IUdR incorporation by the malignant cells into the lungs was measured with a Packard Gamma Spectrometer. The significance of differences between various experimental groups was assessed using the Mann-Whitney U test [35].

RESULTS

In a previous study [19] we found that in vitro sensitization of lymphocytes against monolayers of syngeneic tumors carried out in culture media containing xenogeneic serum such as fetal calf serum (FCS) results in cytotoxic lymphocytes (CL) directed mainly against FCS determinants rather than against the actual cell surface tumor-associated antigens. We therefore studied the generation of CL when sensitization against syngeneic tumors was carried out in the presence of SMS. We demonstrated [19] that sensitization in SMS results in CL manifesting strict specificities against the tumor antigens.

Having found such strict antitumor specificities, we turned to test whether cells of the local growth of the 3LL tumor (L-3LL) possess antigenic specificities different from those of the metastatic population (M-3LL). We examined the specificity of the cytotoxic activity manifested by lymphocytes sensitized against monolayers of M-3LL compared to lymphocytes sensitized against L-3LL monolayers. The results described (Table I), summarizing three separate experiments, indicated that lymphocytes sensitized in fresh syngeneic mouse serum against monolayers of L-3LL lysed L-3LL targets significantly more than they lysed M-3LL cells. The activity against the L-3LL targets was very high, since even at ratios of lymphocytes to targets of 12.5:1 we got high levels of cytotoxicity. Conversely, lymphocytes sensitized against M-3LL cells lysed M-3LL targets significantly more than they lysed L-3LL targets. It appears, therefore, that each of these tumor populations is characterized, in addition to shared determinants, by specific cell surface antigens.

The specificity we obtained against metastatic cells in the experiments outlined above was manifested following sensitization in cell culture. The question arose whether the antigenic differences between M-3LL and L-3LL detected in vitro were not the result of in vitro cultivation of tumor cells. To answer this question, we investigated whether similar immunogenic differences between M-3LL and L-3LL are manifested in vivo, in the tumor-bearing mouse (TBM).

In earlier experiments, we found that freshly removed lymphoid cells from TBM are generally devoid of antitumor cytotoxic activity. Therefore, we incubated the spleen cells derived from TBM grafted with L-3LL or M-3LL cells for 48 h in the absence of sensitizing monolayer, to "unmask" their cytotoxic activity. The "unmasked" cytotoxic lymphocytes were then cross-tested for their cytotoxic activity against M-3LL and L-3LL tumor cells. We found (Table II) that splenic lymphocytes from mice bearing the L-3LL tumor lysed L-3LL targets significantly more than they lysed M-3LL targets. Conversely, cytotoxic lymphocytes from M-3LL TBM manifested an extent of lysis against M-3LL targets that was significantly higher than the lysis obtained against L-3LL targets.

These results indicate that the M-3LL and L-3LL grown in vivo express antigenic differences similar to those demonstrated by the in vitro analysis.

TABLE I. Specificity of Cytotoxic Activity of Syngeneic C57BL/6 Spleen Cells Sensitized In Vitro Against Local (L-3LL) or Metastatic Derived (M-3LL) Tumor Cells

Sensitizing tumor cells	Target tumor cells	Net % lysis at lymphocyte-to-target-cell ratio of:				
		Expt. 1		Expt. 2		Expt. 3
		25:1	12.5:1	25:1	12.5:1	25:1
L-3LL	L-3LL	−54.6	−57.6	−49.3	−31.1	−45.7
L-3LL	M-3LL	−13.1	+ 4.4	− 5.2	− 0.4	− 3.7
M-3LL	M-3LL	−21.5	−31.4	−47.1	−46.5	−37.1
M-3LL	L-3LL	− 9.2	− 4.2	− 7.0	− 9.5	− 8.2

Normal C57BL/6 spleen cells were sensitized in vitro for 5 days on monolayers of L-3LL and M-3LL tumor cells. Negative values of cytotoxicity represent cell-mediated lysis by sensitized lymphocytes above the values obtained by unsensitized spleen cells.

TABLE II. Lytic Activity of Cytotoxic Lymphocytes Generated in M-3LL or L-3LL Tumor-Bearing Mice Against M-3LL and L-3LL Cells

Spleen cell donors[a]	Tumor target cells	Expt. 1		Expt. 2	
		Ratio of lymphocytes to targets	% net lysis	Ratio of lymphocytes to targets	% net lysis
L-3LL TBM	L-3LL	25 :1	−46	20:1	−30
		12.5:1	−25	10:1	− 6
M-3LL TBM	L-3LL	25 :1	− 8	20:1	−17
		12.5:1	− 1.4	10:1	+ 1
L-3LL TBM	M-3LL	25 :1	− 6	20:1	−12
		12.5:1	+ 7	10:1	+14
M-3LL TBM	M-3LL	25 :1	−27	20:1	−21
		12.5:1	− 1.2	10:1	−25

[a]Spleen cells were cultivated for 2 days in vitro without any sensitized monolayer.

The specificity we obtained against metastatic cells, using in vitro cytotoxicity assays, raised the question of whether anti-M-3LL cytotoxic lymphocytes generated in vitro or anti-M-3LL lymphocytes in M-3LL TBM are capable of suppressing the development of metastases in vivo. To test this we injected into the footpad either anti-L-3LL or anti-M-3LL in vitro-sensitized lymphocytes admixed with 2×10^4 L-3LL or M-3LL cells, at lymphocytes-to-tumor cell ratios of 25:1 or 12.5:1. We found no significant differences in growth of the local tumor at these cell ratios. However, when testing for the incidence of lung metastases at 21 days following cell inoculation, we found (Table III) that anti-L-3LL cytotoxic lymphocytes did not reduce the incidence of metastases produced by L-3LL cells (if anything, they increased the number of lung metastases). On the other hand, anti-M-3LL caused a significant reduction of metastases produced following the inoculation with L-3LL. A dramatic reduction was obtained at ratios of 25:1 lymphocytes to tumor cells. The effect of anti-L-3LL and anti-M-3LL cytotoxic lymphocytes on the production of metastases by M-3LL cells was also tested. Here again, anti-L-3LL cells did not reduce the incidence of lung metastases, whereas anti-M-3LL cytotoxic lymphocytes caused a reduction at lymphocyte-to-tumor-cell ratios of 25:1 and 12.5:1.

The "unmasked" cytotoxic lymphocytes obtained from spleens on the 14th day following SC inoculation with 1×10^6 L-3LL or M-3LL tumor cells were tested for their ability to suppress the development of metastases in vivo. "Unmasked" cytotoxic lymphocytes derived from either L-3LL or M-3LL tumor-bearing mice were mixed with 2×10^4 L-3LL or M-3LL cells at a ratio of 50:1 or 25:1 spleen cells to tumor cells and inoculated into the hind footpads of normal syngeneic recipients. When tumors reached 8–10 mm in diameter, the primary tumor was excised by amputation of the tumor-bearing leg. Twelve days following excision, mice were sacrificed and their lungs were examined for metastasis development (Table IV). Metastatic growth in the lungs was assayed by both weighing the lungs and measuring their ^{125}IUdR incorporation. In mice that had been inoculated IFP with L-3LL tumor cells and spleen cells of mice bearing L-3LL tumors (at ratios of 1:25 and 1:50), the metastatic growth in the lungs was accelerated, but the same spleen cells

TABLE III. Anti-M-3LL Lymphocyte Suppression of the Development of Lung Metastases

Sensitizing tumor cells	Transplanted tumor cells		No. of pulmonary metastases at ratios of sensitized lymphocytes to tumor cells equal to:	
			25:1	12.5:1
	Control, L-3LL cells alone			19.6
None	L-3LL		21.7	27.3
L-3LL	L-3LL		28.6	35.2
M-3LL	L-3LL		3[a]	17.8
	Control, M-3LL cells alone			21.1
None	M-3LL		42.4	N.T.
L-3LL	M-3LL		52[a]	42
M-3LL	M-3LL		7.7[a]	3.5[a]

Normal C57BL/6 syngeneic spleen cells were sensitized in vitro for 5 days on monolayers of primary local 3LL (L-3LL) and pulmonary metastasis-derived (M-3LL) carcinoma cells, in the presence of 1% syngeneic mouse serum. Sensitized cells were collected and transplanted at various ratios, together with either M-3LL, or L-3LL tumor cells, intra-footpad. The number of lung metastases was counted 21 days later. Each experimental group contained 10 mice.
[a]Differs significantly from control group according to Mann-Whitney U test (P < 0.05).

inoculated IFP admixed with M-3LL tumor cells failed to influence the development of metastases in the lungs of these mice (Table IV). Conversely, spleen cells originating in M-3LL-bearing mice manifested a slight inhibition of metastases when inoculated together with L-3LL tumor cells, but a high suppressing effect on metastases was observed when these "unmasked" cells were inoculated together with M-3LL tumor cells (Table IV).

Recent studies have suggested that nonspecific mechanisms mediated by cellular components of the immune system, namely naturally occurring killer cells (NK cells), may have a decisive function in controlling tumor development [14–17]. We therefore suggest that metastatic cells are not exempt from the defense mechanism and may be equally susceptible to injury by NK cells. Thus, it is expected that only a resistant fraction of tumor cells which survive in the blood and in various organs or tissues may be the main cellular source for initiation of distant metastases. Hence, it seemed of interest to investigate whether, indeed, cells of tumor metastases and those of the local tumor manifest differences with regard to susceptibility to the cytotoxic activity of NK cells. For that purpose experiments using different in vitro and in vivo approaches were performed to test the relative resistance of M-3LL and L-3LL tumor cells to injury by normal lymphoid cells.

The data described in Table V show that normal spleen cells are capable of killing 3LL tumor cells. The cytotoxic effect was exhibited by both freshly isolated normal spleen cells (Table V) and normal spleen cells cultured in vitro for 2 or 5 days (Tables VI,

TABLE IV. Suppression by Spleen Cells From Mice Bearing M-3LL Tumors, of Metastastic Growth in the Lungs of Tumor-Bearing Recipients

Treatment	Ratio between tumor and spleen cells	No. of mice	Weight of lungs, mg	cpm
L-3LL	–	10	438	13,635
L-3LL + Spleen N	1:25	10	424	12,433
	1:50	10	482	14,008
L-3LL + Spleen L-3LL	1:25	7	706[a]	21,403
	1:50	9	626[a]	25,672[a]
L-3LL + Spleen M-3LL	1:25	9	613	23,858
	1:50	8	355[a]	6,943[a]
M-3LL	–	10	671	25,338
M-3LL + Spleen N	1:25	9	703	29,189
	1:50	10	550[a]	13,467[a]
M-3LL + Spleen L-3LL	1:25	8	660	28,083
	1:50	9	584	17,060
M-3LL + Spleen M-3LL	1:25	10	547	19,759
	1:50	10	476[a]	9,892[a]

L-3LL or M-3LL tumor cells (1×10^6) were inoculated SC. On the 14th day of tumor growth spleen cells originating in these mice were cultivated in vitro for 2 days. These spleen cells were then collected and admixed at the above-described ratio with 2×10^4 L-3LL or 2×10^4 M-3LL tumor cells and inoculated IFP. The subsequently developed local tumors measuring 8–10 mm in diameter were removed, and 11 days following tumor excision mice were inoculated with 1 μCi of ^{125}IUdR, 24 h later mice were killed and both weight of lungs and radioactivity of lungs were determined.
[a]Differs significantly from control group, according to Mann-Whitney U test (P < 0.05).

VII). This cytotoxic effect of normal spleen cells was dose-dependent, eg, a clear increase in cytotoxicity was obtained by increasing the ratio of spleen to tumor cells in the microculture wells.

In parallel, experiments performed with M-3LL target cells presented in Tables V—VII clearly show that metastasis-derived tumor cells (M-3LL) were more resistant to the cytotoxic activity of normal spleen cells than L-3LL tumor cells.

Resistance of M-3LL cells to NK cells of freshly isolated spleen cells was similar to the resistance against spleen cells cultured for 2 or 5 days. In view of numerous works which have demonstrated that the cytotoxic activity of normal lymphoid cells is mainly mediated by NK cells [14—17], experiments were performed to characterize the nature of the effector cells involved in the cytotoxic injury to 3LL tumor cells. Results presented in Table VIII clearly demonstrate that spleen cells derived from either B mice or nude mice, or normal spleen cells treated by anti-Thy 1.2 serum and guinea pig complement, are still efficient in performing their cytotoxic activity against 3LL tumor cells. These characteristics are similar to those described for NK cells by other workers in the field [14, 24]. Thus, these results indicate that natural killer cells directed against the 3LL tumor are present in the spleen of immunologically intact C57BL/6 mice and are not eliminated during 2—5 days of in vitro culturing. The results indicate the existence of differences in the level of cytotoxic activity of NK cells between experiments (Tables V—VII). We attribute these differences to individual shifts in the spleen cell populations.

To test whether the differences in sensitivity of M-3LL and L-3LL tumor cells to the cytotoxic effects of NK cells observed in vitro have any in vivo significance, we tested the capacity of spleen cells derived from normal animals to inhibit the development of

TABLE V. Sensitivity of L-3LL and M-3LL Tumor Cells to the Cytotoxic Action of Fresh Unsensitized Normal Spleen Cells of C57BL/6 Mice

Expt. No.	Ratio between tumor and spleen cells	Target cells	
		L-3LL	M-3LL
1	1:200	−57.5	−19.0
	1:100	−35.6	−21.9
	1:50	−33.6	−14.9
	1:25	−28.8	−18.3
2	1:50	−40.0	−11.4
	1:25	−12.0	− 7.0
3	1:50	−17.0	−14.0
	1:25	− 6.0	+ 0.5
	1:12	+ 0.3	+19.0
4	1:50	−35.8	−16.0
	1:25	−21.9	− 5.2
5	1:200	−29.3	−15.4
	1:100	−23.3	−13.7

Fresh normal spleen cells of C57BL/6 mice were put into the wells on the monolayer of L-3LL or M-3LL tumor cells. Following 18 h survival, part of monolayers were labeled with ^{51}Cr. Negative values represent reduced uptake of isotope in test wells (as a result of cytotoxic activity) compared to control wells. Positive values represent increased uptake of isotope in test wells compared to control wells.

either M-3LL or L-3LL cells in intact syngeneic mice. M-3LL and L-3LL tumor cells were prepared and 2×10^4 cells of each tumor cell suspension were admixed with syngeneic normal spleen cells at a ratio of 1:25–1:200 tumor to spleen cells.

The mixture was inoculated into the hind footpads of syngeneic recipients. The development of tumors was assayed by recording the day of tumor appearance and tumor diameter, at various time intervals (Fig. 1a, b; Fig. 2a, b). The results (Fig. 1a, b) indicate an inhibition of L-3LL tumor growth when the ratio of inoculated tumor to spleen cells was 1:50 and 1:100. On the other hand, spleen cells enhanced the growth of M-3LL tumor cells at tumor to spleen cell ratios of 1:25 and 1:50 and inhibited the growth of M-3LL tumor cells only when the ratio of spleen to tumor cells was 1:100. Yet even at this ratio (1:100) normal spleen cells inhibited L-3LL cells significantly more than they inhibited M-3LL tumor cells. The percentage of inhibition of L-3LL tumors was 51–57%, whereas that of M-3LL tumors was only 25–26%.

In the subsequent experiments, ratios of 1:25–1:50 failed to influence the growth of L-3LL cells (Fig. 2a, b). Inhibition of L-3LL cells was observed only when the ratio between tumor cells and spleen cells reached 1:100–1:200. On the other hand, normal spleen cells mixed with M-3LL cells in a ratio of 1:25 accelerated tumor growth and had no significant influence on the development of M-3LL tumor cells when the ratios were 1:50 and 1:100. Only when the ratios reached 1:200 was a slight retardation of tumor growth obtained. At this high tumor to spleen cell ratio of 1:200, the growth inhibition of L-3LL tumor cells was 40–50% compared to 20–26% for M-3LL cells.

Since hybrid resistance and NK activity have common characteristics [25, 26] and since we aimed at testing the possible role of the MHC system in determining the relative resistance to L-3LL cells and their metastatic descendants, we studied a) in vitro NK activity against L-3LL and M-3LL cells and spleen cells from parental and F_1 origin and b) the

TABLE VI. Sensitivity of L-3LL and M-3LL Tumor Cells to the Cytotoxic Action of Normal Unsensitized Spleen Cells Cultured for 2 Days

Expt. No.	Ratio of tumor-to-spleen cells	Target cells	
		L-3LL	M-3LL
1	1:100	−51.5	−27.4
	1:50	−43.1	−14.0
	1:25	−28.8	−14.4
	1:12	−24.5	− 0.3
2	1:50	−31.7	−17.3
	1:25	−15.3	− 1.4
	1:12	− 7.7	− 1.7
3	1:40	−15.9	−10.2
	1:20	− 3.5	− 0.5
	1:10	− 5.9	− 1.8
4	1:40	−17.6	− 1.6
	1:20	− 5.2	+ 1.8
5	1:50	−35.9	−15.2
	1:25	−22.0	−16.0

Normal spleen cells of C57BL/6 mice were cultivated in RPMI medium + 1% syngeneic mouse serum for 2 days.

growth characteristics of L-3LL and M-3LL tumors in F_1 hosts. M-3LL and L-3LL tumor cells were subjected to lysis by freshly isolated spleen cells from syngeneic, allogeneic, and F_1 mice. The results (Table IX) indicate no H-2 restriction of the NK activity of normal spleen cells. Spleen cells derived from either syngeneic or allogeneic (ie, C3H/eB or BALB/c) and semiallogeneic [ie, F_1 (C3H/eB × C57BL/6) and F_1 (BALB/c × C57BL/6)] mice were equally efficient in their NK activity against 3LL tumor cells. Here again we found the relative resistance to NK cytotoxicity of M-3LL compared to L-3LL cells. Thus, irrespective of the haplotype of the donor, NK cells were more cytotoxic to L-3LL than to M-3LL cells.

We then tested whether the differences in susceptibility of M-3LL cells and L-3LL cells to the semiallogeneic NK cells observed in vitro would be reflected in vivo. Semi-allogeneic recipients and syngeneic controls were inoculated in the hind footpads by either $1 × 10^5$ M-3LL or L-3LL cells, and both tumor appearance and tumor diameter were recorded. Figures 3a, b and 4a, b indicate that there were no significant differences in the growth of either L-3LL or M-3LL tumor cells in syngeneic mice.

On the other hand, in both (BALB/c × C57BL/6) F_1 and (C3H/eB × C57BL/6) F_1 mice, a profound inhibition of L-3LL but not of M-3LL tumor development was observed. On the 15th day following inoculation of $1 × 10^5$ M-3LL tumor cells, 100% of F_1 (BALB/c × C57BL/6) and 85% of F_1 (C3H/eB × C57BL/6) mice had established tumors. On the same day, only 55% of F_1 (BALB/c × C57BL/6) mice and 18% F_1 (C3HeB × C57BL/6) mice bore established L-3LL tumors. Even on the 26th day following the transplantation of L-3LL tumor cells, the percentage of F_1 (BALB/c × C57BL/6) and F_1 C3HeB × C57BL/6) hybrids bearing established L-3LL tumors was 75% and 58%, respectively. When compared with the growth of these tumors in syngeneic C57BL mice, M-3LL tumor growth was uninhibited in F_1 (C3HeB × C57BL/6) hybrids. In F_1 (BALB/c × C57BL/6 hybrids an accelerated growth of M-3LL tumors was observed (Figs. 3, 4).

TABLE VII. Sensitivity of L-3LL and M-3LL Tumor Cells to the Cytotoxic Action of Normal Unsensitized Spleen Cells Cultured for 5 Days

Expt. No.	Ratio of tumor-to-spleen cells	Target cells	
		L-3LL	M-3LL
1	1:50	−15.7	+17.8
	1:25	− 8.2	+ 3.4
	1:12	−17.6	+ 6.5
2	1:50	−21.7	−18.2
	1:25	−22.8	−13.8
	1:12	−20.0	+14.6
	1:6	− 5.6	+13.5
3	1:25	−15.2	+14.6
	1:12	−10.0	+13.5
4	1:25	−27.8	−15.0
	1:12	−14.2	+ 0.3
5	1:25	− 7.7	+ 3.4
	1:12	− 9.5	+10.2

Normal spleen cells of C57BL/6 mice were cultured in RPMI + 1% syngeneic mouse serum for 5 days.

DISCUSSION

In our previous study, we demonstrated that sensitization in culture of syngeneic lymphocytes against 3LL or B-16 tumors in the presence of syngeneic serum instead of the usually used xenogeneic serum, led to the generation of cytotoxic lymphocytes specific to these tumors [19]. In the present study, we applied the same approach to test whether antigenic differences exist between cell populations of the local growth of the 3LL tumor and its lung metastases. The results indicated that lung metastases which develop during the progression of an intra-footpad or SC inoculum of the tumor differ antigenically and immunogenically from the local tumor. Lymphocytes sensitized in culture against M-3LL lysed M-3LL targets more efficiently than they lysed L-3LL targets and vice versa. These differences are not the result of artifacts created by in vitro conditions, since spleen cells derived from L-3LL tumor-bearing mice, once "unmasked" in culture, lysed L-3LL cells, whereas M-3LL targets were relatively resistant. Conversely, spleen cells from M-3LL TBM lysed M-3LL significantly more than they affected L-3LL targets.

These results support the notion that the metastatic cells are indeed phenotypic variants of the local tumor growth. Thus, from a diverse tumor cell population strongly immunogenic migrating variants could be eliminated or suppressed during the early phases of tumor growth, by the immune reaction which they themselves evoke; clones which elicit a low, delayed, or different immune response could be selected out. Alternatively, because we use a serially transplantable tumor, one may assume that in addition to pre-existence of diversity, new antigenic variants may be generated de novo, during the progression of the local tumor. Fidler and Kripke [2, 27], studying the metastatic B-16 melanoma or the UV-induced fibrosarcoma, conducted experiments to test whether tumor cells with high metastatic potency preexist within the tumor cell population. They measured the incidence of lung metastases produced by intravenous inoculation of cell populations derived from different in vitro clones of the tumor cells. The results were that cell populations of different clones differed dramatically in their capacity to produce lung metastases. This suggests that in this tumor, cells with a higher metastatic potency preexist in the initial cell population. If this observation applies also to the 3LL tumor, it may account for the fact that anti-M-3LL CL manifested cytotoxicity against L-3LL

TABLE VIII. Cytotoxic Activity of T-Deprived Nonsensitized Spleen Cells Against 3LL Tumor Cells*

| | % Cytotoxicity | | |
| | Target-to-effector cell ratio | | |
Spleen cells	1:200	1:100	1:50
C57BL	−58	−33.2	−19.5
C57BL after anti-theta + C′ treatment	NT	−51.5	−38.3
B-mice[a] (C57BL)	−56	−40.1	NT
C3H	−43	−40.2	NT
C3H nude	−51	−38.8	NT

[a]B-mice: C57BL/6 mice 2 months old were thymectomized; 1 month later they were irradiated (850 R) and reconstituted with 2×10^6 syngeneic bone marrow cells from normal mice. Two months later, spleen cells of these mice were used in the cytotoxic test against 3LL tumor cells.
*C57BL, C3H (+/+), C3H (nu/nu) mice were 2 months old.

targets, although to a lower extent than against M-3LL (Tables I, II). The preexistence of tumor cells with a high metastatic potency is supported also by our observation that anti-M-3LL CL, when injected into mice admixed with L-3LL, caused a significant reduction in lung metastasis (Tables III, IV). Obviously, metastases produced by a growing subcutaneous tumor such as the tumors we investigated in the present study are determined by factors additional to those which determine the mere growth of metastatic tumor cells when these are injected intravenously. Thus, the very survival of tumor cells that detach from the local growth and migrate via the circulation might depend on their capacity to resist an immune reaction that the host directs against the growing local tumor, which, due to its large antigenic mass, can resist it. Tumor cells that a) can grow progessively in the lungs and b) are antigenically different from the cells of the local growth could be subjected to immune selection by the anti-L-3LL response that is evoked initially in the tumor-bearing animal.

The existence of antigenic differences between a local primary methylcholanthrene-induced tumor and its distant metastases was demonstrated by Sugarbaker and Cohen [29]. Using the method of cross analysis by immunization of mice against primary and metastatic tumors, these authors found that specific antigenic determinants are shared with primary tumor cells by some of the metastases and differ from others. In some cases, metastatic cells derived from the above-mentioned tumors lost their immunogenicity. Schirrmacher et al [30], using a methylcholanthrene-induced nonmetastasizing lymphoma Eb and its metastasizing variant ESb, have reported that these tumor cell lines

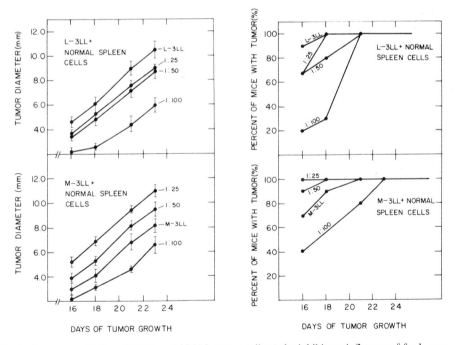

Fig. 1. In vivo sensitivity of L-3LL and M-3LL tumor cells to the inhibitory influence of fresh, unsensitized normal spleen cells of C57BL/6 mice. M-3LL or L-3LL tumor cells (2×10^4) were mixed with fresh normal syngeneic spleen cells at different ratios, as indicated in the figures. These mixtures were inoculated into the hind footpads of normal intact mice. At the indicated time intervals, both the percentage of mice with established tumors (b) and the mean tumor diameter (a) were recorded. Each group consisted of 10 mice.

carry distinct antigens at the responder cell level, the stimulator cell level, and the target cell level. These antigenic differences may be the result of an immunoselection of cells with distinct antigenic properties. This immunoselection may be the result of a specific immune response evoked against the local primary tumor.

Despite the suggestion outlined above our present results do not rule out an attractive assumption, namely, that NK cells themselves may act as an additional and independent selective force and may in fact themselves select antigenic variants manifesting higher resistance to specific and nonspecific cytotoxic effects. Therefore, in our present experiments we tested as well whether cells of the local growth, ie, L-3LL cells, manifest a susceptibility to NK activity which is different from that of M-3LL cells isolated from distant pulmonary metastases. We found that L-3LL cells are highly susceptible to lysis by splenic NK cells (Tables V–VII). In contrast, M-3LL tumor cells are relatively resistant to the cytotoxic activity of the same population of NK cells (Tables V–VII). The activity of NK cells is not directed against or affected by MHC or non-MHC alloantigens, because spleen cells from normal allogeneic or semiallogeneic F_1 hybrid mice are similar to syngeneic cells in their lytic effects and similar differences in susceptibility to allogeneic and semiallogeneic NK cells of L-3LL and M-3LL tumor cells are observed (Table IX). The cultivation of normal spleen cells in vitro for a period of 2 or 5 days did not abolish the cytotoxic function of NK cells (Tables VI, VII).

Experiments performed to characterize the nature of the effector cytotoxic cells present in the normal spleen cell population indicate (Table VIII) that these cells are not T cells and their characteristics are similar to those attributed in the literature to NK cells

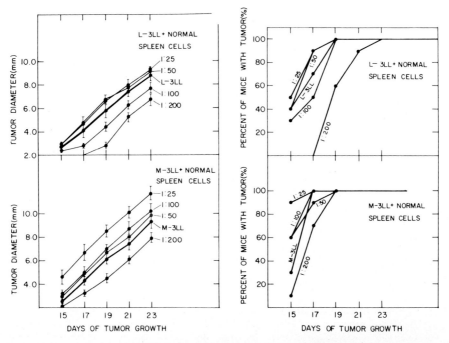

Fig. 2. In vivo sensitivity of L-3LL and M-3LL tumor cells to the inhibitory influence of fresh, unsensitized normal spleen cells of C57BL/6 mice. Conditions of experiment as described in Figure 1.

[17, 24]. Furthermore, we have performed experiments (Tables VI, VII) that strengthen the NK nature of the presently investigated effector cells because depletion of adherent cells failed to diminish the cytotoxic activity of normal spleen cells against the tumor cells. Yet our data so far do not rule out the possible involvement of another recently described population of natural cytotoxic cells (NC cells) which are non-T-cells and have been found to possess a few different characteristics than those attributed to NK cells [31, 32].

The differences in susceptibility of M-3LL and L-3LL tumor cells to the cytotoxic action of NK cells in vitro was also demonstrated in vivo; when spleen cells were admixed with tumor cells and inoculated into syngeneic recipients, the inhibition of L-3LL tumor growth was achieved by NK cells at relatively low doses. To inhibit the growth of M-3LL cells, higher doses of spleen cells were required. The inhibitory effect of M-3LL cells was lower than that obtained with L-3LL cells when admixed with spleen cells at similar ratios (Figs. 1, 2).

Although these results do not exclude the possible involvement of T cells and macrophages in the nonspecific defense against tumor progression in the diseased host, the data obtained in the present investigation indicate that the major nonspecific cytotoxic activity is performed by NK cells.

If indeed the mechanisms underlying NK cell activity and the phenomenon of hybrid resistance have a common basis, one would expect F_1 (BALB/c $\times$ C57BL/6) and F_1 (C3HeB $\times$ C57BL/6) mice to resist L-3LL tumor cells more than M-3LL growth. This, in fact, was the result we obtained (Figs. 3, 4). Our experiments thus clearly indicate that M-3LL and L-3LL tumor cells do differ in their susceptibility to the lytic activity of NK cells. The presently observed resistance of M-3LL tumor cells to NK cells might increase the probability of survival of metastatic cells in the circulation, thus providing an advantage for their spread and progression.

The possible role of NK cells in the elimination of tumor cells is supported by the results of Fidler and Nicolson [33], who demonstrated that following IV inoculation, radiolabeled B-16 melanoma cells that had settled in different organs were rapidly eliminated and only a very small fraction of the inoculated cells finally developed into metastatic foci. They found that 98.2% of the inoculated tumor cells that were arrested

TABLE IX. Cytotoxic Effect of Spleen NK Cells of Different Genotypes on L-3LL and M-3LL Tumor Target Cells

Strain of spleen donor mice	Expt. 1				Expt. 2			
	L-3LL		M-3LL		L-3LL		M-3LL	
	1:200	1:100	1:200	1:100	1:100	1:50	1:100	1:50
C57BL/6	−29.3	−23.3	−15.4	+13.7	−35.6	−33.6	−21.9	−14.9
BALB/c	−46.6	− 9.1	−25.8	− 9.3	−28.7	−37.2	−21.6	− 9.0
C3HeB	−28.8	−26.7	− 5.2	− 3.5	−39.2	−34.7	−20.4	−17.7
F_1 (BALB/c $\times$ C57BL/6)	−51.5	−18.4	+ 9.4	+31.9	−40.0	+ 4.3	−22.9	+ 5.9
F_1 (C3HeB $\times$ C57BL/6)	−46.2	−5.4	−11.6	+ 9.6	−53.6	−42.5	+ 0.4	−2.5

Fresh normal spleen cells obtained from immunologically intact mice of different genotypes were added to monolayers of L-3LL or M-3LL tumor cells for 18 h. The survival fraction of these monolayers was labeled with ^{51}Cr.

in the lungs were eliminated during the first day following inoculation and only 0.2% of transplanted cells developed visible metastases in the lungs [33]. Immunosuppressive procedures such as irradiation or thymectomy and irradiation did not abolish the elimination of the inoculated tumor cells. In fact, the elimination of tumor cells in the lungs and other organs 24 h following their injection was even greater in thymectomized and irradiated than in normal recipients. Although these authors have not considered the involvement of NK cells as part of the mechanism involved in the observed elimination of tumor cells, it is hard to believe that the elimination of tumor cells within a period of 24 h following IV inoculation is due to production of specific immune cytotoxic lymphocytes. On the other hand, it seems plausible that this rapid elimination of tumor cells is performed by preexisting NK cells. This assumption is supported by the fact that irradiation and thymectomy, which prevent the development of immune cytotoxic lymphocytes, failed to abolish activity of NK cells [17, 34].

The possible role of NK cells in tumor progression is further supported by a series of experiments in which Fidler and Nicolson [33] inoculated B-16 melanoma cells IV into allogeneic nude (nu/nu) and nu/+ heterozygote NIH Swiss mice. The allogeneic nu/+

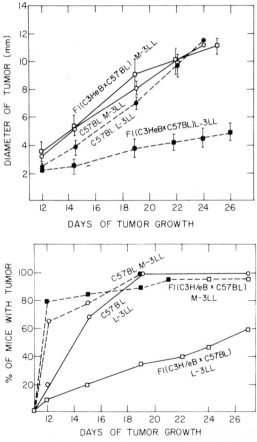

Fig. 3. Capacity of L-3LL and M-3LL tumor cells to grow in syngeneic and semiallogeneic hosts. M-3LL or L-3LL tumor cells (1×10^5) were inoculated into the hind footpads of normal intact F_1 or C57BL/6 control mice. At the indicated time intervals, percent of mice with established tumors (b) and mean tumor diameter (a) were recorded. Each group consisted of 40 mice.

mice killed inoculated tumor cells in a period of 24 h to the same extent as normal syngeneic mice. In the lungs of nude (nu/nu) mice, the percentage of surviving tumor cells was much lower than in normal allogeneic or syngeneic mice. These results are compatible with observations indicating that NK activity in nude mice is increased in comparison to their normal littermates [17, 34].

We therefore suggest that NK cells play an important role in determining metastatic spread and growth. The presently obtained results not only add an additional and new characteristic to the observed biologic differences between primary tumor cells and their metastatic progeny, but they might be of extreme importance and relevant to the mechanisms by which malignant tumors can disseminate their deviant progeny to form metastases in anatomically distant locations in spite of the existence of a protective physiologic mechanism provided by both NK cells and specific cytotoxic immunocytes. Furthermore, our presently described results, as well as those described by others [28], indicate that the development of malignant metastases is the result of a multifactorial process depending on many different phenotypic properties of the tumor cells themselves

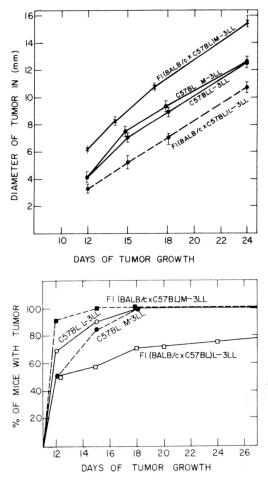

Fig. 4. Capacity of L-3LL and M-3LL tumor cells to grow in syngeneic and semiallogeneic hosts. Conditions of experiment as described in Figure 3.

as well as on a variety of both immunologic and nonimmunologic mechanisms in the diseased host. Whatever the relevance of the different antigenic properties of the metastatic cells to their biologic characteristics, such properties might be of extreme importance with respect to any future rational approach to the problem of immunotherapy of malignancies and may contribute to a better understanding of the unique physiologic characteristics of tumor metastases.

ACKNOWLEDGMENTS

This work was supported by NIH contract No. NO1-CB-74185. The authors are grateful for the excellent technical assistance of Ziona Frenkel and Lea Milgrom.

REFERENCES

1. Rosenberg S, Terry W: Adv Cancer Res 25:323, 1977.
2. Fidler J, Kripke M: Science 197:893, 1977.
3. Coman DR: Cancer Res 13:397, 1953.
4. Fidler J, Nicolson G: J Natl Cancer Inst 57:1199, 1976.
5. Nicolson G, Winkelhake J, Nussey A: In Weiss L (ed): "Fundamental Aspects of Metastases." Amsterdam: North-Holland, 1976, p 291.
6. Fogel M, Gorelik E, Segal S, Feldman M: J Natl Cancer Inst 62:585, 1979.
7. Trope C: Neoplasma 22:171, 1975.
8. Rabotti G: Nature 183:1276, 1959.
9. Chu E, Malmgren R: J Natl Cancer Inst 27:217, 1961.
10. Chatterjee S, Kim U: J Natl Cancer Inst 61:151, 1978.
11. Gershon R, Carter R: Nature 226:368, 1970.
12. Jones P, Castro J: Br J Cancer 35:519, 1977.
13. Alexander P, Eccles S: In Schultz J, Leif E (eds): "Critical Factors in Cancer Immunology." New York: Academic, 1975, p 159.
14. Herberman RB, Nunn ME, Lavrin DH: Int J Cancer 15:216, 1975.
15. Kiessling R, Klein E, Wigzell H: Eur J Immunol 5:112, 1975.
16. Rosenberg EB, McCoy JL, Green SS, Donnelly FC, Siwarski DF, Levine PH, Herberman RB: J Natl Cancer Inst 52:345, 1974.
17. Herberman RB, Holden HT: Adv Cancer Res 7:305, 1978.
18. Treves AJ, Cohen IR, Feldman M: J Natl Cancer Inst 54:977, 1975.
19. Fogel M, Segal S, Gorelik E, Feldman M: Int J Cancer 22:329, 1978.
20. Djeu J, Glaser M, Huang K, Herberman R: Cell Immunol 23:268, 1976.
21. Takasugi M, Klein E: Transplantation 9:219, 1970.
22. More R, Yron I, Ben Sasson S, Weiss D: Cell Immunol 15:382, 1975.
23. Bonmassar E, Houchens D, Fioretti M, Goldin A: Chemotherapy 21:321, 1975.
24. Herberman R, Nunn M, Lavrin D: Int J Cancer 26:230, 1975.
25. Harmon RC, Clar EA, O'Toole C, Wicker LS: Immunogenetics 4:601, 1977.
26. Kiessling R, Hochman PS, Haller O, Shearer GM, Wigzell H, Cudkowicz G: Eur J Immunol 7:655, 1977.
27. Kripke M, Gruys E, Fidler J: Cancer Res 38:2962, 1978.
28. Fidler J, Gersten D, Hart J: Adv Cancer Res 28:150, 1978.
29. Sugarbaker E, Cohen A: Surgery 72:155, 1972.
30. Schirrmacher V, Bosset K, Shantz G, Clauer K, Hubsch D: Int J Cancer 23:256, 1979.
31. Stutman O, Paige C, Figarella E: J Immunol 121:1819, 1978.
32. Paige C, Figarella E, Cuttito M, Cahan A, Stutman O: J Immunol 121:1827, 1978.
33. Fidler IJ, Nicolson GL: Israel J Med Sci 14:38, 1978.
34. Warner N, Woodruff F, Burton R: Int J Cancer 20:146, 1977.
35. Siegel S: "Nonparametric Statistics for the Behavioral Sciences." New York: McGraw-Hill, 1956, pp 116–126.

Journal of Supramolecular Structure 12:403–417 (1979)
Tumor Cell Surfaces and Malignancy 693–707

Analysis of Transmembrane Proteins From Eukaryotic Cells

R.M. Evans, F.G. Grillo, and L.M. Fink

Department of Pathology, University of Colorado Health Sciences Center, Denver, Colorado 80262

The topography and properties of plasma membrane proteins from mouse L-929 cells are studied by comparing their availability for enzymatic labeling on the external and internal surfaces of the membrane. In order to study the internal surface, phagolysosomes are prepared from cells after they ingest latex particles. The plasma membrane surrounding these seems to have an "inside-out" orientation. The sugars of the membrane glycoproteins in intact phagolysosomes are not available for interaction with lectins or available for periodate-borotritide labeling. A comparison of the lectin-binding proteins labeled by lactoperoxidase-catalyzed iodination on the external cell surface with those labeled on the internal cell surface suggests that a variety of plasma membrane glycoproteins span the lipid bilayer.

Using two-dimensional gel electrophoresis it has been shown that selected proteins are labeled at both the internal and external faces of the plasma membrane. Analysis of the 2-D gel electrophoregrams reveals that there are two distinct prominent proteins at 60,000 and 100,000 daltons which are enzymatically iodinated from both sides of the membrane. The partial hydrolysis of the 100,000 dalton protein reveals that different peptides are iodinated when the iodination is performed on intact cells or on the phagolysosomes. These proteins are extensively phosphorylated in cells incubated with inorganic ^{32}P. We conclude that the phagolysosome is probably oriented in an "inside-out" configuration and that this membrane preparation can be used to study the topographic organization of membrane proteins.

The use of oriented membranes, selective labeling of proteins, and affinity separation of proteins in combination with gel electrophoresis to define the position and properties of proteins is discussed.

Key words: mouse L-929 cells, "inside-out" configuration, gel electrophoresis, lectin-binding proteins

Received May 9, 1979; accepted September 10, 1979.

Changes in the composition and structure of the plasma membrane seem to be critical in determining how cells interact with their environment. These changes are probably intimately connected with some of the altered phenotypic characteristics associated with neoplastic transformation. Much of the information on the structure and organization of the plasma membrane comes from studies on red blood cells. However, the anucleate RBC may not be useful as a paradigm for plasma membrane structure in other cells. Because of the complexity of physiologic responses which occur in nucleated replicating cells but not in erythrocytes, we have begun to analyze the protein structure and topography of plasma membrane proteins in fibroblastic mouse cells in culture.

The studies presented are designed to assess the location of proteins in the plasma membrane. A vectoral analysis designates which proteins are available for enzymatic modification a) on the internal surface, b) on the external surface, and c) on both sides of the plasma membrane; the latter thus are candidates likely to have a transmembrane (TMB) configuration. These studies depend upon the selective labeling of the internal and external surfaces of the membranes. One approach has been to saturate all the external labeling sites with an impenetrable probe and then either to permeabilize the cell so that internal labeling can occur [1, 2], or use a permeable probe for internal labeling [3]. Another approach, which is the major method used in the present studies, is to label either "inside-out" or "right-side-out" membranes with an impenetrant probe. Some cells can ingest latex particles to form latex-filled phagolysosomes that appear to have an "inside-out" orientation and a protein composition similar to the plasma membrane from which they are derived.

Hubbard and Cohn [4] iodinated L cells using lactoperoxidase and subsequently prepared phagolysosomes. They showed that the phagolysosomes prepared in this manner contained most of the same iodinated proteins found at the cell surface. Hunt and Brown [5] used the susceptibility of a high-molecular-weight protein in intact cells and phagolysosomes to trypsin hydrolysis to suggest a transmembrane configuration for this protein.

We have used "inside-out" oriented phagolysosomes from mouse cells in conjunction with nonpenetrant enzymatic labeling to orient specific plasma membrane proteins. Our experiments suggest that there are plasma membrane proteins which bridge through the lipid bilayer of the plasma membrane as single polypeptides. Additional experiments show that there are lectin-binding proteins whose carbohydrate moieties are not exposed on the cytoplasmic face of the plasma membrane, that appear to have a transmembrane configuration. Several of the TMB proteins can be identified in high-resolution 2-D gels. Certain TMB proteins are metabolically labeled by $^{32}PO_4 =$ and ^{35}S-methionine and are glysolated. One of the predominant TMB plasma membrane proteins that we have studied has a molecular weight of approximately 100,000 daltons. Some properties of this protein will be described.

METHODS

Cell Culture, Metabolic Labeling of Cell Proteins, Preparation of Phagolysosomes, and Plasma Membranes

Mouse L-929 cells were grown in suspension culture in minimal essential medium (MEM) containing 5% fetal calf serum and 0.15% methylcellulose (15 cps). For analysis of the metabolically labeled proteins the cells are placed in MEM (without methionine) with 5% fetal calf serum and 10 μCi of ^{35}S-methioine per milliliter. After 4 h an equal volume of medium containing 0.2 mM methionine is added and the cells are incubated for 6 h prior to preparation of the plasma membranes. For labeling of the phosphoproteins the cells are incubated for 4 h in phosphate-free MEM containing 1% dialyzed serum and 100 μCi/ml of ^{32}P orthophosphate.

Incubation of cells with 1-μ latex particles and preparation of latex-filled phagolysosomes from these cells was performed as previously described [6].

Plasma membrane was prepared as described by Brunette and Till [7].

Labeling of Cell Surfaces and Phagolysosomes

Cells were rinsed in phosphate buffered saline (PBS) and ^{131}I- or ^{125}I-lactoperoxidase labeled as described by Hynes [8]. After a 10-min labeling period the cells were rinsed in PBS containing 0.5 mM tyrosine. Phagolysosomes were prepared from unlabeled cells and iodinated under similar conditions except that the concentrations of lactoperoxidase and glucose oxidase were reduced to 2.5 and 0.25 μg/ml, respectively.

Phagolysosomes were labeled with dansyl cadaverine using transglutaminase purified from guinea pig liver as previously described [6].

Cells and phagolysosomes were labeled with a periodate-NaB^{3}H$_4$ technique described by Gahmberg and Andersson [9].

Membrane Sample Preparation and Isolation of Specific Membrane Proteins by Affinity Chromatography

The isolation of dansyl cadaverine-labeled proteins on antidansyl IgG affinity columns was performed on phagolysosomes solubilized in Triton X-100 as previously described [6].

Isolation of the iodinatable lectin-binding proteins from intact cells and phagolysosomes was performed by lysing the preparations in 60 mM borate 1% Triton X-100, 1 mM EDTA, 0.5 mM phenylmethylsulfonylfluoride, 2 mM N-ethylmaleimide, 2 mM iodoacetamide, and 2 mM dithiothreitol at pH 7.8. The lysate was clarified at 10,000g for 10 min and chromatographed on a Bio-Rad P-10 column. The excluded proteins were applied to columns containing wheat germ agglutinin (WGA)-Sepharose 6B, Con A-Sepharose 6B, or Lens culinaris-Sepharose 6B. The columns were washed with 0.05 M Tris 1% Triton X-100, pH 7.5, until the effluent radioactivity was essentially at background level. The retained material was eluted with Tris-Triton X-100 containing 0.3 M of the appropriate sugar. The iodinated protein recovered from WGA-Sepharose affinity columns in the presence of N-acetyl-D-glucosamine was dialyzed. The samples from the retained column fractions were precipitated in acidified acetone, washed with ethanol:ether (1:1 v/v), dried under N$_2$, and resuspended in 0.14 M Tris, 22.3% glycerol, 6% sodium dodecylsulfate, 2 mM dithiothreitol, and 0.001% bromphenol blue (pH 6.8). Samples to be analyzed by two-dimensional electrophoresis were resuspended in 9.5 M urea, 2% Triton X-100, 1.6% carrier ampholine (pH 5–7), 0.4% carrier ampholine (pH 3–10), and 2 mM dithiothreitol.

Polyacrylamide Gel Electrophoresis

Discontinuous sodium dodecysulfate-polyacrylamide gel electrophoresis (SDS-PAGE) was carried out as previously described [6]. Two-dimensional electrophoresis was performed essentially as described by O'Farrell [10]. The gels were fixed, stained, and dried, and were either directly autoradiographed or prepared for fluorography as described elsewhere [11].

Studies on the limited proteolysis of membrane proteins recovered from two-dimensional gels were performed essentially as described by Cleveland et al [12].

RESULTS

Studies on the Orientation of the Plasma Membrane Proteins in Phagolysosomes Using Periodate NaB^3H_4 Labeling and Lectin Affinity Columns

When cells were labeled with periodate-borotritide at 4°C, 4×10^5 cpm of ^3H precipitable by 10% cold trichloracetic acid was incorporated per 10^6 cells. In contrast, fewer than 1,000 cpm of acid-precipitable counts were recovered from labeling of phagolysosomes recovered from 10^7 cells.

Both Con A-Sepharose 6MB and WGA-Sepharose 6MB were found to retain intact L cells effectively. This is shown in Table I. The retention of the cells was reduced by running the columns in the appropriate competing sugar. Phagolysosomes containing approximately an equal amount of membrane to the cells showed almost no binding to the lectin affinity columns. The amount of membrane was equalized by matching the iodinatable counts of intact cells with those in the phagolysosomes obtained from cells that had been lactoperoxidase-iodinated.

Double Labeling of Phagolysosomal Proteins

The details of labeling of the external surfaces of cells with lactoperoxidase-catalyzed iodination, preparation of phagolysosomes, and labeling by a transglutaminase-mediated dansyl cadaverine reaction of the inside-out phagolysosomes has been reported [6]. The protocol for these experiments is diagrammed in Figure 1. The enzymatically dansyl cadaverine-labeled proteins from the phagolysosome, which appear to be on the cytoplasmic face, were solubilized and separated from the other iodinatable proteins by affinity chromatography on antidansyl IgG-affinity columns. From these types of analyses and those previously reported [6], we conclude that the plasma membranes in the phagolysosomes have predominantly, if not exclusively, an "inside-out" orientation. The selective vectoral orientation of the membrane in these preparations provides a simple procedure for determining the presence of transmembrane proteins. Figure 2 shows the results of these studies. It can be seen in Figure 2E that there are three major polypeptides of 55,000, 80,000, and 110,000 daltons containing both the dansyl cadaverine and radioactive iodine.

TABLE I. Affinity Chromatography of Lactoperoxidase-Iodinated L Cells and Phagolysosomes on Lectin-Sepharose 6MB

	% Acid-precipitable ^{125}I retained[a]			
	Con A-Sepharose		WGA-Sepharose	
	– Mannose	+ Mannose[b]	– N-AcGlucosamine	+ N-AcGlucosamine[c]
Cells	92	35	98	22
Phagolysosomes	9	11	18	16

[a] Approximately 10^6 cpm of ^{125}I-labeled cells or phagolysosomes prepared from labeled cells were applied to 0.9×8-cm lectin-Sepharose 6MB columns in PBS. Values represent percentage of total trichloroacetic acid-precipitable ^{125}I retained after a 100-ml volume was eluted from the column.

[b] Column run in the presence of 0.1 M mannose.

[c] Column run in the presence of 0.2 M N-acetyl-D-glucosamine.

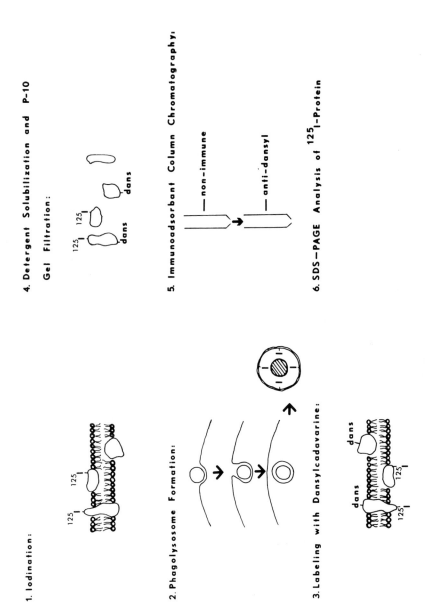

Fig. 1. Diagrammatic representation of labeling and preparation of phagolysosomal proteins. The methods for surface iodination, preparation of phagolysosomes, dansyl cadaverine labeling of proteins using transglutaminase, immune affinity chromatography with antidansyl IgG and SDS-PAGE are given in [6].

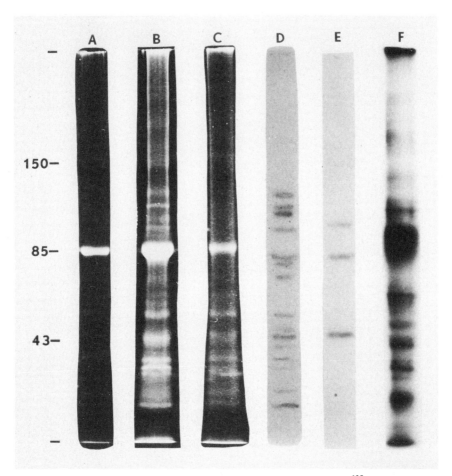

Fig. 2. Sodium dodecylsulfate (5–15%) polyacrylamide gel electrophoresis of ^{125}I-labeled and dansyl cadaverine-labeled cell proteins. Molecular weights ($\times 10^{-3}$) are shown at the left. Lanes A–C are the fluorescent proteins and lanes D–F are autoradiographs of iodinated cell surface proteins. A) Guinea pig liver transglutaminase labeled with dansyl cadaverine. B) Fluorescent proteins solubilized from phagolysosomes labeled with dansyl cadaverine by a transglutaminase-catalyzed reaction after isolation from the cells. C) The fluorescent proteins labeled as described in B that were retained on an antidansyl IgG affinity column. D) Autoradiographic pattern of the cell surface proteins, phagolysosomes; this is an autoradiograph of the proteins in column B. E) Autoradiograph of column C showing the iodinated proteins retained by an antidansyl IgG affinity column. F) Lactoperoxidase-iodinated cell surface proteins from intact L-929 cells.

Lectin Affinity Chromatography of Iodinated Proteins From Cells and Phagolysosomes

The Triton X-100-soluble proteins from iodinated cells, phagolysosomes prepared from labeled cells, and phagolysosomes iodinated directly were chromatographed on Con A and WGA affinity columns. The labeled material was analyzed by SDS-PAGE and the results are shown in Figures 3 and 4.

Figure 3 shows the densitometric tracings of autoradiographs of the SDS-PAGE of ^{125}I-labeled proteins retained by Con A columns. The intact cells have four major protein bands, of 20,000, 100,000, 150,000, and 230,000 daltons. These proteins were also present in the Con A-binding fraction of proteins from phagolysosomes prepared from iodinated cells. The phagolysosomes that were directly iodinated showed Con A-binding proteins of 100,000, 150,000, and 230,000 daltons. A protein of 20,000 daltons was found in the phagolysosomes prepared from iodinated cells but was not present in the phagolysosomes directly iodinated.

The SDS-PAGE analysis of these iodinated preparations retained by WGA affinity columns is shown in Figure 4. The major iodinatable protein of 100,000 daltons found in iodinated intact cells and in phagolysosomes prepared from these cells is not found in directly iodinated phagolysosomes. A 150,000-dalton protein was heavily iodinated in the phagolysosomes that were directly iodinated.

A selected region of the two-dimensional gel analysis of ^{131}I-labeled L cell proteins prepared from lactoperoxidase-iodinated cells and the fraction of this material retained by a WGA affinity column is shown in Figure 5. At least three externally iodinatable proteins which are found in the total phagolysosomal preparation (Fig. 5A) are not detectable in the fraction retained by the WGA affinity column (Fig. 5B). These three proteins are of similar molecular weight to other ^{131}I-labeled proteins retained by the WGA affinity column and are difficult to resolve in one-dimensional SDS-PAGE.

The gels show a string of spots of 85,000 and 115,000 daltons, which form a beads-on-a-string pattern. The mobility of these proteins is markedly affected by affinity purified neuraminidase treatment and probably is related to the glycosylation of these proteins (data not shown).

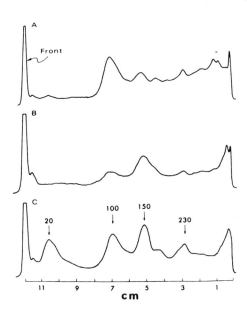

Fig. 3. Sodium dodecylsulfate gel electrophoresis analysis of lactoperoxidase ^{125}I-labeled L-929 proteins eluted from Con A affinity columns. The samples analyzed on 7.5% acrylamide gels were obtained from A) phagolysosomes prepared from iodinated cells, B) directly iodinated phagolysosomes, C) intact cells. The direction of migration is from right to left. The numbers indicated above the densimetric tracings represent approximate molecular weight $\times 10^{-3}$.

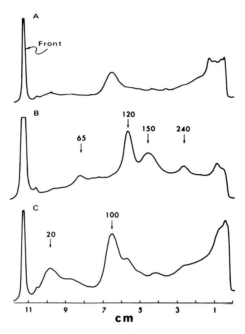

Fig. 4. Sodium dodecylsulfate gel electrophoresis analysis of lactoperoxidase ^{125}I-labeled L-929 proteins eluted from WGA affinity columns. The samples analyzed on 7.5% acrylamide gels were obtained from A) phagolysosomes prepared from iodinated cells, B) directly iodinated phagolysosomes, C) intact cells. For further details see legend to Figure 1.

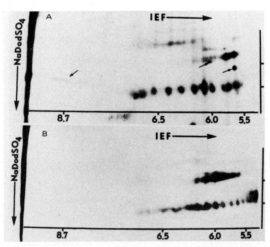

Fig. 5. Two-dimensional gel electrophoresis of lactoperoxidase ^{131}I-labeled L-929 proteins from A) phagolysosomes prepared from iodinated cells and B) phagolysosomes prepared from iodinated cells and retained by a WGA affinity column. The abcissa gives pH values for the first dimension; this figure shows a selected region of a 2-D gel. The arrows denote cell surface iodinatable proteins present in phagolysosomes which were not retained by WGA affinity columns.

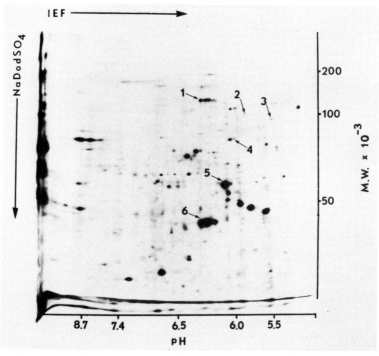

Fig. 6. Two-dimensional gel electrophoresis of phagolysosomal proteins from cells labeled with ^{35}S-methionine. The proteins labeled 1, 3, and 5 are phosphoproteins as shown in Figure 10. The protein 2, 3, and 5 are iodinatable from the outside surface of cells and from the inside surface of isolated phagolysosomes. The protein labeled 6 is actin, which is not iodinatable from the outside surface, as shown in Figure 8.

Two-dimensional Electrophoretic Analysis of the Proteins From Cells and Phagolysosomes

The pattern of phagolysosomal proteins which are metabolically labeled in cells by incubation of the cells with ^{35}S-methionine is shown in Figure 6. Approximately 250 labeled proteins can be detected. The major protein seen at 42,000 daltons is actin. We have prepared membrane from cells by several methods including those described by Allan and Crumpton [13] and Brunette and Till [7]. There are many similarities in the protein composition of these preparations observed in analysis of 2-D gel electrophoresis (data not shown). Therefore, unlabeled membrane from Brunette and Till membrane preparations was added to locate the position of specific proteins in Coomassie blue-stained gels where the mass of the radiolabeled phagolysosomal preparation is too small to be visualized.

The 2-D pattern of the ^{131}I-labeled proteins in phagolysosomes prepared from previously iodinated intact cells is shown in Figure 7. It should be noted that there is extensive labeling of surface proteins which "string out" during isoelectric focusing. Many of these iodinatable cell surface proteins are probably glycoproteins because neuraminidase treatment or endoglycosidase treatment of the cells after the iodination markedly alters the electrophoretic mobility of these proteins following isoelectric focusing (data not shown). The 2-D gels show that there are proteins iodinated on the cell surface to which we cannot find an exact counterpart in the patterns of ^{35}S-methionine-labeled proteins from plasma membranes (Figs. 6 and 7). There is iodination of proteins which exhibit mobility similar to actin, but these do not comigrate with actin as determined by a comparison of the Coomassie blue-stained proteins and the images produced by autoradiography of the iodinated proteins.

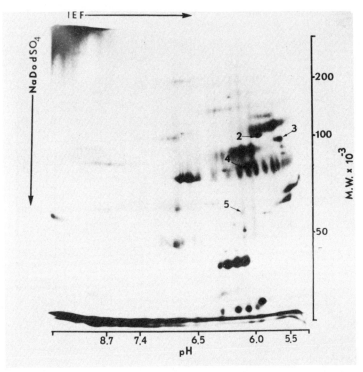

Fig. 7. Two-dimensional gel electrophoresis of the phagolysosomal proteins derived from lactoperoxidase iodinated intact cells. The proteins labeled 2, 3, and 5 are also iodinatable in intact phagolysosomes as shown in Figure 9.

Two-dimensional electrophoresis of phagolysosomes which are iodinated after they are isolated from cells reveals that there are several proteins which have mobilities in iso-electric focusing and SDS-PAGE identical to those of iodinated proteins from the cell surface (Fig. 8). It should be noted that there are marked differences in the proteins labeled by lactoperoxidase when the internal and external surfaces are selectively iodinated (see Figs. 7, 8).

We have selected for further analysis certain specific proteins which are labeled from both the external and the internal side of the plasma membrane. Using 2-D gels we were able to locate an iodinated protein at 100,000 daltons (pI approximately 5.5). The spot corresponding to this protein was punched out of the 2-D gel and was treated separately with papain, chymotrypsin, and Staphylococcal V-8 protease. Limited proteolysis and SDS-PAGE as described by Cleveland et al [12] and shown in Figure 9 reveals that the iodinated peptides are different from the externally labeled and internally labeled protein.

When preparations of plasma membrane from cells metabolically labeled with ^{35}S-methionine and ^{32}PO$_4$ $^=$ are mixed and coelectrophoresed, selective autoradiography with and without a plastic screen reveals that the 100,000 dalton protein is the most heavily phosphorylated protein resolved by 2-D gel electrophoresis of this membrane preparation (Fig. 10).

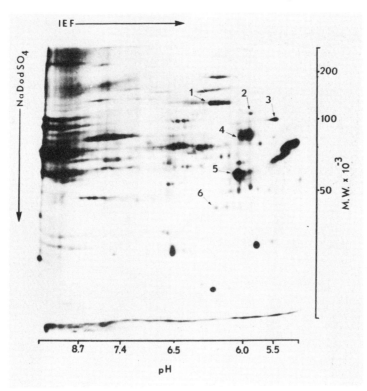

Fig. 8. Two-dimensional gel electrophoresis of the proteins from phagolysosomes which were iodinated after isolation from the cells.

DISCUSSION

Information about the relationships between membrane proteins, and between peripheral membrane proteins and integral proteins, will be important in understanding cellular responses to environmental changes. Because the transduction of signals may be mediated by changes in the distribution or conformation of proteins which span through the lipid bilayer, it is important to determine whether there are a small number of protiens or a wide variety of proteins which have transmembrane properties.

There is extensive indirect evidence suggesting that there are integral membrane proteins in nucleated cells, which are exposed at both the external and internal faces of the plasma membrane [14]. However, only several proteins have been directly characterized as having a TMB orientation [15—18]. A number of different approaches have been used to directly analyze the topographic location of membrane proteins. Walsh and Crumpton [19] have prepared "inside-out" vesicles from lymphocytes and have combined lactoperoxidase iodination of this preparation and immune precipitation with antibodies against cell surface antigens to demonstrate a TMB configuration for HLA antigens. We have used phagolysosomes formed by L cells to obtain plasma membranes in an "inside-out" conformation. This membrane contains most of the cell surface iodinatable proteins, as previously shown by Hubbard and Cohn in 1-D SDS-PAGE [4]. The phagolysosomal membrane

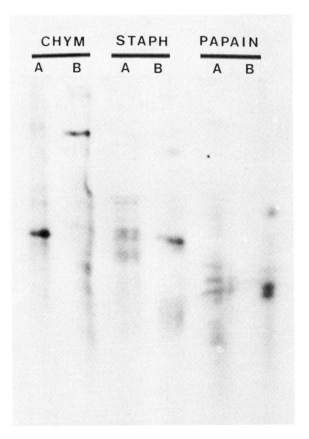

Fig. 9. Sodium dodecylsulfate gel electrophoresis of iodinated peptides from partial proteolytic hydrolysis of the protein designated number 3 in Figures 7 and 8. A) Protein 3 from phagolysosomes labeled after isolation; B) Protein 3 from phagolysosomes derived from iodinated cells.

is also very similar to plasma membrane obtained by other methods [7, 13], with respect to protein composition as analyzed by 2-D gel electrophoresis of either the phagolysosomal proteins from ^{35}S-methionine-labeled cells or the iodinated cell surface proteins in phagolysosomes prepared from previously iodinated intact cells [20].

Several chemical and enzymatic methods have been used to confirm the "inside-out" orientation and the asymmetry of the phagolysosomal membrane preparation. The trypsin insensitivity of lactoperoxidase-iodinated cell surface proteins incorporated into the phagolysosomes has been previously demonstrated [5]. Sandra and Pagano [21] have shown that the asymmetrical distribution of phospholipids in phagolysosomes is consistent with what would be expected in an "inside-out" membrane if there were no major rearrangements during formation and isolation of this membrane.

In the present studies the differential labeling of intact cells and phagolysosomes with periodate-NaB^{3}H$_4$ at 4°C, and the demonstration that intact cells are efficiently retained on lectin affinity columns while phagolysosomes are not, indicate that there is asymmetry of the carbohydrate in phagolysosomes. The results are consistent with evidence showing that glycosylated regions of membrane proteins are asymmetrically distributed and are found only at the exterior cell surface [22–27] if the phagolysosome is "inside-out."

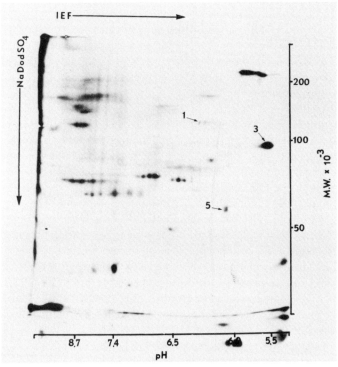

Fig. 10. Two-dimensional gel electrophoresis of the phagolysosomal proteins derived from cells labeled with inorganic $^{32}PO_4 =$.

Because of the asymmetry of the carbohydrates on glycoproteins it is possible to define a glycoprotein as TMB if it is iodinatable on the cytoplasmic surface and reacts with the lectin tested. The experiments show that most of the Con A-binding proteins in phagolysosomes are iodinatable from both sides of the membrane. However, there are WGA-binding proteins which were selectively iodinated at the external or internal cell surface. It is possible that some of these proteins, which are iodinated when isolated phagolysosomes are iodinated, are derived from lysosomes. Another less likely possibility is that these proteins are retained on the WGA lectin affinity column in association with a lectin-binding protein rather than by direct interaction with the WGA. Proteins were reduced and alkylated during the membrane solubilization to decrease the possibility of a protein-protein-lectin interaction. The 2-D gels of WGA proteins show the complexity of proteins at given molecular sizes and illustrate the hazards of suggesting that proteins are identical because they have the same mobility in SDS-PAGE. Even with this caveat, the data are consistent with a TMB configuration for a variety of lectin-binding cell surface proteins.

Another approach to identification of TMB proteins involved iodination of cell surface proteins, internalization of plasma membrane on latex particles by cells, disruption of cells, preparation of phagolysosomes, and labeling of the proteins on the cytoplasmic face of phagolysosomes using transglutaminase to covalently modify the available proteins with the hapten dansyl cadaverine. Using immune affinity chromatography with antidansyl IgG, we can isolate the proteins solubilized from phagolysosomes. We can show that some of these proteins are labeled with iodine. The predominant plasma membrane proteins labeled both externally and with LP iodination and internally with dansyl cadaverine by transglutaminase have molecular weights of 55,000, 80,000, and 100,000. These studies do not prove that these are the only TMB proteins, since the labeling is restrictive in the sense that we can detect only those TMB proteins which have an amino acid iodinatable on their external segment and a glutamine available for the transglutaminase-catalyzed linking of dansyl cadaverine on the internal segment. Because we wanted to analyze TMB proteins further, we have developed other methods of labeling and isolating proteins from the plasma membrane and phagolysosomes.

Another method developed to analyze the proteins available for enzymatic modification on the internal or external face of the plasma membrane is to electrophorese, on O'Farrell 2-D gels, the lactoperoxidase-catalyzed iodinated proteins from phagolysosomes prepared from iodinated intact cells and from directly iodinated phagolysosomes. Using these 2-D gels we have shown that there is marked difference in the proteins exposed to lactoperoxidase at the internal and external surfaces (Figs. 8 and 9) of the plasma membrane. For example, actin is not iodinated at the surface of intact L-929 cells. Cells grown in the absence of serum have similar proteins iodinated as cells washed after growth in the presence of serum, indicating that the pattern is not due to sequestration and labeling of serum proteins. Many of the major iodinatable cell surface proteins are poorly labeled by incubation with radioactive methionine. Compared with the major protein species isolated in phagolysosomes or conventional membrane preparations, many of the most extensively iodinated cell surface proteins give a "beads-on-a-string" pattern in the isoelectric focusing dimension. The mobility of these proteins is markedly altered by neuraminidase or endoglycosidase treatments.

Several proteins which can be identified in 2-D gels are available for lactoperoxidase iodination on both the internal and external surface of the plasma membrane. In Figures 7 and 8 it can be seen that a protein of 100,000 daltons, focusing at approximately pH 5.5, is available for iodination from both sides of the plasma membrane. This protein is very likely a TMB protein. The protein spot was cut out of the 2-D gels and subjected to partial proteolysis. The fragmentation pattern of this protein as shown in Figure 10 suggests that different portions of the same protein are available for iodination at the internal and external faces of the plasma membrane. Since unlabeled carrier membrane proteins are used to localize the iodinated 100,000 dalton protein in the 2-D gels, there is still the unlikely possibility that the discrete spot contains more than one iodinatable plasma membrane protein.

The ability to determine exactly the coordinates for certain proteins in the 2-D gel system allows a comparison of various types of protein labeling. For example, a 2-D analysis of the plasma membrane proteins from cells incubated with $^{32}PO_4^=$ shows that the 100,000 dalton TMB protein is also one of the most phosphorylated proteins in the plasma membrane. Another protein available for iodination at both membrane surfaces has a molecular weight of 60,000 and is extensively phosphorylated. At present the function of these phosphoproteins and the role of the phosphorylation are not known. Experiments are in progress to characterize further the phosphorylation using both proteins from cells labeled with $^{32}PO_4^=$ and proteins from membranes phosphorylated with γ-^{32}P-ATP.

The 100,000 dalton TMB protein is found in membrane preparations from a variety of mouse cell lines, mouse peritoneal macrophages, rat liver cells, and HeLa cells [20]. We speculate that some of the TMB proteins which we are analyzing are structural components of the plasma membrane of a variety of cells in culture.

The studies presented show a variety of approaches to studying the topology of membrane proteins, and they should provide a framework for the future analysis of protein-protein interactions between membrane proteins and for studies of the possible alterations in the orientation of membrane proteins in response to specific stimuli.

ACKNOWLEDGMENTS

This work was supported in part by US Public Health Service grant CA-15823, R. J. Reynolds Industries Inc., and the R. E. Goldberg Foundation. L.M.F. is a recipient of a Career Development Award (CA-00050) from the National Institutes of Health, Bethesda, Maryland. We would like to thank Dr. David Ward of Yale University for his helpful advice on these studies.

REFERENCES

1. Bretscher M: Nature New Biol 231:229, 1971.
2. Schmidt-Ullrich R, Mikelsen RB, Wallach DFH: J Biol Chem 253:6973, 1978.
3. Whiteley NM, Berg HC: J Mol Biol 87:541, 1974.
4. Hubbard AL, Cohn ZA: J Cell Biol 64:461, 1975.
5. Hunt RC, Brown JC: J Mol Biol 97:413, 1975.
6. Evans RM, Fink LM: Proc Natl Acad Sci USA 74:5341, 1977.
7. Brunette DM, Till JE: J Membrane Biol 5:215, 1971.
8. Hynes RO: Proc Natl Acad Sci USA 70:3170, 1973.
9. Gahmberg CG, Andersson LC: J Biol Chem 252:5888, 1977.
10. O'Farrell PH: J Biol Chem 250:4007, 1975.
11. Lasky RA, Mills AD: Eur J Biochem 56:335, 1975.
12. Cleveland DW, Fisher SG, Kirschner MW, Laemmli UK: J Biol Chem 252:1102, 1977.
13. Allan D, Crumpton MJ: Biochem J 120:133, 1970.
14. Ash JF, Louvard D, Singer SJ: Proc Natl Acad Sci USA 74:5584, 1977.
15. Kyte JJ: J Biol Chem 249:3652, 1974.
16. Louvard D, Semeriva M, Maroux S: J Mol Biol 106:1023, 1976.
17. Henning R, Milner R, Reske K, Cunningham BA, Edelman GM: Proc Natl Acad Sci USA 73:118, 1976.
18. Springer TA, Strominger JL: Proc Natl Acad Sci USA 73:2481, 1976.
19. Walsh FS, Crumpton MJ: Nature 269:306, 1977.
20. Evans RM, Fink LM: Unpublished data.
21. Sandra A, Pagano RE: Biochemistry 17:332, 1978.
22. Hirano H, Parkhouse B, Nicolson GL, Lennox ES, Singer SJ: Proc Natl Acad Sci USA 69:2945, 1972.
23. Nicolson GL, Singer JJ: J Cell Biol 60:236, 1974.
24. Pinto da Silva P, Nicolson GL: Biochim Biophys Acta 363:311, 1974.
25. Roos E, Temmick JHM: Exp Cell Res 94:140, 1975.
26. Walsh FS, Barber BH, Crumpton MJ: Biochemistry 15:3557, 1976.
27. Nigam VM, Brailovsky CA: Biochim Biophys Acta 468:472, 1977.

Journal of Supramolecular Structure 12:505–516 (1979)
Tumor Cell Surfaces and Malignancy 709–720

Comparison of the Structures of Human Fibronectin and Plasma Cold-Insoluble Globulin

Gary Balian, Ed Crouch, Eva Marie Click, William G. Carter, and Paul Bornstein

Departments of Biochemistry (G. B., E. C., E. M. C., P. B.) and Medicine (P.B.) University of Washington and, Fred Hutchinson Cancer Research Center (W.G.C.), Seattle, Washington 98195

Human amniotic fluid fibronectin and plasma fibronectin (cold-insoluble globulin) are indistinguishable both immunologically and by amino acid composition. Cyanogen bromide and tryptic peptides also suggest substantial structural homology. However, carbohydrate analysis has demonstrated additional saccharides in fibronectin and an overall increase in carbohydrate content relative to cold-insoluble globulin. Furthermore, limited proteolytic cleavage of the two proteins indicates differences in primary structure or in conformation. Using affinity-purified antibodies to cold-insoluble globulin, a glucosamine-labeled pronase-resistant component, probably proteoglycan, was found to coprecipitate with fibronectin, suggesting an association between these two macromolecules in the connective tissue matrix.

Key words: fibronectin, cold-insoluble globulin, carbohydrate content, proteoglycan, proteolytic cleavage

Fibronectin is a high-molecular-weight glycoprotein that is present in a variety of connective tissues including basement membranes [1]. Fibronectin is also synthesized and secreted by cells in culture and is frequently deposited on the cell surface and in the extracellular matrix produced by these cells [2–6]. A circulating glycoprotein, cold-insoluble globulin (CIG), bears extensive structural and immunologic similarities to fibronectin synthesized by cells and is sometimes referred to as plasma fibronectin [7–10]. Other body fluids, such as amniotic fluid, also contain fibronectin [4, 11].

Fibronectin has been shown to function in cell adhesion [8, 12], in maintenance of cell shape [13, 14] and in cellular movement [15]. The protein interacts with a number of components such as collagen [16–18] and fibrin [19] and can become crosslinked to fibrinogen through the action of plasma transglutaminase [20]. The association of fibronectin with certain cell-surface macromolecules may be necessary for the cell surface functions mediated by fibronectin.

Our objective was to study the similarities and possible differences between CIG and cellular and amniotic fluid fibronectins. Despite the very extensive structural and functional similarities between fibronectin and CIG, a number of findings suggest that the proteins are not identical. Reproducible differences in migration on sodium dodecyl

Received June 26, 1979; accepted November 13, 1979.

sulfate (SDS) gels have been reported; CIG can be resolved as a closely spaced doublet, whereas fibronectin isolated from amniotic fluid, cell culture medium, and cell layer migrates more slowly as a broad band [4, 21–23]. CIG is somewhat less effective in promoting the attachment of virally transformed hamster fibroblasts to a substratum [21], and is considerably less effective in hemagglutination of fixed erythrocytes [24] and in restoring a more normal morphology to transformed cells [24]. In this report we present evidence that fibronectin isolated from human amniotic fluid [4] differs from CIG in its carbohydrate content and in the peptide pattern produced by limited cleavage with two proteases. Preliminary evidence for the interaction of cellular fibronectin with proteoglycans is also provided.

METHODS

Preparation of Cold-Insoluble Globulin

Cold-insoluble globulin was prepared from human plasma cryoprecipitates by a modification of the method described by Mosesson and Umfleet [25]. Frozen plasma was thawed in an ice bath at $0°C$; the residue (cryoprecipitate) was centrifuged and dissolved in 0.2 M NaCl, 0.02 M imidazole buffer (pH 6.8) at room temperature. Glycine was added to a final concentration of 2.1 M, during which the temperature of the mixture dropped to $15°C$. After the precipitate was removed by centrifugation at $15°C$, the supernatant was diluted with an equal volume of cold distilled water and the proteins were precipitated by the addition of 20% v/v ethanol at $-4°$ C. The mixture was maintained at $-4°C$ for 30–60 min and centrifuged at 6,000g for 30 min. The pellet was dissolved in 0.04 M succinate-Tris buffer (pH 7.0) and the CIG was purified by chromatography on DEAE-cellulose using a linear gradient from 0.04–0.1 M succinate-Tris. When necessary, CIG prepared by DEAE-cellulose chromatography was purified further on Biorex-70 (BioRad), using a linear gradient of 0.1–0.3 M succinate-Tris (pH 6.8). CIG preparations produced a characteristic doublet on SDS-polyacrylamide gel electrophoresis when disulfide bonds were reduced. CIG was also prepared from plasma by affinity chromatography on gelatin-Sepharose [16]. A 0.5-mg portion of CIG was reduced and alkylated essentially as described by Crestfield et al [26] using 0.2 mCi [^{3}H] iodoacetic acid.

Preparation of Fibronectin

Second-trimester human amniotic fluid was centrifuged to remove debris, and EDTA (25 mM), phenylmethanesulfonyl fluoride (PMSF, 1 mM), and N-ethylmaleimide (10 mM) were added to minimize proteolysis. Solid ammonium sulfate was added to a final concentration of 20% (w/v) and the precipitate produced was removed by centrifugation and redissolved in 0.05 M Tris-HCl, 0.15 M NaCl (pH 7.5) containing 1 mM PMSF. Further purification was achieved by affinity chromatography on denatured collagen (gelatin)-Sepharose.

Preparation of Antibodies

Fibronectin or CIG (100–200 μg), dissolved in 1 ml phosphate-buffered saline and mixed with an equal volume of Freund's complete adjuvant, was used to immunize rabbits by subcutaneous injection at weekly intervals. Antisera were obtained 4 weeks after the start of the immunization program and after periodic booster injections.

Radioimmunoassays

Inhibition assays were performed as described previously [4] using ^{125}I-CIG or ^{125}I-fibronectin and rabbit antisera to these proteins. The concentration of inhibitor was determined using an absorption coefficient $(E_{1\ cm}^{1\%})$ at 280 nm of 13.

Immune Precipitation of Radiolableled Fibronectin

Rabbit anti-human CIG antibodies were purified by affinity chromatography on CIG linked to Sepharose. Bound IgG was eluted with 0.2 M glycine adjusted to pH 2.8 with HCl and dialyzed against phosphate-buffered saline. Affinity-purified antibody (0.6 mg/ml) was added to radiolabeled culture medium or to cell layer extracts and incubated for 1 h at room temperature. Sheep anti-rabbit gamma globulin antiserum was added and the mixture incubated at 4°C for 16 h. The precipitate was centrifuged and washed with 0.05 M Tris-HCl (pH 7.5). Reduction and alkylation of the immune precipitates was performed essentially as described previously [26].

Metabolic Labeling of Cells in Culture

Amniotic fluid-derived (AF) cells were prepared and maintained as previously described [4]. Cells were labeled with one of the following: 125 μCi/ml [^{35}S] cysteine-HCl, 50 μCi/ml ^{3}H-amino acid mixture, 50 μCi/ml [2 - ^{3}H] mannose, or 50 μCi/ml [1 - ^{14}C] glucosamine. Incubations were performed for 24 h in serum-free medium deficient in the corresponding sugar or amino acid. Culture medium was harvested into protease inhibitors [4]. The cells were first extracted with Hanks's balanced salt solution containing 1 M urea and 0.5 mM PMSF for 15 min at room temperature; cell layers were then suspended in 0.05 M sodium phosphate (pH 11) containing 1% Triton X-100, and were sonicated and centrifuged to remove cell debris. Culture medium, urea extracts, and cell layers were dialyzed into 0.05 M Tris-HCl, 0.15 M NaCl (pH 7.5).

Enzymatic Cleavage

Digestion of a mixture of [^{35}S] cysteine-labeled fibronectin and ^{3}H-CIG with trypsin (Worthington, TPCK) was performed in 0.1 M NH$_4$HCO$_3$ containing 1 mM CaCl$_2$ at 37° for 24 h using an enzyme-to-substrate ratio of 1 to 10 by weight, and the sample was lyophilized. Cation exchange chromatography of tryptic peptides of radiolabeled fibronectin and CIG was performed on a 0.9 - x 50 -cm column of sulphonated polystyrene (UR-30, Beckman) at 55° C using pyridine acetate buffers as previously described [27].

Digestion with cathepsin D (Sigma Chemical Co.) was performed at pH 3.5 and 30°C for 12 h in the presence of 0.2 mM PMSF, using an enzyme-to-substrate weight ratio of 1:250. Reactions were stopped by the addition of a 10-fold molar excess of pepstatin (Peptide Research Institute, Osaka, Japan). Digestion with mast cell protease, an enzyme with chymotrypsin-like specificity purified from rat peritoneal cavity (M. Everett and H. Neurath, in preparation), was performed at pH 7.5 and 30°C for 4 h using an enzyme-to-substrate weight ratio of 1:800. Enzymatic reactions were stopped and protein was precipitated by the addition of trichloroacetic acid (TCA) at 0° C to a final concentration of 10%. Precipitated proteins were prepared for SDS polyacrylamide slab gel electrophoresis by the addition of 0.2% SDS in 0.1 M Tris-HCl buffer (pH 6.8) with or without 50 mM dithiothreitol (DTT). Protein components in gels were stained with a 0.25% solution of Coomassie Brilliant Blue R and radioactive components were visualized by autoradiography [4].

Digestion of immune precipitated fibronectin with pronase (Calbiochem, grade B) was performed in 0.05 M sodium phosphate buffer (pH 7.5) at 37°C with an enzyme-to-substrate weight ratio of 1:30 for 60 h; at this point a second aliquot of enzyme was added and the digestion continued for 24 h. The samples were dialyzed and lyophilized. Chromatography on Sephadex G-50 superfine (Pharmacia) was performed using a 1.2 X 135 cm column eluted with 0.1 M ammonium bicarbonate. Cleavage with cyanogen bromide was performed in 70% formic acid at 30°C for 4 h using an equal ratio, by weight, of cyanogen bromide to protein.

Affinity Chromatography

Salt-soluble collagen, purified from lathyritic rat skin, was denatured by heating at 45°C for 30 min, and coupled to Sepharose CL4B (Pharmacia) using CNBr. Samples were applied to the column in the presence of protease inhibitors in 0.05 M Tris-HCl, 0.15 MNaCl, pH 7.5 at 4°C. Bound fractions were eluted with the above buffer containing 6 M urea.

Amino Acid Analysis

Lyophilized samples were hydrolyzed in vacuo with twice distilled hydrochloric acid at 108°C for 24 h and amino acid compositions were determined on a Durrum D500 analyzer. No corrections were made for hydrolytic losses of individual amino acids. Tryptophan was determined as described by Hugli and Moore [28].

Carbohydrate Analysis

Both fibronectin and CIG were further purified from possible carbohydrate-containing contaminants by molecular sieve chromatography on a column of controlled pore glass (700 Å, Electro Nucleonics Inc.) equilibrated in 0.1% SDS, 1 M urea, 0.025 M Tris-HCl, 0.2 M glycine buffer (pH 8.8). SDS bound to protein was removed by sequential dialysis against 80% acetone and water. Samples were dried to a constant weight and hydrolyzed in 80% acetic acid, 0.5 M H_2SO_4, for 8 h at 80°C and carbohydrate composition was determined by gas-liquid chromatography of the alditol acetate derivatives. Sugars were identified by their positions of elution using an internal standard of inositol; their identification was confirmed by mass spectrometry. Sialic acid was determined by the thiobarbituric acid method using a spectrofluorometric assay [29].

RESULTS

The immunologic cross-reaction of fibronectin and CIG was studied by radioimmunoassay. Purified amniotic fluid fibronectin and CIG inhibited the precipitation of iodinated CIG by anti-CIG antibodies in an identical fashion (Fig. 1). Comparable curves were obtained using culture medium from human amniotic fluid cells or skin fibroblasts as inhibitors of anti-CIG antibodies. Antiserum to amniotic fluid fibronectin was also completely inhibited by both fibronectin and CIG. These experiments indicate complete immunologic cross-reactivity of fibronectin, derived from amniotic fluid or from cells in culture, with plasma CIG.

The amino acid compositions of amniotic fluid fibronectin, culture medium fibronectin, and plasma CIG are shown in Table I. The high degree of similarity among these analyses suggests extensive structural homology between the proteins. Of note is the unusually high amount of threonine present in both proteins. A survey of the level of this amino acid

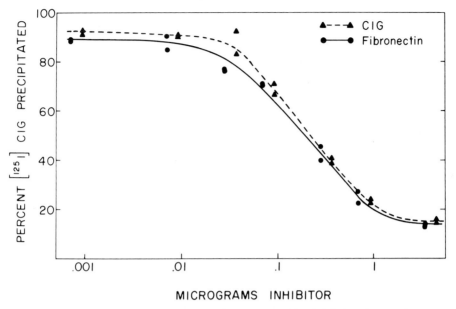

Fig. 1. Radioimmune inhibition curve. Increasing quantities of unlabeled CIG or fibronectin were used to inhibit the precipitation of [^{125}I] CIG by anti-CIG IgG in a double-antibody assay.

TABLE I. Amino Acid Compositions of Human CIG and Amniotic Fluid and Cellular Fibronectins

	Residues/1,000 residues		
	Plasma CIG	Amniotic fluid fibronectin	Cell culture medium fibronectin[a]
Aspartic acid	94	95	92
Threonine	106	101	106
Serine	74	78	78
Glutamic acid	120	122	118
Proline	93	92	71
Glycine	87	88	90
Alanine	42	43	47
Half-cystine[b]	24	25	23
Valine	76	73	77
Methionine	10	11	12
Isoleucine	42	42	45
Leucine	51	56	61
Tyrosine	39	36	40
Phenylalanine	23	25	27
Histidine	21	20	23
Lysine	35	32	37
Arginine	51	50	52
Tryptophan	15	11	ND

[a]From amniotic fluid-derived AF cells.
[b]Determined by performic acid oxidation.
ND: Not determined.

in other proteins shows that a value of about 10% of the total residues is exceeded only by silk fibroin and a few other glycoproteins.

We have previously shown that a cysteine-rich collagen-binding region from fibronectin and CIG migrates differently on SDS-PAGE [18]. Cation exchange chromatography of the tryptic peptides obtained from fibronectin and CIG, radiolabeled at cysteine residues, is shown in Figure 2. There is extensive correspondence and there are no major qualitative differences between the peptides derived from the two proteins, indicating that the cysteine-containing regions are structurally very similar in CIG and fibronectin. The fractions that were not retained by cation exchange chromatography (Fig. 2) were further analyzed by anion exchange chromatography on Dowex-1. The more negatively charged peptides from fibronectin and CIG were also observed to coelute (data not shown).

CIG and fibronectin were separately cleaved with cyanogen bromide and the resulting patterns were analyzed on 15% SDS-acrylamide gels and visualized by staining (data not shown). The pattern of peptides confirmed that extensive similarities exist between the two proteins, as indicated previously using digestion with trypsin. Only minor differences in the pattern of fibronectin- and CIG-derived peptides were apparent. Two proteases were also used to compare the products of partial proteolysis of fibronectin and CIG. The difference in electrophoretic migration between CIG and fibronectin is illustrated in Figure 3 (lanes

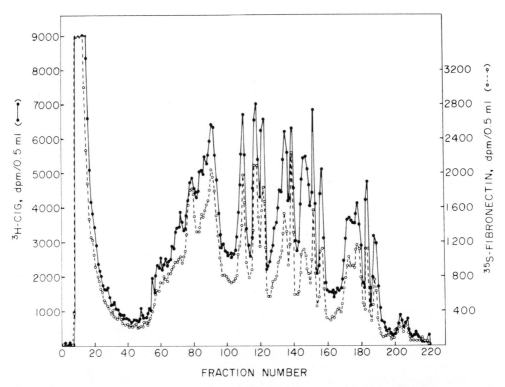

Fig. 2. Cation exchange chromatography of trypsin digests of CIG and fibronectin. [^{35}S] cysteine-labeled fibronectin was purified from amniotic fluid cell culture medium by precipitation with anti-CIG antibody and was reduced and carboxymethylated with iodoacetic acid. CIG was alkylated similarly but using [^{3}H] iodoacetic acid. The preparations of fibronectin and CIG were mixed and cleaved with trypsin, and the resulting peptides were separated on a UR-30 (Beckman) column using a multistep pyridine acetate gradient [27].

1 and 2). The fibronectin band is more diffuse and the average apparent molecular weight of the component chain after reduction of disulfide bonds is 235,000, in contrast to a calculated molecular weight of 220,000 for CIG. The peptides resulting from limited cleavage of CIG and fibronectin with cathepsin D and mast cell protease are also shown in Figure 3. In many instances the peptides derived from fibronectin are more heterogeneous

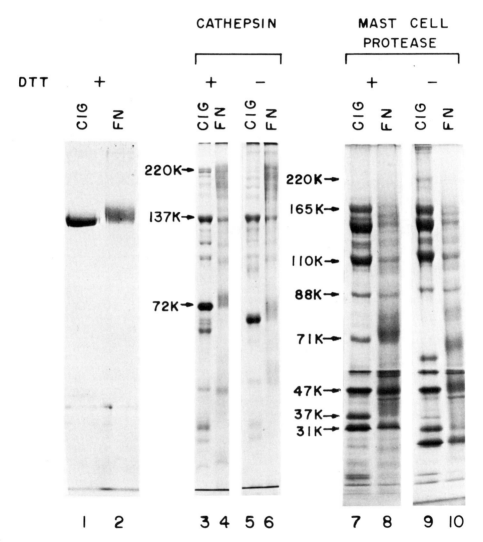

Fig. 3. SDS-polyacrylamide gel electrophoresis of CIG, fibronectin (FN), and their enzymatically derived fragments. Lanes 1, 2: CIG and fibronectin, 5 μg each. Lanes 3–6: Fibronectin and CIG treated with cathepsin D; 20 μg of protein was added to each lane. Lane 7–10: Fibronectin and CIG treated with mast cell protease; 30 μg CIG protein and 40 μg of fibronectin protein was added to each lane. Electrophoresis was performed in the absence (-) or presence (+) of 50 mM DTT on single-layer or composite slab gels. Lanes 1, 2: 5% acrylamide with 10% base; lanes 3–6, 7.5% acrylamide; lane 7–10, 7.5% acrylamide with 12.5% base. Gels were stained with Coomassie blue. The molecular weights indicated by the arrows were obtained by comparison with a mixture of globular proteins of known molecular weights and apply only to lanes 3 and 4 and to lanes 7 and 8.

TABLE II. Carbohydrate Composition of Fibronectin and Cold-Insoluble Globulin Expressed as Percentage Dry Weight

	Amniotic fluid fibronectin	Plasma CIG
Fucose	0.4	Trace
Mannose	1.1	1.0
Galactose	1.7	1.0
N-acetylglucosamine	2.5	1.8
N-acetylgalactosamine	0.7	0.1
Sialic acid	0.6	0.7
Total	7.0	4.6

*Several preparations of each protein were used; the values are an average of at least three determinations.

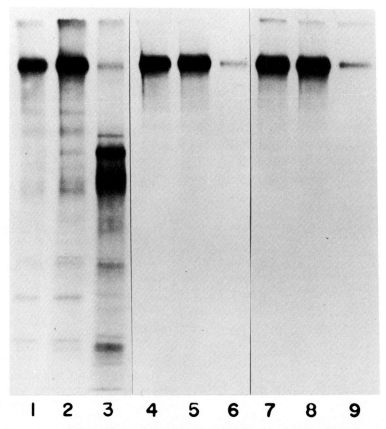

Fig. 4. SDS polyacrylamide gel electrophoresis of amniotic fluid cell fractions. Slab gels were composed of 7% acrylamide with a 10% base and were prepared for autoradiography. Lanes 1–3: [3H] mannose-labeled cells precipitated with trichloroacetic acid; lane 1: culture medium; lane 2: urea extract; lane 3: cell homogenate. Lanes 4–6: [3H] mannose-labeled cells precipitated with anti-fibronectin antibodies; lane 4: culture medium; lane 5: urea extract; lane 6: cell homogenate. Lanes 7–9: [3H] glucosamine-labeled cells precipitated with antifibronectin antibodies; lane 7: culture medium; lane 8: urea extract; lane 9: cell homogenate.

and migrate more slowly than the corresponding peptides from CIG. This behavior is particularly prominent in the case of a 72,000 dalton fragment produced by cathepsin D and the effect is seen whether the gels are run in the absence or presence of a reducing agent (Fig. 3, lanes 3–6). Similar observations have been made using radiolabeled fibronectin from cell culture medium [18]. In addition there are other differences in the cleavage patterns obtained with the two proteases. Notably, at least two low-molecular-weight peptides in digests of CIG do not have prominent counterparts in digests of fibronectin (Fig. 3, compare lanes 3 and 4 and 9 and 10). These results have been reproduced with three different preparations of the two proteins.

Recent experiments have suggested that the electrophoretic heterogeneity of fibronectin can be accounted for by variable glycosylation of the protein [4]. The extent of glycosylation of CIG and fibronectin was therefore compared (Table II). Several differences were observed. Whereas amniotic fluid fibronectin contains significant amounts of fucose and N-acetylgalactosamine, these residues were present in only trace or very low amounts in CIG. Fibronectin also contained increased amounts of galactose and N-acetylglucosamine which contribute to a higher total carbohydrate content of fibronectin.

The polydispersity of fibronectin was further investigated using the glycoprotein isolated from different fractions of cells in culture and by comparing the size of the oligosaccharide-containing peptides. Fibronectin secreted by amniotic fluid cells into culture medium, extracted from cell surfaces with urea or obtained by detergent homogenization of of cell layers, was compared (Fig. 4). A high proportion of the radiolabeled glycoproteins secreted by these cells could be accounted for as fibronectin in the culture medium (Fig. 4, lanes 1, 4, and 7) and in the urea-soluble fractions (Fig. 4, lanes 2, 5, and 8). However, fibronectin constitutes only a small proportion of the total radioactive proteins obtained from the cell layer (Fig. 4, lane 3). Fibronectin could be purified from detergent homogenates of cells by immune precipitation (Fig. 4, lanes 6 and 9).

The oligosaccharide-containing peptides of soluble, immune-precipitated fibronectin were obtained by extensive cleavage of the polypeptide with pronase; the elution pattern of these glycopeptides is shown in Figure 5. The majority of the mannose and glucosamine migrates as a single peak (Fig. 5–1), in agreement with previous reports [30]. The majority of the carbohydrate in fibronectin is therefore in chains of uniform or nearly uniform length. In contrast, carbohydrate from cell layer-derived fibronectin preparations appeared as two major peaks (Fig. 5–2). One peak eluting in the void volume was a glucosamine-rich component containing essentially no mannose; a second peak, containing both glucosamine and mannose, eluted in the same position as the glycopeptides from soluble fibronectin. The glucosamine-rich component is most likely a pronase-resistant core derived from proteoglycan that was coprecipitated with fibronectin by antibodies. Much less proteoglycan was found to precipitate with medium or cell surface fibronectin, as indicated in Figure 5–1.

DISCUSSION

Fibronectin and CIG cross-react immunologically and are indistinguishable by cross-inhibition assays. Chemical and enzymatic cleavage of the two proteins also show extensive structural similarities. Reports from several sources suggest that fibronectin and CIG also share many of their biologic properties. However, as noted earlier, fibronectin is more active in mediating cell attachment [21] and several times more effective in hemagglutination of glutaraldehyde-fixed sheep erythrocytes [24], and in restoring a

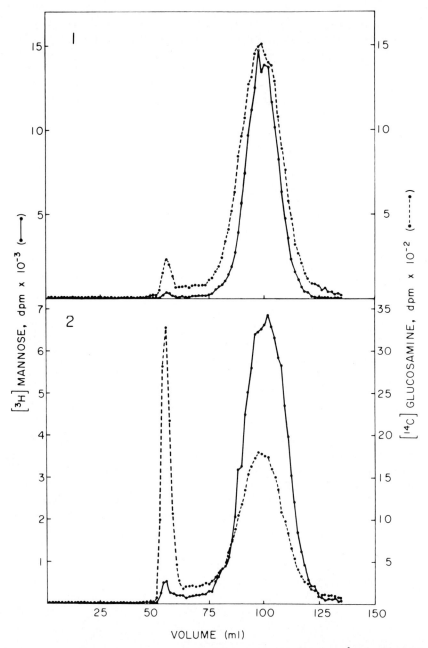

Fig. 5. Sephadex G-50 chromatography. Amniotic fluid cells were labeled with [³H] mannose and [¹⁴C] glucosamine, and culture medium, urea extracts, or cell homogenates were immune-precipitated separately. Mannose- and glucosamine-labeled fractions were mixed and digested with pronase before chromatography. Panel 1: Urea extracts. Panel 2: cell homogenates. The elution pattern of pronase digests of culture medium was the same as that shown in panel 1.

more normal morphology to transformed cells [24]. Recent reports have shown that when fibronectin is synthesized in the presence of tunicamycin, an inhibitor of protein glycosylation, the biological activity of the protein is retained [31]. This indicates that the carbohydrate moiety in fibronectin is not an essential requirement for some of the cell surface properties attributed to the glycoprotein. However, the nonglycosylated protein was shown to be twice as sensitive as the normal protein to proteolysis, both in vitro and using intact cells [31, 32]. These findings suggest that the increased levels of glycosylation of fibronectin could function to protect the protein from premature proteolysis from the cell surface. Differences in peptide pattern obtained after limited enzymatic cleavage of fibronectin and CIG indicate a difference in susceptibility of these two proteins to enzymatic cleavage. Differences in conformation may be responsible for these observations, since additional carbohydrate residues in fibronectin may limit cleavage at specific sites by these proteases. Additional differences in apoprotein structure between fibronectin and CIG, however, cannot be excluded.

A limited amount of proteoglycan may copurify with fibronectin, and although chromatography in SDS-containing buffers would be expected to disrupt the interaction of fibronectin with carbohydrate-containing contaminants, it is difficult to completely eliminate this possibility. Recently a high-molecular-weight, base-stable heteroglycan associated with isolated cell surface fibronectin was described [30]. This oligosaccharide contained galactose, N-acetylglucosamine, and N-acetylgalactosamine as major sugars.

A variety of cell types grown in culture have the ability to synthesize fibronectin or a fibronectin-like molecule that appears as a polydisperse band on SDS gels. The differences that exist between fibronectin and CIG, and the location of CIG in the circulatory system, suggest that the product synthesized and secreted by such cells in tissues could be a precursor to fibronectin found in plasma. Partial deglycosylation could account for the change in migration of fibronectin from a polydisperse band on SDS gels to a doublet represented by the chains of CIG. In this regard, the increased carbohydrate content and slower electrophoretic migration of amniotic fluid fibronectin cannot be attributed to its fetal origin, since human fetal and adult CIG migrate identically on SDS gels (unpublished observations).

Alternatively, CIG may be a synthetic product of cells which are designed to function as a source of plasma proteins, such as hepatocytes or cells associated with the vascular system. This raises the possibility that, depending on their requirements, different cell types may produce different forms of fibronectin. A number of observations have now been made which support the notion that fibronectin is not required by all cells in mediating the interaction of cells with their environment [33]; indeed in the case of epidermal cells and hepatocytes fibronectin does not appear to be required for attachment to a collagenous substratum [34, 35].

Our studies indicate that fibronectin is associated with a pronase-resistant high-molecular-weight glycan, presumably proteoglycan, in amniotic fluid cell layers and that the complex can be precipitated by antibodies to fibronectin. Earlier reports indicate that CIG binds to heparin [36] and that fibronectin is associated with glycosaminoglycan in NIL hamster fibroblasts [37]. We have used amniotic fluid cells to study the incorporation of Na_2 [$^{35}SO_4$]; the uptake of this isotope into a major component, presumably proteoglycan, which is secreted into the culture medium was shown (G. Balian, E. M. Click, and P. Bornstein, unpublished observation). Both fibronectin and proteoglycan are therefore likely to be present in the culture medium of cells but coprecipitation occurs only with homogenates of whole cells. The association of fibronectin and proteoglycan may not occur in culture medium (ie, in solution) or in urea-extractable material because a fibrillar matrix may be required for the alignment of fibronectin and subsequent interaction with proteoglycan.

ACKNOWLEDGMENTS

We thank Mark Powell for performing the carbohydrate analyses and Michael Everitt for providing the mast cell protease. G. B. is an Established Investigator of the American Heart Association. W. G. C. was supported by NIH postdoctoral fellowship GM 06588. This work was supported by NIH grants AM 11248, HL 18645, and AM 00299.

REFERENCES

1. Stenman S, Vaheri A: J Exp Med 147:1054, 1978.
2. Hynes RO: Biochim Biophys Acta 458:73, 1976.
3. Hedman K, Vaheri A, Wartiovaara J: J Cell Biol 76:748, 1978.
4. Crouch E, Balian G, Holbrook K, Duksin D, Bornstein P: J Cell Biol 78:701, 1978.
5. Furcht LT, Mosher DF, Wendelschafer-Crabb G: Cell 13:263, 1978.
6. Chen LB, Murray A, Segal RA, Bushnell A, Walsh ML: Cell 14:377, 1978.
7. Vaheri A, Mosher DF: Biochim Biophys Acta 516:1, 1978.
8. Yamada KM, Olden K: Nature 275:179, 1978.
9. Mosesson MW: Ann NY Acad Sci 312:11, 1978.
10. Vuento M, Wrann M, Ruoslahti E: FEBS Lett 82:227, 1977.
11. Chen AB, Mosesson MW, Solish GI: Am J Obstet Gynecol 125:958, 1976.
12. Grinnell F, Minter D: Proc Natl Acad Sci USA 75:4408, 1978.
13. Yamada KM, Olden K, Pastan I: Ann NY Acad Sci 312:256, 1978.
14. Pena SDJ, Hughes RC: Nature 276:80, 1978.
15. Ali IU, Hynes RO: Cell 14:439, 1978.
16. Engvall E, Ruoslahti E: Int J Cancer 20:1, 1977.
17. Kleinman HK, McGoodwin EB, Martin GR, Klebe RJ, Fietzek PP, Woolley DE:
    J Biol Chem 253:5642, 1978.
18. Balian G, Click EM, Crouch E, Davidson JM, Bornstein P: J Biol Chem 254:1429, 1979.
19. Ruoslahti E, Vaheri A: J Exp Med 141:497, 1975.
20. Mosher DF: J Biol Chem 250:6614, 1975.
21. Hynes RO, Ali IU, Destree AT, Mautner V, Perkins ME, Senger DR, Wagner DD, Smith KK:
    Ann NY Acad Sci 312:317, 1978.
22. Mosher DF: Biochim Biophys Acta 491:205, 1977.
23. Keski-Oja J, Mosher DF, Vaheri A: Biochem Biophys Res Commun 74:699, 1977.
24. Yamada KM, Kennedy DW: J Cell Biol 80:492, 1979.
25. Mosesson MW, Umfleet RA: J Biol Chem 245:5728, 1970.
26. Crestfield AM, Moore S, Stein WH: J Biol Chem 238:622, 1963.
27. Balian G, Click EM, Bornstein P: Biochemistry 10:4470, 1971.
28. Hugli TE, Moore S: J Biol Chem 247:2828, 1972.
29. Hammond KS, Papermaster DS: Anal Biochem 74:292, 1976.
30. Carter WG, Hakomori S: Biochemistry 18:730, 1979.
31. Olden K, Pratt RM, Yamada KM: Proc Natl Acad Sci USA 76:791, 1979.
32. Olden K, Pratt RM, Yamada KM: Cell 13:461, 1978.
33. Kleinman HK, Hewitt AT, Pennypacker JP, McGoodwin EB, Martin GR, Fishman PH: J Supramol
    Struct (In press).
34. Murray JC, Stingl G, Kleinman HK, Martin GR, Katz SI: J Cell Biol 80:197, 1979.
35. Rubin K, Oldberg A, Höök M, Obrink B: Exp Cell Res 117:165, 1978.
36. Stathakis NE, Mosesson MW: J Clin Invest 60:855, 1977.
37. Perkins ME, Ji TH, Hynes RO: Cell 16:941, 1979.

Journal of Supramolecular Structure 12:517–531 (1979)
Tumor Cell Surfaces and Malignancy 721–735

Hormone-Induced Modification of EGF Receptor Proteolysis in the Induction of EGF Action

C. Fred Fox, Michael Wrann, Peter Linsley, and Ron Vale

From the Molecular Biology Institute and Department of Microbiology, University of California at Los Angeles, California 90024

A proposal that EGF action is mediated through enhanced internalization of EGF receptors is modified to account for more recent evidence. EGF receptors turn over at a rapid rate, and the maintenance of a steady state of EGF receptors on the cell surface is provided through a rapid synthesis of EGF receptors, balancing their removal. This rapid turnover of unoccupied receptors may arise through their internalization and proteolysis in the lysosomes, in much the same way as receptors are internalized and degraded when exposed to EGF, which enhances internalization. This provides a dilemma for the endocytic activation concept, since slight enhancement of receptor internalization gives rise to a strong hormone response. This problem may be solved by the observation that EGF induces a change in its receptor, exposing an otherwise unavailable site for proteolytic cleavage. This hormone-dependent modification of receptors may be the critical step in the induction of responses to EGF and other hormones that are internalized with their receptors. Both platelet-derived growth factor (PDGF) and fibroblast growth factor (FGF) are shown to down-regulate EGF receptors, though transiently, placing still more stringent requirements on the specificity by which hormones might act through endocytic activation of their receptors.

Key words: direct labeling of EGF receptors, transient down-regulation of EGF receptors, platelet derived growth factor, receptor proteolysis

Three properties of murine EGF [1] have led several laboratories to select it for studies on the biochemical mechanism of polypeptide hormone-induced stimulation of cell proliferation: 1) EGF can be readily purified by a simple procedure [2]; 2) EGF can be radioiodinated to high specific activity and retain its biological activity [3]; and 3) many cultured cell lines elicit a mitogenic response to EGF (for review see [4]). The mitogenic activity of polypeptide hormones is usually studied in growth-arrested cell monolayers, maintained in culture with a minimal concentration of serum, which is itself rich in mitogens. Addition of nanomolar concentrations of EGF to a monolayer of responsive cells — eg, murine 3T3 cells — induces a sequence of events that ultimately leads to DNA replication. EGF gives rise to these events after binding specifically to high-affinity surface receptors

Michael Wrann's present address is Sandoz Forschungsinstitut, Brunner Strasse 59, A1235 Wien, Austria.

Received September 5, 1979; accepted October 8, 1979.

[3–11]. Studies in which fluorescent and ferritin-labeled EGF derivatives were incubated with cells have shown that EGF enhances the patching of the ferritin or fluorescent labels, and thus presumably the patching of the receptor molecules on the cell surface [12–14].

Shortly after the addition of ferritin or fluorescent EGF probes, the probes begin to appear intracellularly in small vesicles, and their appearance in these vesicles is followed by their incorporation into the lysosomes [12–14]. When EGF and insulin probes, which can be distinguished one from the other by their specific fluorescence properties, are added together both are ultimately detected in the same lysosomal particles [15]. This shows that many hormones, and presumably their receptors as well, share common steps in internalization and/or ultimate deposition in the lysosomes [15]. Das and Fox used photoaffinity probes of EGF to specifically label receptors and showed directly that EGF receptors are internalized [10, 16]. Furthermore, receptor internalization correlates quantitatively with the loss of EGF binding activity that ensues when EGF is added to cells [17]. They also reported that EGF-induced stimulation of DNA synthesis in 3T3 cells is more closely correlated with EGF-induced receptor internalization than with saturation of the EGF receptor [18]. Both EGF receptor down-regulation, which in the cell line studied by Das and Fox is quantitatively equivalent to increased receptor internalization, and EGF-induced stimulation of DNA synthesis are half-saturated at the same level of EGF – a level at which no more than 10% of the EGF receptors are saturated at the steady state of binding. Das and Fox made the important distinction between a steady-state binding level of EGF and the dynamic process of enhanced receptor internalization that is induced by EGF, and they proposed that EGF might stimulate DNA synthesis by a process of "endocytic activation" [16–18]. Their data indicate that the limiting step in EGF-induced stimulation of DNA synthesis in these cells was not EGF binding itself, but rather, a step leading to the internalization and processing of the EGF receptor in the lysosomes, or possibly, internalization and processing itself.

Other recent findings are in essential agreement with these observations. Schechter et al have correlated the local aggregation of EGF:EGF-receptor complexes with the mitogenic activity of EGF [19]. They found that CNBr-treated EGF was antagonistic for EGF binding but biologically far less active. Biological activity of CNBr-treated EGF was restored when it was added to cells together with a carefully controlled concentration of anti-EGF IgG, which promoted aggregation and possibly enhanced the internalization of CNBr-EGF-occupied receptors.

In this review we deal primarily with recent studies from this laboratory which test for possible role(s) of EGF receptor internalization and processing in EGF-induced stimulation of DNA synthesis. We find that EGF receptor down-regulation* can occur in response to a variety of conditions other than EGF addition, and the known rapid turnover of this receptor poses additional constraints on the concept that EGF activity is elicited through a simple endocytic activation of receptor. Normal EGF receptor turnover may also proceed by internalization and proteolysis of EGF receptors in the lysosomes. The specificity problems suggested by these observations may be reconciled by recent observations reported here. We have observed that EGF induces changes in receptor that alter the specific sites that are initially susceptible to proteolytic nicking. These observations show that the susceptibility of the EGF receptor to possible proteolytic activation may occur only when it is occupied by EGF.

---

*In this paper the term "down-regulation" is used to refer to the phenomenon of ligand-induced decrease in ligand-binding activity. Receptor internalization is but one of many processes that could give rise to down-regulation.

MATERIALS AND METHODS

Swiss mouse 3T3 cells, clone 42 from G. Todaro, and human epithilioid carcinoma cells (strain A431 from G. Todaro) [12] were used in these studies. Cells were grown routinely in Dulbecco's modified Eagle's medium (DME) containing 5% (3T3) or 10% (A431) fetal calf serum (FCS) and used on or before the sixth passage from frozen stock. Most experiments were performed on serum-starved cells. These were prepared by growing cells to confluence, and by shifting the serum concentration in the growth medium to 0.5%. The cells were then incubated at 37°C for an additional 24 h to yield the serum-starved cells. The procedures for isolation of EGF from mouse submaxillary glands [1], radio-iodination of EGF [10], assay for EGF binding, EGF receptor down-regulation [20, 21], DNA synthesis [16], protein synthesis [22], "direct" labeling of EGF receptors [23], surface-specific radioiodination, preparation of 3T3 cell membranes, and SDS-polyacryla-mide gel electrophoresis [20] have been described.

RESULTS

EGF-Dependent and EGF-Independent Turnover of EGF Receptors

The experiments described in this section show that a steady state of EGF binding activity is achieved when the rate of receptor synthesis and removal are equal. The experiments described in Figures 1–3 were designed to modify EGF binding activity by modulation of the rate of receptor synthesis or removal. This was accomplished by varying the serum concentration in the growth medium or by incubating cells with cycloheximide and/or EGF.

EGF receptor synthesis is serum dependent. When 3T3 cells are incubated at 37°C at high EGF concentration they lose more than 80% of their EGF binding activity within a few hours, and a new steady-state level of receptors is achieved (Fig. 1). We have studied the recovery of EGF binding activity after removal of EGF (Figs. 1 and 2). EGF binding is restored in a process that requires protein synthesis, and the rate of restoration correlates with the total cellular capacity for protein synthesis (Fig. 2). Both total protein and receptor synthesis are stimulated at high serum concentrations. It therefore appears that the cells constantly synthesize receptors at a rate dependent, among other things, on the serum concentration in the growth medium.

Turnover of unoccupied EGF receptors. If cells synthesize receptors continuously, there must be a mechanism for receptor destruction to account for maintenance of a constant number of receptors on the surface. Upon a shift from 5% to 0.5% serum, 3T3 cells lost 30% of their EGF binding activity within 4 h, and 40% in 12 h (Fig. 1). This loss of binding activity is correlated with a reduced capacity of serum-starved cells to synthesize protein (Fig. 2) or restore EGF binding activity after EGF-induced down-regulation of EGF receptors (Figs. 1 and 2). When serum-starved cells were incubated with cycloheximide to arrest protein synthesis maximally, EGF binding activity declined with a half-time of approximately 7 h (Fig. 3). This is similar to the half-time of receptor recovery after maximal down-regulation of EGF receptors in serum-starved cells (Fig. 2).

Hormone binding enhances internalization and lysosomal degradation of occupied receptors. The experiments treated in the preceding section, and presented in Figures 2 and 3, were done in parallel so that the rate measurements in the different experiments could be compared. In these experiments, the initial rate of loss of EGF binding activity when protein synthesis was arrested maximally by cycloheximide was equal within experi-

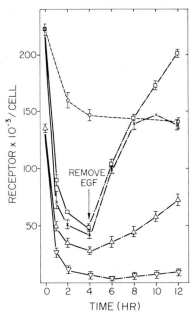

Fig. 1. Effect of serum concentration and cycloheximide on down-regulation of EGF receptors and on the recovery of EGF binding activity following EGF receptor down-regulation. Cells were grown to confluence in medium containing 5% fetal calf serum (FCS). Twenty-four hours prior to time 0, when EGF was added to down-regulate the EGF receptor, the FCS concentration in some dishes was changed to 0.5%. At time 0, the medium of all dishes was changed to fresh DME containing 5% or 0.5% FCS and 50 ng/ml of unlabeled EGF (□,x,△,▽) or no EGF (○). Cycloheximide (2 μg/ml) was added to some samples (▽). At time 4 h, EGF was removed, and the cells were incubated with DME plus FCS, as indicated below. ^{125}I-EGF binding was determined after incubation with 10 nM ^{125}I-EGF for 10 min at 22°C, as described in Materials and Methods. Receptors per cell was calculated directly from the specific binding data. (□ = cells grown and maintained in 5% FCS; ○,x = cells grown in 5% FCS and shifted to 0.5% FCS at time 0; △,▽ = cells starved for 24 h in 0.5% FCS (serum-starved cells) and maintained in 0.5% FCS; - - - - - - = no EGF added; ——— = incubation with EGF added; — · — · — = incubation after EGF removal.)

mental error to the initial rate of restoration of EGF binding activity in cells treated with EGF maximally to down-regulate receptors. Assuming that the loss of EGF binding during cycloheximide treatment of cells is due only to the effects of cycloheximide on receptor synthesis, the rate of EGF receptor synthesis is equal in EGF-treated and EGF-untreated cells. This supports the contention that EGF gives rise to receptor down-regulation by altering the rate of receptor removal from the cell surface. This is obvious from the observations in Figure 3, which show that the rate of disappearance of EGF binding activity induced by 8 nM EGF is 10-fold greater than the maximal rate of loss of EGF binding in the presence of cycloheximide. We therefore propose that the addition of EGF shifts the removal of receptors from an unoccupied mechanism to a more efficient, occupied mechanism, perhaps by lowering the effective "K_m" of receptor for the same removal mechanism that functions in the absence of EGF. In the initial phase after EGF addition, enhanced internalization of EGF and EGF receptors is observed [6, 10, 11, 16]. The rate of enhanced receptor disappearance then declines as the number of receptors (which are considered to be the substrate in this case) declines. A new steady-state level of receptors is then reached when the rates of receptor removal and synthesis become equal.

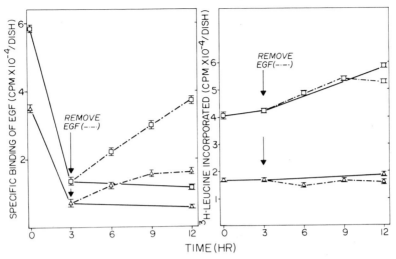

Fig. 2. Comparison of rates of EGF receptor recovery after down-regulation with rates of protein synthesis in serum-starved and unstarved cells. Cells were grown to confluence in medium containing 5% FCS. Twenty-four hours prior to time 0, the FCS concentration in some dishes was changed to 0.5%. At time 0, the medium of all dishes was changed to fresh DME containing 5% or 0.5% FCS and 50 ng/ml of EGF. After a 3 h incubation, EGF was removed from some samples, and DME containing 5% or 0.5% FCS was added to these dishes. ^{125}I-EGF binding (left) and protein synthesis (right) indicated by ^{3}H-leucine uptake into acid-insoluble material were determined as described in Materials and Methods. Cells were incubated in leucine-free minimal essential medium (LF-MEM, Gibco) containing 0.01 mM L-4,5-^{3}H-leucine (New England Nuclear, 5 Ci/mmole) for 60 min at 37°C prior to their being processed for determination of labeled leucine uptake into acid insoluble material. (□ = cells grown and maintained in 5% FCS; △ = cells starved for 24 h in 0.5% FCS and maintained in 0.5% FCS; —— = incubation in the presence of 50 ng/ml of EGF; —·—·— = incubation after EGF removal.)

Identification of the EGF Receptor by Surface-Specific Radioiodination and by "Direct Labeling" with ^{125}I-EGF.

The EGF receptors on murine cells were initially identified by Das et al [10, 16], who observed a high molecular weight ^{125}I-labeled band by SDS-PAGE after cross-linking a specifically bound ^{125}I-EGF photoaffinity probe to the receptor protein. More recent observations show that a small portion of cell-bound ^{125}I-EGF becomes directly attached to its surface receptor on murine 3T3 cells to form a high molecular weight, radioactive band resistant to dissociation in SDS-PAGE [23, 24]. The formation of this direct-labeled hormone-receptor complex is dependent on specific binding of EGF, and the complex can be precipitated with anti-EGF IgG from a Triton X-100 extract of cells incubated with hormone [23]. Upon further incubation at 37°C, this complex is degraded to the same lower molecular weight products described previously for the cross-linking studies [16]. These experiments identify only a small portion of the EGF receptors; direct and photo-affinity labeling with ^{125}I-EGF proceeds to a maximal yield of only a few percent. Since "direct" and photoaffinity-labeling procedures might therefore detect a small, but uncharacteristic fraction of the total receptor population, we turned to surface-specific iodination to label a more sizable, and thus possibly a more representative, fraction of the EGF receptors. Untreated murine 3T3 cells and cells treated with EGF to down-regulate the EGF receptors were labeled by surface-specific iodination. Gel electrophoresis revealed the presence of the murine EGF receptor in the untreated cells as a 170,000 dalton single

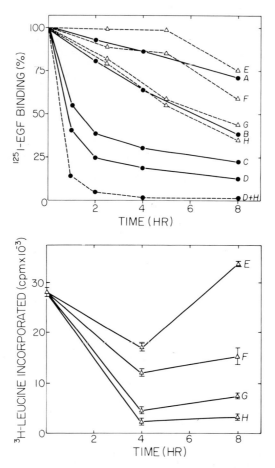

Fig. 3. (Upper) Effect of EGF and/or cycloheximide treatment on EGF binding activity. (Lower) Effect of cycloheximide on protein synthesis. Cells were grown to confluence in DME containing 5% FCS. These cells are from the same batch used for the studies in Figure 2. The FCS concentration was changed to 0.5% and the incubations continued for 24 h. At time 0, 0.4 (A), 2 (B), 10 (C), and 50 (D) ng/ml of unlabeled EGF; 0.04 (E), 0.2 (F), 1.0 (G), and 5.0 (H) μg/ml of cycloheximide; or 50 ng/ml of EGF and 5 μg/ml of cycloheximide (D + H) were added. ^{125}I-EGF binding (upper) and protein synthesis (lower) were determined at the indicated times after the cells had been washed thoroughly to remove EGF and/or cycloheximide.

polypeptide chain [20]. Since the EGF receptor is a minor surface component of these cells, its visualization was possible only when trypsin treatment of cells was used to enrich the cell surface for proteins with a relatively high turnover rate during a brief period of additional growth. In the experiment described in Figures 4 and 5, a surface-labeled band with the electrophoretic mobility of the EFG receptor (M_r = 170,000) was readily detected after a brief period of growth of the trypsin-treated 3T3 cells. This 170,000 dalton band was missing in lane B where EGF had been added to the cells to induce EGF receptor internalization during the brief period of receptor synthesis. Lanes C and D of the same figure show the affinity-labeled EGF: EGF receptor complex produced by direct labeling. The directly labeled receptor migrated more slowly than radiolabeled, unoccupied

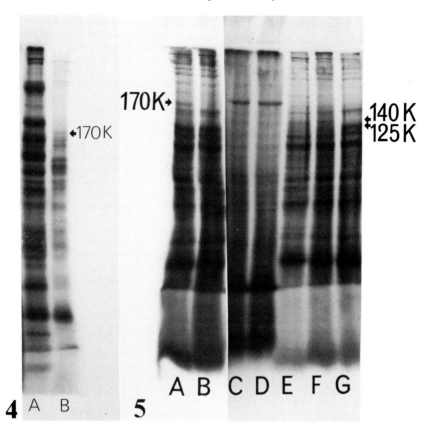

Fig. 4. A,B (left). Effect of trypsin on radioiodinated proteins displayed on surface labeled 3T3 cells. Confluent 3T3 monolayers were radiolabeled by surface-specific iodination [20]. After radiolabeling sample B was incubated with 40 μg/ml of trypsin for 10 min as described in Materials and Methods; sample A received no trypsin treatment. The monolayers were dissolved in buffer containing SDS and processed for SDS polyacrylamide gel electrophoresis on a 5–10% gradient slab gel [20]. Proteins were visualized by autoradiography. The arrow indicates the position of the EGF receptor determined as described for Figure 5.

Fig. 5. A–G, (right). A,B: Effect of EGF on the appearance of proteins subject to surface-specific iodination during the resynthesis of trypsin-sensitive surface proteins. 3T3 monolayers were treated with 40 μg/ml of trypsin, incubated in binding medium containing 50 ng/ml of unlabeled EGF (B) or no EGF (A) for 2 h at 37°C, labeled by surface-specific iodination and processed for gel electrophoresis on a 5–10% gradient slab gel and visualized by autoradiography.

C,D: Direct labeling of EGF receptors. The 3T3 cell monolayers were incubated for 30 min at 37°C in medium containing 50 ng/ml of ^{125}I-EGF. After unbound ^{125}I-EGF was removed, the cells were processed for gel electrophoresis and autoradiography. The relatively high background in these samples is caused by unreacted ^{125}I, which was not removed after the chloroglycoluril-mediated iodination of E,F,G: Effect of EGF-induced EGF receptor down-regulation on the appearance of a 140,000 dalton band produced by trypsin treatment of surface-radioiodinated cells. 3T3 monolayers were labeled by surface-specific iodination, incubated for 0 (E) or 60 (F,G) min in medium containing 50 ng/ml of unlabeled EGF (G) or no EGF (F), treated with 40 μg/ml of trypsin, and processed for gel electrophoresis in SDS solution. Proteins were visualized by autoradiography. Samples A–G were resolved on the same 5–12.5% polyacrylamide gradient slab gel, but samples A and B were phtographed from a different autoradiograph than were samples C-G. From Wrann et al [20].

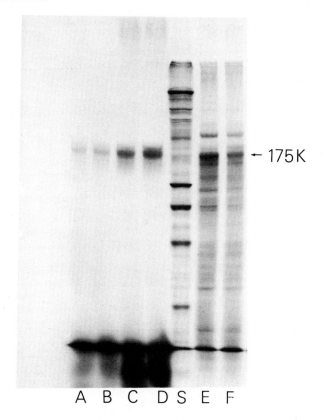

Fig. 6. Identification of the EGF receptor on A431 cells by surface-specific iodination and direct labeling with ^{125}I-EGF. A431 cells or mouse 3T3 cells were grown to confluence in 35 mm culture dishes with DME containing 10% FCS. Direct labeling of the EGF receptor. A431 monolayers were washed twice with medium and incubated in medium containing 100 ng/ml of ^{125}I-EGF prepared by the chloramine-T procedure (lanes A and B) or the chloroglycoluril procedure (lanes C and D) for 30 (lanes A and C) and 90 min (lanes B and D). Unbound EGF was removed, and the cells were dissolved in SDS solution and processed for gel electrophoresis as described under Experimental procedures. Surface labeling. A431 (lanes E and F) cell monolayers were washed twice with binding medium and incubated with medium containing unlabeled EGF 1000 ng/ml (lane F) for 4 h at 37°C to allow for EGF receptor down-regulation. The cell sample for lane E received a similar treatment but was incubated in the absence of EGF. All the monolayers were washed thoroughly, surface iodinated, and processed for gel electrophoresis. Radiolabeled proteins were visualized by autoradiography prior to sampling for direct determination of radioactivity in excised regions of the gels. Lane S, molecular weight standards. From Wrann and Fox [21].

receptor, with an apparent molecular weight of 175,000 daltons. This difference in M_r can be accounted for by the attachment of a single EGF molecule to the 170,000 dalton receptor. Still more convincing evidence for EGF receptor identification by surface-specific iodination was obtained with the human epithelioid carcinoma cell line A431, which has approximately 20 times more surface receptors for EGF than normal fibroblasts [25]. Following surface-specific radioiodination of cells, a 175,000 dalton protein was the most heavily labeled protein band detected after SDS-PAGE and autoradiography of the slab gel (Fig. 6). During EGF-induced EGF receptor down-regulation, the radioactivity in this band decreased in parallel to the loss of surface receptors as determined by ^{125}I-EGF binding. A similar decrease ($\sim$ 50%) was observed in the affinity-labeled EGF receptor band of these cells, which migrated with an apparent M_r = 180,000.

EGF alters a proteolysis-susceptible site on the EGF receptor. The addition of extracellular trypsin in the surface-labeling experiments with 3T3 cells led to an unexpected observation. When the order of reactions in the experiment described in Figure 5 (A, B) was changed so that cells were surface-iodinated first, incubated next in the absence of EGF, and finally treated with trypsin prior to gel electrophoresis, a 140,000 dalton protein was detected. This band was clearly missing in the EGF-treated samples, where an increased amount of a 125,000 dalton protein was found instead (Fig. 5, lanes E–G). This indicates that EGF exposes a new trypsin cleavage site on receptors, giving rise to the 125,000 dalton cleavage product rather than the 140,000 dalton product observed when EGF was not present during trypsin treatment. The observation of the 125,000 dalton protein was also made in studies where ^{125}I-EGF was incubated with isolated membranes to label the receptor directly. As observed with intact cells, a small portion of the membrane-bound ^{125}I-EGF attached to receptor to form a 175,000 dalton component (Fig. 7, lane A). When trypsin was added to the ^{125}I-EGF-treated membranes, the 175,000 dalton complex was degraded to a 125,000 dalton complex, and these data indicate a precursor-product relationship between the 175,000 and 125,000 dalton components. A small quantity of this 125,000 band was also present in the sample not incubated with trypsin. This probably is produced by degradation of EGF receptors by an endogenous membrane protease. Das and Fox [16] had reported earlier that incubation of cells in the presence of chloroquine resulted in some degradation of the 175,000 dalton ^{125}I-EGF:EGF receptor photoaffinity complex to a component of approximately 125,000 daltons. This may be the same component described here.

The observations described in this section support the following scheme of EGF receptor turnover. Receptor removal and degradation in the absence of EGF (unoccupied mode) is accomplished by proteolysis resulting in degradation products that do not give rise to the EGF response(s). The addition of EGF changes the conformation of receptor, shifting receptor removal to the occupied mode and exposing different protease-cleavage sites. Cleavage at these sites may convert receptor to an "activated" form.

Platelet-Derived and Fibroblast Growth Factors Transiently Down-Regulate EGF Receptors and Modify Their Susceptibility to Down-Regulation by EGF.

Transient down-regulation of EGF receptors by PDGF and FGF. Mitogenic concentrations of PDGF (platelet-derived growth factor [26, 27]) or FGF (fibroblast growth factor [28]) modulate EGF binding activity in murine 3T3 cells [29, 30]. In the studies treated in this report, platelet extract (PE) was used as the source of PDGF, and purified bovine pituitary FGF as the source of FGF. Both these hormones stimulated ^{3}H-thymidine uptake by 3T3 cells to a greater extent than did EGF (Fig. 8). Since sensitive radioreceptor assays have not been developed for FGF or PDGF, the influence of these hormones on their own receptors cannot be determined effectively. In fact, we know of no report of a binding assay for PDGF. Though high concentrations of FGF or PDGF do not compete with EGF for binding to the EGF receptor (data not shown), both hormones effectively down-regulate EGF binding activity (Figs. 9 and 10). However, the properties of the down-regulation phenomenon induced by FGF and PDGF differ from the EGF-induced phenomenon. When EGF is added to cells, EGF binding activity is reduced to a new steady-state level and is then maintained at that level. With PDGF or FGF addition, EGF binding

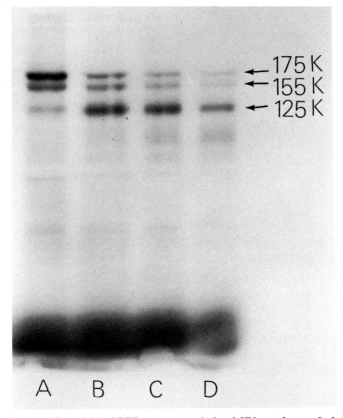

Fig. 7. Tryptic degradation of direct labeled EGF receptors on isolated 3T3 membranes. Isolated surface membranes from 3T3 cells were incubated for 60 min at 23°C in medium containing 50 ng/ml of
^{125}I-EGF to produce direct-labeled EGF receptor [23]. The samples were layered above a 1 ml cushion
of 10% (w:w) sucrose in medium and sedimented for 2 min in a Brinkman microfuge to remove unbound
EGF. The pellets were washed with medium and incubated for 30 min at 0°C with 0 (A), 2.5 (B),
25 (C), or 250 μg/ml (D) of trypsin for 30 min. Trypsin was removed, and the samples were washed
twice with medium, dissolved in SDS solution, and processed for SDS-polyacrylamide gel electrophoresis on a 10% slab gel. The labeled proteins were visualized by autoradiography. From Wrann
et al [20].

activity first decreases but then rebounds to normal or near-normal levels (Figs. 9 and 10).
We call this phenomenon "transient down-regulation." In some experiments, and especially
where cells were treated and maintained with EGF for an extended time to achieve a down-
regulation steady state for the EGF receptor, the EGF binding activity achieved after the
rebound was higher than that encountered prior to addition of FGF (Fig 10). This behavior may be related to inhibition of EGF-induced EGF receptor down-regulation by
FGF and PDGF (Figs. 9 and 10), a phenomenon treated in the next section. With FGF,
the threshold for transient down-regulation of EGF binding was decreased when cells were
previously treated with EGF to achieve a lower steady state of EGF binding activity. We
have not performed tests to determine if the PDGF threshold for PDGF-mediated transient
down-regulation of EGF binding is also decreased by EGF.

Transient down-regulation of EGF binding by FGF or PDGF is dose-dependent for
both these hormones (Fig. 10 and data not shown). Comparison of mitogenesis (Fig. 8)

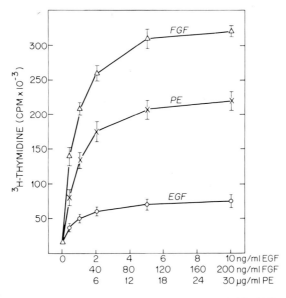

Fig. 8. Stimulation of DNA synthesis of serum-starved 3T3 cells by EGF, FGF, and PE. The indicated amounts of EGF, FGF, and PE were added to cultures of serum-starved 3T3 cells. Uptake of ^{3}H-thymidine into DNA was determined 18 h later.

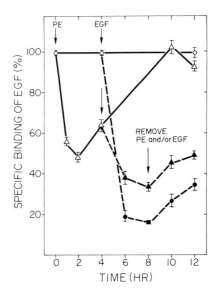

Fig. 9. Effect of PDGF on EGF-induced EGF receptor down-regulation and resynthesis. Serum-starved 3T3 cells were treated with 10 μl/ml of PE (triangles) or nor-PE (circles) at time 0. Unlabeled EGF was added to a final concentration of 50 ng/ml at time 4 h. PE and/or EGF was removed at time 8 h where indicated, and the cells were incubated with 0.5% FCS/DME. ^{125}I-EGF binding was measured on samples processed for assay at the indicated times.

and EGF receptor transient down-regulation induced by FGF or PDGF indicate similar dose-response curves for both these responses. Similarities in the dose-response curves for a membrane perturbation (EGF receptor transient down-regulation) and mitogenesis may indicate that the ability of FGF and PDGF to induce them is closely linked to the abilities of FGF and PDGF to induce obligatory alterations in the target cell membranes, including, but not limited to, internalization of FGF and PDGF receptors. However, we think it is unlikely that transient down-regulation of EGF receptors is linked in any direct, causal way to the abilities of PDGF or FGF to induce DNA synthesis in responsive cells.

Platelet-derived growth factor and fibroblast growth factor inhibit EGF-induced down-regulation of the EGF receptor. The experiments described in Figures 9 and 10 show that the addition of FGF or PDGF leads to transient down-regulation of the EGF receptor, but that EGF binding sometimes rebounds to a level that excedes that observed prior to FGF or PDGF addition. This phenomenon was especially pronounced in cases in which the cells had been maintained at a steady state of partial EGF-induced down-regulation of the EGF receptor, suggesting that incubation of cells with FGF or PDGF might cause inhibition of EGF-induced down-regulation of its receptor. An example of an experiment designed to test this hypothesis directly is given in Figure 9. The experiment in Figure 9 describes the typical pattern of PE-induced transient down-regulation and EGF-induced down-regulation of EGF binding. When EGF was added to the PE- treated (PE is platelet extract, a source of PDGF) cells during the period of EGF receptor rebound, EGF-induced down-regulation of EGF binding was observed, but to a lesser extent than observed with EGF alone. The decreased effectiveness of EGF on down-regulation of EGF binding in PE-treated cells was not due to an effect of PE on EGF receptor turnover. The rate of reappearance of EGF binding activity after EGF-induced down-regulation was the same in PE-treated and untreated cells.

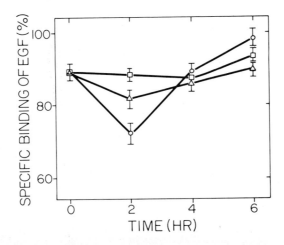

Fig. 10. Transient down-regulation of EGF receptors by FGF. Serum-starved 3T3 cells were treated with 1 ng/ml of EGF for 12 hr prior to time 0, and the EGF remained present in the medium during the subsequent incubations with FGF. At time 0, FGF was added to the cells at 25 (□), 50 (△), and 100 (○) ng/ml, and the cells were incubated for the times indicated and washed thoroughly to remove unlabeled EGF. [125] I-EGF binding was determined using the standard binding assay.

DISCUSSION

The ultimate goal in the study of any receptor system is the identification of the "second messenger" for hormone action and the delineation of the mechanism by which the second messenger functions. In the case of EGF, much is now known about both hormone and receptor, and the fates of the hormone and receptor molecules after their interaction [6, 12–21, 23, 24].

In fact, few hormones or receptors have been studied as extensively as EGF and its receptor. However, the quest for the second messenger still remains. In a recent review, Carpenter and Cohen have listed six possible mechanisms for second messenger generation in an anything but all-inclusive list of hypotheses [4]. Among these are the generation of a second messenger through ligand-induced patching of receptor, through phosphorylation of receptor or other proteins, or through internalization and proteolytic activation of receptor (and/or EGF).

We have selected as our working hypothesis the endocytic activation of receptor, and our reasons for making this selection are twofold: First, in Swiss 3T3 cells, the enhanced internalization and proteolytic processing of receptor induced by EGF has been correlated with the EGF-induced activation of DNA synthesis [18]. Second, a host of biological processes are activated by proteolytic post-translational processing of proenzymes or pro-hormones. Among these are the classical case of the conversion of chymotrypsinogen to chymotrypsin [31], the cleavage events that lead to the blood clotting [32, 33] and complement [34] cascade mechanisms, and the elegant studies of Steiner and his colleagues on the proinsulin to insulin conversion [35]. Additionally, Glenn and Cunningham have obtained evidence linking the stimulation of cell division by thrombin to the proteolysis of the thrombin receptor [36].

The endocytic activation hypothesis applied to EGF action encounters difficulty when examined in the light of evidence indicating that EGF receptors turn over rapidly [11, 37] (Figs. 1–3). Though the fate of receptors removed during normal turnover has not been demonstrated directly, it is conceivable that both normal turnover and EGF-induced loss of EGF binding activity occur by endocytosis and lysosomal processing. If this is the case, it becomes difficult to invision how a mere enhancement of receptor internalization could lead to a specific activation of EGF-induced processes leading to stimulation of DNA synthesis. One answer to this dilemma is the EGF-induced exposure of new protease-sensitive sites on receptor [20] (Fig. 5). This experiment indicates that EGF produces a conformational change in receptor, and this may expose new sites to the proteases existing in the lysosomes or to endogeneous protease(s) that reside on the cell surface and appear to mimic trypsin in their specificity (Figs. 5 and 7). On the basis of these results, we have modified our initially proposed model of endocytic activation to one in which the internalization and processing of receptor is necessary, but not sufficient, for activation of second messenger production. This activation step may also require EGF to alter the sites on receptor sensitive to protease action, wherein the cleavage of the essential protease-sensitive site occurs only when receptor is in the EGF-induced conformation. The observation that hormone-induced modification of receptor occurs in the EGF system (possibly as an obligatory step in the activation process) suggests that enhanced internalization of EGF receptors need not be obligatory for endocytic activation. The turnover of receptors at the rate characteristic of normal, unoccupied receptor turnover could prove adequate for induction of an EGF response in the absence of any change in steady-state receptor level if EGF is internalized with receptor.

Schema 1

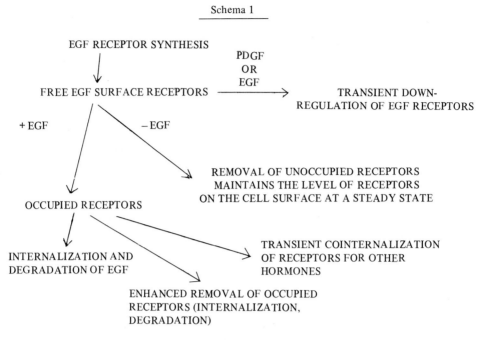

New phenomena that bear on this concept are also described here: the transient down-regulation of receptors induced by PDGF and FGF and the ability of these hormones to inhibit EGF-induced down-regulation of its own receptors. Presuming that the transient down-regulation of EGF receptors observed in these studies (Figs. 9 and 10) constitutes EGF receptor internalization, these data indicate that PDGF and FGF both induce internalization of their own receptors and that, during this process, internalization of EGF receptors in the unoccupied mode (Schema 1) is enhanced. As the receptors for FGF and PDGF achieve a down-regulated steady state, the rates of their internalization decrease, and EGF receptor synthesis restores the level of EGF receptors to the initial or a or a higher level, giving rise to a transiency in EGF receptor down-regulation. The inhibition of EGF-induced EGF receptor down-regulation by FGF and PDGF can be explained by a similar model, in which some common factor (or factors) is involved in the internalization of all these receptors and is limiting for internalization. Since it appears that EGF receptor down-regulation involves clathrin and internalization in coated vesicles [38], other receptors – eg, those for FGF and PDGF – may also be internalized in a process that involves their inclusion into coated vesicles.

Recent ultrastructural observations show that a portion of the EGF receptors resides in a patched configuration prior to EGF addition [13]. In addition, we have observed that in all cell lines tested so far, a considerable portion of the EGF receptors remains in a very high molecular weight form after extraction of membranes with solutions of Triton X-100 [39]. It appears that many of the EGF receptors are already included in organized regions of the membrane. If these regions consist of mixtures of receptors capable of ligand-induced internalization, then the addition of any one of a host of hormones may trigger the transient internalization of a portion of all receptors that share a common organized membrane region in their internalization. If endocytic activation of receptors is a process that functions in an obligatory fashion in activation of second messenger production, this same process may be shared by a wide variety of hormones, which could vary considerably in their effects on cells.

ACKNOWLEDGMENTS

This work was supported by grants from the United States Public Health Service and the American Cancer Society.

Michael Wrann is the recipient of fellowships from Emil Martinez and the Max Kade Foundation.

Peter S. Linsley is a National Cancer Institute trainee (CA09056).

REFERENCES

1. Cohen S: J Biol Chem 237:1555–1562, 1962.
2. Savage CF Jr, Cohen S: J Biol Chem 247:7609–7611, 1972.
3. Carpenter G, Lembach KJ, Morrison MM, Cohen S: J Biol Chem 250:4297–4304, 1975.
4. Carpenter G, Cohen S: Annu Rev Biochem 48:193–216, 1979.
5. Hollenberg MD, Cuatrecasas P: J Biol Chem 250:3845–3853, 1975.
6. Carpenter G, Cohen S: J Cell Biol 71:159–171, 1976.
7. Savage CR Jr, Inagami T, Cohen S: J Biol Chem 247:7612–7621, 1972.
8. Holladay LA, Savage RC Jr, Cohen S, Puett D: Biochemistry 15:2624–2633, 1976.
9. Pruss RM, Herschman HR: Proc Natl Acad Sci USA 74:3918–3921, 1977.
10. Das M, Miyakawa T, Fox CF, Pruss RM, Aharanov A, Herschman HR: Proc Natl Acad Sci USA 74:2790–2794, 1977.
11. Aharonov A, Pruss RM, Herschman HR: J Biol Chem 253:3970–3977, 1978.
12. Haigler H, Ash JF, Singer SJ, Cohen S: Proc Natl Acad Sci USA 75:3317–3321, 1978.
13. Haigler HT, McKanna JA, Cohen S: J Cell Biol 81:382–395, 1979.
14. Schlessinger J, Schechter Y, Willingham MC, Pastan I: Proc Natl Acad Sci USA 75:2659–2663, 1978.
15. Maxfield FR, Schlessinger J, Schechter Y, Pastan I, Willingham MC: Cell 14:805–810, 1978.
16. Das M, Fox CF: Proc Natl Acad Sci USA 75:2644–2648, 1978.
17. Fox CF, Das M: J Supramol Struct 10:199–214, 1979.
18. Fox CF, Vale R, Peterson SW, Das M: Cold Spring Harbor Conferences on Cell Proliferation series, Vol 6, Hormones and Cell Culture, pp. 143–157, 1979.
19. Schechter Y, Hernaez L, Schlessinger J, Cuatrecasas P: Nature 278:835–838, 1979.
20. Wrann M, Linsley P, Fox CF: FEBS Lett 104:415–419, 1979.
21. Wrann M, Fox CF: J Biol Chem 254:8083–8086, 1979.
22. Samson ACR, Fox CF: J Virol 12:579–587, 1973.
23. Linsley PS, Blifield C, Wrann M, Fox CF: Nature 278:745–748, 1979.
24. Baker JB, Simmer RL, Glenn KC, Cunningham DD: Nature 278:743–745, 1979.
25. Fabricant RN, De Larco JE, Todaro GJ: Proc Natl Acad Sci USA 74:565–569, 1977.
26. Pledger WJ, Stiles CD, Antoniades HN, Scher CD: Proc Natl Acad Sci USA 74:4481–4485, 1977.
27. Ross R, Vogel A: Cell 14:203–210, 1978.
28. Gospodarowicz D, Moran JS: Annu Rev Biochem 45:531–558, 1976.
29. Fox CF, Wrann M, Vale R: J Supramol Struct 9 (Suppl 3):176, 1979.
30. Wrann M, Fox CF: Fed Proc 38:301, 1979.
31. Dryer WJ, Neurath H: J Biol Chem 217:527–539, 1955.
32. Rovery M, Poilroux M, Curnier A, Desnuelle P: Biochim Biophys Acta 17:565–578, 1955.
33. Bennet B, Tatnoff OD: Med Clin North Am 56:95–104, 1972.
34. Muller-Eberhard HJ: Annu Rev Biochem 44:697–724, 1975.
35. Steiner DF: Diabetes 26:322–340, 1977.
36. Glenn KC, Cunningham D: Nature 278:711–714, 1979.
37. Carpenter G: J Cell Physiol 99:101–110, 1979.
38. Keen JH, Willingham MC, Pastan IH: Cell 16:303–312, 1979.
39. Linsley P, Fox CF, Iwata K: J Supramol Struct (Suppl 4):113, 1980.

Tumor Cell Surfaces and Malignancy 737–745 (1980)

The Influence of Cell Surface Properties on the Arrest of Circulating Melanoma Cells

George Poste

Department of Experimental Pathology, Roswell Park Memorial Institute, Buffalo, New York 14263

B16 mouse melanoma sublines cultured in vitro spontaneously shed intact vesicles of plasma membrane. These vesicles can be fused with the plasma membrane of cells from homologous and heterologous B16 sublines using polyethylene glycol (PEG) and phytohemagglutinin (PHA). The ability of Fl cells to arrest in the lung and form metastases in this organ is significantly increased by fusion of vesicles from a highly metastatic subline (F10) that localizes exclusively in the lung with cells from another subline (F1) which is poorly metastatic and produce few lung metastases. In contrast, fusion of F1 vesicles with F10 cells does not reduce their ability to localize in the lung of form lung metastases. Vesicle-treated F1 cells revert to their original arrest behavior and metastatic capacity following removal of F10 vesicle components from the plasma membrane. The changes in the arrest and metastatic behavior of F1 cells induced by F10 vesicles are highly specific. Vesicles from other B16 sublines which show limited abilities to localize in the lung (F1, F1^{1r} and F10^{1r}) fail to modify the arrest behavior of F1 cells. These results suggest that the differences in the ability of the F1 and F10 sublines to localize in the lung are determined by differences in surface properties.

Key words: tumor cells, metastasis, malignancy, plasma membrane, plasma membrane vesicles, cell recognition, blood vessels

INTRODUCTION

The invasion of blood vessels by malignant tumor cells and transport of tumor cells to different parts of the body within the circulation represents a major pathway for the metastatic spread of malignant neoplasms. There is a large body of literature describing the distribution and fate of circulating tumor cells [reviews, 1–3], but little is known about the mechanisms responsible for tumor cell arrest in different regions of the microcirculation. In the last few years a number of tumor cell variants have been isolated which differ in their abilities to arrest and/or form metastases in specific organs [4–15]. These

Abbreviations: CMEM, Eagles minimum essential medium plus 10% fetal calf serum; HBSS, Hanks balanced saline solution; ^{125}I-IUDR, ^{125}I-5-iodo-2'-deoxyuridine; IV, intravenous (intravenously); MEM, serum-free Eagles minimum essential medium; PEG, polyethylene glycol (molecular weight 6,000); PHA, phytohemagglutinin-P.

Received for publication August 14, 1979.

cells provide useful experimental systems for studying the factors which determine tumor cell arrest within the microcirculation.

Evidence is presented in this paper which indicates that the marked differences in the ability of various B16 melanoma sublines to arrest in the lung capillary bed [1, 5, 6, 15] result from differences in the surface properties of these cells. This has been demonstrated by showing that transfer of plasma membrane components from cells of a highly metastatic subline (F10) to cells from a poorly metastatic subline (F1) significantly increased the ability of recipient cells to arrest in the lung capillary bed and form metastases in this organ. Plasma membrane components have been transferred between these cells by taking advantage of the recent finding that B16 cells growing in vitro spontaneously shed closed vesicles of plasma membrane into the culture medium [16]. These vesicles can be harvested and fused with the plasma membrane of cultured cells using polyethylene glycol (PEG) to produce temporary alterations in the plasma membrane composition of vesicle-treated cells.

MATERIALS AND METHODS

Cells

The origin and properties of the F1 (low lung metastasis) and F10 (high lung metastasis) sublines of the B16 mouse melanoma cell line and the lymphocyte-resistant variants (F1^{1r}, F10^{1r}) selected from these two sublines have been described in detail elsewhere [5, 15]. All cells were grown in Eagles minimum essential medium (MEM) plus 10% fetal calf serum (CMEM) as described previously [17] and were free of contamination by Mycoplasma species.

Plasma Membrane Vesicles

Plasma membrane vesicles were harvested from the culture medium of actively growing roller bottle cultures of the various B16 sublines and purified as described in detail elsewhere [16]. The protein content of vesicle preparations was measured by the method of Lowry et al [18].

Vesicle-Cell Interactions

Purified vesicle preparations containing 300–400 μg protein were incubated in suspension with 1×10^7 melanoma cells in MEM containing 50 μg/ml PHA (PHA-P; Difco, Detroit, Michigan) and 40% PEG, molecular weight 6,000 (Sigma, St. Louis) (PHA/PEG) for 5 min at 37°C after which the medium was diluted ten fold with MEM and the mixture incubated for a further 15 min at 37°C. Control cells were either not exposed to vesicles or incubated with vesicles in medium without PHA/PEG. For cell arrest experiments, cells were labeled with ^{125}I-5-iodo-2'deoxyuridine (^{125}I-IUDR) (see below) before incubation with vesicles. Vesicle-treated and control cells were then washed three times with prewarmed HBSS and incubated for 10 min at 37°C in 0.2% ethylene diamine tetraacetic (EDTA) in calcium-magnesium-free HBSS to detach adsorbed vesicles and to separate multicellular clumps into single cells.

Because differences in cell size and volume are known to influence the arrest of tumor cells in the microcirculation [1–3], vesicle-treated and control cell populations used for in vivo experiments were matched for these parameters. Cells (5×10^7) were layered onto a sterile density gradient of 10–35% Renograffin 60 (E.R. Squibb, New York) and centrifuged at 13,000 g for 30 min at 4°C in a Beckman L5/50 preoperative ultra-centrifuge using the methods described by Grdina et al [19]. Vesicle-treated and control cells banding at similar densities were recovered and fractionated further by centrifugal elutriation in a Beckman JE-6 elutriation rotor as described elsewhere [19]. The volume distribution of cells in different fractions recovered from the elutriation rotor was measured using a model ZB1 Coulter Counter and a Channelyer II multichannel analyzer (Coulter Electronics, Hialeah, Florida). Vesicle-treated and control cells of similar modal volume were used in all experiments on cell arrest and metastasis formation in vivo. In the present experiments, the modal volume of injected cells was always within the range $1.4-1.6 \times 10^3$ μm^3.

Quantitation of Tumor Cell Arrest

Localization of vesicle-treated and control cells in the lung microcirculation was measured using cells labeled with ^{125}I-IUDR as described previously [14, 15]. Cells were labeled before being incubated with vesicles. The details of the labeling procedure have been described elsewhere [14]. Briefly, actively-growing nonconfluent monolayer cell cultures were incubated in CMEM containing 0.3 $\mu Ci/ml$ ^{125}I-IUDR (New England Nuclear; specific activity, 200 mCi/mmole) for 24 hr. This method labels more than 95% of the cells and does not alter their behavior in vivo [15]. Unanesthetized C57BL/6 mice matched for age, weight and sex were injected in the tail vein with 1×10^5 viable, radio-labeled, vesicle-treated or control cells as a single cell suspension in 0.2 ml HBSS. The radioactivity in 5 representative inocula was measured for each cell preparation using a Packard gamma counter to determine activity/cell number. Mice were killed at intervals from 2 min to 14 days after injection, and their lungs were removed, and placed in vials containing 70% ethanol. The ethanol was changed daily for 3 days to remove alcohol-soluble radioactivity. The remaining radioactivity in the lung represents radiolabel incorporated into the DNA of tumor cells which were viable at the time the animal was killed [15]. The number of viable cells in the lung at defined intervals after injection can then be calculated and expressed as a percentage of the original inoculum.

Metastasis Formation

Vesicle-treated and control cells were injected as a single cell suspension (5×10^4 cells) in 0.2 ml HBSS into the tail vein of 10-week-old unanesthetized C57BL/6 mice matched for weight and sex. The number of pulmonary metastases was measured 18 days later by examining the lungs with a dissection microscope [14, 15].

RESULTS

Vesicle-Cell Interactions

As reported in detail elsewhere [14, 19], plasma membrane vesicles shed spontaneously by different B16 sublines cultured in vitro can be harvested and fused with the plasma membrane of cells from homologous and heterologous B16 sublines using PEG. Fusion of vesicles with the plasma membrane of cultured B16 cells was demonstrated by showing the that B16 cell variants (F1^{1r}, F10^{1r}), which are resistant to killing by lymphocytes from animals immunized against B16 cells, became susceptible to immune lymphocytes after treatment with vesicles from the lymphocyte-sensitive F1 and F10 sublines plus PEG [19]. Killing of target cells by immune lymphocytes requires that the target antigen is an integral component of the plasma membrane [19]. Binding of exogenous target antigens to the cell surface is not sufficient to elicit lymphocyte-mediated cytolysis [1ᶜ]. The ability of vesicles from lymphocyte-sensitive B16 sublines to convert F1[1r] and F10[1r] cells to a sensitive state thus indicates that vesicle-derived antigens have been incorporated into the plasma membrane of acceptor cells in a form still recognized by cytotoxic lymphocytes. Lymphocyte-resistant B16 cells incubated with vesicles from lymphocyte-sensitive sublines in the absence of PEG did not acquire the sensitive phenotype [19]. PEG can, however, be successfully replaced by other agents that induce membrane fusion such as inactivated paramyxoviruses [19]. This suggests that incorporation of vesicle-derived antigens from lymphocyte-sensitive sublines into the plasma membrane of F1[1r] and F10[1r] cells, to render them susceptible to cytotoxic immune lymphocytes, is achieved by fusion of vesicles with the cellular plasma membrane [19].

Vesicle-Induced Modification of Cell Arrest Behavior In Vivo

As described originally by Fidler [5], the F1 and F10 variants of the B16 mouse melanoma cell line differ significantly in their ability to arrest in the lung capillary bed after IV injection into the tail vein of C57BL/6 mice (Fig. 1).

To evaluate the possible role of surface properties in determining these differing arrest patterns, vesicles shed from F1 and F10 cells were fused with cells from heterologous subline prelabeled with ^{125}I-IUDR. These cells were then injected IV to assay their ability to arrest in the lung compared with untreated control B16 sublines or B16 sublines treated with vesicles without PEG. The results (Fig. 1) indicate that PEG-induced fusion of F10 vesicles with F1 cells increases the number of cells that initially arrest in the lung compared with untreated control F1 cells. The vesicle-treated cells are also cleared from the lung more slowly than the control cells (Fig. 1). In contrast, the arrest behavior of F1 cells treated with F10 vesicles in the absence of PEG did not differ from control F1 cells (Fig. 1), suggesting that fusion of vesicles with the plasma membrane is required to modify cell arrest.

The change in the arrest behavior of F1 cells induced by F10 vesicles (plus PEG) is highly specific. Vesicles from poorly metastatic sublines (F1 and F10[1r]) failed to alter the arrest behavior of F1 cells (Fig. 1). This indicates that the changes in F1 cell behavior induced by F10 vesicles do not result from nonspecific alterations in cell surface accompanying the uptake of any type of vesicle.

If F1 cells treated with F10 vesicles plus PEG were cultured in vitro for more than 18 hours before being injected into mice, vesicle-induced changes in cell arrest were no longer detectable (Table I). This suggests that the vesicle components responsible for modifying cell behavior have either been removed completely from the plasma membrane of F1 cells, been inactivated, or are no longer present in sufficient amounts to influence arrest behavior. Reincubation of such cells with F10 vesicles plus PEG for a second time restores the altered arrest pattern (Table I).

In contrast to the ability of vesicles from the highly metastatic F10 subline to alter the arrest of F1 cells, treatment of F10 cells with F1 vesicles plus PEG failed to reduce the arrest or modify the clearance of F10 cells from the lung (Fig. 1).

The long term decay of cell-associated radioactivity in the lung shown in Figure 1. exhibits the biphasic pattern which has been reported previously for pulmonary arrest of wide range of tumor cells injected IV [review, 20]. Liotta and De Lisi [21] have proposed that the initial expontial decay of radioactivity is due to loss (cell death and/or dislodgement) of arrested cells within the microcirculation and that the second portion of the decay curve in which the rate of cell loss decreases is due to the colonization of the lung parenchyma by cells which have successfully escaped from the microcirculation.

Analysis of the data in Figure 1 in terms of this model suggests that PEG-induced fusion of F10 vesicles with F1 cells not only enhances initial cell arrest within the lung capillary bed but also increases the number of cells that reach the extravascular compartment. This enhanced extravasation of cells into the lung parenchyma might therefore be expected to increase the risk of metastasis formation. Experimental investigation of this question revealed that this is indeed the case. As shown in Table II, PEG-induced fusion of F10 vesicles with F1 cells significantly increases their ability to form lung metastases after IV injection. In contrast, the metastatic capacity of F1 cells treated with F10 vesicles without PEG and F1 cells treated with vesicles from F10^{1r} and F1 cells plus PEG was unaltered (Table II). Also, F10 cells incubated with F1 vesicles plus PEG did not show any significant change in metastatic capacity.

DISCUSSION

The present experiments demonstrate that previously reported differences [1, 5, 6 15] in the ability of the F1 and F10 melanoma sublines to arrest in the lung are determined (at least in part) by differences in the surface properties of these cells. The present results indicate that the plasma membrane components responsible for the exclusive localization of the F10 subline in the pulmonary microcirculation can be transferred to F1 cells and increase their capacity to arrest in the lung. This effect is specific for for F10 vesicles and cannot be duplicated by vesicles from the F10^{1r} subline which has a low lung colonizing potential similar to F1 cells.

The increased ability of F1 cells treated with F10 vesicles (plus PEG) to arrest in the lung microcirculation decays rapidly. Vesicle-treated cells injected into the circulation 18 hours or longer after vesicle treatment are indistinguishable from untreated control F1 cells. This suggests that the F10 vesicle components responsible for the altered arrest behavior have either been cleared from the F1 plasma membrane, been inactivated or, if still within the F1 plasma membrane in a functional state, are not present in sufficient amounts to modify cell arrest. The kinetics of the decay of F10 vesicle-induced changes in F1 cell arrest are consistent with other data on the time course for the removal of vesicle components from the plasma membrane measured by biochemical and ultrastructural methods [16]. Similarly, lymphocyte-resistant B16 sublines which have been rendered susceptible to killing by cytotoxic B16-immune lymphocyte by treatment with vesicles from lymphocyte-sensitive sublines revert to their original resistant phenotype 18–24 hours after treatment with vesicles [19].

In contrast to the ability of vesicles from the highly metastatic F10 subline to increase the capacity of F1 cells to arrest in the lung, the converse experiment in which F10 cells were treated with F1 vesicles failed to alter the pattern of cell arrest. This suggests that the ratio of F10 to F1 components in the plasma membrane of these cells is still sufficient to permit expression of the F10 arrest pattern. The incorporation of vesicle components into the plasma membrane and the rate(s) of clearance of vesicle components from cells have yet to be quantitated and it is still possible that the incorporation of greater amounts of F1 vesicle components into the plasma membrane of F10 cells might reduce their ability to localize in the lung.

The present results indicate that the increased arrest of F1 cells in the lung after treatment with F10 vesicles (plus PEG) is accompanied by a significant increase in metastasis formation. At first sight this seems somewhat surprising. As mentioned above, F10 vesicle components do not appear to be present in the plasma membrane (at least in a functional form) for more than 18 hours. How then does treatment of cells with vesicles increase metastasis formation when the proliferation of extravasated cells to form metastases does not begin until 1—2 days after initial cell arrest when vesicle components are no longer present? A possible explanation comes from studies on the extravasation of arrested cells. Vesicle-treated and untreated control cells which arrest in the lung capillary bed begin to invade the blood vessel wall within 4—8 hours after their initial arrest [1, 22, 23]. Once within the vessel wall, tumor cells are less susceptible to injury by hemodynamic forces and circulating host cells and will thus have a greater opportunity of continuing the metastatic process. Treatment of F1 cells with F10 vesicels (plus PEG) would thus be expected to increase the likelihood of metastasis formation simply as a result of increasing the efficiency of tumor cell arrest and invasion within the lung capillary bed. The inability of homologous F1 vesicles and heterologous F10^{lr} vesicles to alter the metastatic capacity of F1 cells is also consistent with this view since these vesicles fail to modify the arrest behavior of F1 cells. These results are thus in agreement with earlier observations showing that the extent of metastasis formation in the lung is proportional to the number of cells that successfully arrest and persist within the lung microcirculation for more than 12 hours [review, 1].

Indirect evidence for the importance of cell surface properties in determining the arrest behavior of circulating tumor cells has been presented in previous studies in which modification of cell surfaces properties by enzymes [24, 25], binding of charged macromolecules [26—28], or treatment with agents that affect cell surface deformability [29] have been found to alter the pattern of cell arrest and metastasis formation in various organs. The present experiments, however, provide the first direct evidence that plasma membrane components affect the arrest behavior of circulating tumor cells. The identity of the F10 vesicle components which enhance the arrest of F1 cells in the pulmonary microcirculation is unknown. Comparison of the composition of F1 and F10 vesicles should eventually resolve this question.

The present experiments also raise several other intriguing questions. For example, would treatment of F1 cells with vesicles from B16 variants that localize preferentially in the ovary [6], the liver [13] and the brain [6] enhance their arrest in these organs in comparable fashion to the effect of vesicles from the lung colonizing F10 variant in promoting arrest of F1 cells in the lung? Also, can vesicles from tumor cells affect the arrest behavior of nonneoplastic cells injected into the circulation? Finally, since the B16 variants used here also shed plasma membrane vesicles when growing in vivo [16], do these structures have any effect on other tumor cells or circulating host cells?

Spontaneous shedding of plasma membrane vesicles is not unique to the B16 melanoma and has been described for several other types of neoplastic cell [30—33]. In addition, shedding of closed plasma membrane vesicles can be readily induced in a variety of cultured cell types by treatment with sulphydryl blocking agents such as formaldehyde and N-ethyl malemide without causing significant cell injury [34]. The ability to fuse such vesicles with the plasma membranes of appropriate target cells in vitro offers a new approach for altering plasma membrane composition in mammalian cells and provides new opportunities for defining functional correlations between membrane composition and specific aspects of cell behavior.

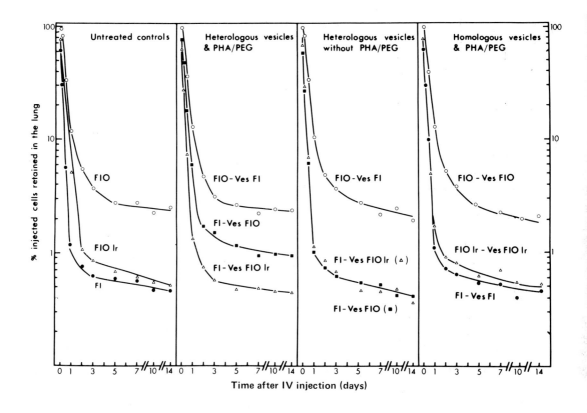

Fig. 1. Arrest and retention of ^{125}I-IUDR labeled B16 sublines and B16 sublines treated with plasma membranes vesicles in the lung after IV injection.

Plasma membrane vesicles (Ves-F1; Ves-F10^{II}; Ves-F10) were harvested from the indicated donor sublines and incubated with ^{125}I-IUDR labeled cells from homologous or heterologous sublines in MEM with or without PHA/PEG as described in the methods. Radiolabeled control cells were incubated in MEM without vesicles. Vesicle-treated and control cell populations were then subjected to density gradient centrifugation and centrifugal elutriation to provide fractions containing cells of similar size and density. These cells were then injected IV into the tail vein of C57BL/6 mice (1 × 10^5 cells/animal) and the lung-associated radioactivity measured at the indicated times after injection and expressed as the percentage of injected cells retained in the lung. Each point represents a mean value derived from measurements on five separate animals.

TABLE I. Arrest Behavior of F1 Cells Treated With F10 Vesicles Following Cultivation In Vitro

Post-vesicle incubation in vitro[a]	Second vesicle treatment[b]	% Injected Cells in the Lung[c] at			
		2 min	1 h	3 h	1 day
none, untreated control F1 cells	–	66.3	57.3	35.1	1.2
none	–	80.3	72.4	58.3	6.2
2 h	–	81.7	67.4	57.6	6.4
4 h	–	77.6	70.3	59.2	6.1
8 h	–	82.1	69.2	55.2	5.6
12 h	–	75.4	67.2	58.1	5.9
18 h	–	70.4	59.3	33.8	1.4
24 h	+	64.1	55.4	33.4	1.3

[a] ^{125}I-UDR labeled F1 cells incubated with F10 vesicles plus PEG as described in the methods after which cells were transferred to CMEM without vesicles and incubated at 37 °C for the indicated times before iv injection into C57BL/6 mice.

[b] ^{125}I-IUDR labeled cells were incubated with F10 vesicles as described above and then incubated for 24 h in CMEM without vesicles after which they were reincubated with F10 vesicles plus PEG and injected immediately into mice.

[c] Measured as described in the legend to Figure 1. The results represent mean values derived from measurements on 5 animals.

TABLE II. Formation of Lung Metastases in C57BL/6 Mice After IV Injection of B16 Melanoma Sublines and B16 Sublines Treated With Plasma Membrane Vesicles*

Cells	Vesicles	PHA/PEG	Average number of lung metastases[a]
F1	–	–	16 ± 7
F1	–	+	14 ± 6
F10	–	–	114 ± 24
F10	–	+	87 ± 16
F10^{1r}	–	+	22 ± 8
F1	F10	–	19 ± 8
F1	F10	+	44 ± 11
F1	F10^{1r}	+	12 ± 6
F10	F1	–	103 ± 16
F10	F1	+	94 ± 19

*Cells were incubated in suspension with or with or without (–) vesicles from the indicated donor cells in the presence (+) or absence (–) of PHA/PEG as described in the methods after which fractions of vesicle-treated and control cell populations were matched for size and density as described in Methods and then injected IV into C57BL/6 mice (5×10^4 cells/animal).

[a] Measured 18 days after injection of cells. The results represent mean values ± SD derived from groups of 5 animals.

ACKNOWLEDGMENTS

This work was supported by grants CA13393 and 18260 to George Poste and NIH Core Support grant CA17609 to Roswell Park Memorial Institute (Cancer Cell Center).

REFERENCES

1. Fidler IJ, Gersten DM, Hart IR: Adv Cancer Res 28:149, 1978.
2. Sugarbaker EV: Curr Prob Cancer 3:3, 1978.
3. Poste G, Fidler IJ: Nature in press.
4. Pilgrim HI: Cancer Res 29:1200, 1969.
5. Fidler IJ: Nature New Biol 242:148, 1973.
6. Nicolson GL, Brunson KW, Fidler IJ: Cancer Res 38:4105, 1978.
7. Liotta A, Vembu D, Saini RK, Boone C: Cancer Res 38:1231, 1978.
8. Suzuki N, Withers R, Koehler MW: Cancer Res 38:3349, 1978.
9. Kerbel RS, Twiddy RR, Robertson DM: Int J Cancer 22:583, 1978.
10. Trope C: Neoplasma 22:171, 1975.
11. Schirrmacher V, Shantz G, Claver K, Domitowski D, Zimmerman HP, Lohman-Matthes ML: Intl J Cancer 23:233, 1979.
12. Briles EB, Kornfeld S: J Natl Cancer Inst 60:1217, 1978.
13. Tao TW, Matter A, Vogel K, Burger MM: Intl J Cancer 23:854, 1979.
14. Poste G, Hart IR, Fidler IJ: Cancer Res, in press.
15. Fidler IJ, Gersten DM, Budmen MB: Cancer Res 36:3160, 1976.
16. Poste G, Nicolson GL: Cancer Res, in press
17. Poste G, Kirsh R, Fogler WE, Fidler IJ: Cancer Res 39:881, 1979.
18. Lowry OH, Rosebrough NJ, Farr AC, Randall RJ: J Biol Chem 193:265, 1951.
19. Poste G, Nicolson GL: Proc Natl Acad Sci USA, in press.
20. Liotta LA, De Lisi C, Vembu D, Boone CC: In Weiss L, Gilbert HA (eds): "Pulmonary Metastasis." Boston: G.K. Hall, 1978, p 62.
21. Liotta LA, De Lisi C: Cancer Res 37:40003, 1977.
22. Poste G, Doll J, Chichester WE, Baier RE, Ackers C: Cancer Res, in press.
23. Warren BA: J Med 4:150, 1973.
24. Hagmar B, Norrby K: Int J Cancer 11:663, 1973.
25. Weiss L, Glaves D, Waite DA: Intl J Cancer 13:850, 1974.
26. Hagmar B: Acta Pathol Microbiol Scand [A] 80:357, 1972.
27. Suemasu K, Watanabe K, Ishikawa S: Gann 62:331, 1971.
28. Tsubura E, Yamashita T, Higouchi T: In Day SB (ed): "Cancer Invasion and Metastasis: Biologic Mechanisms and Therapy." New York: Raven, 1977, p 367.
29. Hagmar B, Ryd W: Intl J Cancer 19:576, 1977.
30. Petitou M, Tuy F, Rosenfeld C, Mishal Z, Paintrand M, Jasnin C, Mathé G, Inbar M: Proc Natl Acad Sci USA 75:2306, 1978.
31. Raz A, Barzilai R, Spira G, Inbar M: Cancer Res 38:2480, 1978.
32. Van Blitterswijk WJ, Emmelot P, Hilkmann HAM, Hilgers G, Feltkamp CA: Intl J Cancer 23:62, 1979.
33. Gasic G, Boettiger D, Catalfamo JL, Gasic TB, Stewart GJ: Cancer Res 38:2950, 1978.
34. Scott RE, Perkins RG, Zschunke MA, Hoerl BJ, Maercklein PB: J Cell Sci 35:229, 1979.

Transforming Gene Product of Avian Sarcoma Viruses and Its Homolog in Uninfected Cells

R. L. Erikson, M. S. Collett, E. Erikson, A. F. Purchio, and J. S. Brugge

Department of Pathology, University of Colorado Health Sciences Center, Denver, Colorado 80262

The product of the avian sarcoma virus (ASV) transforming gene is a 60,000-dalton phosphoprotein, pp60src. Sera from mice and from an occasional rabbit bearing ASV-induced tumors are capable of immunoprecipitating a phosphoprotein of similar, but not identical, structure from normal avian and mammalian cells. This protein is presumed to be the product of the cellular *sarc* gene, and has been tentatively designated pp60sarc. Analysis of the tryptic phosphopeptides reveals that the viral and avian proteins have an apparently identical phosphoserine-containing peptide. They evidently also both have an analogous phosphothreonine residue surrounded by a different amino acid sequence. Immunoprecipitates containing either the viral or normal cellular pp60 protein catalyze the transfer of radiolabeled phosphate from $[\gamma\text{-}^{32}P]$-ATP to the heavy chain of immune rabbit IgG, therefore suggesting that both viral and cellular phosphoproteins may be protein kinases.

Key words: normal cell homolog, avian sarcoma virus, *src* gene product, transformed cells

Cell transformation by avian sarcoma viruses (ASV) results from the expression of a single viral gene, termed *src*, for sarcoma induction [1, 2]. The product of the *src* gene has been shown in this laboratory to be a phosphoprotein with an apparent molecular weight of 60,000, and has been termed pp60src [3–6] in keeping with conventional nomenclature. The identification of pp60src as the product of the ASV *src* gene was based on the use of serum from rabbits bearing ASV-induced tumors (TBR serum) in immunoprecipitation experiments [3, 5, 6], and on the in vitro translation of the region of the ASV genome which encodes *src* [4, 5]. Closely associated with pp60src is a protein kinase activity that is detected by the phosphorylation of the heavy chain of IgG in specific immunoprecipitates [7–9]. This phosphotransferase activity is also found in specific immunoprecipitates of the products synthesized when cell-free lysates are programmed with the region of subgenomic viral RNA that contains the *src* gene [10]. Furthermore, the protein kinase

Received May 22, 1979; accepted May 22, 1979

activity is growth temperature-dependent in cells infected with a mutant virus containing a temperature-sensitive lesion in the src gene [7–9]. Such results suggest that the product of src may produce the transformed phenotype through abnormal phosphorylation of cellular proteins.

It has been shown that normal cells contain DNA sequences, related to src [11, 12], which are termed sarc, and which are transcribed into polyadenylated, polyribosomal-associated RNA [13, 14]. It was not unexpected, then, to find that normal cells contain a phosphoprotein antigenically and structurally related to pp60src, and we have tentatively designated this protein pp60sarc [15, 16]. The detection of this normal cell protein was made possible by the fact that the anti-pp60src antibody produced by some mammals bearing ASV-induced tumors displayed a high degree of cross-reactivity. It is also of interest in this regard that Hanafusa and his co-workers have been able to recover new transforming viruses from tumors induced in chickens with mutant viruses that contain partial deletions of the src gene [17–19]. Apparently, during replication in the chicken the partial deletion mutants undergo recombination with cellular sarc sequences, resulting in the formation of an intact and functional src gene. These newly recovered viruses produce src gene products very similar to that produced by the original wild-type virus used to generate the partial deletion mutant [20].

In this communication, we review some of the similarities and differences of pp60src and pp60sarc.

MATERIALS AND METHODS

Preparation of Antisera and Immunoprecipitation

The preparation of TBR serum, tumor-bearing marmoset (TBM) serum, and tumor-bearing mouse (TBMo) serum has been described [3, 21, 22]. Radiolabeling of cells, preparation of cell extracts, and immunoprecipitation with the use of Staphylococcus aureus, strain Cowan I, to adsorb the immune complexes [23] were carried out as described previously [3, 22].

Cell-Free Protein Synthesis

Cell-free translation was carried out in mRNA-dependent reticulocyte lysates prepared as described by Pelham and Jackson [24], with ^{35}S-methionine (0.5 μCi/μl) as the radiolabel, and 0.5 μg mRNA added per 50-μl reaction. In the experiments described here, the mRNA used was the 3' third of the ASV genome, poly A-containing RNA approximately 21S in size, prepared from both nondefective (nd) ASV and a transformation-defective (td) deletion mutant of ASV [10].

Polyacrylamide Gel Electrophoresis and Autoradiography

Samples were analyzed by electrophoresis through a discontinuous slab gel system (10% acrylamide, 0.27% bis-acrylamide) with the buffer systems described by Laemmli [25]. Fluorography was carried out [26] for ^{35}S-labeled samples. ^{32}P-labeled samples were visualized by autoradiography with the use of DuPont Lightning Plus intensifying screens.

Peptide Mapping and Phosphoamino Acid Analysis

Peptide mapping by limited proteolysis during re-electrophoresis was carried out by the procedure described by Cleveland et al [27]. The two-dimensional analysis of tryptic digests by ascending chromatography followed by electrophoresis at pH 6.5 has been described [28]. For phosphoamino acid analysis, portions of the tryptic digests were dried, dissolved in 30 μl 6 N HCl, and hydrolyzed at $100°C$ for 4 h. The hydrolysates were dried and analyzed by high-voltage paper electrophoresis at pH 1.9 [28].

Assay for Protein Kinase Activity

Protein kinase activity was determined in the bacteria-bound immune complex assay system [7].

RESULTS

In Vitro Synthesis of a Functional Transforming Gene Product

As mentioned in the introduction, evidence about the nature of the ASV transforming gene product was obtained from the cell-free translation of viral RNA containing the *src* gene. When the products of translation of this RNA are compared to those generated by the translation of viral RNA from transformation-defective deletion mutants, the only *src*-specific polypeptide product is pp60src [4, 10]. An illustration of this result is shown in Figure 1. In the panel marked translation, the products synthesized in the cell-free lysate are analyzed directly on a polyacrylamide gel. The prominent pp60src product is seen only when nondefective RNA has been translated. Furthermore, as shown in the panel marked immunoprecipitation, we find that pp60src is specifically immunoprecipitated by TBR serum.

Finally, when these immunoprecipitates are tested for protein kinase activity, we find that only complexes that are formed with TBR serum and contain pp60src reveal

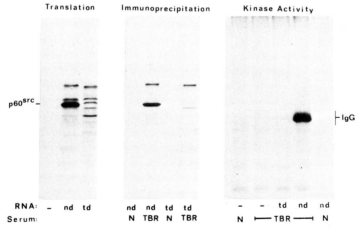

Fig. 1. Left panel: Fluorogram of SDS-polyacrylamide gel analysis of ^{35}S-methionine-labeled polypeptides synthesized in mRNA-dependent reticulocyte lysates programmed by no RNA (−), 21 S poly A-containing RNA from nd ASV (nd), and 21 S poly A-containing RNA from td ASV (td). Middle panel: Fluorogram of SDS-polyacrylamide gel analysis of translation products such as those depicted in the left panel immunoprecipitated with normal rabbit serum (N) or with TBR serum (TBR). Right panel: Autoradiograph of SDS-polyacrylamide gel analysis of the products of phosphotransferase reactions carried out in the bacteria-bound immune complex assay system [7]. A portion of the bacteria-bound immune complexes prepared from the products of translation with either normal rabbit or TBR serum was resuspended in protein kinase reaction mixture and analyzed as described previously.

phosphotransferase activity. The protein phosphorylated in the panel marked kinase activity is the heavy chain of rabbit IgG. These data, as well as other results, have been published, supporting the notion that the transforming gene product is, or is closely associated with, a protein kinase.

Detection of pp60sarc in Normal Cells

Most TBR sera recognize only pp60src encoded by the Schmidt-Ruppin (SR) strain of ASV, the strain used to induce the tumor [29]. Some immune sera from tumor-bearing marmosets recognize pp60sarc in avian cells, but not in mammalian cells [15]. However, we now find that mice bearing tumors induced by injection of SR-ASV-transformed mouse cells (Balb/c) frequently produce antibody that recognizes not only the viral pp60src, but also the endogenous avian cell protein, pp60sarc, and a similar related protein in mammalian cells. In addition, we find an occasional TBR serum that exhibits a similar wide immunoreactivity for pp60sarc. In Figure 2A, the use of these various sera is illustrated. Normal sera from the three types of animals failed to precipitate a phosphoprotein of 60,000 daltons (Fig. 2A, tracks 1, 4, 7). Certain sera from marmosets, mice, and rabbits bearing ASV-induced tumors were able to specifically recognize and immunoprecipitate the normal avian cell protein, pp60sarc (Fig 2A, tracks 2, 5, 8). This 60,000-dalton phosphoprotein is not related to any virion structural proteins because preadsorption of each antiserum with disrupted ASV failed to affect its immunoprecipitation (Fig. 2A, tracks 3, 6, 9). As shown in Figure 2B, TBMo serum (track 4) and cross-reacting TBR serum (track 3) were able to immunoprecipitate a 60,000-dalton phosphoprotein from normal rat embryo fibroblasts as well, whereas normal rabbit serum, TBM serum, and the usual TBR serum (reactive against only pp60src) [tracks 1, 5, and 2, respectively] were unable to recognize normal rat cell pp60sarc.

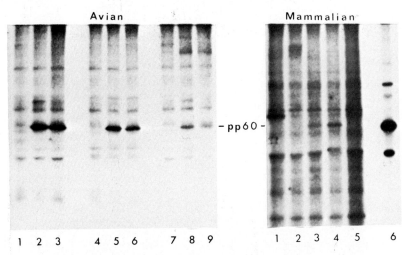

Fig. 2. Autoradiograph of SDS-polyacrylamide gel analysis of ^{32}P-labeled proteins immunoprecipitated from normal uninfected avian and mammalian cells with various sera. Panel A: Extracts of chick embryo fibroblasts immunoprecipitated with the following sera: 1, preimmune marmoset; 2, TBM; 3, TBM preadsorbed with ASV structural proteins; 4, normal mouse; 5, TBMo; 6, TBMo preadsorbed; 6, normal rabbit; 8, cross-reacting TBR; 9, cross-reacting TBR preadsorbed. Panel B: Extracts of rat embryo fibroblasts immunoprecipitated with the following sera; 1, normal rabbit; 2, TBR; 3, cross-reacting TBR; 4, TBMo; 5, TBM. Track 6 depicts the proteins immunoprecipitated from ^{32}P-labeled SR-ASV-infected chick embryo fibroblasts with TBR serum to mark the migration of pp60.

Comparison of Phosphorylation Sites in pp60^{sarc} to Those in pp60^{src}

Our previous studies showed that viral pp60^{src} and pp60^{sarc} are very similar, although not identical, in primary structure [15]. We also have previously shown that pp60^{src} contains two major sites of phosphorylation: one involving phosphoserine, located in the amino terminal two-thirds of the polypeptide, and the other involving phosphothreonine, located in the carboxy terminal one-third [28]. As shown in Figure 3, partial proteolysis by two different proteases reveals that all three phosphoproteins (viral, avian, and mammalian) have remarkably similar structures. The 34,000-dalton V8 fragment originates from the amino terminal portion of pp60^{src} and the 26,000-dalton V8 fragment from the carboxy terminal portion [28]. Other experiments have determined that the elastase-generated fragment of approximately 31,000 daltons is the amino half of pp60^{src}, and the fragment that migrates slightly faster is the carboxy half.

Since similar patterns of digestion are produced by these enzymes on pp60^{sarc}, the origin of the fragments is probably the same as for viral pp60^{src}. The major significant difference is that the electrophoretic mobility of the V8 carboxy terminal fragment of viral pp60^{src} is greater than that of either normal cell protein. It is striking that the phosphopeptide cleavage products of both normal proteins are virtually identical.

That both of the V8 protease peptides from the normal cell proteins contained phosphorus radiolabel implies that the normal cell pp60^{sarc} proteins contain multiple sites of phosphorylation as does viral pp60^{src}. This was confirmed by analysis of the phosphoamino acids present in the intact chick pp60^{sarc} protein and in its two V8 protease fragments. Figure 4 shows that pp60^{sarc} contains both phosphoserine and phosphothreonine, and that the phosphoserine residue is present in the V8 amino terminal fragment and the phosphothreonine in the carboxy end. This pattern of phosphoamino acid occurrence is analogous to that found for viral pp60^{src} [28].

As shown in Figure 5A, B, both the viral pp60^{src} and the normal chicken cell pp60^{sarc} contain two major tryptic phosphopeptides. We have previously shown that the tryptic phosphopeptide from viral pp60^{src} which migrates toward the cathode is derived

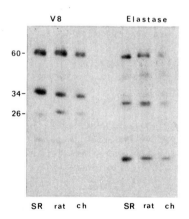

Fig. 3. Analysis of viral, avian, and mammalian pp60 proteins by limited proteolysis. ³²P-labeled pp60 proteins such as those shown in Figure 2A; track 5 and 2B, tracks 4 and 6 were excised from preparative gels, re-run on a second preparative gel, and then subjected to partial proteolysis with Staphylococcus aureus V8 protease (0.005 μg) or with elastase (0.01 μg). The sources of the pp60 proteins analyzed here were SR-ASV-infected chick embryo fibroblasts (SR), rat embryo fibroblasts (rat), and chick embryo fibroblasts (ch).

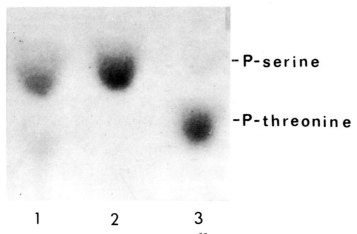

Fig. 4. Analysis of the phosphoamino acids in pp60^{sarc}. ^{32}P-labeled avian pp60^{sarc} and its two major V8 protease cleavage products were excised from preparative gels, eluted, precipitated, and digested with trypsin. Portions of the digests were then hydrolyzed in 6 N HCl and analyzed by high-voltage paper electrophoresis as described in Materials and Methods and in Collett et al [28]. Track 1, avian pp60^{sarc}; track 2, V8 amino fragment; track 3, V8 carboxy fragment.

from the V8 amino terminal portion of the molecule [28]. Figure 5D shows that in avian pp60^{sarc} also, the phosphopeptide that migrates toward the cathode is derived from the V8 amino fragment of this molecule. A mixing experiment (Fig. 5C) demonstrates that these two peptides migrated identically. In contrast, the second tryptic phosphopeptide of pp60^{src}, which is derived from the carboxy terminal portion [28], migrated toward the anode, whereas in the case of pp60^{sarc} the analogous tryptic phosphopeptide remained at the origin during electrophoresis (Fig. 5E). The difference in the electrophoretic mobilities of the carboxy terminal phosphothreonine-containing tryptic peptide of pp60^{src} and of pp60^{sarc} most likely is due to a difference in their amino acid sequences in the region of trypsin-sensitive sites.

Functional Comparison of Normal Cell pp60^{sarc} and Viral pp60^{src}

The presence of a homolog of viral pp60^{src} in normal cells raises a question concerning its possible function in normal growth processes. Previously, it has been shown that the viral pp60^{src} polypeptide has an associated protein kinase activity as judged by its ability to transfer the γ-phosphate from adenosine triphosphate (ATP) to the heavy chain of IgG [7]. In studies on immunoprecipitates of cellular pp60^{sarc}, we find that whenever pp60^{sarc}, whether of avian or mammalian origin, is present in immune complexes formed with immune rabbit IgG, a phosphotransferase activity similar to that of viral pp60^{src} is detectable (Fig. 6); however, when pp60^{sarc} is absent or in an immune complex formed with marmoset or mouse IgG, no such enzymatic activity is observed.

DISCUSSION

These experiments taken together with our past results [5, 6, 28], as well as those of others [8], show that the product of the avian sarcoma virus transforming gene is a phosphoprotein of 60,000 daltons. A similar, but not identical, phosphoprotein is present in normal avian and mammalian cells, in quantities substantially less than that present as the result of viral gene expression [15, 16, 20]. As shown here, both phosphoproteins contain a phosphoserine and a phosphothreonine at analogous locations in the molecules, but the peptide sequence surrounding the phosphothreonine residue in avian pp60^{sarc} confers different behavior on that particular tryptic peptide than the phosphothreonine-containing tryptic peptide in viral pp60^{src}, whereas the phosphoserine-containing tryptic peptide appears identical in viral pp60^{src} and cellular pp60^{sarc}.

Because pp60^{src} and pp60^{sarc} are phosphoproteins, consideration must be given to the possibility that their respective functions will be affected by their state of phosphorylation. We already have evidence that phosphorylation of the serine residue in viral pp60^{src}

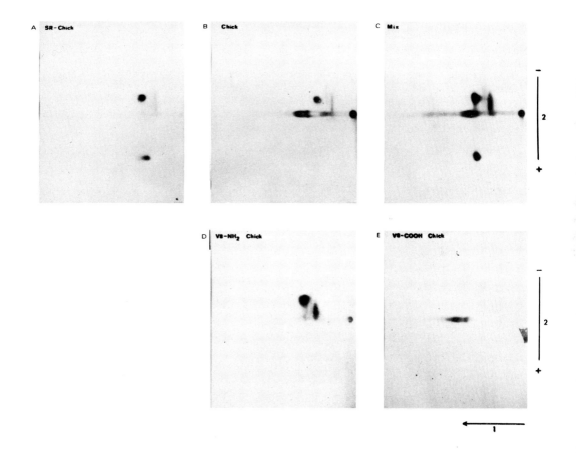

Fig. 5. Two-dimensional analysis of the tryptic phosphopeptides of viral pp60^{src} and avian pp60^{sarc}. ^{32}P-labeled pp60 proteins and the V8 cleavage peptides were excised from preparative gels, eluted, precipitated, and digested with trypsin. The digests were fractionated by ascending chromatography in the first dimension in sec-butanol–n-propanol–isoamyl alcohol–pyridine–H$_2$O (1:1:1:3:3) and electrophoresed at pH 6.5 in the second dimension. A: viral pp60^{src}; B: avian pp60 ^{sarc}; C: mix of viral and avian pp60 proteins; D: V8 amino terminal fragment of avian pp60^{sarc}; E: V8 carboxy terminal fragment of avian pp60^{sarc}.

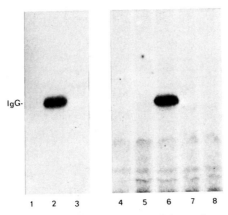

IgG·

1   2   3   4   5   6   7   8

Fig. 6. Autoradiograph of SDS-polyacrylamide gel analysis of the products of phosphotransferase reactions carried out in the bacteria-bound immune complex assay. Extracts of normal avian and mammalian cells were immunoprecipitated and resuspended in kinase reaction mixture, and the transfer of radiolabel from $[\gamma\text{-}^{32}P]$ATP to IgG was analyzed. Left panel: Extracts of normal chick embryo fibroblasts immunoprecipitated with normal rabbit serum (track 1), cross-reacting TBR (track 2), and TBMo (track 3). Right panel: Extracts of normal rat embryo fibroblasts immunoprecipitated with normal rabbit serum (track 4), TBR (track 5), cross-reacting TBR (track 6), TBMo (track 7), and TBM (track 8). The lack of phosphotransferase activity in extracts of normal chick embryo fibroblasts immunoprecipitated with TBR or with TBM has previously been reported [15].

is stimulated by cAMP in cell-free extracts [28]. A summary of our understanding of the general structure of pp60^{src} is diagrammed below.

$$
\begin{array}{ccccc}
 & P & \text{V8 protease} & P & \\
 & & \downarrow & & \\
NH_2 \text{————} & Ser \text{————————} & Thr \text{————} & COOH \\
 & \uparrow & & \uparrow & \\
 & cAMP\text{-} & & cAMP\text{-} & \\
 & stimulated & & independent & \\
\end{array}
$$

It is also clear from work in this laboratory and that of others that both viral and cellular phosphoproteins either are, or are closely associated with, protein kinases [7–9, 16, 22]. More recent, unpublished work in this laboratory has shown that pp60^{src} can be purified extensively by ion-exchange chromatography to yield preparations able to specifically phosphorylate casein, certain cellular proteins, and the purified heavy chain of rabbit IgG, but not histone, phosvitin, or other common kinase substrates. The pp60^{src}-specific phosphorylation of these protein substrates is inhibited by the addition of immune IgG. Comparison of the product of a wild-type and temperature-sensitive (NY68) transforming gene product shows that the temperature-sensitive product is at least five times more thermolabile than the wild-type product. This result is extremely strong evidence that pp60^{src} is itself a protein kinase and that the enzymatic activity described above is not merely due to an associated phosphotransferase. Furthermore, cellular pp60^{sarc} behaves on ion-exchange columns very similarly to pp60^{src}, supporting other data suggesting their close structural similarity.

The presence of a normal cellular protein that appears to be structurally and functionally very closely related to the avian sarcoma virus transforming protein necessarily raises several important points. For example, the structure of this protein has been remarkably conserved, as far as our very preliminary experiments permit such a conclusion, and this implies that it plays a common and essential role in normal cells. Since ASV can produce fibrosarcomas in both avian and mammalian species and transform their cells in culture, perhaps common site(s) of action for pp60^{src} are available in all transformation-sensitive cells. One might also speculate that all three proteins (viral, avian, and mammalian) function via the same circuits. Transformation by the viral protein may occur, then, merely because it is present in substantially greater quantities than is the cellular pp60^{sarc} in normal cells [15].

It is clear that additional studies using both purified normal and viral proteins must be pursued in order to obtain additional insights into the roles of these two proteins in normal cell growth and viral transformation.

ACKNOWLEDGMENTS

This research was supported by grants CA-21117 and CA-21326 from the National Cancer Institute and grant VC243 from the American Cancer Society. M.S.C. was a fellow in cancer research supported by a grant from the Damon Runyon–Walter Winchell Cancer Fund, and J.S.B. was supported by Fellowship Award CA-05534 from the National Institutes of Health.

We thank Hidesaburo Hanafusa and his co-workers for helpful discussions and communication of their unpublished results, as well as J.M. Bishop and his colleagues' communication of unpublished results. The SR-ASV-transformed Balb/c mouse cells used to produce the tumor-bearing mouse sera used in this study were originally obtained from J.T. Parsons.

REFERENCES

1. Hanafusa H: In Fraenkel-Conrat H, Wagner RP (eds): "Comprehensive Virology." New York: Plenum, 1977, vol 10, p 401.
2. Vogt PK: in Fraenkel-Conrat H, Wagner RP (eds): "Comprehensive Virology." New York: Plenum, 1977, vol 9, p 341.
3. Brugge JS, Erikson RL: Nature 269:346, 1977.
4. Purchio AF, Erikson E, Erikson RL: Proc Natl Acad Sci USA 74:4661, 1977.
5. Purchio AF, Erikson E, Brugge JS, Erikson RL: Proc Natl Acad Sci USA 75:1567, 1978.
6. Brugge JS, Erikson E, Collett MS, Erikson RL: J Virol 26:773, 1978.
7. Collett MS, Erikson RL: Proc Natl Acad Sci USA 75:2021, 1978.
8. Levinson AD, Oppermann H, Levintow L, Varmus HE, Bishop JM: Cell 15:561, 1978.
9. Rübsamen H, Friis RR, Bauer H: Proc Natl Acad Sci USA 76:967, 1979.
10. Erikson E, Collett MS, Erikson RL: Nature 274:919, 1978.
11. Stehelin D, Varmus HE, Bishop JM, Vogt PK: Nature 260:170, 1976.
12. Wang SY, Hayward WS, Hanafusa H: J Virol 24:64, 1977.
13. Spector DH, Smith K, Padgett T, McCombe P, Roulland-Dussoix D, Moscovici C, Varmus HE, Bishop JM: Cell 13:371, 1978.
14. Spector DH, Baker B, Varmus HE, Bishop JM: Cell 13:381, 1978.
15. Collett MS, Brugge JS, Erikson RL: Cell 15:1363, 1978.
16. Oppermann H, Levinson AD, Varmus HE, Levintow L, Bishop JM: Proc Natl Acad Sci USA 76:1804, 1979.
17. Hanafusa H, Halpern CC, Buchhagen DL, Kawai S: J Exp Med 146:1735, 1977.
18. Halpern CC, Hayward WS, Hanafusa H: J Virol 29:91, 1979.
19. Wang L-H, Halpern CC, Nadel M, Hanafusa H: Proc Natl Acad Sci USA 75:5812, 1978.
20. Karess RE, Hayward WS, Hanafusa H: Proc Natl Acad Sci USA 76:3154, 1979.

21. Marczynska B, Deinhardt F, Schubien J, Tischendorf P, Smith RD: J Natl Cancer Inst 51:1225, 1973.
22. Collett MS, Erikson E, Purchio AF, Brugge JS, Erikson RL: Proc Natl Acad Sci USA 76:3159, 1979.
23. Kessler SW: J Immunol 115:1617, 1975.
24. Pelham HRB, Jackson RJ: Eur J Biochem 67:247, 1976.
25. Laemmli UK: Nature 227:680, 1970.
26. Bonner WM, Laskey RA: Eur J Biochem 46:83, 1974.
27. Cleveland DW, Fischer SG, Kirschner MW, Laemmli UK: J Biol Chem 252:1102, 1977.
28. Collett MS, Erikson E, Erikson RL: J Virol 29:770, 1979.
29. Brugge JS, Steinbaugh PJ, Erikson RL: Virology 91:130, 1978.

Tumor Cell Surfaces and Malignancy 757–764 (1980)

Gene Expression of Abelson Murine Leukemia Virus

O. N. Witte, N. Rosenberg, and D. Baltimore

Department of Biology and Center for Cancer Research, Massachusetts Institute of Technology, Cambridge, Massachusetts 02139 (O.N.W., D.B.), and Cancer Research Center, Tufts University School of Medicine, Boston, Massachusetts 02111 (N.R.)

Abelson murine leukemia virus (A-MuLV) represents a simple genetic system with which to study genes capable of transforming specific lymphoid target cells. A-MuLV encodes a single known protein of 120,000 molecular weight (P120). A portion of this molecule is expressed at the cell surface but its function is not known. Serological reagents specific for P120 can be produced in mice regressing A-MuLV syngeneic tumors. Such sera identify a protein in normal mouse lymphoid tissues which may represent the cellular gene from which A-MuLV was derived.

Key words: leukemia, transforming gene product, Abelson murine leukemia virus

CHARACTERISTICS OF DEFECTIVE TRANSFORMING RETROVIRUSES

Abelson murine leukemia virus (A-MuLV) is a member of the replication-defective, rapidly transforming (DT) group of retroviruses. Included among this group are the murine and feline sarcoma viruses, the murine spleen focus-forming virus, and the avian erythroblastosis and myelocytomytosis virus strains [1, 2]. DT viruses have structural and genetic features which distinguish them from the prototype transforming retroviruses — avian sarcoma viruses (ASV). ASV contains genes for both replicative functions (packaging proteins, virion enzyme) and the transforming protein (*src*) within a single RNA molecule. All members of the DT retroviruses described to date have lost all functional proteins necessary for replication but have retained regions (mainly at the 3' and 5' ends of the genome) required for appropriate reverse transcription and packaging by a helper virus. New genetic information, presumably derived from the host cell genome by a recombination mechanism, is inserted into the DT virus genome and is responsible for the altered transforming potential of the new virus. Currently available data suggest that the various DT viruses represent unique cellular gene(s) and hence could show varying transformation potentials and mechanisms of action.

Received April 18, 1979; accepted April 18, 1979.

A-MuLV GENOME STRUCTURE AND GENE EXPRESSION

A-MuLV was derived by Abelson and Rabstein [3] from the replication-competent Moloney MuLV (M-MuLV) by in vivo passage through a steroid-treated mouse. The parental M-MuLV strain normally induced thymomas. The A-MuLV (isolated with M-MuLV as the helper virus) gave rise to non-T-cell lymphoid tumors. The demonstrated oncogenic potential of A-MuLV now includes B lymphoid stem cells from adult bone marrow and spleen, fetal liver, some macrophage-like cells, plasmacytomas, and even some strains of established fibroblasts in culture [4–7].

Recent heteroduplex mapping [8] demonstrated that the A-MuLV genome RNA (5,500 bases) has retained regions of homology to M-MuLV at the 5' (1,320 bases) and 3' (750 bases) ends of the genome. The center of the A-MuLV genome has a 3,500-base insert presumably derived from the mouse genome.

The only known protein and candidate for the transforming function encoded by A-MuLV is a fusion protein of 120,000 molecular weight called P120 [9, 10]. This protein contains an N-terminal region of about 30,000 molecular weight derived from the M-MuLV *gag* gene-retained sequences and a 90,000 molecular weight region from the A-MuLV-unique sequences (Fig. 1). With the use of serologic reagents against the M-MuLV *gag* gene, protein P120 was found in all cells transformed by A-MuLV and could be translated in vitro from A-MuLV genomic RNA [9].

Although this protein contains sequences homologous to the virion core protein precursor of M-MuLV, $Pr65^{gag}$, P120 is much more stable during pulse chase experiments than the helper virus precursors (Fig. 2). P120 is not readily detectable in extracellular virions released from transformed mouse cells. P120 is a phosphoprotein [9] and binds or aggregates with the membrane pellet during cell fractionation experiments. P120 represents about 0.05–0.1% of the cellular protein recovered during a pulse label.

Currently, no conditional or deletion mutants of the P120 protein have been characterized to the extent which would definitively link P120 to the transformation process.

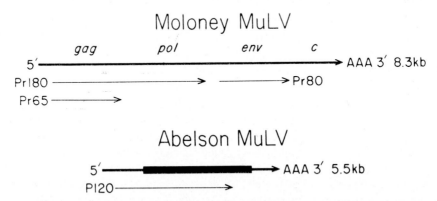

Fig. 1. Genome structure of Moloney and Abelson MuLV RNAs. The single-stranded RNA genomes of M-MuLV and A-MuLV and their known protein gene products and genetic regions are shown. A-MuLV retains 1,320 bases at its 5' end and 750 bases at its 3' end homologous to the ends of the M-MuLV genome [8]. The center of the A-MuLV genome (represented by the thicker bar) is not homologous to M-MuLV. It represents the unique sequences of A-MuLV derived from the mouse genome. The A-MuLV P120 protein is a fusion protein. Its amino-terminal region is derived from the M-MuLV *gag* gene and its carboxy-terminal region from the A-MuLV-unique sequences [9, 14].

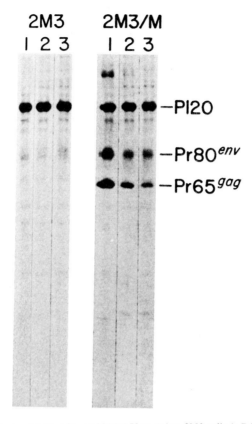

Fig. 2. Pulse chase analysis of A-MuLV and M-MuLV proteins. 2M3 cells (a BALB/c lymphoid A-MuLV-transformed nonproducer line) and 2M3/M (superinfected with M-MuLV) were pulse-labeled (30 min) with ^{35}S-methionine [9]. Cells from the pulse period (lane 1) or aliquots washed and chased in complete media for 1 h (lane 2) or 3 h (lane 3) were extracted for immunoprecipitation with a polyvalent goat anti-MuLV serum. Precipitates were collected with S. aureas [19] and analyzed on SDS–10% polyacrylamide gels [20] and developed by fluorography [21].

PREPARATION OF ANTI-ABELSON TUMOR SERUM

To further characterize this protein we sought to prepare serologic reagents with specificity to the A-MuLV-unique region of P120. Because of the successful application by immune sera in the avian sarcoma virus system [11, 12] and the recent description of an A-MuLV cell surface antigen [13], we prepared syngeneic tumor regressor serum against A-MuLV in vitro transformed mouse lymphoid cell lines [5, 14].

Mice of the C57L/J strain were able to reject syngeneic A-MuLV in vitro transformed lymphoid cell lines. These cell lines expressed the A-MuLV-specific P120 as well as the M-MuLV helper virus precursor proteins. Analysis of serum samples from such regressor animals by immunoprecipitation demonstrated antibody prominently reactive with the P120 protein and the Pr80^{env} precursor of M-MuLV. The activity to the helper virus protein determinants could be competed with unlabeled M-MuLV virion protein (Fig. 3), but most of the anti-P120 activity was not absorbed, suggesting that a unique antigenic determinant had been recognized. This antibody reactivity to P120 could not

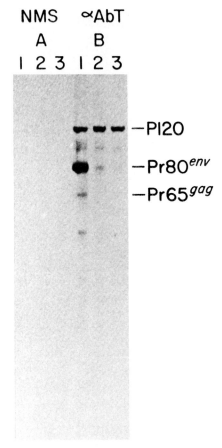

Fig. 3. Demonstration of activity for the unique region of P120 in anti-AbT serum. Extracts of 2M3/M cells labeled for 30 min with ^{35}S-methionine were immunoprecipitated with 2.5 μl of (A) normal mouse serum (A) or (B) anti-Abelson tumor serum (B). Lane 1 had no competing protein; lane 2 had 50 μg and lane 3 150 μg of M-MuLV virion proteins included in the lysates. Samples were collected and analyzed as in Figure 2.

be competed with extracts of M-MuLV-infected fibroblasts, Moloney sarcoma virus-transformed NIH/3T3 cells, spleen focus-forming virus-infected NIH/3T3, or polyoma virus-transformed mouse cells. Anti-P120 activity could be competed with all of the A-MuLV-transformed cell lysates we have examined (unpublished observations). No additional A-MuLV-specified proteins have been found with such sera [14].

Pr80^{env} is the precursor of the M-MuLV virion glycoprotein gp70 and a small non-glycosylated protein, p15E, both found on the external surface of the virion envelope and cell membrane [15, 16]. Pr80^{env} is synthesized on membrane-bound polysomes and is apparently nascently or very rapidly glycosylated by the en bloc addition of high-mannose carbohydrate units [17]. As the Pr80^{env} undergoes proteolytic cleavage, the carbohydrate is processed to the complex form (containing sialic acid and fucose) found on the finished gp70. Thus Pr80^{env} and its products gp70 and p15E have a pattern of synthesis and processing similar to other external or peripheral cell membrane glycoproteins, and it is not

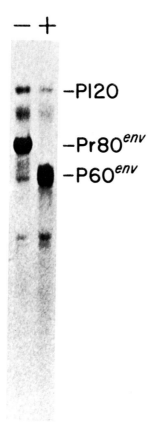

Fig. 4. Endoglycosidase H sensitivity demonstrates carbohydrate on Pr80^{env} but not on P120. An extract of ^{35}S-methionine-labeled (30 min) 2M3/M cells was immunoprecipitated with polyvalent goat anti-M-MuLV protein serum. One-half (+ lane) was digested with endoglycosidase H [17] prior to electrophoresis. Samples were analyzed as in Figure 2.

unexpected that they would represent a prominent tumor antigen. P120, however, does not become glycosylated, as judged by lack of incorporation of glycoprotein precursors like ^{3}H-mannose or ^{3}H-D-glucosamine [14] and lack of sensitivity to endoglycosidase H (Fig. 4), an enzyme that cleaves the high-mannose groups from recently synthesized Pr80^{env} and shifts its electrophoretic mobility [17].

DETECTION OF AN A-MuLV-SPECIFIED CELL SURFACE ANTIGEN

Risser and co-workers [13] have described an A-MuLV-specified cell surface antigen detected by antibody-mediated cytoxicity employing a similar syngeneic regressor serum; no data on the molecular species carrying this antigen was shown.

Since our anti-Abelson tumor serum (anti-AbT serum) contained precipitating antibody specific for the A-MuLV-unique region of P120 we tested for the presence of this antigen at the cell surface by a two-stage immunofluorescence assay. Viable A-MuLV-transformed nonproducer fibroblast lines — A2 (NIH/3T3) and lymphoid in vitro-derived

2M3 (BALB/c bone marrow) — were used as test cells to direct attention to A-MuLV gene expression in the absence of helper virus (Table I). Only the anti-AbT serum could stain the cells. Sera against M-MuLV p15 and p30 that could precipitate P120 from cell lysates [9] were unable to stain the nonproducer cells.

Absorption of anti-AbT serum with M-MuLV proteins coupled to Sepharose, M-MuLV-infected NIH/3T3 cells, or Moloney sarcoma virus-transformed NIH/3T3 cells did not remove the ability to stain the cell membrane of A-MuLV-transformed cells. However, absorption with one A-MuLV-transformed cell line could both remove the staining activity when tested on another A-MuLV-transformed cell line and reduce the ability to precipitate P120 from labeled cell lysates [14]. These studies suggest that a region of P120 unrelated to the MuLV *gag* gene is expressed at the cell membrane and induces a serologic response during A-MuLV tumor regression.

USE OF ANTI-AbT SERUM TO SEARCH FOR THE NORMAL CELLULAR GENE PRODUCT REPRESENTED IN A-MuLV

Erikson and co-workers [18] have successfully used tumor regressor serum to identify a normal cellular protein with homology to the ASV *src* gene from normal in vitro fibroblasts. In their case, the ASV *src* protein and normal cellular *src* protein were of identical size and shared extensive homology. Since A-MuLV P120 is a fusion protein containing about 90,000 molecular weight of protein sequence derived from the host cell, we expected that a large protein (>90,000 molecular weight) would be implicated. Initial attempts to identify a normal cellular protein from BALB/c/3T3 cells or freshly explanted tissues from nonlymphoid organs such as liver were negative. However, pulse-labeled tissue explants of thymus, spleen, and bone marrow from BALB/c or C57BL6/J mice all revealed a large protein (150,000 molecular weight) when precipitated with anti-AbT (Fig. 5). This protein represents a very small fraction of the total labeled protein and may be more abundant in thymus owing to a higher cell viability during the labeling procedure. We are currently investigating the cellular and tissue distribution of this 150K protein and comparing it to the A-MuLV-encoded P120 protein. We suspect this 150,000 molecular weight protein represents the normal cellular gene product with which M-MuLV recombined to produce A-MuLV.

TABLE I. Cell Surface Fluorescence on A-MuLV-Transformed Cells*

Serum	A2 (NIH/3T3 nonproducer)	2M3 (BALB/c lymphoid nonproducer)	2M3/M (2M3 superinfected with M-MuLV)
Normal mouse serum	−	−	−
Anti-AbT	++	+++	++++
Normal rabbit serum	−	−	−
Rabbit anti-M-MuLV p15	−	−	−/+
Rabbit anti-M-MuLV p30	−	−	++
Rabbit anti-M-MuLV gp70	−	−	++++

*Viable cells [$(1-2) \times 10^6$] were stained for cell surface antigens in suspension at 4°C with 50 μl normal or immune sera at a final 1:20 dilution. Fluoresceinated goat anti-mouse IgG or goat anti-rabbit IgG at 1:15 or 1:40 dilutions, respectively, were used for the second stage. Wet mounts and fixed smears were examined. A subjective quantitation of + (dull) to ++++ (very bright) is shown; −, no fluorescence.

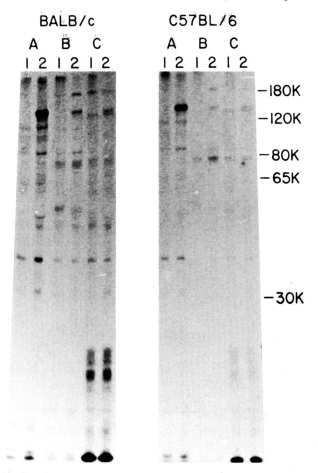

Fig. 5. Detection of a normal mouse protein cross reactive to the unique region of P120. Cell suspensions of thymus (A), spleen (B), and bone marrow (C) from BALB/c and C57BL6/J mice were labeled for 1 h with ^{35}S-methionine (100 μCi/10^7 cells). Labeled cells were extracted and immunoprecipitated with normal mouse sera (lane 1) or anti-AbT (lane 2). Precipitates were collected and analyzed as in Figure 2.

ACKNOWLEDGMENTS

This work was supported by grant VC-4J from the American Cancer Society and grants CA-24220 and CA-14051 from the National Cancer Institute. O.N.W. is a Helen Hay Whitney Fellow. N.R. is a Research Scholar of the American Cancer Society, Massachusetts Division. D.B. is a Research Professor of the American Cancer Society.

REFERENCES

1. Graf T, Beug H: Biochim Biophys Acta 516:269, 1978.
2. Van Zaane D, Bloemers HPJ: Biochim Biophys Acta 516:249, 1978.
3. Abelson HT, Rabstein LS: Cancer Res 30:2213, 1979.
4. Potter M, Sklar MD, Rowe WP: Science 182:592, 1973.
5. Rosenberg N, Baltimore D, Scher CD: Proc Natl Acad Sci USA 72:1932, 1975.

6. Raschke WC, Baird S, Ralph P, Nakoinz I: Cell 15:261, 1978.

7. Scher CD, Siegler R: Nature 253:729, 1975.

8. Shields A: PhD thesis, MIT, 1979.

9. Witte ON, Rosenberg N, Paskind M, Shields A, Baltimore D: Proc Natl Acad Sci USA 75:2488, 1978.

10. Reynolds FH, Sacks TL, Deobagkar DN, Stephenson JR: Proc Natl Acad Sci USA 75:3974, 1978.

11. Brugge JS, Erikson RL: Nature 269:346, 1977.

12. Purchio AF, Erikson E, Brugge JS, Erikson RL: Proc Natl Acad Sci USA 75:1567, 1978.

13. Risser R, Stockert E, Old LJ: Proc Natl Acad Sci USA 75:3918, 1978.

14. Witte ON, Rosenberg N, Baltimore D: J Virol (in press).

15. Witte ON, Weissmann IL: Virology 69:464, 1976.

17. Witte ON, Wirth DF: J Virol 29:735, 1979.

18. Collett MS, Brigge JS, Erikson RL: Cell 15:1363, 1978.

19. Kessler SJ: Immunol 115:1617, 1975.

20. Laemmli UK: Nature 227:680, 1970.

21. Bonnar WM, Laskey RA: Eur J Biochem 46:83, 1974.

Tumor Cell Surfaces and Malignancy 765–772 (1980)

On the Biochemistry of Transformation by Rous Sarcoma Virus

S. J. Singer, J. F. Ash, Roger C. Carroll, Michael H. Heggeness, and
Peter K. Vogt

*Department of Biology, University of California at San Diego, La Jolla, California 92093,
and Department of Microbiology, University of Southern California School of Medicine,
Los Angeles, California 90033*

In order to isolate those biochemical events associated specifically with transformation of fibroblasts, we have been investigating a system involving a normal
rat kidney (NRK) cell line infected with a temperature-sensitive mutant (LA23)
of Rous sarcoma virus (RSV). At $33°$, the permissive temperature, the cells exhibit the transformed phenotype (but do not produce infectious virus), while
at $39°$, the non-permissive temperature, the cells exhibit the normal phenotype.
The phenotypic characteristics studied were cell morphology, the cytoskeletal
structure, the mobility of surface receptors, aerobic glycolysis, and glucose
transport. The apparent increase in the mobility of surface receptors upon
transformation of cultured fibroblasts, which is very likely responsible for the
more ready agglutinability by lectins of transformed compared to normal fibroblasts, was shown to be directly associated with a breakdown of the cytoskeleton
upon transformation.

With the hypothesis in mind that transformation by RSV might be due to a
pleiotypic and reversible enzymic modification of cytoskeletal and metabolic
components of the normal cell, we grew LA23-NRK cells *at the permissive temperature* in the presence of inhibitors of protein synthesis. Within hours, the
phenotypic characteristics mentioned above reverted from transformed to normal, as was anticipated from the hypothesis. The recent findings of Collett and
Erikson, that the protein product of the transforming *src* gene of RSV is associated with a protein kinase enzymic activity, is entirely consistent with this
hypothesis. We have begun to look for those proteins in the transformed cell
which might be affected in vivo by such an activity, and have so far concluded
that the cytoskeletal proteins filamin and myosin are not altered, within a factor
of 2, in their degree of phosphorylation by RSV transformation.

The proposal is discussed that transformation by RSV may be the consequence
of permanently placing a cell into a new steady-state program differing from that
of the normal cell.

Key words: oncogenic viruses, pleiotypic modifications, transmembrane interactions, altered steady-state

Received July 25, 1979; accepted July 25, 1979.

This is a very exciting period in tumor biology, in part because of a joining together that has already taken place of two approaches to the problem of viral transformation. Investigators who have been interested in the genomes and molecular genetics of oncogenic viruses — genotypers — and investigators who have worked on the biochemical and cell biological characteristics of virally transformed cells — phenotypers — have heretofore carried on their activities so independently of one another as to be almost in separate worlds. But recent developments have created a firm linkage between the genotypers and phenotypers that is certain to develop into a well-traveled bridge between the two.

Our own entree into the fraternity of phenotypers arose some years ago from interests in the areas of membrane structure and function. That the surface properties of normal and transformed cells might be different, reflecting the different social behavior of these cells, has been a long-standing belief in tumor biology. Burger [7, 8] and Sachs [20] and their colleagues provided important evidence that supported this belief in the case of normal and transformed fibroblasts. They showed that lectins more readily agglutinated transformed fibroblasts than normal fibroblasts, but that if the normal cells were trypsinized they also became readily agglutinable. From these experiments there arose the concept of "cryptic sites"; that the surface of the normal fibroblast contained lectin receptor sites that were somehow shielded or cryptic, and that either trypsinization or the processes of transformation resulted in their exposure to binding by the lectins.

In developing the fluid mosaic model of the molecular organization of membranes [36], it was realized that a quite different explanation of these differential agglutination results was possible. It was suggested that the *numbers* of lectin binding sites on the surfaces of normal and transformed fibroblasts need not be substantially different [cf 26, 32], but their *distribution* might be. If these sites were clustered on the transformed cell, but dispersed on the normal cell, lectin-bridging between clusters on two transformed cells would be more efficient than between dispersed sites on two normal cells [Fig. 7, 35], and lectin agglutinability of the transformed cells would therefore occur at lower lectin concentrations than with normal cells. This hypothesis seems to be substantially correct, with the important additional feature that the clusters of lectin receptors on transformed fibroblasts are *induced* to form by the binding of the multivalent lectin itself, a process that does not occur to a significant extent on normal fibroblasts [21, 24, 25, 30]. In other words, it appears that the lectin receptors are more mobile in the plane of the membrane of the transformed cell than of the normal cell.

The question then became: What factor(s) is responsible for this apparent difference in receptor mobility? Over the ensuing years several classes of molecular mechanisms were advanced to account for the difference. One was that the lipid viscosity of the transformed fibroblast was lower than that of the normal fibroblast [34]. A second class of mechanism was that external surface components, such as fibronectin, were present on normal fibroblasts but not on the transformed cells, and such external proteins restricted the lateral motions of membrane receptors [13, 17, 18, 41, 46, 47]. A third class was that internal cytoskeletal proteins are in different structural states in normal and transformed cells [3, 27, 28] and, in the former, they inhibit receptor mobility [27, 35]. This last type of mechanism was given strong support by our studies of transmembrane interactions in flat cells such as normal fibroblasts as compared to round cells such as transformed fibroblasts [1, 2, 5, 6, 14]. A summary of our investigations with normal fibroblasts has been presented [37], and recent studies are described elsewhere in this volume (see Ash et al).

Briefly, what we have found is that when any one of several independent integral proteins in the membranes of normal fibroblasts is treated with lectins or their specific antibodies (usually followed by secondary antibodies), the integral protein is induced to aggregate specifically into small clusters, which appear to line up precisely over the actin-myosin-containing stress fibers that lie immediately under the membrane. This process then effectively immobilizes these clusters; ie, they do not exhibit any further significant clustering or mobility. On the other hand, as is well known from other studies (for review, see ref 31), when round cells are similarly treated with specific antibodies to individual integral proteins in their surface membranes, capping of the proteins often occurs. In the process of capping, we have found [5, 6, 14] that the antibody-induced clusters of membrane protein always become associated with actin, myosin, and α-actinin on the underside of the membrane. It therefore appears that a unifying concept of what generally occurs on flat and on round cells upon antibody-induced clustering of a surface receptor is as follows: the clusters of the receptor somehow become linked in either case to actin/myosin across the membrane.* If the actin and myosin are organized into extended stress fibers, however, such transmembrane linkage effectively immobilizes the clusters. If, on the contrary, the actin and myosin are relatively disorganized and stress fibers are broken down, such transmembrane linkage produces a complex of the receptor cluster and actin/myosin, which is relatively small, still mobile in the plane of the membrane, and capable of being collected into a cap.

Thus, the results of Burger [7, 8] and Sachs [20] and their collaborators can be explained by the following proposal. Either trypsinization of normal fibroblasts or the processes of transformation causes a breakdown of the intracellular stress fibers (by mechanisms not yet clear). Addition of lectins to the normal fibroblasts cross-links the lectin receptors to form small clusters that become linked across the membrane to the actin/myosin in stress fibers and are thereby immobilized. Addition of lectins to transformed fibroblasts produces a clustering of the (essentially same number of) lectin receptors, and the clusters again become linked across the membrane to actin/myosin, but the actin/myosin is largely disaggregated. The resultant transmembrane complexes are then collected into large patches on the cell surface. It is the formation of lectin bridges between such patches on two neighboring transformed cells that results in more efficient agglutination than between two normal cells.

If this proposal was correct, another question arose: How does the process of transformation of fibroblasts cause a breakdown of the intracellular stress fibers (among the many other possible changes produced)? In approaching this question, we were much influenced by studies on the cytoskeleton of the erythrocyte. This cytoskeleton consists of a complex of two high molecular weight proteins (bands 1 and 2), together called spectrin, along with a lower molecular weight protein (band 5), which is an actin (for review, see ref 22). It is known that the band 2 component, but not band 1, can be phosphorylated in vivo (for review, see ref 12). Our laboratory provided evidence some years ago that the reversible phosphorylation of band 2 protein was associated with a reversible aggregation of the spectrin complex on the cytoplasmic face of the membrane [4, 33]. Pursuing what we considered to be the analogous roles of the spectrin-actin complex in erythrocytes and the membrane-associated myosin-actin complex of fibroblasts [27], we therefore considered the possibility that the breakdown of the stress fibers of normal fibroblasts upon transformation was due to a change in the state of phosphorylation of some critical component(s) of the stress fibers. We reasoned that this or a similar enzymatic process should be reversible in vivo, and therefore we undertook the following experiments.

*An alternative view, that the clusters of receptors become linked to some external surface component rather than across the membrane to actin/myosin, is ruled out at least in the case of fibronectin. While the fibronectin on the surfaces of normal fibroblasts is organized into fibrils that line up directly over the actin/myosin stress fibers, as demonstrated by Heggeness et al [16] and confirmed by Hynes and Destree [19], the distribution of fibronectin is extremely pauci-disperse, completely unlike the regular distribution of clustered receptors on the normal fibroblast surface.

In order to isolate phenotypic changes that were specifically associated with the transformation of fibroblasts, an experimental system was chosen that involved a temperature-sensitive mutant (LA23) of Rous avian sarcoma virus (RSV) infecting a normal rat kidney (NRK) continuous cell line. LA23-NRK cells grown at the permissive temperature (33°C) exhibit the transformed phenotype with respect to cell morphology and cytoskeletal characteristics, and at the nonpermissive temperature (39°C) they exhibit the normal phenotype. They can be shifted from one to the other phenotype within hours after the appropriate temperature shift. At neither temperature is virus progeny produced. It was then shown [3] that if LA23-NRK cells were grown *at the permissive temperature* in the presence of cycloheximide or other inhibitors of protein synthesis, the cells reverted within hours from the transformed to the normal phenotype. It was then remarked [3]:

> . . . these results show that: a) protein synthesis is required to maintain the transformed state in LA23-infected cells at the permissive temperature; and b) protein synthesis is *not* required for the myosin-containing structures to revert from the transformed to normal state. . . . These findings are therefore consistent with the hypothesis that the product of the viral *src* gene [which is responsible for the transformation process (45)] is directly or indirectly involved in a reversible chemical modification of components of the myosin-containing complex inside the cells.

If it is indeed true that the components of the cytoskeleton of the normal cell were in some manner reversibly modified upon transformation, such modification might be pleiotypic and would affect many other components of the normal cell as well. Accordingly, the glycolytic properties of the LA23-NRK cells were then investigated. It was found [9] that the rate of aerobic glycolysis (lactate production) by these cells was significantly higher at the permissive than at the non-permissive temperatures, unlike uninfected NRK cells, where the rates were the same at the two temperatures. Furthermore, the enhanced rate at the permissive temperature was affected by dinitrophenol and oligomycin in characteristically different ways than the rate at the non-permissive temperature, as if the mitochondria in the cells at the permissive temperature were more uncoupled than at the non-permissive temperature. The finding of greatest interest, however, was that if cells growing at the permissive temperature were treated with cycloheximide or other inhibitors or protein synthesis, their rate of aerobic glycolysis, and the sensitivities of that rate to dinitrophenol and oligomycin, reverted rapidly from the transformed phenotype to the normal.

The facts that the metabolic properties, as well as the cytoskeletal properties, of the transformed phenotype were reverted to normal by the inhibition of protein synthesis at the permissive temperature were therefore consistent with the idea that the *src* gene product was somehow responsible for a pleiotypic reversible modification of normal cell components upon transformation by RSV.

At about this time, the striking results of Collett and Erikson [10, 11] were published, providing strong evidence that the *src* gene product was associated with a protein kinase activity. This work is discussed elsewhere in this volume (see Erikson). The results and hypotheses we have derived are clearly entirely consistent with the association of the *src* gene product with such a potentially pleiotypic enzymic activity.

This demonstration of an *src* gene-coded protein kinase activity, however, was carried out in vitro in an immunoprecipitate containing the *src* gene product, in which the heavy chain of the antibody was phosphorylated in the presence of γ^{32}P-ATP. The in vivo substrates for the *src* gene product are not known. In fact, if the *src* gene product is a very highly specific enzyme, it may phosphorylate and activate some other pleiotypic enzyme with an activity different from phosphorylation (such as phosphatase, an acetylase, etc). We and others have therefore proceeded to attempt to detect and identify in vivo substrates for the *src* gene product's activity. There are two general ways of doing this: one is to look for the appearance in extracts of transformed cells of new phosphorylated components, or for components with significantly increased ^{32}P-specific activity, in 1-D or 2-D electrophoresis gels, irrespective of the identity of these proteins; the other is to investigate whether specific identifiable components have an altered ^{32}P-specific activity associated with the transformed phenotype. The latter approach could be carried out, for example, using specific antibodies to immunoprecipitate individual known proteins from cell extracts, and determining their specific activities.

At this juncture it is important to note that normal uninfected cells contain a gene homologous to the viral *src* gene (called the *sarc* gene) [40], which codes for a protein product that is antigenically cross-reactive with the viral *src* gene product and that exhibits a protein kinase activity in immunoprecipitates (see Erikson, this volume). It is therefore a strong possibility that the in vivo activity of the *src* gene product is to alter the level of phosphorylation of one or more cellular proteins in the transformed as compared to the normal cell, rather than to cause the phosphorylation of components that are not phosphorylated in the normal cell. If this is true, then the search for the in vivo effects of the *src* gene product must be designed to detect quantitative (as well as qualitative) changes in protein phosphorylation.

Our first efforts in this direction have concentrated on the cytoskeletal proteins filamin and myosin. Filamin was chosen for a number of reasons. It is a protein found in smooth muscle and non-muscle cells [44], which when mixed with F-actin filaments cross-links the latter into fiber bundles [43]. These fiber bundles are morphologically similar to the stress fibers seen in normal fibroblasts and other flat cells, and the suggestion was made [43] that the interaction between filamin and F-actin could be important in the in vivo formation of the stress fibers. Furthermore, filamin is capable of being phosphorylated [42], and it has been reported [29] that its level of phosphorylation is correlated with its capacity to interact with F-actin. Finally, its large molecular weight gives it a unique mobility in SDS-PAGE gels and allows the protein band to be sliced from the gel relatively free from contaminating components.

In experiments to be reported in detail elsewhere, LA23-NRK cells were grown at the permissive and non-permissive temperatures in low phosphate-F12 medium containing ^{32}P-P$_i$. Two types of experiments have been performed with this system. 1) Hot detergent extracts of the cells, after removal of nucleic acids, were subjected to SDS-PAGE, and parallel gels were either Coomassie blue-stained, autoradiographed, or sliced and counted. 2) Detergent extracts of the cells were immunoprecipitated using rabbit antibodies to chicken gizzard filamin or to pig or human uterine myosin. The precipitates were dissolved in SDS, subjected to SDS-PAGE, and parallel gels were either Coomassie blue-stained, autoradiographed, or the antigen band was sliced out for counting. In addition, the former type of experiment was carried out with chick embryo fibroblasts (CEF) and CEF infected with a wild-type RSV (B77). These experiments are difficult because the level of radioactivity in individual protein components is low, and the background radioactivities on the gels show some variability. The results of many experiments, however, have convinced us that, although both filamin and the heavy chain of myosin are phosphorylated in vivo in these cells [23], within a factor or two there was no difference in the ^{32}P specific activity of these proteins between the transformed and the normal phenotypes.

Many similar experiments are contemplated with other specific cellular components, but at present we have no information about the possible in vivo protein substrates of the *src* gene protein kinase activity.

The picture that is emerging of the biochemical nature of transformation by RSV is both novel and extremely interesting. In the past, phenotypers interested in the transformed cell have concentrated on one or another purported parameter of transformation — eg, the disappearance of fibronectin from fibroblast cell surfaces, the appearance of plasminogen activator, changes in glycolipid and glycoprotein profiles, and so forth. That transformed cells differ from their normal counterparts in a myriad of biochemical features is clear, but the interrelationships among these features is largely obscure, because we do not know enough about the metabolic pathways of cells and their interconnections to derive a coherent scheme to account for the origin of these differences between the transformed and normal phenotypes.

Transformation by RSV may be thought of as the consequence of permanently placing a cell into a new steady-state program differing from that of the normal cell. The normal cell is characterized by a genetically determined program that controls the steady-state of the cell as a function of external conditions. This program somehow determines the operation of the normal cell cycle and the steady-state distribution of normal cell constituents at different stages in the cell cycle. If at any state in the cell cycle the normal cell is subjected to a transient perturbation — eg, by a hormone or growth factor — the steady state is transiently perturbed, but upon removal of the perturbing agent or its metabolic sequelae, the normal cell will eventually return to its steady-state program. The integration of the *src* gene into the genome of the RSV-infected cell, however, apparently permanently changes the steady-state program. The presence of the *src* gene protein kinase activity must allow the metabolic machinery of the cell *partially to escape* the regulatory mechanisms that operate in the normal cell. This places the cell into a new steady state and a new steady-state program. The key word here is "partially." Let us suppose, for example, that the viral *src* gene and the normal *sarc* gene protein kinases have parallel pleiotypic phosphorylating activities. In the normal cell these activities are kinetically balanced by dephosphorylating activities to achieve a steady-state level of phosphorylation of each of the protein substrates at a given stage in the cell cycle. The introduction of the *src* gene kinase, however, might then increase the rate of phosphorylation of these substrates, either because of a dosage effect (because many more copies of the *src* gene kinase than of the normal *sarc* gene kinase are present in the infected cell), or perhaps because the *src* gene kinase is a mutated form of the normal, which has lost one or more of its allosteric regulatory sites, which are used to control the activity of the normal enzyme. The normal dephosphorylating activities might then be unable kinetically to return the level of phosphorylation of these protein substrates to that of the normal cell, and a new steady state would develop [38]. Although such a new steady state was permanent in the sense that it was genetically determined, in principle it would be reversible if the new enzymatic activities introduced by transformation could be suitably manipulated or repressed.

If this picture is basically correct, transformation by Rous sarcoma virus might then be thought of as a "steady-state disease." Identification of those cellular components which are enzymically modified upon RSV transformation could shed much light on the mechanisms of regulation of normal cell growth and development.

The question of the relevance of this picture to cancer in general is a fascinating one to contemplate. It would be of interest, for example, to carry out experiments similar to those we have discussed above, with temperature-sensitive transformed cells that were transformed by agents differing from RSV [eg, 39, 15, 48], to see if at the permissive temperature the addition of cycloheximide or other inhibitors of protein synthesis causes a reversion from the transformed to the normal phenotype. If experiments of this kind did result in such reversion, a pleiotypic and reversible enzymatic modification process might be implicated in the mechanism of transformation by these agents.

ACKNOWLEDGMENTS

The original studies that are discussed in this paper were supported by grants CA-22031 and GM-15971 from the National Institutes of Health to S.J.S., and by research contract NO1 CP53518 from the National Cancer Institute to P.K.V.

REFERENCES

1. Ash JF, Singer SJ: Proc Natl Acad Sci USA 73:4575, 1976.
2. Ash JF, Louvard D, Singer SJ: Proc Natl Acad Sci USA 74:5584, 1977.
3. Ash JF, Vogt PK, Singer SJ: Proc Natl Acad Sci USA 73:3603, 1976.
4. Birchmeier W, Singer SJ: J Cell Biol 73:647, 1977.
5. Bourguignon LYW, Singer SJ: Proc Natl Acad Sci USA 74:5031, 1977.
6. Bourguignon LYW, Tokuyasu KT, Singer SJ: J Cell Physiol 95:239, 1978.
7. Burger MM: Proc Natl Acad Sci USA 62:994, 1969.
8. Burger MM, Goldberg AR: Proc Natl Acad Sci USA 57:359, 1967.
9. Carroll RC, Ash JF, Vogt PK, Singer SJ: Proc Natl Acad Sci USA 75:5015, 1978.
10. Collett MS, Erikson RL: Proc Natl Acad Sci USA 75:2021, 1978.
11. Erikson E, Collett MS, Erikson RL: Nature 274:919, 1978.
12. Fairbanks G, Avruch J, Dino JE, Patel VP: J Supramol Struct 9:97, 1978.
13. Gahmberg CG, Kiehn D, Hakamori S: Nature 248:413, 1974.
14. Geiger B, Singer SJ: Cell 16:213, 1979.
15. Graf T, Ade N, Beug H: Nature 275:496, 1978.
16. Heggeness MH, Ash JF, Singer SJ: Ann NY Acad Sci 312:414, 1978.
17. Hogg NM: Proc Natl Acad Sci USA 71:488, 1974.
18. Hynes RO: Proc Natl Acad Sci USA 70:3170, 1973.
19. Hynes RO, Destree AT: Cell 15:875, 1978.
20. Inbar M, Sachs L: Proc Natl Acad Sci USA 63:1418, 1969.
21. Inbar M, Sachs L: FEBS Lett 32:124, 1973.
22. Marchesi VT, Furthmayr H, Tomita M: Ann Rev Biochem 45:667, 1976.
23. Muhlrad A, Oplatka A: FEBS Lett 77:37, 1977.
24. Nicolson GL: Nature New Biol 243:218, 1973.
25. Noonan KD, Burger MM: J Cell Biol 59:134, 1973.
26. Ozanne B, Sambrook J: Nature 232:156, 1971.
27. Painter RG, Sheetz M, Singer SJ: Proc Natl Acad Sci USA 72:1359, 1975.
28. Pollack R, Osborn M, Weber K: Proc Natl Acad Sci USA 72:994, 1975.
29. Rosenberg S, Stracher A, Detwiler TC, Lucas RC: Fed Proc 37:1790, 1978.
30. Rosenblith JZ, Ukena TE, Yin HH, Berlin RD, Karnovsky MJ: Proc Natl Acad Sci USA 70:1625, 1973.
31. Schreiner GF, Unanue ER: Adv İmmunol 24:37, 1976.
32. Sela B, Lis H, Sharon N, Sachs L: Biochim Biophys Acta 249:564, 1971.
33. Sheetz MP, Singer SJ: J Cell Biol 73:638, 1977.
34. Shinitzky M, Inbar M: J Mol Biol 85:603, 1974.
35. Singer SJ: Adv Immunol 19:1, 1974.
36. Singer SJ, Nicolson GL: Science 175:720, 1972.
37. Singer SJ, Ash JF, Bourguignon LYW, Heggeness MH, Louvard D: J Supramol Struct 9:373, 1978.
38. Stadtman ER, Chock PB: Curr Topics Cell Regul 13:53, 1978.
39. Stéhelin D, Graf T: Cell 13:745, 1978.
40. Stéhelin D, Varmus HE, Bishop JM, Vogt PK: Nature 260:170, 1976.
41. Stone KR, Smith RE, Joklik WK: Virology 58:86, 1974.

42. Wallach D, Davies PJA, Pastan I: J Biol Chem 253:3328, 1978.
43. Wang K, Singer SJ: Proc Natl Acad Sci USA 74:2021, 1977.
44. Wang K, Ash JF, Singer SJ: Proc Natl Acad Sci USA 72:4483, 1975.
45. Wang LH, Duesberg PH, Kawai S, Hanafusa H: Proc Natl Acad Sci USA 73:447, 1976.
46. Wickus G, Branton P, Robbins PW: In Clarkson B, Beserga R (eds): "Cold Spring Harbor Conference on Control of Proliferation in Animal Cells." Cold Spring Harbor, New York: Cold Spring Harbor Laboratory, 1974, p 541.
47. Yamada KM, Weston JA: Proc Natl Acad Sci USA 71:3492, 1974.
48. Yamaguchi N, Weinstein IB: Proc Natl Acad Sci USA 72:214, 1975.

Plasminogen Activator and the Membrane of Transformed Cells

James P. Quigley, Ronald H. Goldfarb, Clifford Scheiner, Jill O'Donnell-Tormey, and Tet Kin Yeo

Department of Microbiology and Immunology (J.P.Q., R.H.G., C.S.), and Department of Cell Biology (J.P.Q., J.O'D-T.,T.K.Y.), SUNY — Downstate Medical Center, Brooklyn

Studies have been conducted on the enzyme plasminogen activator (PA) in cultures of RSV transformed CEF. The enzyme exists in two forms, a soluble extracellular form (PA_{ex}) and a cell-associated form that is firmly bound to specific membranes (PA_{mem}) when cell homogenates are subfractionated. Both forms of the enzyme are induced in a synergistic fashion by treatment of RSVCEF with the tumor promoter phorbol myristate acetate (PMA). The induction of the enzyme by PMA has allowed for the purification of PA_{ex}. In addition, PMA treatment of RSVCEF causes pronounced morphological alterations in culture. The use of protease inhibitors, [³H] -DFP, and a direct fluorometric assay for PA indicate that the morphological changes are due to the direct catalytic action of PA, independent of plasminogen, until now its only known natural substrate. Recent experiments suggest that PA_{mem} is responsible for the morphological changes and that residual amounts of LETS protein are lost from the cell surface and substratum coincident with the morphological changes. The possible role of serine proteases in regulatory cellular behavior in transformed or tumor promoter-treated cells is discussed.

Key words: plasminogen activator, proteases, tumor promoters, membranes, LETS, cell surface

A serine protease that is assayed as an activator of plasminogen has been shown to be elevated in primary tumor cells, in cells transformed by oncogenic viruses and in a number of tumorgenic cell lines [see reviews 1–3]. The early appearance of elevated levels of this enzyme has been correlated with malignant transformation in culture through the use of viral mutants that are temperature-sensitive for transformation [4, 5]. Plasminogen activatory (PA) catalytically converts the serum zymogen, plasminogen, to the active protease, plasmin, which in turn has the capacity to degrade fibrin and other protein substrates, including cell surface proteins [6, 7]. Furthermore, plasmin can activate other protease zymogens by highly efficient cascade mechanisms, thereby generating additional proteolytic activity within the cellular microenvironment [2, 8]. A correlative relationship between PA activity plasmin generation, and malignant transformation has been demonstrated in several different laboratories [9–14]. It appears, however, that in some specific cell lines

Ronald H. Goldfarb's present address is Laboratory of Immunodiagnosis, National Cancer Institute, Bethesda, MD 20205.

Received August 27, 1979; accepted October 26, 1979.

and clonal isolates, elevation of PA levels does not always accompany oncogenic transformation [15–17]. Enhanced PA activity in malignant cells is therefore not an absolute rule. Nevertheless, studies with primary transformants such as RSV-infected chick embryo fibroblasts (CEF) have clearly indicated that oncogenic transformation en masse is closely correlated with enhanced levels of PA [4, 5, 18].

PA from cultures of RSV-transformed cells has been shown to be a serine protease of approximately 50,000 daltons with an apparent catalytic specificity toward specific arginine residues [19, 20]. Other molecular weight forms of the enzyme exist in different transformed systems, but these molecular weight differences depend on cell type and not the transforming agent [2, 21, 22].

PA is actively released from the cells into the culture medium and exists as a soluble enzyme. The cell-associated form of the enzyme, however, exists in a particulate form and appears to be firmly bound to specific membranes [18]. Defining the relationship between the extracellular, soluble form of the enzyme and the cell-associated, particulate form will require detailed studies on the purified forms of the enzyme and antibodies directed against them. Studies on purified PA from cultured cells and antibodies to PA, however, have been described for only a few cases [23, 24] because of the limited amount of actual enzyme in culture supernatants, the problems encountered in purifying small quantities of self-digesting proteolytic enzymes, and the difficulties in obtaining high-titer antibody against proteases. Detailed knowledge of the biochemistry of the PAs from transformed cells awaits the solutions to these problems.

Some normal cells also synthesize and secrete PA. In many cases, it appears that the production of the enzyme fluctuates with the physiological developmental or hormonal state of the cells [25–27]. The expression of PA in both normal cells and malignant cells can be modulated by a variety of compounds, including steroid hormones, cyclic nucleotides, lymphoid products, and growth factors [29–32]. Control of PA expression by these natural products may be related to specialized cellular functions requiring extensive or limited proteolysis at defined times during the life-span of the specific cell.

Phorbol esters are a class of compounds known as tumor promoters that can also modulate PA expression in different cell types [33, 34]. Phorbol myristate acetate (PMA), is a potent inducer of tumor formation in the well-established two-stage carcinogenesis system [35, 36]. PA activity in normal CEF can be induced 10-fold by low concentrations of PMA [33]. More recent studies have shown that PMA synergistically enhances the elevated levels of PA in the already transformed RSVCEF [37]. Thus the PA level of RSVCEF, which is 40–100-fold greater than that of CEF, can be elevated further (up to 1,000 fold) by continuous treatment of RSVCEF cultures with nanogram quantities of PMA [37]. It has not yet been determined whether this induction of proteolytic activity is involved in the mechanism of tumor promotion by phorbol esters. The finding that protease inhibitors suppress in vivo tumor formation when added in conjunction with PMA in the two-stage carcinogenesis system [38, 39] suggests, however, that specific proteolytic enzymes, possibly PA, may indeed be involved in tumor initiation or formation.

Work in our laboratory has focused on the response of RSVCEF cultures to PMA, and the resulting modulation of both cell-associated PA and extracellular PA in the treated cells. We have demonstrated [37] that RSVCEF cultures, maintained in PMA-containing serum-free medium, secrete high levels of PA for up to four days. This effect is observed with only viable, intact cells and is suppressed by inhibitors of macromolecular synthesis. The PA induced by PMA is identical in molecular weight and catalytic specificity to the

PA produced by the untreated RSVCEF. It has therefore been possible to obtain PA-enriched culture fluid from PMA-treated RSVCEF cultures for the purification of PA (R.H. Goldfarb and J.P. Quigley, manuscript submitted).

PMA-treated RSVCEF cultures also exhibit pronounced morphological changes not observed in PMA-treated normal CEF cultures [40]. The cells become clustered and dense cellular aggregates are formed. We have now demonstrated that the formation of the clustered aggregates is a result of the high levels of PA activity in the cultures [40]. The protease-mediated morphological changes, however, are not due to generation of plasmin from plasminogen, even though plasminogen is the only known natural substrate of PA. The results indicate that direct catalytic activity of PA itself is responsible for protein alterations that mediate the morphological changes. In addition, recent experiments suggest that the membrane-associated form of PA is responsible for the morphological alterations and that residual amounts of a 250,000 dalton protein is lost from both the cell surface and cell substratum during the protease-mediated alterations.

MATERIALS AND METHODS

Cell Culture

Cultures of fibroblasts from 11-day-old chick embryos (CEF) and their viral transformants (RSVCEF) were prepared, infected, and maintained as described previously [18, 37]. Eagle's minimal essential medium (MEM) supplemented with 10% fetal bovine serum (FBS) was used throughout unless otherwise noted. All experiments were performed only on second, third, or fourth passage cultures of CEF or RSVCEF.

Membrane Isolation

Subcellular fractionation of RSVCEF cell homogenates and the measurement of marker activities was performed as described previously [18]. The B band membrane fraction was removed from the sucrose gradient at the 20–40% interface [18], washed 1 time by high-speed centrifugation, resuspended in homogenizing medium, frozen, and subsequently used as the source of PA and for all membrane treatment experiments.

Plasminogen Activator (PA) Measurements

The preparation of plasminogen, plasminogen-depleted serum, and fibrinogen, as well as the assay procedure for plasminogen activator (PA) using ^{125}I-labeled, fibrin-coated Linbro wells, was performed as previously described [18, 37]. The direct measurement of PA using a fluorescent substrate (Z-gly-gly-arg-AMC) and a recording spectrofluorometer was carried out as previously described [20].

PMA Treatment of Cells

Procedures for treatment of cultures with PMA, measurement of extracellular and cell-associated PA from PMA-treated cultures, and morphological characterization of the cultures have been described previously [37].

Protease Inhibitor Studies

The addition of protease inhibitors to cell cultures and enzyme assay systems, as well as the concentrations employed, was as described previously [40].

Measurement of Serine Enzymes by [^{3}H]-DFP Labeling and Gel Electrophoresis

Labeling of culture fluid with [^{3}H]-DFP in the presence or absence of protease inhibitors and analysis of the labeled enzymes by SDS-polyacrylamide gel electrophoresis and fluorography were as described previously [40] and will be described in detail elsewhere (C.J. Scheiner and J.P. Quigley, manuscript in preparation).

Analysis of PA activity on SDS-polyacrylamide gels was as described previously [37].

Lactoperoxidase (LPO) Catalyzed Iodination of Cells and Substratum

Cultures were washed one time with PBS and incubated with 1 ml of PBS + 200 μCi/ml of carrier-free Na^{125}I + 20 μg of LPO. 10 μl of dilute H$_2$O$_2$ (18 μl of 30% H$_2$O$_2$ in 100 ml of PBS) was added every 20 sec to a total of 100 μl. After 15 min of incubation at 22°C, 3 ml of PBS was added, and the cells were scraped from the dishes and washed by centrifugation 3 times. The washed cell pellet was dissolved in gel sample buffer. The substratum was prepared by adding 1% SDS and sample buffer to the cell-denuded dishes.

Materials

The initial stock of PMA was a gift of Dr. W. Troll. Subsequently PMA has been purchased from Dr. P. Borchert (University of Minnesota). Leupeptin, antipain, chymostatin, and elastatinal were gifts of Dr. W. Troll and the Japanese-American Cancer Program. Diisopropylfluorophosphate (DFP), p-nitrophenylguanidobenzoate (NPGB), hirudin, soybean trypsin inhibitor (SBTI), and N-α-tosyl-L-lysyl-chloromethane (TLCK) were purchased from Sigma. Benzamidine and ϵ-aminocaproic acid (ϵACA) were purchased from Aldrich Chemical. Human plasmin was a gift from Dr. J. Fenton. Trypsin and chymotrypsin were purchased from Worthington Biochemical. Trasylol was a gift from Dr. M. Mosesson. Na^{125} iodide was purchased from New England Nuclear, and [^{3}H]-DFP was from Amersham. Sera were obtained from both Grand Island Biological and Flow Laboratories, and tissue culture plasticware was obtained from Falcon.

RESULTS

Membrane-Associated PA

Plasminogen activator (PA) exists in two forms; a soluble, extracellular form that is released into cell culture medium and a cellular form that is associated with particulate material [18, 19]. The subcellular distribution of the cell-associated form of PA from cultures of RSVCEF has been examined using differential centrifugation and sucrose gradient centrifugation. The activities and the percent distribution of a series of marker enzymes specific for different subcellular organelles were compared to that of PA in the different fractions isolated by the subfractionation procedures [18]. The results of the study are summarized in Table I.

Greater than 80% of the cell-associated form of PA is located in a postnuclear fraction that sediments at 100,000g (membrane + granule fraction, Table I). Further fractionation of this material by sucrose gradient centrifugation demonstrates that the majority of cell-associated PA can be isolated in a membrane fraction that contains less than 10% of the total cellular protein (fraction B, Table I). This fraction contains the majority of the plasma membrane marker Na$^+$-K$^+$ ATPase. In addition, this fraction contained the bulk of the enzyme 5$^\prime$nucleotidase and tritium-labeled fucose, but little or no nuclear and cytoplasmic material, and was contaminated only to a small degree with mitochondria, rough

TABLE I. Subcellular Distribution of Plasminogen Activator in Virus Transformed Cells

		% Protein	% PA	% Na^+-K^+ ATPase
I. Differential centrifugation	Homogenate	100	100	100
	Crude nuclear fraction	10	8	14
	Membrane + granule fraction	31	83	85
	Soluble cytoplasmic fraction	58	9	1
II. Sucrose gradient centrifugation	A band	3	4	13
	B band	8	61	51
	C band	7	12	15
	D band	2	3	3
	Soluble released	11	3	2

Cultures of RSVCEF were washed 2 times with medium, and the cells were scraped from the culture dishes and washed 2 times by centrifugation. A cell homogenate was prepared by breaking cells in a Dounce homogenizer in 0.25 M sucrose-0.01 M Tris-0.001 M EDTA, pH 7.4. Cell fractions were prepared by differential centrifugation as described previously [18]. The membrane and granule fraction was further subfractionated by layering it on a preformed discontinuous sucrose gradient containing equal volumns of 60%, 40%, and 20% sucrose and centrifuging it at 100,000g for 3 h. Material was collected from the gradient and analyzed for protein and a number of enzymes as described [18].

endoplasmic reticulum, and lysosomes [18]. The appearance of this fraction in the electron microscope, its buoyant density, and the relatively high specific activities of Na^+-K^+ ATPase, [^{3}H] fucose, and 5'-nucleotidase indicate that the fraction is enriched in surface membrane [18].

Further purification of fraction B by equilibrium centrifugation on a shallow sucrose gradient reduces further the lysosomal contaminating activities and results in a PA distribution that closely parallels the distribution of the membrane enzyme, 5'-nucleotidase (Fig. 1). Thus it appears that cellular PA is isolated and closely associated with smooth, plasma membrane-like elements of the transformed cell.

In order to examine the nature of the association of PA with membranes, fraction B was subjected to a number of physical and chemical treatments and then centrifuged at 100,000g for one hour. The distribution of PA and other marker enzymes in the resulting supernatant and pellet was monitored. Table II indicates that after vigorous sonication or hypotonic extraction in the presence of the chelating agent EDTA, PA activity remains sedimentable and rebands in a sucrose gradient at approximately its original density. The plasma membrane marker, 5'-nucleotidase, behaves similarly under the same conditions. The small amount of the lysosomal enzyme β-D-glucosaminidase which contaminates fraction B, serves as internal control for the behavior of granule-enclosed enzymes following such treatments. Table II demonstrates that the two procedures result in a substantial solubilization of the β-D-glucosaminidase activity, indicating that granule-enclosed enzymes can be released by these treatments. The sedimentation, however, of 80–90% of the PA activity following these treatments, and its subsequent rebanding on a sucrose gradient, indicate that PA, as isolated, is not enclosed within membrane granules but is firmly associated with membrane components.

In order to further examine the nature of PA's association with cellular membrane, fraction B was treated with 2 M salt solutions of the chaotropic series, centrifuged, and analyzed for any solubilization of PA activity. The chaotropic series of salt solutions can be arranged in relative hydrophobic disrupting ability [41] and therefore give an indication

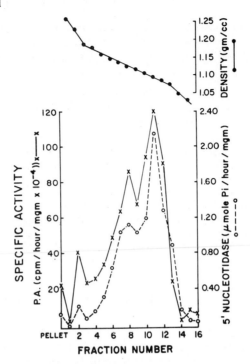

Fig. 1. Equilibrium centrifugation of fraction B on a continuous sucrose gradient. Fraction B (3.1 mg protein) was layered on a continuous 20–45% sucrose gradient, preformed on a 60% sucrose cushion. The gradient was centrifuged at 40,000 rpm for 18 h in an SW41 rotor. The gradient was punctured and fractions were analyzed for PA activity and 5'nucleotidase activity. The refractive index of each fraction was determined and the density was calculated for a standard curve.

TABLE II. Distribution of PA and Membrane and Granule-Associated Enzymes in a High-Speed Supernate and Pellet After Various Treatments and Extractions of Fraction B*

Treatment	Fraction	Distribution (%)		
		PA	5'-Nucleotidase	β-D-glucosaminidase
Control-homogenizing medium	Pellet	90	91	83
	Supernate	10	9	17
Sonication in homogenizing medium	Pellet[a]	81	83	34
	Supernate	19	17	66
Extraction in 0.001 M EDTA	Pellet	85	87	57
	Supernate	15	13	43

*Fraction B was divided into aliquots. One aliquot was diluted with homogenizing medium and served as a control. Another aliquot was diluted with homogenizing medium and was sonicated three times for 10 sec each time. A third aliquot was diluted with distilled water containing 1 mM EDTA and homogenized in a Dounce homogenizer. All three samples were centrifuged at 50,000 rpm for 1 h in a SW50.1 rotor. The resulting pellets and supernatants were analyzed for the indicated enzymes as described [18].

[a] Pellet was rebanded on a discontinuous sucrose gradient, and 87% of the PA activity and 81% of the 5'-nucleotidase activity were recovered at the sucrose interface corresponding to the position of the original B band.

of the forces that maintain PA's associations with membranes. Figure 2 shows the results of these experiments and indicates that treatment with simple 2 M salt solutions, such as KCl, does not release PA from its membrane association. Only those salts that have high hydrophobic disrupting ability bring about solubilization of PA. The close correlation of PA solubilization from membranes with the hydrophobic disrupting ability of the chaotropic salts indicates that PA is not bound to membranes by just simple electrostatic means, but is tightly associated with the membranes.

Unanswered Questions Concerning the Membrane-Associated PA and Extracellular PA — Need for a Purified Molecule

The previous experiments establishing the firm association of PA with specific membranes of the transformed cell raises some fundamental questions concerning the nature of PA, the control of PA production and release, and the role of PA in malignant transformation. Although the above-described studies indicate that PA, as isolated, is tightly associated with plasma membrane-like elements of the cell, the exact membrane location of PA remains unanswered. The chemical relationship of the membrane associated form of PA (PA_{mem}) with the soluble, extracellular form of PA (PA_{ex}) and the biochemical mechanism whereby PA_{mem} is processed for release into the extracellular milieu are also unknown. In addition, the possible existence of an inactive PA zymogen and the control of PA biosynthesis in the normal and transformed cell also remain unknown. Finally, although enhanced PA synthesis in RSV-transformed cultures is well established [5, 18, 19], the exact role of PA in the manifestation of the transformed phenotype, and whether PA_{mem} or PA_{ex} or both play a major part in this role, remain as unanswered questions.

It appeared to us that any experimental approach that might be successfully used in answering these questions would have to involve a purified form of PA and a monospecific antibody made against the purified PA. Purification of PA from RSVCEF cultures how-

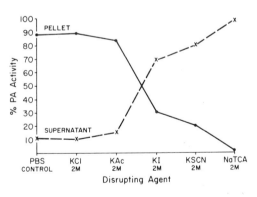

Fig. 2. Isolation of high-speed supernatant and pellet following disruption of B band membranes in 2 M salt. Fraction B was divided into 6 aliquots. An aliquot was diluted in PBS (phosphate buffered saline) and served as control. Five other aliquots were brought to 2 M salt concentration with stock solutions of the chaotropic series of salts. Each of the samples was mixed, incubated at room temperature for 15 min, and centrifuged at 40,000 rpm for 1 h. The resulting supernatant and pellet from each sample were analyzed for PA activity.

ever, would be a logistically difficult task. Although PA activity in RSVCEF cultures is 40–100-fold higher than in normal CEF cultures, it has been estimated that the actual amount of PA secreted over 8–12 hours into RSVCEF culture supernatant is only 1 ng/ml [19]. Therefore, extremely large amounts of culture fluid (500–1,000 liters) would have to be accumulated in order to even begin purification attempts. The accumulation of such large amounts of culture supernatant would also take considerable time. This logistical block to purification of RSVCEF PA, however, has been circumvented by the use of a tumor promoter.

Phorbol Myristate Acetate and Its Effect on PA Activity

PMA is a potent inducer of tumor formation in the well-established two-stage carcinogenesis system [35, 36]. Although the mechanism of tumor promotion by PMA is unknown, it has been shown that protease inhibitors suppress tumor formation when added in conjunction with PMA in the 2-stage carcinogenesis experimental system [38, 39], suggesting a role for proteolytic enzymes in tumor promotion. Wigler and Weinstein [33] have demonstrated that PA activity in normal CEF can be induced 10-fold by low concentrations of PMA. We have recently confirmed this important finding and have also demonstrated that PMA synergistically enhances the elevated levels of PA in the already transformed RSVCEF [37]. These findings are summarized in Figure 3. The pronounced synergistic effect of PMA on the transformed cultures has been examined in detail [37]. PMA was effective in inducing both PA_{mem} and PA_{ex} activity at concentrations as low as

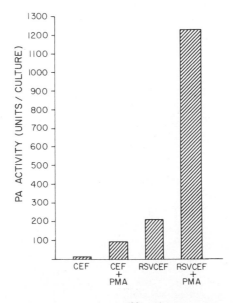

Fig. 3. Effect of PMA on the production of PA_{ex} activity in cultures of CEF and RSVCEF. Parallel cultures of CEF and RSVCEF, pregrown for 2 days in plasminogen-free fetal bovine serum, were washed and incubated in 5 ml of serum-free MEM in the presence and absence of PMA (100 ng/ml). After 20 h of incubation, the culture fluid was removed and centrifuged to remove cells, and the supernatant was acidified to pH 3.5. to stabilize PA. PA activity in the acidified supernatant was determined using the ^{125}I-fibrin plate assay. Cell number per 10 cm tissue culture dish was 6.5×10^6 for CEF, 7.6×10^6 for CEF + PMA, 8.1×10^6 for RSVCEF, and 8.9×10^6 for RSVCEF + PMA.

1 ng/ml (1.7×10^{-9}M) and was maximally effective between 25 and 100 ng/ml. The induction of PA_{mem} could be detected as early as 1 hour after PMA treatment, followed by an increase in PA_{ex} between 2 and 4 hours. The induction of both forms of PA was sensitive to cycloheximide, indicating that new protein synthesis was required. Analysis by SDS-polyacrylamide gel electrophoresis (Fig. 4) demonstrated that the PA that was induced by PMA was identical in molecular weight with that of PA produced by untreated RSVCEF cultures.

The latter experiment indicated that the PMA-treated cultures could be used as source material for the purification of RSVCEF PA. Harvesting conditions have been developed that represent new modifications for obtaining enhanced yields of PA-enriched culture supernatants [37]. The modifications included 1) initial growth of the cultures in plasminogen-free serum to eliminate plasminogen/plasmin contamination; and 2) after confluence, keeping the cultures in serum-free, PMA-containing medium and harvesting them two times a day for up to 3–5 days in order to eliminate serum contaminants in the culture supernatants. An analysis of 6 separate harvesting experiments is summerized in Table III. It can be seen that after three days of harvesting and PMA treatment, the PA activity of the culture supernatants is 20-fold higher than the untreated RSVCEF cultures

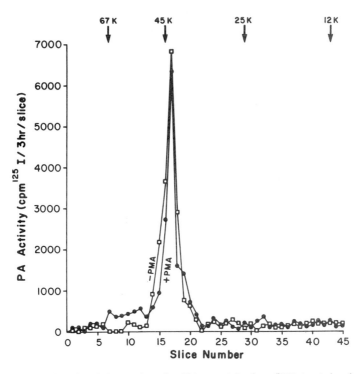

Fig. 4. SDS-polyacrylamide gel electrophoresis of PA_{ex} activity from PMA-treated and nontreated cultures of RSVCEF. Five units of concentrated PA_{ex} from PMA-treated (●——●) and nontreated (□——□) companion cultures of RSVCEF was subjected to electrophoresis in adjacent lines of a slab gel. The gels were sliced and assayed for PA activity as previously described [37]. Molecular weight standards were run on the same slab gel, and their positions are indicated by arrows at the top of the figure. Recovery of PA activity from the gels was 78% and 74%, respectively.

TABLE III. Secretion of PA From Serum-Free Cultures of PMA-Treated RSVCEF*

Culture conditions[a]	Extracellular PA activity (units/culture)
CEF (untreated)	0.9 (0–1.2) [b]
RSVCEF (untreated)	51 (29–58)
RSVCEF (PMA-treated)	
Day 1	
a	346 (256–525)
b	524 (367–589)
Day 2	
a	538 (437–746)
b	860 (799–1,268)
Day 3	
a	724 (625–959)
b	1,057 (820–1,273)
Day 4	
a	1,059 (907–1,208)
b	910 (804–1,112)
Day 5	
a	815 (597–959)

*Cell cultures were incubated for 12 h in MEM supplemented with plasminogen-depleted fetal calf serum (5%), with or without PMA (100 ng/ml). The cultures were then washed 2 times with PBS and 1 time with MEM and were incubated in serum-free MEM with or without PMA. After 12 h, the culture supernatants were removed, centrifuged, acidified, and assayed for PA activity. The RSVCEF cultures that had been treated with PMA were further incubated in fresh MEM containing PMA and were harvested twice a day for 5 days. The culture medium was replaced each time with MEM containing PMA.
[a]The a and b designations refer to morning and evening harvestings; the duration between harvestings varied between 8 and 14 h.
[b]The values represent the average of 6 separate experiments, for which the range of activities is given in parentheses.

and 1,000-fold higher than untreated normal CEF cultures. These advances have shortened considerably the time required to accumulate sufficient quantities of crude PA for purification.

A method for purifying the enzyme from these PA-enriched supernatants, employing affinity ligands, ion-exchange chromatography, and molecular sieving chromatography has now been established. The results of such a study will be reported in a separate communication (R.H. Goldfarb and J.P. Quigley, manuscript submitted).

Effects of PMA on the Morphology of RSVCEF Cultures

During the harvesting of PA-enriched culture supernatants from the serum-free cultures of RSVCEF, distinct morphological alterations in the cultures occurred [37, 40]. Figure 5 illustrates these morphological changes. Following initial treatment with PMA (100 ng/ml), RSVCEF cultures undergo cellular elongation, followed by cell clustering in which cell–cell adhesion appears to be enhanced (Fig. 5B). Continued incubation with PMA results in the formation of colonial-like aggregates of cells (Fig. 5C), and networks of these aggregates are present throughout the entire dish (Fig. 5D). This pattern of

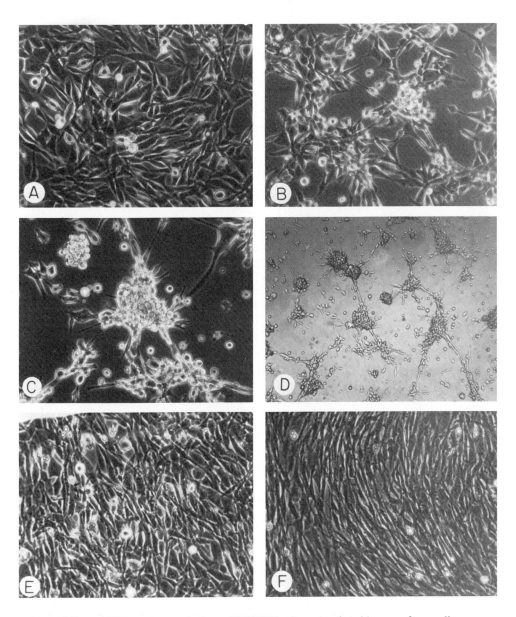

Fig. 5. Effect of PMA on the morphology of RSVCEF cultures incubated in serum-free medium. Culture conditions and treatment with PMA were as described in Figure 3. (A) initial cultures of RSVCEF; (B) RSVCEF after 6 h of PMA treatment; (C) RSVCEF after 23 h of PMA treatment; (D) same as C, except that magnification is 33 ×; (E) RSVCEF after 23 h in the absence of PMA; (F) CEF cultures after 23 h of PMA treatment. Magnification of D 33 ×; all others, 117 ×.

morphological alterations is not observed in transformed cultures incubated in serum-free medium without PMA (Fig. 5E) or in normal cultures incubated with PMA (Fig. 5F), although cellular elongation does take place in PMA-treated normal cultures.

The cells in the clustered aggregates are viable as determined by both trypan blue dye exclusion and the ability of the cells to grow when the clusters are passaged and plated in serum-supplemented media [40]. The cells in the clusters are also metabolically active, since they synthesize and secrete relatively large amounts of PA, as the peak of PA activity in the cultures correlates with the time of maximum clustering.

Effect of Protease Inhibitors on PMA-Induced Morphological Changes

During the harvesting of PA-enriched culture supernatants from PMA-treated cultures a number of different RSV strains and stocks were employed, and it was observed that the higher the PA levels of the starting RSV-transformed cultures, the more rapid were the morphological changes. Since these morphological alterations are also reminiscent of changes in culture that occur when CEF are treated with exogenous serine proteases (J.P. Quigley, unpublished observations), it was of interest to determine whether the observed morphology was a direct result of the enhanced, endogenous protease activity in the PMA-treated cultures.

Several specific protease inhibitors were added to RSVCEF cultures at the time of PMA-addition. The effect of this treatment on the morphological arrangement of the cultured cells was determined at 25 h and is shown in Figure 6. The RSVCEF cultures treated with PMA display the above-described distinct morphological changes (Fig. 6b) when compared with untreated RSVCEF cultures (Fig. 6a). The PMA-induced formation of cell clusters and dense cellular aggregates is prevented by specific protease inhibitors, including DFP, the active site inhibitor of serine enzymes (Fig. 6c); NPGB, an ester that is an active site titrant of specific serine enzymes (Fig. 6e); benzamidine, an arginine analog (Fig. 6g); and leupeptin an arginine-containing peptide aldehyde (Fig. 6i). Other protease inhibitors, however, fail to inhibit the PMA-induced morphological changes; these include trasylol, an inhibitor of plasmin (Fig. 6d), and ϵACA, a lysine analog (Fig. 6f). Soybean trypsin inhibitor (SBTI), a general inhibitor of trypsin-like enzymes, and antipain, a peptide aldehyde with a different structure than leupeptin [42], partially inhibit cell cluster formation (Fig. 6h and 6j).

More extensive protease inhibitor experiments are summarized in Table IV. The data confirm the morphological studies illustrated in Figure 6 and extend the list of effective and ineffective protease inhibitors. Leupeptin, DFP, NPGB, and benzamidine inhibit the morphological changes at the indicated concentrations. In addition to ϵACA and trasylol, chymostatin, and inhibitor of chymotrypsin-like enzymes, elastatinal, an inhibitor of elastase-like enzymes, and hirudin, a specific inhibitor of thrombin, also have no inhibitory action on the PMA-induced changes. Antipain has some inhibitory capacity and TLCK at 200 μM partially inhibits the morphological changes, but this is due to the toxic effects of TLCK at this concentration. If the concentration of TLCK is reduced to 50 μM, no inhibition of morphology occurs (Table IV). SBTI shows a graded response, low concentrations fail to inhibit, while the morphological changes are inhibited at relatively high SBTI concentrations.

It should be noted that none of the inhibitors prevent PMA-induced cellular elongation (Table IV), an early alteration observed in PMA-treated cultures. The subsequent alterations in morphology are the most sensitive to protease inhibitors. The data therefore

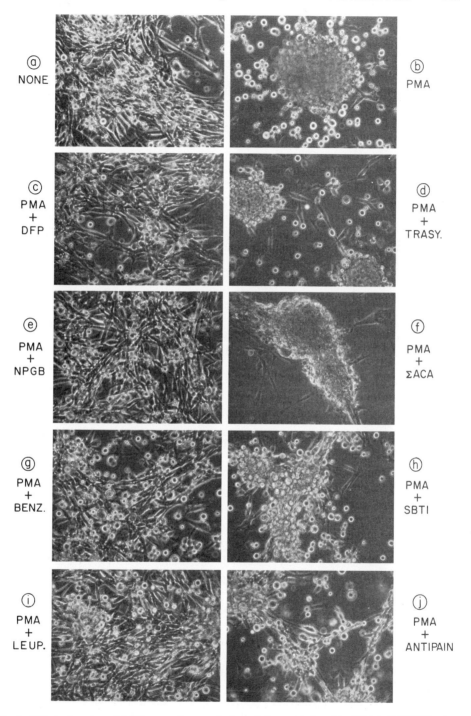

Fig. 6. Effect of protease inhibitors on the morphological changes induced by PMA in RSVCEF cultures. Culture conditions were as described in Figure 1. RSVCEF cultures in serum-free medium were either left untreated (a), treated with PMA alone (b), or treated with PMA plus the indicated inhibitor (c–j). Photographs were taken after 25 h. The concentrations of inhibitors were as follows: DFP, 4×10^{-4} M; trasylol, 20 U/ml; NPGB, 1×10^{-5} M; ϵACA, 2×10^{-3} M; benzamidine, 2×10^{-3} M; SBTI, 10 μg/ml; leupeptin, 5×10^{-4} M; antipain, 5×10^{-4} M.

TABLE IV. Effect of Protease Inhibitors on PMA-Induced Morphological Changes in Cultures of RSVCEF*

Addition to culture		Morphological changes	
		Elongation	Clustering
None		−	−
PMA (100 ng/ml)		+	+++/++++
PMA + leupeptin	$(5 \times 10^{-4}M)$	+	−
PMA + DFP	$(4 \times 10^{-4}M)$	+	−/+
PMA + NPGB	$(1 \times 10^{-5}M)$	+	−
PMA + benzamidine	$(2 \times 10^{-3}M)$	+	−/+
PMA + ϵACA	$(1 \times 10^{-2}M)$	+	+++
PMA + trasylol	(100 U/ml)	+	++++
PMA + chymostatin	$(5 \times 10^{-4}M)$	+	++++
PMA + elastatinal	$(5 \times 10^{-4}M)$	+	++++
PMA + hirudin	(10 U/ml)	+	+++
PMA + antipain	$(5 \times 10^{-4}M)$	+	+/++
PMA + TLCK	$(5 \times 10^{-5}M)$	+	++++
PMA + TLCK	$(2 \times 10^{-4}M)$	+	++
PMA + SBTI	$(1-5 \mu g/ml)$	+	+++
PMA + SBTI	$(5-20 \mu g/ml)$	+	++
PMA + SBTI	$(20-100 \mu g/ml)$	+	−/+

*Cultures of RSVCEF, pregrown in medium containing plasminogen-depleted serum, were washed and incubated in medium plus the indicated additions. After 8 h, the cultures were scored for elongated cells, and after 24 h, the cultures were scored for the appearance of cell clusters or dense aggregates. Scoring of (−) through (++++) is based on the extent of cell cluster formation. The results represent a composite of 4 separate experiments.

suggest that a serine protease (DFP-sensitive) is responsible for the clustered morphology elicited by treatment of transformed cultures with PMA. The results also suggest that this serine enzyme is sensitive to NPGB and the arginine analogs benzamidine and leupeptin, but relatively insensitive to the lysine analogs ϵACA and TLCK and also insensitive to inhibitors of plasmin, trypsin, chymotrypsin and thrombin.

Evidence that the inhibition of PMA-induced morphological changes by the specific protease inhibitors is not due to relative toxicity of the compounds is indicated by viability of the cells (trypan blue exclusion) cell growth studies, and macromolecular synthesis experiments in the presence and absence of the protease inhibitors. Further evidence that the inhibitory effect of these specific compounds is due to their protease inhibitory potential and not their relative toxicity is presented elsewhere [40].

Effect of Protease Inhibitors on the Direct Catalytic Activity of PA.

Since PA is elevated in PMA-treated cultures and is a serine protease with arginine specificity [19], it could be responsible for proteolytic changes that mediate the observed morphological alterations in culture. Although a substrate for PA other than plasminogen has not been previously described, there was no reason to assume that a protease such as PA has a single substrate. It was therefore conceivable that cellular or extracellular proteins are cleaved directly by PA, resulting in the morphological changes. To examine this possibility, it was necessary to test the inhibitors used in the morphological study for their effect on the direct catalytic activity of PA. This posed a difficult problem, since the

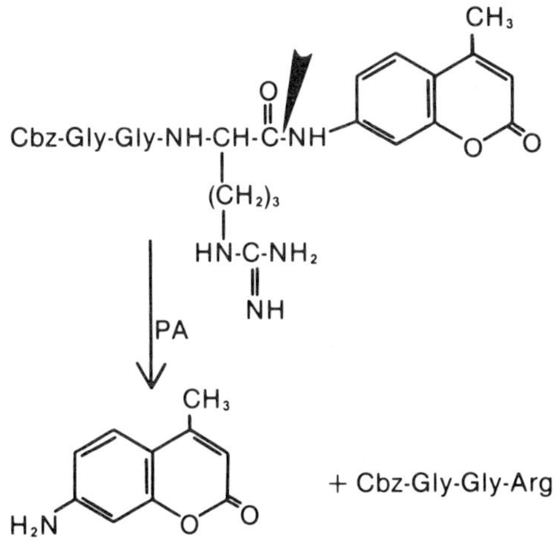

	Maxima (nm)	
	Excitation	Emission

A. Substrate Cbz-Gly-Gly-NH-CH-C-NH ... 325   395

B. Product ... + Cbz-Gly-Gly-Arg   345   445

C. Optimum difference for assay purposes   383   455

Fig. 7. Structure and fluorescence properties of substituted 4-methylcoumarins. The amide bond (arrow), resembling a peptide bond, is cleaved by proteases with arginine specificity, such as PA, resulting in the release of a highly fluorescent product, AMC. The presence of the gly-gly in the tripeptide moiety adds to the specificity of the substrate.

standard assay for PA is an indirect two-step procedure involving the conversion of plasminogen to plasmin and the subsequent measurement of plasmin-mediated fibrinolysis. The presence of more than one protease (PA and plasmin) in the two-step assay would preclude the screening of potential PA inhibitors. However, a direct assay for PA using a fluorescent substrate was developed in collaboration with M. Zimmerman and W. Troll [20]. The substrate is an arginine-containing tripeptide linked by an amide bond to a highly fluorescent leaving group (Fig. 7). The amide bond can be cleaved by PA, resulting in the release of the fluorescent product. Nanogram quantities of PA can be detected by this assay system [20]. Using this substrate, several inhibitors were examined for their effect on the catalytic activity of PA isolated from PMA-treated RSVCEF cultures. The results are shown in Figure 8. Leupeptin, NPGB, DFP, and benzamidine all inhibit PA activity at concentrations consistent with their inhibitory effect on cell morphology. Trasylol and ϵACA, which have no effect on morphology, do not inhibit PA activity, but do inhibit plasmin activity. Hirudin and TLCK, inhibitors of thrombin and trypsin, respectively, have no effect on PA activity or on morphology. SBTI has little effect on PA activity between 1 and 5 μg/ml, but does inhibit PA at higher concentrations; this closely parallels the effect of SBTI on morphology (Table IV).

     The effect of protease inhibitors on both the PMA-induced morphological changes and the direct catalytic activity of PA isolated from PMA-treated cultures is summarized in Table V. The results are completely consistent with the notion that PA, independent of plasminogen, catalytically alters the morphology of transformed cells.

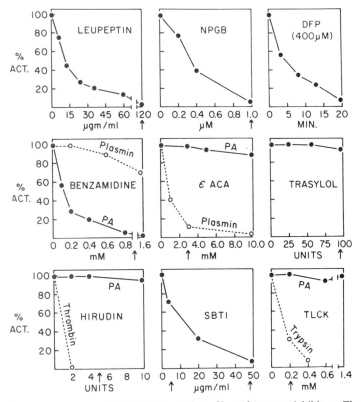

Fig. 8. Direct fluorometric assay of RSVCEF PA activity: effect of protease inhibitors. The cultures were harvested, centrifuged, acidified to pH 3.5 and used as the source of PA activity. The assay procedure was that of Zimmerman et al. [20], using the fluorescent substrate Z-gly-gly-arg-AMC. All fluorometric determinations were performed on a Perkin Elmer 204A spectrofluorometer equipped with a chart recorder. Inhibitors were rapidly mixed with buffer 0.05 M Tris (pH 7.4); substrate (5×10^{-4}M); and 75 μl of culture fluid in a total assay volume of 500 μl. The release of the fluorescent product was measured over a 30 min time span. Thrombin was assayed using the same fluoremetric procedure. Trypsin and plasmin were assayed directly by the release of radiolabeled peptides from ^{125}I-labeled fibrin. (●——●) PA activity; (○——○) activity of the other encymes as indicated. Arrows represent concentrations of inhibitors that were tested in culture and were part of the composite experiments presented in Table IV.

Identification of PA as the Major NPGB-Sensitive TLCK-Insensitive Serine Enzyme in RSVCEF Cultures.

Since DFP, a specific inhibitor of all serine enzymes, is an inhibitor of the morphological changes induced by PMA, it was of interest to determine the number of serine enzymes in the PMA-treated RSVCEF cultures. Culture supernatants were removed from PMA-treated cells at the time of maximum morphological change, preincubated with various protease inhibitors, treated with [³H]-DFP, and analyzed on SDS-polyacrylamide gels. Since DFP covalently labels serine enzymes, autoradiography of the gels allows for the identification of the major DFP-labeled enzymes. An aliquot of the culture supernatant, not treated with inhibitors of [³H]-DFP, was co-electrophoresed in an adjacent lane of the slab gel for parallel determination and identification of PA activity. The results are shown in Figure

TABLE V. Effect of Protease Inhibitors on Morphological Changes and Catalytic Activity of Plasminogen Activator

Inhibitor	Morphological change	PA activity
Leupeptin	Inhibition	Inhibition
DFP	Inhibition	Inhibition
NPGB	Inhibition	Inhibition
Benzamidine	Inhibition	Inhibition
ϵACA	No inhibition	No inhibition
Trasylol	No inhibition	No inhibition
Chymostatin	No inhibition	No inhibition
Elastatinal	No inhibition	No inhibition
Hirudin	No inhibition	No inhibition
SBTI 5 μg/ml	Partial inhibition	Partial inhibition
SBTI 100 μg/ml	Inhibition	Inhibition
TLCK	No inhibition	No inhibition

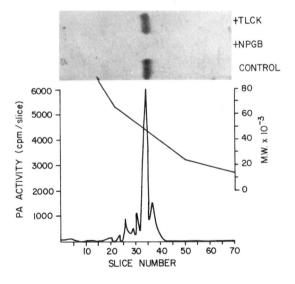

Fig. 9. SDS-polyacrylamide gel electrophoretic analysis of [^{3}H]-DFP-labeled serine enzymes in PMA-treated RSVCEF culture fluids. Equal amounts of culture fluid from PMA-treated RSVCEF were pre-incubated with DMSO (control), NPGB, or TLCK, and then reacted with [H^3]-DFP. Samples were dialyzed, lyopholized, and coelectrophoresed on a 10% slab gel, along with appropriate molecular weight standards and 50 μl of untreated culture fluid. The gel lane containing the untreated culture fluid was excised, washed, sliced and assayed for PA activity. The remainder of the gel was stained, destained, and fluorographed for visualization of [^{3}H]-labeled serine enzymes.

9. The major serine enzyme in the culture supernatant, as determined by autoradiography, is a molecule of approximately 48,000 daltons.* Incorporation of [^{3}H]-DFP into this molecule is prevented by pretreatment of the sample with NPGB but not by pretreatment with TLCK, indicating that the active site of this molecule is sensitive to the former but not the latter inhibitor. PA activity directly coincides with the 48,000 dalton [^{3}H]-DFP-labeled species.

A similar experiment was carried out using membranes from PMA-treated RSVCEF cultures. [^{3}H]-DFP labeling of membranes with and without preincubation with NPGB and TLCK was carried out followed by fluorometric and enzymatic analysis of polyacrylamide gels (results not shown). Fluorometry of the gel indicated that a number of [^{3}H]-DFP-labeled species were present in the RSVCEF membranes. However, only 1 species (a doublet at 48,000 and 51,000 daltons) was both sensitive to NPGB and insensitive to TLCK. The position of this molecular species was coincident with the peak of PA activity as determined by enzymatic analysis of a parallel lane of the polyacrylamide gel, which contained untreated membranes.

These results correlate precisely with previous findings (Table V) which showed that NPGB inhibited both PA activity and morphological changes, while TLCK inhibited neither. The data from polyacrylamide gel analysis, therefore provide further evidence that PA is the DFP-sensitive enzyme responsible for the morphological changes.

PA$_{mem}$ as a Mediator of Cellular Morphological Changes

Although the evidence presented above (Table V, Fig. 9) strongly indicates that PA is the serine enzyme responsible for the PMA-induced morphological changes, none of the experiments indicated which form of the enzyme, PA$_{mem}$ or PA$_{ex}$, was responsible for the alterations. Our initial interpretation was that PMA induced enhanced synthesis and secretion of PA and that when sufficient catalytic quantities of PA$_{ex}$ built up in the culture medium, it enzymatically altered a cell surface or extracellular protein(s), thereby initiating the morphological changes. To test this hypothesis, small coverslips containing RSVCEF cells were placed in tissue culture dishes of varying sizes and incubated in serum-free medium ranging from 1 ml up to 35 ml in the presence or absence of PMA. Release of PA$_{ex}$ from the small amount of cells on the coverslips (approximately 10^5 cells) into a relatively large extracellular volume (1 ml vs 35 ml) would be a sufficient dilution of PA$_{ex}$ to prevent its build-up and subsequent catalytic activity. The morphology of the cells was monitored during the PMA-treatment. The results are illustrated in Figure 10. To our surprise the cells on the coverslips incubated in either 1 ml, 7 ml, or 35 ml of PMA-containing media underwent similar morphological alterations (control coverslips in PMA-free medium did not undergo any changes). The PA$_{ex}$ activity was relatively high in the 1 ml of medium and was barely detectable in the 35 ml of medium, while the cell-associated PA activity was found to be approximately equal when the cells from the experimental coverslips were scraped and assayed (data not shown). These results suggest that it is the enhanced levels of PA$_{mem}$ that is responsible for the morphological changes.

---

*Upon prolonged exposure of the gel to the x-ray film, other minor DFP-labeled species can be detected. These proteins, however, represent either multiple forms of PA, trace levels of serine enzymes that are not sensitive to NPGB, or proteins that have been labeled nonspecifically with [^{3}H]-DFP (C. Scheiner and J.P. Quigley, manuscript in preparation).

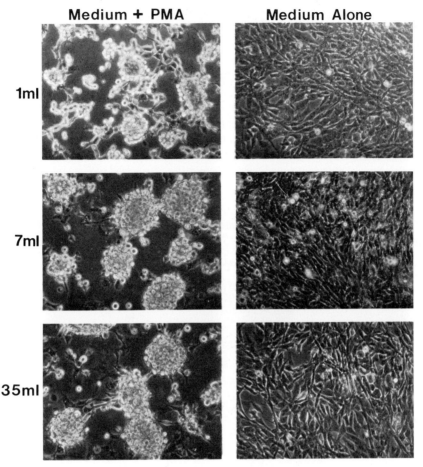

Fig. 10. Morphological observations on coverslips containing RSVCEF incubated in different volumes of medium ± PMA. RSVCEF were grown on coverslips (20 mm) until confluent ($1-2 \times 10^5$ cells). The coverslips were washed 2 times in medium and transferred to Petri dishes of 3.5 cm, 10 cm, and 15 cm diameter. Medium ± PMA was added to the dishes (1 ml, 7 ml or 35 ml, respectively) and then incubated. After 24 h of incubation, photographs were taken (140 × magnification).

Cellular Substratum and Surface Proteins as Substrates for the Direct Catalytic Activity of PA.

The identity of the exact cellular substrate for PA, whose catalytic alteration mediates some or all of the PMA-induced morphological changes is unknown. It was reasonable to assume initially that it was a cell surface or extracellular protein, since the morphological changes appeared to involve cell–cell and/or cell–substratum interaction. Therefore, cultures incubated in medium alone (no clustering), in medium plus PMA (cluster formation), and in medium, plus PMA, plus the protease inhibitor leupeptin (cluster formation prevented), were analyzed for changes in polypeptide pattern by the surface-labeling technique of lactoperoxidase catalyzed iodination. Following iodination, cells were scraped from the culture dish and analyzed by SDS-polyacrylamide gels. The proteins remaining on the cell-denuded culture dish (substratum) were also solubilized in SDS and analyzed by gel electrophoresis. The results of an initial experiment are illustrated in Figure 11. Although preliminary, the data indicate that a polypeptide of approximately 250,000 daltons is reduced on the cell surface following PMA treatment, and this reduction is prevented by leupeptin treatment of the PMA-containing cultures (lanes 1–3). The sensitivity of this protein to PMA treatment and its protection by leupeptin treatment is even more pronounced when substratum proteins are analyzed (lanes 4–6). There may be other polypeptide alterations that occur during the morphological alterations, but more detailed analysis of internal, cell surface, and substratum proteins under a variety of conditions is needed and is now being conducted.

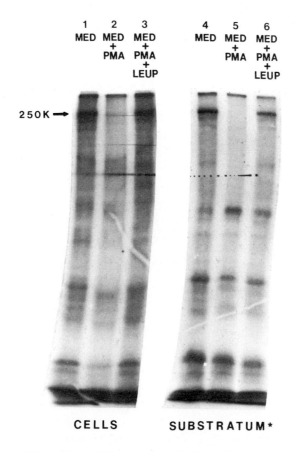

Fig. 11. Analysis of the ^{125}I-labeled surface and substratum proteins from RSVCEF cultures incubated ±PMA ±leupeptin. Cultures of RSVCEF were incubated in medium alone (med.), or in medium + PMA (100 ng/ml) until cell clusters had formed or in medium + PMA + leupeptin (5×10^{-4}M), which prevented cell cluster formation. The cell surface and substratum proteins from the 3 different cultures were labeled with ^{125}I using lactoperoxidase catalyzed iodination as described in Materials and Methods. The samples were electrophoresed on an SDS-7.5% polyacrylamide slab gel along with molecular weight standards and human cold-insoluble globulin (250,000 daltons). The gel was dried and processed for autoradiography.

DISCUSSION

Numerous in vivo and in vitro studies have indicated that proteolytic enzymes are involved in cellular alterations that are related to malignant transformation [3]. The activity of one specific protease, plasminogen activator (PA) has been shown to be elevated in primary tumor cells, cells transformed by both oncogenic virus and chemical carcinogens, and in a number of tumorigenic cell lines [1–3, 9–14]. Although a number of exceptions have been reported [15–17], it appears that an enhanced level of PA often accompanies or precedes malignant transformation. This has been clearly shown in the case of well-characterized Rous sarcoma virus-induced transformation of embryonic fibroblasts, where studies with mutants, temperature-sensitive for malignant transformation, have indicated a direct correlation between transformation and enhanced PA production [4, 5]. For this reason our lab has focused on the RSVCEF culture system for the purpose of chemically defining the biological role for PA in the altered behavior of the transformed cell. Studies from this and other laboratories [3] have already suggested that PA activity and/or the plasmin activity generated by PA may be involved in the altered morphology, migration, growth potential, glycoprotein composition, microfilament pattern, and adhesive properties of malignantly transformed cells. More detailed studies, however, on the molecular and catalytic properties of PA, its location in the cell, and control of its production and release are obviously needed before the enzyme's role is clearly defined.

Although the released, extracellular form of PA exists as a soluble enzyme, the cell-associated form, as isolated, is bound to specific membranes (Table I, Fig. 1). It does not appear to be loosely bound to membranes, since sonication, salt extraction, and chelating agents are unable to release it from its membrane-bound state (Table II). Only hydrophobic disrupting agents are capable of solubilizing it (Fig. 2).

The subcellular fractionation studies presented in Table I and Figure 1, although suggestive, do not prove that PA is a plasma membrane enzyme. They only demonstrate that a majority of the cell–associated PA is isolated in a membrane fraction that is highly enriched in plasma membrane. This fraction has many of the properties of a surface membrane, including a 1.08–1.14 g/cc buoyant density; a smooth appearance in electron micrographs; significant enrichment in [^{3}H]-fucose; and a relatively high specific activity of Na$^+$-K$^+$ ATPase and 5′-nucleotidase. PA is clearly bound to membranes in this fraction. Nevertheless, it is possible that PA is associated with a membrane that is not part of the plasmalemma but is similar to it in its physical and chemical properties and is therefore isolated in the same subcellular fraction. Conversely, cell-associated PA might exist as a soluble enzyme in situ but upon homogenization becomes firmly bound to specific, plasma membrane-like elements of the cell, and is therefore isolated as an apparent membrane enzyme. In situ localization studies on RSVCEF cultures using specific reagents such as monospecific antibodies in combination with temperature shifts from nonpermissive to permissive conditions are needed to resolve these possibilities.

The studies with the tumor promoter, PMA, showing an induction of PA in normal cell culture and a synergistic enhancement of PA in the already transformed cell culture (Fig. 3), give further credence to the notion that PA is a rapidly inducible enzyme, is highly sensitive to cellular perturbations, and because of its catalytic nature, possesses unique regulatory potential. This induction of PA may indeed be related to the mitogenic and growth-promoting ability of PMA shown in other cellular systems [43, 44]. Serine proteases exogenously added to normal cells have clearly demonstrated that these specific enzymes are capable of dramatically altering cellular behavior, therefore the induction of an endogenous serine protease could offer the malignant cell or the tumor promoter-treated cell a distinct phenotypic advantage for unlimited growth and altered cellular behavior. In addition, the suggestion that tumor promoters act in vivo by causing an expanding outgrowth of initiated or premalignant cells [46, 47] is also consistent with protease induction being a distinctly important feature of tumor promotion.

The specific PMA-induced morphological changes observed in the treated RSV-transformed CEF cultures (Fig. 5) in which colonial-like aggregates of viable, actively secreting cells are formed, may or may not be related to the mechanism of tumor-promoting action: but they definitely have allowed for the detection of a new catalytic activity of PA. The morphological changes brought about by PMA can be prevented by protease inhibitors (Fig. 6). Both the nature of the inhibitors and the concentrations used to prevent the morphological changes (Table IV) correlate exactly with the inhibitory pattern of these compounds on PA activity as measured in a direct fluorometric assay (Fig. 8). The pattern of inhibition is *inconsistent* with the possibility that the causative enzyme catalyzing the morphological alterations is plasmin. These studies therefore indicate that PA, present in relatively high concentrations in PMA-treated cultures, can itself act catalytically on a cellular or extracellular protein substrate to bring about these morphological changes independent of plasminogen – until now PA's only known natural substrate.

The evidence that PA itself is responsible for the morphological changes is strengthened by the observation that DFP and NPGB inhibit the changes, whereas TLCK does not (Table V), and that PA is the only detectable NPGB-sensitive, TLCK-insensitive, [^{3}H]-DFP labeled enzyme in the PMA-treated cultures (Fig. 9). Since these results indicate that PA acts catalytically on substrates other than plasminogen, it is no longer possible to rule out the involvement of PA in the manifestation of specific phenotypic properties of transformed cells by simply removing plasminogen from the culture system [48, 49]. The catalytic potential of PA itself will also have to be taken into account.

Although it has not been conclusively shown which form of PA (PA_{mem} or PA_{ex}) in the PMA-treated cultures is responsible for the catalytic induction of the morphological changes, the coverslip experiment described in Figure 10 suggests that PA_{mem} may be the enzyme form responsible. Since a build-up of PA_{ex} is prevented by having a relatively small amount of cells secrete PA_{ex} into a large volume of extracellular medium; and since the morphological change still takes place, it would appear that PA_{mem}, whose specific activity under such conditions remains unchanged, catalytically alters a membrane protein or a protein juxtaposed to the membrane, giving rise to the morphological change. If in fact this proves to be true, then the PA_{mem} is not just a simple transitory or intermediate form of PA with no catalytic potential. It will have to be considered as a potential intrinsic modifier of biological membranes that is enhanced upon malignant transformation or tumor-promoting treatment.

The nature of the protein substrate for PA is also unclear at present. The iodinated protein pattern observed in the experiment described in Figure 11 indicates that a 250,000 dalton protein, possibly the LETS protein, is altered prior to or during the morphological change. It has already been shown by others that the LETS protein is lost from cell surfaces upon malignant transformation of normal CEF [6, 48] or PMA treatment of normal CEF [47]. Indeed, the amount of 250,000 dalton protein present on the transformed cells or substratum (lanes 1 and 4, Fig. 11) represents only 10–30% of that which would be detected in cultures of normal CEF cells (normal cell data not shown).It therefore appears that the residual amount of LETS remaining on RSV-transformed CEF is further diminished upon treatment of the RSVCEF with PMA (lanes 2 and 5, Fig. 11). This almost complete removal of the LETS-like protein is coincident with the PMA- induced morphological change and is prevented by treatment with protease inhibitors (lanes 3 and 6, Fig. 11). It therefore is conceivable that PA itself catalytically removes LETS from the cells and substratum, or PA catalytically cleaves a protein that is itself responsible for the attachment of LETS to the cell surface and substratum. In either case, more detailed studies on the relationship of PA's catalytic specificity with cell surface and substratum protein are now ongoing in the laboratory.

Finally, the synergistic induction of PA by PMA in RSV-transformed cultures has had enormous practical value. The enhancement of the enzyme has allowed for the accumulation of PA-enriched harvest fluid and the purification of the enzyme. Although only $5-20$ μg of the enzyme can be purified from 1 liter of culture fluid, large-scale batch purification procedures have now been designed, and sufficient quantities of PA will soon be available to perform some limited biochemical experiments. These will include determining the mitogenic capacity of RSVCEF PA for normal CEF, the ability of PA to induce morphological changes, the catalytic ability of purified PA to cleave LETS and other membrane proteins, and the effect of purified PA on the biological properties of cultured CEF. In addition, purified PA will be used as an antigen for the eventual production of a specific anti-PA antibody. Such an antibody can be used to determine the precise location of cell-associated PA, the relationship between PA_{mem} and PA_{ex}, the possible existence of PA zymogens, and the control of PA biosynthesis. If it is a catalytic inhibitory antibody, then the role of PA in malignant transformation can be examined directly. Nevertheless, for the present, the sensitivity of RSVCEF cultures to PMA and the newly demonstrated catalytic function for PA, provide a system to examine the role of PA in malignant transformation, PMA in tumor promotion, and serine proteases as modulator of cellular function.

ACKNOWLEDGMENTS

This work was supported in part by grant BC163 from The American Cancer Society and NIH grant CA 16740. The authors acknowledge Ms Gisela Venta-Perez, Ms Marie Towle, and Mr. Angelo Albano for their skilled technical assistance and Ms Roseann Lingeza for her unending patience and skill in preparing this manuscript.

REFERENCES

1. Reich E: In Reich E, Rifkin DB, Shaw E (eds): "Proteases and Biological Control." Cold Spring Harbor New York: Cold Spring Harbor Laboratory, 1975, pp 333–342.
2. Christman JK, Silverstein SC, Acs G: In Barrett AJ (ed): "Proteinases in Mammalian Cells and Tissues." Amsterdam: North-Holland, 1977, pp 90–149.
3. Quigley JP: In Hynes RO (ed): "Surfaces of Normal and Malignant Cells." Chichester: John Wiley & Sons, 1979, pp 247–285.
4. Unkeless JC, Tobia A, Ossowski L, Quigley JP, Rifkin DB, Reich E: J Exp Med 137:85, 1973.
5. Rifkin DB, Beal LP, Reich E: In Reich E, Rifkin DB, Shaw E (eds): "Proteases and Biological Control." Cold Spring Harbor, New York: Cold Spring Harbor Laboratory, 1975, pp 841–847.
6. Hynes RO: Proc Natl Acad Sci USA 11:3170, 1973.
7. Blumberg PM, Robbins PW: Cell 6:137, 1975.
8. Neurath H, Walsh K: Proc Natl Acad Sci USA 73:3825, 1976.
9. Ossowski L, Quigley JP, Kellerman GM, Reich E: J Exp Med 138:1056, 1973.
10. Pollack R, Risser R, Conlon S, Rifkin DB: Proc Natl Acad Sci USA 71:4792, 1974.
11. Laug WE, Jones PA, Benedict WF: J Natl Cancer Inst 54:173, 1975.

12. Christman JK, Silagi SS, Newcomb EW, Acs G, Silverstein S: Proc Natl Acad Sci USA 72:47, 1975.
13. Nagy B, Ban J, Brdar B: Int J Cancer 19:614, 1977.
14. Howett MK, High CS, Rapp F: Cancer Res 38:1075, 1978.
15. Mott DM, Fabisch PH, Sani BP, Sorof S: Biochem Biophys Res Commun 61:621, 1974.
16. Wolf BA, Goldberg AR: Proc Natl Acad Sci USA 73:3613, 1976.
17. Montesano R, Drevon C, Kuroki T, Saint Vincent L, Handleman S, Sanford KK, Defeo D, Weinstein IB: J Natl Cancer Inst 59:1651, 1977.
18. Quigley JP: J Cell Biol 71:472, 1976.
19. Unkeless JC, Dano K, Kellerman GM, Reich E: J Biol Chem 249:4295, 1974.
20. Zimmerman M, Quigley JP, Ashe B, Dorn C, Goldfarb RH, Troll W: Proc Natl Acad Sci USA 75:750, 1978.
21. Vetterlein D, Young PL, Bell TE, Roblin R: J Biol Chem 254:575, 1979.
22. Granelli-Piperno A, Reich E: J Exp Med 148:223, 1978.
23. Christman JK, Silverstein SC, Acs G: J Exp Med 142:419, 1975.
24. Astedt B, Holmberg L: Nature 261:595, 1976.
25. Unkeless JC, Gordon S, Reich E: J Exp Med 139:834, 1974.
26. Beers WH, Strickland S, Reich E: Cell 6:387, 1975.
27. Strickland S, Reich E, Sherman MI: Cell 9:231, 1976.
28. Rifkin DB: J Cell Physiol 97:421, 1978.
29. Strickland S, Beers WH: J Biol Chem 251:5694, 1976.
30. Vassalli JD, Reich E: J Exp Med 145:429, 1977.
31. Werb Z: J Exp Med 147:1695, 1978.
32. Lee LS, Weinstein IB: Nature 274:696, 1978.
33. Wigler M, Weinstein IB: Nature 259:232, 1976.
34. Christman JK, Copp RP, Pedrinan L, Whalen CE: Can Res 38:3854, 1978.
35. Van Duuren BL: Prog Exp Tumor Res 11:31, 1969.
36. Berenblum I: In Becker FF (ed): "Cancer 1." New York: Plenum, 1975, pp 323–344.
37. Goldfarb RH, Quigley JP: Cancer Res 38:4599, 1978.
38. Troll W, Klassen A, Janoff A: Science 169:1211, 1970.
39. Hozumi M, Ogawa M, Sugemura T, Takeuchi T, Umezawa H: Cancer Res 32:1725, 1972.
40. Quigley JP: Cell 17:131, 1979.
41. Hatefi Y, Hanstein WG: In Fleischer S, Packer L (eds): "Methods in Enzymology," vol 31. New York: Academic Press, 1974, pp 770–790.
42. Aoyagi T, Umezawa H: In Reich E, Rifkin DB, Shaw E (eds): "Proteases and Biological Control." Cold Spring Harbor New York: Cold Spring Harbor Laboratory, 1975. pp 429–454.
43. Estensen RD, Haddon JW, Touraine F, Touraine JL, Haddox MK, Goldberg ND: In Baserga R (ed): "Control of Proliferation of Animal Cells." Cold Spring Harbor, New York: Cold Spring Harbor Laboratory, 1973, pp 627–634.
44. Dicker P, Rozengurt E: Nature 276:723, 1978.
45. Noonan KD: Curr Topics Membr Transp 11:397, 1978.
46. Sivak A, Van Duuren BL: J Natl Cancer Inst 44:1091, 1970.
47. Dreidger PE, Blumberg PM: Cancer Res 37:3257, 1977.
48. Hynes RO, Wyke JA, Bye JM, Humphreys KC, Pearlstein ES: In Reich E, Rifkin DB, Shaw E (eds): "Proteases and Biological Control." Cold Spring Harbor, New York: Cold Spring Harbor Laboratory, 1975, pp 931–944.
49. Chen LB, Buchanan JM: Proc Natl Acad Sci USA 72:1132, 1975.

Tumor Cell Surfaces and Malignancy 797—819 (1980)

Structure and Function of the Fibronectins

Kenneth M. Yamada, Liang-Hsien E. Hahn, and Kenneth Olden

Laboratory of Molecular Biology, National Cancer Institute, Bethesda, Maryland 20205

The fibronectins are high-molecular-weight, adhesive glycoproteins present on the cell surface and circulating in blood. The cellular form of fibronectin is often decreased after malignant transformation, and its loss is associated with altered cell adhesion, morphology, and cell-cell interactions. We have explored the mechanisms by which fibronectin acts by a) comparing the biologic activities and structure of plasma and cellular fibronectins, b) examining the role of its asparagine-linked carbohydrate moiety in biologic activity and metabolism, and c) characterizing and isolating specific binding regions for extracellular macromolecules.

Direct comparisons of purified cell surface and plasma fibronectins from chicken and man reveal identical biologic activities in cell attachment to collagen and in cell spreading. However, cellular fibronectin is 50 times more active in restoring a more normal morphology to transformed fibroblasts than plasma fibronectin, and it is over 150 times more effective as a hemagglutinin. These differences in biologic activity are accompanied by structural differences as revealed by sodium dodecyl sulfate gel electrophoresis of plasma fibronectins versus cellular fibronectins from cell surfaces or culture medium.

The role of carbohydrates in the function of fibronectin was analyzed with the drug tunicamycin to inhibit glycosylation. Nonglycosylated fibronectin is not significantly less active than normal fibronectin in several biologic assays, including hemagglutination and capacity to restore a more normal morphology and alignment to transformed fibroblasts. However, the absence of carbohydrate does result in a twofold to threefold increase in susceptibility to proteolytic degradation both in vivo and in vitro. These and earlier results indicate that the carbohydrate moiety of fibronectin is not required for its synthesis, secretion, or biologic function, but instead helps to protect the protein against proteolytic attack.

A polypeptide fragment of 40K daltons containing the binding site for collagen was isolated from cellular fibronectin after proteolysis by chymotrypsin; a homologous but not identical site is present in plasma fibronectin. A second fragment of 160K daltons lacks the collagen-binding site but posseses cell surface-binding site(s) that are active in hemagglutination and cell spreading, and are inhibitory to cell attachment to collagen. A third fragment, of 205K daltons, possesses both cell- and collagen-binding sites and can mediate attachment of cells to collagen.

Separate, high-affinity binding sites for the glycosaminoglycans hyaluronic acid and heparin are also present on fibronectin; some interaction with heparin sulfate was also found. The 160K fragment contains the heparin-binding site, and a smaller heparin-binding domain of 50K daltons was isolated with pronase.

Received June 6, 1979; accepted June 8, 1979.

Our studies suggest that fibronectin acts in various cellular and extracellular matrix interactions by utilizing specific, structurally distinct polypeptide domains that can be isolated and characterized.

Key words: fibronectin, cell surface glycoprotein, cellular adhesion, transformation, hemagglutination, oligosaccharides, collagen, glycosaminoglycans, heparin, hyaluronic acid, proteolytic fragments

INTRODUCTION

Cellular fibronectin is a major cell surface glycoprotein that is usually decreased after malignant transformation (see Yamada and Olden [1] and Hynes [2] for reviews). Previous work has shown that fibronectin is an adhesive protein that is implicated in a wide variety of cellular interactions including cell-cell adhesion, cell adhesion to substrata, cell spreading, and the parallel cell alignment characteristic of fibroblasts. Fibronectin is also thought to be an important regulator of cell morphology, cell surface architecture, and the organization of intracellular microfilament bundles. The biologic activities of fibronectin are summarized in Table I.

This abundance of activities provides a major challenge: to determine how fibronectin acts in each event at the molecular level. The simplest hypothesis for its overall mechanism of action has been that cellular fibronectin acts via a combination of cell-cell and cell-substratum adhesiveness [1, 3–5] (Fig. 1). This concept is supported by antibody inhibition experiments with antifibronectin [6], by analyses of mutants in cell adhesion [7], and by a number of classical studies of cell rounding and of cells cultured on substrata of low adhesiveness, all of which can mimic the effects of loss of fibronectin. However, to understand how fibronectin acts as an adhesive glycoprotein will require careful biochemical dissection of the structure and the functions of fibronectin.

MATERIALS AND METHODS

Fibronectin Isolation

Chicken and human cellular and plasma fibronectins were prepared as described [8, 9]. ^{14}C-labeled cellular fibronectin was prepared by incubation of chick embryo fibroblast cultures with 5 μCi/ml ^{14}C-glycine (Amersham, 54 mCi/mmole) for 24 h prior to urea extraction.

Electrophoresis

Sodium dodecyl sulfate-polyacrylamide slab gel electrophoresis was performed as previously described [9–12]. Disulfide bonds were reduced by inclusion of 0.1 M dithiothreitol (Calbiochem). For higher resolution of high-molecular-weight proteins, 3%/4% polyacrylamide gels were prepared as usual, except that a 3% solution of prepolymerized polyacrylamide (BDH Chemicals, MW > 5,000,000) in water was added prior to the addition of ammonium persulfate to achieve a *final* concentration of 0.5% polyacrylamide (note that the original reference, Yamada and Kennedy [9], contains a typographical error concerning the final concentration). The 0.5% prepolymerized polyacrylamide does not become cross-linked in the gel, and it therefore has little effect on mobilities; however, it markedly decreases lateral protein diffusion, resulting in sharper bands. It also stiffens the gels, which reduces the risk of tearing when handled.

Bioassays

Hemagglutination [13], effects on cell morphology [3], cell spreading [14], and cell attachment to collagen [15, 16] were assayed as described in the references cited. The attachment of cells to collagen was found to be subject to substantial variations in background (cells attaching in the absence of fibronectin) and reproducibility between samples or between experiments. We therefore selected a strain of Chinese hamster ovary (CHO) cells that survived two cycles of the following selection: Cells were trypsinized and plated in serum-free medium, as described [16], on nonwettable petri dishes. After 1.5 h, the attached cells were discarded. The cells in suspension were permitted to attach to dishes coated with type I collagen (sterilized by ultraviolet light) in the presence of 10 $\mu g/ml$ cellular fibronectin for 1.5 h at 37°C. The attached cells were subcultured, then frozen and stored in liquid nitrogen. Assays were not performed with cells maintained in culture for

---

TABLE I. Biologic Activities of Fibronectin

   I.   Cell-cell aggregation (agglutination)
       A. Fixed erythrocytes
       B. Live cells (chick embryo, BHK)
  II.   Cell-substratum adhesiveness
       A. Collagen substratum
       B. Plastic substratum
       C. Cell spreading
 III.   Reversion of transformed phenotype
       A. Cell alignment and overlapping
       B. Fibroblastic morphology
       C. Microvilli and ruffles
       D. Microfilament bundles
 IV.   Rate and directionality of cell motility
  V.   Reticuloendothelial system clearance of colloids
 VI.   Binding to collagen, fibrin, and heparin

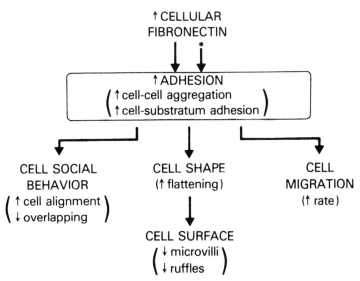

Fig. 1. Postulated biologic model of action of fibronectin. Asterisk indicates contributions of other adhesive mechanisms, such as other adhesive molecules or regulators of cytoskeletal function.

more than a month after defrosting. This strain had low nonspecific attachment with good reproducibility and a high sensitivity to fibronectin; even 0.1 μg/ml fibronectin was reliably measured [22].

Nonglycosylated Fibronectin

Nonglycosylated fibronectin was isolated by immunoaffinity chromatography from cultures of chick embryo fibroblasts treated with tunicamycin. Primary cultures were preincubated for 3.5 h in culture medium with or without 0.5 μg/ml tunicamycin (a gift from Dr. Gakuzo Tamura). Cells were passaged with 0.25% trypsin, then replated at the same cell density in the appropriate preincubation medium and incubated for another 24 h. Control and tunicamycin-treated cultures were homogenized separately in pH 11 phosphate buffer containing 1% Triton X-100 and ultracentrifuged, then diluted and neutralized [12, 17]. Fibronectin was isolated from the homogenates by affinity chromatography using affinity-purified goat anti-fibronectin antibodies coupled covalently to Sepharose 4B (Pharmacia) [6, 17]. Nonspecifically adsorbed protein was eluted with 0.1 M borate buffer (pH 8.5) containing 0.5 M NaCl. Fibronectin was then eluted from the resin with 0.2 M acetic acid (pH 2.9) containing 0.5 M NaCl. The eluates were immediately adjusted to pH 11.0 with NaOH, then dialyzed against buffer A [0.15 M NaCl, 1 mM CaCl$_2$, 10 mM cyclohexylaminopropane sulfonic acid (CAPS), pH 11.0].

Protease digestions of ^{14}C-leucine-labeled nonglycosylated and glycosylated fibronectins were performed with 50 μg of each in 0.05 μg/ml pronase (Calbiochem) in 0.1 M sodium phosphate buffer (pH 7.4) at 37°C. Aliquots of 100 μl were removed at specified intervals, and radioactivity in soluble and acid-precipitable fractions was determined after precipitation with trichloroacetic acid [17].

Amino sugar analyses [18] or labeling with ^{3}H-mannose and ^{14}C-glucosamine were performed as described elsewhere [17, 19].

Affinity Columns

Gelatin (from Sigma or Nutritional Biochemicals) was washed exhaustively to deplete glycosaminoglycans, first with deionized water at 4°C (four changes over 18 h), then with 3 M NaCl plus 10 mM ethylenediaminetetraacetic acid (EDTA), then three more times with water at 4°C. It was solubilized by heating to 100°C, cooled to 45°C, then diluted into coupling buffer and coupled to CNBr-Sepharose (Pharmacia).

Heparin (Sigma, grade I, 169.7 USP units/mg) was coupled to agarose as described [20].

Collagen-Binding Fragment

The 40K collagen-binding fragment was detected and isolated exactly as previously described [21]. The fragment was further purified by chromatography on a 1.5 × 85.5 cm Sephacryl S-200 column (Pharmacia) in buffer B (100 mM NaCl, 1 mM CaCl$_2$, 50 mM CAPS, pH 11.0). The 160K fragment was purified from the material that did not bind to gelatin-agarose on a 1.6- × 94.5-cm column of Sephacryl S-300 [22]. The 205K fragment was produced by digestion of intact cellular fibronectin bound to gelatin with 0.4% chymotrypsin for 2 or 3 min, then purified on a Sephacryl S-300 column [22]. All fragments were homogeneous by sodium dodecyl sulfate (SDS) gel electrophoresis except for the 205K fragment, which contained a small amount of a 200K band. There was no detectable intact fibronectin (240K in this Laemmli gel system) in any of the fragment preparations [22].

Heparin-Binding Fragment

[3]H-heparin was purchased from New England Nuclear (sodium salt, reduced by ^{3}H-sodium borohydride, 0.332 mCi/mg), and purified on a 1.5-$\times$ 60-cm Sephadex G-100 column (Pharmacia) in 0.15 M NaCl, 10 mM sodium phosphate, pH 7.4. The high-molecular-weight fraction was pooled and rechromatographed on this column in comparison with unlabeled glycosaminoglycans of known size (a generous gift from Drs. M. B. Mathews and J. A. Cifonelli, University of Chicago). The marker glycosaminoglycans were detected by the phenol sulfuric acid assay [23], and the average molecular weight of the labeled heparin was calculated to be 12,000.

To isolate heparin-binding fragments, 0.25 mg of fibronectin was diluted into 100 mM NaCl, 10 mM CaCl$_2$, 50 mM Tris-HCl, pH 7.0 (buffer E), and applied to 1 ml heparin-agarose columns (0.8 $\times$ 2.1 cm), washed with five column volumes of buffer E, then incubated in 6 μg/ml chymotrypsin (Worthington) or pronase in buffer E for 2 h at 23°C. The columns were eluted with 1 volume of 10 mM sodium phosphate, pH 7, containing 2 mM phenylmethanesulfonic acid (PMSF), and the eluate was adjusted to 2% in SDS and heated to 100°C for 2 min. After washing with five column volumes of buffer E and two volumes of the phosphate-PMSF solution, the gel beads were transferred to glass tubes and centrifuged to sediment the beads. The beads were incubated in 0.5 ml of a 3$\times$ homogenization buffer (final concentrations were 2% SDS, 2 mM PMSF, 10 mM sodium phosphate, pH 7.0) at 100°C for three 2-min periods separated by vortexing. The beads were sedimented and the supernatant was analyzed on SDS gels.

RESULTS AND DISCUSSION

We shall review the results and implications of a series of recent experiments analyzing how fibronectin acts as an adhesive glycoprotein in a variety of cellular events. We have approached this problem of molecular mechanisms of action by using three general approaches: 1) Investigating whether all fibronectins are identical, or whether some forms are missing certain structures and functions; 2) determining the role of the carbohydrate moiety in fibronectin's biologic function; and 3) identifying, isolating, and purifying active site regions of the molecule.

Biologic Assays

For these studies, we utilized four different assays of biologic activity (shown in Fig. 2), each of which appears to quantitate a slightly different aspect of fibronectin's activity.

a. Hemagglutination of fixed erythrocytes is a model system for measuring cell-cell adhesive interactions. It is quantitated by standard hemagglutination procedures using microtiter plates, in which biologic activity is defined as the lowest concentration of protein that can produce half-maximal agglutination [13]. For a molecule to cause hemagglutination, there must be both interaction with the cell surface and multivalency of the binding molecule to link together more than one cell.

b. The cell morphology assay utilizes transformed test cells derived from a mouse tumor. A series of serial dilutions of fibronectin is added to replicate cultures of these cells [3, 9]. The end point is defined as the lowest concentration of fibronectin at which there is a detectable difference in cell shape and parallel alignment of cell bodies compared with controls in "blind" evaluations of sets of 4–6 phase-contrast photomicrographs of random fields. This assay evaluates the capacity of a protein to enhance cell spreading in the presence of serum and to alter cell-cell interactions involved in parallel alignment of cells. The former effect probably reflects increased cell-substratum adhesion, since enhanced cell spreading can be mimicked by polylysine and collagen. Parallel alignment of cells, however, probably also involves lateral cell-cell adhesiveness between adjacent cells.

c. Cell spreading of BHK cells onto plastic substrata in serum-free salt solutions is quantitated according to the method of Grinnell et al [14]. The end point is the concentration of protein that permits spreading of 50% of the cells in 45 min. This assay requires that the adhesive molecule interact with both the cell surface and the substratum. It is less specific than the other assays in that a variety of molecules than can bind to the cell surface by different means are all quite effective in promoting cell spreading [24]. The assay is performed in the absence of serum, since the plasma fibronectin normally present in serum can mediate cell spreading.

d. Cell attachment to collagen is assayed by the procedure of Kleinman et al [16], modified from the original Klebe assay [15]. CHO cells require fibronectin to attach to type I collagen adsorbed onto nonwettable plastic petri dishes. These cells cannot normally attach to this type of dish, nor to collaten-coated dishes, unless fibronectin is present. The attachment mediated by fibronectin involves both binding to the collagen and to the cells. Both this assay and the cell spreading assay can be performed by pretreating the substratum with fibronectin, then washing extensively prior to the assay. In both assays, fibronectin remains bound to the substratum and readily mediates cell attachment or spreading.

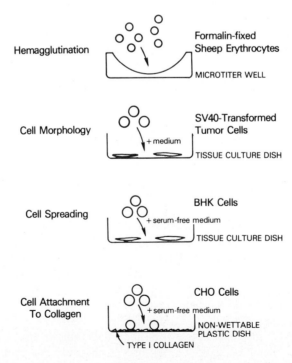

FIBRONECTIN BIOLOGICAL ASSAYS

Fig. 2. Biologic assays for fibronectin activity. See text for discussion.

Are All Fibronectins Identical?

We first compared cellular and plasma fibronectins in the series of four bioassays. A summary of the recently published results [9] is shown in Figure 3. Fibronectins purified from plasma or from fibroblast cell surfaces of both chicken and man are of equal specific activity in the two assays involving cell attachment to substrata. All proteins have half-maxima for attachment to collagen and for cell spreading of $1-1.5$ μg/ml.

In contrast, the plasma fibronectins were 50 to 200 times less effective than cellular fibronectins in hemagglutination or in restoring a more normal morphology to transformed cells. We note parenthetically that these differences in biologic activity cannot be explained by contamination of cellular fibronectin by proteoglycans or glycosaminoglycans, since 1) purified cellular fibronectin preparations contain very little xylose [8] (one xylose for each chain of contaminating complex carbohydrate would be expected), and also are free of N-acetyl galactosamine; 2) hemagglutination or these effects on cell morphology are not induced by hyaluronic acid, chondroitin sulfate, or heparin [13, 25]; 3) the effects of fibronectin on hemagglutination or cell morphology are not blocked by treatment with testicular hyaluronidase (effective against hyaluronic acid and chondroitin sulfates) or chondroitinase ABC [5, 13, 25], but are blocked by proteases [5, 13] and by antibody specific to the fibronectin monomer eluted from preparative SDS gels [3, 5, 13]; and 4) there is no glucosamine-labeled material sensitive to exhaustive treatment with chondroitinase ABC or to nitrous acid in our fibronectin preparations (K. Kimata, personal communication).

We investigated whether structural differences between plasma and cellular fibronectins accompany these differences in certain biologic activities. In a high-resolution SDS gel system (described in Methods) in which high-molecular-weight proteins differing by 10,000 apparent molecular weight can be separated by several millimeters, we see substantial differences in electrophoretic migration between plasma and cellular fibronectins of both chicken and man. Plasma fibronectins from both species are resolved into doublet

CELLULAR VS. PLASMA FIBRONECTINS

BIOLOGICAL ACTIVITY	RELATIVE SPECIFIC ACTIVITIES
RECONSTITUTION OF NORMAL CELL MORPHOLOGY AND ALIGNMENT	50X
HEMAGGLUTINATION	150-200X
CELL ATTACHMENT TO COLLAGEN	1X
CELL SPREADING ON PLASTIC	1X

Fig. 3. Comparison of in vitro biologic activities of human and chicken cellular and plasma fibronectins. The activities of cellular fibronectin relative to the specific activities of plasma fibronectin are listed (see Yamada and Kennedy [9] for documentation). From Yamada and Kennedy [9], with permission.

bands with apparent sizes 5,000–10,000 daltons less than the corresponding cellular fibronectins, which migrate as single bands (eg, see Fig. 4). These differences are probably caused by true differences in polypeptide size rather than by anomalies in migration due to differing carbohydrate content, since fibroblast cell surface fibronectin and plasma fibronectin have very similar carbohydrate content and composition [8, 26–28].

These size differences are retained after cleavage of the molecules with trypsin to form fragments of 200,000–205,000 daltons [9]. There are consequently no major size differences in the cleaved regions of these molecules that contain the interchain disulfide bonds that link together the subunits of each molecule.

A highly schematic summary of these results is presented in Figure 5. Cellular fibronectin is the larger molecule, and it has all four biologic activities. Plasma fibronectin is apparently shorter and is deficient in two activities, hemagglutination and capacity to restore a normal morphology to transformed fibroblasts. These missing activities involve cell-cell adhesion and (in the morphology assay) probably an increased level of cell-substratum adhesiveness in the presence of serum (note that in the other assays involving cell-substratum adhesiveness, serum is omitted). One uncertainty is whether the doublet band of the plasma form is due to differences in size between the subunits of each fibronectin dimer, or to two different-size classes of plasma fibronectin dimer. We currently favor the idea that each molecule has subunits of different length, since the unreduced dimeric molecule migrates in SDS-polyacrylamide gels as a single band.

In other respects, the plasma and cellular forms of fibronectin arc very similar. They have similar amino acid and carbohydrate compositions, subunit organization, secondary and tertiary structure indicated by spectrophotometry, peptide maps, and immunologic

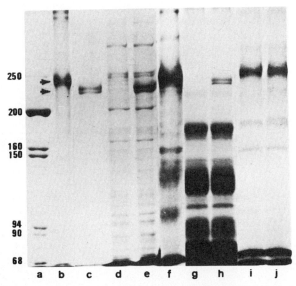

Fig. 4. Comparison of electrophoretic mobilities of human cellular and plasma fibronectins. Samples were analyzed in a 3%/4% polyacrylamide gel containing 0.5% linear polyacrylamide. a) Protein molecular weight standards ($\times$ 10^{-3} daltons). b) Human cell-surface fibronectin. c) Human plasma fibronectin. d) Humogenate of confluent culture of human WI38 cells labeled with ^{125}I. e) Same as previous lane plus plasma fibronectin. f) Autoradiogram of lane e. g) Conditioned cultured medium collected after labeling of WI38 cells for 24 h with ^{14}C-leucine. h) Same as previous lane plus plasma fibronectin marker. i) Autoradiogram of lane g. j) Autoradiogram of lane h. From Yamada and Kennedy [9].

cross-reactivity (review in Yamada and Kennedy [9] and Alexander et al [29]). The nature of the peptide region accounting for the size differences between the forms of fibronectin is therefore important, since it may account for the two unique biologic activities of cellular fibronectin. Preliminary results to be presented later suggest that this difference region may be internal rather than at the amino terminus. We conclude that not all fibronectins are identical and that a molecular explanation must account for these structural and functional differences between plasma and cellular fibronectins.

Role of Fibronectin's Carbohydrate

The carbohydrate moiety of cellular fibronectin is primarily, if not entirely, of only one type [8, 19, 28]. It consists of a core region of N-acetyl glucosamine and mannose attached to asparagine residues, plus peripheral sugars characteristic of the "complex" class of asparagine-linked oligosaccharide commonly found in serum proteins. This fact is important, since a new inhibitor of glycosylation, tunicamycin, can selectively block the synthesis of this class of oligosaccharide by inhibiting dolichol pyrophosphate-mediated transfer of the core oligosaccharide to proteins.

We had previously characterized the effects of inhibiting glycosylation on fibronectin metabolism [19]. Nonglycosylated fibronectin was synthesized at normal rates, and its initial secretion onto the cell surface was almost entirely normal. However, its rate of protein turnover (primarily while on the cell surface) was increased twofold to threefold, resulting in an approximately threefold overall decrease in levels of the protein on the cell surface. In contrast, total protein turnover was not significantly altered. These experiments suggested that the oligosaccharide on fibronectin is not required for its synthesis or secretion, but might instead be involved in controlling turnover rates [19].

One important possibility still remaining was that the carbohydrate was required for biologic function. To test this hypothesis, nonglycosylated and glycosylated chick cellular fibronectins were isolated by affinity chromatography on agarose columns to which affinity-purified anti-fibronectin was covalently coupled [17]. The source of nonglycosylated fibronectin was chick fibroblasts pretreated for 3.5 h with high levels of tunicamycin to deplete internal pools of glycosylated fibronectin; previous studies of the kinetics of fibronectin secretion had shown that the molecule first appears on the cell surface after 30–45 min and secretion is complete within 3 h. The pretreated cells were then trypsinized with high concentrations of trypsin (250 times the amount required to remove cell surface fibronectin), then replated and cultured in the presence of tunicamycin for another 24 h. The fibronectin that was subsequently synthesized was isolated by affinity chromatography. Nonglycosylated fibronectin was 98% free of carbohydrate by direct chemical analysis (amino sugar analyses) and showed 98% decreases in the incorporation of ^{14}C-glucosamine

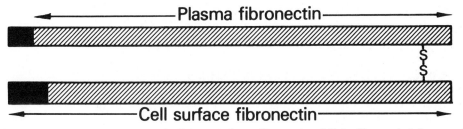

Fig. 5. Schematic comparison of cellular and plasma fibronectins. Cellular fibronectin is longer and has subunits of equal apparent size. Plasma fibronectin is shorter, and may have subunits of unequal size.

and ^{3}H-mannose compared to nonglycosylated fibronectin [17]. In addition, the nongly-cosylated protein lost its capacity to bind to concanavalin A columns, to which all of the native molecule binds [19].

Surprisingly, nonglycosylated fibronectin is as active as glycosylated fibronectin in all four assays of biologic activity [17]. There are no differences in specific activities, nor in the dose-response curves for each assay. An example of the identical activities of the two molecules in cell spreading is shown in Figure 6.

However, one major difference does exist. The isolated nonglycosylated molecule is approximately two times more sensitive to proteolysis by the broad-spectrum protease pronase than glycosylated fibronectin (Fig. 7). This result is important in confirming that the nonglycosylated molecule is inherently more susceptible to proteolysis than the fully glycosylated molecule, and that the twofold to threefold increase in turnover rates reported previously is probably due to this change rather than to some unusual alteration in the protein degradation system of tunicamycin-treated cells [17, 19].

We conclude from these experiments that there is no evidence that the carbohydrate moiety of fibronectin is required for its synthesis, secretion, or in vitro biologic activity. Instead, the carbohydrate appears to stabilize the protein against proteolytic attack and regulates its turnover rate. In terms of function, it appears that even though carbohydrate might be present in the parts of fibronectin that interact with the cell surface or with substrata such as collagen, it is not required for activity. Attention should therefore be focused on the polypeptide portion of the molecule to determine its mechanisms of biologic activity.

Isolation of Active Sites: Rationale

Fibronectin's action as an adhesive molecule can be conceptually divided into the series of binding interactions listed in Table II. Each interaction (for example, binding to the cell surface), may be mediated by a specific active site. Adhesive interactions would then involve a combination of such active sites. For example, two or more cell surface bind-ing sites might be used for cell-cell adhesion, or one cell surface-binding and one collagen-binding site for attachment to collagen. Cellular fibronectin may also have a self-association site that is absent from plasma fibronectin, since it is dramatically more insoluble at neutral pH and tends to form aggregates or fibrils on the cell surface.

How might such active sites be isolated? One attractive possibility is that each active site is in a separate structural domain of the molecule, and that such domains can be isolated separately. A spectrophotometric study of isolated chick cellular fibronectin utilizing circular dicroism and fluorescence suggested that the molecule consists of domains of structure connected by flexible polypeptide chains. It proved possible to melt out (denature) the domains by heating, and the loss of structure occurred at temperatures similar to those which destroy its hemagglutinating activity [13, 30].

A simple, general method for isolating structural domains is to subject proteins to limited proteolysis. Extended polypeptide chains are more accessible to proteases and are readily hydrolyzed, whereas the cleavage sites located within folded polypeptide domains tend to be buried or inaccessible owing to steric hindrance to the protease. Proteolysis might therefore generate specific fragments of fibronectin that retain structurally and functionally intact domains.

Our general approach is depicted in Figure 8. Fibronectin is first permitted to bind to an interacting molecule, eg, collagen. The complex is digested by various proteases, eg, chymotrypsin. After extensive washing, the fragments that remain bound are eluted with

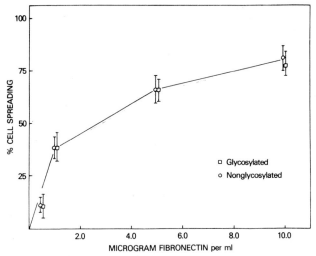

Fig. 6. Comparison of cell spreading activities of glycosylated and nonglycosylated fibronectins isolated by immunoaffinity chromatography. The percentage of total BHK cells that were fully spread on plastic tissue culture dishes after 45 min is plotted as a function of protein added to the 1-ml assay mixture [14, 17].

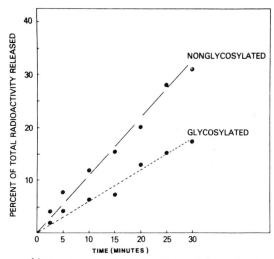

Fig. 7. Rates of release of ^{14}C-leucine after digestion of labeled glycosylated or nonglycosylated fibronectin by pronase. Aliquots (50 μg/ml) of each protein were digested for the indicated times by pronase (0.05 μg/ml) at 37°C, then precipitated with trichloroacetic acid. The acid-soluble radioactivity is plotted as the percentage of original cpm released into supernatants.

TABLE II. Possible Binding Interactions of Fibronectin

1. Collagen
2. Glycosaminoglycans and proteoglycans
3. Fibrin and fibrinogen
4. Cell surface
5. Self-association

8 M urea for further purification, or with boiling 2% SDS for examination on SDS-poly-acrylamide gels. Such fragments should still contain the binding site, whereas those that pass through the column would not.

Active Sites: Collagen Binding

Both cellular and plasma fibronectins bind to collagen and can mediate the attachment of cells to collagen. The results of limited chymotryptic hydrolysis of fibronectin bound to gelatin (denatured collagen) are shown in Figure 9. Within 2 min of treatment with 3% (w/w) chymotrypsin:fibronectin, a 205K dalton fragment is generated that remains bound on the column. This intermediate is further cleaved to a stable 40K dalton fragment that persists for at least 20 h of digestion [21]. This 40K fragment is a single polypeptide chain, since it migrates with the same mobility before or after reduction with dithiothreitol; the anomalous mobility changes noted by others for a collagen-binding 72K fragment from plasma fibronectin [31] are not characteristic of this fragment. Seventy percent of purified preparations of this 40K fragment labeled with ^{14}C will rebind to gelatin affinity columns, confirming that it contains a collagen-binding site. Thirty percent of the radioactivity will bind to columns with covalently attached native type I collagen [21]. This lower capacity to bind to native type I collagen compared to denatured collagen is also characteristic of the intact molecule [32, 33].

This collagen-binding polypeptide region may contain an average of one asparagine-linked oligosaccharide per mole, since it contains approximately 20% of total incorporated ^{14}C-glucosamine [21], and since fibronectin has an average of five oligosaccharide units

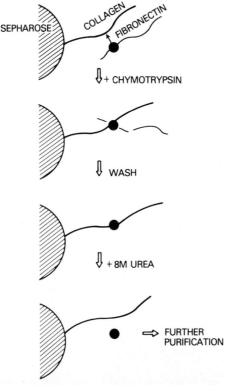

Fig. 8. Procedure for isolation of active sites. See text for discussion.

per monomer [8, 28]. Preliminary analyses suggest that this fragment has an unusual amino acid composition, with glycine constituting nearly 15% of the residues and an enrichment in cysteine.

Does plasma fibronectin possess an analogous binding site? Binding of chicken or human plasma fibronectin to gelatin affinity columns followed by similar chymotryptic digestions produce similar fragments of 41K or 42K daltons [21]. All of the fibronectins tested, therefore, appear to possess homologous binding regions. However, one surprising finding is that although intact chicken plasma fibronectin is apparently smaller than the cell surface form by 5,000–10,000 daltons, its collagen-binding fragment is slightly larger than that from cellular fibronectin. This difference is reproducible in coelectrophoresis experiments in which the two fragments are found to migrate with different mobilities even after mixing together prior to electrophoresis [21]. Since the 40K fragment is probably an internal fragment (see below), this difference strongly suggests that differences between plasma and cellular fibronectins are internal, rather than amino terminal differences due to simple protein processing. This concept, if correct, further suggests that these two forms of fibronectin are from separate genes. This possibility should be explored further by more detailed peptide mapping and sequencing experiments.

The 205K collagen-binding fragment produced after brief proteolysis by chymotrypsin is similar to the 205K fragments produced by trypsinization or plasminolysis (reviewed in Yamada and Olden [1]). These 205K fragments lacks a 15K–30K polypeptide region that

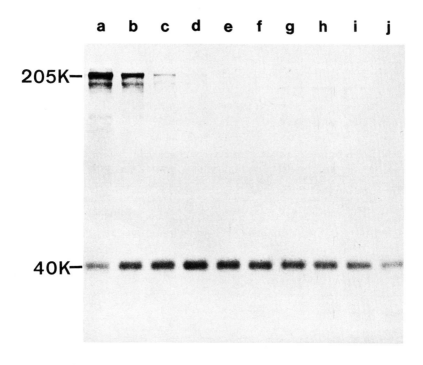

Fig. 9. Autoradiogram of fibronectin fragments remaining bound to gelatin-agarose after digestion by chymotrypsin. ^{14}C-glycine-labeled fibronectin was permitted to bind to gelatin-agarose, then incubated with α-chymotrypsin for 10 min to 20 h. The gelatin-agarose was washed extensively; then bound polypeptides were eluted with boiling 2% SDS. a) 10 min of digestion; b) 25 min; c) 50 min; d) 80 min; e) 2 h; f) 3 h; g) 5 h; h) 7.5 h; i) 10 h; j) 20 h.

contains all of the interchain disulfide bond(s) holding fibronectin subunits in dimers and multimers. The chymotryptic 205K fragment was recovered from gelatin affinity columns using 8 M urea, then purified by molecular sieve chromatography on Sephacryl S-300 columns at alkaline pH. This large purified fragment was tested for other activities in studies of the second type of active site described below.

Active Sites: Cell Surface Interaction

Although the 40K collagen-binding fragment readily attaches to collagen, it cannot mediate the attachment of cells to collagen (discussed below). This finding suggests that the cell surface binding site is missing, and that it might have been lost in the material that does not bind to the gelatin affinity columns after proteolysis. The major chymotryptic fragment in such eluates has been isolated by chromatography in Sephacryl S-300, and is a homogeneous species on SDS-polyacrylamide gel electrophoresis with an apparent molecular weight of 160,000.

The 40K, 160K, and 205K fragments were compared with the intact molecule in the series of in vitro bioassays. A summary of the most pertinent results is shown in Table III (the detailed results will be presented elsewhere [22, 34]).

The 40K fragment is inactive in all bioassays. However, it is capable of competitively inhibiting fibronectin-mediated attachment of cells to collagen (eg, 5 µg produces a 73% inhibition of attachment mediated by 0.15 µg of intact fibronectin). These results are important in indicating that the 40K fragment is the functionally important binding region of fibronectin, since it will competitively bind to collagen to prevent intact fibronectin from binding [22].

In contrast, the 160K fragment itself is capable of mediating hemagglutination, although with low activity (half-maximal at 188 µg/ml), and is nearly as active as the intact molecule in mediating cell spreading on plastic dishes. By itself, it is inactive in cell attachment to collagen. However, it can competitively inhibit fibronectin-mediated cell attachment to collagen if preincubated with the cells (14 µg/ml inhibits 0.15 µg/ml of intact fibronectin by 93%). Importantly, the 160K fragment is not inhibitory if it is first preincubated with the collagen-coated dish, then washed [22].

The 205K fragment was moderately active in hemagglutination (10% of the activity of intact fibronectin), fully active in the cell spreading assay, and most interestingly, active in mediating cell attachment to collagen (70% of the activity of the intact molecule).

The most straightforward interpretation of these results is that the 40K fragment contains the collagen-binding site of fibronectin, the 160K fragment contains the cell surface-binding site(s), and the 205K fragment contains both active sites. As expected,

TABLE III. Summary of Biologic Activities of Fibronectin Fragments

	40K	160K	205K
Hemagglutination	−	+[a]	+[b]
Cell spreading	−	+	+
Cell attachment to collagen	−	−	+
Competitive inhibition of cell attachment of collagen	+[c]	+[d]	

[a]Retains 2% activity of intact fibronectin.
[b]Retains 10% activity.
[c]Much lower activity if preincubated with cells.
[d]No activity if preincubated with collagen-coated dish.

the 160K and 40K fragments can be generated from the 205K fragment after more extensive proteolysis with chymotrypsin. These conclusions support the concept that fibronectin consists of domains of structure that are resistant to proteases, and that these domains contain functionally important binding sites for collagen or for the cell surface receptor(s) for fibronectin.

Active Sites: Glycosaminoglycan Binding

The identification of collagen- and cell surface-binding regions suggested that fibronectin might possess other active site regions. For example, plasma fibronectin was previously known to interact with heparin [35], although this binding was thought to be relatively nonspecific in terms of the classes of glycosaminoglycan with which interactions occurred.

To evaluate this type of interaction, we developed the simple filter-binding assay shown in Figure 10. This assay depends on the finding that purified fibronectin becomes insoluble and aggregated when transferred from the usual alkaline CAPS buffer to conditions of physiologic salt and pH [8]. We incubate purified fibronectin with various tritiated glycosaminoglycans for 1 h in Dulbecco's phosphate-buffered saline (PBS), then trap the fibronectin and any bound glycosaminoglycans on nitrocellulose filters. The fibronectin is trapped on such filters with >98% efficiency as determined by experiments with ^{14}C-glycine-labeled fibronectin, and glycosaminoglycans remain on the filter only in the presence of fibronectin.

We first compared the efficiency of binding of a series of complex carbohydrates isolated by Robert Pratt (National Institute of Dental Research) from ^{3}H-glucosamine-labeled chick embryo fibroblasts following standard pronase digestion and DEAE cellulose chromatography procedures. Chondroitin sulfate and glycopeptides isolated from either the cell monolayer or conditioned culture medium did not bind to fibronectin (Fig. 11). Heparan sulfate from the cell layer did bind reproducibly to fibronectin in a number of experiments, but only 3–4% of the total could bind. The most effective binding was found with hyaluronic acid (Fig. 11). Other experiments to be described later also indicated that commercially available ^{3}H-heparin also bound well to fibronectin.

It is important to note parenthetically that the specific radioactivity of a ligand can affect the proportion bound, if the total concentration of ligand is close to the dissociation constant. For example, recent use of hyaluronic acid preparations of higher specific activity has permitted binding of 80–90% of total input counts to fibronectin. The poor binding

GLYCOSAMINOGLYCAN BINDING ASSAY

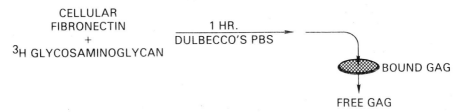

Fig. 10. Filter binding assay for glycosaminoglycan binding to fibronectin. Purified fibronectin (275 μg/ml) is incubated for 1 h in the presence of various isolated glycosaminoglycans labeled with ^{3}H, then filtered through nitrocellulose filters (Millipore), washed with PBS, and counted in a scintillation spectrometer.

of other glycosaminoglycans could be due to a very weak binding affinity (their specific activities were fortunately greater than four times higher than this preparation of hyaluronic acid) or to complete absence of such sites. Our results do, however, suggest specificity of binding of only certain glycosaminoglycans to fibronectin that does not correlate with simple electrostatic charge.

Are the glycosaminoglycan-binding sites saturable? We compared the capacity of three glycosaminoglycans to compete for the binding of ^{3}H-hyaluronic acid or ^{3}H-heparin to fibronectin. The binding of hyaluronic acid was competable by 80% with 1 μg/ml of unlabeled hyaluronic acid, and was maximally competed at only 20 μg/ml (Fig. 12). This site is therefore saturable. In contrast, the binding of hyaluronic acid was only slightly affected by even 100 μg/ml of chondroitin sulfate or heparin.

The converse results were obtained with ^{3}H-heparin binding. Only heparin could compete for this site, with 80% inhibition of binding with 10 μg/ml of unlabeled material; this site therefore appears to be of somewhat lower affinity than the hyaluronic acid site. Hyaluronic acid and chondroitin sulfate do not compete for binding at the heparin site even at concentrations of 100 μg/ml (Fig. 13). The hyaluronic acid and heparin sites are therefore both saturable, and they are separate binding sites since they do not cross-compete.

The filter binding assay also permits an estimate of binding affinities. We purified high-molecular-weight heparin from the mixture of chain lengths present in commercial ^{3}H-heparin and determined its size by comparison with glycosaminoglycans of known size (see Methods). A Scatchard plot of its binding to fibronectin is shown in Figure 14. Three other repeats of this experiment with different preparations and concentrations of fibronectin and heparin confirmed that the binding curve is biphasic; the best estimates of

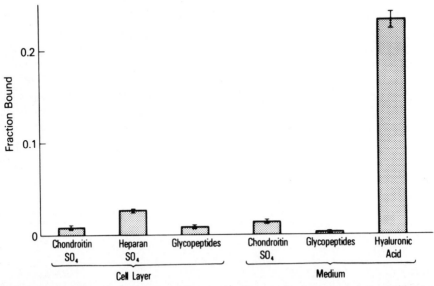

Fig. 11. Binding of glycosaminoglycans to fibronectin. Glycosaminoglycans and glycopeptides were isolated from the cell layer or from conditioned medium of chick embryo fibroblasts labeled for 24 h with ^{3}H-glucosamine. The cell monolayer or culture medium was digested exhaustively with pronase, then chromatographed on DEAE cellulose; these fractions were provided by Dr. Robert Pratt. The proportion of total counts (minus nonspecific binding in the absence of fibronectin) that bind to fibronectin is indicated for each fraction ± SE. From [41].

affinity are $K_{D_1} = 4.2 \times 10^{-9}$ M and $K_{D_2} = 1.1 \times 10^{-7}$ M. Thus, the binding site for heparin is saturable and of high affinity [41].

By extrapolating the curves to the abscissa, the average number of binding sites per fibronectin monomer is estimated to be approximately 0.1. Although this result may suggest that only a subpopulation of fibronectins binds heparin, the more likely explanation is that this result is a consequence of using a multiple-site ligand. Specifically, the purified heparin has an average molecular weight of 12,000, or roughly 25 repeated disaccharide units. As shown for hyaluronic acid [36], a large number of repeating units probably result in multiple possible binding sites on each molecule. Several fibronectins might then bind to each heparin molecule, resulting in a nonlinear Scatchard plot and an underestimate of binding sites. Independent evidence described below indicates that there is approximately one heparin binding site per fibronectin monomer.

Active Sites: Heparin Binding

The approach utilized previously to isolate the collagen-binding region was modified to isolate the heparin-binding site. Heparin was coupled to agarose, then fibronectin was permitted to bind to the heparin and was proteolytically digested. Of five proteases tested, the most interesting results were obtained with chymotrypsin and pronase (Fig. 15). Chymotrypsin digestion produces a series of fragments that remain bound to heparin, the most prominent of which is a single peptide of 160K daltons (Fig. 15d). This polypeptide is the same fragment described previously that contains cell surface interaction site(s). Subsequent digestion of this fragment with pronase or, in fact, digestion of entire original molecule with pronase produces a much smaller peptide of 50K daltons that remains bound to heparin (Fig. 15c). This 50K fragment is assumed to be the heparin-binding domain of fibronectin.

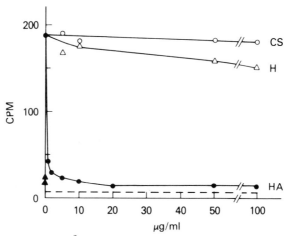

Fig. 12. Competitive inhibition of ^{3}H-hyaluronic acid binding to fibronectin by unlabeled glycosamino-glycans. ^{3}H-glucosamine-labeled hyaluronic acid isolated from chick embryo fibroblasts (medium + cell layer) was incubated for 1 h with fibronectin in the presence of the unlabeled glycosaminoglycans chondroitin sulfate (CS), heparin (H), or hyaluronic acid (HA), then collected on nitrocellulose filters. Dotted line indicates radioactivity bound to filters if the fibronectin is omitted. Triangles on Ordinate axis indicates radioactivity bound after ^{3}H-hyaluronic acid plus fibronectin mixtures are treated with testicular hyaluronidase (10 μg/ml).

In contrast to the results obtained with collagen affinity columns, the 40K chymotryptic fragment does not bind to these heparin affinity columns and is recovered in the material that washes through the columns (Fig. 15a,b). The material recovered after pronase digestion of intact fibronectin is of particular interest. It contains the same 40K fragment and a new fragment of 90K daltons (Fig. 15a). The presence of the 40K fragment after digestion by even this broad spectrum protease suggests that this fragment is a tightly organized domain with no unfolded peptide regions that would be readily accessible to proteases in general. The 90K fragment presumably represents most of the difference region between the 50K fragment and the remainder of the 160K fragment.

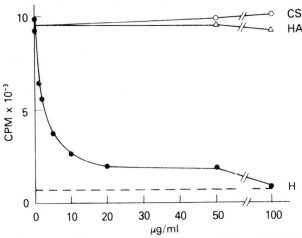

Fig. 13. Competitive inhibition of ^{3}H-heparin binding to fibronectin by unlabeled glycosaminoglycans. ^{3}H-heparin (New England Nuclear) was incubated for 1 h with fibronectin in the presence of unlabeled chondroitin sulfate (CS), hyaluronic acid (HA), or heparin (H) at the indicated final concentrations. From [41].

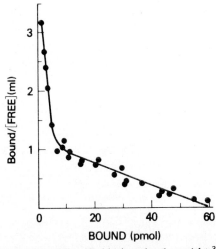

Fig. 14. Scatchard analysis of binding of purified high-molecular-weight ^{3}H-heparin to fibronectin.

We estimated the number of heparin-binding sites per fibronectin molecule by determining the molar recovery of the 50K heparin-binding fragment. The original efficiency of binding of ^{14}C-fibronectin to the heparin affinity columns is 90%. Digestion of bound fibronectin with pronase, followed by extensive washing, results in 25% retention of radioactivity on the column. Densitometry of gels stained with Coomassie blue provides a similar figure of 21% remaining in the 50K band. Therefore, from the original fibronectin applied to the column, approximately 21% of the molecule is recovered in the 50K fragment. If the molecular weight of fibronectin is assymed to be 240K on SDS gels, there is 1.0 heparin-binding site per fibronectin molecule.

Mapping of Sites on Fibronectin

Figure 16 summarizes our data concerning the fibronectin fragments, and Figure 17 presents a tentative scheme for the organization of these active sites of fibronectin. The

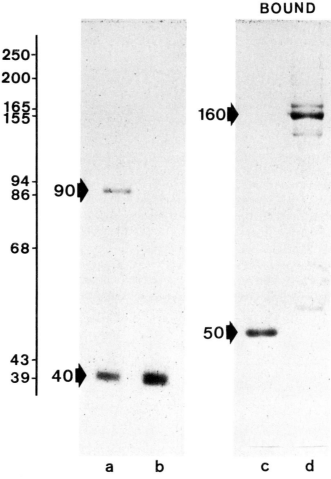

Fig. 15. Heparin-binding fragments of fibronectin. Chick cellular fibronectin (250 μg) was permitted to bind to 1-ml columns of heparin-Sepharose, then digested with pronase (a, c) or chymotrypsin (b, d) at 6 μg/ml for 1 h at 23°C. Nonbound material was eluted (a, b); then after extensive washing the materials remaining bound were eluted with 2% SDS (c, d). All samples were brought to 2% in SDS, then analyzed on a 4%/7.5% polyacrylamide-SDS gel and stained for protein with Coomassie blue.

intact fibronectin molecule is composed of multiple subunits linked by interchain disulfide bonds that are confined to one end of each subunit of 220,000–240,000 daltons. Although it has been suggested that these disulfide bonds are at the carboxyl terminus, in analogy with the reported organization of plasma fibronectin (see refs. 31, 37–39; but see ref. 40), this assignment must be considered entirely tentative until N-terminal determinations have been performed on fragments from this form of fibronectin. Cleavage at a highly protease-sensitive site near these disulfides creates a 205K fragment that still retains the cell surface interaction site(s) for cell spreading, attachment to collagen, and hemagglutination. This fragment also still retains collagen-binding and heparin-binding sites.

Further cleavage with chymotrypsin or pronase generates the 40K collagen-binding fragment, which is now devoid of cell surface- and heparin-binding sites. These sites are found in the 160K chymotryptic fragment, which can still mediate cell spreading and has weak hemagglutinating activity. However, it has lost the ability to mediate attachment of cells to collagen. The relative order of the 160K and 40K fragments seems to be as indicated in Figure 17, according to preliminary pactamycin mapping experiments. This protein synthesis inhibitor rapidly blocks the initiation of translation. Experiments in which the fibronectin is labeled at various times after blocking initiation, followed by proteolysis of the fibronectin on gelatin affinity columns and determination of specific activity of labeling in various fragments at various times, permit an estimate of which fragment is closer to the amino terminus; the 160K fragment appears to be the closest. The 50K heparin-binding fragment can be generated by pronase digestion of the 160K fragment; the functional activity of the 90K fragment has not yet been examined.

Functional Consequences of Active Sites

Figure 18 presents a speculative model of fibronectin organization. This adhesive molecule can be envisioned as consisting of domains of polypeptide structure connected by flexible, unfolded polypeptide strands. The flexible regions can account for the highly asymmetric, floppy overall structure of the molecule [8, 30], and they are susceptible to proteolysis. The structural domains defined by proteolysis experiments appear to contain active sites, and these include specific collagen-, cell surface-, and heparin-binding sites.

Adhesive or binding interactions between cells and extracellular macromolecules such as collagen or glycosaminoglycans can be explained in terms of combinations of appropriate active sites. One prediction of this model is that cell-substratum interactions

	240	205	40	160	50
Multimeric	+	–	–	–	–
Collagen binding	+	+	+	–	–
Heparin binding	+	+	–	+	+
Cell attachment to collagen	+	+	–	–	ND
Cell spreading	+	+	–	+	ND
Hemagglutination	+	(+)	–	(+)	ND

Fig. 16. Summary of results of analyses of fibronectin proteolytic fragments compared to the intact molecule. See text for documentation.

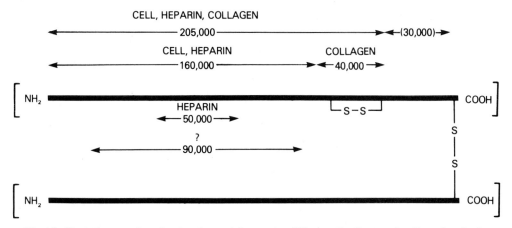

Fig. 17. Tentative mapping of active sites and fragments of fibronectin. See text for discussion. Both amino and carboxyl termini are blocked. The 30,000 dalton region containing the interchain disulfide bonds is cleaved by proteases. It is indicated by parentheses because it is placed at the carboxyl terminus only by analogy with the organization of bovine plasma fibronectin [37], and because chick cellular fibronectin is different from bovine and human plasma fibronectins in that an intact 30K fragment cannot be recovered readily.

INTERACTIONS OF FIBRONECTIN

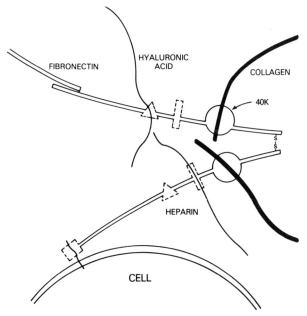

Fig. 18. Speculative summary of the interactions of fibronectin mediated by specific domains. Such domains appear to include cell surface-, collagen-, heparin-, and hyaluronic acid-binding, and fibronectin self-binding regions. The arrangement of sites is arbitrary; eg, the cell surface and self-association sites are not meant to be in the same domain.

might require only the monomer of fibronectin. This notion is supported by the finding of nearly full activity of the 250K fragment in cell attachment to collagen and in cell spreading. On the other hand, cell-cell adhesion should require at least a dimer to permit the attachment of one cell to another. Hemagglutinating activity of the monomeric 205K fragment is decreased by 90% compared to the intact molecule. The residual 10% activity may be due to noncovalent fibronectin-fibronectin interactions between monomeric 205K fragments attached to adjacent cells, since cellular fibronectin is known to possess strong noncovalent aggregating properties at neutral pH.

One other consequence of this model should be emphasized. When fibronectin is secreted into extracellular spaces, it should still be capable of binding both collagen and glycosaminoglycans. Fibronectin may therefore help to organize such macromolecules present in extracellular spaces and in basement membranes into extended collagen-hyaluronic acid or collagen-proteoglycan matrices.

In conclusion, fibronectin appears to act as an adhesive molecule involved in a wide variety of cellular activities. Its mechanisms of action can now be analyzed at the molecular level in terms of combinations of a remarkable variety of specific active sites that can be isolated for study. This approach should help to simplify studies of several complex biologic events by permitting analysis at the level of individual binding reactions, which are more amenable to characterization by conventional biochemical and biophysical techniques.

ACKNOWLEDGMENTS

We thank Dorothy W. Kennedy for valuable assistance and Robert M. Pratt for productive collaborations.

REFERENCES

1. Yamada KM, Olden K: Nature 275:179, 1978.
2. Hynes RO: Biochim Biophys Acta 45:73, 1976.
3. Yamada KM, Yamada SS, Pastan I: Proc Natl Acad Sci USA 73:1217, 1976.
4. Willingham MC, Yamada KM, Yamada SS, Pouyssegur J, Pastan I: Cell 10:375, 1977.
5. Ali IU, Mautner VM, Lanza R, Hynes RO: Cell 11:115, 1977.
6. Yamada KM: J Cell Biol 78:520, 1978.
7. Pouyssegur J, Willingham MC, Pastan I: Proc Natl Acad Sci USA 74:243, 1977.
8. Yamada KM, Schlesinger DH, Kennedy DW, Pastan I: Biochemistry 16:5552, 1977.
9. Yamada KM, Kennedy DW: J Cell Biol 80:492, 1979.
10. Laemmli UK: Nature 227:680, 1970.
11. Studier FW: J Mol Biol 79:237, 1973.
12. Olden K, Yamada KM: Cell 11:957, 1977.
13. Yamada KM, Yamada SS, Pastan I: Proc Natl Acad Sci USA 72:3158, 1975.
14. Grinnell F, Hays DG, Minter D: Exp Cell Res 110:175, 1977.
15. Klebe RJ: Nature 250:248, 1974.
16. Kleinman HK, McGoodwin EB, Rennard SI, Martin GR: Anal Biochem 94:308, 1979.
17. Olden K, Pratt RM, Yamada KM: Proc Natl Acad Sci USA 76:3343, 1979.
18. Ashwell G: Methods Enzymol 3:95, 1957.
19. Olden K, Pratt RM, Yamada KM: Cell 13:461, 1978.
20. Fujikawa K, Thompson AR, Legaz ME, Meyer RG, Davie EW: Biochemistry 12:4938, 1973.
21. Hahn LE, Yamada KM: Proc Natl Acad Sci USA 76:1160, 1979.
22. Hahn LE, Yamada KM: Cell (In press).
23. Ashwell G: Methods Enzymol 8:85, 1966.
24. Grinnell F, Hays DG: Exp Cell Res 116:275, 1978.

25. Yamada KM, Ohanian SH, Pastan I: Cell 9:241, 1976.
26. Mosesson MW, Chen AB, Huseby RM: Biochim Biophys Acta 386:509, 1975.
27. Vuento M, Wrann M, Ruoslahti E: FEBS Lett 82:227, 1977.
28. Carter WG, Fukuda M, Hakomori S: Ann NY Acad Sci 312:160, 1978.
29. Alexander SS, Colonna G, Edelhoch H: J Biol Chem 254:1501, 1979.
30. Alexander SS, Colonna G, Yamada KM, Pastan I, Edelhoch H: J Biol Chem 254:5820, 1978.
31. Balian B, Click EM, Crouch E, Davidson JM, Bornstein P: J Biol Chem 254:1429, 1979.
32. Dessau W, Adelmann BC, Timpl R, Martin GR: Biochem J 169:55, 1978.
33. Engvall E, Ruoslahti E, Miller EJ: J Exp Med 147:1584, 1978.
34. Hahn LE, Yamada KM: Fed Proc 38:798, 1979.
35. Stathakis NE, Mossesson MW: J Clin Invest 60:855, 1977.
36. Hascall VC, Heinegard D: J Biol Chem 249:4242, 1974.
37. Iwanaga S, Suzuki K, Hashimoto S: Ann NY Acad Sci 312:56, 1978.
38. Hynes RO, Ali IU, Destree AT, Mautner V, Perkins ME, Senger DR, Wagner DD, Smith KK: Ann NY Acad Sci 312:317, 1978.
39. Yamada KM, Olden K, Pastan I: Ann NY Acad Sci 312:256, 1978.
40. Furie M, Rifkin DB: J Cell Biol 79:54a, 1978.
41. Yamada KM, Kennedy DW, Kimata K, Pratt RM: Submitted for publication.

Molecular Interactions of Fibronectin

Erkki Ruoslahti, Edward G. Hayman, and Eva Engvall

Division of Immunology, City of Hope National Medical Center, Duarte, California 91010

Fibronectin mediates attachment of cells to surfaces *in vitro,* and its abundance in basement membrane structures suggests that it serves a similar function *in vivo.* The cell attachment promoting activity of fibronectin depends on its capacity to interact with a number of other macromolecules. These include collagen, fibrin(ogen), glycosaminoglycans, and as yet unidentified receptors on the surfaces of various mammalian and avian cells and on the surfaces of Staphylococci.

Denatured collagens bind more avidly to fibronectin than the native forms. Of the latter, type III is the most active one. The collagen-binding is inhibited by fibrinogen and vice versa, indicating that the same (or overlapping) binding sites are responsible for the binding of fibronectin to collagen and fibrinogen. The binding site for collagen in fibronectin can be localized in a homogeneous fragment with a molecular weight of 30,000. This binding site is distinct from the one interacting with cell surfaces, since the cell attachment promoting activity is found associated with collagen-nonbinding fragments of fibronectin. These same fragments also bind to Staphylococci, suggesting that the cell surface receptor in these bacteria may be similar to that of eukaryotic cells.

Glycosaminoglycans bind to collagen-fibronectin complexes resulting in a complex more stable to disruption with urea than complexes of any two of the components. This phenomenon may be important in the formation of the fibronectin-containing, adhesive, extracellular matrix, and its significance to the apparent disturbance that many malignant cells have in forming such a matrix in particular, warrants further study.

Key words: fibronectin, collagen, glycosaminoglycans, cell surface, cell attachment

Recent findings implicate the ubiquitous cell surface, tissue, and blood glycoprotein fibronectin [for review see 1, 2] in mediation of adhesion of cells to basement membranes and extracellular matrix. Fibronectin, when attached to the surface of culture dishes through binding to collagen or directly to plastic, strongly promotes attachment and spreading of cells to the surface [3–6]. Immunofluorescence studies have localized fibronectin to connective tissue and in basement membranes in particular [7–9], providing indirect evidence for the assumption that the function of fibronectin is that of a cell attachment protein. The role of fibronectin in cell attachment depends on specific interactions of fibronectin with other macromolecules such as collagens, fibrin(ogen), glycosaminoglycans, and possibly with an as yet unidentified component(s) on cell surfaces. The purpose of this chapter is to review recent information on the characteristics and specificity of these

Supported by grants CA 22108 and CA 16434 from the National Cancer Institute, DHEW.
Received April 9, 1979, accepted April 11, 1979.

molecular interactions and their role in the cell attachment promoting activity of fibronectin.

BINDING OF FIBRONECTIN TO FIBRINOGEN AND COLLAGEN

It has been known for a long time that the plasma form of fibronectin, "cold-insoluble globulin," tends to coprecipitate with fibrinogen in the cold [10]. This depends on a direct binding of fibronectin to fibrinogen, demonstrable by chromatography of fibronectin on Sepharose to which fibrinogen or fibrin monomer is coupled [11, 12]. The binding is not readily demonstrable unless the temperature is lowered. This probably depends on the weakness of the interaction.

Fibronectin also binds to collagen [12–16]. The avidity of this binding is much higher than that to fibrinogen [16]. Denatured collagens are more efficient binders of fibronectin than their native forms. Of the native forms of the different genetic types of collagen, type III is the most active (Table I). Studies with fragments of the individual collagen chains show that binding sites for fibronectin are found in several locations along the polypeptide chain [16], but one particular site may be more active than the others [17]. This site contains the only region cleaved by mammalian collagenase in collagen. In type III collagen, this site is also susceptible to trypsin, suggesting that it has structural features different from those of other collagens. It will be interesting to see whether this relates to the higher activity of native type III collagen in binding of fibronectin and whether this site is the only location to which fibronectin binds in native collagen. Considering the fact that fibronectin is particularly abundant in various basement membranes [7–9], it was somewhat surprising that the collagen(s) containing the AB chains was less active in binding of fibronectin than the interstitial collagens [16] since this collagen presumably is a basement membrane collagen, at least in muscle tissue [18]. This suggests that the binding of fibronectin may be a specialized function type III collagen. In fact, fibronectin in tissues is codistributed with reticulin, connective tissue material which also contains

TABLE I. Relative Activities of Fibrinogen and Different Genetic Types of Collagen in Binding to Fibronectin*

Protein	Concentration required for 50% inhibition of fibronectin to gelatin (μg/ml)
Fibrinogen	> 1,000
Native collagens	
type I	100
type II	100
type III	1
AB	70
Denatured collagens	
type 1	0.15
type II	0.15
type III	0.15
AB	4

*From Engvall et al [16].

type III collagen [9]. The binding of fibronectin to fibrinogen and collagen is apparently mediated by the same (or overlapping) binding sites, since the binding of fibronectin to fibrinogen is inhibited by denatured collagen (gelatin) and vice versa [18]. The biological significance of the weak binding of fibronectin to fibrin(ogen) is not known, but since fibronectin mediates cell attachment, it seems reasonable to assume that fibronectin bound to a fibrin clot would provide an adhesive temporary matrix for cells to grow in. Fibronectin is known to become incorporated in a blood clot, where it is cross-linked to fibrin by the transglutaminase (factor XIII) [19]. The cross-linking could compensate for the weakness of the interaction between fibronectin and fibrin.

INTERACTION OF FIBRONECTIN AND FIBRONECTIN–COLLAGEN COMPLEXES WITH GLYCOSAMINOGLYCANS

Fibronectin has been reported to bind directly to heparin [20], and addition of heparin to plasma brings about precipitation of a complex of heparin, fibrinogen, and fibronectin [20–22]. Recent studies in our laboratory have disclosed a strong binding of heparin and other glycosaminoglycans to fibronectin–collagen (gelatin) complexes. It was found that fibronectin-loaded gelatin-Sepharose bound ^{35}S-heparin. Treatment of fibronectin-loaded gelatin-Sepharose with nonradioactive heparin resulted in a tighter binding of fibronectin in the column, as evidenced by the need for higher concentrations of urea to elute fibronectin from such a column than from a column that was not treated with heparin (Fig. 1). Some, but not all, of the other glycosaminoglycans also are active in interacting with fibronectin–gelatin complexes (Table II). The interaction of heparin, heparin sulfate, and hyaluronic acid with fibronectin–gelatin complexes was confirmed by another assay: The effect of glycosaminoglycans on the

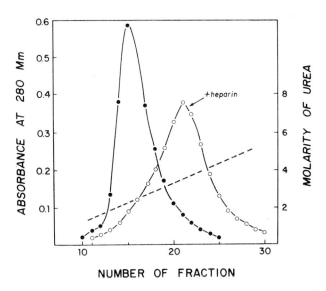

Fig. 1. Effect of heparin on the elution of fibronectin bound to gelatin-Sepharose. Two 5 ml columns of gelatin-Sepharose [13] were loaded with fibronectin from 15 ml plasma and washed with phosphate buffered saline (PBS). A solution of heparin (5 ml 0.5 mg/ml, –○–) or PBS (–●–) was then passed through the column. After washing with PBS, the columns were eluted with a linear gradient (– – –) consisting of 20 ml PBS and 20 ml 8 M urea.

TABLE II. Interaction of Glycosaminoglycans With Fibronectin–Gelatin Complexes*

Glycosaminoglycan	Fibronectin in 4 M urea eluate/ fibronectin in 3 M urea eluate
None	0.34
Heparin	0.94
Heparin sulfate with 17% sulfate	0.75
Heparin sulfate with 9% sulfate	0.37
Hyaluronic acid	0.43
Chondroitin sulfate (A, B, and C)	0.34

*Gelatin-Sepharose columns were loaded with fibronectin and washed. One column volume of glycosaminoglycan solution (0.5 mg/ml) was passed through the columns and, after washing, the columns were eluted with increasing concentrations of urea. The treatment of the columns with active glycosaminoglycans caused elution of fibronectin at higher concentrations of urea [23].

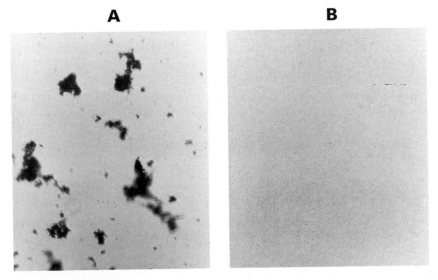

Fig. 2. Agglutination of gelatin-coated polystyrene beads [23] in the presence of fibronectin (200 μl) with (A) and without (B) heparin (50 μg/ml).

agglutination of gelatin-coated beads with fibronectin (Fig. 2). The gelatin-coated beads did not agglutinate in the presence of fibronectin or glycosaminoglycan alone, but did agglutinate in the presence of both. The same glycosaminoglycans–heparin, highly sulfated heparin sulfate, and hyaluronic acid that interacted with fibronectin-loaded gelatin columns — were active in bringing about the agglutination. The agglutination-promoting effect of these glycosaminoglycans was evident between 20 and 200 μg/ml. Larger amounts (> 300 μg/ml) did not support the agglutination [23].

The interaction of glycosaminoglycans with fibronectin–collagen complexes has several important implications to the understanding of the significance of extracellular matrix to the behavior of cells. Cultured transformed cells often, but not always, lack cell layer-associated fibronectin [see 1, 2]. While such cells can produce less fibronectin and collagen than normal cells [24]. the difference is not large enough to account for the lack of surface fibronectin. It will be important to look into the possibility that the defect in transformed cells would be in the quantity or quality of the glycosaminoglycans produced. Transformation-associated changes in glycosaminoglycans have been reported. Particularly interesting in this respect is heparin sulfate, because of its ubiquitous distribution and the fact that it has, in association with fibronectin, been implicated in cell attachment [25]. It is possible that our agglutination assay can be regarded as a model for the formation of extracellular matrix. Based on this model, it seems that the three components, collagen, fibronectin, and glycosaminoglycans, may all be needed for the proper formation of matrix. Furthermore, since different glycosaminoglycans were not equally active in interacting with fibronectin—collagen complexes, both the type of glycosaminoglycans produced and the nature of their postsynthetic modification, could be important in determining the properties and quantity of matrix formed. Determination of the quantity and type of the glycosaminoglycans interacting with fibronectin—collagen complexes in cultures of various normal and transformed cells may provide answers to some of these questions.

Our findings on the relationship of glycosaminoglycans and fibronectin also have important implications with regard to some earlier work on the functional properties of fibronectin. It has been found that cell-derived fibronectin is more active than plasma fibronectin in causing transformed cells to assume normal morphology upon addition of fibronectin [26]. Our results show that glycosaminoglycans (and presumably also proteoglycans) would copurify with fibronectin on gelatin-Sepharose. Since samples from cell cultures would be more likely to contain these substances than plasma, it will be necessary to study whether the observed differences between cellular and plasma fibronectin are due to the presence of different contaminants in the two types of fibronectins. In other studies it has been found that gelatin-coated particles are taken up by slices of liver if fibronectin is present [27]. The uptake requires heparin to be present also. This has been interpreted as enhancement of phagocytosis by fibronectin, and it has been suggested that plasma fibronectin may serve to promote removal of effete tissue (collagen binding) and small blood clots (fibrin binding). Our results show that gelatin-coated particles are agglutinated in the presence of fibronectin and heparin. It will be necessary to show that the uptake of the particles is due to phagocytosis and not simply agglutination of the particles on the liver slices before conclusions can be drawn on the functional significance of the uptake phenomenon.

INTERACTION OF FIBRONECTIN WITH CELL SURFACES AND ITS RELATIONSHIP TO COLLAGEN BINDING

Attachment and spreading of cells to surfaces coated with fibronectin is greatly enhanced compared to surfaces devoid of protein or coated with other proteins [3–6, 17, 28]. This implies an interaction of fibronectin with cell surfaces. The molecular nature of this interaction is unknown. Variant cell lines that show poor attachment to fibronectin-coated surfaces have been described [29]. We have studied the relation of the cell attachment-promoting and collagen-binding activities of fibronectin and have shown that the interactions are independent of one another. Using digestion of fibronectin with trypsin followed by affinity chromatography on gelatin-Sepharose, we have isolated fragments of fibronectin that retain the collagen-binding property of fibronectin [30]. One of the fragments obtained is a 30,000 mol wt glycopeptide that is homogeneous by electrophoretic and N-terminal analysis. The collagen-binding peptides are not active in promoting cell attachment when used to coat culture dishes, whereas such activity is found in the fragments that do not bind to gelatin-Sepharose [31]. These results show that fibronectin has two different kinds of binding sites, one that binds to collagen [and fibrin(ogen)] and one that interacts with cell surfaces.

It has recently been shown in our laboratory that fibronectin also binds to Staphylococci [31]. A specific enrichment of fibronectin is found when plasma is incubated with commercial, fixed Staphylococci, and the bound proteins eluted from the bacteria. [125] I-labeled fibronectin also binds to Staphylococci, and this binding is inhibited by unlabeled fibronectin. We have used this assay to show that the collagen nonbinding peptides are as inhibitory in this assay as whole fibronectin, while the collagen-binding peptides are inactive (Fig. 3). This suggests that the binding to Staphylococci is mediated by the same region in the fibronectin molecule that interacts with cell surfaces. It is possible that Staphylococci possess the same or similar receptors for fibronectin as the one presumably present on the surface of fibroblasts and other cells. Such binding could be of pathogenetic importance for the relationship of Staphylococci to their hosts. If, indeed, the staphylococcal receptor is related to the cell surface receptor, the assay could be useful in the identification and isolation of the receptor in mammalian cells. Such work is now in progress in our laboratory.

In conclusion, fibronectin seems to have a common binding site for collagen and fibrin and another one for an as yet unidentified receptor on the surface of many vertebrate cells and perhaps also on Staphylococci. Glycosaminoglycans stabilize the fibronectin—collagen interaction and possibly also the fibronectin—fibrin interaction. Our current views on the structure—function relationships of fibronectin are presented schematically in Figure 4. Elucidation of the molecular interactions of fibronectin will further under-

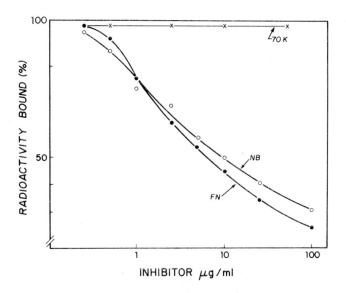

Fig. 3. Inhibition of binding of [125] I-labeled human plasma fibronectin to Staphylococci by unlabeled human plasma fibronectin (FN) and its collagen-binding (70K) and collagen-nonbinding (NB) fragments. The assay was performed using fixed Staphylococci (Pansorbin, Calbiochem) according to Kuusela [31]. The collagen-binding and nonbinding fragmnets have been described [6, 30].

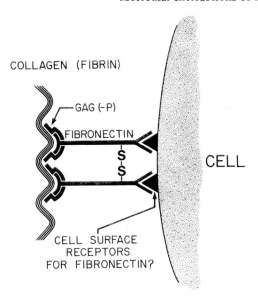

COLLAGEN (FIBRIN)

GAG (-P)

FIBRONECTIN

CELL

CELL SURFACE
RECEPTORS
FOR FIBRONECTIN?

Fig. 4. A model for the molecular interactions of fibronectin as mediator of cell attachment. For discussion of the model, see text. GAG = glycosaminoglycan; P = protein subunit of proteoglycan.

standing of the role of the fibronectin matrix in physiological processes such as various morphogenetic events and of the disturbances of the fibronectin attachment system in malignancy and other disease processes.

ACKNOWLEDGMENTS

We thank Dr. Alfred Linker for the heparin sulfate samples and Aulikki Pekkala for technical assistance. This was supported by grants CA 22108 and CA 16434 from the National Cancer Institute, DHEW.

REFERENCES

1. Vaheri A, Ruoslahti E, Mosher D (eds): Ann NY Acad Sci 312, 1978.
2. Yamada KM, Olden K: Nature 275:179, 1978.
3. Klebe RJ: Nature 250:248, 1974.
4. Pearlstein E: Nature 262:497, 1976.
5. Grinnell F, Minter D: Proc Natl Acad Sci USA 75:4408, 1978.
6. Ruoslahti E, Hayman EG: FEBS Lett 97:221, 1979.
7. Linder E, Vaheri A, Ruoslahti E, Wartiovaara J: J Exp Med 142:41, 1975.
8. Quaroni A, Isselbacher KJ, Ruoslahti E: Proc Natl Acad Sci USA 75:5548, 1978.
9. Stenman S, Vaheri A: J Exp Med 147:1054, 1978.
10. Morrison PR, Edsall JT, Miller SG: J Am Chem Soc 70:3103, 1948.
11. Ruoslahti E, Vaheri A: J Exp Med 141:497, 1975.
12. Stemberger A, Hörmann H: Hoppe-Seylers Z Physiol Chem 357:1003, 1976.
13. Engvall E, Ruoslahti E: Int J Cancer 20:1, 1977.
14. Dessau W, Adelmann BC, Timpl R, Martin GR: Biochem J 169:55, 1978.
15. Jilek F, Hormann H: Hoppe-Seylers Z Physiol Chem 359:247, 1978.
16. Engvall E, Ruoslahti E, Miller EJ: J Exp Med 147:1584, 1978.

17. Kleinman HK, McGoodwin EB, Klebe RJ: Biochem Biophys Res Commun 72:426, 1976.
18. Duance VC, Restall DJ, Beard H, Bourne FJ, Bailey AJ: FEBS Lett 79:248, 1977.
19. Mosher DF: J Biol Chem 250:6614, 1975.
20. Stathakis NE, Mosesson MW: J Clin Invest 60:855, 1977.
21. Fyrand O, Solum NO: Thrombosis Res 8:659, 1976.
22. Matsuda M, Saida T, Hasegawa R: Thrombosis Res 9:541, 1976.
23. Ruoslahti E, Engvall E: (in preparation).
24. Adams SL, Sobel ME, Howard BH, Olden K, Yamada KM, de Crombrugghe B, Pastan I: Proc Natl Acad Sci USA 74:3399, 1977.
25. Culp LA, Rollins BJ, Buniel J, Hitri S: J Cell Biol 79:788, 1978.
26. Yamada KM, Kennedy DW: J Cell Biol 80:492, 1979.
27. Blumenstock F, Weber P, Saba TM: J Biol Chem 252:7156, 1977.
28. Höök M, Rubin K, Oldberg Å, Öbrink B, Vaheri A: Biochem Biophys Res Commun 79:726, 1977.
29. Pena SDJ, Hughes RC: Nature 276:80, 1978.
30. Ruoslahti E, Hayman EG, Kuusela P, Shively JE, Engvall E: J Biol Chem (in press).
31. Kuusela P: Nature 276:718, 1978.

Ascorbate-Induced Fibroblast Cell Matrix: Reaction of Antibodies to Procollagen I and III and Fibronectin in an Axial Periodic Fashion

L. T. Furcht, G. Wendelschafer-Crabb, D. F. Mosher, and J. M. Foidart

Department of Laboratory Medicine and Pathology, University of Minnesota, Minneapolis (L.T.F., G.W.-C.), Department of Medicine, University of Wisconsin Medical School, Madison, Wisconsin (D.F.M.), Laboratory of Developmental Biology and Anomalies, National Institute of Dental Research, Bethesda, Maryland (J.M.F.)

Fibronectin and procollagen types I and III are constituents of the extracellular matrix of human fibroblasts. Ultrastructural immunocytochemistry using the peroxidase anti-peroxidase method showed fibronectin and procollagen antibodies reacting in continuous fashion on 10 nm diameter extracellular fibrils on human fibroblasts. Intracellular localization showed an intense accumulation of procollagen within cells cultured under routine conditions. This accumulation appeared almost as if there were a blockade in secretion of procollagen under routine culture conditions. Cells treated with ascorbic acid do not have the dense intracellular accumulation of procollagens seen with the apparent blockade of secretion in cells cultured under routine conditions. Ascorbate treated cells also have a more pronounced extracellular accumulation of matrix fibronectin and procollagen constituents. At the electronmicroscopic level a new 40 nm diameter fibril is formed after ascorbic acid treatment of human fibroblasts. Antibody to fibronectin and procollagen I and III are seen binding to the 40 nm diameter fibrils in a periodic or stuttered appearance. The fibronectin and procollagen antibodies react with a 70 nm axial repeat along these 40 nm fibrils formed after ascorbate treatment. These studies suggest that under routine culture conditions "precursor" fibrils of fibronectin and procollagen are formed. Ascorbic acid treatment leads to enhanced matrix formation. Ultrastructural studies clearly show antibodies to fibronectin bind to fibronectin on native collagen fibrils formed by human fibroblasts cultured with ascrobic acid. Lastly there is an asymmetric or 70 nm axial periodic distribution of fibronectin along these definitive or mature collagen fibrils formed after ascorbic acid treatment.

Abbreviations: PBS = phosphate-buffered saline; PBS-NSS = phosphate-buffered saline + 1% normal sheep serum; PAP = peroxidase anti-peroxidase complex; RaFN = rabbit antibody to fibronectin; RaProcol I = rabbit antibody to procollagen type I; RaProcol III = rabbit antibody to procollagen type III.

Received May 25, 1979; accepted November 13, 1979.

Key words: fibronectin, collagen, immunoelectronmicroscopy, axial periodicity, ascorbic acid,
            human fibroblasts

The fibroblast cell matrix consists of highly structured glycoproteins, collagen, and proteoglycans. Fibronectin is a 220,000 dalton glycoprotein that is secreted by numerous cultured cells in vitro and is associated with basal lamina in vivo [1–3]. Fibronectin is thought to be important for cell adhesion, especially to collagen [4, and reviewed in 5]. Fibronectin and types I and III collagen and procollagen are major components of the cell matrix of connective tissue cells and occur largely as extracellular fibrils [6–9]. These matrix components also occur in a soluble form secreted into the medium and as a diffusely arranged membrane component [9, 10; additional manuscript in preparation]. Fibronectin interacts with collagen type III more than with type I [11, 12], and specific cyanogen bromide fragments of collagen are responsible for the interaction with fibronectin [13]. Fibronectin is extensively disulfide bonded on the cell surface [14] and is able to be cross-linked to itself and collagen by transglutaminase [15].

Collagen is secreted by fibroblasts cultured in vitro in the form of procollagen [16], and one cell is capable of synthesizing multiple collagens – ie, types I and III [17]. Procollagen has been shown to be a component of the cell matrix by immunofluorescence and biochemical studies [6, 8]. After synthesis, multiple modifications of procollagen occur that lead to the final cross-linked fibrillar structure. For example, procollagen peptidase cleaves nonhelical segments from terminal components of the procollagen chain. Post-translational processing also involves cross-linking following the action of lysyl hydroxylase and prolyl hydroxylase. A number of cofactors have been shown for the latter enzymes, including oxygen [19], iron [20], and ascorbic acid [21, 22].

There has been considerable interest in the possibility that posttranslational prolyl hydroxylation may regulate either procollagen synthesis or secretion. The activity of prolyl hydroxylase changes as a function of cell density or ascorbate treatment [22]. At confluence, when there is the largest accumulation of collagen [23], fibronectin, and fibrils, the activity of prolyl hydroxylase is highest. In certain cases prolyl hydroxylase may be a rate-limiting factor in secretion of procollagen [18, 21, 22, 24].

Cultured fibroblasts are incapable of producing ascorbate, even when derived from species capable of synthesizing vitamin C in vivo and therefore synthesis under-hydroxylated collagen. The lack of vitamin C has been suggested by some to play a role in the altered synthesis and organization of collagen in cells cultured in vitro [21, 22]. Addition of ascorbate causes enhanced synthesis and secretion of collagen in vitro [21, 22]. It would therefore appear that there is a possible interrelationship among cell density, collagen, and fibronectin secretion, ascorbate treatment, and fibrillogenesis. In this paper we report the results of ascorbate treatment on the evolution of the extracellular matrix using intra- and extracellular immunocytochemical localization of fibronectin and procollagen I and III.

METHODS

Cell Culture

Human skin fibroblasts, passage (5–20) were grown in Dulbecco's minimal essential medium with 10% fetal calf serum (DMEM+S) on 60 mm Falcon tissue culture plates or Lab Tek chamber slides as described elsewhere [9]. For ascorbate treatment, upon reaching stationary phase, cells were treated with freshly prepared sodium ascorbate (50 μg/ml) (Sigma) in DMEM+S every other day for seven days, with controls receiving medium changes only.

Antigen and Antibody Purification

Fibronectin was affinity purified from fresh frozen plasma by affinity chromatography on immobilized gelatin [25, 26] with antiserum prepared with affinity purification as described [27, in preparation].

Procollagen type I was purified from dermatosporactic fetal calf skin (kindly provided by Dr. Charles M. LaPière, University of Liège, Belgium), and type III procollagen was purified from fetal calf skin by DEAE cellulose chromatography [28, in preparation]. Purity of the antigens was determined by amino acid analysis and migration of component chains on sodium dodecyl sulfate (SDS) polyacrylamide gels with and without reduction with 2-mercaptoethanol, before and after pepsin digestion [29]. Immunization and specific affinity adsorption to remove cross-contaminating antibodies and final isolation of affinity-purified type-specific procollagen antibody was performed [30, 31; in preparation].

Light Microscopic Immunocytochemical Localization

Samples for light microscopy were grown in 60 mm culture dishes of Lab Tek chamber slides to the desired density and were then fixed with 0.2% glutaraldehyde for 20 min. To render the cells permeable to antibodies without completely disrupting membranes, fixed cells were first dehydrated and then rehydrated in a graded series of ethanol ranging from 10% to 95%, similar to the method of DeMey et al [32]. Once cells were dehydrated they were washed with 0.05 M glycine in phosphate-buffered saline (PBS), and then incubated in PBS with 1% normal sheep serum (PBS-NSS). Cultures were incubated in antibodies (at dilutions determined by previous titration) for 30 min each, with constant rotation. Primary antibodies included affinity-purified RaFN (1/500), affinity-purified RaProcol type I (1/50), affinity-purified RaProcol type III (1:100), and RaFN with the antibodies adsorbed out with affinity-purified fibronectin. The secondary (linking) antibody was goat antirabbit gamma globulin used at 1/500 dilution (Cappel). The detecting antibody complex, peroxidase antiperoxidase (PAP) (Cappel), was used at a 1/1,000 dilution. Cultures were washed and agitated for 30 min before and between antibody steps with PBS-NSS. After PAP incubation, cells were washed with PBS for 30 min and then reacted with 3–3′-diaminobenzidine tetrahydrochloride (DAB) and 0.0025% H_2O_2 in PBS pH 7.6 for 6 min, rendering bound antibody brown via the complexed peroxidase. Cultures on Lab Tek slides were mounted in permount, and cultures in 60 mm dishes were viewed through buffer with an Olympus BH microscope and photographed with an automatic camera system.

Electron Microscopy

For extracellular immunocytochemical localization, cells were treated as described elsewhere [9, 10]. Briefly, cells were grown to desired density and then fixed with 1% glutaraldehyde (Electron Microscopy Sciences) for 20 min at $37°C$. Samples were washed with PBS, treated with 0.05 M glycine (Sigma) in PBS, and then rinsed with PBS + 1% normal sheep serum. Antibody incubations were done for 10 min with agitation following the protocol listed above. After PAP incubation samples were rinsed with PBS and developed with the DAB-H_2O_2 mixture for 6 min, after which samples could be photographed for light microscopy. Samples were then post-fixed with 1% OsO_4 (Polyscience) in PBS for one-half hour at room temperature and embedded in Epon 812 (Pelco). Sixty to eighty nm thin sections were viewed and photographed without heavy metal counterstain with a Philips EM 300 electron microscope operated at 40 kV.

Cells for routine morphological examination were fixed with 1% glutaraldehyde and then 1% OsO_4, embedded, and sectioned as described above. Thin sections were stained with uranyl acetate (aqueous saturated) (Sigma) for 20 min and then with Reynold's lead citrate for 5 min before viewing at 60 kV with a Philips EM 300.

RESULTS

Light Microscopic Localization on Subconfluent Fibroblasts

Immunocytochemical localization of fibronectin, type I procollagen, and type III procollagen after glutaraldehyde fixation and dehydration and rehydration in ethanol yields information on the dynamics of their intracellular synthesis, movement, and secretion, as well as their involvement in the extracellular matrix. In subconfluent cultures of human fibroblasts viewed by bright-field light microscopy, fibronectin is located in the peripheral zones of the cytoplasm in globular foci that appear to run along cytoskeletal structures. At this stage a small amount of extracellular localization in the form of a matrix is seen (Fig. 1A).

Procollagen type I has quite different intracellular localization compared to fibronectin in subconfluent cultures. Rather than being peripherally localized in the cytoplasm, procollagen type I is located in intensely reacting perinuclear granules that do not appear to stream all the way out to the cell margins. Essentially no extracellular distribution of type I procollagen is seen at this point (Fig. 1B).

Procollagen type III has an intracellular distribution quite similar to that of type I in low-density cultures, with the majority of staining being perinuclear. The staining is not as it is for type I procollagen, and some reaction is also localized peripherally near the plasmalemma, with a small amount of extracellular staining in the form of a matrix also present (Fig. 1C).

A fibronectin adsorption control, which is free of staining, demonstrates the specificity of the reaction (Fig. 1D).

Light Microscopy of Post-Confluent Fibroblasts

Cells cultured for one week beyond confluence develop a dense extracellular filamentous matrix of fibronectin (Fig. 2A), type I procollagen (Fig. 2B), and type III procollagen (Fig. 2C). Intracellular staining for fibronectin and type III collagen is diminished (Figs. 2A and C). Matrix formation for type I procollagen, although present, is not as heavily stained as for fibronectin and type III procollagen, suggesting a smaller amount of antigen present. Intracellular perinuclear granules remain heavily stained (Fig. 2B). Adsorption controls are negative (Fig. 2D).

Light Microscopy of Ascorbate-Treated Post-Confluent Fibroblasts

Treatment of confluent cultures with 50 μg/ml ascorbate for 1 week results in no profound changes in the light microscopic localization pattern of either fibronectin (Fig. 3A) or type III procollagen (Fig. 3C). However, it appears that type I procollagen is transported from the perinuclear granules to the exterior of the cells, where it is released into the medium and incorporated extracellularly (Fig. 3B). Adsorption controls are negative (Fig. 3D).

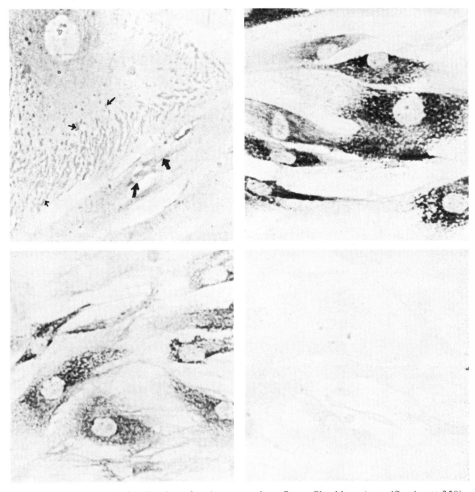

Fig. 1. Light microscopic localization of antigens on subconfluent fibroblasts (magnification × 350). A. Fibronectin localization of well-spread, low-density cells. Intracellular fibronectin staining is compartmentalized in structures near the plasmalemma (small arrows). Some extracellular staining is seen forming a matrix between adjacent cells (large arrows). B. Type I procollagen localization in subconfluent cells reveals a dense packaging of the antigen in perinuclear granules. No extracellular matrix is visualized. C. Type III procollagen localization in subconfluent cultures reveals dense perinuclear staining as well as some extracellular matrix formation. D. Control in which antifibronectin is preadsorbed with fibronectin is free of reaction product.

Electron Microscopy of Post-Confluent Fibroblasts With and Without Ascorbate

Ultrastructural studies on cells grown with and without ascorbate and prepared for extracellular localization of fibronectin, type I procollagen and type III procollagen reveal dramatic changes in the type of fibrils and the distribution of all three antigens on the fibrils.

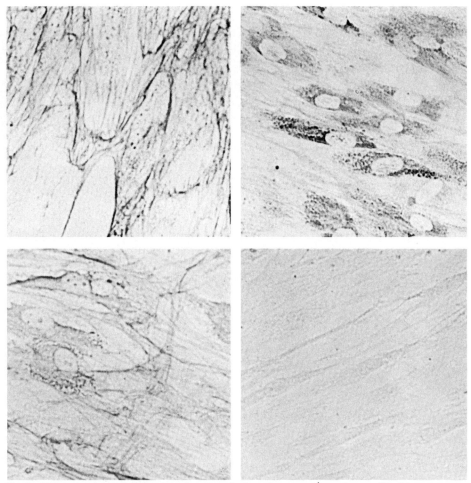

Fig. 2. Light microscopic localization of antigens in 1 week postconfluent human fibroblasts (magnification, × 350). A. Fibronectin forms a dense extracellular matrix, which surrounds cells. Some intracellular staining is seen, but the bulk of the antigen is present in the matrix. B. Type I procollagen is present in perinuclear granules, with little extracellular matrix seen. C. Type III procollagen is present throughout the cytoplasm of the cells, as well as in the extracellular matrix. D. Fibronectin adsorption control is free of staining.

In cultures that are one week postconfluent (no ascorbate treatment) the filaments are approximately 10 nm in diameter, and all three antigens are localized in a nonperiodic fashion on these filaments. In general all filaments are positive for all three antigens, suggesting that fibronectin (Fig. 4), type I procollagen (Fig. 5), and type III procollagen (Fig. 6) are all components of the nonperiodic filaments. Very frequently the filaments form at sites of apparent invagination of the cell, or where cells appear to overlap. Controls are free of reaction product (Fig. 7).

When similar cultures are not treated with antibodies, but are instead stained with uranyl acetate and lead citrate after sectioning, the filaments are nonperiodic and appear to range in diameter from 10–15 nm and course lengths of cells (Fig. 8). The lack of easily recognizable periodicity when sections are stained with heavy metals shows that the

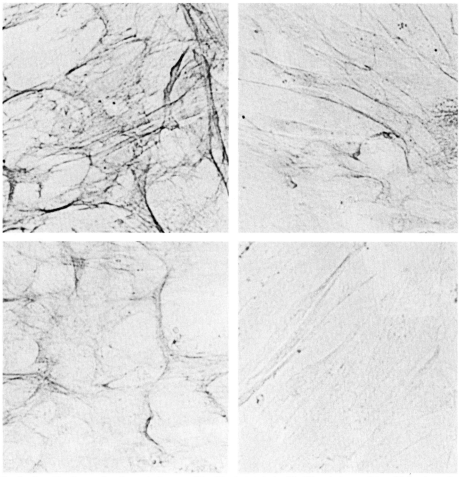

Fig. 3. Localizations of antigens in human fibroblasts treated with 50 µg/ml ascorbic acid for 1 week
after confluence (magnification, × 350). A. Fibronectin localization reveals dense extracellular
matrix with minimal intracellular staining (much as seen in Fig. 2A). B. Type I procollagen is present
in an extracellular matrix, and intracellular staining is greatly diminished as compared with nonascorbate-
treated cultures (Fig. 2B). C. Type III procollagen is present in the extracellular matrix, and intracellular
staining has diminished in comparison with Figure 2C. D. Fibronectin adsorption control is free of
staining.

periodic peroxidase reaction product in antibody studies is related to the periodicity of
antibodies reacting along the fibrils (see below).

In cultures grown to confluence and then treated daily with 50 µg/ml ascorbate for
1 week, a new, larger diameter (40 nm) fibril appears that is distinct from the nonperiodic
thinner filaments. Antibodies to fibronectin, and procollagen I and III react with an axial
periodicity of approximately 70 nm repeat on these larger diameter fibrils (Figs. 9–11),
and antibodies continue to react in a nonperiodic fashion to the smaller diameter
(10 nm filaments. Inserts on figures clearly illustrate the periodicity of the antibody
reaction product. Adsorption controls are free of peroxidase reaction product in ascorbate-
treated cells (Fig. 12).

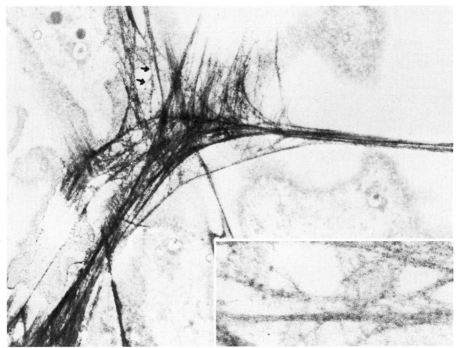

Fig. 4. Electron micrograph of extracellular fibronectin localization on 1 week post-confluent fibroblasts. The extracellular matrix, which stains for fibronectin, is composed of long filaments that course singly or form bundles. Inset is higher magnification of area indicated by arrows (magnification, × 9,900; inset × 29,700).

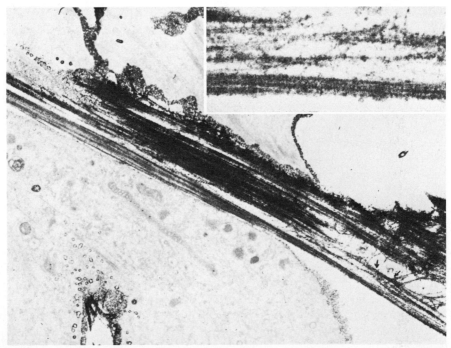

Fig. 5. Electron micrograph of type I procollagen localization on 1 week post-confluence human fibroblasts. The extracellular matrix stains for type I procollagen, much as is seen in Figure 4. Inset is higher magnification of area indicated by arrows (magnification, × 9,900; inset × 29,700).

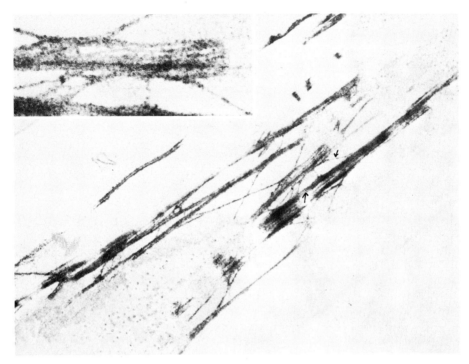

Fig. 6. Electron micrograph of type III procollagen localization on 1 week post-confluent fibroblasts. Staining is very similar to that seen in Figures 4 and 5. Inset is higher magnification of area indicated by arrows (magnification, × 9,900; inset × 29,700).

Fig. 7. Filaments are free of reaction product in electron micrograph of fibronectin adsorption control (magnification, × 9,900).

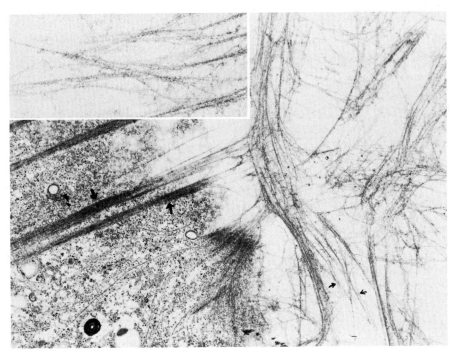

Fig. 8. Electron micrograph of heavy metal-counterstained thin section of 1 week post-confluent fibroblasts reveals ultrastructural morphology of the filaments. The filaments range in diameter from 10–15 nm and often appear juxtaposed with intracellular actin filaments (large arrow). Inset is higher magnification of area indicated by small arrows (magnification, × 9,9000; inset × 29,700).

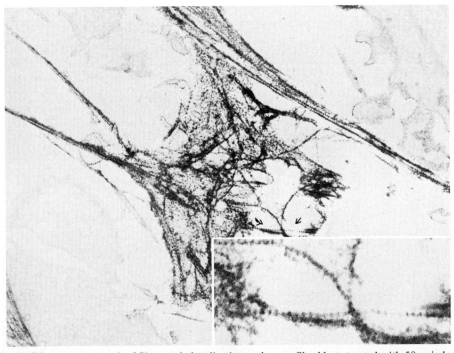

Fig. 9. Electron micrograph of fibronectin localization on human fibroblasts treated with 50 μg/ml ascorbate for 1 week after confluence. Periodic fibrils, which bind to fibronectin antibodies, develop after ascorbate treatment and constitute a large portion of the extracellular matrix. Inset is higher magnification of periodic (40 nm diameter) fibril from area indicated by arrow (magnification, × 9,900; inset × 29,900).

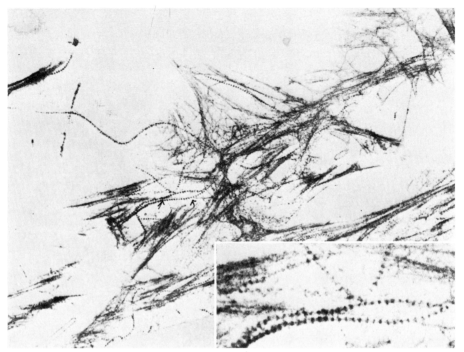

Fig. 10. Type I procollagen localized on ascorbate-treated fibroblasts, visualized by electron microscopy. Many periodic fibrils are present in the matrix, which stains for type I procollagen. The periodic fibrils are thicker (40 nm) than filaments seen in non-ascorbate-treated cultures and often curve throughout the matrix. Inset is higher magnification of periodic fibrils in area indicated by arrows (magnification, X 9,900; inset X 29,700).

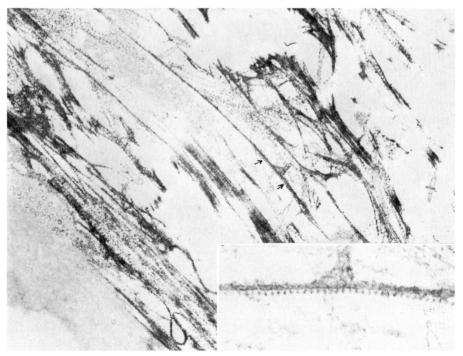

Fig. 11. Type III procollagen also develops periodic fibrils within matrix of ascorbate-treated fibroblasts. The localization pattern is indistinguishable from that seen in Figures 9 and 10. Inset is higher magnification of area indicated by arrows (magnification, X 9,900; inset X 29,700).

Fig. 12. A fibronectin adsorption control of ascorbate-treated fibroblasts is free of staining (magnification, × 9,900).

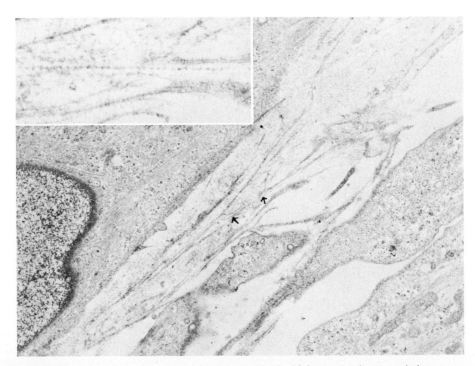

Fig. 13. Thin section of ascorbate-treated fibroblasts stained with heavy metals to reveal ultrastructural morphology. Periodic fibrils, seen in the matrix, are 40–50 nm thick and the 60–70 nm axial periodicity characteristic of mature collagen. Inset is higher magnification of area indicated by arrows (magnification, × 9,900; inset × 29,700).

Ascorbate-treated cells that are counterstained with heavy metals also show 70 nm periodicity in some fibrils which are 40–50 nm in diameter (Fig. 13). But this is generally not seen unless cells are first reacted with antibody. In these cultures there is also apparent periodicity of extracellular material that can not clearly be described as filamentous (Fig. 13). This most likely represents areas where fibrils are forming or are dipping in and out of the thin section. Adsorption of collagen antibodies with fibronectin yielded identical patterns, as seen with affinity-purified collagen antibody alone, suggesting that the collagen antibody reactions were not due to any possibly contaminating fibronectin antibodies.

DISCUSSION

These studies have examined the development of the extracellular matrix and the effects of ascorbic acid on human skin fibroblasts cultured in vitro. The studies used immunocytochemical localization of fibronectin, procollagen I and III intra- and extra-cellularly at the light microscopic level and localization of these same antigens extra-cellularly at the electron microscopic level. At low cell density very little if any cell matrix is seen. As cells increase contact with each other, and more so at confluence, a dense extracellular matrix of fibronectin and procollagen I and III appears. There is a distinct change in the intracellular distribution of these proteins destined to be in the cell matrix as a function of density and ascorbate treatment. At low cell density there are small amounts of fibronectin within cells that appears to be moving out to the periphery of the cell in dense intracellular globules. These seem to be near microfilament regions, and an association of extracellular fibronectin and extracellular actin has been shown by others [33, 34]. As the matrix is being laid down extensively in confluent cultures, not very many cells have this dense globular intracellular fibronectin accumulation.

The intracellular localization of both procollagen I and III is quite distinct from that of fibronectin. In both low and higher density cells, procollagen I and III are located in dense perinuclear areas probably analogous to the endoplasmic reticulum shown in earlier studies [35]. As cell density increases, the matrix forms, and initially more procollagen III relative to procollagen I appears extracellularly on these cells. It appears that, prior to matrix formation, there is possibly a partial block in secretion leading to an intracellular accumulation of procollagen I and III. As the procollagen I or III appears in the extra-cellular matrix, there is correspondingly less of the particular procollagen type intra-cellularly. The apparent partial blockade of secretion is best evidenced by Figure 2B, which shows high-density confluent cultures reacted with procollagen I antibody; signi-ficant intracellular localization is seen, and there is little procollagen I in the matrix at this point. At the same time, considerable fibronectin and procollagen III are seen in the matrix. The disparity between extracellular procollagen I and III could be due to more complete processing of procollagen I to collagen type I than procollagen III to collagen type III. Since the particular antibody we are using (RaProcol I) recognizes specific sites on the amino terminal extension of procollagen that are not present on collagen, less antibody reaction would be seen with a more complete processing of pro-collagen to collagen. This is a potential explanation for seeing less procollagen I than procollagen III in the extracellular matrix at this point.

Electron microscopic studies show that in confluent cultures, nonperiodic fibrils are formed that are composed of fibronectin and procollagen I and III. These filaments are lacy by light microscopy, have a diameter of 10–15 nm, and appear to form at or near the cell surface, sometimes at sites where there is an invagination of the cell. They are similar to fibrils demonstrated by routine heavy metal staining [36] of cultured cells shown by other investigators [23].

The effects of ascorbate are quite dramatic. Very low density logarythmically growing human cells are killed by ascorbate at concentrations (50 $\mu g/ml$) that have no effect on quiescent or near-confluent cultures. At high cell density ascorbate appears to result in the movement of intracellular procollagen I, more than procollagen III, out of cells and an enhanced matrix formation. This is most evident when one compares procollagen I intracellularly at the light level in ascorbate versus control cultures. Most likely one could find cell densities where there is a more profound shift of procollagen III in the presence of ascorbate.

The effects of ascorbate are even more dramatic on the extracellular fibrils. With heavy metal counterstaining, the periodic fibrils induced in ascorbate-treated cultures are significantly larger in diameter (40–50 nm) than the nonperiodic thinner filaments (10 nm) seen in control cultures. Most surprisingly, there is an unequivocal reaction of fibronectin and procollagen I and III antibodies in an axial periodic fashion, with a repeat of approximately 70 nm on the 40–50 nm diameter fibrils in ascorbate-treated cultures. This is precisely analogous to the axial periodicity seen in negative-stained collagen fibrils [reviewed in 37]*.

We refer to these large diameter periodic fibrils as the definitive collagen fibril. This clearly is not artifact, since no such reaction is observed when antibody is absorbed with specific antigen, and since no such reaction is seen in control samples untreated with ascorbate. Additionally, if one were to argue that we are simply adding more protein around the fibril that leads to the staining, it should be noted that 1) samples for immunocytochemical localization are not stained with heavy metals, only with osmium tetroxide, which leads to the perioxidase coupled antibody reaction product to become electron dense, and 2) there are routinely many more bands seen in positive heavy metal-stained collagen fibrils formed from isolated components or in vivo [23, 36]. Based on this, it is clear that the antibodies to fibronectin and procollagen I and III are reacting to antigenic determinants arranged with axial periodicity along the fibril. This apparent periodicity (approximately 70 nm) is reminiscent of the ¼ to ¾ staggered arrangement of independent collagen molecules within the microfibril [reviewed in 37]. Perhaps relative to this, studies have shown that there is a particular cyanogen bromide fragment, CB7, of the alpha$_1$ (I) chain that reacts with fibronectin [13]. Also, there is a characteristic proeolytic fragment of fibronectin with a molecular weight of 42,000 that binds collagen [38]. In sum, there is documented biochemical segregation of the fibronectin-collagen interaction, and we appear to be demonstrating a type of segregation of fibronectin and procollagen antigenic determinants along the definitive collagen fibril by immunocytochemical techniques. We have also observed that extended culture of fibroblasts for 4–8 weeks or more in the absence of ascorbate leads to the development of the definitive collagen fibril, which has an axial periodic arrangement of fibronectin and procollagen type I antigenic determinants along its length [Furcht et al, in preparation].

These studies suggest that in human fibroblasts precursor filaments are formed at early confluence, and that they are nonperiodic filaments composed of at least fibronectin, procollagen III, and procollagen I. By inference these must all codistribute, because when we react any of the affinity-purified antibodies — fibronectin, procollagen I, or procollagen

---

*Recently we have observed a periodic reaction of antibodies to helical determinants of collagen types I and III similar to that shown using the procollagen antibodies with specificities for the amino terminal extensions [Furcht, Wendelschafer-Crabb, Mosher, and Foidart, in preparation].

III — we see that for any given antibody all of the fibrils seen ultrastructurally react positively. Since these are all specific reactions, it would imply that there is codistribution along the nonperiodic filaments. Under the influence of ascorbate or very extended time in culture (4–8 weeks) [Furcht et al, in preparation], definitive collagen and fibronectin fibrils are formed. Importantly, these definitive collagen fibrils have an assymetric organization of fibronectin and procollagen types I and III, as evidenced by periodic reaction products of the antibodies.

REFERENCES

1. Hynes RO: Biochim Biophys Acta 458:73, 1976.
2. Vaheri A, Mosher DF: Biochim Biophys Acta 516:1, 1978.
3. Yamada KM, Olden K: Nature 275:179, 1978.
4. Klebe RJ: Nature 250:248, 1974.
5. Grinnell F: Int Rev Cytol 53:65, 1978.
6. Bornstein P, Ash JF: Proc Natl Acad Sci USA 74:2480, 1977.
7. Hedman K, Vaheri A, Wartiovaara J: J Cell Biol 76:748, 1978.
8. Vaheri A, Kurkinen M, Lehto VP, Linder E, Timpl R: Proc Natl Acad Sci USA 75:4944, 1978.
9. Furcht LT, Mosher DF, Wendelschafer-Crabb G: Cell 13:262, 1978.
10. Furcht LT, Mosher DF, Wendelschafer-Crabb G: Cancer Res 38:4616, 1978.
11. Jilek F, Hörmann H: Hoppe Seylers Z Physol Chem 359:247, 1978.
12. Engvall E, Ruoslahti E, Miller EJ: J Exp Med 147:1584, 1978.
13. Kleinman HK, McGoodwin ER, Martin GR, Klebe RJ, Fietzek PP, Woolley DE: J Biol Chem 253:5642, 1978.
14. Hynes RO, Destree A: Proc Natl Acad Sci USA 74:2855, 1977.
15. Mosher DF: J Biol Chem 250:6614, 1975.
16. Bornstein P: Ann Rev Biochem 43:567, 1974.
17. Gay S, Martin G, Miller EJ, Timpl R, Kuhn K: Proc Natl Acad Sci USA 73:4037, 1976.
18. Prockop DJ, Berg RA, Kivirikko KI, Uitto J: In Ramachandran GN, Reddi AH (eds): "Biochemistry of Collagen." New York: Plenum, 1976, pp 163–273.
19. Uitto J, Prokop DJ: Biopolymers 13:4586, 1974.
20. Juva K, Prokop D, Cooper GN, Lash J: Science 152:92, 1966.
21. Peterkofsky B: Biochem Biophys Res Commun 49:1343, 1972.
22. Peterkofsky B: Arch of Biochem and Biophys 152:318, 1972.
23. Goldberg G, Green H: J Cell Biol 22:225, 1964.
24. Switzer BR, Summer GK: J Nutrition 102:721, 1972.
25. Engvall E, Ruoslahti E: Int J Cancer 20:1, 1977.
26. Dessau W, Jilek F, Adelmann BC, Hörmann H: Biochim Biophys Acta 533:227, 1978.
27. Furcht LT, Mosher DF, Wendelschafer-Crabb G, Woodbridge P, Foidart JM: Nature 277:393, 1979.
28. Smith BD, Byers PH, Martin G: Proc Natl Acad Sci USA 69:3260, 1972.
29. Furthmayer H, Timpl R: Anal Biochem 41:510, 1971.
30. Foidart JM, Abe S, Martin GR, Zizic TM, Barnet EV, Lawley TJ, Katz SI: N Engl J Med 299:1203, 1978.
31. Timpl R In Ramachandran GN, Reddi AH (eds): "Biochemistry of Collagen." New York: Plenum, 1976.
32. DeMey J, Hoekeke J, DeBander M, Guens G, Joniau M: Nature 264:273, 1976.
33. Hynes RO, Destree AT: Cell 15:875, 1978.
34. Singer II: Cell 16:675.
35. Olson BP, Prokop DJ: Proc Natl Acad Sci USA 71:2033, 1974.
36. Bruns RR, Gross J: Biopolymers 13:931, 1976.
37. Miller A: In Ramachandran GN, Reddi AH (eds): "Biochemistry of Collagen." New York: Plenum, 1976, pp 85–136.
38. Ruoslahti E, Hayman EG, Kuusela P, Shively JE, Engvall E: J Biol Chem 254:6054, 1979
39. Balian G, Click EM, Crouch E, Davidson JM, Bornstein P: J Biol Chem 254:1429, 1979.

Tumor Cell Surfaces and Malignancy 845–855 (1980)

Transglutaminase and ε- (γ-Glutamyl) Lysine Isopeptide Bonds in Eukaryotic Cells

Paul J. Birckbichler and M.K. Patterson, Jr.

Biomedical Division, The Samuel Roberts Noble Foundation, Inc., Ardmore, Oklahoma 73401

Transglutaminase activity was reduced in malignant hepatoma, virus-transformed human and hamster cells, and chemically transformed mouse cells when compared to normal counterparts. The reduction in enzyme activity reflected the presence of fewer transglutaminase molecules in transformed cells. Greater amounts of the enzyme activity were particulate-associated in confluent and arrested normal human cells. Indirect immunofluorescence studies with antibody to cellular transglutaminase demonstrated the presence of transglutaminase in Triton X-100-insoluble material. A parallel between pericellular fibronectin and transglutaminase (TGase) was demonstrated. Normal human and mouse cells that elicited contact inhibition of growth and had the high TGase activity also had more ε-(γ-glutamyl) lysine isopeptide bonds than transformed counterparts. Similarly nonproliferating human cells had higher transglutaminase activity and isopeptide levels than did proliferating populations. These results suggest that isopeptide bond formation stabilizes the cell membrane and contributes to a nonproliferating state. Inhibition of isopeptide formation should therefore lead to a mitogenic response. Preliminary results support such a relationship. A model depicting control of isopeptide formation at either enzyme or substrate level is presented.

Key words: transglutaminase, isopeptide, fibronectin, cytoskeleton, proliferation

The enzyme transglutaminase (TGase) and its product, the isopeptide ε-(γ-glutamyl) lysine, have drawn considerable attention during the past two decades. Both have been the subject of recent reviews [1–3]. The purpose of this article is to elaborate on the occurrence and possible biologic role of cellular TGase and its product, ε-(γ-glutamyl) lysine isopeptides, in eukaryotic cells. Emphasis will be placed on our work using normal and transformed cells, particularly the human embryonic lung system maintained in cell culture.

Transglutaminase catalyzes a Ca^{2+}-dependent acyl transfer reaction between peptide-bound glutaminyl moieties and various primary amines producing new γ-amide bonds of glutamic acid and ammonia [4]. When the primary amine is the ε-amino group of peptide-

Received April 23, 1979; accepted November 9, 1979.

bound lysine, inter- and/or intramolecular ϵ-(γ-glutamyl) lysine crosslinks are produced. While TGase and ϵ-(γ-glutamyl) lysine isopeptides have been localized in a variety of materials [5–27], a definitive role for either in cells is still unclear.

We initially became interested in this area with the report that stabilization of fibrin clots was the result of TGase-catalyzed formation of isopeptide bonds [5–7]. Subsequently we showed that proteolytic digests of proteins from plasma membrane and endoplasmic reticulum membranes of mouse L cells possessed ϵ-(γ-glutamyl) lysine bonds [10]. Since many properties that distinguish malignant and normal cells are mediated at the cell surface [28], we began an investigation to ascertain if differences in TGase and/or isopeptide crosslinks might explain some of the differential properties of these cells.

MATERIALS AND METHODS

Details concerning cells [24] and procedures for cell culture [24], cell enumeration [24], isopeptide analysis [13], and protein determination [24] have been described. Cystamine (Sigma) when added to cultures was incorporated into the medium.

Cells were washed three times with cold (4°C) balanced salt solution (116 mM NaCl, 5.4 mM KCl, 1 mM NaH_2PO_4, 0.8 mM $MgSO_4$, 26 mM $NaHCO_3$, pH 7.4), scraped lightly into 5 ml cold (4°C) calcium-free homogenization buffer (250 mM sucrose, 0.2 mM $MgSO_4$, 5 mM Tris-HCl, pH 7.4), and homogenized with a mechanically driven Potter-Elvehjem homogenizer. Where appropriate, the homogenate was centrifuged at 105,000 g for 1 h. In some instances the washed cells (still attached to the flask) were extracted with 5 ml of calcium-free homogenization buffer containing 0.5% (v/v) Triton X-100 for 10 min at room temperature. The liquid was removed and the residue scraped into 3 ml of calcium-free homogenization buffer.

TGase activity was determined by measuring the amount of 0.5 mM, 1,4-^{14}C-putrescine (0.7 μCi/μmole) that was incorporated into trichloroacetic acid-insoluble material following incubation of cell preparation and exogenous substrate [24]. A unit of enzyme activity is defined as the nanomoles of putrescine incorporated per hour with 10 mg of casein as acceptor. Specific activity is expressed as units per milligram protein.

Cells for immunofluorescence studies were grown on coverslips (10.5 × 35 mm). The coverslips were removed, washed three times with phosphate-buffered saline (137 mM NaCl, 2.7 mM KCl, 8 mM Na_2HPO_4, 1 mM KH_2PO_4, pH 7.4), fixed with 3.5% formaldehyde (20 min, 20°) and acetone (20 min, −20°). In some instances washed cultures were incubated for 10 min at room temperature with phosphate-buffered saline containing 0.5% (v/v) Triton X-100, the liquid was removed, and the residue was washed prior to fixation. The fixed material was then incubated with nonimmune rabbit or rabbit anti-guinea pig liver trans-glutaminase serum (1:10 dilution) and stained with fluorescein-conjugated goat anti-rabbit IgG (Cappel Labs, 1/10 dilution). The stained coverslips were examined with a Leitz fluorescence microscope using transmitted dark field illumination and a 54 × objective. Photographs were taken on Kodak Tri X-pan film using an exposure time of 1 min.

Antiserum to guinea pig liver transglutaminase purified to homogeneity [24] was produced by injection of female rabbits at multiple sites with 0.5 mg transglutaminase on five separate occasions 14 days apart.

The proliferative capactiy of the culture was examined by determining the ^{3}H-thymidine that was incorporated into trichloroacetic acid-insoluble material at various times following subculture. ^{3}H-thymidine (New England Nuclear, 50 Ci/mmole) was added to the culture medium at a final level of 0.1 μCi/ml. After incubation for 1 h at

37°, the liquid was removed and the cell layer washed with phosphate-buffered saline containing 4 mM thymidine. The cell layer was extracted for 30 min at room temperature with 10% trichloroacetic acid, the liquid was removed, and the residue was extracted again with 10% trichloroacetic acid for 1 h at 4°. The residue was dissolved in 0.5 N NaOH by incubation for 2 h at 37°. Aliquots were taken for liquid scintillation counting and protein determination.

RESULTS AND DISCUSSION

Transglutaminase Activity

Assays of transformed cells had lower TGase activity than normal counterparts [23, 24]. The systems included primary (3'-methyl-4-dimethylaminoazobenzene induced) and serially propagated (Novikoff) rat hepatoma, virus-transformed human (WI-38 VA13A) and hamster (PyBHK-21/C13) cells, and chemically transformed mouse (C3H 10T1/2 CL8 MCA CL15) cells. Mixing experiments have previously shown that free molecules endogenous to the homogenate are not responsible for the lower activity [23, 24]. Kinetic studies demonstrated that the affinity of the enzyme for the amine donor putrescine was unchanged following transformation, and the reason for the lower activity was a decrease in the number of active sites in the preparation [23]. Immunofluorescence studies with antibody to guinea pig liver TGase suggested this was probably a result of fewer TGase molecules in the preparation [29].

Recent studies suggest that the method of cell harvest affects the level of TGase activity and distribution of activity found in the human cell. This finding has resulted in a reevaluation of our earlier report [24] on TGase activity and distribution in the human cell and has necessitated development of a revised method for processing cells grown in monolayer culture. This newer procedure eliminates the centrifugation and resuspension steps originally used. In contrast to our previous report of lower TGase activity in preconfluent cultures, the revised method gave similar values for preconfluent (day 3) and confluent (day 7) cultures (Table I). It appears that the differences previously observed between preconfluent and confluent populations in our earlier report reflected the loss of soluble TGase activity from preconfluent cells due to the method of cell collection.

While the lack of a difference in TGase activity between preconfluent and confluent cultures would appear to negate a relationship between growth and TGase activity as previously proposed [24], closer examination has revealed that as the proliferative population decreased, as evidenced by ^{3}H-thymidine incorporation, TGase activity was increasing (Table I). The divergence of the two parameters was enhanced in cultures arrested by low serum medium. Other investigators likewise have established proliferative differences among preconfluent, confluent, and arrested cultures [30, 31].

Perhaps more significant than the apparent increase in TGase activity as cells enter a nonproliferative state was the observation of a differential in TGase distribution (Table I). More of the TGase activity was particle-associated after 7 days in culture. This was demonstrated in cells mechanically disrupted or extracted with Triton X-100. The possible functional significance of this differential distribution will be discussed later.

Transformed WI-38 VA13A cells had lower TGase activity irrespective of the method used for cell harvest. Although distribution studies in the transformed cell are tenuous at best because of the low activity, WI-38 VA13A cells appeared to have the majority of their activity in the cytosol fraction. Analysis of the baby hamster kidney cell system

TABLE I. Transglutaminase Activity, Distribution and Thymidine Incorporation in WI-38 Cells

State	Days after subculture	[³H]-Thymidine incorporation[a]	TGase activity (units/mg protein)	% Activity insoluble Homogenization[b]	% Activity insoluble Extraction[c]
Preconfluent[d]	3	1.0	8.7 ± 1.0^f (6)[g]	6 ± 1 (3)	20 ± 4 (5)
Confluent[d]	7	0.44, 0.31	9.4 ± 0.9 (19)	34 ± 5 (8)	49 ± 3 (4)
Confluent[d]	10	0.34, 0.29	10.0 ± 0.9 (4)	ND[h]	ND
Arrested[e]	10	0.06, 0.06	13.2, 11.2	ND	ND
Arrested[e]	14	0.07	24.5 ± 2.2 (11)	38 ± 5 (8)	49 ± 4 (4)

[a]Day x (dpm/mg protein)/Day 3 (dpm/mg protein).
[b]105,000 × gh residue.
[c]0.5% (v/v) Triton X-100 residue.
[d]Medium = McCoy's CM5a + 10% fetal bovine serum [24].
[e]Medium = McCoy's CM5a + 0.5% fetal bovine serum.
[f]Mean ± SEM.
[g]Number of preparations assayed.
[h]Not determined.

using the revised method confirmed our initial report of a differential in TGase activities between normal and polyoma-transformed baby hamster kidney cells.

As illustrated in Table I, some of the TGase activity resisted solubilization when WI-38 cells were extracted with the nonionic detergent Triton X-100. This detergent had essentially no effect on TGase activity. About 80% of the activity was solubilized in preconfluent, growing cultures while 50% resisted solubilization in confluent and arrested cultures. Indirect immunofluorescence staining with antibody to guinea pig liver TGase confirmed these data. A general intracellular fluorescence was evident when WI-38 cultures were stained for TGase (Fig. 1A,C). When extracted with 0.5% Triton X-100 and then stained, a fluorescent fibrous network was observed in confluent (Fig. 1D) and arrested (Fig. 1F) WI-38 populations, while the fibrous pattern was not observed in preconfluent populations (Fig. 1B). Specificity of the antisera was demonstrated by adsorption with purified guinea pig TGase (Fig. 1E) and the absence of fluorescence when nonimmune serum was used. The antiserum produced one precipitin band by immunodiffusion analysis. Transformed cells showed weak fluorescence (Fig. 2) and did not show significant amounts of activity or fluorescence staining following Triton X-100 extraction. Triton treatment failed to enhance TGase activity in these cells, suggesting that the enzyme was not present in an inaccessible form. The differential in (a) distribution of TGase activity and in (b) immunofluorescent staining with antiserum to TGase between preconfluent growing and confluent or arrested WI-38 cultures suggests the possibility of multiple forms of TGase in these cells. Whether this reflects TGase isozymes or posttranslational modification of a single gene product is presently unknown. The use of monoclonal antibodies would appear to be invaluable in the elucidation of such differences.

Pericellular Fibronectin

Numerous observations suggested that there was an interrelationship between TGase and the pericellular matrix protein fibronectin [32, 33] in WI-38 cells. These included the observation that (a) normal cells had higher TGase activity and more bound fibronectin than

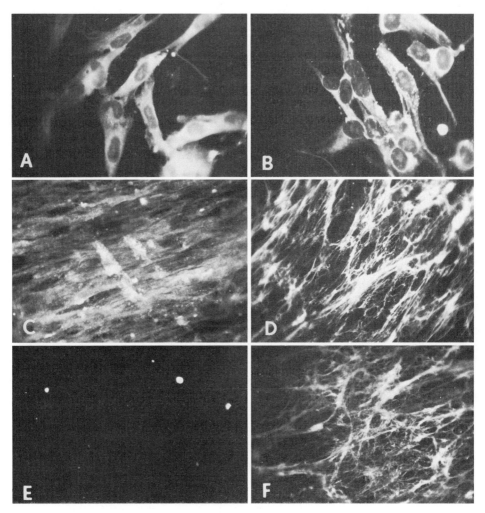

Fig. 1. Transglutaminase immunofluorescence of WI-38 fibroblasts. Coverslip cultures were washed three times with phosphate-buffered saline. The residue was fixed with formaldehyde-acetone, and studied by indirect immunofluorescence with rabbit anti-TGase. In some instances cultures were incubated for 10 min at RT with phosphate-buffered saline that contained 0.5% (v/v) Triton X-100, the liquid was removed, and the residue was washed prior to fixation. A, preconfluent, no Triton X-100; B, preconfluent, Triton X-100; C, confluent, no Triton X-100; D, confluent, Triton X-100; E, arrested, Triton X100, adsorbed with guinea liver pig TGase; F, arrested, Triton X-100.

did transformed counterparts [34, 35]; (b) TGase activity and TGase distribution paralleled pericellular fibronectin (when one was low the other was low; when one was high the other was high); (c) cells treated with trypsin showed no fibrous fibronectin [36] or TGase [29] by immunofluorescence staining but did elicit solubilized and activated particulate TGase activity [24, 29]; (d) fibronectin was a substrate for TGase [37–41].

The latter observation suggested that pericellular fibronectin was linked via TGase-catalyzed isopeptide bonds to the cell, another protein such as collagen, or itself [42]. Attempts to detect such a linkage have been unsuccessful. While polymeric fibronectin

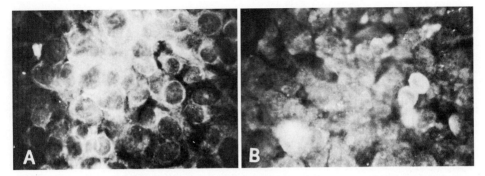

Fig. 2. Transglutaminase immunofluorescence of WI-38 VA13A fibroblasts. Coverslip cultures were washed three times with phosphate-buffered saline. The residue was fixed with formaldehyde-acetone and studied by indirect immunofluorescence. A, confluent, rabbit anti-TGase; B, confluent, rabbit serum.

has been reported in cells [38, 43] and while incubation of WI-38 cultures with activated human plasma Factor XIII led to a selective polymerization of fibronectin [37], apparently via isopeptide crosslink formation, fibronectin as isolated from plasma was devoid of isopeptide [3, 29]. Plasma fibronectin, however, could be polymerized in vitro via isopeptide formation with activated Factor XIII or guinea pig liver TGase [29, 41]. Cellular fibronectin has not to our knowledge been examined for isopeptide bonds. Human and chick fibronectin reportedly are similar to but not identical with plasma fibronectin by several criteria [44]. In our experience incubation of WI-38 cells with 50 μg trypsin for 1 h, which released fibronectin from the cell surface, did not release significant amounts of isopeptide from the cell. Thus if fibronectin is bound to the cell via an isopeptide bond, it would be in a region of the molecule that remains attached to the cell. The existence of such a fragment has been suggested [44]. If plasma fibronectin arises from cellular fibronectin by protease cleavage as suggested, then our findings with trypsin would appear consistent with plasma fibronectin having no isopeptide linkage and a lower molecular weight than cellular fibronectin.

Another possible explanation for the lack of isopeptide in trypsin-released material is the activation of an isopeptidase that directly cleaves the isopeptide bond. While most interactions between fibronectin and the cell surface are thought to occur by disulfide and hydrogen bonding interactions [43, 45], an isopeptide bond could still exist in a portion of the molecule where even disulfide cleavage would leave it attached to the cell.

The possibility of fibronectin being linked to collagen has not been extensively studied although collagen and fibronectin codistribute when examined by immunofluorescence microscopy [46]. Fibronectin has recently been crosslinked to collagen by activated plasma Factor XIII in vitro [47]. Collagen itself has not been found to contain significant levels of isopeptide [P.J. Birckbichler, unpublished observation].

Cellular Isopeptides

The ϵ-(γ-glutamyl) lysine content in proteolytic digests of WI-38 cells was higher than in digests of Simian virus-transformed clones WI-38 VA13A and WI-38 VA13-2RA [13]. Differentials were independent of whether the data were expressed on a per cell, per milligram protein, or per amino acid equivalent. Serum-arrested normal cells had the

TABLE II. Isopeptide Content in Cell Protein[a]

Cell	State[b]	pmole ϵ-(γ-Glutamyl)lysine 10^6 cells
Human		
WI-38	Preconfluent	489 ± 67[c] (11)[d]
	Confluent	641 ± 42 (19)
	Arrested	1,483 ± 148 (15)
WI-38 VA13A	Confluent	34 ± 5 (15)
WI-38 VA13-2RA	Confluent	34, 37
Mouse		
C3H 10T½ CL8	Confluent	201 ± 24 (5)
C3H 10T½ CL8 MCA CL15	Confluent	73 ± 8 (4)
Hamster		
BHK-21/C13	Confluent	55
PyBHK-21/C13	Confluent	62, 72

[a]Digestion procedure [13].
[b]Days after subculture: Preconfluent = 3, Confluent = 7, Arrested = 14.
[c]Mean ± SEM.
[d]Number of preparations assayed.

highest level of isopeptide (Table II). Examination of other paired systems showed that normal mouse embryo cells had more isopeptide bonds than methylcholanthrene-transformed counterparts, but differences were not readily apparent between normal and polyoma-transformed baby hamster kidney cells. In our hands, however, the normal hamster kidney cell did not exhibit contact inhibition of growth, while the normal human and mouse cells did. The normal hamster kidney cell has been reported to produce tumors when inoculated into hamsters [48].

Transformed cells do not appear to acquire the higher isopeptide levels of normal cells following attempts to inhibit growth. While lowering the serum concentration in the medium to 0.1% appeared to increase TGase activity and isopeptide content of WI-38 VA13A cells about twofold, the intrinsic low level of both TGase and isopeptide product in these cells makes this apparent increase questionable. Experiments using synchronous populations might better address this question.

Preliminary fractionation studies show that approximately 70% of the isopeptide in the normal cell sediments at 105,000 g h. This would appear consistent with the concentration of amine acceptor sites (potential isopeptide crosslinks) in the 105,000 g h pellet [24]. As previously mentioned, significant isopeptide was not released from the cell by incubation of confluent or arrested cells with trypsin under conditions that result in pericellular fibronectin removal and activation of TGase activity.

Biologic Role

The presence of TGase in Triton X-100-insoluble material suggests that TGase (a) is a membrane protein, (b) is associated with a membrane protein, (c) is associated with cytoskeletal components, or (d) is associated with pericellular fibronectin. Possibility (a) seems unlikely because of low particulate TGase activity and low immunofluorescence staining with antitransglutaminase antibody in preconfluent proliferating populations. The possibility still exists, however, that upon homogenization TGase is released from the membrane unless anchored by another component. The other three possibilities, separately or in combination, appear more likely. One possible mechanism is that the affinity of TGase for a membrane protein increases as cells become confluent and the fibronectin and cytoskeletal network builds up. Such an interaction could cause the TGase to be associated with the cell surface and possibly even be drawn into the membrane. The lower number of active sites in particle-associated TGase and their exposure by trypsin treatment lend support to such an interaction [24]. This association of TGase with the membrane would bring it into juxtaposition to a protein(s) and enable isopeptide crosslink formation essential for the stabilization of the membrane or extramembrane matrix. Attempts to demonstrate surface or extracellular TGase activity have been unsuccessful. This suggests that external TGase, if present, is not readily accessible to the exogenous reagents. The observation of a fibrous TGase pattern with antitransglutaminase after extraction with Triton X-100 also supports such a contention.

A unique possibility is that TGase is the transmembrane protein suggested by Hynes [49, 50] that links fibronectin on the cell exterior with actin microfilaments on the cell interior. The absence or removal of fibronectin from the cell surface or destruction of actin microfilaments would destroy the complex, perhaps resulting in the release of TGase to the cell cytosol. This complex of actin, transmembrane protein, and fibronectin is more prevalent in the confluent populations [50].

The existence of transmembrane proteins and consequent interactions between external surface proteins and cytoskeletal components have been shown in several systems [51–66]. Preliminary studies in our laboratory showing incorporation of the biologically active amine putrescine into Triton X-100-insoluble protein with consequent blockage of isopeptide bond formation would appear consistent with such a transmembrane interaction.

The higher level of isopeptide bonds in arrested human cells suggests a relationship between isopeptide crosslinks of the cellular architecture and a nonproliferating state. Rice and Green [25] have shown that nonproliferating keratinocytes form an insoluble envelope under the plasma membrane that consists of protein crosslinked by ϵ-(γ-glutamyl) lysine bonds. Thus the TGase activity and isopeptide level may reflect more the proliferation state of these cells than the transformed state, as was first thought. If this is true, inhibition of isopeptide formation would lead to a mitogenic response. One manner in which inhibition can be accomplished is by inactivation of TGase [15, 67]. Preliminary results showed that confluent WI-38 cells had reduced TGase activity concomitant with an increased ^{3}H-thymidine incorporation following 24 hr incubation with 0.01–1 mM cystamine. Within 72 hr the cystamine-treated cultures had more cells, DNA, and protein than untreated cells.

Figure 3 is a diagram of a proposed model designed to incorporate our findings. Under normal proliferating conditions, isopeptide bonds are maintained at a minimal level (A). In reaction 1 as cells cease to proliferate, TGase activity increases, and the cell is stabilized as a result of increased isopeptide bonding (B). Possible control mechanisms for maintaining cellular membrane in a nonrigid state and thereby "divisionable" during mitosis are depicted in reactions 2 and 3. In reaction 2 an increase in a substrate competitor, eg, putrescine, blocks isopeptide formation via production of a nonlysine isopeptide (C). In reaction 3 inhibition of enzyme activity occurs by an endogenous inhibitor, eg, cystamine, or by modulation of the enzyme by intracellular Ca^{2+} concentration (D). Current data do not allow selection of either alternative. The relationship of increased putrescine levels to pro

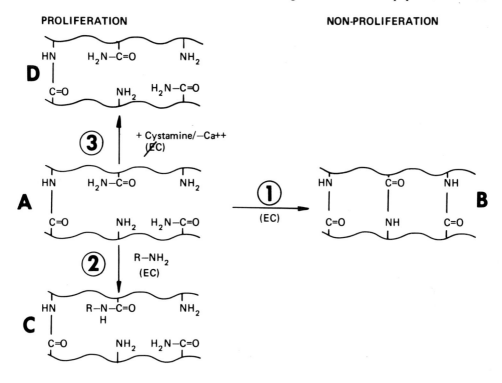

Fig. 3. Model depicting isopeptide control by proliferating and nonproliferating cells. A, lower level of isopeptide under proliferating conditions; B, stabilization of cell by isopeptide formation under nonproliferating conditions; C, maintenance of low isopeptide by control at substrate level. A substrate competitor, eg, putrescine, vies for the carboxamide site producing a nonlysine isopeptide; D, maintenance of low isopeptide by control at enzyme level. Inhibition of enzyme activity by direct inhibition of enzyme, eg, cystamine or low levels of calcium. EC, enzyme complex consisting of transglutaminase with an essential sulfhydryl group and calcium. ĔC, inhibition of the enzyme complex.

liferating tissues is well established [68, 69] and would tend to favor control of isopeptide formation via substrate competition. Transglutaminase-catalyzed incorporation of putrescine into cellular proteins has been reported [23, 24, 70, 71]. The formation of cystamine at the cellular level, however, has not been thoroughly studied and Ca^{2+} flux as a control at the enzyme level is a viable possibility [67, 72–77].

While the emphasis of discussion has centered on control of the system relative to enzyme and amine donor moieties, it should be noted that the conformation of the amine acceptor protein likewise might play a crucial role in any control mechanism [3].

ACKNOWLEDGMENTS

We thank Gerald R. Orr, Engene Conway, Henry A. Carter, Merle D. Maxwell, and Hazel Johnson for their technical assistance.

REFERENCES

1. Folk JE, Chung SI: Adv Enzymol 38:109, 1973.
2. Lorand L, Stenberg P: In Fasman GD (ed): "Handbook of Biochemistry and Molecular Biology. Proteins." Cleveland: CRC Press, 1976, vol 2, p 669.
3. Folk JE, Finlayson JS: Adv Protein Chem 31:1, 1977.
4. Clarke DD, Mycek MJ, Neidle A, Waelsch H: Arch Biochem Biophys 79:338, 1959.
5. Matacic S, Loewy AG: Biochem Biophys Res Commun 30:356, 1968.
6. Lorand L, Rule NG, Ong HH, Furlanetto R, Jacobsen A, Downey J, Oner N, Bruner-Lorand J: Biochemistry 7:1214, 1968.
7. Pisano JJ, Finlayson JS, Peyton MP: Science 160:892, 1968.
8. Harding HWJ, Rogers GE: Biochemistry 10:624, 1971.
9. Williams-Ashman HG, Notides AC, Pabalan SS, Lorand L: Proc Natl Acad Sci USA 69:2322, 1972.
10. Birckbichler PJ, Dowben RM, Matacic S, Loewy AG: Biochim Biophys Acta 291:149, 1973.
11. Abernethy JL, Hill RL, Goldsmith LA: J Biol Chem 252:1837, 1977.
12. Rice RH, Green H: Cell 11:417, 1977.
13. Birckbichler PJ, Carter HA, Orr GR, Conway E, Patterson MK Jr: Biochem Biophys Res Commun 84:232, 1978.
14. Siefring GE, Lorand L: In Kruckenberg WC, Eaton JW, Brewer GJ (eds): "Progress in Clinical and Biological Research." New York: Alan R Liss, 1978, vol 20, p 25.
15. Lorand L, Siefring GE Jr, Lowe-Krentz L: J Supramol Struct 9:427, 1978.
16. Matacic SS, Loewy AG: Biochim Biophys Acta 576:263, 1979.
17. Wajda IJ, Lee JM, Waelsch H: J Neurochem 14:389, 1967.
18. Harding HWJ, Rogers GE: Biochemistry 11:2858, 1972.
19. Lorand L, Shishido R, Parameswaran KN, Stech TL: Biochem Biophys Res Commun 67:1158, 1975.
20. Dutton A, Singer SJ: Proc Natl Acad Sci USA 72:2568, 1975.
21. Goldsmith LA, Martin CM: J Invest Dermatol 64:316, 1975.
22. Buxman MM, Wepper KD: J Invest Dermatol 65:107, 1975.
23. Birckbichler PJ, Orr GR, Patterson MK Jr: Cancer Res 36:2911, 1976.
24. Birckbichler PJ, Orr GR, Conway E, Patterson MK Jr: Cancer Res 37:1340, 1977.
25. Rice RH, Green H: J Cell Biol 76:705, 1978.
26. Novogrodsky A, Quittner S, Rubin AL, Stenzel KH: Proc Natl Acad Sci USA 75:1157, 1978.
27. Plishker MF, Thorpe JM, Goldsmith LA: Arch Biochem Biophys 191:49, 1978.
28. Patterson MK Jr: J Natl Cancer Inst 53:1493, 1974.
29. Birckbichler PJ, Patterson MK Jr: Ann NY Acad Sci 312:354, 1978.
30. Cristofalo VJ, Sharf BB: Exp Cell Res 76:419, 1973.
31. Dell'Orco RT, Mertens JG, Kruse PF Jr: Exp Cell Res 77:356, 1973.
32. Vaheri A, Ruoslahti E, Westermark B, Ponten J: J Exp Med 143:64, 1976.
33. Mosher DF, Saksela O, Keski-Oja J, Vaheri A: J Supramol Struct 6:551, 1977.
34. Hynes RO: Biochim Biophys Acta 458:73, 1976.
35. Vaheri A, Mosher DF: Biochim Biophys Acta 516:1, 1978.
36. Teng NNH, Chen LB: Proc Natl Acad Sci USA 72:413, 1975.
37. Keski-Oja J, Mosher DF, Vaheri A: Cell 9:29, 1976.
38. Keski-Oja J: FEBS Lett 71:325, 1976.
39. Mosher DF: Biochim Biophys Acta 491:205, 1977.
40. Mosher DF: Ann NY Acad Sci 312:38, 1978.
41. Mosher DF: J Biol Chem 250:6614, 1975.
42. Vaheri A, Alitalo K, Hedman K, Keski-Oja J, Kurkinen M, Wartiovaara J: Ann NY Acad Sci 312:343, 1978.
43. McConnell MR, Blumberg PM, Rossow PW: J Biol Chem 253:7522, 1978.
44. Yamada KM, Kennedy DW: J Cell Biol 80:492, 1979.
45. Ali IU, Hynes RO: Biochim Biophys Acta 510:140, 1978.
46. Vaheri A, Kwikinen M, Lehto V, Linder E, Timpl R: Proc Natl Acad Sci USA 75:4944, 1978.
47. Mosher DF, Schad PE, Kleinman HK: J Clin Invest 64:781, 1979.
48. Macpherson I, Stoher M: Virology 16:147, 1962.
49. Hynes RO: Cell 1:147, 1974.
50. Hynes RO, Destree AT: Cell 15:875, 1978.
51. Ji TH, Nicolson GL: Proc Natl Acad Sci USA 71:2212, 1974.

52. Albertini DF, Clark JI: Proc Natl Acad Sci USA 72:4976, 1975.
53. Yu J, Branton D: Proc Natl Acad Sci USA 73:3891, 1976.
54. Nicolson GL: J Supramol Struct 5:65, 1976.
55. Nicolson GL: Biochim Biophys Acta 457:57, 1976.
56. Nicolson GL: Biochim Biophys Acta 458:1, 1976.
57. Ash JF, Singer SJ: Proc Natl Acad Sci USA 73:4575, 1976.
58. Bourguignon LYW, Singer SJ: Proc Natl Acad Sci USA 74:5031, 1977.
59. Ash JF, Louvard D, Singer SJ: Proc Natl Acad Sci USA 74:5584, 1977.
60. Gabbiani G, Chaponnier C, Sumbe A, Vassalli P: Nature 269:697, 1977.
61. Schreiner GF, Fujiwara K, Pollard TD, Unanue ER: J Exp Med 145:1393, 1977.
62. Liu SC, Fairbanks G, Palek J: Biochemistry 16:4066, 1977.
63. Koch GLE, Smith MJ: Nature 273:274, 1978.
64. Flanagan J, Koch GLE: Nature 273:278, 1978.
65. Yahara I, Kahimoto-Sameshima F: Cell 15:251, 1978.
66. Moore PB, Ownby CL, Carraway KL: Exp Cell Res 115:331, 1978.
67. Siefring GE Jr, Apostol AB, Velasco PT, Lorand L: Biochemistry 17:2598, 1978.
68. Russell DH, Durie BGM (eds): Prog Cancer Res Ther 8:1–172, 1978.
69. Jaane J, Poso H, Raina A: Biochim Biophys Acta 473:241, 1978.
70. Schrode J, Folk JE: J Biol Chem 253:4837, 1978.
71. Birckbichler PJ, Orr GR, Carter HA, Patterson MK Jr: Biochem Biophys Res Commun 78:1, 1978.
72. Lorand L, Weissmann LB, Epel DL, Bruner-Lorand J: Proc Natl Acad Sci USA 73:4479, 1976.
73. Anderson DR, Davis JL, Carraway KL: J Biol Chem 252:6617, 1977.
74. King LE Jr, Morrison M: Biochem Biophys Acta 471:162, 1977.
75. Vannucchi S, Del Rosso M, Cella C, Urbano P, Chiarugi V: Biochem J 170:185, 1978.
76. Lessin LS, Kurantsin-Mills J, Wallas C, Weems H: J Supramol Struct 9:537, 1978.
77. Maxfield FR, Willingham MC, Davies PJA, Pastan I: Nature 277:661, 1979.

Tumor Cell Surfaces and Malignancy 857–872 (1980)

Processing of Cell Surface Glycoproteins in Normal and Transformed Fibroblasts

R.J. Ivatt, S.C. Hubbard, and P.W. Robbins

Department of Biology and Center for Cancer Research, Massachusetts Institute of Technology, Cambridge, Massachusetts 02139

I. OVERVIEW: ASSEMBLY OF A LARGE LIPID-LINKED OLIGOSACCHARIDE AND ITS SUBSEQUENT MODIFICATIONS AFTER TRANSFER TO PROTEIN

Changes in the structure of complex carbohydrates at the cell surface, during both differentiation and neoplasia, have emphasized the importance of the correct expression of these components for normal development. The overall picture of the biosynthesis of cell surface glycoproteins has been built up from the results of a large number of investigations (reviewed in references 1–7). However, an understanding of how this expression is regulated requires a more detailed knowledge concerning the mechanism of their synthesis than we have at present.

A major class of cell surface glycoproteins contains oligosaccharide chains linked to asparagine residues via the sugar N-acetylglucosamine. This class can be further subdivided on the basis of composition into high-mannose and complex-type chains (Fig. 1) [5]. In spite of the large difference in composition these two oligosaccharide types share a common pentasaccharide core. In 1977 this laboratory made the unexpected finding [8] that the pentasaccharide cores of complex chains were not derived by the apparently more straightforward sequential addition of five sugars, but rather by extensive degradation of high-mannose chains. This conclusion was also reached by other workers [9, 10]. Since that time it has been a working hypothesis in this laboratory that the controlled degradation of high-mannose structures regulates the availability of core structures for subsequent conversion to complex-type chains and thereby controls the composition of the glycoproteins at the cell surface. The factors that determine whether an oligosaccharide chain should remain as a high-mannose structure or be more extensively processed to form the core structure for a complex chain are both intriguing and of fundamental importance when considering the regulation of glycoprotein assembly.

Asparagine-linked carbohydrates are assembled along the complex multistep pathway outlined in Figure 2. A large mannose-rich oligosaccharide is first assembled as a dolichol-pyrophosphate-linked intermediate in the rough endoplasmic reticulum [6], where it is trans-

Received August 20, 1979; accepted August 20, 1979.

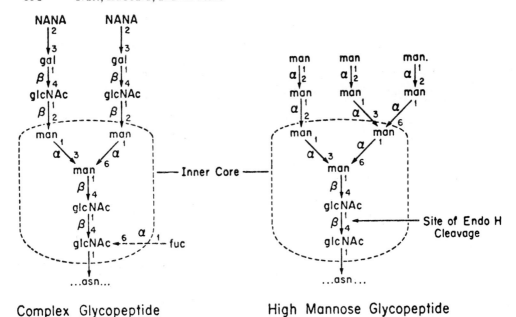

Complex Glycopeptide   High Mannose Glycopeptide

Fig. 1. Representative structures for the complex-type and high-mannose oligosaccharides of glycoproteins. The dashed perimeter encloses the common pentasaccharide core that contains either external mannose residues (usually an additional two to six mannoses) for high-mannose structures or external N-acetylglucosamines, galactoses, and sialic acids for complex-type oligosaccharides. The presence of fucose on the proximal N-acetylglucosamine is unique to complex-type oligosaccharides. Also identified is the site of endo H cleavage of high-mannose oligosaccharides.

ferred en bloc to nascent polypeptide chains [11]. The oligosaccharide at this stage contains extra glucose and mannose residues [12] that are subsequently removed as the glycoproteins migrate through the endoplasmic reticulum to the Golgi apparatus [13, 14]. The extent of this selective removal determines whether the oligosaccharide chains remain as high-mannose structures or are more extensively processed to provide the core structures for complex-type chains. The complex chains are formed by the addition of N-acetylglucosamine, galactose, sialic acid, and fucose to the pentasaccharide core [3, 4]. This group of sugars is incorporated by a family of specific enzymes in the Golgi apparatus and does not appear to involve lipid-linked intermediates [15–18]. In this presentation we will discuss the assembly of the lipid-linked precursor (Section II), its transfer to protein (Section III), and its subsequent modifications (Section IV). The final section describes parallel studies that have compared the processing of cell surface glycoproteins in normal and transformed fibroblasts.

II. ASSEMBLY OF THE MAJOR LIPID-LINKED OLIGOSACCHARIDE

The major lipid-linked oligosaccharide contains three glucose, nine mannose, and two N-acetylglucosamine residues arranged as shown in Figure 3. This arrangement was first reported by Li et al [12] and contains the mannose structure reported by Ito et al [19] for the major type A chain of thyroglobulin. Similar structures for the major oligosaccharide have been described by Spiro et al [20] and Parodi and Leloir [21], but they differ in containing

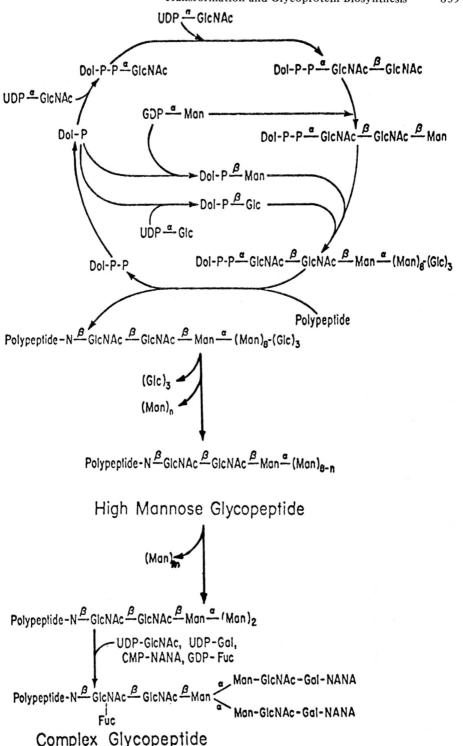

Fig. 2. Scheme for the assembly of the lipid-linked precursor oligosaccharide and its possible fates after transfer to protein. The assembly of the oligosaccharides occurs in the endoplasmic reticulum. Transfer from lipid to protein occurs in the rough endoplasmic reticulum and glucose residues are removed during its migration to the Golgi apparatus. The mannose residues if removed are probably cleaved in the Golgi apparatus. The addition of the N-acetyllactosamine branches and the terminal sugars is by Golgi enzymes.

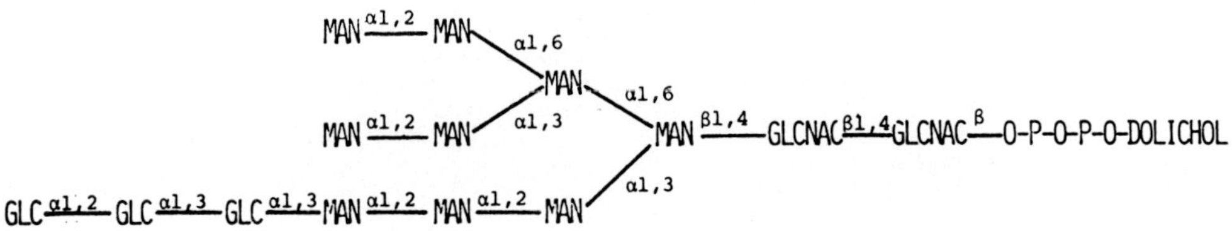

Fig. 3. Structure of the major lipid-linked oligosaccharide precursor [12, 22].

either two glucose and ten mannose or four glucose and nine mannose residues, respectively. It is not clear at this stage whether this reflects different sources of the oligosaccharide or different analytical approaches. The arrangement of the glucose residues reported in Figure 3 for the major oligosaccharide from CHO cells is identical to that determined for Nil 8 cells in this laboratory [22].

We have addressed the synthesis of the lipid-linked oligosaccharide using two complementary approaches. One approach has utilized a microsome preparation from Nil 8 cells which has proved to be a very flexible system for investigating the lipid-linked intermediates in the assembly process. The second approach has studied the products formed when intact Nil 8 cells are labeled in culture. The former system will be referred to as in vitro labeling and the latter system will be referred to as in vivo labeling.

The in vivo system has, in addition to demonstrating the relevance of the in vitro results, provided an appreciation of the kinetics of the assembly pathway and the steady-state levels of the intermediates. The profiles of the lipid-linked oligosaccharides shown in Figure 4 illustrate this point. A 1-min pulse with $[^3H]$ mannose reveals the rapid isotopic labeling of a structure containing five mannose residues and two N-acetylglucosamine residues and the subsequent slower appearance of isotope into larger molecules. A 3-min pulse illustrates the relative levels of these intermediates at steady state and a 10-min pulse followed by a 5-min chase demonstrates the precursor-product relationship of these intermediates and the completed $Glc_3Man_9GlcNAc$ species. Another feature revealed by these labeling patterns is the absence of substantial amounts of a $Man_9GlcNac_2$ structure. From these results one makes the inference that as soon as the $Man_8GlcNac_2$ structure gains the ninth mannose residue, it is rapidly glucosylated.

In a typical experiment with the in vitro system the microsome preparation is preincubated with GDP-mannose and UDP-glucose to complete any partially completed oligosaccharide chains and then is washed with GDP and UDP to remove any unused monosaccharide precursors. If the microsome preparation is then preincubated with UDP-N-acetylglucosamine, a procedure which provides a large number of lipid-linked acceptor sites for mannose, a brief (30 sec) reexposure to $[^{14}C]$ GDP-mannose results in the rapid formation of lipid-linked oligosaccharides containing one to five mannose residues. This ability to collect the small intermediates has allowed the early stages of oligosaccharide assembly to be investigated. At progressively later times of incubation these intermediates are increased, both in amount and in length. After 4 min of incubation the profile of intermediates in the in vitro system resembles that in the in vivo system, with a rapid accumulation of $Man_5GlcNac_2$ and its slower elongation (Fig. 5). The initiated chains can be chased into $Man_9GlcNac_2$ by addition of cold GDP-mannose and then into $Glc_3Man_9GlcNac_2$ by addition of UDP-glucose. The latter species is slowly transferred to endogenous polypeptide

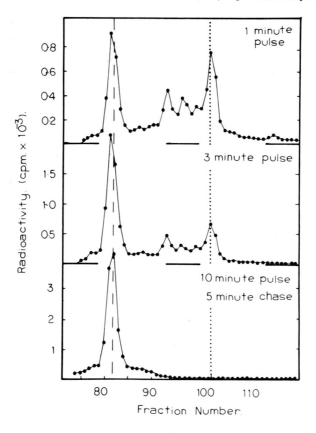

Fig. 4. Metabolism of dolichyl-pyrophosphate oligosaccharides. Intact fibroblasts were labeled for 1 min, 3 min, and 10 min with (2-^{3}H)mannose, and the dolichyl-linked oligosaccharides were examined. The 1-min pulse demonstrates the rapidity with which the smaller oligosaccharides approach isotopic equilibrium. After a 3-min pulse the smaller oligosaccharides have attained their steady distribution (which is very similar to the distribution after a 1-min pulse) and the accumulation of label into the largest species, $Glc_3Man_9GlcNAc_2$, has increased. This species continues to accumulate radiolabel for several more minutes and does not attain isotopic equilibrium until 15 min. The 10-min pulse that was followed by a 5-min chase with unlabeled mannose demonstrates the precursor-product relationship of the smaller oligosaccharides and $Glc_3Man_9GlcNAc_2$. The dashed line identifies the elution position of $Glc_3Man_9GlcNAc_2$ and the dotted line identifies the elution position of $Man_5GlcNAc_2$. The identification of these species was reported previously [11, 22].

chains. The membrane preparation therefore allows, by judicial choice of experimental conditions, all the intermediate species to be acquired in good yield and also allows the addition of glucose and mannose residues to be examined independently. The chemical structures of these intermediately glycosylated species have been examined and the relationship between them suggests the sequential pathway of addition shown in Figure 6.

In contrast to the controversy over the structure of the major lipid-linked oligosaccharide, there is general agreement over the manner of addition of the first three sugar residues. The two N-acetylglucosamine residues are donated by UDP-N-acetylglucosamine [23–25]. A phosphate is transferred with the first sugar to form dolichyl-pyrophosphate-

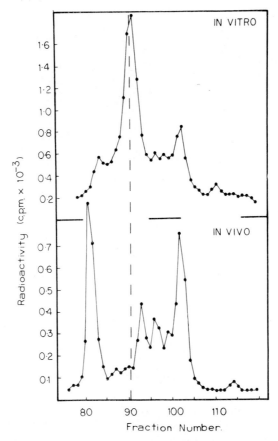

Fig. 5. Comparison of the metabolism of dolichyl-pyrophosphate-oligosaccharides in the in vivo and in vitro model systems. The upper profile illustrates the distribution of the lipid-linked oligosaccharides produced by the microsomal preparation after a 5-min incubation with GDP-[^{14}C] mannose, and the lower profile illustrates the distribution of the lipid-linked oligosaccharides produced by intact fibroblasts after a 1-min incubation with [2-^{3}H] mannose. The microsomal preparation was washed after incubation with UDP to deplete the Dol-P-Glc pool, and therefore the major product is Man$_9$GlcNAc$_2$, identified by the dashed line; however, there are small amounts of larger oligosaccharides, which reflect incomplete removal of Dol-P-Glc, and a spectrum of smaller oligosaccharides (Man$_8$GlcNac$_2$) left incomplete as a result of the depletion of GDP-[^{14}C] mannose by the endogenous GDP-mannose hydrolase activity. The lower profile is described in the legend to Figure 4.

N-acetylglucosamine, to which the second sugar is transferred directly. This disaccharide is the acceptor for all subsequent additions. The β-mannose is also transferred from a nucleotide-sugar, GDP-mannose, to form the trisaccharide β-mannose-di-N-acetylchitobiose [26], referred to as M-K in Figure 6. The subsequent mannose residues have the α-configuration and are transferred with inversion from dolichyl-phosphate-β-mannose. The order of addition is as follows: The Man$_2$GlcNac$_2$ species contains a 1-3 linkage, the Man$_3$GlcNAc$_2$ species is branched, and the fourth and fifth mannoses extend the 1-3 branch. It is an intriguing observation that the Man$_5$GlcNAc$_2$ species already contains the acceptor for the glucose residues but is not glucosylated until the remaining mannoses have been added. The

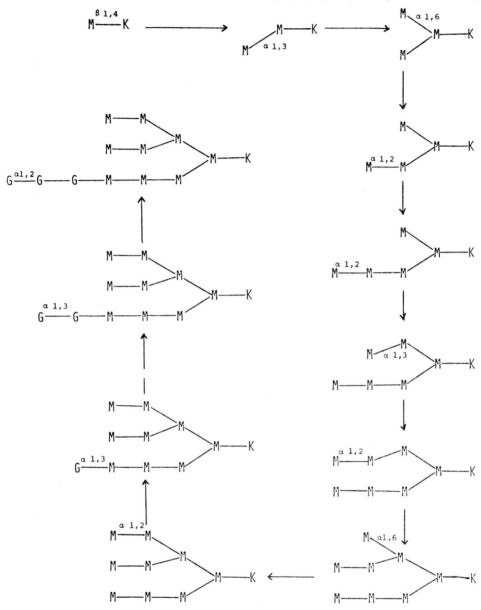

Fig. 6. The pathway for the assembly of the lipid-linked precursor oligosaccharide $Man_2GlcNAc_2$ is resistant to acetolysis and provides $ManGlcNAc_2$ on Smith degradation. $Man_3GlcNAc_2$ provides $Man_2GlcNAc_2$ and free mannose on acetolysis and $ManGlcNAc_2$ on Smith degradation. $Man_4GlcNAc_2$ provides $Man_3GlcNAc_2$ and free mannose on acetolysis and $ManGlcNAc_2$ on Smith degradation. $Man_5GlcNAc_2$ provides $Man_4GlcNAc_2$ and free mannose on acetolysis and $ManGlcNAc_2$ on Smith degradation. $Man_6GlcNAc_2$ provides $Man_4GlcNAc_2$ and a mannose dimer sensitive to β elimination on acetolysis and $Man_2GlcNAc_2$ on Smith degradation. $Man_7GlcNAc_2$ provides $Man_4GlcNAc_2$ and a mannose trimer sensitive to β elimination on acetolysis and $Man_2GlcNAc_2$ on Smith degradation. $Man_8GlcNAc_2$ provides the same products as $Man_7GlcNAc_2$ and in addition free mannose on acetolysis. $Man_9GlcNAc_2$ provides the same products as $Man_7GlcNAc_2$ and in addition a mannose dimer on acetolysis. An identical sequence of additions for the mannose residues has been established for the lipid-linked oligosaccharides in Chinese hamster ovary cells by Chapman and Kornfeld [50].

sixth and seventh mannoses complete the 1-6 branch, and the eight and ninth mannoses form a second -16 branch. The glucoses are added sequentially at this point. The role of the glucose residues and the timing of their addition is discussed in the next section.

III. TRANSFER OF THE OLIGOSACCHARIDE FROM LIPID TO PROTEIN AND ROLE OF THE GLUCOSE RESIDUES

The occurrence of glucose residues on the dolichyl-linked intermediates was initially an embarrassment, as very few glycoproteins have been demonstrated to contain covalently bound glucose. It is a working hypothesis in this laboratory that these glucose residues are a signal for the major transferase which is responsible for transferring the oligosaccharide from dolichyl-pyrophosphate to suitable polypeptides. If, as is currently believed [27], glycosylation of glycoproteins is a cotranslational event, it would require the transferase to scan nascent polypeptide chains as they are translocated into the lumen of the rough endoplasmic reticulum for appropriately located asparagine residues — the general sequences asn-x-ser and asn-x-thr are glycosylated [28]. To scan simultaneously both the polypeptide chains for the appropriate sequence and the oligosaccharide for its completed structure would probably require prohibitively extensive binding sites. The involvement of the glucose residues as a signal for of completeness of the $Man_9 GlcNAc_2$ structure would considerably simplify recognition of completed oligosaccharide chains by the transferase. Three glucose residues on a single branch provide a binding determinant that is simple enough to be readily recognized yet complex enough to be unambiguous. The pathways for the assembly and degradation of the major oligosaccharide presented in this study are consistent with the glucose residues acting as a signal, as they demonstrate that the glucose are the last residues added and the first removed. The role of the glucose residues has been tested in this laboratory [29] by comparing the relative efficiency of transfer, from lipid to protein, of fully glucosylated and unglucosylated $Man_9 GlcNAc_2$ oligosaccharides. The results of simultaneously incubating these two lipid-linked species with membrane preparations from Nil 8 cells containing endogenous polypeptide acceptors demonstrated that the glucosylated $Man_9 GlcNAc_2$ structure is transferred five times more efficiently than the unglycosylated one. This aspect has been confirmed by an alternative approach that observed the structure of the glycopeptide-bound oligosaccharides after a short pulse labeling of intact cells [11]. These studies revealed that the major glycopeptide-bound oligosaccharide after a 1-h labeling period is $Man_9 GlcNAc_2$ but that at earlier time points the glucosylated species was more heavily represented. This result indicates that the species that is actually transferred is fully glucosylated and that subsequently hexose residues are removed from it. After a 1-min pulse there was virtually no unglucosylated material and 80% of the glycopeptide-bound fraction contained at least two glucose residues. There is therefore good experimental evidence for believing that the glucose residues are important for transfer of the lipid-linked oligosaccharide to protein and that, on the basis of the timing of their addition and removal, they provide an important binding determinant/signal for the transferase.

IV. SELECTIVE REMOVAL OF GLUCOSE AND MANNOSE RESIDUES AND SUBSEQUENT ADDITION OF OTHER SUGARS TO THIS CORE

The major oligosaccharide containing three glucose and nine mannose residues is, after transfer to protein, processed so that all of the glucose and up to six of the mannose residues are removed. The extent of removal of the mannose residues determines the availability of the pentasaccharide core structures that can be converted to complex-type chains and thereby controls the composition of the glycoproteins at the cell surface. As a result, the molecular details of processing are of considerable interest, as they should provide some important answers regarding the regulation of glycoprotein biosynthesis.

A. Kinetics of Sugar Removal

The rate of removal of the hexose residues has been investigated by study of the size of the high-mannose chains attached to glycoproteins at various stages of processing [11]. This study has revealed that after a 10-min pulse the bulk of the oligosaccharide chains have lost at least two hexose residues and that with increasing chase times the average size of the chains decreases even further; after two hours the profile resembles that of mature high-mannose structures. However, even after substantially longer periods of time there is very little material containing fewer than five hexose residues. The reason for this absence is discussed in Section IVC; it was revealed by an elegant series of studies from Stuart Kornfeld's laboratory [30] that demonstrate that the $Man_5 GlcNAc_2$ species receive an external N-acetylglucosamine residue before the remaining two mannose residues are removed. Recently, we have isolated and characterized the intermediates in the processing pathway; these studies have demonstrated that the pathway described in the next section is the major route for the sequential removal of sugar residues.

B. Sequence of Sugar Removal

The pathway for the removal of hexose residues begins with the $Glc_3 Man_9 GlcNAc_2$ compound and proceeds to a $Man_5 GlcNAc_2$ compound. In order to determine the order of hexose removal the intermediately glycosylated species in the processing pathway were isolated. Nil-8 cells were cultured in the continuous presence of [^3H] mannose for 24 h. The glycopeptide fraction was obtained by exhaustive pronase digestion of the protein residue left after extraction of the cells with chloroform/methanol 2:1; and chloroform/methanol/water 10:10:3, and then subsequently digested with Endo-H to release the high-mannose chains. These oligosaccharides were isolated by column chromatography and characterized by acetolysis, Smith degradation, and glycohydrolase digestion. The order of removal of the hexose residues, suggested by comparison of the structures of sequentially related compounds, is shown in Figure 7.

The first three residues to be removed are the glucose residues. At the $Hex_9 GlcNac_2$ stage there is less than 5% of the α-mannose residue in a form resistant to α-mannosidase, ie, containing one or more external glucose residues that would block this exoenzyme. Therefore greater than 98% of the glucose residues are removed before the removal of a single mannose residue is detected. The four α 1-2-linked mannose residues are then sequentially removed. First, the residue on the middle branch is removed; then the last-added mannose, which we earlier suggested to be the signal for the attachment of the glucose residues, and finally the two residues on the α 1-3 branch are removed. This pathway is consistent with the high-mannose structures reported by Li and Kornfeld [32] for Chinese hamster ovary cells, yet is different from the pathway inferred from the 1gM glycopeptides characterized by Chapman and Kornfeld [31].

The material characterized during this study was derived from a long continuous labeling experiment, and consequently the bulk of the oligosaccharide chains represent mature high-mannose structures that will not be processed further. The possibility exists that there are two pathways for the processing of high-mannose structures, one of which provides the core regions for complex-type chains and another that produces the various

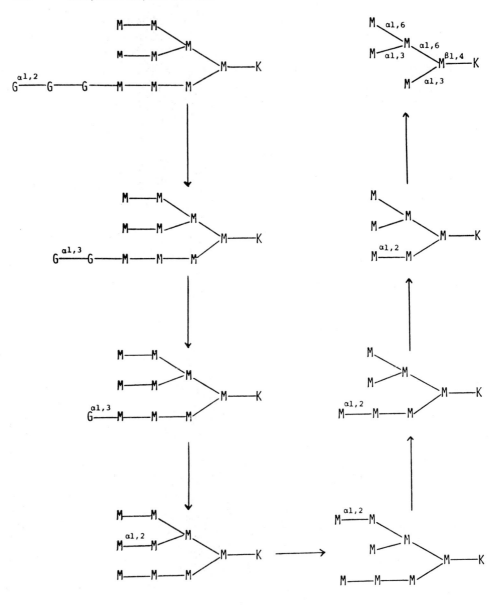

Fig. 7. A possible pathway for the processing of the precursor oligosaccharide after transfer to protein. $Man_9GlcNAc$ loses 95% of the expected α-mannose on α-mannosidase and is substantially uncontaminated with terminal glucose residues. It yields a mannose dimer, a mannose trimer, and $Man_4GlcNAc$ on acetolysis. $Man_8GlcNAc$ yields $Man_4GlcNAc$ and two mannose dimers on acetolysis; one dimer is sensitive to β elimination. $Man_7GlcNAc$ yields free mannose, a mannose dimer, and $Man_4GlcNAc$ on acetolysis. $Man_6GlcNAc$ yields free mannose, a mannose dimer, and $Man_3GlcNAc$ on acetolysis. $Man_5GlcNAc$ yields free mannose, a mannose dimer, and $Man_2GlcNAc$ on acetolysis.

high mannose structures. If there are two pathways, they converge at the $Man_5GlcNAc_2$ stage. An intriguing question, therefore, is: Do the oligosaccharides travel along different processing pathways from the start or does the decision to make complex-type chains occur late, at the $Man_5GlcNAc_2$ stage?

C. Conversion From High Mannose to Complex-Type Chain

The molecular details of the conversion from high-mannose to complex-type chains have been derived from a detailed study of a mutant Chinese hamster ovary cell line 15B. This line has a greatly reduced production of complex-type chains associated with its phenotype and, and, on examination, was found to be deficient in an N-acetylglucosaminyl transferase. The unexpected finding was that the major product was not the $Man_3GlcNAc_2$ core illustrated in Figure 1, but a structure containing five mannose residues! Subsequent examination revealed the sequence outlined in Figure 8. The removal of the remaining two mannose residues is preceded by the addition of an external N-acetylglucosamine residue and the substrate for the final mannohydrolase(s) is this $GlcNAcMan_5GlcNAc_2$ structure. Ironically, the common pentasaccharide core of the high-mannose and complex-type chains is therefore not thought to exist as such without additional mannose or N-acetylglucosamine residues.

D. Completion of the Complex-Type Oligosaccharides

The completion of the complex-type oligosaccharides has been recently reviewed [3, 4], so the purpose of this paragraph is to provide a background for Section V, rather than extensively review this area. The addition of the sugars N-acetylglucosamine, galactose, and sialic acid occurs in the Golgi apparatus [15–18]. The sugars are added one at a time directly from the nucleotide sugar by a family of specific glycosyl transferases. This phase is then in complete contrast to the en bloc transfer of the lipid-linked oligosaccharide that occurs in the rough endoplasmic reticulum [6]. The routes currently believed to be responsible for the completion of complex-type oligosaccharides are shown in Fig. 9. After the $GlcNAcMan_5GlcNAc_2$ structure has two of its mannose residues removed, a second external N-acetylglucosamine residue is added by an enzyme distinct from the one that glycosylated the α 1-3 branch [33]. These terminal N-acetylglucosamine residues are galactosylated and finally sialylated [1, 2]. However, the extent of these last two processes is not always complete (eg, In Kuda and Hakomori [34]) and there is no clear explanation yet why this should be. The addition of fucose is thought to follow the addition of at least one external N-acetylglucosamine residue [35]. There are more complex structures which contain three (eg, fetuin [36] and VSV G protein [37]) and even four N-acetyllactosamine branches (eg, orosomucoid [38]) with either the α 1-3, or more usually, the α 1-6 mannose residue being doubly substituted [36, 37]. The galactosyl transferase has been the most extensively investigated enzyme because of its availability from milk and its apparently relaxed substrate requirements [39], since free N-acetylglucosamine, any terminal N-acetylglucosamine, and even glucose will accept galactose. This contrasts to the N-acetylglucosaminyl transferases, which appear to be very stringent in their substrate requirements [3, 4, 33] – see section IV. Sialyl transferases have been isolated by Hill and his coworkers [40] and their substrate requirements are being established [41].

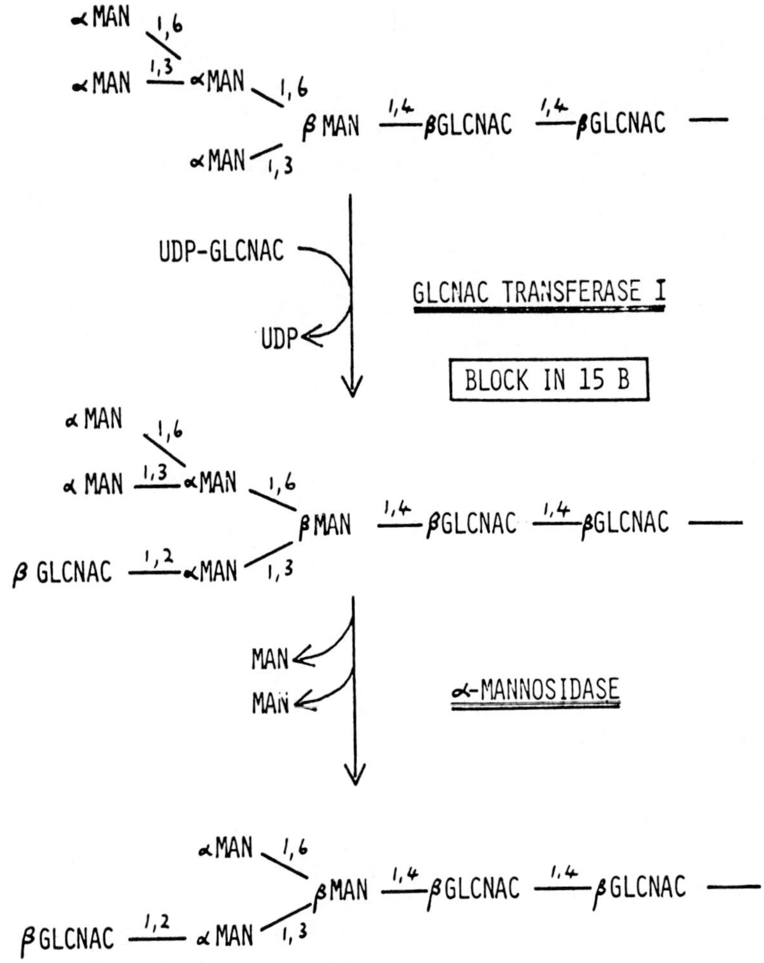

Fig. 8. Conversion of high-mannose oligosaccharides to complex types. The major asparagine-linked oligo-saccharide produced by the CHO mutant cell line 15B has the structure Man₅GlcNAc₂ [30], and this has now been shown to be the acceptor for the first external N-acetylglucosamine residue. The α-mannosidase(s) which reduce the manose composition from 5 to 3 residues are present in the 15B mutant, yet are not expressed as the preferred substrate for the(se) α-mannosidase(s), GlcNAC₁ Man₅GlcNAc₂, is not formed [49]. The removal of the six mannose residues from Man₉GlcNAC₂ to produce the pentasaccharide core, Man₃GlcNAc₂, therefore occurs in two phases, which are interrupted by the addition of an external N-acetylglucosamine residue.

V. EFFECT OF TRANSFORMATION ON PROCESSING OF CELL SURFACE GLYCO—PROTEINS IS RESTRICTED TO A LATE EVENT IN THEIR BIOSYNTHESIS

The occurrence of highly sialylated cell surface glycoproteins is one of the most reproducible biochemical correlates with transformation [42–44]. With the molecular details for the overall pathway of glycoprotein processing now available, we have investigated the molecular basis for this increase in complex-type oligosaccharides, which occurs at the expense of high-mannose structures. The experimental system we chose was another rodent embryonic fibroblast

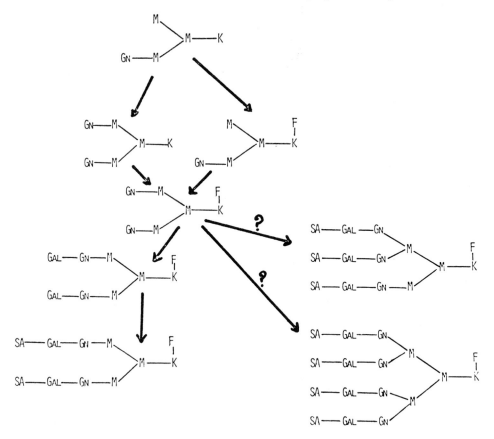

Fig. 9. Possible fates for the mannose-three core. The proximal N-acetylglucosamine of the di-N-acetylchitobiose core (K) may or may not become fucosylated; if this occurs, it may come before or after the second N-acetylglucosamine residue (GN) is added. The galactose residues (Gal) which are added to these N-acetylglucosamine residues may or may not become sialylated. A further area of variation that is poorly understood in terms of its biosynthesis, yet is well documented in final structures, is the formation of tri- and tetra-antenary N-acetyllactosamine branches.

line, Rat-1, which was transformed with an avian sarcoma virus. One attractive feature of this system for us is that the virus is defective and therefore does not complicate the comparison of the host glycoprotein patterns in the normal and transformed phenotypes. A second feature that makes this an attractive system is that transformation is temperature-sensitive, the change in phenotype taking a few hours.

Initial experiments revealed that the influx of labeled mannose into the lipid-linked oligosaccharide precursor and the transfer of this oligosaccharide from lipid to protein occurred at very similar rates in the normal and transformed phenotypes. Further investigation of the processing of cell surface glycoproteins has compared the kinetics of processing of the high-mannose structures. This study revealed identical kinetics for the normal and transformed phenotypes. Glycopeptides labeled briefly with mannose and chased for increasing lengths of time reveal in the two phenotypes identical distributions of high-mannose structures. After a 10-min pulse the predominant species contain nine mannose residues and either one or no glucose residue. With increasing periods of chase time, the glucose is removed and species containing less mannose are observed. The kinetics are very similar to those reported for Hamster embryonic fibroblasts [11].

In contrast to the similarity in the processing of high-mannose structures there was a clearly discernible difference in the distributions of complex-type glycopeptides. This difference was observed during the pulse-chase experiments but is most clearly revealed in the distributions of mannose in the glycopeptides derived from cells labeled in the continuous presence of [³H] mannose for 15 h (Fig. 10). One observes the large increase in the complex-type glycopeptides routinely reported. The contribution of this investigation is to emphasize two points: First, the difference between the normal and transformed phenotypes is restricted

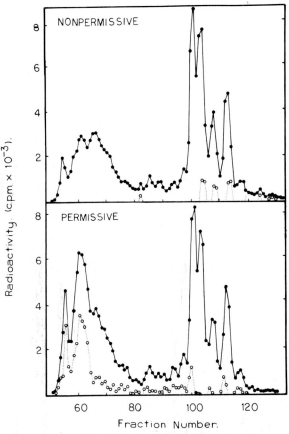

Fig. 10. Comparison of the mature oligosaccharide chains attached to glycoproteins in normal and transformed fibroblasts. The upper profile illustrates the distribution of mature oligosaccharides attached to glycoprotein by ts-Rat-1 B77 cells at the nonpermissive temperature (41°) (closed circles), and the lower profile illustrates these oligosaccharides produced by ts-Rat-1-B77 at the permissive temperature (34°) (closed circles). The differences in the relative distributions of the various glycopeptide species in cells grown at the permissive and nonpermissive temperatures are shown in the profiles with open circles and dashed lines. Mannose label eluting between fractions 98 and 120 is in typical high-mannose structures (Fig. 7): Man₉GlcNAc, 102; Man₈GlcNAc, 104; Man₇GlcNac, 108; Man₆GlcNAc, 112; Man₅GlcNAc, 117. The mannose label eluting near the exclusion limit is in complex-type structures (Fig. 9) and the species more highly represented at the permissive temperature are tentatively identified as tri- and tetraantennary species.

to a late event in glycoprotein processing and is localized to just two highly sialylated species (open symbols, Fig. 10), not a general increase in the sialylated glycopeptides. Second, this increase — which occurs against a background of enormous differences in the phenotypes (changes in the morphology of the cells [45], reorganization of their cytoskeleton [46], changes in composition of their cell surface and secreted proteins [47] and in rates of glycosis [48]) — is produced by a biosynthetic machinery that conserves the ratios of adjacent intermediates, eg, the ratio of $Man_8GlcNAc_2$ to $Man_7GlcNAc_2$, etc. As the processing of glycoproteins occurs with the hydrolytic cleavage of residues or with the transfer of activated sugars — steps that are not readily reversible — the conservation of the ratio of adjacent intermediates most probably reflects a highly conserved organization of the enzymes involved in glycoprotein biosynthesis, making it one of the very few pathways not disrupted on transformation.

CONCLUSIONS

Our conclusion is that the processing of cell surface glycoproteins is very similar in both normal and transformed fibroblasts, with a similar large mannose-rich oligosaccharide being transferred en bloc from a lipid carrier to nascent proteins and with the subsequent removal of glucose and mannose residues to provide the core structures for complex-type oligosaccharides having the same kinetics and structural pathway. The transformed phenotype has associated with it an enhanced capacity to produce the more highly sialylated glycopeptides. Our tentative identification of these glycopeptides as tri- and tetra-antennary complex-type oligosaccharides (Fig. 9) suggests to us that it is not solely the ability to sialylate that is enhanced upon transformation but the ability to make the more highly branched oligosaccharides with their attendant extra sialylation sites. Our hypothesis is that the most important enzymatic activity involved in the assembly of cell surface glycoproteins that is enhanced upon transformation is the β-1,4-N-acetylglucosaminyl transferase(s) that introduce(s) these branches.

REFERENCES

1. Spiro RG: Adv Protein Chem 27:349–467, 1973.
2. Spiro RG: Methods Enzymol 8:3–26, 1966.
3. Sturgess J, Moscarello M, H. Schachter H: Curr Top Membranes Transport 11:15–105, 1978.
4. Schacter H, Narasimhan S, Wilson JR: "Glycoproteins and Glycolipids in Disease Processes." American Chemical Society, 1978, pp 21–46.
5. Kornfeld R, Kornfeld S: Ann Rev Biochem 45:217–237, 1976.
6. Waechter CJ, Lennarz WJ: Ann Rev Biochem 45:95–112, 1976.
7. Gottschalk A: "Glycoproteins." Amsterdam: Elsevier, 1972.
8. Robbins PW, Hubbard SC, Turco SJ, Wirth DF: Cell 12:893–900, 1977.
9. Tabas I, Schlesinger S, Kornfeld S: J Biol Chem 253:716–722, 1978.
10. Hunt LA, Etchison JR, Summers DF: Proc Natl Acad Sci USA 75:754–758, 1978.
11. Hubbard SC, Robbins PW: J Biol Chem 254:4568–4576, 1979.
12. Li E, Tabas I, Kornfeld S: J Biol Chem 253:7762–7770, 1978.
13. Grinna L, Robbins PW: J Biol Chem 254:8814–8818, 1979.
14. Tabas I, Kornfeld S: Fed Proc 38:355, 1979.
15. Neutra M, Leblond CP: J Cell Biol 30:137–144, 1966.
16. Bennett G, Leblond CP: J Cell Biol 46:409–416, 1970.
17. Fleischer B, Fleischer S, Ozawa H: J Cell Biol 43:59–65, 1969.
18. Schachter H: Biochem Soc Symp 40:57–71, 1974.
19. Ito S, Yamashita K, Spiro RG, Kobata A: J Biochem 81:1621–1631, 1977.
20. Spiro RG, Spiro NJ, Bhoyroo VD: J Biol Chem 251:6409–6419, 1976.

21. Parodi AJ, Leloir LF: Biochim Biophys Acta 559:1–37, 1979.
22. Liu T, Stetson B, Turco SJ, Hubbard SC, Robbins PW: J Biol Chem 254:4554–4559, 1979.
23. Behrens NH, Parodi AJ, Leloir LF, Krisman CR: Arch Biochem Biophys 143:375–383, 1971.
24. Ghalambor MA, Warren CD, Jeanloz RW: Biochem Biophys Res Commun 57:407–414, 1974.
25. Palamarczyk G, Hemming FW: Biochem J 148:245–251, 1975.
26. Levy JA, Carminatti H, Cantarella AI, Behrens NH, Leloir LF, Tabora E: Biochem Biophys Res Commun 60:118–125, 1974.
27. Rothman JE, Lodish HF: Nature 269:775–780, 1977.
28. Marshall RD: Ann Rev Biochem 41:673–702, 1972.
29. Turco SJ, Stetson B, Robbins PW: Proc Natl Acad Sci USA 74:4411–4414, 1977.
30. Li E, Kornfeld S: J Biol Chem 253:6426–6431, 1978.
31. Chapman A, Kornfeld R: J Biol Chem 254:824–828, 1979.
32. Li E, Kornfeld S: J Biol Cehm 254:1600–1605, 1979.
33. Narasimhan S, Stanley P, Schachter H: J Biol Chem. 252:3926–3933, 1977.
34. Fukuda M, Hakomori SI: J Biol Cehm 254:3458–3465, 1979.
35. Wilson JR, Williams D, Schachter H: Biochem Biophys Res Commun 72:909–916, 1976.
36. Baenziger J, Fiete D: J Biol Chem 254:789–795, 1979.
37. Etchison JR, Robertson JS, Summers DF: Virology 78:375–392, 1977.
38. Wagh PV, Bornstein I, Winzler RJ: J Biol Chem 244:658–665, 1969.
39. Morrison JF, Ebner KE: J Biol Chem 246:3977–3984, 1971.
40. Sadler JE, Rearick J, Paulson JC, Hill RC: J Biol Chem 254:4434–4443, 1979.
41. Rearick J, Sadler JE, Paulson JC, Hill RC: J Biol Chem 254:4444–4451, 1979.
42. Buck CA, Glick MC, Warren L: Biochemistry 9:4567–4576, 1970.
43. Warren L, Critchley D, Macpherson I: Nature 235:275–277, 1972.
44. Van Beck WP, Smets LA, Emmelot P: Cancer Res 33:2913–2922, 1973.
45. Kawai S, Hanafusa H: Virology 46:470–479, 1971.
46. Pollack R, Osborn M, Weber K: Proc Natl Acad Sci USA 72:994–998, 1975.
47. Hynes R: Biochim Biophys Acta 458:73–107, 1976.
48. Racker E: J Cell Physiol 89:697–701, 1976.
49. Tabas I, Kornfeld S: J Biol Chem 253:7779–7786, 1978.
50. Chapman A, Kornfeld R: J Biol Chem (In press).

Tumor Cell Surfaces and Malignancy 873–886 (1980)

Possible Role of Glycolipid in Development, Cell Growth Regulation, and Transformation

Sen-itiroh Hakomori

Department of Pathobiology and Microbiology, University of Washington, Seattle, Washington 98195

1) A progressive branching of lacto-N-glycosyl carbohydrate chain linked to glycolipid and to band 3 protein has been observed during the development of fetal to adult human erythrocytes. A linear repeating structure of $Gal\beta1\rightarrow4GlcNAc\beta1\rightarrow3Gal$ was converted to a branched structure $Gal\beta1\rightarrow4GlcNAc\beta1\rightarrow3(Gal\beta1\rightarrow4GlcNAc\beta1\rightarrow6)Gal\beta1\rightarrow4GlcNAc$. Some of the linear structure represents i-antigen, and some of the branched structure represents I-antigen. Such changes of carbohydrate structure in membrane coincide with the switch from fetal hemoglobin (HbF) to adult hemoglobin (HbA) synthesis, and may define the stage of differentiation in cellular function.

2) Cell-to-cell contact induces enhancement of a particular type of glycolipid synthesis (contact response). A mimic "contact response" of GM_3 synthesis was observed when sparse growing culture was treated with the affinity purified anti-GM_3 ganglioside Fab. The synthesis of GM_3 ganglioside was enhanced severalfold, but not the synthesis of GM_2, GM_1, and GD1a. Growth of antibody-treated 3T3 cells was inhibited and showed reduced cell saturation density. Some cellular proteins which had specific affinity with glycolipids were released by ethidium bromide. Addition of such cellular proteins in 3T3 cell culture induced a reduction of cell saturation density. These results suggest that a particular glycolipid (contact-sensitive glycolipid) could be a receptor for a particular cell surface protein that may induce "contact inhibition." Some carbohydrate chains such as $Gal\beta1\rightarrow3GalNAc\beta1\rightarrow4Gal\rightarrow R$, which is common both to glycolipid and glycoprotein may be receptor growth stimulation from serum in vitro. Therefore, growth inhibition induced by anti-glycolipid Fab or by cell surface protein could be due to a block of the recepting growth stimulation through serum factors.

Key words: glycolipid, carbohydrate chain, human erythrocyte

This is a summary of our recent studies on two topics: 1) changes of glycolipid and glycoprotein carbohydrate chains during the ontogenic development of human erythrocytes and 2) possible role of glycolipid in "contact inhibition" and cell growth regulation.

Membrane changes associated with the process of ontogenesis have been suggested through the orderly appearance or disappearance of antigen markers such as F_9 [1], blood group ABH [2], and Forssman [3] and Ii-antigens [4], although chemical structural change has not been clearly demonstrated. The antigen i could be converted to I during the development of fetal to adult erythrocytes [4], although a rare individual with a genetic

Received March 18, 1979; accepted April 5, 1979.

defect cannot develop I-antigen (adult i) [5]. The Ii-antigens have been regarded as the precursors of blood group ABH antigens [6].

In the first part of this chapter the changes in carbohydrate structure closely related to a conversion of antigen i to I during ontogenetic development are presented.

The biochemical basis of cell surface changes associated with cell contact is important not only for understanding the growth control of normal cell proliferation (density-dependent growth inhibition, or contact inhibition, [7—9]) but also for elucidating the mechanism of cell recognition involved in processes of histogenesis and morphogenesis as well as in responses of immune cell systems. An intriguing phenomenon is the significant increase in chemical concentration and synthesis of a certain glycolipid when cell population density of contact inhibitable cells increases [10—13]. The cell biological implication of glycolipid response on cell contact has been studied through cellular and glycolipid response to the specific anti-glycolipid antibodies and to the cell surface proteins released by chaotropic reagent. On the other hand, a possible role of some glycolipid carbohydrate chains in receiving serum growth stimulation has been disclosed [14], and its cell biological significance is to be discussed.

MATERIALS AND METHODS

All the materials and experimental methods have been described in the quoted references in Results or in footnotes to figures and tables.

RESULTS AND DISCUSSION

Structural Changes of a Common Carbohydrate Chain in Glycolipids and Glycoproteins Associated With Development of Human Erythrocytes

Recently we have identified the minimum essential structure required for expression of i-antigens and I-antigens as seen in Table I; namely, a linear, twice repeated Galβ1→4GlcNAcβ1→3Gal structure for i [15] and a branched Galβ1→4GlcNAcβ1→3 (Galβ1→4GlcNAcβ1→6) Gal structure for various I-specificities [16]. The presence of

TABLE I. Structures of i- and I-Determinants

1. i-Active determinant
   Galβ1→4GlcNAcβ1→3Galβ1→4GlcNAcβ1→3Galβ1→4Glc→Cer
   (Determinant Dench, Tho, Hog, McC, and McDon monoclonal anti-i antibodies)
2. I-Active determinant
   Galβ1→4GlcNAcβ1
   $\qquad\qquad\qquad\searrow$ $^6_3$Galβ1→4GlcNAcβ1→3Galβ1→4Glcβ→Cer
   Galβ1→4GlcNAcβ1 $\qquad\nearrow$
   (active with all anti-I monoclonal antibodies)
   Galβ1→4GlcNAcβ1
   $\qquad\qquad\qquad\searrow$ $^6_3$Galβ1→4GlcNAcβ1→3Galβ1→4Glcβ→Cer
   GlcNAcβ1 $\qquad\nearrow$
   (active with Ma, Woj, Step, and Gra monoclonal I-antibodies)
   GlcNAcβ1
   $\qquad\qquad\qquad\searrow$ $^6_3$Galβ1→4GlcNAcβ1→3Galβ1→4Glcβ→Cer
   Galβ1→4GlcNAcβ1 $\qquad\nearrow$
   (active with Step, Gra, Ver, Ful, anti-I antibodies)

Galβ1→4GlcNAcβ1→6 branch confers I-activity and, simultaneously, suppresses i-activity, therefore, i to I conversion during the development of erythrocytes represents the branching process [16, 17].

A similar progressive branching process in carrier carbohydrate chains for blood group glycolipids A- and H-determinants has been implicated as being associated with the developmental process [18]. As seen in Table II, we have isolated and identified three to four sets of glycolipid carbohydrate chains from human erythrocyte membranes [19, 20]; these are H_1, H_2, H_3, and A^a, A^b, and A^c, according to the order of the complexity of the carbohydrate chain. As shown in Table III, surface-labeled activities of blood group A glycolipid variants A^c and A^d in fetal erythrocytes were considerably lower than those of adult erythrocytes. Antibodies directed against H_3 glycolipid, which do not cross-react with a

TABLE II. Structures of Blood Group Glycolipids Isolated From Human Erythrocytic Membranes

A-active structures

A^a　　GalNAcα1
$$\searrow \overset{3}{\underset{2}{}}\text{Gal}\beta1\to4\text{GlcNAc}\beta1\to3\text{Gal}\beta1\to4\text{Glc}\to\text{Ceramide}$$
　　　L-Fucα1 ↗

A^b　　GalNAcα1
$$\searrow \overset{3}{\underset{2}{}}\text{Gal}\beta1\to4\text{GlcNAc}\beta1\to3\text{Gal}\beta1\to4\text{GlcNAc}\beta1\to3\text{Gal}\beta1\to4\text{Glc}\to\text{Ceramide}$$
　　　L-Fucα1 ↗

A^c　　　L-Fucα1
$$\searrow \overset{2}{\underset{3}{}}\text{Gal}\beta1\to4\text{GlcNAc}\beta1$$
　　GalNAcα1 ↗ 　　　　　　　　　　　$\searrow \overset{3}{\underset{6}{}}\text{Gal}\beta1\to4\text{GlcNAc}\beta1\to3\text{Gal}\beta1\to4\text{Glc}\to\text{Ceramide}$
　　　L-Fuc1 　　　　　　　　　　　　　　↗
$$\searrow \overset{2}{\underset{3}{}}\text{Gal}\beta1\to4\text{GlcNAc}\beta1$$
　　GalNAcα1 ↗

A^d　　Similar to A^c but with an additional branching structure, exact structure undetermined.

H-active structures

H_1　　L-Fucα1-2Galβ1→4GlcNAcβ1→3Galβ1→4Glc→Ceramide

H_2　　L-Fucα1→2Galβ1→4GlcNAcβ1→3Galβ1→4GlcNAcβ1→3Galβ1→4Glc→Ceramide

H_3　　L-Fucα1→2Galβ1→4GlcNAcβ1
$$\searrow \overset{3}{\underset{6}{}}\text{Gal}\beta1\to4\text{GlcNAc}\beta1\to3\text{Gal}\beta1\to4\text{Glc}\to\text{Ceramide}$$
　　L-Fucα1→2Galβ1→4GlcNAcβ1 ↗

H_4　　Similar to H_3 but with an additional branching structure, exact structure undetermined.

TABLE III. Surface-Labeled Activities of Blood Group A Glycolipids Variant: Percent of Activity of Newborn Erythrocytes to that of Adult Erythrocytes

	Percent activity of newborn erythrocytes to adult erythrocytes			
	A^a	A^b	A^c	A^d
Experiment 1	95	65	24	20
Experiment 2	84	92	45	30
Experiment 3	110	96	46	35

A erythrocytes of adult and newborn were surface labeled by galactose oxidase and tritiated borohydride, membranes were isolated, glycolipid fractions were prepared by DEAE-Sephadex chromatography, and the nonradioactive standard A variants glycolipids were added, and A^a, A^b, A^c, and A^d fractions were separated on thin-layer chromatography. Activities of each variant obtained from newborn erythrocytes were compared with those of adult erythrocytes. Values were expressed as percent of adult erythrocytes.

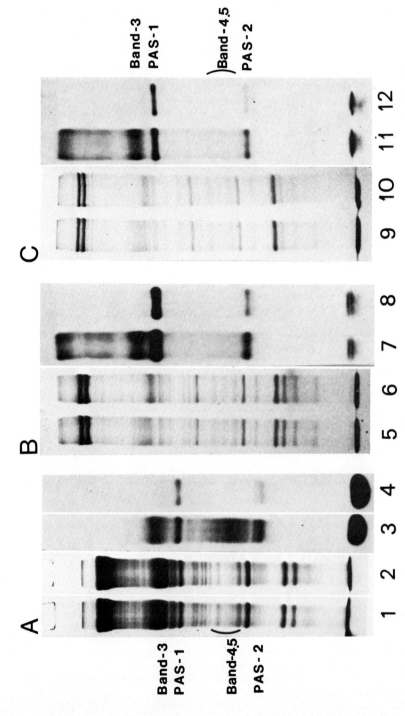

Fig. 1. SDS-polyacrylamide gel electrophoresis of erythrocyte membrane proteins of adult I-active erythrocytes (A), adult i-active erythrocytes (B), and umbilical cord i-active erythrocytes (C) labeled by the galactose oxidase-NaB[^{3}H]$_4$ method. Lanes 2, 4, 6, 8; and 10, 12 are the labeled erythrocytes after endo-β-galactosidase treatment, whereas Lanes 1, 3; 5, 7; and 9, 11 are the labeled erythrocytes without enzyme treatment. Lanes 1, 2; 5, 6; and 9, 10 are Coomassie blue stained gels, Lanes 3, 4; 7, 8; and 11, 12 are fluorographs of the gels 1, 2; 5, 6; and 9, 10, respectively. Note the disappearance of Band 3 and Band 4.5 after enzyme treatment (Lanes 4, 8, 12 compared to Lanes 3, 7, 11). Reproduced from Fukuda, Fukuda, and Hakomori [26].

straight chain H_1 and H_2, reacted with adult erythrocytes much more strongly than with fetal erythrocytes. In contrast, the antibodies directed to precursor structure, lacto-N-triosylceramide, reacted very weakly to adult erythrocytes but showed a clearly higher reactivity with newborn and fetal erythrocytes [18].

Recently, band 3, the major intrinsic membrane glycoprotein of human erythrocytes [for review see 21, 22], has been assigned as I-antigen carrier [23]. We have also found that endo-β-galactosidase from Escherichia freundii [24], whose substrate specificity has been established [25], directly modifies specific cell surface glycoproteins and glycolipids. The following antigenic changes were particularly remarkable by treatment of human erythrocytes with the endo-β-galactosidase: 1) abolition of Ii-antigenic activity, 2) decrease of the reactivity with anti-ABH blood group and anti-paragloboside antibodies, and 3) a slight but distinct increase of the reactivity with anti-lacto-N-triosylceramide antibodies [26]. Accompanying these antigenic changes, surface-labeled carbohydrates in band 3 and band 4.5 glycoproteins and in glycolipids with longer carbohydrates such as H_2, H_3, and H_4 were strikingly reduced or were eliminated completely, as shown in Figures 1, and 2. Thus,

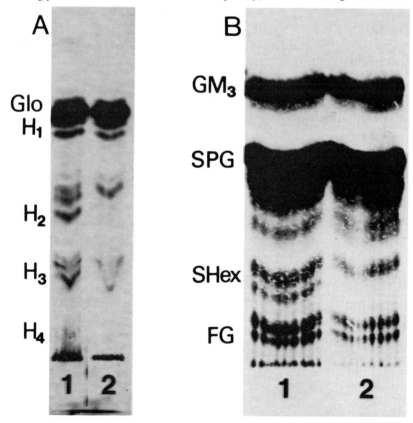

Fig. 2. Fluorography pattern of thin-layer chromatogram of the surface-labeled neutral glycolipids (A) and gangliosides (B). A, lane 1, upper phase neutral glycolipids from adult I erythrocytes; lane 2 the same glycolipid fraction prepared from endo-β-galactosidase-treated adult I erythrocytes. Cells were labeled by galactose oxidase-NaB[^{3}H]$_4$, extracted, and fractionated as described [26]. Glo, H_1, H_2, H_3, H_4 indicate the position of authentic reference glycolipid; structures of H_1 to H_4 (see Table II). Note that reduction or elimination of H_4, H_3, and H_2 glycolipid after endo-β-galactosidase treatment. Glo: globoside, GM_3: hematoside, SPG: sialylparagloboside, SHex: sialyllacto-N-norhexaosylceramide [15], FG: fucoganglioside [36], H_1, H_2, H_3, H_4: H-active glycolipids with respective structures as shown in Table II. Reproduced from Fukuda, Fukuda, and Hakomori [25].

it was concluded that the major I-antigens and i-antigens of human erythrocytes are associated with bands 3 and 4.5, and with long-chain glycolipids [26].

A large variety of heterogeneous oligosaccharides with different molecular sizes were released by the enzyme treatment from adult I-active erythrocytes in a striking contrast to the homogeneous small-sized oligosaccharides released from i-active umbilical cord erythrocytes and i-active adult erythrocytes [26]. A linear carbohydrate chain such as R→GlcNAc β1→3*Gal*β1→4GlcNAcβ→R can be readily hydrolyzed by endo-β-galactosidase into di- and trisaccharides, whereas the galactoside linkage at a branching structure such as R→GlcNAc β1→6(R→GlcNAcβ1→3)*Gal*β1→4GlcNAc was hardly hydrolyzed by this enzyme [25]. This accounts for the release of oligosaccharides with various molecular sizes from adult I-erythrocytes, which are probably derived from the heterogeneous branched structures. In contrast, a homogeneous small-sized oligosaccharide probably can be released from a linear structure.

Methylation analysis of glycopeptides isolated from band 3 glycoprotein from adult, newborn, and adult i-erythrocytes showed a striking difference and confirmed the above proposal. Namely, a much higher quantity of 2,3,4,6-tetra-0-methylgalactose and 2,4-di-0-methylgalactose was yielded from adult glycopeptides than from newborn glycopeptides and adult i-variant glycopeptides [27]. Thus, fetal to adult development in the band 3 carbohydrate chain is identical to that found in blood group glycosphingolipids, as shown in Figure 1. An idealized version of the developmental change of the carbohydrate chain is shown in Figure 3. The structural relationship between Ii, ABH blood group antigen, and gangliosides is explained in Figure 4.

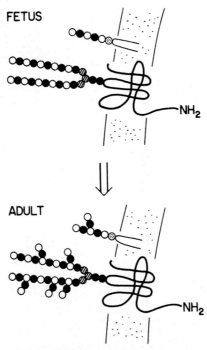

Fig. 3. Idealized version of the structural changes in carbohydrates linked to lipid (ceramide) and Band 3 protein of human erythrocytes (○: Gal, ●: GlcNAc, ⊗: Glc, ⊖: Man). A linear straight chain, Gal-GlcNAc repeating units are linked to Glc-Cer or to mannosylGlucNAc core of Band 3 protein in fetal erythrocytes. When fetal erythrocytes are converted to adult erythrocytes the linear chains are converted to those having Gal-GlcNAc branchings.

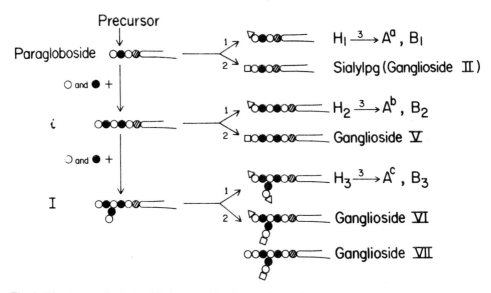

Fig. 4. The structural relationship between blood group I, i, A, B, H active glycolipids and various types of gangliosides in erythrocyte membranes. Paragloboside is converted to i antigen by addition of Gal-GlcNAc branch. Paragloboside, i and I structures are, respectively, converted by fucosylation (indicated by route 1), to H_1, H_2, and H_3 glycolipids [19, 20]. These H structures are further converted to A^a, A^b, and A^c glycolipids [19], or B_1, B_2 glycolipids by α-N-acetylgalactosaminylation/ or α-galactosylation (route 3). On the other hand, paragloboside, i, and I active glycolipids are sialylated and converted to sialosylparagloboside (ganglioside II), ganglioside V, ganglioside VI, or ganglioside VII, respectively (route 2). Ganglioside V is sialyl-lacto-N-norhexaosylceramide [15], and ganglioside VI is a new type of ganglioside recently isolated from human erythrocytes [35]. Ganglioside VII is the branched ganglioside containing α-Gal [16]. The i activities are associated with repeating Gal-GlcNAc structure, but the activity is completely suppressed by fucosylation, therefore no i activities are found in H_2, A^b, and B_2 (Watanabe and Hakomori, unpublished observation). However, i activities are not completely suppressed by sialylation, for some activities are detectable in ganglioside V [15]. I activities are associated with the branched octaosylceramide [16]. The activity is greatly suppressed by fucosylation, for H_3 showed a very minimum I activity and A^c did not show any activity (Watanabe and Hakomori unpublished observation). I activities were only partially suppressed by sialylation or galactosylation, for ganglioside VII showed considerable I activity [16]. When one of the terminal chains of ganglioside VI was fucosylated, there was only minimum I activity [35]. The branched structures H_3, A^c are present in much higher concentration in adult than in fetal erythrocytes [18] ($\circ$: Gal, $\bullet$: GlcNAc, $\otimes$: Glc, $\triangle$: Fuc, $\square$: Sialic acid). Ganglioside I is GM_3 (hematoside); gangliosides III and IV are not identified.

Possible Role of Glycolipids in Cell Growth Regulation, "Contact Inhibition," and Transformation

The phenomena, as described in the following subsections, indicate that certain specific glycolipids on cell surfaces may regulate cell growth through receiving the growth inhibitory as well as the growth stimulatory ligands. Metabolism of the receptor glycolipid itself could be regulated by either inhibitory or stimulatory ligands.

Cell Contact-Dependent Glycolipid Response. A glycolipid response on cell contact was considered to be related to "contact inhibition" of cell growth since contact inhibitability and contact-dependent glycolipid synthesis showed parallelism in various cells [10–12, 29], although the contact-dependent glycolipid response may not be correlated with tumorigenicity [28]. The loss of contact inhibition was closely associated with the loss of contact-dependent glycolipid response [10–13]. Highly contact-inhibitable cells showed contact response of glycolipid synthesis at the early stage (touching stage) rather than at the later stage (confluency) of cell contact [29]. The concentration of higher ganglioside (GDla) of contact-inhibitable 3T3 cells increased severalfold at the touching stage and decreased to a normal level when cells were contact-inhibited at confluency [29]. Similarly, "GDla ganglioside" of muscle cells increased severalfold at the touching stage before cell fusion is initiated [30].

The cell-contact response of neutral glycolipids such as ceramide trihexoside was correlated with the enhancement of α-galactosyltransferase activity. Only the activity of UDP-galactose:lactosylceramide-α-galactosyl-transferase but not UDP-galactose: glucosylceramide-β-galactosyltransferase of both BHK and NIL cells increases severalfold at the contact-inhibited stage as compared to sparse growing cells. A similar enzyme response on cell contact was not observable in transformed cells [13, 29]. Based on these observations, a model was presented in the first NCI-UCLA Symposium in 1971 [31], in which a surface ektoprotein that recognizes glycolipid was postulated. The summary of this model is reproduced in Figure 5.

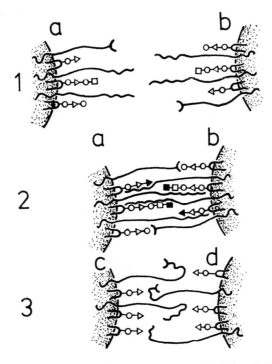

Fig. 5. A model for ektoprotein that recognized "contact-sensitive" glycolipid of contact-inhibitable cells. 1) Growing cells, a certain proportion of glycolipids and proteins (or glycoproteins), arranged in a certain order. The structures and the order of carbohydrates and proteins should be complementary. 2) Confluent cells, when cell a and b meet, the carbohydrates and proteins are linked together through complementary structure, and some carbohydrates can extend their chain for the better linkages between complementary proteins. These linkages should be noncovalent, and possibly mediated by bivalent cations as cells are dissociable by EDTA. 3) Transformed malignant cells; carbohydrate chains are incomplete, consequently no complementary structures were found between glycolipids and proteins. Intercellular linkages were therefore not formed.

A Mimic Contact Response of Glycolipid and Growth Inhibition Induced by Anti-Glycolipid Fab. If the model presented in Figure 5 is true, anti-glycolipid antibodies, particularly directed to a "contact-sensitive glycolipid," applied on cell surfaces should induce growth inhibition and mimic contact response of glycolipid synthesis.

The affinity purified anti-GM_3 ganglioside Fab inhibited cell growth and reduced cell saturation density of NIL and 3T3 cells to a great extent; however, cell growth of transformed NIL and 3T3 cells was not inhibited and saturation density was not reduced in the presence of anti-GM_3 antibodies' Fab. The affinity-purified anti-globoside Fab did not induce cell growth inhibition and did not reduce cell saturation density for either NIL or 3T3 cells [32].

The enhanced synthesis of GM_3 ganglioside, but not GD1a, or GD1b and GM_1 gangliosides, was induced by anti-GM_3 antibodies' Fab (see Fig. 6). This enhancement of GM_3 synthesis was most remarkable when sparse cells were treated with anti-GM_3 antibodies' Fab, but to a lesser extent when crowded cells were treated [32]. Therefore, the effect of anti-ganglioside antibodies to ganglioside synthesis varied depending on the cell saturation density.

These observations suggested further that contact-dependent glycolipid response as well as the process of "contact inhibition." could be based on a possible interaction between antibody-like ektoprotein and contact-sensitive glycolipid. This assumption has been supported by the demonstration that 1) anti-glycolipid antibodies' Fab enhance synthesis of contact-sensitive glycolipid, and 2) the antibody Fab induces a similar state of growth inhibition, as seen in contact-inhibited cells, but fails to induce growth inhibition for

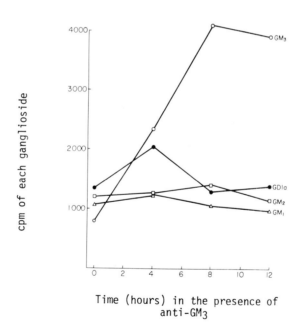

Time (hours) in the presence of
anti-GM_3

Fig. 6. Effect of anti-GM_3 Fab on ganglioside synthesis in 3T3 cells. 3T3 cell cultures (10 cm plate; 4×10^4 cells/cm^2) were inhibited in the presence of [^{14}C]-galactose (1 μCi/ml) for a total of 12 h. Fab anti-GM_3 was added (3 μg/ml) to each culture at 0, 4, and 8 h of incubation. At 12 h cells were washed, harvested, and radiolabeled gangliosides were extracted and analyzed on TLC. The activities of each ganglioside were determined [32].

transformed cells [32]. The putative ektoprotein has not been isolated or characterized, but a preliminary result, as described below and elsewhere [33], suggests that such a protein may indeed exist.

A Reduction of Cell Saturation Density Induced by Cell Surface Proteins. Cell surface proteins (CSP), metabolically labeled with [^{35}S]-methionine, were released on incubation of a cell sheet with phosphate buffered saline containing ethidium bromide (10 μg/ml, 37°C, 30 min). The protein fraction will bind to trypsinized cells and the binding of released CSP fraction from 3T3 cells was reduced to 50–60% by preincubation of CSP with GM$_3$ prior to the addition of CSP to the cells. About 30–40% of total CSP binding on trypsinized 3T3 cells was reduced on incubating CSP with GM$_3$ prior to incubation of CSP with 3T3 cells. [^{35}S]-CSP bound to 3T3 cells was 280 cpm/10^6 cells, whereas that preincubated with GM$_3$ was 150 cpm/10^6 cells by mean values of triplicate experiment (Lingwood and Hakomori, unpublished data). In a previous study, various glycolipids covalently linked to an amino propyl glass column were used to study which component of CSP would bind to glycolipid-glass columns. A specific elimination of two components with molecular weights of 200,000 and 150,000 was observed when CSP was passed through a GM$_3$ column. These components were not eliminated by lactosylceramide, Forssman, and globoside columns. However, those proteins that bound to a specific glyco-lipid column were difficult to elute by various chaotropic reagents and detergents [33]. Although these results are preliminary, some of the ethidium-bromide released protein has a specific affinity to GM$_3$ ganglioside and some other glycolipids as well.

Addition of such cellular proteins to 3T3 cell culture induced a remarkable reduction of cell saturation density for 3T3 cells but not for Kirsten virus transformed 3T3 cells (see Fig. 7; Lingwood and Hakomori unpublished observation). This indicates that the CSP present in the ethidium-bromide released fraction could recognize GM$_3$ and some other cell surface glycolipids and then induce the enhanced susceptibility of contact inhibition. This result is compatible with the finding that anti-GM$_3$ Fab induces enhanced susceptibility to contact inhibition.

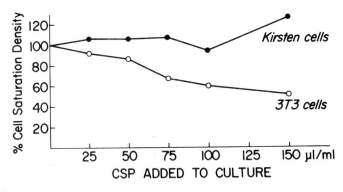

Fig. 7. Effect of cellular proteins ("CSP") released by ethidium bromide on cell growth. Cell surface proteins (CSP) released by incubating 3T3 cell sheets in a glucose-containing basic salt solution con-taining 10 μg/ml of ethidium bromide at 37°C for 30 min. Some cells detached from the culture dishes but are viable. The solution was separated by centrifugation and extensively dialyzed and concentrated through membrane filtration. Cells were cultured in medium containing 25–150 μg/ml of cell surface protein. Cell saturation density was determined after 3 days for 3T3 cells and after 4 days for 3T3 cells transformed by murine sarcoma virus Kirsten strain (Kirsten cells). Note that cell saturation density was reduced as much as 40–50% in a medium containing 150 μg/ml of CSP. Kirsten cell growth was unaltered. Each point is the mean value of triplicate. The determination is of two separate experiments.

Glycolipid Carbohydrate Chain as a Serum Growth Factor Receptor. Serum growth factors are essential to maintain cell growth in vitro, although the significance of such factors in vivo is not known. We found that the major activity in cell growth stimulation of fetal calf serum was specifically eliminated through affinity columns composed of a specific glycolipid covalently linked to Sepharose [34] or a glycolipid-liposome entrapped in polyacrylamide [35]. The growth-stimulating activity was trapped most strongly and specifically by the ganglio-N-tetraosylceramide (asialo GM_1)-column, but was not eliminated by lactosylceramide, α-galactosyllactosylceramide, globoside, ganglio-N-triosylceramide, hematoside, hematosidol (sialic acid carboxyl of hematoside was reduced to alcohol) see Fig. 8). The column containing GM_1 ganglioside and GM_1 gangliosidol (sialic acid carboxyl of GM_1 ganglioside was reduced to alcohol) reduced the activity. Both the increase of cell numbers and [^{3}H] thymidine incorporation into cells were inhibited by culturing cells in the media containing fetal calf serum, which was treated with a ganglio-N-tetraosylceramide or a GM_1 ganglioside-polyacrylamide column.

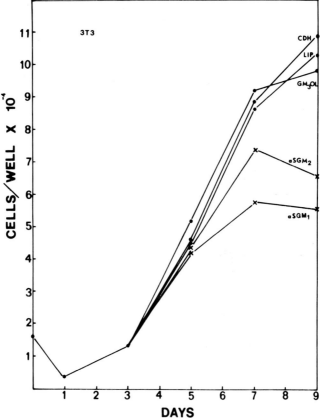

Fig. 8. Growth curve of 3T3 cells grown in medium containing fetal calf serum which was passed through glycolipid affinity columns. Balb 3T3 cells were plated in 24 well plates (each well diameter 1.5 cm) at the cell number indicated for day 0. On day 2 the medium was removed, cells were washed with Dulbecco-modified Eagle's (DME) medium without serum, and 1 ml of DME containing 0.4% fetal calf serum was added. On day 3 the medium was removed and 1 ml of the indicated medium was added. Values are the mean of triplicate measurement of trypsinized cells from wells and counted by a Coulter counter at the indicated time. CDH: liposomes containing ceramide dihexaside (lactosylceramide), GM_3OL: GM_3-ganglioside whose sialic acid carboxyl residue is reduced to primary alcohol, $aSGM_2$: asialo-GM_2, $aSGM_1$: asialo GM_1, LIP: a plain cholesterol lecithin liposome without glycolipid inclusion.

The active factor was recovered by eluting the column with 2 M potassium thiocyanate or with 8 M urea, followed by dialysis and concentration through membrane filtration (Table IV). However, the activity was not fully recovered from the column during the treatment in most of the experiment. Furthermore, pretreatment of 3T3 cells with monovalent antibodies to ganglio-N-tetraosylceramide or to GM_1-ganglioside inhibits growth stimulation by serum (Table V). These findings suggest that a specific carbohydrate chain Galβ1→3GalNAcβ1→4Galβ1→R may function as a receptor of serum growth stimulation. Cell growth inhibition induced by monovalent antibodies to GM_3 and GM_1 and by cell surface protein-recognizing glycolipid, as described in the previous section, could be due to the block of receptor serum growth factor.

TABLE IV. Stimulation of 3T3 Cell Growth by Eluate From Ganglio-N-Tetraosylceramide-Sepharose 4B Column

	Cells/well	
	I	II
DME	44,640 ± 2,700	35,290 ± 1,540
FCS	60,456 ± 15,950	110,520 ± 28,890
Lactose (0.2M)	36,170 ± 2,230	42,234 ± 4,310
KSCN (2M)	42,340 ± 5,456	42,880 ± 1,640
Urea (6M)	64,636 ± 12,150	70,500 ± 3,080

30 ml of fetal calf serum diluted with the same volume of phosphate-0.14 M NaCl was passed slowly through a 10 ml column volume of ganglio-N-tetraosylceramide covalently bound to Sepharose 4B. The column was washed with phosphate 0.14 M NaCl until normal ultraviolet absorption material was washed off. Then the column was sequentially eluted with the indicated solutions. The eluates (50 ml) were dialyzed extensively against 0.15 M saline and then phosphate buffered 0.14 M NaCl, and concentrated to 5 ml. Cells were seeded in Falcon 24 well plates (1.5 cm diameter for each well) in 1% fetal calf serum plus 50 μl eluates. Values are 2 separate experiments, I and II. In both experiments, triplicate wells were counted in a Coulter cell counter after 5 days of incubation at 37°C.

TABLE V. Inhibition of Serum Stimulation by Preincubation with Anti-Asialo GM_1-Fab

Condition	[^{3}H]-Thy Incorp. ± SD (n = 5)
Control	13,620 ± 2,400
Preincubated with phosphate 0.14 M NaCl	11,420 ± 1,400
Preincubated with 20 μl Fab[a]	7,270 ± 1,800
Preincubated with 50 μl Fab	4,760 ± 430
Unstimulated	2,530 ± 1,030

Balb/c 3T3 cells were seeded in multi-well plates (2,000–3,000 cells per well; each had a diameter 0.9 cm). Two days later the medium was changed to the one containing 0.4% FCS. 40 h later, the medium was aspirated and the wells were washed with phosphate 0.14 M NaCl. The wells were then incubated for 6 h with the indicated amount of purified anti-asialo GM_1-Fab or phosphate 0.14 M Nacl. The cells were then washed once in warm Dulbecco modified Eagle's medium without serum and then a fresh 1% FCS was added. Sixteen hours later, 1 μCi of [^{3}H]-thymidine was added and the incubation was continued for 5–6 h. The cells were then processed to determine [^{3}H]-thymidine incorporation into trichloroacetic acid insoluble material.

A Working Hypothesis for a Possible Role of Glycolipids in Regulating Cell Growth.
Several pieces of knowledge which suggest a possible function of a specific glycolipid in regulation of cell proliferation have been discussed, yet a correlation between the pieces of knowledge is unknown. However, a working hypothesis may be helpful, at this stage, to visualize a common background on which the various phenomena are based. To summarize our knowledge:

1) Some glycolipids on the cell surface membrane are sensitive to cell contact and transformation; ie, their synthesis increases on cell contact, disappears on transformation.

2) Monovalent antibodies directed to contact-sensitive glycolipids induce a "mimic contact response" of glycolipid – ie, increase its synthesis and induce growth inhibition.

3) Cell surface proteins that recognize contact-sensitive glycolipids may exist on the cell surface, which may induce growth inhibition upon cell-to-cell contact.

4) A carbohydrate sequence similar to that found in contact-sensitive glycolipid could be a common receptor for serum growth factor. Therefore, serum growth factor could be competitive with a putative cell surface protein (ektoprotein), which may inhibit cell growth.

It is possible that a common glycolipid structure is a receptor of growth inhibitor as well as growth stimulator. Serum growth stimulation was inhibited by pretreatment of cells with monovalent antibodies directed to ganglio-N-tetraosylceramide. On exogenous addition of gangliosides in culture medium, the cell growth was inhibited, possibly because the activities of growth factors were blocked. Two phenomena, contact response for glycolipid synthesis and mimic contact response induced by anti-glycolipid antibodies, suggested that metabolism of the receptor glycolipid itself could be regulated by either inhibitory or stimulatory ligands on the cell surface. Transformed cells may be lacking in either growth inhibitory ektoprotein or another mechanism, receptor growth inhibitor and stimulator. Deficiency in ektoprotein that recognizes glycolipid or a defect in glycolipid synthesis in transformed cells led to a failure of "functional cell contact" as well as a failure of receptor serum growth factor. Normal cells are receptors of the serum growth factor when they are growing as sparse culture, whereas they cease to receive growth stimulation at a certain cell contact stage because the receptor may be preoccupied or inactivated with the growth inhibitory ektoprotein. It is of crucial importance, therefore, to demonstrate the specificity and function of putative ektoproteins that are directed to glycolipid.

REFERENCES

1. Artzt K, Dubois P, Bennett D, Condamine H, Daninet C, Jacob F: Proc Natl Acad Sci USA 70:2988–2992, 1973.
2. Szulman AE: In Human Blood Groups. 5th International Convocation of Immunologists, Buffalo, NY. Basel: Karger, 1976, pp 426–436.
3. Willison KR, Stern TL: Cell 14:785–793, 1978.
4. Marsh WL: Br J Haematol 7:200–209, 1961.
5. Wiener AS, Unger LJ, Cohen L, Feldman J: Ann Intern Med 44:221–240, 1956.
6. Feizi T, Kabat EA, Vicari G, Andersson B, Marsh WL: J Immunol 106:1578–1592, 1971.
7. Todaro G, Green H: J Cell Biol 17:299–303, 1963.
8. Stoker M, Rubin H: Nature 215:171, 1967.
9. Dulbecco R: Nature 227:802, 1970.
10. Hakomori S: Proc Natl Acad Sci USA 67:1741–1747, 1970.
11. Sakiyama H, Gross SK, Robbins PW: Proc Natl Acad Sci USA 69:872–876, 1972.
12. Critchley DR, MacPherson I: Biochim Biophys Acta 246:145–159, 1973.
13. Kijimoto S, Hakomori S: Biochem Biophys Res Commun 44:557–563, 1971.
14. Patt LM, Hakomori S: Fed Proc 37:1827 (abstr #3058), 1978.

15. Niemann H, Watanabe K, Hakomori S, Childs RA, Feizi T: Biochem Biophys Res Commun 81:1286–1293, 1978.
16. Watanabe K, Hakomori S, Childs RA, Feizi T: J Biol Chem 254:3221–3228, 1979.
17. Feizi T, Childs RA, Watanabe K, Hakomori S: J Exp Med 149:975–980, 1979.
18. Watanabe K, Hakomori S: J Exp Med 144:644–653, 1976.
19. Hakomori S, Watanabe K, Laine RA: Pure Appl Chem 49:1215–1227, 1977.
20. Hakomori S, Watanabe K, Laine RA: Human Blood Groups, 5th International Convocation Immunologists, Buffalo, NY. Basel: Karger, 1976, pp 150–163.
21. Steck TL: J Cell Biol 12:12–19, 1974.
22. Marchesi VT, Furthmayer H, Tomita M: Annu Rev Biochem 45:667–698, 1976.
23. Childs RA, Feizi T, Fukuda M, Hakomori S: Biochem J 173:333–336, 1978.
24. Fukuda MN, Matsumura G: J Biol Chem 251:6218–6225, 1976.
25. Fukuda MN, Watanabe K, Hakomori S: J Biol Chem 253:6814–6819, 1978.
26. Fukuda MN, Fukuda M, Hakomori S: J Biol Chem 254:5458–5465, 1979.
27. Fukuda M, Fukuda MN, Hakomori S: J Biol Chem 254:2700–3703, 1979.
28. Sakiyama H, Robbins PW: Fed Proc 32:86–90, 1973.
29. Yogeeswaran G, Hakomori S: Biochemistry 14:2151–2156, 1975.
30. Whatley R, Ng SK-C, Roger J, McMurray WC, Sanwal BD: Biochem Biophys Res Commun 70:180–185, 1976.
31. Hakomori S, Kijimoto S, Siddiqui B: In Fox F (ed): "Membrane Research." New York: Academic Press, 1972. pp 253–277.
32. Lingwood CA, Hakomori S: Exp Cell Res 108:385–390, 1977.
33. Carter WG, Fukuda M, Longwood CA, Hakomori S: Ann NY Acad Sci 312:160–177, 1978.
34. Young WW Jr, Laine RA, Hakomori S: Meth Enzymol 50:137–140, 1978.
35. Marcus DM: In Witting LA (ed): "Glycolipid Methodology." 1976, pp 233–246.
36. Watanabe K, Powell ME, Hakomori S: J Biol Chem 253:8962–8967, 1978.

observed to form mainly on cells moving on flat substrata and represent a conformation of the cell to that substratum. Generally, they are very thin — only 0.1–0.4 μm thick in fibroblasts — and appear to contain no other cytoplasmic organelles than a meshwork of actin-containing microfilaments, particularly in their thinnest peripheral portions. Ruffles often form at and near the margins of lamellipodia, as a result of uplift of the margin or directly from the upper surface. However, they should not be considered special protrusions; they are merely upward extensions of a lamellipodium. *Filopodia* are long, thin, tapering protrusions that are often branched and adhere to the substratum mainly or entirely at their tips. They are particularly characteristic of cells moving in a three-dimensional fibrous matrix, but by no means entirely limited to them. They have also been observed on cells moving on flat substrata, especially in vivo. Like lamellipodia, filopodia also appear to contain only a meshwork of microfilaments, but if they are straight and under tension, their microfilaments may be oriented into a bundle. *Microspikes* are short, spike-like versions of filopodia, formed occasionally by both fibroblasts and epithelial cells and universally by the tips of extending neurites. Often they are quite straight and bend only at their base, giving the impression that they are hinged when they move about in the medium. *Lobopodia* are long, mostly unbranched, finger-like projections from the cell surface that are much thicker and usually shorter than the much more attenuated filopodia. They have been observed thus far only in vivo in early embryos, where they may be commonplace. They too are filled with microfilaments.

Blebs stand in contrast to all these other protrusions in that they have a highly standardized form, which is invariably hemispheric. All blebs look alike. In keeping with their hemispheric form, they are unstructured [2]. They lack the meshwork of microfilaments that invariably fills all the other protrusions just described, and in thin sections they appear to be empty blisters of plasma membrane, arising above and protruding outside the intact underlying microfilamentous cortex [3–5]. Characteristically, blebs form and recede rapidly in a matter of seconds. They have not been observed to have a locomotor function in vitro. Within the embryo during early embryogenesis, however, they frequently become true organs of locomotion. Rather than quickly receding, they continue to protrude, nourished by an abundant flow of cytoplasm from the main body of the cell, which gives them structure [6]. The cell literally pours itself into the advancing bleb and thus moves itself along [7].

Each of these cell protrusions, including blebs, extends actively from the cell surface and in one way or another has been shown to be an essential part of the locomotor apparatus. Another kind of cell protrusion, *retraction fibers,* also deserves attention, even though they are not actively involved in locomotion, because they are routinely confused with filopodia (even in the best of journals). Retraction fibers [8] are long, taut, exceedingly thin, absolutely straight cell extensions that are formed when a portion or all of the margin of the cell retracts. Their tips, which adhere firmly to the substratum, represent some of the previous focal contacts of the adhering marginal part of the cell. Like other nonhemispheric protrusions, they too are filled with microfilaments. This is not surprising, for they are really derived from lamellae or filopodia or other adhering regions of the cell margin. The essential point to be made is that retraction fibers are formed passively, as a result of retraction, not protrusion, even though they appear to be able to exert active contractile force. They tell where the cell has been, not where it is going. It is vital, therefore, to avoid the common mistake of confusing them with filopodia and microspikes.

This rough classification is legitimate in that all of these protrusions are usually morphologically distinctive. However, each may also grade into another. A receding lamella may form blebs as well as ruffles. Filopodia may broaden and spread on the substratum as lamellipodia. And lamellae may form microspikes at their edges. Even hemispheric blebs may extend to form elongated structured lobopodia that adhere at their tips and shorten, or that adhere to and spread out on a substratum and become lamellae.

STRUCTURE OF SURFACE PROTRUSIONS

In order to operate effectively as organs of locomotion, these various protrusions must of course have purchase on some topographically stable substratum in order to gain traction. Although this is a matter of crucial importance that is being investigated in a number of laboratories and that must one day be understood if we are to understand cell movement, it is a most intractable problem. I have therefore chosen in this essay to ignore it in favor of a consideration of how the cells form the various kinds of surface protuberances that serve in one way or another as their organs of locomotion, regardless of how they adhere to the substratum.

A significant feature of all these protrusions, excepting blebs, is the fibrous cytoskeletal ultrastructure of the cytoplasm. They are packed with a meshwork of microfilaments, composed mainly of F-actin and associated proteins, and they lack cytoplasmic organelles. Since these microfilaments are continuous with the meshwork of microfilaments found more or less universally in the cortical cytoplasm of tissue cells, it is not unreasonable to think of these protrusions as extensions of the cell cortex. Further, since all of these protrusions, excepting blebs, vary in some way from the form of a sphere and have a certain stability, they must be structured [2, 9]. The obvious candidate for this structuring is the meshwork of microfilaments. It is an excellent candidate not only because it is there (it is the only structure evident in the electron microscope), but because in addition we now have increasing chemical and physical reasons to assign a structural as well as a contractile role to the cytoplasmic contractile proteins [10, 11]. Moreover, their close contact with the inner surface of the plasma membrane [12–14] provides a structural basis for an interaction between these two major constituents of the cell periphery. The best evidence for this postulated structural role for the microfilaments, however, would be a demonstrated loss or lack of structure in their absence. Such an experiment has been provided by Nature in the form of blebs. Their invariable hemispheric form and high degree of instability (they are always short-lived, retracting within seconds after they have appeared) are always associated with a hyaline cytoplasm that in thin sections is characteristically structureless. Blebs seem to be devoid of microfilaments and indeed of all other cytoplasmic organelles, such as microtubules, mitochondria, Golgi, and endoplasmic reticulum [3–5].

How a meshwork of microfilaments might operate to give each kind of structured protrusion its distinctive form is, of course, a complete mystery and one of the fundamental questions in research on cell movement. It is relatively easy to imagine how a contractile cortical meshwork might cause constriction of a portion of a cell, as during cytokinesis, but how could it be responsible for the reverse – the extension of a portion of a cell? The best models at hand have been provided by the beautiful work of Tilney and his associates [10, 15, 16] on the extension of the acrosomal filament of certain spermatozoa. It seems that actin, without interaction with myosin, can cause extension of these elongate protrusions by a process involving either rapid polymerization of nonfilamentous actin into F-actin or changes in packing arrangement of filaments within a bundle. Once the acrosomal extension is formed, the actin filaments then provide the needed skeletal support. Unfortunately for tissue cells (ie, for us who work on them), however, this polymerization model seems at present to be of limited use. At least some of the actin in the cortical cytoplasm of tissue cells is already present in its filamentous form before protrusions form. If, therefore, polymerization of actin were involved in protrusive activity of tissue cells, it could account for only part of the process. And, furthermore, given the polarity of actin filaments attached to the plasma membrane, protrusive activity of the cell surface cannot be mediated by interaction of these filaments with myosin (see Mooseker et al [17] for discussion).

Two other cytoplasmic components of great structural importance are microtubules and intermediate (100-Å) filaments. The former have been exhaustively investigated and are certainly important in the genesis and maintenance of the overall shape of many cells and of course of specialized protrusions such as cilia and flagella, but they do not seem to be directly involved in the protrusive activities of the kinds of cells I discuss in this essay. In fact, as Abercrombie et al [18] have emphasized, fibroblasts seem to lack an effective cytoskeleton in the strict sense. When a fibroblast detaches from its surroundings, it does not retain its extended shape but retracts to a spheroid shape, which is maintained until new adhesions are formed. Moreover, when microtubules are disrupted by colchicine or colcemide, protrusive activity continues. However, the cell polarity is destroyed, for protrusive activity continues all around the periphery of the cell, giving the cell a pancake-like appearance [19, 20]. This suggests that microtubules somehow reinforce the polarity of the cell and therefore the dominance of the leading lamella, probably by their orientation along the long axis of the cell. Thus, they play a role in the maintenance of an elongate cell shape, once it is established by the protrusive and adhesive activity of the cell.

Intermediate filaments have only recently been subjected to intensive study and it does seem that they too have some kind of structural role [21]; but like microtubules, they do not in themselves maintain the shapes of fibroblasts. And there is certainly no evidence that they have any direct function in protrusive activity. It is probably significant that they appear to be particularly abundant in epithelial cells, where microtubules are either absent or present only in vanishingly small numbers [22–24]. Some intermediate filaments are of course associated with desmosomes as tonofilaments, which no doubt have some kind of structural function.

SOURCE OF CELL SURFACE FOR PROTRUSIVE ACTIVITY

Although detachment of the trailing edge of an extending cell is necessary for displacement of the whole cell, it is in considerable part a passive activity [25]. The business end of the operation is the front. For it is there, at the leading edge, that the protrusive activity that thrusts the cell forward is taking place. It is to this fascinating process that I wish now to devote my attention.

Inasmuch as the remainder of this essay will be concerned with protrusive activities of the cell surface, I am obligated to define what I mean by this commonplace but often ambiguous term. It is now well established 1) that the plasma membrane and the cytoskeletal proteins of the cortical cytoplasm are both structurally and functionally linked and 2) that in consequence it no longer makes sense to speak of them separately, as if they were separate entities. Together they constitute a unit. Accordingly, when henceforth I refer to the "cell surface" I encompass in this term the plasma membrane, including both its peripheral and integral components, and the cortical cytoplasm with which it is intimately linked.

A number of lines of evidence now support an intriguing and useful working hypothesis: that tissue cells have enough cell surface material (as just defined) already present at the surface of the cell at any given moment during interphase of the mitotic cycle to satisfy their requirements for the local increases in surface area that accompany protrusive activity.

Even though cell growth and protein synthesis, including of course the synthesis and assembly of new cell surface material, take place continually during G-1 up to the restriction point, as the daughter cells double their volume [26–28], it is proposed that this synthetic activity is not required for protrusive activity and thus not for cell movement. And, indeed, it has been shown that enucleated fibroblasts and epithelial cells continue to spread and move about [29–31], even in the presence of cyclohexamide [31], demonstrating conclusively that this kind of protrusive activity does not depend on protein synthesis.

If fabrication of new cell surface is not required for protrusive activity, the additional cell surface of a protrusion must naturally be derived from already existent cell surface in another part of the cell. Cell surface must move from one place to another, presumably by surface flow. One would predict, therefore, that the local increase in surface area that occurs in a locus of protrusive activity would be accompanied by a corresponding decrease in surface area elsewhere. Thus, formation of new protrusions or expansion of protrusions already present will necessarily require retraction of other protrusions. Moreover, the amount of surface area retracted should be roughly equivalent to the amount protruded. In a word, during all of this moving about, the total surface area of the cell should remain unchanged. It should be emphasized, incidentally, that when I speak of "cell surface," I mean surface materials at the periphery of the cell, not those that might be added from the interior, by exocytosis, for example.

This hypothesis is certainly not original. Indeed, in a sense it is a logical extension of the proposal of Weiss and Garber [32] that there is a competition among lamellar protrusions of fibroblasts in locomotion, based on the acute observation that as one lamella assumes dominance others recede. The dominant one appears to expand at the expense of the others. And anyway it is a common observation that protrusive activity and retractive activity of fibroblasts in culture are somehow balanced, in the sense that for brief periods of time they always yield a cell of roughly standard spread area; and a rounded cell that respreads always expands again to about the same area as before.

Finally, a word is in order concerning the possible relevance of certain studies of surface flow to this hypothesis. Wolpert and Gingell, with characteristic insight, already suggested some years ago [33] that membrane flow lies at the basis of protrusion formation, a notion that is completely consistent with the proposed hypothesis, if one includes flow of the cytoskeletal cortex along with that of the surface membrane to which it is linked. Direct evidence of a kind of surface flow in fibroblasts and epithelial cells has come from marking the edge of an advancing lamella with various small particles [22, 34–37] (but see Bretscher [38]). Particles attached to the surface at the edge of a lamella invariably move centripetally, toward the nucleus, in a kind of capping. It has been proposed that such unidirectional particle transport is due to a continuous and exceedingly rapid flow of cell surface away from the margin, new surface being assembled rapidly at the advancing margin. Leaving aside the possibility that such flow is wholly or partially induced by the multivalent particles themselves, the possible significance of such a unidirectional flow is not clear, especially in the light of the evidence on protrusive activity that I am about to present. I intend, therefore, to bypass these interesting findings temporarily, until such time as we better understand their significance and can find a way of integrating them with other evidence at hand.

Mobility of the Cell Surface in Relation to Protrusive Activity

On theoretical grounds, we have every reason to assume that plasma membrane can flow from one part of the cell surface to another, because of its fluidity at physiological temperatures [39–41]. Moreover, morphological studies of the cell surface during different phases of cellular activity have yielded results that are thoroughly consistent with this. Fully spread fibroblasts tend to have smooth surfaces, as viewed in the scanning electron microscope, whereas rounded ones are covered with a forest of microvilli and tiny blebs [42–45]. And when measurements are made of the total area of cell surface, taking the areas of these protuberances into account, rounded early mitotic cells and fully spread cells turn out to have approximately the same surface area [45]. It is not surprising, therefore, that when such a rounded cell begins to spread and its microvilli disappear, they disappear first in the marginal regions, where spreading first starts and lamellae are first evident, and then continue to disappear progressively submarginally as the whole cell becomes involved in the spreading and flattening process. These results clearly imply that much of the surface of these cells is conserved in the abundant tiny protrusions that cover all or much of the surface of rounded cells. Such a reserve could conceivably provide a ready supply of surface on which the cell could draw for the rapid formation or expansion of filopodia and lamellipodia, rather than having to depend on the assembly or exocytosis of entirely new cell surface.

A number of observations on other systems suggest that this is not an artifact of culture conditions but a general phenomenon that occurs in vivo within organisms as well. For example, microvilli disappear in the region of the furrow during cleavage of hydromedusa eggs [46] and decrease in size and number as the yolk syncytial layer of a teleost egg expands in epiboly [23]. Further, in this same egg, folds on the surface cells of the blastoderm disappear as these cells also flatten and expand in epiboly; and folds on the surface of Xenopus epidermal cells also disappear as these cells spread during wound closure [24].

Since microvilli and folds of the cell surface are invariably packed with a meshwork of contractile microfilaments, flattening or unfolding of them must involve a redistribution of the cortical cytoplasmic material, as well as of plasma membrane. And, indeed, there is now considerable evidence suggesting that cortical microfilaments can in fact move from one part of a cell to accumulate in another part and that when they do this they have a profound effect on surface activity. A few examples will suffice. Microfilaments accumulate or become ordered at the equator during mitosis, where they soon become involved in the furrowing of cytokinesis (see, for example, Schroeder [47, 48]). There is also evidence that microfilaments accumulate at the apical ends of cells of the neural plate, where they become involved in constriction of this part of the cell during neurulation (see the review by Karfunkel, [49]). Capping of Con A by amoebae of Dictyostelium is accompanied by a movement of cortical actin and myosin with a resultant accumulation of them beneath the cap [50]. Macrophages treated with colchicine concentrate their microfilamentous cortex at one end of the cell, with an accompanying concentration of phagocytic activity in that region [51]. And, finally, when the surface of the external yolk syncytial layer of the Fundulus egg folds during epiboly, the meshwork of microfilaments in the cortical cytoplasm beneath the folds becomes vastly thickened [23].

In view of these results, we have every reason to propose that the disappearance of marginal microvilli of a fibroblast during the formation of marginal lamellar protrusions is a sign that these tiny protuberances are contributing their plasma membrane and its associated microfilament meshwork to the formation of the spreading lamella.

If so, these observations also imply that, once a fibroblast is completely spread and all microvilli and blebs have disappeared, a new source of cell surface material must be provided; else how could such a cell continue to expand its current protrusions or form new ones, as it moves over the substratum? There seem to be two possible sources of such a supply: addition of new cell surface from the interior of the cell or flow of material already at the cell surface, which is made available by the retraction of other protrusions. A number of lines of evidence favor the latter possibility.

Contact Inhibition of Protrusive Activity

Of all the social activities among cells moving on plane substrata in culture the best known is contact inhibition of cell movement [52]. Although this important phenomenon is usually dealt with in terms of the temporary inhibition of protrusive and ruffling activity that occurs where a lamellipodium contacts and adheres to another cell, a subsequent and equally important consequence of this adhesion is an *augmentation* of protrusive activity, either of the free, uncontacted part of the same lamella or elsewhere on the cell surface [53–56]. As a matter of fact, it is this dual effect — inhibition of protrusive activity and hence of spreading (and ruffling), followed by augmented protrusive activity elsewhere along the free border of the cell — that accounts for the directional movement of fibroblasts centrifugally from an explant. Clearly, if protrusive activity of the leading and therefore dominant lamella is inhibited, it will lose its competitive advantage, so to speak, and other regions of the cell surface, particularly other free, uncontacted regions of the same lamella, will gain advantage and increase their protrusive activity. Although no one appears to have made the requisite measurements, it seems most likely that during contact inhibition cell surface that would have been utilized for continued protrusion of the inhibited cell border is now available for protrusive activity elsewhere. If it is thus utilized and flows from the inhibited region to the region of increased protrusive activity, the overall area of the cell surface should not change.

An invariable, but often ignored, accompaniment of contact inhibition is a retraction of the region of the lamella in contact with the other cell. This is called contact retraction [57]. It involves retraction of the contacted part, which, since it is stuck to the other cell, does not break away (at least, not immediately) and is thereby placed under tension. The cause and significance of this interesting reaction are not known, but it suggests that contact might stimulate contractile activity in the microfilament system in the cortical cytoplasm, a not surprising result in view of the linkage of this system to the plasma membrane. In addition, since protrusive activity soon accelerates nearby, one might speculate that such a withdrawal might be a means of diverting cell surface away from the region of contact and making it available for adjacent protrusive activity.

Antagonism Between Blebbing and Spreading

Although the phenomenon has never been studied quantitatively, many of us who work on the mechanism of tissue cell locomotion on plane substrata in culture have often remarked that spread fibroblasts or epithelial cells seldom form blebs, except under special circumstances (see below), and when actively blebbing cells begin to spread, they cease to bleb. Fundulus deep cells, for example, bleb much less frequently, if at all, if spread (both in vivo and in vitro) [58]. There seems to be an antagonism between spreading and blebbing.

A case in point is contact-induced spreading. Certain cells tend to remain rounded and form blebs actively in culture as long as they remain separate. When they contact other cells, however, they adhere to them and quickly spread. Significantly, as they spread, blebbing ceases. Good examples of this are deep cells of the early Fundulus gastrula [59; Shure and Trinkaus, unpublished observations], corneal epithelial cells of the chick embryo [22], and retinal pigment cells of the chick embryo [60–62]. It is not understood how contact with another cell might induce spreading, a matter of much interest in its own right, but the arresting feature of this phenomenon in the present context is that cells actively involved in the formation of one kind of protrusion (blebs) cease forming that protrusion when they form another kind of protrusion, in this case lamellipodia. It seems that these cells must choose between one kind of protrusive activity and another. Could this be due to the availability of only a given amount of cell surface?

Another striking and, at present, more instructive example of such an antagonism is that between spreading, with its accompanying ruffling, and blebbing of fibroblasts. Harris [63] found that one can induce a fibroblast to bleb merely by detaching the edge of one of its lamellae from the substratum. Being under tension, the detached margin retracts immediately and then blebs actively, often precisely in that lamellar region. Also, in these fibroblasts blebbing frequently alternates with ruffling. Thus, as cells respread after being detached, their margins first bleb; then, as the cell becomes more flattened, ruffling replaces the blebbing. There is clearly an antagonism between lamellar protrusive activity at the leading edge (whether it be spreading or ruffling, which seem to be basically the same protrusive activity) and blebbing. This could be the result of competition for a given amount of cell surface.

Retraction-Induced Spreading

The most impressive evidence that protrusive activity of one region of the surface of a tissue cell depends on retractive activity in another comes from a recently discovered phenomenon that Chen has termed "retraction induced spreading" [64–66]. In brief, when the tapering, taut trailing edge of a moving chick heart fibroblast detaches from the plane substratum in culture (whether naturally or artificially upon the intervention of a microneedle) and quickly retracts, an immediate consequence is a spurt of protrusive activity at the leading edge of the cell, ie, at its opposite end.

Ordinarily, a lamellipodium at the leading edge of a chick heart fibroblast advances on a glass substratum at an average rate of about 21 μm^2/min [65]. Upon abrupt retraction of the trailing edge, however, its rate of advance increases dramatically. During the first 8 sec period after detachment of the trailing edge, when it is retracting at a rate of 1,800 μm^2/min, the speed of advance of the leading edge increases to a new accelerated rate of from 132 μm^2/min to 618 μm^2/min, for an average speed of 240 μm^2/min. This represents a tenfold increase in the rate of protrusion of the leading lamellipodium. After this initial fast retraction, the trailing portion of the cell retracts much more slowly and is completely retracted by 2–3 min after detachment [25]. Interestingly, the rate of spreading at the leading edge also gradually declines after its initial burst, but it does not regain its normal rate until 10–15 min after detachment. Significantly, planimetric measurements of total spread area of such retracting fibroblasts give the same values at the beginning and the end of this sequence. The overall decrease in spread area of the trailing portion of the cell is compensated for exactly by the overall increase in spread area at the leading edge.

Immediately after detachment of the trailing edge, however, there is a transitory decrease in total spread area. During the first 8 sec after detachment, the rate of decrease in the area of the trailing portion is clearly greater than the rate of increase of the leading portion (see above). This is a fascinating discrepancy, for it appears to be a case of the exception proving the rule. Examination of the cell surface with scanning electron microscopy (SEM) at this time reveals that surface folds appear over the nucleus, immediately after retraction, probably representing excess cell surface derived from the retracted trailing portion of the cell [25]. Such folds would of course not be detected in planimetric measurements of whole living cells and so would show up as a decrease in total surface area. Predictably, when these folds disappear, about 10 min later, planimetric measurements show that the previous total surface area has been restored. It seems possible, therefore, that with retraction of the trailing portion of the cell the cell surface is transferred toward the leading edge, where it is utilized in the accelerated protrusive activity. Moreover, it seems highly probable that some of this cell surface passes from the rear to the front by way of transitory surface folds, which would thus represent a temporary reserve of cell surface.

Observations demonstrating that increased protrusive activity very similar to this can also be induced in very different cells — extending neurites in culture — suggest that we may be dealing with a general phenomenon of universal importance. Wessells and Nuttall [67] have found that if the central part of the tip of an extending neurite (growth cone) is lifted off the substratum with a microneedle so that it retracts, the two sides will protrude in divergent directions. This leads to branching and demonstrates that one can induce neuronal branching at will. By the same token, one can cause a tip to extend preferentially to the left or to the right merely by lifting the microspikes of the other side from the substratum. Upon detachment, they of course retract, and the consequence is increased protrusive activity on the other side. By this means, Wessells and Nuttall are able to "steer" neurite extension at will, first in one direction and then in another.

Competition between protrusive activities in different regions of a cell has also been observed in an epithelial sheet from the chick amnion spreading in culture [68]. When a gap appears in the sheet just in back of the spreading leading edge, it never seems to be closed by retrogade movement of a cell at the leading edge. Thus, an already established spreading lamella at one end of the cell seems to prevent spreading elsewhere on the surface of the cell, possibly because of competition for a given amount of cell surface.

In another entirely different system, the epidermis of the transparent fin of the tadpole of Xenopus laevis, Radice [24] has shown that when basal epidermal cells spread to close a wound in vivo, extension of a lamellipodium on the free edge of a cell at the edge of a wound is compensated for, at least in part, by retraction of the rear end of the same cell. In this instance, however, the retraction of another part of the cell is not the stimulus for further spreading at the leading edge, as in the experiments just described for spread fibroblasts and extending neurites. The stimulus is the creation of a free edge, by the artificial imposition of a wound. Retraction of the trailing edge comes somewhat later, after the leading edge has spread and thinned considerably. This reversed sequence of events is correlated with two facts. In the intact epidermis, prior to wounding, the basal cells are relatively thick and thus have plenty of cell surface available right there at the leading edge for initial spreading and thinning. And the margins of these basal cells always retract somewhat upon wounding. It is only after this retracted marginal material is entirely spread out over the wound surface and thus "used up," as it were, that retraction of the trailing edge occurs. It is as if further advance at the front cannot take place unless reinforcements are brought up from the rear.

Because of technical difficulties, measurements of surface area have not yet been made in these spreading Xenopus epidermal cells, nor in extending neurites; however, since the relationship between retraction and protrusion in these cells seems basically the same as in moving fibroblasts, the observations also support the hypothesis that retraction of one part of the cell is a precondition for continued protrusion of another part.

Retraction-induced protrusive activity in fibroblasts and neurites is of great interest not only because it constitutes the most vivid and direct evidence of a competition for cell surface among the various protrusions of the cell surface, but also because this provides the experimentalist with direct control over protrusive activity. A particularly frustrating aspect of research on tissue cell movement has been the impossibility of predicting precisely where and when new protrusive activity will occur. Now, for the first time, one can induce rapid protrusive activity in one area of the cell surface at will, merely by causing retraction of another area. This crucial aspect of cell movement has therefore become open for analysis and many questions have come to the surface. In particular, it would be of great interest to know whether there is in fact surface flow (of plasma membrane and cortical cytoplasm) toward the region of increased protrusive activity, as we would now predict. Perhaps marking the cell surface with monovalent antibodies or lectins will provide a partial answer [37].

Relevance of Bleb Formation

We understand no better the mechanism of the formation of unstructured blebs than of structured protrusions. However, here too, there is evidence that there is surface flow involved. To appreciate how this might happen and its possible relation to bleb formation, we must look at the structure and behavior of blebs in some detail. A curious and important feature of blebs is that the meshwork of cortical microfilaments appears to remain essentially intact at the base of a bleb, rather than move out into it as in structured protrusions [3, 5]. It looks as if the plasma membrane of the bleb has separated from the microfilamentous cortex of the cytoplasm. If this fine-structural picture is an accurate representation of what happens, then separation of the plasma membrane from the cortical microfilament meshwork could well be a crucial event in the formation of a bleb and be responsible for two of its primary characteristics — clear, hyaline cytoplasm and hemispheric form. The hyaline nature of the cytoplasm is obviously a consequence of the absence of cytoplasmic organelles such as mitochondria, etc., which are apparently sieved out by the intact microfilamentous cortex at the base of a bleb. The hemispheric form could also be due to this separation, because if the plasma membrane is no longer anchored to the cortical meshwork of microfilaments, it is probably incapable of resisting the thrust of the normal internal hydrostatic pressure of the cell (turgor). Since this pressure is exerted evenly in all directions, the result would be a ballooning outward as a hemispheric blister.

Strong evidence that cortical microfilaments can indeed have such an anchoring effect on the cell periphery has come from the deformability studies of Wolpert [69] on cleaving sea urchin eggs. As the furrow forms and its thickened band of cortical microfilaments becomes obvious [48], its resistance to deformation by the application of negative pressure on the cell surface increases. Strong evidence that blebbing of the cell surface is associated with weakening or absence of the microfilamentous cortex has come from recent studies of the capping of concanavalin A by amoebae of Dictyostelium discoideum. Condeelis [50] has found that capping is accompanied by a concentration of much of the cell's myosin-like and actin-like microfilaments underneath the cap (see p. 893). This, of course, causes a marked thinning of the microfilament cortex at the other end of the cell, with the result — of much interest in the present context — that the cell surface bulges to form a number of rounded protrusions (blebs?). Blebs also form at the poles of many dividing cells during anaphase, precisely when there is a great accumulation of microfilaments in the furrow. Could this be due to a thinning or weakening of the microfilamentous cortex at the poles [70]?

Harris [36] has produced support for the hypothesis that blebbing is due to the momentary release of the hydrostatic pressure within the cell at weak points in the cell surface by immersing cells in medium made strongly hypertonic with sorbitol. This reverses the pressure differential across the cell surface, with the result that further blebbing ceases and existing blebs collapse. The effect is reversible. Of course, decreasing the internal hydrostatic pressure of the cell in this way would also have other effects, such as increasing the concentration of various dissolved molecules like soluble enzymes. The possible influence of such a consequence on protrusive activity has not been explored.

Although local separation of the plasma membrane from the cortical cytoplasm could well be the primary event in the formation of a bleb, it is not sufficient to explain the quick local increase in cell surface that such a protuberance represents. This must depend on either a stretching of the plasma membrane at that locus or the addition of new membrane. It seems unlikely that stretching is involved. The only plasma membrane that has been studied in detail for this possibility, that of the human erythrocyte, appears to stretch little if at all; its surface area remains constant throughout osmotic hemolysis [71, 72]. Although it may be justly protested that the plasma membrane of the erythrocyte is hardly comparable to that of a rapidly deforming tissue cell, still it is all we have to go on. And anyway, as we shall see, present information appears to render an assumption of stretchability of the plasma membrane unnecessary.

But if we assume that the plasma membrane does not stretch, the increase in area in one of these moving tissue cells must be due to assembly of new membrane at the site, insertion of new membrane from the cytoplasm below by exocytosis, or movement of membrane into the site from elsewhere on the cell surface. Although there is clear evidence of the assembly of much new membrane in the formation of the acrosomal filament of Thyone sperm [15], there is no evidence of it during the formation of the protrusions of tissue cells. Nor is there any evidence of the addition of already formed membrane by exocytosis. Hogan and I [73] studied thin sections of motile, blebbing Fundulus deep cells and never found membrane vesicles subjacent to or fused with cell surface (but, of course, if there were such vesicles it would be easy to miss them). This leaves us with the last possibility — movement of cell surface into the site of the prospective bleb from elsewhere on the cell surface.

Tickle and I [6] tried to get information on this matter by marking the surface of Fundulus deep cells with carbon particles near a normally forming bleb or a bleb formed artificially by exertion of negative pressure by means of a micropipette on a localized area of the cell surface. In each case, the marks moved toward the protrusion as it formed. This suggests that there is a flow of nearby cell surface toward the forming protrusion, ie, that the protrusion gets its extra area by recruitment of nearby uninvolved cell surface. The source of this flow is rather puzzling, however, since the surfaces of these cells are quite smooth, there being no microvilli or microblebs that could serve as a reserve source of cell surface [3; Trinkaus and Erickson, unpublished observations]. This is not an insignificant matter. Since the diameter of a bleb of one of these embryonic blastomeres is rather large, a quarter to a third that of the whole cell, the surface flow involved must be considerable. Measurements of particle movement elsewhere on the cell surface during bleb formation have not been made; hence, we do not know whether there is a concomitant decrease in surface area on the other side of the cell, although this would not be surprising since volumetric measurements have shown that the cell body decreases distinctly in volume as a bleb expands to form a large protrusion [6]. The hypothesis that extra membrane is involved in bleb formation is supported by the observation [36] that when a bleb on a fibroblast retracts it crenates or wrinkles — as if, when drained of its fluid contents, the extra surface, having nowhere to go, simply folds up like an accordion. This has also been observed to occur normally upon retraction of blebs of Fundulus blastomeres [7].

Since blebs often form in spread fibroblasts in the lamellar region close to where a local retraction has just occurred, the sudden local availability of retracted cell surface could be a determining factor in their localization. In rounded embryonic cells, however, where blebs seem to form anywhere on the cell surface, we have no inkling as to what might be the localizing factors. In fact, whatever these localizing factors might be, they often break down, as when a bleb spreads over the cell surface in a circus or limnicola movement. Nor do we understand what causes the cell surface to move toward the site of bleb formation from the sides. Perhaps the extra surface is moved in by a concentric contraction of its cortical meshwork of microfilaments. But this is pure speculation.

ANTAGONISM BETWEEN PROTRUSIVE ACTIVITY AND CYTOKINESIS

A number of lines of evidence now suggest that there is not only a competitive relationship among different protrusive activities but also an antagonism between the protrusive activities of cell movement and cytokinesis. This is not surprising, since both plasma membrane and contractile cortical cytoplasm are utilized in both. An important aspect of cell division is the accumulation of cortical cytoplasm at the equator to form a "contractile ring" of circumferentially oriented cortical microfilaments in the furrow. The thickening of this ring as the furrow deepens has been taken as evidence that this contraction is a major force in the formation and deepening of the furrow, and therefore in cytokinesis [47, 48, 70, 74, 75]. Clearly, the activity of the actomyosin cortical microfilament system is heavily involved in both cytokinesis and cell movement (although in the latter case, we still do not know how). It seems inevitable, therefore, that when the cell engages in one of these activities the other will be reduced or precluded.

Another common feature of protrusive activity associated with cell movement and cytokinesis is increase in surface area — local during protrusive activity and general during cytokinesis. Increase in surface area during cytokinesis is based in part on simple geometry. When a sphere is divided into two spheres with the same total volume, the surface required to cover the unchanged volume increases by about 26%. However, this does not necessarily require addition of new surface. This calculation assumes that the spheres involved are smooth-surfaced, like billiard balls. But many spheroid cells, such as fibroblasts that are about to divide, are in fact not at all smooth on the surface; they are covered with a forest of microvilli, folds, and microblebs which increases their true surface area enormously [43–45]. Thus, if the increased surface required during furrowing is drawn from these surface protrusions, no new surface would be required. However, as a consequence, the amount of surface available for a locomotor protrusive activity, such as spreading, would be correspondingly reduced, and by this token cytokinesis and protrusive activity would compete for cell surface. It is therefore of much interest that microvilli on the surface of the egg of the hydromedusa Aequoria disappear in the actively furrowing region but remain intact in the noncleaving portion of the egg surface [46]. This result is clearly consistent with the hypothesis that the new surface required during the formation of the daughter cells is provided by the unfolding of old surface already there on the mother cell. It is not yet known whether this unfolding provides all of the requisite 26% increase in cell surface area; this is clearly a matter deserving more attention than it has yet received. Nor is it known where the 26% comes from in smooth-surfaced cells like Fundulus deep cells.

After cytokinesis of a fibroblast or epithelial cell is complete, the daughter cells are freed of this competitive relationship and spreading is once again possible. It begins almost immediately and seems to get the extra cell surface required from the remaining microvilli and microblebs [45]. There must of course be addition of new cell surface, as the daughter cells gradually grow during G-1 and eventually double their volume. For, with this increase in volume, the surface area inevitably increases. But, as I have shown (see p. 892), this slow addition of new cell surface is not required for protrusive activity and cell movement.

Antagonism Between Cell Spreading and Cytokinesis

Even though, for unknown reasons, untransformed fibroblasts will not synthesize DNA and divide in culture unless they spread on the substratum during interphase [76], nevertheless when they do divide they apparently must assume a spheroid form. One rarely sees normal cells dividing in the spread state. Everyone who has watched cultures of fibroblasts closely has marveled at how they suddenly retract from the substratum and "round up" to go into mitosis, remaining attached to the substratum solely at their focal sites of adhesion by long, thin retraction fibers. (Indeed, such rounded early mitotic cells are so easily detached from the substratum, because of the tenuousness of these retraction fibers, that this is the basis of a practical method of collecting synchronously dividing cells, merely by shaking them off the substratum.) Clearly, even though spreading during interphase is a precondition for division of a fibroblast, when the act itself is about to occur the cell must become spheroid in order to perform. There is obviously an antagonism between the protrusive activity of spreading and cytokinesis; and it is only when cytokinesis is fully complete that the daughter cells begin to spread again, given the proper substratum. It seems probable that this antagonism is based at least in part on competition for contractile machinery and plasma membrane, ie, for that given amount of cell surface that is essential for both.

It may be objected that this antagonism between spreading and cytokinesis could as well be due merely to simple geometric considerations — there being insufficient space in a thin, highly spread cell for the spindle, the asters, and the movement of chromosomes. This could be so. However, since there is also an antagonism between another protrusive activity (blebbing) and cytokinesis in large spheroid, embryonic blastomeres (see below), this possibility seems improbable. In any case, whatever the reasons may be for this important antagonism between spreading and cytokinesis, for some curious reason there appears to have been no systematic study of it.

Antagonism Between Phagocytosis and Cytokinesis

Phagocytosis also ceases during cytokinesis. For example, phagocytosis of IgG-opsonized erythrocytes by the macrophage line J774 stops completely during all phases of cell division between midprophase and early G-1 [77]. These cells show rapid phagocytosis at all other stages of the cell cycle. This antagonism is of interest in the present context because of the basic resemblance of phagocytosis and spreading. In both cases, lamellar cytoplasm spreads over a solid or semisolid substratum. The only differences are probably trivial — the size of the particle over which the spreading occurs and whether it is anchored or not. If the particle is small and unanchored, it is engulfed. If it is large and firmly anchored, it serves as a substratum for spreading. Indeed, spreading fibroblasts also show phagocytosis, although it is usually called "pinocytosis," and, as in phagocytosis by macrophages, lamellar cytoplasm is involved. It takes place on the upper surface of the leading lamella and is associated with ruffling. Further, the cortical meshwork of microfilaments somehow participates in both spreading and phagocytosis. If microfilaments are caused to concentrate at one end of a leukocyte by treatment with colchicine, phagocytic activity also concentrates at that end [51]. In view of the basic similarity of phagocytosis and cell spreading, it is little wonder that cytokinesis is antagonistic to both. This is no doubt due in part to the common need of these processes for contractile microfilaments and plasma membrane.

Antagonism Between Blebbing and Cytokinesis

Study of the behavior of deep blastomeres of the teleost blastoderm has revealed another antagonism between protrusive activity and cytokinesis that in its own way is just as striking. If cells of blastulae and early gastrulae of the teleosts Oryzias and Fundulus are cultured on a lowly adhesive substratum such as bacteriological plastic in the presence of serum, they remain spherical and continually form large blebs that have a diameter about a third that of the cell. When such a cell is about to enter upon mitosis, however, this incessant blebbing ceases, with the result that the cell becomes completely spherical and quiescent (Fujinami, unpublished observations; Shure and Trinkaus, unpublished observations). It remains so in Fundulus for about 15 min and then enters upon cytokinesis. The resulting daughter cells also remain quiescent for a short time and desist from blebbing. But about 8 min after cytokinesis they resume normal, frequent blebbing and continue like this until shortly before the next cytokinesis. There is clearly an antagonism between blebbing and cytokinesis. Since we do not understand how blebs form, we can only guess that this antagonism is based, as spreading and phagocytosis seem to be, on a competition for contractile cortical cytoplasm and plasma membrane. In any case, it seems certain that when this particular antagonism is understood, we will understand much more about the mechanism of blebbing (and perhaps cytokinesis as well) than we now do.

ADDENDUM

I would like now to discuss briefly the possible implications of these thoughts for our understanding of two fundamental developmental problems — the commencement of gastrulation and directional cell movements during morphogenesis.

Cleavage and the Commencement of Gastrulation

In view of this antagonism between protrusive activity of the cell surface and cytokinesis, one would predict that there would be little or no cell movement in the embryo during periods of development when all of the cells are undergoing rapid division. And, indeed, this is precisely the case at the very beginning of development, when *all* the blastomeres are engaged in the rapid divisions of cleavage. Cleaving blastomeres are legendary for their geographical stability. They do not move. Quite the contrary: They remain so nicely in place after each succeeding cleavage division that in certain eggs the exact location of the daughter cells of each succeeding cleavage is entirely predictable. And because of this cytokinetic regimentation, the lineage of early blastomeres in such eggs can be traced with precision to quite advanced stages. Witness the famous studies of cell lineage in the mosaic eggs of the annelids, molluscs, and tunicates. But even in nonmosaic embryos, such as those of echinoderms and vertebrates, where the typical patterning of the earliest cleavages is soon blurred, cell movements do not begin until after the rate of cleavage has drastically declined. Indeed, insofar as is known, gastrulation, the next phase of development, with its massive and often extensive cell movements, does not begin in any embryo until after the rapid divisions of cleavage have almost or entirely come to a halt. Moreover, once gastrulation has started, the rate of cell division remains at an exceedingly low level [eg, 23].

A striking example of the antagonism between cleavage and gastrulation is found in the echinoderms. Because of their exquisite transparency, echinoderm embryos have been the material of choice in many studies of cleavage and gastrulation. The rapidity of their cleavage in some instances is truly astonishing. In Paracentrotus lividus, for example, each succeeding division occurs just 30 min after the last, at a normal summer temperature of $27°$ in Marseille. (And in Xenopus laevis, cleavage is even faster, the interval being $15-30$ min at $22-24°$ [78]). This is a generation time far shorter than that of the most rapidly dividing cell lines in culture and actually comparable to that of many bacteria! In point of fact, the interval between divisions is so short that the S period for the next division begins already in telophase of the preceding division. With each cleavage division coming along like this, right on the heels of the last, the cytoskeletal apparatus of cleavage — microtubules for the asters and spindle and contractile microfilaments for furrowing — is bound to be totally and constantly involved [70, 74, 75]. For this reason, it seems most improbable that this apparatus could be made available for cell locomotion between divisions. And indeed there is none. Why these cleaving blastomeres are so obsessed with the matter at hand that often they do not even undulate in between!

Several workers have taken advantage of the stellar qualities of these beautiful embryos to follow the fate of the various kinds of blastomeres right up to and during gastrulation [79]. Thus we know the early development of echinoderms in truly precise detail. In considering the relation between cleavage and cell movement, however, the fate of the four micromeres formed at the vegetal pole by the fourth cleavage is of most interest. For most of the descendants of these small blastomeres develop into the primary mesenchyme cells of the gastrula [80, 81], the very first cells to move during gastrulation. Later on, these cells form the spicules of the pluteus larva [80, 81]. The morphogenesis of these delicate and distinctive skeletal elements by chains of these cells has been the subject of a series of elegant studies by Okazaki (see, eg, ref 82), but for now it is their locomotion that is our primary concern. Well before the onset of the invagination of the archenteron they move out of the tightly packed vegetal plate of the blastocoel wall and migrate extensively on the inner surfaces of the lateral walls of the blastocoel. It is arresting, therefore, that the ancestors of these cells are the first blastomeres to cease cleavage. After their first appearance as four small blastomeres at the vegetal pole of the 16-cell stage, the micromeres undergo but three more cleavages to form a total of 32 cells. The number appears to vary somewhat from one species to another, but it is always of this order of magnitude. Okazaki, for example, counted about 30 of them shortly after their release from the vegetal wall in Clypeaster and Mespilia [83, 84]. After this, as they are migrating about, they either do not divide [85] or divide very little [81, 83, 86, 87]. In contrast to the micromeres, the mesomeres and macromeres of the 16-cell stage continue to divide for upwards of six more cleavages [81, 88], ceasing much later than the micromeres, and, significantly, their descendants, which form the rest of the embryo, do not engage in locomotion until a considerably later time than the descendants of the micromeres. If there is antagonism between cleavage and the onset of the normal cell movements of gastrulation, we should expect to find exactly what has been found — that those blastomeres that cease dividing first are the first to move and those that cease last are the last to move.

This antagonism no doubt explains at least in part how it happens that the cell movements of gastrulation do not begin sooner. Rapid division of the zygote by cleavage is surely necessary to provide the large number of cells required for the mass cell movements of gastrulation and for later organogenesis and histogenesis, as we have all been taught, but as long as these rapid cleavages go on, tying up the machinery of cell movement, gastrulation cannot begin. As cleavage wanes, that machinery is released and becomes available for other activities, such as cell locomotion. Interestingly, in the only two instances where the first surface activities associated with cell movement have been observed in situ during early development, in sea urchins [85] and teleosts [7, 89, 90], the first sign of this is the appearance of blebs, a protrusive activity that ceases abruptly as the preparations for cytokinesis begin.

Directional Cell Movements During Morphogenesis

One of the distinctive features of morphogenetic cell movements during embryogenesis is their extraordinary directionality. Although there may be minor deviations along the way, the net movement of the cells engaged in any particular morphogenetic movement is along the same paths toward the same destination. In spite of the crucial importance of this directionality in the construction of the organism, however, we still do not understand how it occurs [91].

The most popular idea has been that it is the environment of these moving cells within the embryo that somehow imparts their patterns of migration, including their directionality. Until recently this has been no more than a reasonable idea. Now, there is solid evidence on the matter. A number of clever studies of the neural crest have established that the migratory pathways traced by these remarkable cells are determined in large part by the embryonic environment through which they migrate. If neural crest cells are transplanted to a new site, along the neural tube, either heterochronically or heterotopically, they move to the destinations typical of the new site [92–94]. In consequence, the question for neural crest cells is no longer whether the environment may have a determining influence, but how.

Chemotaxis has often been proposed, but the only firm evidence for it is in vitro, where polymorphonuclear leukocytes respond readily and predictably to chemotactic attractants. All evidence in the embryo is equivocal. Another ancient and popular idea, stemming from the days of Harrison, has been *contact guidance*: that cells could be guided by orientations in their substrata within the embryo, as they are in culture [95, 96]. Even though there is no unambiguous evidence that this occurs in situ, there is much that is suggestive [97]. Here again the neural crest, that most studied of migratory primordia, is instructive. Since these cells emigrate from the dorsal aspect of the neural tube through a highly complex mixture of cells and various constituents of extracellular matrix (ECM) [98], it comes as no surprise that the onset of emigration of certain cells of the neural crest is apparently dependent on the appearance of an ECM substratum in the region to be invaded. Thus the migration of the cranial crest is preceded by the appearance of a large cell-free space filled with ECM into which the cells migrate [99]. That such ECM could provide an oriented substratum for migrating crest cells gains support from the observations of Löfberg and Ahlfors [100] that fibrils of ECM on the sides of the neural tube have the same orientation as the neural crest cells migrating in that region. But even if contact guidance is at work, giving orientation to the migration of neural crest cells and to other cells elsewhere in the embryo, it cannot in and of itself give directionality. It can only give orientation. That is, it can keep a cell moving either forward *or* backward with a certain orientation and prevent it from moving sideways, but it cannot guarantee forward movement only. This would require additional factors. *Contact inhibition of cell movement* can and does certainly give directionality to the movement of cells migrating from a cell mass in culture [52] and has been shown to operate in vivo as well [101, 102]. But when there are no more cells coming up from behind to inhibit cells from moving backward, they would be free to move in that direction as well. Accordingly, it is difficult to see how contact inhibition could give directionality in situ for long-distance embryonic migrations like those of the neural crest, after the cells have moved well away from their source. Another way in which cells behind might possibly influence the forward movement of cells in front is by contact-induced blebbing.

Fundulus deep cells in culture respond to nudging by forming a bleb at the opposite side of the cell [58, 103]. Finally, it has also frequently been suggested that if *gradients in adhesiveness* of the substratum existed within the embryo, cells would tend to move along these, from regions of lesser to regions of greater adhesiveness. And here too there are excellent in vitro model systems where cells have been shown to do just that [104–106]. But, once again, there is no evidence that such gradients exist within the organism, where they might be utilized by moving cells. In sum, even though a number of eminently reasonable ways of imposing directionality upon moving cells has been proposed, and demonstrated to work in vitro, none at present is at the same time a sufficient mechanism in itself *and* unequivocally demonstrated to be operative in vivo. We must therefore pose the question again: How might migrating cells gain directionality during morphogenesis?

I suggest that with the discovery of retraction-induced spreading an exciting new factor has been added — a force generated by the cells themselves — that in combination with other factors might move cells surely and inexorably toward their destinations. If so, we will have taken a long stride toward understanding directionality of cell movement. For, when the trailing edge of a moving fibroblast detaches and retracts in the course of its locomotion in vitro, the forward spreading of its dominant leading lamella is always accelerated [64–66]. That is to say, detachment and retraction at the rear of one of these moving cells *reinforces* movement at the front in the same direction as it was traveling before. This no doubt explains why an individual fibroblast tends to continue moving in vitro in a given direction for extended periods in the absence of collision with other cells [107]. Now then, if retraction-induced spreading operates in vivo (and there seems at present to be no a priori reason why it should not), this could conceivably provide just that added factor which together with certain environmental influences could keep a cell moving in a given direction. I can best illustrate what I mean by a simple speculation. Let us imagine that once cells are set in motion (whatever the stimuli) they tend to move away from their source as a result of their contact inhibiting properties. If their substratum is oriented, the guidance that it imparts will tend to keep them from moving sideways. At first, they will be inhibited from moving backward by contact with cells coming from behind. However, already at this early stage in their emigration, and continuously throughout their movement, their initial forward movement on their oriented substrata will be reinforced by retraction-induced protrusive activity at the leading edge. In other words, once cells are moving in a particular direction, they will tend to continue in that direction simply because detachment and retraction will tend to occur at the rear end, with a consequent acceleration of protrusive activity and continued forward movement at the front end. Thus, by retraction-reinforced protrusive activity of the existing leading edge, combined with responses to contact with other cells and orientations of the substratum that have been well-established for in vitro conditions, cells may achieve the genuine directionality of movement on which much morphogenesis rests. Now, what is needed are comparable studies of cells moving in vivo, within the embryo.

ACKNOWLEDGMENTS

I am indebted to W-T. Chen, M. S. Mooseker, G. P. Radice, and M. S. Shure for many stimulating discussions. My recent research has been supported by grants from the NIH (US PHS-HD-7137 and CA-22451).

REFERENCES

1. Clark ER: Am J Anat 13:351, 1912.
2. Rayleigh L: Phil Mag (Ser 5) 34:145, 1892.
3. Lentz TL, Trinkaus JP: J Cell Biol 32:121, 1967.
4. Trinkaus JP, Lentz TL: J Cell Biol 32:139, 1967.
5. Fujinami N: J Cell Sci 22:133, 1976.
6. Tickle C, Trinkaus JP: J Cell Sci 26:139, 1977.
7. Trinkaus JP: Devel Biol 30:68, 1973.
8. Taylor AC, Robbins E: Dev Biol 7:660, 1963.
9. Harvey EN: Protoplasmatologia 2(5):1, 1954.
10. Tilney LG, Hatano S, Ishikawa H, Mooseker MS: J Cell Biol 59:109, 1973.
11. Pollard TD: J Supramolec Struct 5:317 (269), 1976.
12. Pollard TD, Korn ED: J Biol Chem 248:448, 1973.
13. Pollard TD, Weihing RR: CRC Crit Rev Biochem 2:1, 1974.
14. Weihing RR: Methods Achiev Exp Pathol 8:42, 1979.
15. Tilney LG: In Brinkley BR, Porter KR (eds): "International Cell Biology." New York: Rockefeller Press, 1977, p 388.
16. Tilney LG: J Cell Biol 64:289, 1975.
17. Mooseker MS, Pollard TD, Fujiwara K: J Cell Biol 79:444, 1978.
18. Abercrombie M, Dunn GA, Heath JP: In Lash JW, Burger MM (eds): "Cell Tissue Interaction." New York: Raven Press, 1977, p 57.
19. Vasiliev JM, Gelfand IM, Domnina LV, Ivanova OY, Komm SG, Olshevskaja LV: J Embryol Exp Morphol 24:625, 1970.
20. Goldman RD: J Cell Biol 51:752, 1971.
21. Eriksson A, Thornell L-E: J Cell Biol 80:231, 1979.
22. DiPasquale A: Exp Cell Res 94:191, 1975.
23. Betchaku T, Trinkaus JP: J Exp Zool 206:381, 1978.
24. Radice GP: (Submitted.)
25. Chen W-T: J Cell Biol 75, No. 2, Pt2:416a, 1977.
26. Pardee AB: Proc Natl Acad Sci 71:1286, 1974.
27. Baserga R: "Multiplication and Division in Mammalian Cells." New York: Marcel Dekker, 1976, p 239.
28. Pardee AB, Dubrow R, Hamlin JL, Kletzien RF: Ann Rev Biochem 47:715, 1978.
29. Goldstein L, Cailleau R, Crocker T: Exp Cell Res 19:332, 1960.
30. Shay JW, Porter KR, Krueger TC: Exp Cell Res 105:1, 1977.
31. Goldman RD, Pollack R, Hopkins NH: Proc Natl Acad Sci USA 70:750, 1973.
32. Weiss PA, Garber B: Proc Natl Acad Sci USA 38:264, 1952.
33. Wolpert L, Gingell D: "Asp Cell Motil." Cambridge: Cambridge U Press, 1968, p 169.
34. Abercrombie M, Heaysman JEM, Pegrum SM: Exp Cell Res 62:389, 1970.
35. Harris AK, Dunn GA: Exp Cell Res 73:519, 1972.
36. Harris AK: Ciba Found Symp 14:3, 1973.
37. Harris AK: Nature 263:781, 1976.
38. Bretscher MS: Nature 260:21, 1976.
39. Frye LD, Edidin M: J Cell Sci 7:319, 1970.
40. Singer SJ: In Rothfield (ed): "Structure and Functions of Biological Membranes." New York: Academic, 1971, p 145.
41. Singer SJ, Nicolson GL: Science 175:720, 1972.
42. Wolpert L, Gingell D: Ciba Found Symp 10:241, 1969.
43. Follett EAC, Goldman RD: Exp Cell Res 59:124, 1970.
44. Knutton S, Sumner MCB, Pasternak CA: J Cell Biol 66:568, 1975.
45. Erickson CA, Trinkaus JP: Exp Cell Res 99:375, 1976.
46. Szollosi D: J Cell Biol 44:192, 1970.
47. Schroeder TE: Z Zellforsch Mikrosk Anat 109:431, 1970.
48. Schroeder TE: J Cell Biol 53:419, 1972.
49. Karfunkel P: Int Rev Cytol 38:245, 1974.

50. Condeelis J: J Cell Biol 80:751, 1979.
51. Berlin RD, Oliver JM: J Cell Biol: 789, 1978.
52. Abercrombie M, Heaysman JEM: Exp Cell Res 5:111, 1953.
53. Abercrombie M, Ambrose EJ: Exp Cell Res 15:332, 1958.
54. Trinkaus JP, Betchaku T, Krulikowski LS: Exp Cell Res 64:291, 1971.
55. Partridge T, Davies PS: J Cell Sci 14:319, 1974.
56. Erickson CA: Exp Cell Res 115:303, 1978.
57. Abercrombie M, Dunn GA: Exp Cell Res 92:57, 1975.
58. Trinkaus JP: Zoon 6:51, 1978.
59. Trinkaus JP: Dev Biol 7:513, 1963.
60. Middleton CA: Ciba Found Symp 14:251, 1973.
61. Middleton CA: Nature 259:311, 1976.
62. Middleton CA: Exp Cell Res 109:349, 1977.
63. Harris AK: Dev Biol 35:97, 1973.
64. Chen W-T: J Cell Biol 79, No. 2, Pt2:83a, 1978.
65. Chen W-T: J Cell Biol 81:684, 1979.
66. Dunn GA: BSCB Symp Adhes Motil. Cambridge: Cambridge U Press, (In press).
67. Wessells NK, Nuttall RP: Exp Cell Res 115:111, 1978.
68. Vaughan RB, Trinkaus JP: J Cell Sci 1:407, 1966.
69. Wolpert L: Exp Cell Res 41:385, 1966.
70. Sanger JW, Sanger JM: Methods Achiev Exp Pathol 8:110, 1979.
71. Canham PB, Parkinson DR: Can J Physiol Pharmacol 48:369, 1970.
72. Jay AWL: Biophys J 13:1166, 1973.
73. Hogan JC Jr, Trinkaus JP: J Embryol Exp Morphol 40:125, 1977.
74. Rappaport R: Int Rev Cytol 31:169, 1971.
75. Arnold JM: Cell Surf Rev 1:55, 1976.
76. Folkman J, Moscona A: Nature 273:345, 1978.
77. Berlin RD, Oliver JM, Walter RJ: Cell 15:327, 1978.
78. Nieuwkoop PD, Faber J: "Normal Tables of Xenopus laevis." Amsterdam: North-Holland, 1975.
79. Hörstadius S: "Experimental Embryology of Echinoderms." Oxford: Clarendon, 1973, p 192.
80. Boveri T: Zool Jahrb Abt Anat Ont 14:630, 1901.
81. Endo Y: Dev Diff (Tokyo, Iwanami Shoten) 1–66, 1966.
82. Okazaki K: Symp Cell Biol (Japan) 22:163, 1971.
83. Okazaki K: Embryologia 5:283, 1960.
84. Okazaki K: Exp Cell Res 40:585, 1965.
85. Gustafson T, Wolpert L: Exp Cell Res 24:64, 1961.
86. Agrell I: Ark Zool 6:213, 1954.
87. Paresi E, Filosa S, DePetrocellis B, Monroy A: Devel Biol 65:38, 1978.
88. MacBride EW: "Textbook of Embryology." London: MacMillan, 1914, vol 1, p 504.
89. Wourms JP: J Exp Zool 182:169, 1972.
90. Kageyama T: Devel Growth Diff 19:103, 1977.
91. Trinkaus JP: Cell Surf Rev Amsterdam: North-Holland, 1:225, 1976.
92. Weston JA, Butler SL: Dev Biol 14:246, 1966.
93. LeDouarin NM, Teillet MAM: Dev Biol 41:162, 1974.
94. Noden DM: Dev Biol 42:106, 1975.
95. Harrison RG: J Exp Zool 17:521, 1914.
96. Weiss PA: J Exp Zool 100:353, 1945.
97. Trinkaus JP: In Locke M (ed): "Major Problems in Developmental Biology." New York: Academic, 1966, p 125.
98. Weston JA, Derby MA, Pintar JE: Zoon 6:106, 1978.
99. Pratt RM, Larson MA, Johnson MC: Dev Biol 44:298, 1975.
100. Löfberg J, Ahlfors K: Zoon 6:87, 1978.
101. Lesseps R, Hall M, Murnane MB: J Exp Zool 297:459, 1979.
102. Van Haarlem R: Devel Biol 70:171, 1979.
103. Tickle C, Trinkaus JP: Nature 261:413, 1976.
104. Carter SB: Nature 208:1183, 1965.
105. Harris AK: Exp Cell Res 77:285, 1973.
106. Letourneau PC: Devel Biol 44:92, 1975.
107. Gail MH, Boone CW: Biophys J 10:980, 1970.

The Association of α-Actinin and Clathrin With the Plasma Membrane

Keith Burridge, James Feramisco, and Stephen Blose

Cold Spring Harbor Laboratory, Cold Spring Harbor, New York

The role of α-actinin in the attachment of actin to plasma mebranes has been investigated. Double-label indirect immunofluorescence has been used to show that in lymphocytes α-actinin will concentrate beneath caps of aggregated surface Ig, confirming the recent report by Geiger and Singer [23]. Specific antibody-staining of SDS gels has indicated that α-actinin is a major component in isolated plasma membranes prepared from three different cell types by two different procedures. A fraction of this α-actinin is readily dissociated from these membranes with relatively little parallel release of actin. The remaining α-actinin is more resistant to extraction but can be removed by prolonged dialysis against low ionic-strength buffers which also dissociate most of the actin. The dissociation characteristics of α-actinin from the plasma membrane lead us to suggest that α-actinin does not form a direct link between actin and the membrane, although it may promote and stabilize actin attachment by cross-linking adjacent actin filaments close to the membrane.

During the course of our work with isolated plasma membranes we have tentatively identified a prominent component of these membranes as clathrin, the major protein of coated vesicles [8].

Key words: α-actinin, clathrin, plasma membranes, actin attachment, immunoautoradiography on gels

During the last few years much has been learned about the proteins involved in the force generation required for cell movement, but the question of how these force generating elements, such as actin, are attached to cell membranes remains unanswered. Much of the thinking about nonmuscle motility has been influenced by the knowledge of the structure of muscle and the properties of the muscle-contractile elements. In striated muscles the actin filaments within each sarcomere insert into the Z-line and emerge from either side of a Z-line with opposite polarities [1]. A major component of the Z-line throught to be involved in actin attachment is the protein α-actinin, which in vitro has the properties of binding to and cross-linking actin filaments [2–4]. The discovery of α-actinin in non-muscle cells [5, 6] led to the suggestion that it might also mediate actin attachment to

Abbreviations: ATP) adenosine triphosphate; EGTA) ethyleneglycol bis (β aminoethylether)-N,N'-tetraacetic acid; EDTA) (ethylenedinitrilo) – tetraacetic acid; MES) 2 (N-Morpholino) ethane sulfonic acid; PBS) Dulbecco's phosphate buffered saline; SDS) sodium dodecylsulfate.

Received May 2, 1979; accepted August 13, 1979.

membranes in these cells [5]. This suggestion gained indirect support from immuno-fluorescent micrographs which revealed that α-actinin was found not only with a periodic distribution along the microfilament bundles but also appeared to be at the terminations of these bundles in regions of cell-substrate adhesion and cell-to-cell contact [5]. Such regions in electron micrographs have frequently increased electron density [7] and this together with the associated filaments is reminiscent of a muscle Z-line.

This paper is directed towards investigating the possible role of α-actinin in the attachment of actin filaments to nonmuscle plasma membranes. Direct analysis of isolated plasma membranes indicates the presence of α-actinin as a major component. Some evidence is obtained from the dissociation of α-actinin from these membranes that is more consistent with α-actinin having an indirect role in actin attachment, with α-actinin possibly promoting and stabilizing the attachment by cross-linking adjacent filaments rather than providing a direct link in the attachment itself.

While working with isolated plasma membranes our attention was drawn to a major component of these membranes with an approximate molecular weight by SDS gel electrophoresis of 175,000. This we have tentatively identified as the protein clathrin, the major protein of coated vesicles and coated pits [8, 9].

MATERIALS AND METHODS

Cells

Hela cells were grown suspended in Dulbecco's modified Eagle's medium (DME) supplemented with 10% calf serum. Mouse myeloma cells, P3 X63 Ag8, were a generous gift of Dr. G. Kohler and were grown suspended in DME with 9% fetal-calf serum (FCS). Gerbil fibroma cells (IMR-33) which have a fibroblast morphology were obtained from the American Type Culture Collection and were grown in 10 cm plastic petri dishes in DME with 9% FCS.

Mouse lymphocytes were obtained from the spleens of Balb/c mice and were suspended in DME containing 2% FCS that had been inactivated for complement at $56°C$ for 30 minutes. In several preparations the red blood cells were lysed by incubating in 0.85% NH_4Cl, 10mM Tris Cl, pH 7.4 for 10 minutes on ice. The cells were then washed twice in DME containing 2% FCS.

Antibody Against α-Actinin

An antiserum was raised in rabbits against beef cardiac α-actinin which was the generous gift of Dr. D. Goll in 1973. The protein was further purified by elution from preparative-SDS-polyacrylamide gels. The initial two injections were given ten days apart at multiple subcutaneous sites in Freund's complete adjuvant. These were followed by a series of four intravenous injections every seven to ten days, with the final two being of α-actinin that had not been eluted from the preparative gels.

For immunofluorescence studies, the antibody against α-actinin was affinity purified. For this α-actinin was purified by a new method [Feramisco and Burridge, submitted for publication] from chicken gizzards. The protein was eluted from preparative SDS gels and coupled to Sephadex G-50 (fine) by the cyanogen bromide method [10]. A crude IgG fraction, prepared by a 40%-saturated ammonium sulphate precipitation of the whole serum, was applied to the column equilibrated in buffer A (0.15M NaCl), 0.1% sodium azide, 50mM Tris HCl, pH 7.5). The column was washed extensively in Buffer A until the OD_{280} of the eluate returned to baseline and the bound antibody was then eluted with 0.3M sodium citrate (pH 3.0). After rapid neutralization this was dialyzed against Buffer A.

Capping and Double-Label Immunofluorescence

For the capping of mouse splenic lymphocytes, the freshly prepared cells were incubated in fluorescein-labelled goat anti-mouse IgG (Cappel) for 30 minutes to one hour at 4°C. The cells were used at about 10^7/ml and the commercial antibody was used at 1/10 dilution after dialysis against Dulbecco's phosphate buffered saline (PBS). After the initial incubation the cells were washed with an excess of cold PBS, then suspended in 1 ml of PBS at room temperature, and allowed to cap at this temperature. At pre-determined time points the cells were fixed by addition of an equal volume of 3% formaldehyde in PBS. After at least five minutes fixation, the cells were washed and resuspended in PBS and then plated onto polylysine coated coverslips. The cells were then permeabilized by incubating the coverslips in PBS containing 0.5% Triton X-100. After approximately five minutes the cells were rinsed in PBS and then treated with the affinity purified anti-α-actinin antibody used at a concentration of about 100 μg/ml. After a one hour incubation at 37°C the coverslips were washed in PBS for 30 minutes and then incubated with the second antibody, a rhodamine conjugated goat anti-rabbit IgG (Cappel) diluted 1/50 in PBS. After one hour at 37°C the coverslips were washed again for 30 minutes, rinsed in deionized water, and then mounted in gelvatol.

For the staining of the gerbil fibroma cells, the coverslips were fixed in 3% formaldehyde and then permeabilized and treated with the antibodies under identical conditions used for staining the coverlips of the mouse lymphocytes.

Cells were photographed on a Zeiss photomicroscope III with a Zeiss 63X oil-phase 3 lens on an epifluorescence nose piece. Fluorescein was analyzed with a Zeiss dichroic-excitation filter BP 485/20 and barrier filter LP520, and rhodamine with a G546 (narrow band, pass interference filter, 546nm±2nm) excitation filter and LP590, barrier filter. Photomicrographs were recorded on Kodak Tri-X film (5063), EI 400, or Ektachrome-400 film (5074), EI 800. 100% of the light was diverted to the film plane for exposure. Image magnification at the film plane was 270X.

Reaction of Gels With Antibodies

Analytical SDS-slab gels were run using the discontinuous buffer system of Laemmli [11]. The separating gels contained 10% acrylamide and 0.13% bisacrylamide, or 7.5% acrylamide and 0.195% bisacrylamide, while the stacking gels contained 5% acrylamide and 0.13% bisacrylamide.

Gels were treated with the crude antiserum against α-actinin diluted 1/30th in Buffer A essentially as described previously [12, 13]. One major modification, however, was in the preparation of the second radio-iodinated antibody. This was purified and iodinated as follows. An immunoadsorbent was prepared by covalently coupling column purified rabbit IgG to Sepharose 4B, using cyanogen bromide to activate the Sepharose 4B [10]. After an overnight incubation with the rabbit IgG, the column was washed and any unreacted groups were blocked with 1M ethanolamine, pH 8.5. The column was then washed with 0.1M glycine-HCl, pH 2.3.to elute noncovalently bound protein. After washing in this buffer the column was re-equilibrated in Buffer A, before incubating with goat anti-rabbit IgG (purchased from either Calbiochem or Miles). The column was washed with buffer A until the OD_{280} of the eluate returned to the background level, at which point the specific goat anti-rabbit IgG was eluted with 0.1M glycine-HCl, pH 2.3. The eluted IgG was immediately neutralized with 1M Tris buffer, pH 8.8 and then dialyzed against Buffer A. For iodination a peak fraction of the eluted protein (approximately 9 mg/ml) was dialyzed against 0.1M sodium borate pH 8.6, and was then reacted with 1 millicurie of ^{125}I-labelled Bolton-Hunter reagent [14] (New England Nuclear) as described previously [13]. Typically, activities of between 5×10^8 and 8×10^8 cpm/mg protein have been obtained. The iodinated antibody was separated from the iodinated, low-molecular-weight, reaction products on a small Sephadex G50 (fine) column, equilibrated in Buffer A, and the iodinated protein was stored frozen together with 10 mg/ml of BSA. For reacting on gels, the antibody was used at 10^7 cpm/ml in Buffer A to which an additional 10 mg/ml human hemoglobin (Sigma) had been added. Reaction with gels was for about 12 hours with three to four day washings in Buffer A, both between the first and second antibodies, and after the second antibody prior to staining the gel with Coomassie blue, drying, and autoradiography.

Plasma Membrane Reparation

Plasma membranes were prepared from Hela cells and the cultured myeloma cells by the Brunette and Till procedure [15] with a modification that has been described previously [16] to decrease nuclear contamination. This procedure was also used to isolate plasma membranes from the substrate adherent gerbil fibroma cells after these were suspended by treatment with PBS containing EDTA. The procedure of Thom et al [17] was also used to isolate plasma membranes from the gerbil fibroma cells.

Electron Microscopy

Isolated membranes were fixed with 2% glutaraldehyde and 2% tannic acid in PBS at 4°C for 1 hour, then centrifuged into a pellet. The pellet was washed three times in PBS and postfixed in 1% OsO_4 in PBS for 30 minutes at 20°C. The pellets were then stained with saturated aqueous uranylacetate for 20 minutes, dehydrated in graded alcohol over 15 minutes, and embedded in Epon 812. Thin sections were prepared and stained with lead citrate.

Membrane fractions were prepared for negative staining by placing a 10μl sample on a Formvar-carbon coated grid for two to three minutes and then removing excess buffer. The grid was stained with 2%-aqueous uranylacetate for 30 seconds and air dried. Membrane fractions were decorated with heavy meromyosin after the method of Ishikawa et al [18].

Purification of Clathrin

Coated vesicles were purified from frozen calf brain (Pel-freez) by the procedure of Keen et al [19]. Clathrin was dissociated from the coated vesicles and purified by gel filtration on Sepharose C1-4B [19].

RESULTS

Characterization of the α-Actinin Antibody

The antibody used in this study was similar to one which we have used previously [5], and like that one gave specific staining of myofibril Z-lines in indirect immuno-fluorescence (data not shown). We have tested this antibody further by using it to stain SDS gels of both pure proteins and complex mixtures such as cell lysates. In Figure 1 purified chicken gizzard α-actinin and chicken breast phosphorylase were electrophoresed in parallel gel slots. The proteins were compared by conventional staining with Coomassie blue, and the gels were also reacted with the anti-α-actinin which specifically labelled the α-actinin gel-band but not that corresponding to phosphorylase. Figure 2 shows an SDS gel of whole Hela cells stained for protein and a parallel autoradiograph of a similar gel reacted with the same antibody. A single band at 100,000 molecular weight is labelled with this antibody. On some gels with enhanced resolution this band could be resolved clearly as a doublet, as was reported previously [5], and this was not affected by the presence of protease inhibitors during the gel sample preparation.

For immunofluorescence studies anti-α-actinin antiserum was further purified by affinity chromatography. When the resulting antibody was applied to fixed and per-meablized fibroblasts and used for indirect immunofluorescence, the staining pattern illustrated in Figure 3 was typically observed. A periodic distribution of α-actinin along the microfilament bundles is seen, frequently with bright regions where the filament bundles end. The cell shown in this figure had been plated for about eight hours and was still spreading. Visible in this cell and others during the spreading process are fluorescent foci corresponding to α-actinin in the centers of the microfilament polygonal networks, transitory structures characteristic of spreading cells, and described originally by Lazarides [20] and studied subsequently by Gordon [21].

Concentration of α-Actinin Beneath Lymphocyte Caps

Balb/c mouse-splenic lymphocytes were capped with fluorescein-labelled goat anti-mouse IgG. At time points during the course of capping, the cells were fixed, plated on polylysine-coated coverslips, permeabilized, and reacted with the affinity purified rabbit anti-α-actinin antibody. The staining of lymphocytes with anti-α-actinin is shown in Figure 4 and was performed at the same time and under identical conditions as those used for staining the fibroblast in Figure 3. The α-actinin is preferntially concentrated beneath the lymphocyte cap. It should be noted that in most lymphocytes that have not been stimulated to cap, the distribution of α-actinin appears fairly uniform throughout the cell. With capping, most of the α-actinin as measured by immunofluorescence, moved into one pole of the cell in apparent association with the fluorescent cap. However, some staining could still be detected in the rest of the cell and in some cells a detectable increase was sometimes noted at the opposite pole to the cap. This second point of localization was usually much smaller than the cap and may indicate a new point of assembly of cytoskeletal proteins in the "front" of the cell opposite the uropod over which the cap is formed.

α-Actinin as a Component of Isolated Plasma Membranes

The Brunette and Till [15] procedure has been used to isolate plasma membranes from several different cell types. A typical preparation of plasma membranes isolated in this way from Hela cells is shown in Figure 5. The inset shows a low magnification phase micrograph of the membranes in suspension. They can be seen to consist of sheets, en-velopes, or rolls of plasma membrane. When a section of a pellet of these membranes is examined by transmission electron microscopy, little contamination by other organelles can be observed. One face of the membrane appears "fuzzy" with particulate and fila-mentous material attached, and we presume this to be the cytoplasmic face. Occasionally, discrete filaments can be seen to emerge from this submembranous cortex, and these filaments will bind HMM confirming that they are actin. In some regions structures with the appearance and dimensions of coated vesicles or coated pits can also be seen and have been indicated.

Such membranes were routinely purified further by centrifugation over a sucrose gradient or by placing in dense sucrose beneath a sucrose gradient and then by centrifuging up the gradient. Reducing agents (either dithiothreitol or β-mercaptoethanol) were included in the gradients to reduce any disulphide bonds that had been formed by the

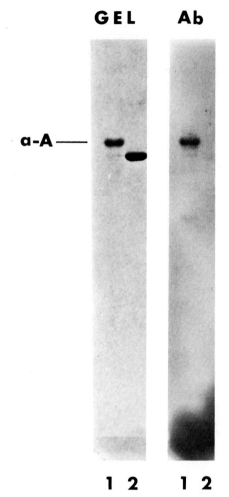

Fig. 1. Immunological detection of α-actinin in an SDS gel. Purified chicken gizzard α-actinin and chicken breast phosphorylase were electrophoresed in adjacent slots of a 10% polyacrylamide SDS slab-gel. A photograph is shown of the Coomassie blue stained dried-down gel together with the corresponding autoradiograph of the same gel after it had been reacted first with anti-α-actinin and secondly with ^{125}I-labelled goat anti-rabbit IgG. The anti-α-actinin antibody labels only the band corresponding to the α-actinin and not the phosphorylase.

presence of zinc in the membrane isolation. The membranes band at a density of about 1.17 g/ml. When membranes that have been spun up a gradient are analyzed by SDS gel electrophoresis, a complex pattern of bands is seen (Fig. 6a). When such a gel is analyzed by indirect immunoautoradiography with antibody against α-actinin labelling of a single band (or tight doublet of bands) with a molecular weight of about 100,000 occurs (Fig. 6a). This labelled band corresponds to a band in the Coomassie blue-stained gel and comigrates with purified rat skeletal muscle α-actinin but has a slightly faster mobility when compared with the α-actinin from chicken gizzard. Several of the other prominent bands in the gels of these plasma membrane preparations we have tentatively identified as cytoskeletal elements, including actin, myosin, and filamin, either by their comigration with the purified proteins or by their reaction with the corresponding antibodies (data not shown).

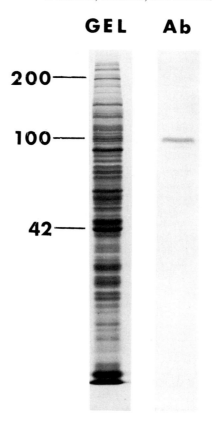

Fig. 2. Detection of α-actinin in a gel of whole Hela cells by reaction with specific antibody. Whole Hela cells were dissolved and electrophoresed in SDS. The photograph of a gel slice stained with Coomassie blue is shown, together with the autoradiograph of a parallel gel slice that was reacted first with anti-α-actinin and then with the iodinated second antibody, as described in Materials and Methods. A single band, that can sometimes be resolved into a tight doublet, is labelled with a molecular weight of approximately 100,000.

When preparations of the Hela plasma membranes were placed above continuous sucrose gradients and subjected to prolonged centrifugation, then SDS gel analysis of fractions across the gradient (Fig. 6b) indicated that several prominent proteins partially dissociate from the plasma mebranes and remain at the top of the gradient. One of these proteins we have identified as α-actinin by its reaction with the anti-α-actinin antibody (Fig. 6c). In this gel, equal volumes of a fraction at the top of the gradient and one corresponding to the position of the peak of the membranes were compared. More α-actinin is detected in the fraction at the top of the gradient. Usually, however, the membranes were collected in about three fractions, whereas only a single fraction at the top of the gradient was enriched for α-actinin. When the membranes were resedimented on a second identical gradient, α-actinin was not detected at the top of the gradient by Coomassie blue staining of a gel of the gradient fractions. For the extraction experiments described below the membranes were either taken off a gradient or were washed in buffer such that the readily dissociable components would have been removed before the extraction were started.

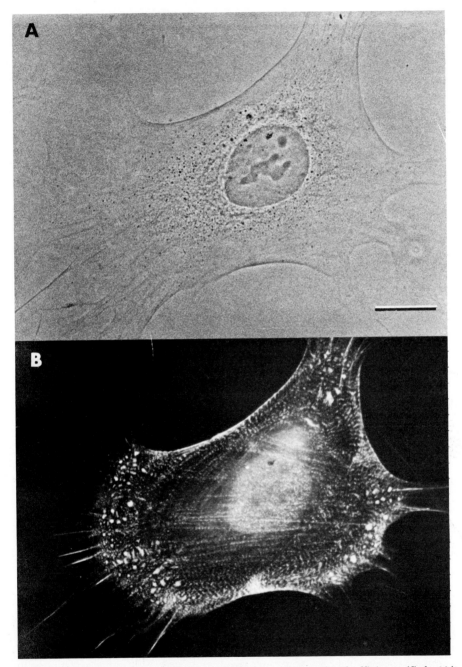

Fig. 3. Phase and fluorescent micrographs of a gerbil fibroma cell stained with affinity purified rabbit anti-α-actinin approximately eight hours after plating. The cell was fixed and processed for indirect immunofluorescence as described in Materials and Methods. Bar = 20μm.

Plasma membranes have been isolated from a myeloma cell line and from gerbil fibroma cells (cells with a fibroblastic morphology) by the producedure of Brunette and Till [15], and from the gerbil fibroma cells also by the procedure of Thom et al [16]. In each case SDS gels of these membranes have revealed a prominent band by Coomassie blue staining at 100,000 which was reacted with the α-actinin antibody. Human red blood cell membranes isolated by hypotonic lysis and centrifugation were also analyzed for α-actinin. Of all the plasma membranes examined these alone did not yield a band at 100,000 molecular weight that reacted with the anti-α-actinin antibody (data not shown).

Identification of Clathrin in Isolated Plasma Membranes

One of the prominent bands in the gels of isolated plasma membranes has an approximate molecular weight of 175,000. This comigrates with purified brain clathrin (Fig. 7). In two-dimensional gels [22] the purified brain clathrin also appears to comigrate with this component although both enter the isoelectric focusing dimension poorly and tend to streak (data not shown). Preliminary data suggests that both the purified brain clathrin and the plasma-membrane protein contain similar tryptic peptides when the tyrosine-containing peptides are compared after radio-iodination.

In the analysis of the plasma membranes on sucrose gradients (Fig. 6b), one of the bands that remained at the top of the gradient comigrates with purified clathrin. It should be noted that a significant proportion continues to move with the plasma membranes in the sucrose gradient. Further evidence that this band is indeed clathrin has been obtained by electron microscopic analysis of this material at the top of the gradient. Initial examination failed to reveal recognizable coated-vesicle structures, but after a 48 hour dialysis into a buffer promoting the formation of coated vesicles [19], these characteristic structures were observed quite frequently (Fig. 8).

Extraction of α-Actinin and Other Proteins From Isolated Plasma Membranes

The nature of the association of α-actinin with the plasma membranes was investigated by extraction of the membranes with various buffers. For the extraction experiments, the membranes were taken either from the sucrose gradients, or after washing the membranes from the Brunette and Till preparation in PBS containing 0.2% β-mercaptoethanol. Either treatment effectively removed most of the proteins that would dissociate readily from the membranes. When such Hela plasma membranes were incubated with, or dialyzed against, physiologically isotonic buffers around neutral pH rather few proteins were extracted when analyzed by gel electrophoresis. Brief extraction (90 minutes) at low ionic strength also had little effect on the protein composition of these membranes. When the membranes were extracted with a myosin extraction buffer (high salt containing MgATP) most of the band comigrating with purified muscle myosin was selectively extracted from these membranes (Fig. 9). Reacting such a gel with the anti-α-actinin antibody revealed a slight decrease in the amount of α-actinin but most remained associated with the plasma membranes.

A brief incubation (30 minutes) with either an actin depolymerization buffer (2mM Tris, 0.2mM ATP, 0.1% β-mercaptoethanol, pH 7.4) or a buffer that will extract α-actinin from muscle (2mM Tris, 0.2mM EDTA, 0.1% β-mercaptoethanol, pH 8.8) had little effect on the pattern of membrane proteins as judged by SDS gels. Prolonged extraction by dialysis against these buffers for 36 hours at 4°C had a marked effect on the membranes. The latter buffer caused the membranes to vesiculate and give rise to small vesicles with the release of most of the proteins detected by Coomassie blue staining (Fig. 10). The actin depolymerization buffer caused less disruption of the membranes but also resulted in extensive extraction of many of the proteins. Both buffers caused most of the actin to remain in the supernatant after the membranes were pelleted at 145,000g for 1 hour. The α-actinin was also largely removed from the membranes by both buffers and was found in the supernatants by antibody staining of the gels of the resulting pellets and

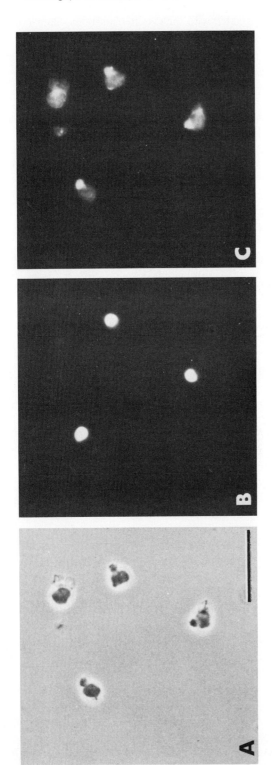

Fig. 4. Double-label immunofluorescent micrographs of mouse lymphocytes to show the distribution of α-actinin relative to capped surface Ig. Lymphocytes were processed for capping and staining with anti-α-actinin as described in the text. A) Four lymphocytes are shown in a phase micrograph after capping for 15 minutes at room temperature with fluorescein-labeled anti-Ig. B) The same lymphocytes viewed under selective optics for the fluorescein fluorescence to reveal the distribution of the surface Ig. Only 3 of the cells were B-lymphocytes as judged by binding of the fluorescein-labeled antibody. In these 3 cells it was concentrated over the uropods of each cell. C) The same cells were viewed with optics specific for the rhodamine fluorescence to detect the distribution of the anti-α-actinin. It should be noted that the same conditions were used for staining these cells with anti-α-actinin as for the staining of the fibroblast in Figure 3. The α-actinin is concentrated beneath the 3 fluorescent caps, although some is also evident in the rest of the cell body. In two of the cells a smaller concentration of α-actinin can also be detected at the opposite pole of the cell to the caps. Bar = 20μm.

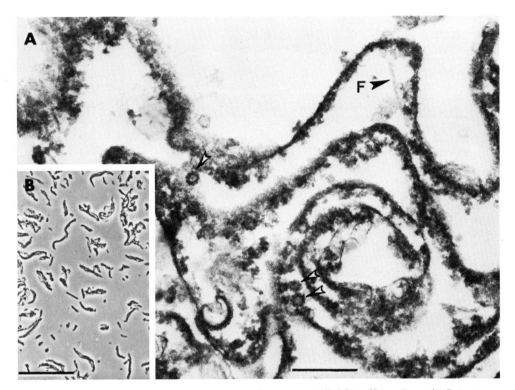

Fig. 5. Light and electron micrographs of plasma membranes purified from Hela cells by the Brunette and Till procedure. The inset B) shows a phase micrograph of freshly prepared membranes in suspension. (Bar = 50μm.) A) shows an electron micrograph of a section through a pellet of these membranes after their reaction with heavy meromyosin. A decorated filament is indicated by the arrow marked F. Three structures resembling coated vesicles or coated pits have also been marked with arrows. Bar = 0.5μm.

supernatants (Fig. 10). It should be noted that the myosin continued to sediment with the membranes or vesicles under these extraction conditions and was one of the few prominent bands remaining in the membrane pellets. This may be due to the low ionic strength conditions promoting myosin filament formation and aggregation, such that it would sediment with the membranes without necessarily being associated with them.

DISCUSSION

Using double-label immunofluorescence we have demonstrated that α-actinin will accumulate beneath the region of a lymphocyte cap. Similar, but more detailed results, were recently presented by Geiger and Singer [23]. Previously it has been shown that both actin [24–30] and myosin [31] will concentrate beneath areas where cell surface molecules have been patched or capped by externally applied multivalent ligands. The finding that α-actinin is also concentrated in such regions could merely reflect the accumulation of actin at these sites since α-actinin is an actin-binding protein. However, it is also consistent with a possible role for α-actinin in the attachment of actin to membranes [5].

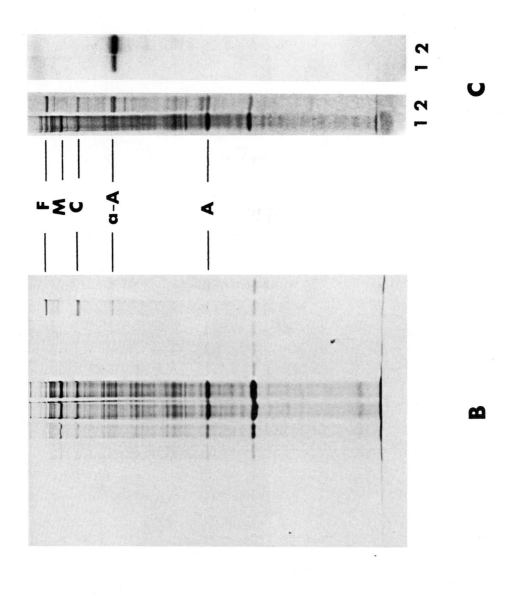

To investigate whether α-actinin could have a role in the attachment of actin to membranes, we have analyzed the association of α-actinin with isolated plasma membranes. Using specific antibody staining of SDS gels as an assay for α-actinin, we have demonstrated this protein in isolated plasma membranes prepared from three different cell types using two different preparative procedures. Only with red-blood-cell membranes did we not find evidence for the presence of α-actinin. It should be noted that in a previous report α-actinin was also tentatively identified in plasma membrane preparations isolated from sarcoma 180 ascites cells by comigration of a band in SDS gels with purified muscle α-actinin [32]. To quantitate the amount of α-actinin in association with the plasma membranes, we developed a radioimmunoassay, but this was not successfully applied to the plasma membranes because the nonmuscle α-actinin only partially cross-reacted with the muscle α-actinin standards against which the antibody had been raised.

To determine how the α-actinin is associated with the membranes, we have tried a series of extractions with different buffers. The principle of selective extraction is well illustrated for myosin (Fig. 9), which could be extracted from the membranes by brief incubation in a buffer which will dissociate actin-myosin interactions. The release of myosin from the membranes was not accompanied by an equivalent actin extraction, demonstrating that the association of myosin with these membranes was via actin and not the other way around as was suggested some years ago [33]. Could the same approach be applied to actin and α-actinin to determine whether the α-actinin mediates actin attachment to the membranes or vice versa? Several different buffers were tried but two were of particular interest: one, an actin depolymerizing buffer and the other, a solution that will extract α-actinin from muscle. Both these extraction buffers removed many proteins from the membranes and effectively stripped the membranes of both actin and α-actinin, such that it was not possible to determine whether the actin was bound via the α-actinin, or the other way around.

Fig. 6. SDS gel analysis of plasma membranes isolated from Hela cells. A) Plasma membranes isolated by the Brunette and Till procedure were further purified by floatation up a 30–55% sucrose density gradient (containing 50mM $NaPO_4$, pH 7.0, 0.1% β-mercaptoethanol). Centrifugation at 40,000 rpm in a Beckman SW50.1 rotor caused the membranes to float up to their buoyant density of about 1.17 gm/ml. About 20 μg of protein from the peak membrane fraction was electrophoresed in one slot of a 10%-polyacrylamide gel. A photograph of the gel stained with Coomassie blue is shown, together with a corresponding autoradiograph after reacting a parallel gel slice with anti-α-actinin followed by ^{125}I-labelled second antibody. The antibody reacts with a tight doublet of bands with a molecular weight of about 100,000. B) Plasma membranes purified by the Brunette and Till procedure were resuspended in PBS + 0.2% β-mercaptoethanol and layered above a linear gradient of 30–55%-sucrose containing 50mM $NaPO_4$, pH 7.0, 0.1% β-mercaptoethanol, with an underlying cushion of 60% sucrose. The gradient was centrifuged in a Beckman SW27.1 rotor at 25,000 rpm for 15 hours. Equal volume fractions were collected and 25 μl of each fraction (except the bottom two which were not analyzed) were electrophoresed in successive slots of a 10%-polyacrylamide SDS gel. The top fraction of the gradient is on the right of the figure. C) The identification of α-actinin in two fractions of a sucrose gradient in which plasma membranes had been sedimented. A gradient such as that shown in B was run and 25 μl of the peak membrane fraction and a fraction at the top of the gradient (fraction 14, where 15 were collected) were electrophoresed in adjacent slots (1 and 2, respectively) of a 10%-polyacrylamide gel. The photograph of the Coomassie blue-stained, dried-down gel and the corresponding autoradiograph after the same slice had been reacted first with anti-α-actinin and then with the second ^{125}I-labelled antibody are shown. More α-actinin is detected in the fraction at the top of the sucrose gradient than that corresponding to the peak membrane fraction. The positions of migration of the purified proteins filamin (F), myosin (M), clathrin (C), α-actinin (a-A), and actin (A) are indicated for the gels shown in B and C. It should be noted that gels electrophoresed in A, B, and C were run on different occasions and slight differences in protein migration can be detected.

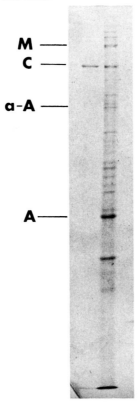

Fig. 7. SDS gel analysis of purified brain clathrin and Hela plasma membranes. A sample of purified brain clathrin was electrophoresed on a 10%-polyacrylamide gel adjacent to a sample of plasma membranes taken from the peak membrane fraction off a sucrose gradient. A photograph is shown of a dried down gel stained with Coomassie blue. Note the close migration of the purified clathrin (C) with a polypeptide migrating in the gel of whole membranes. The positions of migration of the purified proteins myosin (M), clathrin (C), α-actinin (a-A), and actin (A) are indicated on the left side of the gel.

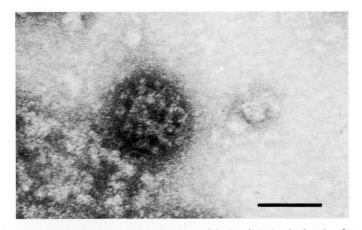

Fig. 8. An electron micrograph of a coated vesicle formed during dialysis of a fraction from a sucrose gradient of Hela plasma membranes. Plasma membranes isolated by the Brunette and Till procedure were sedimented on a sucrose gradient as described for Figure 6. The fraction second from the top of the gradient (fraction 14) was dialyzed against 0.1M sodium MES (pH 6.5), 1mM EGTA, 0.5mM $MgCl_2$, and 0.02% sodium azide. After 48 hours an aliquot was placed on a Formvar-coated grid and stained with 2% uranyl acetate. The electron micrograph shows a structure typical of isolated coated vesicles. Bar = 0.1μm.

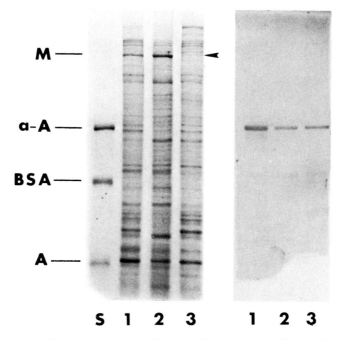

Fig. 9. SDS gel analysis of plasma membranes before and after incubation with extraction buffers. 0.2 ml of Hela cell plasma membranes, isolated by the Brunette and Till procedure, were extracted at 4°C with either 4 ml of 2mM Tris HCl, 0.2mM EDTA, 0.1% β-mercaptoethanol, pH 8.8, or 0.6M NaCl, 0.1M NaPO$_4$, 1mM MgCl$_2$, 4mM ATP, 0.1% β-mercaptoethanol, pH 6.5. After 1.5 hours the membranes were sedimented at 27,000g for 20 minutes. The pellets were dissolved in SDS and compared with a sample of the starting membranes on a 7.5%-polyacrylamide gel. The first sample (1) was the starting membranes, the second (2) had been extracted with the low ionic-strength buffer, and the third (3) had been extracted with the high ionic strength ATP-containing buffer. A photograph of a dried down gel stained with Coomassie blue is shown. Approximately 40μg of protein of the 3 membrane samples were electrophoresed in parallel slots next to a sample of standards (S), which contained the purified proteins α-actinin, BSA, and ovalbumin. The positions of migration of the proteins myosin (M), α-actinin (a-A), BSA, and actin (A) are indicated next to the gel. The position of the myosin heavy chain is also marked with an arrow next to the third membrane sample indicating its absence or marked extraction from this sample. An autoradiograph is also shown of a parallel gel of the three membrane samples after it was reacted with the anti-α-actinin antibody followed by the ^{125}I-labelled second antibody.

One set of circumstances, however, was routinely observed in which a portion of the α-actinin appeared to be preferentially released from the membranes without an equivalent loss of the actin. Whenever the freshly prepared membranes were washed in the presence of isotonic phosphate buffered saline containing reducing agents, or such membranes were placed over a sucrose gradient, some α-actinin appeared to be released together with certain other gel bands. This was best illustrated by the analysis of fractions across a sucrose gradient. Here it was found that a significant portion of the α-actinin did not sediment with the plasma membranes but rather remained at the top of the gradient (Fig. 6b). The amount of actin in these fractions at the top of the gradient varied between experiments, but frequently was lower than the amount of α-actinin, indicating that at least a fraction of the α-actinin will dissociate from these membranes without an equivalent loss of actin. A possible explanation for the α-actinin that dissociates readily is that it is

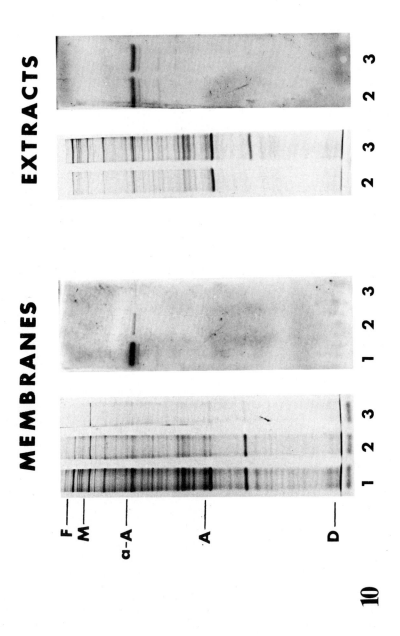

binding to single actin filaments, whereas the α-actinin which is only extracted by prolonged dialysis against low ionic strength buffers is cross-linking filaments and as a result is more tightly associated with the membranes. That much of the α-actinin will dissociate from the plasma membrane without an equivalent dissociation of actin suggests that this fraction, at least, is not linking actin to the membrane. We are, therefore, led to conclude that much of the α-actinin present in the membrane preparations is there because it is bound to actin, rather than the other way around. If it does have a role in actin attachment, we believe it is indirect and the result of its ability to crosslink actin filaments, a property which would tend to promote and stabilize actin attachment if there is an equilibrium between free actin filaments and those bound to receptors at the membrane.

The other proteins that dissociate readily from the plasma membranes and remain at the top of the sucrose gradients are also interesting. Two of the prominent ones have been tentatively identified as filamin and clathrin. The clathrin that dissociates does appear capable of reconstituting "baskets" as seen in the EM which are reminiscent of the purified coated vesicles of which clathrin is a major component. This and other evidence suggests that this protein is indeed clathrin. Since the isolation of coated vesicles by Pearse and her discovery of clathrin [8, 9], most work on this protein has been directed towards its role in the coated vesicle. Coated vesicles, however, do arise from the plasma membrane via coated pits and are probably important in the internalization of aggregated membrane components. Does the clathrin detected in this study represent material that has already formed coated pits or vesicles, or is some of it associated with the plasma membrane in a nonaggregated form? Electron micrographs of the plasma membrane preparations certainly reveal structures that could be coated vesicles or pits (Fig. 5) but how much of the clathrin is in such structures cannot be answered at the moment. It has recently been reported that clathrin has an affinity for both actin and α-actinin [34]. If further work confirms this, then the finding of clathrin in plasma membrane preparations becomes particularly relevant to the question of actin attachment to membrane components.

Fig. 10. SDS gel analysis of plasma membranes after extraction with low ionic strength buffers. Hela cell plasma membranes were isolated by the Brunette and Till procedure and were extracted by dialysis against either 2mM Tris Cl, 0.2mM ATP, 0.1% β-mercaptoethanol, pH 7.4 (sample 2), or 2mM Tris, 0.2mM EDTA, 0.1% β-mercaptoethanol, pH 8.8 (sample 3). After 36 hours of dialysis the membranes were sedimented at 145,000g for 1 hour and the supernatants and pellets were compared by electrophoresis in SDS on a 10%-polyacrylamide gel. A photograph of the stained gel of the pellets (membranes) is shown on the left together with its corresponding autoradiograph after reacting the gel with the anti-α-actinin antibody, followed by the second iodinated antibody. On the right a photograph of the stained gel of the extract supernatants is shown together with their corresponding autoradiograph after reaction with the same antibodies. Sample 1 is the starting membrane preparation, while samples 2 and 3 were the pellets and supernatants after dialysis against the buffers described above. Equal volumes were loaded in the gel slots, not equal protein concentrations. Each pellet was dissolved in 1 ml of gel sample buffer and 25µl was loaded in the respective gel slots. Similarly equal volumes of the supernatants were electrophoresed. The autoradiograph indicates very little α-actinin remaining in these membranes after extraction and most can be seen in the gels of the supernatants. The autoradiograph of the supernatant gels reveals some minor bands reacting with the α-actinin antibody which probably correspond to minor proteolytic degradation products since during the dialysis no protease inhibitors were included.

ACKNOWLEDGMENTS

The authors thank Dr. J.D. Watson for his support of this work, Dr. G. Kohler for his generous gift of mouse myeloma cells, and Dr. D. Goll for his gift of beef-cardiac α-actinin. We gratefully acknowledge the skilled technical assistance of Lois Jordan. We thank Anne Bushnell for help with the electron microscopy and Ted Lukralle for photographic assistance. Madeline Szadkowski patiently typed several versions of this manuscript. This work was supported by the Robertson Research Fund, a Cancer Center grant from the National Cancer Institute to the Cold Spring Harbor Laboratory (CA13106), by grants from the NIH (GM26298-01 and HL23848-01), and by a postdoctoral fellowship from the Muscular Dystrophy Association to J.F.

REFERENCES

1. Huxley HE: J Mol Biol 7:281, 1963.
2. Ebashi S, Ebashi F: J Biochem 58:7, 1965.
3. Holmes GR, Goll DE, Suzuki A: Biochim Biophys Acta 253:240, 1971.
4. Podlubnaya ZA, Tskhovrebova LA, Zaalishvili MM, Stefanenko GA: J Mol Biol 92:357, 1975.
5. Lazarides E, Burridge K: Cell 6:289, 1975.
6. Schollmeyer JE, Furcht LT, Goll DE, Robson RM, Stromer MH: In Goldman R, Pollard T, Rosenbaum J (eds): "Cell Motility." New York: Cold Spring Harbor Laboratory, 1976, pp 361.
7. Heaysman JEM, Pegrum SM: Exp Cell Res 78:71, 1973.
8. Pearse BMF: J Mol Biol 97:93, 1975.
9. Pearse BMF: Proc Natl Acad Sci USA 73:1255, 1976.
10. Porath J, Axen R, Emback S: Nature 215:1491, 1967.
11. Laemmli UK: Nature 227:680, 1970.
12. Burridge K: Proc Natl Acad Sci USA 73:4457, 1976.
13. Burridge K: Methods Enzymol 50:54, 1978.
14. Bolton AE, Hunter WM: Biochem J 133:529, 1973.
15. Brunette DM, Till JE: J Membr Biol 5:215, 1971.
16. Gruenstein E, Rich A, Weihing RR: J Cell Biol 64:223, 1975.
17. Thom D, Powell AJ, Lloyd CW, Rees DA: Biochem J 168:187, 1977.
18. Ishikawa H, Bischoff R, Holtzer H: J Cell Biol 43:312, 1969.
19. Keen JH, Willingham MC, Pastan IH: Cell 16:303, 1979.
20. Lazarides E: J Cell Biol 68:202, 1976.
21. Gordon WE, Bushnell A: Exp Cell Res 120:335, 1979.
22. O'Farrell PH: J Biol Chem 250:4007, 1975.
23. Geiger B, Singer SJ: Cell 16:213, 1979.
24. Ash JF, Singer SJ: Proc Natl Acad Sci USA 73:4575, 1976.
25. Toh BH, Hard GC: Nature 269:695, 1977.
26. Gabbiani G, Chapponier C, Zumbe A, Vassali P: Nature 269:697, 1977.
27. Oliver JM, Lalchandani R, Becker EL: J Reticuloendothel Soc 21:359, 1977.
28. Ash JF, Louvard D, Singer SJ: Proc Natl Acad Sci USA 74:5584, 1977.
29. Bourguignon LYW, Singer SJ: Proc Natl Acad Sci USA 74:5031, 1977.
30. Bourguignon LYW, Tokuyasu KT, Singer SJ: J Cell Physiol 95:239, 1978.
31. Schreiner GF, Fujiwara K, Pollard TD, Unanue ER: J Exp Med 145:1393, 1977.
32. Moore PB, Ownby CL, Carraway KL: Exp Cell Res 115:331, 1978.
33. Willingham MC, Ostlund RE, Pastan I: Proc Natl Acad Sci USA 71:4144, 1974.
34. Schook W, Puszkin S, Bloom W, Ores C, Kochwa S: Proc Natl Acad Sci USA 76:116, 1979.

Interactions Between the Plasma Membrane and Cytoskeleton of Cultured Fibroblasts

J. F. Ash, D. Louvard, and S. J. Singer

Department of Biology, University of California at San Diego, La Jolla, California 92093 (J.F.A., S.J.S.) and the European Molecular Biology Laboratory, Heidelberg (D.L.)

Observations of cultured cells made by double-fluorescence staining indicate that regions of the plasma membrane which are in close contact with actin-containing cytoplasmic fibers have characteristics different from other regions of the membrane. On fixed cells it is found that several integral membrane proteins are excluded from these regions of membrane-fiber apposition. If, however, these same integral proteins are clustered by their specific antibodies, the patches produced are rapidly lined up over the cytoplasmic fibers, resulting in a transmembrane linkage of clustered membrane proteins to the actin cytoskeleton.

These observations have led us to predict the existence of a class of integral membrane proteins, X proteins, which are associated with actin fibers and are responsible for both the initial exclusion and then the transmembrane linkage of clusters of other integral membrane proteins. In an attempt to identify X proteins we have produced antisera against purified plasma membranes prepared from porcine intestinal brush borders. These antisera detect surface antigens on fixed human fibroblast cells which are initially lined up over actin fibers. These antigens are, thus, candidates for the hypothesized X proteins. Using the fluorescence microscope, we are attempting to isolate the potential X antigens with a staining absorption assay.

Key words: surface receptors, transmembrane interactions, actin

We have previously reported results on the lectin- or antibody-induced transmembrane linkage of plasma membrane proteins to adjacent cytoplasmic actin-containing fibers [1—3]. These experiments demonstrated that while several specific integral membrane proteins are initially excluded from regions of the membrane rich in adjacent actin fibers, clusters of these same integral proteins produced before fixation by their specific antibodies became quickly lined up at these membrane sites adjacent to actin [2]. This induced transmembrane linkage is not inhibited by colchicine or azide treatment. Newly displayed fibronectin is spontaneously lined up over these actin adjacent membrane sites

Received July 25, 1979; accepted July 25, 1979.

[4], although the limited extent of the fibronectin distribution described in Heggeness et al [4] rules out a direct role of fibronectin in either producing the exclusion or inducing the lining up of other clustered membrane proteins. These results have led us to predict the existence of a class of membrane proteins we have called "X proteins" [2, 3]. The X proteins are assumed to be integral membrane proteins associated directly or indirectly with cytoplasmic actin fibers. Other classes of membrane proteins do not interact with X proteins until they are clustered by external agents such as lectins [1], antibodies [2, 3], or perhaps by hormones [5, 6]. The proposed interaction of clustered membrane proteins with X proteins thus leads to a special organization of these clusters relative to other, unclustered membrane proteins. This could allow for subsequent specific processing of the clusters, for instance, by endocytosis via coated pits [7].

The identification of integral membrane proteins for candidates as X proteins is, therefore, of considerable interest for studies of a variety of membrane processes involving receptor clustering and transmembrane signaling as well as for studies of general membrane structure. Our approach to the problem of identifying X proteins has been to generate antisera against purified plasma membranes or membrane fractions and test the ability of these sera to recognize integral membrane proteins which are initially distributed over adjacent cytoplasmic actin fibers. This analysis has been performed on cultured fibroblasts with the fluorescence microscope using indirect two-color staining to localize the membrane antigens exposed on the surface and then the actin fibers inside the cells. The initial results of these studies will be reported here.

METHODS

Immunofluorescence Microscopy

We have described the procedures and reagents used for two-color localizations of surface components and cytoplasmic actin [2, 8]. Human WI-38 lung fibroblasts were used for all analyses and were cultured as previously described [2].

Preparation of Antisera Directed Against Intestinal Brush Border Membranes

Closed vesicles from porcine intestinal brush border were prepared as described in Louvard et al [8]. Rabbits were immunized with 1–2 mg of total vesicle protein in an emulsion with 50% complete Freund's adjuvant. The antigen was injected directly into both hind leg popliteal lymph nodes and intradermally into the back skin using a total volume of 1 ml per rabbit. The animals were boosted with 1 mg of antigen in saline or incomplete Freund's adjuvant intradermally and subcutaneously 2–3 weeks following the primary injection. Sera were collected 10 days after the second injection and at 1-week intervals following the first bleeding.

Absorption of Antisera

The intact intestinal vesicles (5 mg/ml protein) were treated overnight with 2.5% Emulphogen BC-720 (GAF, New York), a nonionic detergent, in 10 mM KPO_4 (pH 7.5) at 4°C. The detergent-treated vesicles were then centrifuged at 45,000 rpm in a Beckman (Palo Alto, California) Ti-50 rotor for 30 min and the supernatant containing the solubilized proteins was collected. The ability of this detergent-solubilized antigen, or fractions of it, were tested for their ability to absorb the surface-staining capacity on WI-38 cells of the rabbit antisera prepared against the intact vesicles. Dilutions of a serum which gave detectable, but submaximal, staining were first determined. Then aliquots of serum were diluted with various concentrations of solubilized vesicle protein to twice this predetermined level. After an overnight incubation at 4°C the aliquots were shaken for 2 h at room temperature with Biobeads SM-2 (BioRad, Richmond, California) (50 mg SM-2/mg BC-720) to remove the detergent. The beads were allowed to settle and the solution removed and centrifuged at 45,000 rpm for 30 min to remove the remaining antigen-antibody precipitates. The absorbed aliquots were then diluted with equal volumes of phosphate-buffered saline and tested for their ability to stain the surface of WI-38 cells. This staining was compared with that produced by sera which were initially diluted with detergent buffer containing no antigen and processed in parallel. Usually a series of 1:2 dilutions of antigen were used and the antigen concentration which was judged to reduce the staining intensity to 50% of the unabsorbed serum was determined. Solubilized vesicle protein concentrations were determined spectrophotometrically by assuming $A280_{(1\ mg/ml)} = 1.0$.

RESULTS AND DISCUSSION

Antibody production, as judged by immunofluorescence staining or antigen precipitation, was detected as early as 9 days after the primary injection. After boosting, the sera from animals injected with intact vesicles would give detectable staining at dilutions up to 1:200 and yielded patterns such as those seen in Figure 1. Surface stripes of staining were observed to stand out against a dim uniform background. These stripes were found to be initially displayed on membrane regions lying above actin cables (Fig. 1; contrast with initial distributions of beta-2-microglobulin or aminopeptidase found by Ash and co-workers [2, 3]). Treatment of cells with these sera or IgG fractions before fixation yielded the same staining patterns as seen in Figure 1 and had no apparent effect on the cells.

Antigen absorption experiments were conducted with one batch of serum which gave slightly submaximal staining at a dilution of 1:100. The surface stripes on fixed cells were the predominant feature observed at this serum dilution. When intact vesicles were extracted with the nonionic detergent Emulphogen BC-720, the solubilized proteins were effective in absorbing the staining capacity of this serum (1:100) at a minimum concentration of 1 mg/ml.

Attempts to fractionate the complex detergent extract by DEAE cellulose chromatography are illustrated by the experiment shown in Figure 2. When the extract is fractionated on Whatman DE-52 columns, a peak of absorbing activity is revealed which is five times more effective than the original extract. This result indicated that the assay system can be used to follow the purification of antigens capable of absorbing the staining activity of the serum. Difficulties in finding techniques adequate to resolve the components of this extract have not allowed the precise identification of X antigens as yet, but our attention has focused on a peptide which migrates on sodium dodecyl sulfate (SDS) gels with an apparent molecular weight of 90,000 (Fig. 2). A protein of this molecular weight is present in all fractions effective in absorbing the staining, and it is depleted in or absent from all fractions that are ineffective.

The rationale for producing antisera against such a complex antigen as the intestinal brush border plasma membrane comes from the observation that these membranes are derived from microvilli which are enriched in actin [10]. It is possible to purify large quantities of vesicles from these membranes free of contaminating intracellular membranes and cytoplasmic structures [9]. Since these vesicles contain actin, we could assume that the membranes are likely sources of actin-associated integral membrane proteins. These mem-

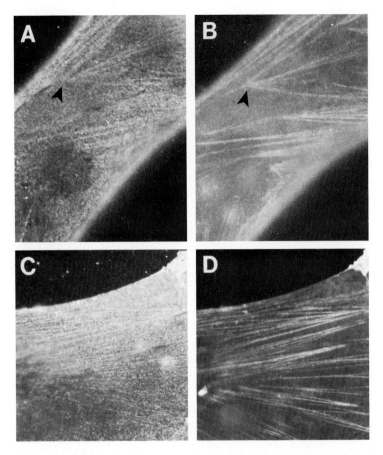

Fig. 1. WI-38 human fibroblasts stained with an antiserum produced against porcine intestine brush border membranes (A, C) and for intracellular actin (B, D). The cells were fixed before staining. Surface staining with the rabbit antiserum was detected by rhodamine-labeled goat anti-rabbit IgG antibodies. The cells were then briefly treated with detergent, and the cytoplasmic actin fibers were stained with a fluorescein system based on rabbit muscle heavy meromyosin [8]. The stripes of stain on the surface (A, C) are superimposable on the actin fibers located inside the cells close to the membrane (B, D). Contrast this initial distribution of membrane proteins with those seen in Ash et al [2] and Singer et al [3].

branes, of course, also contain a large quantity of hydrolytic enzymes [9], which are unlikely candidates for X proteins. Purified antibodies to one of these enzymes, aminopeptidase, were previously used in a study of the surface of WI-38 cells in which it was found that WI-38 aminopeptidase is excluded from membrane regions overlying actin filaments [2]. It was also clear from this previous study that the amount of aminopeptidase on the surface of WI-38 cells is low, since two layers of indirect fluorescent antibodies were necessary to detect the antiaminopeptidase. We expected that if the brush border membranes contained X proteins which were antigenic in rabbits, then the antisera should give relatively strong staining of X proteins on the fibroblasts, since X should be present in much larger amounts than hydrolytic enzymes such as aminopeptidase. This staining should be detectable against the weak staining for the relatively rare (on WI-38) antigens such as aminopeptidase.

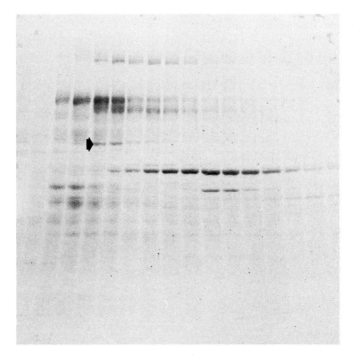

Fig. 2. Gradient SDS-polyacrylamide gels of detergent-solubilized porcine brush border membrane proteins fractionated on Whatman DE-52 DEAE cellulose. The column was equilibrated with 10 mM NaPO$_4$ (pH 6.0) and eluted with a linear gradient (0–0.3 M) of NaCl in the phosphate buffer. Successive fractions were tested for their ability to absorb the surface-staining capacity of the antiserum to the whole brush border. Those fractions containing a 90,000-dalton peptide (marked with an arrow) were five times more effective in absorbing the staining than the original extract. Other fractions had little or no detectable activity.

The fact that the sera described here gave strong surface staining on WI-38 cells when visualized by a single layer of indirect fluorescent antibodies demonstrates that there are some antigens in the brush border which are more commonly represented on WI-38 cells than aminopeptidase. The fact that this staining was enhanced in membrane regions over actin on fixed cells suggests further that these antigens are of a different class than those represented by aminopeptidase. We therefore assume that some of the antibodies produced against the brush border membranes recognize what we have defined as X proteins on the surface of WI-38 cells. This assumption is based on the staining patterns produced by these antisera and not on any functional criteria such as association with other clustered membrane proteins. The ability to differentially stain membrane regions overlying actin fibers, however, strongly supports the hypothesis that there are membrane proteins specific to regions of actin-membrane association.

The use of the staining absorption assay described here should eventually allow the identification and isolation of these new X protein antigens from the intestinal brush border. This should allow the production of monospecific antisera to these proteins. These new sera would then become powerful tools for further detailed structural and functional studies of this important membrane region. An immediate application of such an anti-X serum would be in the investigation of the role of X proteins in the capping of membrane antigens in lymphocytes. We have previously speculated [3, 11] that X proteins are involved in capping. The antibody-induced clustering of a surface receptor on round cells is proposed to produce a linkage of such clusters with X proteins, and hence to actin, as in the case of fibroblasts. In round cells, however, the actin/myosin filaments are much smaller than in flat cells, and these transmembrane complexes of clustered receptor—X—actin/myosin are still mobile in the plane of the membrane, and can be collected into a cap. We could therefore test two important predictions about the role of X proteins in capping reactions with an anti-X serum: 1) X proteins should be present in all caps [3, 11] and 2) prior capping of X proteins should perturb or inhibit capping of other membrane antigens. Information from these experiments will demonstrate the extent of the involvement of membrane-cytoskeleton interactions in transmembrane signaling events.

ACKNOWLEDGMENTS

The original studies that are discussed in this paper were supported by grants CA-22031 and GM-15971 from the National Institutes of Health to S. J. S.

REFERENCES

1. Ash JF, Singer SJ: Proc Natl Acad Sci USA 73:4575, 1976.
2. Ash JF, Louvard D, Singer SJ: Proc Natl Acad Sci USA 74:5584, 1977.
3. Singer SJ, Ash JF, Bourguignon LYW, Heggeness MH, Louvard D: J Supramol Struct 9:373, 1978.
4. Heggeness MH, Ash JF, Singer SJ: Ann NY Acad Sci 312:414, 1978.
5. Haigler H, Ash JF, Singer SJ, Cohen S: Proc Natl Acad Sci USA 75:3317, 1978.
6. Maxfield FR, Schlessinger J, Schecter Y, Pastan I, Willingham MC: Cell 14:805, 1978.
7. Anderson RGW, Vasile E, Mello RJ, Brown MS, Goldstein JL: Cell 15:919, 1978.
8. Heggeness MH, Ash JF: J Cell Biol 73:783, 1977.
9. Louvard D, Maroux S, Baratti J, Desnuelle P, Mutaftschiev S: Biochim Biophys Acta 291:747, 1973.
10. Bretscher A, Weber K: Exp Cell Res 116:397, 1978.
11. Bourguignon LYW, Singer SJ: Proc Natl Acad Sci USA 74:5031, 1977.

Cell Mutants as a Tool to Study Malignant Transformation of Fibroblasts

Jacques Pouysségur, Arlette Franchi, and Patrick Silvestre

Centre de Biochimie, Université de Nice, Parc Valrose, 06034 Nice, France

From 3T3 Balb/c cells, mutants with low adhesiveness to plastic substratum were selected. One of these clones, AD6, was found to be deficient in glucosamine-6-phosphate N-acetylase. A result of this block is a decrease by 60–70% of cell surface carbohydrates, and as a consequence there is a general reduction in the exposure of glycoproteins at the cell surface. This biochemical defect is fully reverted to normal, simply by growing the mutant cells in presence of 10 mM N-acetylglucosamine. This specific and reversible enzymatic block allows us to conclude that the abnormal properties of AD6 cells — low adhesion, round shape, increased agglutinability by lectins, loss of directional locomotion, and absence of microfilament bundles — are the result of the surface carbohydrate defect, since reversion of glycoprotein synthesis to normal results in the general reversion of the altered phenotype. However, in spite of this apparent transformed phenotype, AD6 cells have normal growth control and are not tumorigenic.

Using $[^3H]$-2-deoxyglucose suicide, we selected from a spontaneously transformed clone of Chinese hamster lung fibroblasts a mutant (DS7) impaired in glucose metabolism. DS7 has a fourfold to fivefold decreased ability to transport either 2-deoxyglucose or 3-O-methylglucose and produces 14 times less lactic acid than the wild-type when grown on 5 mM glucose. This block in aerobic glycolysis, which is located at the level of phosphoglucose isomerase, makes that cell line dependent exclusively on respiration for its energy requirement. The parental line grows at low serum concentration, is anchorage-independent, and is tumorigenic in *nude* mice. The derived DS7 cells have retained both the in vitro transformed phenotype and the tumor-forming capability.

A general conclusion of these studies is that the altered properties and cell behavior of transformed fibroblasts, such as low adhesiveness, round morphology, increased agglutinability by lectins, altered motility, absence of microfilament bundles, and increase in hexose transport and in aerobic glycolysis, are dissociable from malignant transformation. These phenotypic alterations should therefore be considered as events secondary to the mechanism that leads to the loss of growth control.

Key words: malignant transformation, surface carbohydrate-deficient fibroblast mutant, phosphoglucose isomerase-free mutant, glucose uptake- and glycolysis-deficient fibroblast
mutant, growth control, tumorigenicity

Received July 16, 1979; accepted July 16, 1979.

INTRODUCTION

Among the various properties which accompany in vitro transformation of fibro-blasts [1–4], it has been very difficult to assign to any particular altered function a primary role in the establishment or the maintenance of the malignant phenotype. In an attempt to dissect this very complex phenotype and to analyze the causal relationship between alterations of cell surface, membrane glycoproteins, hexose transport, aerobic glycolysis, and malignant transformation, we have chosen a genetic approach.

Our first objective in this approach was to isolate, either from normal or from transformed fibroblasts, mutants specifically altered in one of the transformed properties. The second objective was to analyze the molecular basis of the altered cellular function and to determine whether other alterations in cell behavior that have not been selected for are expressed.

In this paper we report the analysis of the properties of two cell mutants. One, mutant AD6, derived from Balb 3T3 cells, is impaired in the synthesis of cell surface carbohydrates. The unique properties of that cell line led us to propose that surface changes such as round shape, low adhesion, high agglutinability by lectins, loss of actin bundles, and directionality of locomotion, which are often encountered in transformed cells, are dissociable from abnormal growth control [5–7]. The second mutant, DS7, derived from a spontaneous transformed fibroblast line, has a low glucose transport activity and a block in glycolysis. Its in vitro and in vivo properties indicate that, at least in Chinese hamster fibroblasts, increased hexose transport and aerobic glycolysis, do not seem to be required for the expression of 1) the in vitro transformed phenotype and 2) the tumorigenicity.

MATERIALS AND METHODS

Cell Lines and Culture Conditions

Balb/c 3T3 fibroblasts and the derivative mutant cells AD6 were grown as previously reported [5]. Chinese hamster lung fibroblasts were subcloned from the established line CC139 (American Type Culture Collection) generously provided by Dr. G. Buttin. From that cell line we selected a clone (023) resistant to 3 mM ouabain. These cells and the derivative mutant DS7 were maintained in Dulbecco's minimum essential medium (DMEM) (Gibco, catalog No. 21) supplemented with 10% fetal calf serum, penicillin (50 units/ml) and streptomycin (50 μg/ml). All cells were grown at 37°C in an atmosphere of 95% air/5% CO_2.

Mutagenesis

Mutagenesis and the method of selection of the mutant AD6 have been previously described [5]. For the selection of hexose uptake-deficient cells, exponentially growing cells ($10^4 - 2 \times 10^4$ cells/cm^2) were treated with 0.25 μl/ml of ethyl methane sulfonate (EMS) in Dulbecco's MEM for 16 h. The cells were washed twice with Dublecco's phosphate-buffered saline (PBS), cultured, and passaged for 6 days in Falcon flasks before the selection outlined in Figure 3 was applied.

2-Deoxyglucose and 3-O-Methylglucose Transport Assays

Cells were planted in 35-mm dishes, cultured 2–3 days near confluency and assayed for hexose uptake 1 day after medium change. The medium was aspirated and the cells were washed twice with 2 ml of PBS kept at 37°C. Cells were incubated in a water bath regulated at 37°C for 2-deoxyglucose and at 20°C for 3-O-methylglucose in presence of the radiolabeled sugar in 1 ml of PBS. At appropriate times, the medium was aspirated and cells were washed four times with 2 ml of ice-cold PBS. Cells were homogenized in 1 ml of 0.1 N NaOH and on each homogenate radioactivity and protein were determined.

Assays of Glycolytic Enzymes and Aerobic Glycolysis

Cells were grown to confluency in a 100-mm dish and the monolayer was washed three times with ice-cold PBS. The cells were removed in 1 ml of 10 mM phosphate, pH 7.5, with a rubber policeman and homogenized with a Dounce homogenizer (20 strokes). Homogenates were centrifuged 20 min at 20,000g and the supernatant was kept for enzyme assays. Hexokinase, glucose-6-P-dehydrogenase and glucose-6-P-isomerase were measured at room temperature in 50 mM phosphate pH 7.5, 2 mM adenosine triphosphate (ATP), 2 mM $MgCl_2$, 1 mM $NADP^+$, and 5 mM substrate (glucose or glucose-6-P or fructose-6-P). For hexokinase and phosphoglucose isomerase assays, an excess of purified glucose-6-P-dehydrogenase was added. Phosphofructokinase was measured as in Schneider et al [8].

For lactic acid assays, DS7 and 023 cell lines were respectively planted at 5×10^5 and 2.5×10^5 cells per 60-mm dish. One day later the cells were washed twice with PBS and the assay was initiated by addition of growth medium containing 5 mM glucose and 10% dialyzed fetal calf serum. Aliquots were assayed for glucose content with the Sigma glucose assay kit and for lactate using lactate dehydrogenase coupled to the glutamate/pyruvate transaminase [9]. Cell number was determined on duplicate dishes.

Growth in Soft Agar

The method used was essentially that described by Macpherson and Montagnier [10]. We substituted agar for agarose.

Tumorigenicity Assays

Cells were harvested by trypsinization and 6×10^6 washed cells suspended in 0.2 ml of medium were injected at a single subcutaneous site into each nude mouse.

RESULTS

Analysis of a Cell Surface Carbohydrates Defective Cell Line

Biochemical defect of the mutant AD6. The method of isolation and the biochemical and biologic characterization of this fibroblast mutant have been already published [5,6]. We will briefly report here the main results and conclusions.

AD6 cells derive from the contact-inhibited cell line Balb 3T3, after selection for low-adherence cells [5]. Most of the clones we have isolated after four cycles of selection have a very low adhesiveness to substratum (glass, polystyrene) and display a round morphology.

Biochemical analysis of the surface of AD6 cells has revealed 1) a decrease in the exposure of glycoproteins at the outer surface measured by their accessibility to lactoperoxidase; and 2) a general decrease in the total amount of membrane carbohydrates: mannose, galactose, N-acetylglucosamine, N-acetylgalactosamine, and sialic acid [11]. We have shown that this glycoprotein synthesis defect of AD6 cells is due to a block in the acetylation of glucosamine-6-phosphate (Fig. 1). Three lines of evidence support this conclusion: 1) instead of the uridine diphosphate-acetylated sugar, glucosamine-6-phosphate accumulates in AD6 when a trace amount of glucosamine is given to the cells; 2) addition of 10 mM N-acetylglucosamine to the medium totally reverses the biosynthesis defect of surface carbohydrates

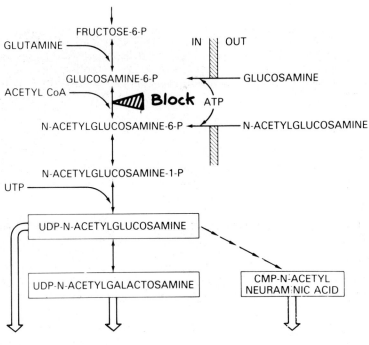

FRUCTOSE-6-P

GLUTAMINE

GLUCOSAMINE-6-P   IN ‖ OUT

ACETYL CoA   GLUCOSAMINE

Block   ATP

N-ACETYLGLUCOSAMINE-6-P ◄   N-ACETYLGLUCOSAMINE

N-ACETYLGLUCOSAMINE-1-P

UTP

UDP-N-ACETYLGLUCOSAMINE

UDP-N-ACETYLGALACTOSAMINE   CMP-N-ACETYL NEURAMINIC ACID

PRECURSORS FOR TRANSFER REACTIONS IN GLYCOPROTEINS,
GLYCOLIPIDS, HETEROSACCHARIDES

Fig. 1. Metabolic pathway of amino sugars. Arrow indicates position of the block in AD6.

and the exposure of glycoproteins at the surface [6]; 3) glucosamine-6-phosphate N-acetylase has been found to be strongly decreased in AD6 cells [12].

The reduction in the exposure of some glycoproteins at the surface seems to be a
consequence of the defect in the biosynthesis of amino sugars. Indeed we have shown that,
one of the major iodinizable surface polypeptides (apparent mol wt 97,000 daltons) in
Balb 3T3 accumulates in the membrane of AD6 cells as a nonglycosylated or partially glycosylated precursor of lower mol wt (95,000 daltons) that is no more accessible to lactoperoxidase and fails to bind to a concanavalin A column. However, restoration of normal biosynthesis of amino sugars by growing AD6 with N-acetyglucosamine restores after 3–4 generations 1) the correct molecular weight of the 95,000-dalton polypeptide, 2) its capacity to
bind concanavalin A, and 3) its exposure at the cell surface [13].

The fact that N-acetylglucosamine is able to reverse the overall biochemical surface
alterations of the mutant suggests strongly that AD6 cells derive from the parental Balb 3T3
by a single mutation at the level of the acetylase (Fig. 1). Therefore AD6 cells provide a
"clean" system in which the amount of surface carbohydrates and the exposure of glycoproteins at the cell surface can be manipulated simply by altering the concentration of N-
acetylglucosamine in the medium. Such a system makes it possible to ask what is the role
of cell surface carbohydrates in cell behavior and do these carbohydrates play a role in
growth control?

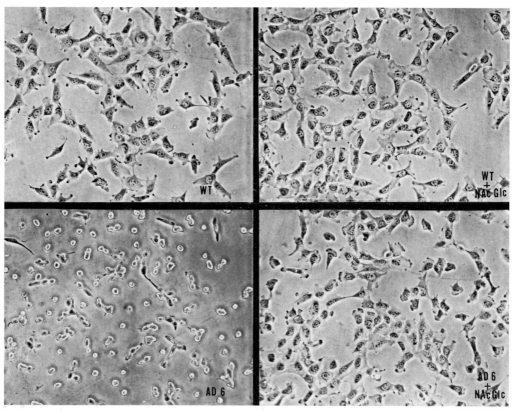

Fig. 2. Morphology of AD6 and wild-type cells. Effect of N-acetylglucosamine. Pictures were taken 3 days after planting and 1 day after medium change. N-acetylglucosamine (+ NAcGlc) was added at 10 mM in the culture medium at the time of planting. WT, Balb 3T3 cells; AD6, mutant AD6.

Biologic Properties of AD6 Cells

Morphology. The first apparent change of the mutant AD6 is its very round shape when grown at low cell density. This compact and round shape of AD6 cells reverts to the flat and asymmetric morphology of the wild-type Balb 3T3 after 3–4 days of culture with 10 mM N-acetylglucosamine (Fig. 2). This effect on the morphology is specific for the mutant AD6 [6].

Adhesion. Low adhesion to substratum is the phenotype selected for the isolation of AD6 cells. Indeed, the detachment of these cells, either mechanically or by trypsin, was found to be very easy compared to the detachment of wild-type cells [5]. The restoration of cell surface carbohydrates to normal with N-acetylglucosamine restores the high adhesivity of the parent cell [6].

Agglutinability and surface microvilli. Other characteristics of transformed fibroblasts such as increase in the number of surface microvilli and increase in agglutinability by lectins [14,15] have also been observed in AD6 cells. However, when AD6 was grown with

N-acetylglucosamine, the number of microvilli and the index of agglutinability by concanavalin A fell to values close to those of wild-type cells [6].

Actin bundles. Transformation of fibroblasts usually led to a disorganization of the packed 60 Å actin-containing microfilaments and this disappearance of actin bundles was correlated with the loss of growth control [16, 17]. It has been shown, by means of an antibody against myosin, that AD6 has no microfilament bundles [7]. Here again, the restoration of the flat morphology of AD6 cells with the acetylated sugar restores the formation of these actin cables [7].

Motility. Using time-lapse cinematography we have analyzed the locomotion of AD6 cells across the substratum. No alteration in the rate of locomotion was observed, but in contrast to wild-type cells, AD6 cells have lost the directionality of locomotion. This aberrant locomotion, which resembles that of some transformed cells [18], is due to a failure in the stabilization of the poorly developed leading edge. Restoration of adhesion sites, either by addition of purified fibronectin or by growing AD6 with N-acetylglucosamine reverses the directionality of locomotion [19].

Anchorage dependence for growth and tumorigenicity. The biologic properties of AD6 mentioned above are characteristic of many transformed fibroblasts. This phenotype prompted us to analyze the growth control of AD6 cells. We have found that this mutant has kept the dependence for high serum concentration, the low saturation density, and the anchorage dependence for growth that characterize the parent Balb 3T3. Indeed AD6 cells are unable to grow either in soft agarose or in bacteriologic Petri dishes in which they cannot adhere. However, if AD6 cells are supplemented with N-acetylglucosamine and plated in bacteriologic dishes, they will again show enough adhesion to initiate DNA synthesis and to grow as well as in tissue culture dishes. This last result points out that, like the parent, AD6 shows an absolute anchorage dependence for growth.

The injection of 1×10^6 cells (AD6, Balb 3T3 and SV40-3T3 Balb transformed lines) to Balb/c mice did not give rise to tumors (0/8) in the case of AD6 and parent cells. Only the SV40 transformed derivative was found to be tumorigenic (8/8) [6].

Conclusion. A summary of the biologic properties of AD6 are reported in Table I. Two conclusions can be drawn from this study. First, we have shown that a single mutation affecting the biosynthesis of surface carbohydrates is enough to mimic the abnormal behavior of transformed fibroblasts in culture. This conclusion is mainly based on the fact that correction of the single enzymatic defect of AD6 cells restores adhesion, morphology agglutinability, actin bundles, and directionality of locomotion to normal.

Secondly, this morphologic phenotype of transformed cells appears to be secondary to the mechanism which controls cell division since we have been able to uncouple it from growth control in AD6 cells (Table I).

Analysis of a Fibroblast Mutant Defective in Hexose Transport and Glycolysis

Besides alterations in surface properties and social behavior, transformed fibroblasts display pronounced increases in nutrient uptake [20,21]. The stimulation of glucose metabolism (increase in hexose transport and in aerobic glycolysis) which accompany malignant transformation has been extensively studied and considered as a general feature of cancer cells. Moreover, this hexose metabolism is shut off in quiescent fibroblasts and any event which will lead to the reinitiation of DNA synthesis and proliferation will be preceded by a stimulation of glucose entry and lactic acid production.

In order to evaluate the importance of the link between hexose transport/aerobic gly-

TABLE I. Biologic Properties of Cell Lines

Properties	Cell Lines			
	SV40-3T3	AD6	AD6 + NAcGlc	Balb 3T3
Surface alterations				
Adhesion	Low	Low	High	High
Morphology	Round	Round	Flat	Flat
Agglutinability by lectins	High	High	Low	Low
Actin Bundles	–	–	++	++
Directionality of locomotion	+/–	–	++	++
Growth control				
Saturation Density	High	Low	Low	Low
Growth in agarose	++	–	–	–
Tumorigenicity	++	–	–	–

colysis and malignant transformation, we attempted to introduce a unique mutation to block glycolysis and to reduce glucose transport in a tumorigenic cell line of Chinese hamster. The isolation and transformed properties of such a mutant are described in the following sections:

Isolation of the mutant DS7. The spontaneous transformed Chinese hamster cell line 023 (derived from CC139) was mutagenized and treated for a short time with tritiated 2-deoxyglucose. After a period of storage in liquid nitrogen, wild type cells which have accumulated labeled 2-deoxyglucose-6-phosphate were killed. However, any mutant with a defect either in glucose transport or in hexokinase activity was expected to survive this radiation suicide. Fig. 3 shows the schema of that selection in which DS7 was isolated. After several days of storage, by which time survival had severely decreased, most of the surviving clones were found to have a decreased ability to take up 2-deoxyglucose.

Biochemical Characterization of the Mutant DS7. The uptake of 2-deoxyglucose or the transport of 3-O-Methylglucose, a nonmetabolizable glucose analog, are reduced fourfold or fivefold in DS7 cells (Fig. 4). Besides this alteration in the transport activity, DS7 cells also have a decreased ability to phosphorylate 2-deoxyglucose. After 2 min of incubation with labeled 2-deoxyglucose, only 10% of this sugar is phosphorylated in the mutant cells, whereas parent cells accumulate more than 90% of the phosphorylated form. Transport of amino acids measured with α-aminoisobutyric acid was found to be unaltered. This result demonstrates the high specificity of the method of selection for glucose uptake-deficient cells. The hexose transport and phosphorylation defect is found in DS7 cells when grown in regular medium (25 mM glucose). However, if DS7 cells are grown in glucose-free medium or at low glucose concentration (0.1 mM), in vivo phosphorylation resumes normal values in the first hour and glucose transport activity returns to that of the wild-type cells after 24 h(Franchi A, Silvestre P, Pouysségur J, in preparation). These results suggest that the

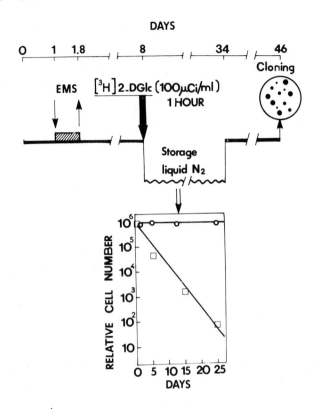

Fig. 3. Scheme of the "tritium suicide" method for selection of glucose uptake-deficient mutants.
Cells were mutagenized as described in Methods with ethyl methane sulfonate (EMS), grown for
6 days, and resuspended after trypsinization at a density of 8×10^6 cells/ml. This cell suspension
was incubated 1 h at 37°C in glucose-free medium containing 2-deoxy-[1-^{3}H]-glucose (17 Ci/mmole,
100 μCi/ml). The cells were centrifuged to eliminate the labeled sugar, frozen in 10% dimethylsulfoxide (10^6 cells/ml) and stored in liquid N_2. Periodically samples were thawed and the cells plated to
analyze survivors. □, cells incubated with radioactive sugar; ○, cells incubated with 10 μM of unlabeled
2-deoxyglucose.

hexose transport and phosphorylation defect of DS7 cells are due to an inhibition or a
repression secondary to the accumulation of a glucose metabolite. Indeed we have found
that when growing in glucose, DS7 cells accumulate an unusual pool of glucose-6-phosphate
(Fig. 5). This over accumulation of glucose-6-phosphate (10 mM) was due to a mutation
abolishing the activity of phosphoglucose isomerase (Table II).

As is to be expected, owing to this enzymatic defect of the glycolytic pathway, DS7
cells do not produce lactic acid (14 times less than the wild-type) and their consumption
of glucose is very low (Fig. 6). The implication of this glycolytic block is that DS7 derives
its energy from respiration. Accordingly, we have observed that in contrast to the parent
cells, DS7 is very sensitive to oligomycin. Incubated with 0.1–1 μg/ml of this metabolic
inhibitor, they die within minutes, whereas the wild-type cells can survive and proliferate
in these conditions, in which synthesis of mitochondrial ATP is prevented. This observation
is in agreement with the existence of a specific glycolytic block in DS7 cells and points up
the specific requirement for respiration in this particular cell line.

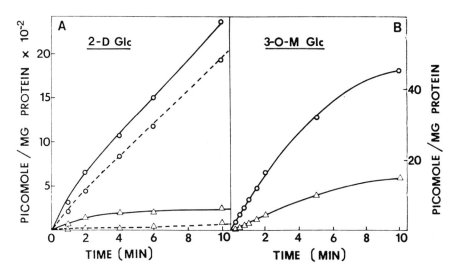

Fig. 4. Uptake of 2-deoxyglucose and transport of 3-O-methylglucose in 023 and DS7 cell lines. DS7 (△) and 023 (○) in monolayers were incubated with 50 μM 2-deoxy-[1-^{3}H]-glucose (A) or 1.2 μM 3-O-methyl-[1-^{3}H]-glucose (B). The rates of transport were measured as described under Methods. At indicated times, aliquots of homogenates were taken for protein determination, scintillation counting, and determination of intracellular phosphorylated 2-deoxyglucose (dashed line) by BaSo$_4$ precipitation. 2-deoxyglucose uptakes were run at 37°C; 3-O-Methylglucose transport was run at 20°C with cells precharged with 50 mM, 3-O-methylglucose.

Anchorage Dependence and Tumorigenicity of DS7 Cells. The parent clone 023, which we have used for this study, has the growth properties of a transformed cell line in that it has low serum dependence for growth, it is able to grow at a high rate in soft agarose, and it is tumorigenic in nude mice. Interestingly, these three characteristics of abnormal growth control are still observed in the hexose transport-deficient and glycolysis-deficient mutant cell line. A summary of these properties is presented in Table III. Besides its ability to grow at low serum concentration (0.5%), DS7 has kept the anchorage independence for growth of the parent (15% of the cells vs 25% in the wild-type form colonies in agarose). Ten of these colonies were picked up from agarose plates, grown in monolayers, and tested for glucose transport and aerobic glycolysis. All of them displayed the phenotype of DS7.

Finally, the preliminary tests for tumorigenicity in nude mice were positive. Three of six of the animals injected with DS7 cells gave rise to tumors. The only noticeable difference between 023 and DS7 is that in the case of DS7 the lag of tumor formation was longer and the growth rate of the tumor slower. A more quantitative analysis of tumorigenicity is in progress.

The conclusion of this second analysis is that increase in hexose transport and in aerobic glycolysis, which are known to be tightly associated with the high proliferation state of transformed and cancer cells, can be dissociated from the mechanism that leads to altered growth control. Moreover, we have surprisingly found that not only a high rate of glycolysis but also glycolysis per se is not required for the expression of the malignant transformed phenotype.

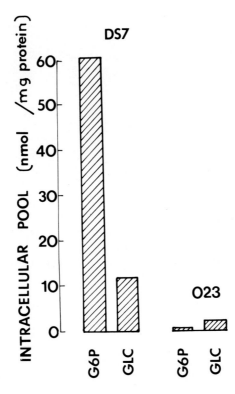

Fig. 5. Intracellular pools of glucose and glucose-6-phosphate in DS7 and 023 cell lines. Soluble pools were determined on confluent cells grown on the usual medium containing 25 mM glucose. Glucose and glucose-6-phosphate were analyzed enzymatically with purified hexokinase and glucose-6-phosphate dehydrogenase.

TABLE II. Glycolytic Enzyme Activities (nmoles/min/mg protein)

| | Cell Lines | |
Enzymes	Wild-type 023	Mutant DS7
Glucose transport (2-deoxyglucose)	40	8
Hexokinase	25	30
Phosphoglucose isomerase	1,100	< 5
Phosphofructokinase	145	90
Glucose-6-P-dehydrogenase	95	70
Lactate dehydrogenase	2,200	1,750

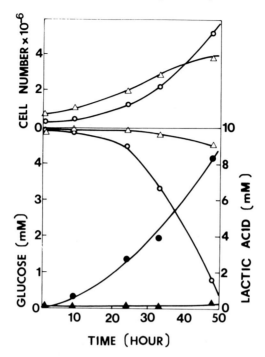

Fig. 6. Glucose consumption and lactic acid production in exponentially growing 023 and DS7 cells. Glucose (open symbols) and lactic acid (filled symbols) present in the culture medium were assayed starting 24 h after cell plating as indicated under Methods. Cell numbers were determined in parallel dishes. △, ▲, DS7; ○, ●, 023.

TABLE III. Growth Characteristics of DS7 and Wild-Type Cells

Cell Lines	Growth in Monolayer (generation time, h)		Growth in agarose[a] (frequency,%)	Tumorigenicity[b]
	10% serum	0.5% serum		
WT (023)	12	65–70	24	5/6
DS7	15	70–75	16	3/6

[a]For determination of colony-forming ability the number of colonies was measured after 12 days. Values were expressed as percentage of cell input (8×10^3 cells) from duplicate dishes.
[b]No. of mice that developed tumors/No. of mice injected. Cells were scored as tumorigenic if a palpable nodule appeared at the site of injection within 10 weeks.

DISCUSSION

In this study we have used a genetic approach to investigate the relationship between, on the one hand, altered growth control and tumorigenicity and, on the other, a set of transformed properties such as low adhesion, round morphology, increased agglutinability, decreased actin bundles, altered cell locomotion, and increased glucose transport and aerobic glycolysis.

The general picture that can be drawn from this analysis is summarized in Figure 7. The primary effect of malignant transformation is altered growth. In fibroblasts, an additional effect is decreased adhesiveness. This decreased adhesiveness results in a set of surface and behavior changes that has been called "the morphologic phenotype of transformation" [3]. A decrease in cyclic AMP levels [22], a deficiency in fibronectin [23], and a defect in cell surface carbohydrates (the present study with AD6) are three distinct mechanisms that lead to decreased adhesiveness and therefore to the "morphologic phenotype of transformation." However, this phenotype is separable from altered growth. This conclusion is based on the properties of AD6 and on reconstruction experiments in which purified fibronectin was added to various transformed cells [23,24].

An additional effect of malignant transformation that we have investigated in this report is increased hexose uptake and aerobic glycolysis. This metabolic feature of cancer cells is also separable from altered growth and from the "morphologic phenotype of transformation." The dissociation from altered growth control results from the fact that the mutant DS7, which has a low glucose transport activity and a block in glycolysis, is still able to express independence of anchorage for growth and tumorigenicity. This dissociation from the "morphologic phenotype of transformation" is established by the fact that AD6 exhibits glucose metabolism (transport and glycolysis) of normal cells (unpublished data).

Since the original observation that aerobic glycolysis is enhanced in malignantly transformed cells [25], there has been considerable interest of the role of glycolysis in the control of cell proliferation. It has been suggested that aerobic glycolysis is not unique to malignantly transformed cells, but is instead a requirement for normal cell proliferation [26]. The phosphoglucose isomerase-free mutant described in this report offers an interesting approach to that problem. Surprisingly, we have found that the high rate of glycolysis of the fibroblast line 023 (99% of glucose is converted to lactic acid) can be abolished 1) without changing seriously the proliferation rate (12 h generation time in 023 vs 15–17 h in DS7) and 2) without blocking the expression of the malignant phenotype.

These results therefore raise the question of the role of glycolysis in cell proliferation. Our preliminary observations on tumorigenicity would suggest that high aerobic glycolysis might be considered a "helper function" in tumor formation and expansion. The very high sensitivity to anaerobiosis of nonglycolytic cells such as DS7 may explain the lag of tumor formation (DS7) as a consequence of local anoxia before vascularization has taken place. A more quantitative study on cell proliferation and on tumorigenicity comparing glycolytic and nonglycolytic cells may facilitate a better understanding of the role of this ubiquitous metabolic function in cell growth.

In conclusion, this report shows the use of somatic cell genetics to be a powerful approach in dissecting the very complex phenotype of malignant fibroblasts.

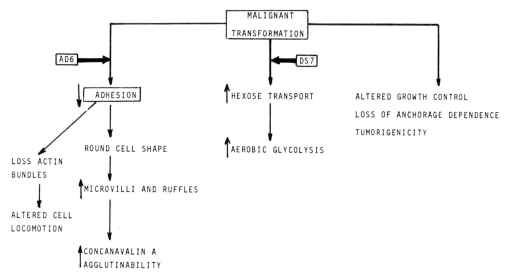

Fig. 7. Proposed relationship between altered growth control and some transformed properties in fibroblasts.

ACKNOWLEDGMENTS

J. Pouysségur thanks Dr. Ira Pastan and Kenneth Yamada for invaluable advice, helpful discussions, and material support concerning the first part of this work. The authors are indebted to Professor G. Ailhaud for interest and support in the second part of this research, to Professor G. Fareed for reviewing this work, and to M. Coppin for typing the manuscript. This work was funded by the CNRS (LP 7300) and the DGRST (Membranes Biologiques, contract No. 77.7. 1269). C.N.R.S. (Centre National de la Recherche Scientifique). D.G.R.S.T. (Délégation Générale à la Recherche Scientifique et Technique).

REFERENCES

1. Robbins JC, Nicolson GL: In Becker FF (ed): "Cancer: A Comprehensive Treatise." New York: Plenum, 1975, Vol 4, pp 3–54.
2. Hynes RO: Biochim Biophys Acta 458:73–107, 1976.
3. Pastan I, Willingham M: "Nature 274:645–650, 1978.
4. Yamada KM, Pouysségur J: Biochimie 60:1221–1233, 1978.
5. Pouysségur J, Pastan I: Proc Natl Acad Sci USA 73:544–548, 1976.
6. Pouysségur, J, Willingham M, Pastan I: Proc Natl Acad Sci USA 74:243–247, 1977.
7. Willingham M, Yamada K, Yamada S, Pouysségur J, Pastan I: Cell 10:375–380, 1977.
8. Schneider JA, Diamond I, Rozengurt E: J Biol Chem 253:872–877, 1978.
9. Lowry O, Passoneau J: In "A Flexible System of Enzymatic Analysis." New York: Academic, 1972, p 194.
10. MacPherson I, Montagnier L: Virology 23:291–294, 1964.

11. Pouysségur J, Pastan I: Biol Chem 252:1639–1646, 1977.
12. Neufeld E, Pastan I: Arch Biochem Biophys 188:323–327, 1978.
13. Pouysségur J, Yamada K: Cell 13:139–150, 1978.
14. Burger MM: Proc Natl Acad Sci USA 62:994–1001, 1969.
15. Willingham M, Pastan I:Proc Natl Acad Sci USA 72:1263–1267, 1975.
16. Pollack R, Osborn M, Weber K:Proc Natl Acad Sci USA 72:994–998, 1975.
17. Edelman GM, Yahara I: Proc Natl Acad Sci USA 73:2047–2051, 1976.
18. Ponten J: In Becker FF (ed): "Cancer:A Comprehensive Treatise." New York:Plenum, 1975, Vol 4, p 55.
19. Pouysségur J, Pastan I:Exp Cell Res 121:373–383 (1979).
20. Hatanaka M: Biochim Biophys Acta 355:77–104, 1974.
21. Pardee AB, Jimenez de Asua L, Rozengurt E: In Clarkson B, Baserga R (eds): "Control of Proliferation In Animal Cells. " Cold Spring Harbor, New York: Cold Spring Harbor Laboratory, 1974, pp 547–561.
22. Pastan I, Johnson GS, Anderson WB: Annu Rev Biochem 44:491–522, 1975.
23. Yamada KM, Yamada SS, Pastan I: Proc Natl Acad Sci USA 73: 1217–1221, 1976.
24. Ali IU, Mautner V, Lanza R, Hynes RO:Cell 11:115–126, 1977.
25. Warburg O: Science 123:309–314, 1956.
26. Wang T, Marquadt C, Foker J: Nature 261:702, 1976.

Author Index

Subject Index